Imaging Brain Diseases

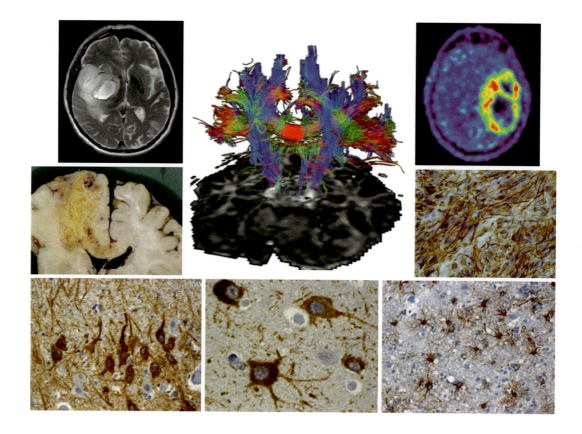

Serge Weis • Michael Sonnberger
Andreas Dunzinger • Eva Voglmayr
Martin Aichholzer • Raimund Kleiser
Peter Strasser

Imaging Brain Diseases

A Neuroradiology, Nuclear Medicine, Neurosurgery, Neuropathology and Molecular Biology-based Approach

Volume III

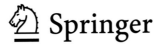

Serge Weis
Division of Neuropathology
Neuromed Campus
Kepler University Hospital
Johannes Kepler University
Linz
Austria

Michael Sonnberger
Department of Neuroradiology
Neuromed Campus
Kepler University Hospital
Johannes Kepler University
Linz
Austria

Andreas Dunzinger
Department of Neuro-Nuclear Medicine
Neuromed Campus
Kepler University Hospital
Johannes Kepler University
Linz
Austria

Eva Voglmayr
Department of Neuroradiology
Neuromed Campus
Kepler University Hospital
Johannes Kepler University
Linz
Austria

Martin Aichholzer
Department of Neurosurgery
Neuromed Campus
Kepler University Hospital
Johannes Kepler University
Linz
Austria

Raimund Kleiser
Department of Neuroradiology
Neuromed Campus
Kepler University Hospital
Johannes Kepler University
Linz
Austria

Peter Strasser
PMU University Institute for Medical &
Chemical Laboratory Diagnostics
Salzburg
Austria

ISBN 978-3-7091-1543-5   ISBN 978-3-7091-1544-2   (eBook)
https://doi.org/10.1007/978-3-7091-1544-2

© Springer-Verlag GmbH Austria, part of Springer Nature 2019
This work is subject to copyright. All rights are reserved by the Publisher, whether the whole or part of the material is concerned, specifically the rights of translation, reprinting, reuse of illustrations, recitation, broadcasting, reproduction on microfilms or in any other physical way, and transmission or information storage and retrieval, electronic adaptation, computer software, or by similar or dissimilar methodology now known or hereafter developed.
The use of general descriptive names, registered names, trademarks, service marks, etc. in this publication does not imply, even in the absence of a specific statement, that such names are exempt from the relevant protective laws and regulations and therefore free for general use.
The publisher, the authors, and the editors are safe to assume that the advice and information in this book are believed to be true and accurate at the date of publication. Neither the publisher nor the authors or the editors give a warranty, expressed or implied, with respect to the material contained herein or for any errors or omissions that may have been made. The publisher remains neutral with regard to jurisdictional claims in published maps and institutional affiliations.

This Springer imprint is published by the registered company Springer-Verlag GmbH, AT part of Springer Nature.
The registered company address is: Prinz-Eugen-Str. 8-10, 1040 Wien, Austria

Dedicated
to my late mother Louise and my Aunt Marie-Antoinette
for their lifelong generous support and
to Denisa for our future adventures
(Serge Weis)

to my brother Geri
(Michael Sonnberger)

Dedicated
to my parents for their support and encouragement and
to my daughter Ella the sunshine of my life
(Andreas Dunzinger)

For my wife, my sons, and my daughter.
Thank you for being here with me, you make my life
worth living …
(Peter Strasser)

Preface

The present book deals with picturing various diseases of the human nervous system using different imaging modalities. The appearances of the diseases are visualized on computerized tomography (CT) scans, magnetic resonance imaging (MRI) scans, nuclear medicine scans, surgical intraoperative pictures, gross anatomy, histology, and immunohistochemistry pictures. It is aimed at attracting the interest of neurologists, neuroradiologists, neurosurgeons, and neuropathologists as well as all allied neuroscientific disciplines. The information provided should facilitate the understanding of the disease processes in their daily routine work.

There exist many good and detailed books on the neuroradiologic aspects of brain diseases. Although these books contain hundreds of CT and MR scans, no histologic picture disclosing the microscopic features of the disorders dealt with is included. On the other hand, there exist excellent books describing the neuropathological features of brain disorders. Again, many light and electron microscopic pictures are included; however, the neuroradiologic scans are sparse or lacking. The correlative combination of nuclear medicine scans with either neuroradiologic scans or neuropathology images is nearly absent. The present book is, hence, an attempt to bridge the gap between neuro-clinicians, neuro-imagers, and neuropathologists.

It is our intention to present the brain disorders in a very systematic way allowing the reader to easily find the topics in which she or he is particularly interested. Although it might be considered monotonous, we feel that this approach is an effective didactic way in presenting data which can quickly be retrieved.

The book starts with a description of the various imaging modalities, i.e. computerized tomography and nuclear magnetic resonance imaging (Chap. 1). Here, the tremendous advances achieved during the last two decades are illustrated with the wealth of new imaging techniques available for daily routine diagnosis like spectroscopy, perfusion imaging, diffusion weighted imaging, and diffusion tensor imaging. Nuclear medicine imaging (Chap. 2) aims at representing the functional/metabolic state of the brain using different techniques (SPECT, PET) and applying various tracers like methionine, fluordeoxyglucose, fluorethyltyrosine, etc. in order to visualize various biochemical pathways (i.e., transmitter, amino acids, glucose). Chapter 3 describes the neuropathological approach for analyzing brain diseases. The cellular and tissue components of the normal nervous system are presented. The immunohistochemical typing of the various cells which make up the nervous system is presented in detail. A detailed description of the normal human brain and its vascular supply is provided in Chaps. 4–14 of Part II.

The subsequent chapters (Chaps. 15–83) of Part III to Part X deal with the various disorders involving the nervous system which can be grouped into the following disorders: hemodynamic (Chaps. 15 and 16), vascular (Chaps. 17–24), infectious (Chaps. 25–29), neurodegenerative (Chaps. 30–40), demyelination (Chaps. 41–43), epilepsy (Chaps. 44 and 45), trauma and intoxication (Chaps. 46–48), and the vast field of tumors (Chaps. 49–83).

The approach in presenting a brain disease entity is in the following order: brief definition of the entity, relative incidence, age incidence, sex incidence, predilection sites of the lesion, description of the characteristic CT findings with representative CT scans, description of the characteristic MRI findings with representative MRI scans, nuclear medicine findings, macroscopic features including intraoperative findings, microscopic features, ultrastructural features, immunohistochemical staining characteristics, spectrum of reactivities to proliferation markers, differential diagnosis, pathogenesis and molecular biological characteristics, treatment, and biologic behavior, prognosis, and prognostic factors.

Although molecular biology was and is undoubtedly the scientific trendsetter during the last decades and for the forthcoming years, however, some doubts about the promises made by medical molecular biologists are appropriate. In the future, people will see bands on blots, but they will not see anymore the cell, the tissue, and the organism and finally not anymore the patient. Okazaki in his *Fundamentals of Neuropathology* expressed the same opinion as follows: "Many residents are intelligent and well versed in the latest molecular biologic concepts or neurochemical advances, but they often have difficulties in recognizing actual brain lesions or interpreting histologic findings."

Furthermore, we want to impart to our young colleagues a sound and comprehensive knowledge on diseases involving the nervous system. Through this schematic, straightforward presentation, the aspiring clinical neuroscientist in training will hopefully not undergo the same frustrations that we experienced.

Special thanks are expressed to Johannes Trenkler, M.D. (Head, Department of Radiology); Robert Pichler, M.D., Ph.D. (Head, Department of Nuclear Medicine); and Prof. Andreas Gruber, M.D., Ph.D. (Head, Department of Neurosurgery), at the Neuromed Campus of the Kepler University Hospital (formerly Landes-Nervenklinik Wagner-Jauregg) for their fruitful collaboration. Dr. Weis thanks his medical team including Ognian Kalev, M.D. (senior consultant); Karoline Ornig, M.D. (trainee); and Dave Bandke, M.D., B.S.A. (trainee), for providing interesting cases. The help of Michaela Gnauer, clinical psychologist, for reviewing Chap. 14 is highly appreciated.

Finally, the authors acknowledge the skillful technical help of the following medical technologists (in alphabetical order):

- In neuropathology: Sabine Engstler, Susanne Fiedler, Gabriele Göberl, Christina Keuch, Anna Kroiss, Monika Lugmayr, and Christa Winter-Schwarz. Special thanks are necessary to appreciate the diligent work of Stefan Pirngruber as best mortuary technician and archivist of the histological blocks and sections. Birgit Kronfuss helped with secretarial work.
- In Neurosurgery: Hans-Peter Dahl, Franz Knogler, and Thomas Wimmer for registering the intraoperative images. Hans-Peter was very helpful with annotating some images.
- In neuroradiology: to the whole team of radiotechnologists (too many to name).
- In neuronuclear medicine: to the whole team of radiotechnologists (especially Silke Kern for her technical knowledge and her good memory of patients).

The authors thank Mag. Barbara Pfeiffer (Vienna), Claus-Dieter Bachem (Heidelberg), Andrea Ridolfi (Turin), Abha Krishnan, Jeyaraj Allwynkingsly, and Shanjini Rajasekaran (Chennai) from Springer-Verlag Wien, New York, for a smooth and perfect collaboration.

Linz, Austria	Serge Weis
Linz, Austria	Michael Sonnberger
Linz, Austria	Andreas Dunzinger
Linz, Austria	Eva Voglmayr
Linz, Austria	Martin Aichholzer
Linz, Austria	Raimund Kleiser
Salzburg, Austria	Peter Strasser

Contents

Volume I

Part I   The Techniques

1   Imaging Modalities: Neuroradiology 3
   1.1   Introduction 3
   1.2   CT-Imaging 4
      1.2.1   Equipment 4
      1.2.2   Image Presentation........................... 5
      1.2.3   Characteristics of CT-Imaging................. 6
      1.2.4   Contrast and Details Resolution................ 6
      1.2.5   Artifacts 6
      1.2.6   Contrast Medium 6
      1.2.7   Recent Developments and Trends 6
      1.2.8   CT-Angiography 7
      1.2.9   CT-Perfusion 7
   1.3   MR Imaging.. 9
      1.3.1   Equipment 9
      1.3.2   Image Presentation........................... 9
      1.3.3   Characteristics of MR Imaging 11
      1.3.4   Contrast and Details Resolution................ 13
      1.3.5   Imaging Protocols 13
      1.3.6   Artifacts 14
      1.3.7   Contrast Medium 14
      1.3.8   Recent Developments and Trends 15
      1.3.9   MR Spectroscopy............................. 15
      1.3.10 MR Angiography 16
      1.3.11 MR-Perfusion Imaging 18
      1.3.12 MR Diffusion-Weighted Imaging (DWI).......... 19
      1.3.13 MR Diffusion Tensor Imaging (DTI)............. 19
      1.3.14 Functional MRI (fMRI)....................... 20
      1.3.15 Neuronavigation and Intraoperative MRI 22
      1.3.16 Imaging Protocol Lists........................ 27
   Selected References 28

2	**Imaging Modalities: Nuclear Medicine**	29
2.1	Introduction	29
2.2	SPECT: Single Photon Emission Computed Tomography	39
2.3	PET—Positron Emission Tomography	42
2.4	FDG-PET	44
2.5	Amino Acid PET	48
2.6	123I-FP-CIT	49
2.7	D2 Receptor Ligands	50
2.8	Brain Perfusion SPECT	51
2.9	Amyloid Imaging	53
2.10	Indications for Nuclear Medicine Examinations	54
	Selected References	55
3	**Imaging Modalities: Neuropathology**	57
3.1	Introduction	57
3.2	Removal, Fixation, and Cutting of the Brain and Spinal Cord	58
	3.2.1 Removal and Fixation of the Brain	58
	3.2.2 Removal and Fixation of the Spinal Cord	63
	3.2.3 Brain Cutting	65
	3.2.4 Gross Anatomical Examination of the Cut Brain	74
	3.2.5 Sampling of Brain Regions for Microscopic Examination	75
	3.2.6 Handling of Surgical Specimens	75
3.3	Fixation and Processing of Tissue	76
	3.3.1 Fixation of Sampled Tissue	76
	3.3.2 Processing of Tissue	78
3.4	Staining of Tissue	79
	3.4.1 Classical Stain	79
	3.4.2 Special Stains	83
	3.4.3 Special Neuro-stains	84
	3.4.4 Special Stains for Connective Tissue	87
	3.4.5 Other Special Stains	89
3.5	Immunohistochemistry	89
	3.5.1 General Principles	89
	3.5.2 Neuronal Markers	92
	3.5.3 Synaptic Markers	95
	3.5.4 Astroglial Markers	96
	3.5.5 Oligodendroglial Markers: Myelin Markers	97
	3.5.6 Microglial Markers	99
	3.5.7 Markers for Neurodegeneration	100
	3.5.8 Tumor Markers	102
	3.5.9 Vascular Markers	103
	3.5.10 Hematopoietic and Lymphatic Markers	105
	3.5.11 Proliferation Markers in Tumors	105
	3.5.12 Markers for Infectious Agents	107
	3.5.13 Immunohistochemical Panels	108

3.6	Other Techniques	108
	3.6.1	Electron Microscopy	108
	3.6.2	Fluorescence Microscopy	108
	3.6.3	Enzyme Histochemistry	108
	3.6.4	*In Situ* Hybridization (ISH)	111
	3.6.5	Molecular Biology	111
	3.6.6	Other Imaging Techniques	114
Selected References	114

Part II The Normal Human Brain

4 Subdivisions of the Nervous System 121
- 4.1 Central Nervous System (CNS) and Peripheral Nervous System (PNS) 121
  - 4.1.1 Central Nervous System (CNS) 121
  - 4.1.2 Peripheral Nervous System (PNS) 122
- 4.2 Cerebrospinal and Autonomic Nervous System 122
  - 4.2.1 Cerebrospinal Nervous System 122
  - 4.2.2 Autonomic Nervous System 123
- 4.3 Cortical Areas 123
  - 4.3.1 Somatotopic Organization 123
  - 4.3.2 Primary Cortical Areas 123
  - 4.3.3 Secondary Cortical Areas 123
- 4.4 Gray and White Matter 125
  - 4.4.1 Gray Matter 125
  - 4.4.2 White Matter 125
  - 4.4.3 Nuclei and Ganglia 125
  - 4.4.4 Tracts 125
  - 4.4.5 Neuropil 125
- Selected References 127

5 Gross Anatomy of the Nervous System 129
- 5.1 Subdivisions of the Central Nervous System 129
- 5.2 Telencephalon 129
  - 5.2.1 Superolateral Surface 131
  - 5.2.2 Medial Surface 135
  - 5.2.3 Inferior Surface 136
- 5.3 Limbic System 137
- 5.4 Hippocampal Formation 138
- 5.5 Amygdala 142
- 5.6 Basal Ganglia 143
  - 5.6.1 Caudate Nucleus 144
  - 5.6.2 Globus Pallidus 145
  - 5.6.3 Putamen 145
  - 5.6.4 Nucleus Accumbens 145
- 5.7 White Matter 146
  - 5.7.1 Projection Fibers 147
  - 5.7.2 Association Fibers 147
  - 5.7.3 Commissural Fibers 148

		5.8	Diencephalon	150
			5.8.1 Thalamus	150
			5.8.2 Hypothalamus	153
			5.8.3 Subthalamus	155
			5.8.4 Epithalamus	155
		5.9	Mesencephalon	156
		5.10	Pons	156
		5.11	Medulla Oblongata	160
		5.12	Cerebellum	162
		5.13	Spinal Cord	163
		5.14	Pituitary Gland	164
		5.15	3D Reconstructions of the Brain and Cutplanes	166
		Selected References		168
6	**Ventricular System: Cerebrospinal Fluid (CSF)—Barriers**			169
	6.1	Introduction		169
	6.2	Ventricular System		169
		6.2.1	Lateral Ventricles	169
		6.2.2	Third Ventricle	174
		6.2.3	Fourth Ventricle	174
	6.3	Cerebrospinal Fluid (CSF)		174
	6.4	Choroid Plexus		176
	6.5	Barriers		176
		6.5.1	The Blood–Brain Barrier (BBB)	176
		6.5.2	The Brain–Liquor Barrier (BLB)	176
		6.5.3	The Blood–Liquor Barrier	176
	Selected References			177
7	**Meninges**			179
	7.1	Introduction		179
	7.2	Dura Mater		179
	7.3	Dural Sinuses		182
	7.4	Arachnoidea		186
	7.5	Pia Mater		186
	7.6	The Meningeal Spaces		188
	7.7	Arachnoidal Granulations		188
	Selected References			189
8	**Arterial Supply of the Brain**			191
	8.1	Introduction		191
	8.2	Carotid System		191
	8.3	Vertebro-Basilar System		199
	8.4	Clinical Vascular Syndromes		202
		8.4.1	Anterior Cerebral Artery Syndrome	202
		8.4.2	Middle Cerebral Artery Syndrome	208
		8.4.3	AICA Syndrome (Lateral Pontine Syndrome)	208
		8.4.4	Posterior Inferior Cerebellar Artery Syndrome (PICA Syndrome)	208
		8.4.5	Posterior Cerebral Artery Syndrome	209
	Selected References			209

Contents

9 Venous Drainage of the Brain 211
    9.1 Introduction 211
    9.2 Venous System 211
    9.3 Dural Venous Sinuses 218
    Selected References 224

10 Histological Constituents of the Nervous System 225
    10.1 Neuron 225
        10.1.1 Classification of Neurons 229
        10.1.2 Size of Neurons 231
        10.1.3 Types of Neuronal Connection 231
    10.2 Synapse 232
        10.2.1 The Presynaptic Membrane 232
        10.2.2 The Postsynaptic Membrane 234
        10.2.3 The Synaptic Cleft 234
        10.2.4 Types of synapses 234
        10.2.5 Classification of synapses 235
    10.3 Nerve Fibers and Peripheral Nerve 236
        10.3.1 Morphological Features of Nerve Fibers 236
        10.3.2 Classification of Nerve Fibers 238
        10.3.3 Structure of Peripheral Nerves 238
    10.4 Glial Cells 239
    10.5 Astroglia (Astrocytes) 240
    10.6 Oligodendroglia (Oligodendrocytes) 245
    10.7 Microglia 247
    10.8 Ependymal Cells 249
    10.9 Tanycytes 250
    10.10 Molecular Composition of White Matter Myelin 250
        10.10.1 Lipids 250
        10.10.2 Myelin Basic Protein (MBP) 250
        10.10.3 Proteolipid Protein (PLP) 250
        10.10.4 Myelin-Associated Glycoprotein (MAG) 250
        10.10.5 Myelin Oligodendrocyte Glycoprotein (MOG) .. 251
        10.10.6 2′,3′-Cyclic Nucleotide 3′-Phosphodiesterase (CNP) 251
        10.10.7 Myelin Oligodendrocyte Basic Protein (MOBP) 251
        10.10.8 Other CNS Myelin Proteins 252
    10.11 Meninges 252
        10.11.1 Dura mater 252
        10.11.2 Arachnoidea 252
        10.11.3 Pia Mater 252
        10.11.4 Sinuses 254
    10.12 Choroid Plexus 254
    10.13 Vessels 254
        10.13.1 Artery 255
        10.13.2 Arteriole 255
        10.13.3 Capillary 256
        10.13.4 Venule and Vein 258

		10.13.5 Endothelium	258
		10.13.6 Glymphatic System	259
	10.14	Neurovascular Unit	259
	Selected References		261

11 Microscopical Buildup of the Nervous System 267
	11.1	Cerebral Cortex	267
		11.1.1 Architectonics	269
		11.1.2 Layers and Networks of the Cerebral Cortex	282
	11.2	Hippocampus	294
		11.2.1 Cornu Ammonis (Hippocampus Proper)	295
		11.2.2 Gyrus Dentatus (Fascia Dentata, Gyrus Involutus)	299
		11.2.3 Entorhinal Cortex	300
		11.2.4 Nucleus Basalis Meynert	300
	11.3	Amygdala	300
	11.4	White Matter	301
	11.5	Basal Ganglia	301
		11.5.1 Caudate Nucleus and Putamen	301
		11.5.2 Globus Pallidus	304
	11.6	Diencephalon	305
		11.6.1 Thalamus	305
		11.6.2 Hypothalamus	306
	11.7	Mesencephalon	306
		11.7.1 Substantia Nigra	307
		11.7.2 Nucleus Ruber	308
	11.8	Pons	310
	11.9	Medulla Oblongata	311
		11.9.1 Area Postrema	312
		11.9.2 Pyramis	312
		11.9.3 Inferior Olivary Complex	313
	11.10	Cerebellum	313
	11.11	Spinal Cord	318
	11.12	Ventricular System	321
		11.12.1 Ventricular Lining	321
		11.12.2 Choroid Plexus	321
	Selected References		323

12 Functional Systems 325
	12.1	Introduction	325
	12.2	Sensory System: Visual System	325
	12.3	Motor System: Central Motor System	333
		12.3.1 Corticospinal Tract	333
	12.4	Motor System: Basal Ganglionic System	333
	12.5	Sensory System: Somatosensory System	333
	12.6	Cerebral Cortex	341
	12.7	Limbic System	342
	12.8	Hippocampal System	345
		12.8.1 Polysynaptic Intrahippocampal Pathway	345
		12.8.2 Direct Intrahippocampal Pathway	348
		12.8.3 Regulatory Circuits	348

	12.9	Amygdalar System.	349
	12.10	Cerebellum.	349
	12.11	Thalamic System	351
	12.12	Hypothalamus and Hypophyseal System.	351
	12.13	Two-stream Hypothesis	355
		12.13.1 Visual System: Two-Stream Hypothesis	355
		12.13.2 Ventral Stream	357
		12.13.3 Dorsal Stream.	360
	12.14	The Connectome	360
	12.15	Rich-Club Organization.	363
	Selected References		366
13	**Neurotransmitter Systems**		**369**
	13.1	Acetylcholine.	373
	13.2	Catecholamines Monoamines	376
		13.2.1 Dopamine.	376
		13.2.2 Noradrenaline.	381
		13.2.3 Monoamines: Adrenaline.	384
		13.2.4 Monoamines: Serotonin.	385
	13.3	Amino Acids	388
		13.3.1 γ-Aminobutyric Acid (GABA)	388
		13.3.2 Glutamic Acid (Glu)	391
	Selected References		395
14	**Localization of Brain Function**		**401**
	14.1	Frontal Cortex	403
		14.1.1 Primary Motor Cortex	403
		14.1.2 Supplementary Motor Area	403
		14.1.3 Premotor Cortex.	403
		14.1.4 Prefrontal Cortex (Frontal Association Cortex)	403
		14.1.5 Frontal Pole: Orbitofrontal Area	404
		14.1.6 Mesial Aspect: Cingulate Gyrus	404
	14.2	Parietal Cortex	404
		14.2.1 Primary Somatosensory Cortex	404
		14.2.2 Secondary Somatosensory Cortex	405
		14.2.3 Somatosensory Association Area.	405
		14.2.4 Postcentral Gyrus.	405
		14.2.5 Superior and Inferior Parietal Lobules.	405
		14.2.6 Supramarginal and Angular Gyri	405
		14.2.7 Angular Gyrus	406
		14.2.8 Mesial Aspect: Cuneus.	406
	14.3	Occipital Cortex.	406
		14.3.1 Primary Visual Cortex	406
		14.3.2 Visual Association Cortex	406
		14.3.3 Mesial Aspect.	406
		14.3.4 Lateral Aspect	407
	14.4	Temporal Cortex	408
		14.4.1 Primary Auditory Cortex	408
		14.4.2 Auditory Association Cortex	408

		14.4.3	Inferomedial Aspect (Amygdala and Hippocampus)	408
		14.4.4	Anterior Tip (Including Amygdala; Bilateral Lesions)	408
		14.4.5	Latero-inferior Aspect	408
		14.4.6	Latero-superior Aspect	408
		14.4.7	Non-localizing	409
		14.4.8	With Epileptogenic Lesions	409
	14.5	Language Areas		409
	14.6	Cortical Syndromes		412
	14.7	Limbic System		413
		14.7.1	Hippocampus	413
		14.7.2	Amygdala	413
		14.7.3	Stria Terminalis	413
		14.7.4	Septal Nuclei	413
		14.7.5	Cingulate Cortex	413
	14.8	Corpus Callosum		413
	14.9	Basal Ganglia		415
	14.10	Thalamus		416
	14.11	Hypothalamus		417
	14.12	Cerebellum		418
	14.13	White Matter		419
	Selected References			422

Part III The Brain Diseases: Edema and Hydrocephalus

15	**Brain Edema: Intracranial Pressure—Herniation**		427
	15.1	Definition	427
	15.2	Epidemiology	427
	15.3	Localization	428
	15.4	General Imaging Findings	428
	15.5	Neuropathology Findings	434
		15.5.1 Microscopic Features	439
		15.5.2 Ultrastructural Features	440
	15.6	Molecular Neuropathology	440
	15.7	Treatment and Prognosis	441
	Selected References	441

16	**Hydrocephalus**		443
	16.1	Definition	443
	16.2	Clinical Signs and Symptoms	443
	16.3	Epidemiology	443
	16.4	General Imaging Findings	444
	16.5	Neuropathology Findings	449
	16.6	Molecular Neuropathology	451
	16.7	Treatment and Prognosis	451
	Selected References	451

Part IV The Brain Diseases: Vascular system

17 Vascular Disorders: Hypoxia 455
    17.1   Introduction 455
    17.2   Clinical Signs 456
    17.3   Epidemiology 456
    17.4   Neuroimaging Findings 456
    17.5   Neuropathology Findings 463
    17.6   Molecular Neuropathology 466
    17.7   Treatment and Prognosis 470
    Selected References 470

18 Vascular Disorders: Ischemia–Infarction–Stroke 473
    18.1   Introduction 473
    18.2   Clinical Signs and Symptoms 473
    18.3   Epidemiology 474
    18.4   Neuroimaging Findings 477
    18.5   Neuropathology Findings 484
    18.6   Molecular Neuropathology 489
    18.7   Treatment and Prognosis 496
    Selected References 496

19 Vascular Disorders: Hemorrhage 499
    19.1   General Considerations 499
    19.2   Intracerebral Hemorrhage 500
        19.2.1   Clinical Signs and Symptoms 500
        19.2.2   Epidemiology 500
        19.2.3   Neuroimaging Findings 500
        19.2.4   Neuropathology Findings 501
        19.2.5   Molecular Neuropathology 501
        19.2.6   Treatment and Prognosis 503
    19.3   Subarachnoid Hemorrhage (SAH) 505
        19.3.1   Clinical Signs and Symptoms 505
        19.3.2   Epidemiology 505
        19.3.3   Neuroimaging Findings 505
        19.3.4   Neuropathology Findings 510
        19.3.5   Molecular Neuropathology 514
        19.3.6   Treatment and Prognosis 514
    19.4   Subdural Hemorrhage 520
        19.4.1   Clinical Signs and Symptoms 520
        19.4.2   Epidemiology 520
        19.4.3   Neuroimaging Findings 520
        19.4.4   Neuropathology Findings 521
        19.4.5   Molecular Neuropathology 522
        19.4.6   Treatment and Prognosis 524
    19.5   Epidural Hemorrhage (EDH) 529
        19.5.1   Clinical Signs and Symptoms 529
        19.5.2   Localization 529
        19.5.3   Neuroimaging Findings 529

		19.5.4	Neuropathology Findings.	530
		19.5.5	Molecular Neuropathology	530
		19.5.6	Treatment and Prognosis	533
	Selected References			533
20	**Vascular Disorders: Arteriosclerosis**			**537**
	20.1	Introduction		537
	20.2	Epidemiology		537
	20.3	Neuroimaging Findings		538
	20.4	Neuropathology Findings.		538
	20.5	Molecular Neuropathology		540
	20.6	Treatment and Prognosis		542
	Selected References			548
21	**Vascular Disorders: Aneurysms**			**551**
	21.1	Definition		551
	21.2	Epidemiology		551
	21.3	Neuroimaging Findings		551
	21.4	Neuropathology Findings.		552
	21.5	Molecular Neuropathology		558
	21.6	Treatment and Prognosis		570
	Selected References			576
22	**Vascular Disorders: Malformations**			**577**
	22.1	Introduction		577
	22.2	Arteriovenous Malformation (AVM)		577
		22.2.1	Epidemiology	577
		22.2.2	Neuroimaging Findings	577
		22.2.3	Neuropathology Findings.	578
		22.2.4	Molecular Neuropathology	584
		22.2.5	Treatment and Prognosis	585
	22.3	Cavernous Hemangioma (Cavernoma)		585
		22.3.1	Epidemiology	585
		22.3.2	Neuroimaging Findings	585
		22.3.3	Neuropathology Findings.	586
		22.3.4	Molecular Neuropathology	586
		22.3.5	Treatment and Prognosis	586
	22.4	Capillary Telangiectasia		593
		22.4.1	Epidemiology	593
		22.4.2	Neuroimaging Findings	596
		22.4.3	Neuropathology Findings.	596
		22.4.4	Molecular Neuropathology	596
		22.4.5	Treatment and Prognosis	596
	22.5	Dural AV-Fistula		599
		22.5.1	Neuroimaging Findings	599
	Selected References			603
23	**Vascular Disorders: Angiopathies**			**605**
	23.1	Introduction		605
	23.2	Cerebral Amyloid Angiopathy		605
		23.2.1	Clinical Signs and Symptoms	605
		23.2.2	Epidemiology	606

		23.2.3	Neuroimaging Findings.................	606
		23.2.4	Neuropathology Findings..............	607
		23.2.5	Molecular Neuropathology	607
		23.2.6	Treatment and Prognosis	615
	23.3	Binswanger Disease............................		615
		23.3.1	Clincal Signs and Symptoms	615
		23.3.2	Epidemiology........................	616
		23.3.3	Neuroimaging Findings................	616
		23.3.4	Neuropathology Findings	616
		23.3.5	Molecular Neuropathology	622
		23.3.6	Treatment and Prognosis	622
	23.4	Fahr Disease................................		622
		23.4.1	Clinical Signs and Symptoms	622
		23.4.2	Localisation	622
		23.4.3	Neuroimaging Findings................	622
		23.4.4	Neuropathology Findings..............	622
		23.4.5	Molecular Neuropathology	626
		23.4.6	Treatment and Prognosis	626
	23.5	Cerebral Autosomal Dominant Arteriopathy (CADASIL)...		626
		23.5.1	Clinical Signs and Symptoms	626
		23.5.2	Epidemiology.......................	627
		23.5.3	Neuroimaging Findings................	627
		23.5.4	Neuropathology Findings..............	628
		23.5.5	Molecular Neuropathology	632
		23.5.6	Treatment and Prognosis	632
	Selected References			633
24	**Vascular Disorders: Vasculitis**........................			635
	24.1	Definition................................		635
	24.2	Clinical Signs and Symptoms		636
	24.3	Epidemiology..............................		637
	24.4	Neuroimaging Findings		637
	24.5	Neuropathology Findings.......................		641
	24.6	Molecular Neuropathology		641
	24.7	Treatment and Prognosis		649
	Selected References			649

Part V The Brain Diseases: Infections

25	**Infections: Bacteria**................................		653
	25.1	Clinical Signs and Symptoms	653
	25.2	Classification of Bacteria.........................	653
	25.3	General Aspects	655
	25.4	Epidemiology................................	655
	25.5	Imaging Features	657
		25.5.1 Meningitis	657
		25.5.2 Encephalitis	661
		25.5.3 Brain Abscess...........................	661
		25.5.4 Subdural Empyema	663

	25.6	Neuropathology Findings.	666
	25.7	Molecular Neuropathology	687
	25.8	Treatment and Prognosis	690
	Selected References		691

26 Infections: Viruses. 693
	26.1	Clinical Signs and Symptoms	693
	26.2	Classification of Viruses.	693
	26.3	Epidemiology.	693
	26.4	Neuroimaging Findings	696
	26.5	Neuropathology Findings.	697
	26.6	Molecular Neuropathology	698
	26.7	Treatment and Prognosis	699
	26.8	Unspecified Nodular Encephalitis	699
	26.9	RNA Viruses: Human Immunodeficiency Virus (HIV)-1.	700
		26.9.1 HIV-1 Encephalitis (HIVE)	702
		26.9.2 HIV-1 Leukoencephalopathy (HIVL)	703
		26.9.3 Lymphocytic Meningitis (LM) and Perivascular Lymphocytic Infiltration (PLI)	703
		26.9.4 Vacuolar Myelopathy (VM) and Vacuolar Leukoencephalopathy (VL)	706
		26.9.5 Neuropathological Changes in Early Stages of HIV-1 Infection	706
		26.9.6 Neuropathological Changes in HIV-1-Infected Children	708
		26.9.7 Therapy: HAART Effects and Therapy-Induced Immune Restitution Inflammatory Syndrome (IRIS).	710
		26.9.8 The Sequalae of HIV-1 Infection of the Nervous System.	715
		26.9.9 Pathogenetic Mechanisms	717
	26.10	DNA-Virus: Cytomegalovirus Infection (CMV)	720
		26.10.1 Neuroradiology Findings.	720
		26.10.2 Neuropathology Findings.	720
	26.11	Progressive Multifocal Leukoencephalopathy (PML).	722
		26.11.1 Clinical Signs and Symptoms	722
		26.11.2 Neuroimaging Findings	725
		26.11.3 Neuropathology Findings.	725
		26.11.4 Molecular Nauropathology	730
	26.12	Herpes Simplex Virus (HSV) Encephalitis	731
		26.12.1 Clinical Signs and Symptoms	731
		26.12.2 Neuroimaging Findings	731
		26.12.3 Neuropathology Findings.	736
		26.12.4 Molecular Neuropathology	736
		26.12.5 Treatment and Prognosis	736
	26.13	Tick-Borne Encephalitis	736
		26.13.1 Clinical Signs and Symptoms	736
		26.13.2 Epidemiology.	737
		26.13.3 Neuroimaging Findings	737

		26.13.4	Neuropathology Findings.	739
		26.13.5	Molecular Neuropathology	741
		26.13.6	Treatment and Prognosis	742
	Selected References			742

27 Infections: Parasites ... 749
- 27.1 Classification of Parasitic Agents. ... 749
- 27.2 Clinical Signs and Symptoms ... 749
- 27.3 *Toxoplasma gondii* ... 749
  - 27.3.1 Clinical Signs and Symptoms ... 749
  - 27.3.2 Epidemiology. ... 751
  - 27.3.3 Neuroimaging Findings. ... 752
  - 27.3.4 Neuropathology Findings. ... 752
  - 27.3.5 Molecular Neuropathology ... 752
  - 27.3.6 Treatment and Prognosis ... 756
- 27.4 Taeniasis: Coenurosis/Cysticercosis ... 762
  - 27.4.1 Cysticercosis: Clinical Signs and Symptoms. ... 762
  - 27.4.2 Coenurosis: Clinical Signs and Symptoms ... 762
  - 27.4.3 Epidemiology. ... 763
  - 27.4.4 Neuroimaging Findings. ... 763
  - 27.4.5 Neuropathology Findings. ... 767
  - 27.4.6 Molecular Neuropathology ... 768
  - 27.4.7 Treatment and Prognosis ... 771
- Selected References ... 771

28 Infections: Fungi. ... 773
- 28.1 General Aspects ... 773
  - 28.1.1 Clinical Signs and Symptoms ... 773
  - 28.1.2 Epidemiology. ... 773
  - 28.1.3 Classification of Fungi. ... 773
  - 28.1.4 Neuroimaging Findings. ... 775
  - 28.1.5 Neuropathology Stains. ... 776
  - 28.1.6 Molecular Neuropathology ... 776
  - 28.1.7 Treatment. ... 776
- 28.2 *Aspergillus Fumigatus* ... 777
  - 28.2.1 Neuroimaging Findings. ... 777
  - 28.2.2 Neuropathology Findings. ... 778
  - 28.2.3 Molecular Neuropathology ... 781
- 28.3 *Cryptococcus Neoformans* ... 782
  - 28.3.1 Neuroimaging Findings. ... 782
  - 28.3.2 Neuropathology Findings. ... 785
  - 28.3.3 Molecular Neuropathology ... 785
- 28.4 *Candida Albicans*. ... 787
  - 28.4.1 Neuropathology Findings. ... 787
  - 28.4.2 Molecular Pathology ... 787
- Selected References ... 793

29 Prion Encephalopathies ... 797
- 29.1 General Aspects ... 797
  - 29.1.1 Clinical Signs and Symptoms ... 799
  - 29.1.2 Neuroimaging Findings. ... 799
  - 29.1.3 Neuropathology Findings. ... 804

		29.1.4	Treatment and Prognosis	816
		29.1.5	Molecular Neuropathology	816
	29.2	Creutzfeldt–Jakob Disease (CJD)		818
		29.2.1	Clinical Signs	818
		29.2.2	Macroscopic Features	819
		29.2.3	Microscopic Features	819
	29.3	Variant CJD		820
		29.3.1	Clinical Signs and Symptoms	820
		29.3.2	Microscopic Features	821
		29.3.3	Molecular Neuropathology	821
	29.4	Gerstmann–Sträussler–Scheinker Disease (GSS)		821
		29.4.1	Clinical signs	821
		29.4.2	Microscopic Features	821
	29.5	Fatal Familial Insomnia (FFI)		822
		29.5.1	Clinical signs	822
		29.5.2	Microscopic Features	822
	29.6	Kuru		822
		29.6.1	Clinical signs	822
		29.6.2	Macroscopical Features	822
		29.6.3	Microscopical Features	822
	Selected References			823

Volume II

Part VI The Brain Diseases: Aging and Neurodegeneration

30 Neurodegeneration: General Aspects 827

30.1	Introduction		827
30.2	Clinical Signs and Symptoms		827
	30.2.1	Dementia	828
	30.2.2	Motor Disorders	830
30.3	Neuropathologic Changes		830
	30.3.1	Gross-anatomical Changes	830
	30.3.2	Microscopical Changes	830
	30.3.3	Amyloid Deposits	830
	30.3.4	Neurofibrillary Changes: Tauopathies	838
	30.3.5	Neuropil Threads	839
	30.3.6	Lewy Bodies	839
	30.3.7	Granulovacuolar Degeneration	840
	30.3.8	Ballooned Neurons	840
	30.3.9	Histological Visualization of Amyloid Deposits and Tangles	841
	30.3.10	Immunohistochemical Pattern in the Differential Diagnosis	844
	30.3.11	Frequencies of Neuropathology Diagnoses	844
30.4	Comparisons		844
30.5	Molecular Neuropathology		844
	30.5.1	Concepts of Neurodegenerative Diseases	844
	30.5.2	Relevant Proteins	846

	30.5.3	Amyloid and the Amyloid Cascade Hypothesis	847
	30.5.4	Tau	849
	30.5.5	Synuclein (α-Syn)	849
	30.5.6	TDP-43	851
	30.5.7	FUS	851
	30.5.8	Nucleotide Repeat Diseases	853
30.6	Biomarkers		853
30.7	Brief Sketch of the Differential Diagnoses		856
30.8	Differential Diagnoses: Lobar Atrophies		856
	30.8.1	Pick Disease	856
	30.8.2	Primary Progressive Aphasia (PPA)	856
	30.8.3	Motor Neuron Disease with Dementia	857
	30.8.4	Dementia Lacking Distinctive Histopathology (DLDH)	857
30.9	Differential Diagnoses: Subcortical Dementias		857
	30.9.1	Progressive Subcortical Gliosis (PSG)	857
	30.9.2	Parkinson Disease with Dementia	857
30.10	Differential Diagnoses: Rare Cortical Dementias		857
	30.10.1	Chromosome 17-Associated Dementia	857
	30.10.2	Familial Presenile Dementia with Tangles (FPDT)	858
	30.10.3	Meso-Limbo-Cortical Dementia	858
30.11	Differential Diagnoses: Down Syndrome		858
30.12	Differential Diagnoses: Diffuse Neurofibrillary Tangles with Calcifications (DNTC)		859
30.13	Differential Diagnoses: Rare Neurodegenerative Disorders		859
	30.13.1	Thalamic Degeneration	859
	30.13.2	(Non) Hereditary Bilateral Striatal Necrosis	860
	30.13.3	Neuroacanthocytosis	860
	30.13.4	Pallidal Degenerations	860
	30.13.5	Dentato-Rubro-Pallido-Luysian Degeneration	860
	30.13.6	Substantia Reticularis degeneration	861
30.14	Differential Diagnoses: Argyrophilic Grain Disease (AG)		861
30.15	Differential Diagnoses: Adult Polyglucosan Body Disease (APBD)		863
30.16	Differential Diagnoses: Normal Pressure Hydrocephalus (NPH)		863
30.17	Differential Diagnoses: Mitochondrial Encephalomyopathies		864
	30.17.1	Clinical Signs of Mitochondrial Encephalopathies	864
	30.17.2	Neuropathology Findings	864
30.18	Differential Diagnoses: Metabolic and Traumatic Disorders		866
	30.18.1	Hallervorden-Spatz Disease	866
	30.18.2	Leukodystrophies	866

	30.18.3 Wilson Disease: Hepato-Lenticular Degeneration	867
	30.18.4 Dementia Pugilistica	867
	Selected References	867

31 Normal Aging Brain ... 871
- 31.1 Introduction ... 871
  - 31.1.1 WHO Definition of Well-Being ... 871
- 31.2 Clinical Signs and Symptoms ... 872
- 31.3 Epidemiology ... 872
- 31.4 Neuroimaging Findings ... 872
- 31.5 Neuropathology Findings ... 874
- 31.6 Incidental White Matter Changes ... 877
- 31.7 Molecular Neuropathology ... 881
  - 31.7.1 Astrocytes ... 882
  - 31.7.2 Microglia ... 882
  - 31.7.3 Autophagy ... 883
  - 31.7.4 Unfolded Protein Response (UPR): Endoplasmic Reticulum Stress—Stress Response Pathways ... 883
  - 31.7.5 Mitochondria ... 884
  - 31.7.6 Advanced Glycation End-Product (AGE) ... 885
  - 31.7.7 cAMP Response Element Binding Protein (CREB) ... 885
  - 31.7.8 Ion Channels and ROS ... 885
  - 31.7.9 Sirtuins ... 885
  - 31.7.10 Translocator Protein (TSPO) ... 886
  - 31.7.11 Cathepsins ... 886
  - 31.7.12 Ghrelin ... 886
  - 31.7.13 Klotho ... 886
  - 31.7.14 Iron ... 886
  - 31.7.15 Insulin ... 887
  - 31.7.16 Signaling ... 887
- 31.8 Genetics of Successful Aging ... 887
- 31.9 Non-coding RNAs ... 888
- 31.10 DNA Damage ... 890
- 31.11 Treatment and Prognosis ... 890
- Selected References ... 892

32 Neurodegenerative Diseases: Alzheimer Disease (AD) ... 897
- 32.1 Clinical Signs and Symptoms ... 897
- 32.2 International Working Group (IWG) Clinical Criteria ... 897
- 32.3 Early-Onset AD Versus Late-Onset AD ... 900
- 32.4 Neuroimaging Findings ... 900
- 32.5 Neuropathology Findings ... 903
- 32.6 The Proposed Diagnostic Criteria ... 903
  - 32.6.1 Ball Criteria: The Hippocampal Criteria ... 903
  - 32.6.2 Newcastle Criteria (Tomlinson, Roth, Blessed) ... 915
  - 32.6.3 NIH Criteria (Khachaturian) ... 915

		32.6.4	NINCDS-ADRA	916
		32.6.5	CERAD Criteria	917
		32.6.6	NIH/Reagan	918
	32.7	Staging of Neurofibrillary Tangle Development		919
	32.8	Phases of Aß-deposition by Thal et al. (2002)		923
	32.9	Molecular Neuropathology		923
		32.9.1	Genetics	923
		32.9.2	Aberrations in Mitochondrial DNA (mtDNA)	926
		32.9.3	Epigenetics	927
	32.10	Treatment and Prognosis		928
	Selected References			928
33	**Neurodegenerative Diseases: Lewy Body Dementia**			**933**
	33.1	Clinical Signs and Symptoms		933
	33.2	Epidemiology		933
	33.3	Neuroimaging Findings		935
	33.4	Neuropathology Findings		939
	33.5	Molecular Neuropathology		939
	33.6	Treatment and Prognosis		939
	Selected References			943
34	**Neurodegenerative Diseases: Fronto-temporal Lobar Degeneration**			**945**
	34.1	Clinical Signs and Symptoms		945
	34.2	Epidemiology		945
	34.3	Neuroimaging Findings		945
	34.4	Neuropathology Subgroups		953
	34.5	Types of FTLD		954
		34.5.1	Fronto-temporal Lobar Degeneration with TDP-43 Proteinopathy	954
		34.5.2	Fronto-temporal Lobar Degeneration with Motor Neuron Disease Type Inclusions	956
		34.5.3	Fronto-temporal Lobar Degeneration with *GRN* Mutation	958
		34.5.4	Fronto-temporal Lobar Degeneration with *VCP* Mutation	959
		34.5.5	Fronto-temporal Lobar Degeneration with *C9ORF* Mutation	959
		34.5.6	Fronto-temporal Lobar Degeneration with Ubiquitin-Positive Inclusions (FTLD/UPS)	960
		34.5.7	Fronto-temporal Lobar Degeneration with Tauopathy	960
		34.5.8	Pick Disease	960
		34.5.9	Cortico-basal Degeneration	962
		34.5.10	Progressive Supranuclear Palsy	962
		34.5.11	Argyrophilic Grain Disease	962
		34.5.12	Sporadic Multiple System Tauopathy with Dementia	962

		34.5.13	White Matter Tauopathy with Globular Glial Inclusions	964
		34.5.14	Tangle-Only Dementia.....................	964
		34.5.15	Fronto-temporal Lobar Degeneration with *MAPT* Mutation	965
		34.5.16	Fronto-temporal Lobar Degeneration with FUS Proteinopathy....................	965
		34.5.17	Neuronal Intermediate Filament Inclusion Disease (NIFID)...........................	966
		34.5.18	Basophilic Inclusion Body Disease (BIBD)	966
		34.5.19	Atypical Fronto-temporal Lobar Degeneration with Ubiquitin-Positive Inclusions (FTLD-U).......................	967
		34.5.20	Fronto-temporal Lobar Degeneration with No Inclusions........................	967
	34.6	Molecular Neuropathology		968
	34.7	Treatment and Prognosis		968
	Selected References			968
35	**Neurodegenerative Diseases: Progressive Supranuclear Palsy (PSP)–Cortico-Basal Degeneration (CBD)**............			973
	35.1	Introduction		973
	35.2	Progressive Supranuclear Palsy (PSP).................		973
		35.2.1	Clinical Signs..........................	973
		35.2.2	Epidemiology..........................	973
		35.2.3	Neuroimaging Findings	974
		35.2.4	Neuropathology Findings.................	976
		35.2.5	Molecular Neuropathology	978
		35.2.6	Treatment and Prognosis	978
	35.3	Cortico-Basal Degeneration (CBD)....................		978
		35.3.1	Clinical Signs..........................	978
		35.3.2	Neuroimaging Findings	978
		35.3.3	Neuropathology Findings.................	981
		35.3.4	Molecular Neuropathology	984
		35.3.5	Treatment and Prognosis	984
	Selected References			984
36	**Neurodegenerative Diseases: Vascular Dementia**			987
	36.1	Introduction		987
	36.2	Clinical Signs and Symptoms		988
	36.3	Diagnostic Criteria................................		989
	36.4	Epidemiology.....................................		989
	36.5	Neuroimaging Findings		989
	36.6	Neuropathology Findings...........................		991
	36.7	Leuko-araiosis		995
	36.8	Morbus Binswanger................................		995
	36.9	Cerebral Amyloid Angiopathy.......................		995
	36.10	CADASIL		995
	36.11	Molecular Neuropathology		995
	36.12	Treatment and Prognosis		995
	Selected References			1000

37 Neurodegenerative Diseases: Parkinson Disease 1001
- 37.1 Clinical Signs and Symptoms 1001
- 37.2 Epidemiology..................................... 1003
- 37.3 Neuroimaging Findings 1003
- 37.4 Neuropathology Findings........................... 1007
- 37.5 Molecular Neuropathology 1012
  - 37.5.1 Pathogenesis................................ 1012
  - 37.5.2 Genetics 1013
  - 37.5.3 Epigenetics................................. 1017
- 37.6 Treatment and Prognosis........................... 1018
- Selected References 1019

38 Neurodegenerative Diseases: Multiple System Atrophy (MSA)....................................... 1021
- 38.1 Introduction 1021
- 38.2 Clinical Signs and Symptoms 1021
- 38.3 Epidemiology..................................... 1022
- 38.4 Neuroimaging Findings 1022
- 38.5 Neuropathology Findings........................... 1027
- 38.6 Molecular Neuropathology 1034
- 38.7 Treatment and Prognosis 1034
- Selected References 1035

39 Neurodegenerative Diseases: Motor Neuron Diseases......... 1037
- 39.1 Introduction 1037
- 39.2 Clinical Signs and Symptoms 1037
- 39.3 Diagnostic Criteria................................ 1037
- 39.4 Epidemiology..................................... 1039
- 39.5 Neuroimaging Findings 1039
- 39.6 Neuropathology Findings........................... 1042
- 39.7 Molecular Neuropathology 1045
  - 39.7.1 Pathogenetic Mechanisms 1045
  - 39.7.2 Genes...................................... 1050
- 39.8 Treatment and Prognosis 1055
- Selected References 1056

40 Neurodegenerative Diseases: Huntington Disease 1059
- 40.1 Introduction 1059
- 40.2 Clinical Signs and Symptoms 1059
- 40.3 Epidemiology..................................... 1059
- 40.4 Neuroimaging Findings 1059
- 40.5 Neuropathology Findings........................... 1063
- 40.6 Molecular Neuropathology 1065
  - 40.6.1 Genetics 1067
  - 40.6.2 Epigenetics................................. 1067
- 40.7 Treatment and Prognosis 1067
- Selected References 1067

Part VII The Brain Diseases: Myelin Disorders

41 Demyelinating Diseases: Multiple Sclerosis 1071
    41.1   Introduction 1071
    41.2   Clinical Signs and Symptoms 1071
    41.3   Epidemiology 1073
    41.4   Neuroimaging Findings 1073
    41.5   Neuropathology Findings 1077
    41.6   Molecular Neuropathology 1087
    41.7   Treatment and Prognosis 1092
    Selected References 1093

42 Demyelinating Diseases: Neuromyelitis Optica Spectrum Disorder 1097
    42.1   Clinical Signs and Symptoms 1097
    42.2   Epidemiology 1098
    42.3   Neuroimaging Findings 1098
    42.4   Neuropathology Findings 1101
    42.5   Molecular Neuropathology 1101
    42.6   Treatment and Prognosis 1103
    Selected References 1103

43 Demyelinating Diseases: Acute Demyelinating Encephalomyelitis (ADEM) 1105
    43.1   Introduction 1105
    43.2   Clinical Signs and Symptoms 1105
    43.3   Epidemiology 1105
    43.4   Neuroimaging Findings 1105
    43.5   Neuropathology Findings 1106
    43.6   Molecular Neuropathology 1115
    43.7   Treatment and Prognosis 1115
    Selected References 1115

Part VIII The Brain Diseases: The Epilepsies

44 Epilepsies: General Aspects 1119
    44.1   Introduction 1119
    44.2   Definitions 1119
    44.3   Classification of the Epilepsies 1121
        44.3.1   International League Against Epilepsy (ILEA) Classification-1981 1121
        44.3.2   International League Against Epilepsy (ILEA) Classification-1989 1121
        44.3.3   International League Against Epilepsy (ILEA) Classification-2010 1122
        44.3.4   International League Against Epilepsy (ILAE) Classification-2017 1122
        44.3.5   International Classification of Diseases Classification (ICD)-2012 1123
        44.3.6   Electroclinical Syndromes 1123

	44.4	Neuroimaging Findings 1124
		44.4.1 Transient Seizure Related Imaging Features 1124
	44.5	Etiological Classification of Epilepsies 1129
	44.6	Neuropathological Lesions Associated with the Epilepsies 1129
	44.7	Molecular Neuropathology 1132
	44.8	Malformations Due to Genetic Changes 1135
	44.9	Treatment 1138
	Selected References 1139

45 Epilepsies: Temporal Lobe Epilepsy 1143
    45.1 Introduction 1143
    45.2 Clinical Signs. 1143
    45.3 Neuroimaging Findings 1143
    45.4 Neuropathology Findings. 1147
    45.5 Molecular Neuropathology 1153
    45.6 Treatment and Prognosis 1154
    Selected References 1154

46 Epilepsies: Malformations of Cortical Development—Focal Cortical Dysplasia (FCD) 1157
    46.1 Introduction 1157
    46.2 Neuroimaging Findings 1157
    46.3 Neuropathology Findings. 1158
    46.4 Historical Classification. 1165
    46.5 Molecular Neuropathology 1168
    Selected References 1168

47 Epilepsies: Malformations of Cortical Development—Heterotopia 1171
    47.1 Definition 1171
    47.2 Neuroimaging Findings 1171
    47.3 Neuropathology Findings. 1171
        47.3.1 White Matter Heterotopia 1171
        47.3.2 Nodular Heterotopia. 1175
        47.3.3 Periventricular Nodular Heterotopia 1176
        47.3.4 Subcortical Laminar Heterotopias 1178
    47.4 Molecular Neuropathology 1179
    Selected References 1179

Part IX The Brain Diseases: Trauma and Intoxication

48 Trauma. 1185
    48.1 Definition 1185
    48.2 Epidemiology. 1185
    48.3 Clinical Signs and Symptoms 1185
    48.4 Classification of TBI 1186
    48.5 Neuroimaging Findings 1192
        48.5.1 Cerebral Contusions. 1192
        48.5.2 Chronic Traumatic Brain Injury. 1192

	48.6 Focal Injuries 1196
	48.7 Diffuse Injuries 1207
	48.8 Chronic Traumatic Encephalopathy................... 1212
	48.9 Molecular Neuropathology 1214
	48.10 Treatment and Prognosis 1218
	Selected References 1220

49 Intoxication: Alcohol................................. 1223
   49.1 Introduction 1223
   49.2 Ethanol: Acute and Chronic Alcoholism 1223
       49.2.1 Clinical Signs and Symptoms 1223
       49.2.2 Epidemiology................................. 1223
       49.2.3 Neuroimaging Findings 1224
       49.2.4 Neuropathology Findings...................... 1224
   49.3 Wernicke–Korsakoff Encephalopathy 1228
       49.3.1 Clinical Signs............................... 1228
       49.3.2 Neuroimaging Findings 1228
       49.3.3 Neuropathology Findings...................... 1230
       49.3.4 Molecular Neuropathology 1230
   49.4 Cerebellar Degeneration 1230
       49.4.1 Clinical Signs............................... 1230
       49.4.2 Neuropathology Findings...................... 1230
   49.5 Central Pontine Myelinolysis........................ 1233
       49.5.1 Clinical Signs............................... 1233
       49.5.2 Neuroimaging Findings 1233
       49.5.3 Neuropathology Findings...................... 1233
       49.5.4 Molecular Neuropathology 1233
   49.6 Marchiafava–Bignami Disease 1235
       49.6.1 Clinical Signs............................... 1235
       49.6.2 Neuroimaging Findings 1235
       49.6.3 Neuropathology Findings...................... 1238
   49.7 Fetal Alcohol Spectrum Disorders (FASD) 1238
       49.7.1 Clinical Signs............................... 1238
       49.7.2 Neuropathology Findings...................... 1239
       49.7.3 Molecular Neuropathology 1240
   Selected References 1240

50 Intoxication: Street Drugs 1243
   50.1 Introduction 1243
       50.1.1 General Aspects.............................. 1243
       50.1.2 Clinical Signs and Symptoms 1243
       50.1.3 Neuroimaging Findings 1244
   50.2 Opiates 1244
       50.2.1 Neuroimaging Findings 1244
       50.2.2 Neuropathology Findings...................... 1245
       50.2.3 Molecular Neuropathology 1247
   50.3 Cocaine 1253
       50.3.1 Clinical Signs and Symptoms 1253
       50.3.2 Neuroimaging Findings 1254

Contents

50.3.3 Neuropathology Findings. 1254
50.3.4 Molecular Neuropathology 1254
50.4 Cannabis. 1255
50.4.1 CNS Complications of Cannabis. 1255
50.4.2 Neuroimaging Findings 1256
50.4.3 Neuropathology Findings. 1256
50.4.4 Molecular Neuropathology 1256
50.5 Amphetamine and Methamphetamine. 1257
50.5.1 Clinical Signs and Symptoms 1257
50.5.2 Neuroimaging Findings 1257
50.5.3 Neuropathology Findings. 1257
50.5.4 Molecular Neuropathology 1257
50.6 Designer Drugs 1258
50.6.1 Substances 1258
50.6.2 Modes of Action. 1258
50.6.3 Molecular Neuropathology 1259
50.6.4 Outcome. 1259
Selected References 1259

Volume III

Part X The Brain Diseases: Tumors

51 Tumors of the Nervous System: General Considerations 1263
51.1 Clinical Signs and Symptoms 1263
51.2 Definitions 1264
51.2.1 Neuro-oncology 1264
51.2.2 Tumor. 1264
51.2.3 Neoplasia 1264
51.2.4 Brain Tumor. 1264
51.2.5 Malignant Versus Benign. 1264
51.2.6 Seeding and Metastases 1264
51.2.7 Various Modalities of Therapy. 1265
51.2.8 Endpoints on Clinical Trials 1265
51.3 Histologic Tumor Characteristics 1266
51.3.1 Cellularity 1266
51.3.2 Anaplasia 1266
51.3.3 Metaplasia 1266
51.3.4 Pleomorphism 1266
51.3.5 Mitoses. 1266
51.3.6 Reactive Versus Neoplastic 1267
51.3.7 Endothelial Proliferation and Neovascularity 1268
51.3.8 Necrosis 1268
51.3.9 Encapsulation and Invasion 1269
51.3.10 Rosettes 1269
51.3.11 Palisades and Pseudopalisades. 1270
51.3.12 Desmoplasia. 1270
51.3.13 Reactive Astrogliosis 1271
51.3.14 Microglial Activation. 1271

51.3.15	Perivascular Lymphocytic Cuffing	1271
51.4	WHO Classification of Tumors of the Central Nervous System	1271
51.5	Grading Systems for Brain Tumors	1273
51.5.1	WHO Grading System	1273
51.5.2	Kernohan et al. (1949)	1273
51.5.3	Ringertz (1950)	1273
51.5.4	St. Anne/Mayo	1274
51.5.5	Smith Grading for Oligodendroglioma	1274
51.6	Frequencies of Brain Tumors	1275
51.7	Molecular Neuropathology: The Hallmarks of Cancer	1275
51.8	Molecular Neuropathology: Cell Cycle	1277
51.8.1	The Cell Cycle in Normal Cells	1277
51.8.2	The Cell Cycle in Cancer Cells	1280
51.9	Molecular Neuropathology: DNA Damage Response	1281
51.9.1	Mechanisms of DNA Damage Recognition	1281
51.9.2	Mechanisms of DNA Damage Repair	1282
51.10	Molecular Neuro-oncology: Oncogenes	1285
51.11	Molecular Neuropathology: Tumor Suppressors	1286
51.12	Molecular Neuropathology: Cell Death	1289
51.12.1	Apoptosis	1289
51.12.2	Autophagy	1293
51.12.3	Necroptosis	1296
51.12.4	Ferroptosis	1296
51.12.5	Pyroptosis	1296
51.12.6	Parthanatos	1297
51.12.7	NETosis	1297
51.12.8	Caspase-Independent Cell Death	1297
51.13	Molecular Neuropathology: Genomic Instability	1300
51.14	Molecular Neuropathology: Signal Transduction Pathways	1302
51.14.1	PKC	1305
51.15	Molecular Neuropathology: Epigenetic Changes	1305
51.16	Molecular Neuropathology: Telomeres and Telomerase	1306
51.17	Molecular Neuropathology: Angiogenesis	1306
51.17.1	Features of Tumor Endothelial Cells	1307
51.18	Molecular Neuro-oncology: Glioma Invasion and Microenvironment	1310
51.19	Molecular Neuro-oncology: MicroRNAs	1315
51.20	Molecular Neuro-oncology: Stem Cell Hypothesis	1315
51.21	Carcinogenic Agents	1317
51.22	Common Molecular Changes in Brain Tumors	1318
51.23	Treatment for Brain Tumors	1325
	Selected References	1327

52 Diffuse Astrocytoma WHO Grade II 1333
    52.1 Epidemiology 1333
    52.2 Neuroimaging Findings 1334
    52.3 Neuropathology Findings 1334

		52.4	Molecular Neuropathology	1344
			52.4.1 Pathogenesis	1344
			52.4.2 Genetics	1344
			52.4.3 Epigenetics	1344
			52.4.4 Gene Expression	1345
		52.5	Treatment and Prognosis	1345
		Selected References		1345
53	**Anaplastic Astrocytoma WHO Grade III**			**1347**
		53.1	Epidemiology	1348
		53.2	Neuroimaging Findings	1348
		53.3	Neuropathology Findings	1352
		53.4	Molecular Neuropathology	1358
		53.5	Treatment and Prognosis	1358
		Selected References		1359
54	**Glioblastoma**			**1361**
		54.1	Epidemiology	1362
		54.2	Neuroimaging Findings	1362
		54.3	Neuropathology Findings	1374
		54.4	Molecular Neuropathology	1389
			54.4.1 Pathogenesis	1389
			54.4.2 Genetics	1390
			54.4.3 Epigenetics	1395
			54.4.4 Gene Expression	1395
		54.5	Treatment and Prognosis	1398
			54.5.1 Treatment: State of the Art	1398
			54.5.2 Treatment: Historical Aspects	1399
		Selected References		1400
55	**Gliosarcoma WHO Grade IV-Giant Cell Glioblastoma WHO Grade IV**			**1403**
		55.1	Gliosarcoma WHO Grade IV	1403
			55.1.1 Epidemiology	1403
			55.1.2 Neuroimaging Findings	1403
			55.1.3 Neuropathology Findings	1406
			55.1.4 Molecular Neuropathology	1406
			55.1.5 Treatment and Prognosis	1410
		55.2	Giant Cell Glioblastoma WHO Grade IV	1410
			55.2.1 Epidemiology	1411
			55.2.2 Neuroimaging Findings	1411
			55.2.3 Neuropathology Findings	1411
			55.2.4 Molecular Neuropathology	1414
			55.2.5 Treatment and Prognosis	1414
		Selected References		1414
56	**Gliomatosis Cerebri**			**1417**
		56.1	Epidemiology	1417
		56.2	Neuroimaging Findings	1418
		56.3	Neuropathology Findings	1421

	56.4	Molecular Neuropathology	1421
	56.5	Treatment and Prognosis	1421
	Selected References		1423

57 Pilocytic Astrocytoma WHO Grade I ... 1425
- 57.1 Epidemiology ... 1425
- 57.2 Neuroimaging Findings ... 1426
- 57.3 Neuropathology Findings ... 1426
- 57.4 Molecular Neuropathology ... 1435
  - 57.4.1 Pathogenesis ... 1435
  - 57.4.2 Genetics ... 1435
  - 57.4.3 Epigenetics ... 1436
- 57.5 Treatment and Prognosis ... 1436
- Selected References ... 1437

58 Oligodendroglioma WHO Grade II-Anaplastic Oligodendroglioma WHO Grade III ... 1439
- 58.1 Oligodendroglioma WHO Grade II ... 1439
  - 58.1.1 Epidemiology ... 1439
  - 58.1.2 Neuroimaging Findings ... 1440
  - 58.1.3 Neuropathology Findings ... 1440
  - 58.1.4 Molecular Neuropathology ... 1446
  - 58.1.5 Treatment and Prognosis ... 1450
- 58.2 Anaplastic Oligodendroglioma WHO Grade III ... 1450
  - 58.2.1 Epidemiology ... 1451
  - 58.2.2 Neuroimaging Findings ... 1451
  - 58.2.3 Neuropathology Findings ... 1454
  - 58.2.4 Molecular Neuropathology ... 1454
  - 58.2.5 Treatment and Prognosis ... 1458
- Selected References ... 1458

59 Oligo-astrocytoma WHO Grade II-Anaplastic Oligo-astrocytoma WHO Grade III ... 1461
- 59.1 Oligo-astrocytoma WHO Grade II ... 1461
  - 59.1.1 Epidemiology ... 1461
  - 59.1.2 Neuroimaging Findings ... 1461
  - 59.1.3 Neuropathology Findings ... 1464
  - 59.1.4 Molecular Neuropathology ... 1468
  - 59.1.5 Treatment and Prognosis ... 1468
- 59.2 Anaplastic Oligo-astrocytoma WHO Grade III ... 1468
  - 59.2.1 Epidemiology ... 1469
  - 59.2.2 Neuroimaging Findings ... 1469
  - 59.2.3 Neuropathology Findings ... 1469
  - 59.2.4 Molecular Neuropathology ... 1478
  - 59.2.5 Treatment and Prognosis ... 1478
- Selected References ... 1478

60 Ependymal Tumors ... 1481
- 60.1 General Aspects ... 1481
  - 60.1.1 Clinical Signs and Symptoms ... 1481
  - 60.1.2 Nuclear Medicine Imaging Findings ... 1481

Contents

		60.1.3	Molecular Neuropathology	1481
	60.2	Ependymoma WHO Grade II		1483
		60.2.1	Epidemiology	1484
		60.2.2	Neuroimaging Findings	1484
		60.2.3	Neuropathology Findings	1486
		60.2.4	Treatment and Prognosis	1491
	60.3	Anaplastic Ependymoma WHO Grade III		1491
		60.3.1	Epidemiology	1492
		60.3.2	Neuroimaging Findings	1492
		60.3.3	Neuropathology Findings	1492
		60.3.4	Treatment and Prognosis	1497
	60.4	Myxopapillary Ependymoma (WHO Grade I)		1497
		60.4.1	Epidemiology	1498
		60.4.2	Neuroimaging Findings	1498
		60.4.3	Neuropathology Findings	1498
		60.4.4	Treatment and Prognosis	1499
	60.5	Subependymoma (WHO Grade I)		1502
		60.5.1	Epidemiology	1503
		60.5.2	Neuroimaging Findings	1503
		60.5.3	Neuropathology Findings	1503
		60.5.4	Treatment and Prognosis	1510
	Selected References			1510
61	**Choroid Plexus Tumors**			1513
	61.1	General Aspects		1513
		61.1.1	Epidemiology	1513
		61.1.2	Nuclear Medicine Imaging Findings	1513
		61.1.3	Differential Diagnosis	1514
		61.1.4	Molecular Neuropathology	1514
		61.1.5	Treatment and Prognosis	1514
	61.2	Choroid Plexus Papilloma WHO Grade I		1514
		61.2.1	Neuroimaging Findings	1515
		61.2.2	Neuropathology Findings	1515
	61.3	Atypical Choroid Plexus Papilloma (WHO Grade II)		1521
		61.3.1	Neuroimaging Findings	1522
		61.3.2	Neuropathology Findings	1522
	61.4	Choroid Plexus Carcinoma WHO Grade III		1522
		61.4.1	Neuroimaging Findings	1526
		61.4.2	Neuropathology Findings	1526
		61.4.3	Molecular Neuropathology	1526
	Selected References			1531
62	**Dysembryoplastic Neuroepithelial Tumor (DNT)**			1533
	62.1	Epidemiology		1533
	62.2	Neuroimaging Findings		1534
	62.3	Neuropathology Findings		1534
	62.4	Molecular Neuropathology		1537
	62.5	Treatment and Prognosis		1542

Selected References 1542

63 Desmoplastic (Infantile) Astrocytoma/Ganglioglioma (DIA/DIG) 1545
- 63.1 Epidemiology..................................... 1545
- 63.2 Neuroimaging Findings 1546
- 63.3 Neuropathology Findings........................ 1546
- 63.4 Molecular Neuropathology 1549
- 63.5 Treatment and Prognosis 1551
- Selected References 1551

64 Ganglioglioma/Gangliocytoma 1553
- 64.1 Ganglioglioma 1553
  - 64.1.1 Epidemiology............................... 1554
  - 64.1.2 Neuroimaging Findings 1554
  - 64.1.3 Neuropathology Findings................... 1556
  - 64.1.4 Molecular Neuropathology 1558
  - 64.1.5 Treatment and Prognosis 1563
- 64.2 Anaplastic Ganglioglioma 1563
  - 64.2.1 Epidemiology............................... 1563
  - 64.2.2 Neuroimaging Findings 1564
  - 64.2.3 Neuropathology Findings................... 1564
  - 64.2.4 Molecular Neuropathology 1564
  - 64.2.5 Treatment and Prognosis 1565
- Selected References 1565

65 Neurocytoma: Central—Extraventricular 1567
- 65.1 Epidemiology..................................... 1567
- 65.2 Neuroimaging Findings 1568
- 65.3 Neuropathology Findings........................ 1570
- 65.4 Molecular Neuropathology 1572
- 65.5 Treatment and Prognosis 1574
- Selected References 1574

66 Rosette-Forming Glioneuronal Tumor (RGNT) 1575
- 66.1 Epidemiology..................................... 1575
- 66.2 Neuroimaging Findings 1575
- 66.3 Neuropathology Findings........................ 1579
- 66.4 Molecular Neuropathology 1583
- 66.5 Treatment and Prognosis 1583
- Selected References 1584

67 Pineal Parenchymal Tumors 1587
- 67.1 General Aspects 1587
  - 67.1.1 Epidemiology............................... 1587
  - 67.1.2 Nuclear Medicine Imaging Findings 1587
  - 67.1.3 Differential Diagnosis 1587
  - 67.1.4 Molecular Neuropathology 1587
- 67.2 Pineocytoma..................................... 1588
  - 67.2.1 Neuroimaging Findings 1588

		67.2.2	Neuropathology Findings. 1591
		67.2.3	Treatment and Prognosis 1595
	67.3	Pineal Parenchymal Tumor of Intermediate Differentiation 1595
		67.3.1	Neuropathology Findings. 1595
		67.3.2	Treatment and Prognosis 1597
	67.4	Pineoblastoma 1597
		67.4.1	Neuroimaging Findings 1597
		67.4.2	Neuropathology Findings. 1599
		67.4.3	Treatment and Prognosis 1599
	Selected References 1601
68	**Medulloblastoma**. 1605
	68.1	Epidemiology. 1606
	68.2	Neuroimaging Findings 1606
	68.3	Neuropathology Findings. 1609
	68.4	Molecular Neuropathology 1621
		68.4.1	Pathogenesis. 1621
		68.4.2	Molecular Classification of Medulloblastomas . . . 1621
		68.4.3	Epigenetics. 1623
	68.5	Treatment and Prognosis 1623
	Selected References 1626
69	**Embryonal Tumors: Other CNS Embryonal Tumors** 1629
	69.1	General Aspects 1629
	69.2	CNS Embryonal Tumor, NOS 1630
		69.2.1	Epidemiology. 1631
		69.2.2	Neuroimaging Findings 1631
		69.2.3	Neuropathology Findings. 1631
		69.2.4	Molecular Neuropathology 1636
		69.2.5	Treatment and Prognosis 1636
	69.3	Embryonal Tumors with Multilayered Rosettes, C19MC-Altered 1636
		69.3.1	Epidemiology. 1636
		69.3.2	Neuropathology Findings. 1636
		69.3.3	Molecular Neuropathology 1638
		69.3.4	Treatment and Prognosis 1639
	69.4	Medulloepithelioma. 1639
		69.4.1	Epidemiology. 1639
		69.4.2	Neuropathology Findings. 1639
		69.4.3	Molecular Neuropathology 1640
		69.4.4	Treatment and Prognosis 1640
	Selected References 1640
70	**Embryonal Tumors: Atypical Teratoid/Rhabdoid Tumor (ATRT)**. 1643
	70.1	Epidemiology. 1643
	70.2	Neuroimaging Findings 1643

		70.3	Neuropathology Findings.	1645
		70.4	Molecular Neuropathology	1648
		70.5	Treatment and Prognosis	1649
	Selected References			1649
71	**Tumors of the Peripheral Nervous System**			1651
	71.1	General Aspects		1651
		71.1.1	Clinical Signs and Symptoms	1651
		71.1.2	Classification of Tumors of the Peripheral Nervous System.	1651
		71.1.3	Nuclear Medicine Imaging Findings	1652
	71.2	Schwannoma		1654
		71.2.1	Epidemiology.	1654
		71.2.2	Neuroimaging Findings	1654
		71.2.3	Neuropathology Findings.	1657
		71.2.4	Molecular Neuropathology	1665
		71.2.5	Treatment and Prognosis	1665
	71.3	Neurofibroma.		1665
		71.3.1	Epidemiology.	1665
		71.3.2	Neuroimaging Findings	1666
		71.3.3	Neuropathology Findings.	1666
		71.3.4	Molecular Neuropathology	1668
		71.3.5	Treatment and Prognosis	1670
	71.4	Perineurioma		1670
		71.4.1	Epidemiology.	1672
		71.4.2	Neuroimaging Findings	1672
		71.4.3	Neuropathology Findings.	1674
		71.4.4	Molecular Neuropathology	1674
		71.4.5	Treatment and Prognosis	1674
	71.5	Hybrid Nerve Sheath Tumors		1675
		71.5.1	Neuropathology Findings.	1675
	71.6	Malignant Peripheral Nerve Sheath Tumor (MPNST)		1675
		71.6.1	Epidemiology.	1678
		71.6.2	Neuroimaging Findings	1678
		71.6.3	Neuropathology Findings.	1679
		71.6.4	Molecular Neuropathology	1681
		71.6.5	Treatment and Prognosis	1682
	71.7	Neurofibromatosis Type 1 (NF1).		1682
		71.7.1	Incidence and Diagnostic Criteria	1682
		71.7.2	Neuroimaging Findings	1683
		71.7.3	Neuropathology Findings.	1683
		71.7.4	Molecular Neuropathology	1683
	71.8	Neurofibromatosis Type 2 (NF2).		1683
		71.8.1	Incidence and Diagnostic Criteria	1686
		71.8.2	Neuroimaging Findings	1688
	71.9	Schwannomatosis.		1688
		71.9.1	Incidence and Diagnostic Criteria	1688
	71.10	Molecular Neuropathology		1688

		71.10.1 Neurofibromatosis Type 1 (NF1)	1689
		71.10.2 Neurofibromatosis Type 2 (NF2)	1689
		71.10.3 Schwannomatosis	1690
		71.10.4 Malignant Peripheral Nerve Sheath Tumor (MPNST)	1691
		71.10.5 Epigenetics	1692
	Selected References		1692
72	**Tumors of Meningothelial Cells: Meningiomas**		**1695**
	72.1	Introduction	1695
	72.2	General Aspects	1695
		72.2.1 Clinical Signs and Symptoms	1695
		72.2.2 Epidemiology	1695
		72.2.3 Neuroimaging Features	1696
	72.3	Meningioma	1705
		72.3.1 Neuropathology Findings	1707
	72.4	Atypical Meningioma	1727
		72.4.1 Neuropathology Findings	1727
	72.5	Anaplastic (Malignant) Meningioma	1729
		72.5.1 Microscopic Features	1729
	72.6	Common Neuropathology Aspects	1729
	72.7	Molecular Neuropathology	1733
		72.7.1 Pathogenesis	1733
		72.7.2 Genetics	1733
		72.7.3 Signaling Pathways	1733
		72.7.4 Hh (Hedgehog) Pathway	1733
		72.7.5 Wnt (Wingless) Pathway	1734
		72.7.6 Chromosomal Aberrations and Mutations	1734
		72.7.7 Epigenetics	1735
		72.7.8 Gene Expression	1736
	72.8	Treatment and Prognosis	1736
	Selected References		1738
73	**Tumors of the Sellar Region**		**1741**
	73.1	Classification of Tumors of the Sellar Region	1741
	73.2	Craniopharyngioma	1741
		73.2.1 Clinical Signs and Symptoms	1742
		73.2.2 Epidemiology	1742
		73.2.3 Neuroimaging Findings	1742
		73.2.4 Neuropathology Findings	1743
		73.2.5 Molecular Neuropathology	1752
		73.2.6 Treatment and Prognosis	1753
	73.3	Pituicytoma	1753
		73.3.1 Epidemiology	1753
		73.3.2 Neuroimaging Findings	1753
		73.3.3 Neuropathology Findings	1754
		73.3.4 Molecular Neuropathology	1755
		73.3.5 Treatment and Prognosis	1755

	73.4	Granular Cell Tumor of the Sellar Region............ 1757
		73.4.1 Epidemiology............................. 1758
		73.4.2 Neuroimaging Findings.................... 1758
		73.4.3 Neuropathology Findings.................. 1758
		73.4.4 Molecular Neuropathology................. 1762
		73.4.5 Treatment and Prognosis.................. 1762
	73.5	Spindle Cell Oncocytoma........................ 1763
		73.5.1 Epidemiology............................. 1763
		73.5.2 Neuroimaging Findings.................... 1763
		73.5.3 Neuropathology Findings.................. 1763
		73.5.4 Molecular Neuropathology................. 1764
		73.5.5 Treatment and Prognosis.................. 1764
	Selected References.................................... 1764

74 Tumors of the Pituitary Gland........................ 1767
- 74.1 Epidemiology..................................... 1767
- 74.2 Classification of Pituitary Tumors.................... 1767
  - 74.2.1 Clinical Classification of Pituitary Tumors...... 1768
  - 74.2.2 Radiologic Classification of Pituitary Tumors.... 1768
- 74.3 Radiological Features of Pituitary Tumors............. 1769
  - 74.3.1 Microadenoma............................ 1769
  - 74.3.2 Macroadenoma........................... 1770
- 74.4 Neuropathology Classification of Pituitary Tumors...... 1774
  - 74.4.1 Historical Histological Classification of Pituitary Tumors....................... 1774
  - 74.4.2 Immunohistochemical Classification of Pituitary Tumors....................... 1774
- 74.5 Molecular Neuropathology.......................... 1774
- 74.6 Treatment.. 1780
- 74.7 Prognostic Clinicopathological Classification of Pituitary Tumors................................ 1781
- 74.8 Pituitary Adenomas................................ 1781
  - 74.8.1 Somatotroph Adenoma..................... 1781
  - 74.8.2 Lactotroph Adenoma...................... 1785
  - 74.8.3 Thyrotroph Adenoma...................... 1787
  - 74.8.4 Corticotroph Adenoma..................... 1789
  - 74.8.5 Gonadotroph Adenoma..................... 1790
  - 74.8.6 Null Cell Adenoma........................ 1792
  - 74.8.7 Plurihormonal and Double Adenoma.......... 1794
- 74.9 Atypical Pituitary Adenoma......................... 1796
- 74.10 Pituitary Carcinoma............................... 1798
  - 74.10.1 Clinical Signs and Symptoms............... 1798
  - 74.10.2 Epidemiology............................ 1798
  - 74.10.3 Neuroimaging Findings.................... 1798
  - 74.10.4 Neuropathology Findings.................. 1798
  - 74.10.5 Molecular Neuropathology................. 1800
  - 74.10.6 Prognosis............................... 1800
- 74.11 Pituitary Blastoma................................ 1800

		74.11.1	Clinical Signs and Symptoms	1801
		74.11.2	Epidemiology	1801
		74.11.3	Neuropathology Findings	1801
		74.11.4	Molecular Neuropathology	1801
		74.11.5	Prognosis	1801
	74.12	Apoplexia of the Pituitary		1802
		74.12.1	Clinical Signs and Symptoms	1802
		74.12.2	Epidemiology	1802
		74.12.3	Neuroimaging Findings	1802
		74.12.4	Neuropathology Findings	1802
		74.12.5	Molecular Neuropathology	1802
		74.12.6	Treatment and Prognosis	1805
	Selected References			1808
75	**Cystic Lesions**			**1811**
	75.1	Introduction		1811
	75.2	General Aspects		1811
	75.3	Epidermoid Cyst		1811
		75.3.1	Epidemiology	1811
		75.3.2	Neuroimaging Findings	1812
		75.3.3	Neuropathology Findings	1812
		75.3.4	Molecular Neuropathology	1817
		75.3.5	Treatment and Prognosis	1817
	75.4	Dermoid Cyst		1817
		75.4.1	Epidemiology	1819
		75.4.2	Neuroimaging Findings	1821
		75.4.3	Neuropathology Findings	1821
		75.4.4	Molecular Neuropathology	1825
		75.4.5	Treatment and Prognosis	1825
	75.5	Rathke's Cleft Cyst		1825
		75.5.1	Epidemiology	1825
		75.5.2	Neuroimaging Findings	1829
		75.5.3	Neuropathology Findings	1829
		75.5.4	Molecular Neuropathology	1833
		75.5.5	Treatment and Prognosis	1833
	75.6	Colloid Cyst of the Third Ventricle		1833
		75.6.1	Epidemiology	1834
		75.6.2	Neuroimaging Findings	1834
		75.6.3	Neuropatholog Findings	1834
		75.6.4	Molecular Neuropathology	1838
		75.6.5	Treatment and Prognosis	1838
	75.7	Enterogeneous cyst		1841
		75.7.1	Epidemiology	1841
		75.7.2	Neuroimaging Findings	1841
		75.7.3	Neuropathology Findings	1841
		75.7.4	Molecular Neuropathology	1844
		75.7.5	Treatment and Prognosis	1844
	75.8	Arachnoidal Cyst		1845

		75.8.1	Epidemiology..................................	1845
		75.8.2	Neuroimaging Findings......................	1845
		75.8.3	Neuropathology Findings....................	1845
		75.8.4	Molecular Neuropathology	1849
		75.8.5	Treatment and Prognosis	1849
	Selected References			1851
76	**Germ Cell Tumors**.......................................			**1855**
	76.1	General Aspects		1855
		76.1.1	Epidemiology.................................	1855
		76.1.2	Nuclear Medicine Imaging Findings...........	1856
		76.1.3	Immunophenotype...........................	1856
		76.1.4	Differential Diagnosis	1857
		76.1.5	Molecular Neuropathology	1857
		76.1.6	Treatment and Prognosis	1857
	76.2	Germinoma		1858
		76.2.1	Neuroimaging Findings......................	1858
		76.2.2	Neuropathology Findings....................	1858
	76.3	Yolk Sac tumor.......................................		1861
		76.3.1	Neuropathology Findings....................	1863
	76.4	Embryonal Carcinoma................................		1865
		76.4.1	Neuroimaging Findings......................	1865
		76.4.2	Neuropathology Findings....................	1865
	76.5	Choriocarcinoma		1869
		76.5.1	Neuroimaging Findings......................	1870
		76.5.2	Neuropathology Findings....................	1870
	76.6	Teratoma		1870
		76.6.1	Neuroimaging Findings......................	1872
		76.6.2	Neuropathology Findings....................	1874
	Selected References			1878
77	**Lymphomas**...			**1881**
	77.1	Introduction		1881
	77.2	Primary CNS Lymphoma:		1884
		77.2.1	Clinical Symptoms and Signs	1884
		77.2.2	Epidemiology.................................	1884
		77.2.3	Neuroimaging Findings......................	1884
		77.2.4	Neuropathology Findings....................	1885
		77.2.5	Molecular Neuropathology	1894
		77.2.6	Treatment and Prognosis	1903
	77.3	Intravascular Lymphoma		1904
		77.3.1	Clinical Signs and Symptoms	1904
		77.3.2	Epidemiology.................................	1904
		77.3.3	Neuroimaging Findings......................	1904
		77.3.4	Neuropathology Findings....................	1904
		77.3.5	Molecular Neuropathology	1908
		77.3.6	Treatment and Prognosis	1908
	77.4	Post-Transplant Lymphoproliferative Disorder (PTLD) ...		1909
		77.4.1	Epidemiology.................................	1909

		77.4.2	Neuroimaging Findings 1909
		77.4.3	Neuropathology Findings. 1910
		77.4.4	Molecular Neuropathology 1910
		77.4.5	Treatment and Prognosis 1910
	77.5	Plasmacytoma 1914	
		77.5.1	Epidemiology............................. 1914
		77.5.2	Neuroimaging Findings 1915
		77.5.3	Neuropathology Findings. 1915
		77.5.4	Molecular Neuropathology 1920
		77.5.5	Treatment and Prognosis 1920
	Selected References 1920		

78 Histiocytic Tumors 1923

	78.1	General Considerations 1923	
		78.1.1	Definitions 1923
		78.1.2	Epidemiology............................. 1923
		78.1.3	Nuclear Medicine Imaging Findings 1924
	78.2	Langerhans Cell Histiocytosis (LCH) 1924	
		78.2.1	Clinical Signs and Symptoms 1924
		78.2.2	Epidemiology............................. 1924
		78.2.3	Neuroimaging Findings 1925
		78.2.4	Neuropathology Findings. 1927
		78.2.5	Molecular Neuropathology 1930
		78.2.6	Treatment and Prognosis 1930
	78.3	Non-Langerhans Cell Histiocytoses 1930	
		78.3.1	Epidemiology............................. 1930
		78.3.2	Neuroimaging Findings 1931
		78.3.3	Neuropathology Findings. 1931
		78.3.4	Molecular Neuropathology 1934
		78.3.5	Treatment and Prognosis 1934
	Selected References 1941		

79 Soft Tissue Tumors: Mesenchymal, Non-meningothelial Tumors 1943

	79.1	General Aspects 1943	
		79.1.1	Classification of Soft tissue tumors 1943
		79.1.2	Grading of Soft Tissue Tumors 1943
		79.1.3	Incidence 1944
		79.1.4	Pathogenesis............................. 1944
	79.2	Solitary Fibrous Tumor/Hemangiopericytoma 1944	
		79.2.1	Epidemiology............................. 1945
		79.2.2	Neuroimaging Findings 1945
		79.2.3	Neuropathology Findings. 1948
		79.2.4	Molecular Pathology 1952
		79.2.5	Treatment and Prognosis 1952
	79.3	Hemangioblastoma 1956	
		79.3.1	Epidemiology............................. 1956
		79.3.2	Neuroimaging Findings 1956
		79.3.3	Neuropathology Findings. 1959

		79.3.4	Molecular Pathology	1960
		79.3.5	Treatment and Prognosis	1961
	79.4	Lipoma..		1961
		79.4.1	Definition................................	1961
		79.4.2	Neuroimaging Findings	1962
		79.4.3	Neuropathology Findings...................	1962
	79.5	Undifferentiated High-Grade Pleomorphic Sarcoma: Malignant Fibrous Histiocytoma (MFH)................		1967
		79.5.1	Neuropathology Findings...................	1967
	79.6	Other Mesenchymal Tumors		1967
		79.6.1	Hemangioma	1967
		79.6.2	Epithelioid Hemangioendothelioma	1967
		79.6.3	Angiosarcoma	1970
		79.6.4	Kaposi Sarcoma..........................	1970
		79.6.5	Ewing Sarcoma/Peripheral Primitive Neuroectodermal Tumor	1970
		79.6.6	Angiolipoma	1972
		79.6.7	Hibernoma...............................	1972
		79.6.8	Liposarcoma..............................	1972
		79.6.9	Desmoid-Type Fibromatosis	1972
		79.6.10	Myofibroblastoma	1972
		79.6.11	Inflammatory Myofibroblastic Tumor	1973
		79.6.12	Benign Fibrous Histiocytoma	1973
		79.6.13	Fibrosarcoma	1973
		79.6.14	Undifferentiated Pleomorphic Sarcoma/Malignant Fibrous Histiocytoma	1973
		79.6.15	Leiomyoma	1973
		79.6.16	Leiomyosarcoma	1973
		79.6.17	Rhabdomyoma...........................	1974
		79.6.18	Rhabdomyosarcoma.......................	1974
	Selected References			1974
80	**Bone Tumors**			1977
	80.1	General Aspects of Bone Tumors		1977
		80.1.1	Classification of Bone tumors	1977
		80.1.2	Incidence	1977
		80.1.3	Nuclear Medicine Imaging Findings	1977
		80.1.4	Molecular Pathogenesis......................	1977
		80.1.5	Treatment and Prognosis	1984
	80.2	Osteoma..		1985
		80.2.1	Localization	1985
		80.2.2	Neuroimaging Findings	1985
		80.2.3	Pathology Findings	1985
	80.3	Osteoid Osteoma		1986
		80.3.1	Localization	1986
		80.3.2	Neuroimaging Findings	1986
		80.3.3	Pathology Findings	1987
	80.4	Osteoblastoma.....................................		1992

		80.4.1	Localization 1992
		80.4.2	Pathology Findings 1992
	80.5	Osteosarcoma................................... 1992
		80.5.1	Localization 1992
		80.5.2	Imaging Findings......................... 1992
		80.5.3	Pathology Findings 1994
	80.6	Chondroma...................................... 1996
		80.6.1	Localization 1996
		80.6.2	Pathology Findings 1996
	80.7	Chondrosarcoma 1998
		80.7.1	Localization 1998
		80.7.2	Imaging Findings......................... 1998
		80.7.3	Pathology Findings 2000
	80.8	Fibrous Dysplasia................................ 2005
		80.8.1	Localization 2005
		80.8.2	Imaging Findings......................... 2005
		80.8.3	Pathology Findings 2005
	80.9	Chordoma....................................... 2005
		80.9.1	Localization 2010
		80.9.2	Imaging Findings......................... 2010
		80.9.3	Pathology Findings 2010
	80.10	Giant Cell Tumor................................ 2010
		80.10.1	Localization 2010
		80.10.2	Imaging Findings......................... 2014
		80.10.3	Pathology Findings 2014
	80.11	Aneurysmal Bone Cyst 2016
		80.11.1	Localization 2017
		80.11.2	Imaging Findings......................... 2017
		80.11.3	Pathology Findings 2018
	Selected References 2020
81	**Metastatic Tumors** 2025
	81.1	General Aspects................................. 2025
		81.1.1	Epidemiology............................. 2025
		81.1.2	Neuroimaging Findings.................... 2025
		81.1.3	Neuropathology Findings................... 2038
		81.1.4	Histologic Features 2038
		81.1.5	Molecular Neuropathology 2041
		81.1.6	Treatment and Prognosis 2041
		81.1.7	Immunohistochemical Approach............ 2045
	81.2	Lung Tumors 2051
		81.2.1	General Aspects.......................... 2051
		81.2.2	Neuropathology Findings................... 2051
		81.2.3	Immunophenotype........................ 2051
	81.3	Breast Tumors 2051
		81.3.1	General Aspects.......................... 2051
		81.3.2	Neuropathology Findings................... 2051
		81.3.3	Immunophenotype........................ 2061

81.4	Skin Tumors: Melanoma		2061
	81.4.1	General Aspects	2064
	81.4.2	Neuropathology Findings	2064
	81.4.3	Immunophenotype	2070
81.5	Renal Tumors		2073
	81.5.1	General Aspects	2073
	81.5.2	Neuropathology Findings	2073
	81.5.3	Immunophenotype	2073
81.6	Urinary Tract Tumors		2073
	81.6.1	General Aspects	2073
	81.6.2	Neuroimaging Findings	2073
	81.6.3	Immunophenotype	2073
81.7	Prostate Tumors		2076
	81.7.1	General Aspects	2076
	81.7.2	Neuropathology Findings	2076
	81.7.3	Immunophenotype	2082
81.8	Testicular Tumors		2082
	81.8.1	General Aspects	2082
	81.8.2	Neuropathology Findings	2082
	81.8.3	Immunophenotype	2084
81.9	Gastro-Intestinal Tumors		2084
	81.9.1	General Aspects	2084
81.10	Colon Carcinoma		2085
	81.10.1	Neuropathology Findings	2085
	81.10.2	Immunophenotype	2085
81.11	Esophageal Carcinoma		2085
	81.11.1	Neuropathology Findings	2085
81.12	Gastric Carcinoma		2085
	81.12.1	Neuropathology Findings	2085
	81.12.2	Immunophenotype	2085
81.13	Liver Carcinoma		2085
	81.13.1	Neuropathology Findings	2085
	81.13.2	Immunophenotype	2085
81.14	Pancreas		2093
	81.14.1	Neuropathology Findings	2093
	81.14.2	Immunophenotype	2093
81.15	Female Genital Tract		2093
	81.15.1	General Aspects	2093
81.16	Ovarian Carcinoma		2093
	81.16.1	Neuropathology Findings	2095
	81.16.2	Immunophenotype	2099
81.17	Carcinoma of the Vagina and Cervix		2099
	81.17.1	Neuropathology Findings	2099
	81.17.2	Immunophenotype	2101
81.18	Uterine Carcinoma		2101
	81.18.1	Neuropathology Findings	2101
	81.18.2	Immunophenotype	2101
Selected References			2104

82	**Therapy-Induced Lesions**		2107
	82.1	Introduction	2107
	82.2	General Imaging Findings	2107
	82.3	Radiation Necrosis	2107
		82.3.1 Epidemiology	2108
		82.3.2 Neuroimaging Findings	2108
		82.3.3 Neuropathology Findings	2108
		82.3.4 Molecular Neuropathology	2114
		82.3.5 Treatment and Prognosis	2116
	82.4	Therapy-Induced Leukoencephalopathy	2116
		82.4.1 Clinical Signs	2116
		82.4.2 Neuroimaging Findings	2116
		82.4.3 Neuropathology Findings	2116
		82.4.4 Molecular Neuropathology	2117
	82.5	Therapy-Induced Secondary Neoplasms	2117
		82.5.1 Molecular Neuropathology	2117
	Selected References		2117
83	**Tumor Progression– Pseudoprogression**		2119
	83.1	Introduction	2119
	83.2	Neuroimaging Findings	2119
	83.3	Neuroimaging Criteria for Therapeutic Outcome	2122
		83.3.1 RANO Response Criteria for *Low-Grade Glioma*	2122
		83.3.2 The Immunotherapy Response Assessment in Neuro-Oncology (iRANO) Criteria	2125
	83.4	Nuclear Medicine Findings	2125
	83.5	Molecular Neuropathology	2125
	Selected References		2137
84	**Autoimmune Encephalitis: Paraneoplastic Syndromes**		2139
	84.1	Definitions	2139
	84.2	Epidemiology	2139
	84.3	Clinical Signs	2139
	84.4	Autoimmune Encephalitides	2142
		84.4.1 Limbic Encephalitis (LE)	2142
		84.4.2 Paraneoplastic Limbic Encephalitis (PLE)	2142
		84.4.3 NMDA-R Encephalitis	2142
		84.4.4 Voltage-Gated Potassium Antibody Syndromes	2143
		84.4.5 Morvan Syndrome	2145
		84.4.6 AMPAR (GluR1, GluR2) Antibody Syndrome	2145
		84.4.7 Glycine Receptor Antibody Syndrome	2146
		84.4.8 Dopamine 2 Receptor Antibody Syndrome (D2RA)	2146
		84.4.9 GABA Receptor Ab Syndrome	2146
		84.4.10 Metabotropic Glutamate Receptor Antibody Syndrome	2147
		84.4.11 IgLON5 Ab Syndrome	2147

	84.5	Neuroimaging Findings............................ 2148
		84.5.1 General Imaging Findings................... 2148
	84.6	Neuropathology Findings........................... 2148
	84.7	Molecular Neuropathology 2151
		84.7.1 Predisposition to Autoimmunity.............. 2153
	84.8	Treatment and Prognosis.......................... 2155
		Selected References 2164

Appendix A: WHO Classification of Tumors of the Central Nervous System............................... 2167

Appendix B: WHO Classification of Tumors................... 2181

References 2209

Index.. 2215

About the Authors

Serge Weis is the head of the Division of Neuropathology at the Neuromed Campus of the Kepler University Hospital, Johannes Kepler University, Linz, Austria. He is a native of Luxembourg and studied medicine at the University of Vienna (Austria). He was trained in neuropathology at the Ludwig Maximilians University, Munich, Germany. He was deputy director at the Department of Neuropathology, Otto von Guericke University Magdeburg, (Germany) and director of neuropathology at the Stanley Medical Research Institute, Bethesda, MD, USA. His scientific interests are focused on brain tumors, neurodegeneration, and biological psychiatry. He edited the largest book in German-speaking countries on Alzheimer disease and wrote a book, published in 1993, on 3D reconstruction of the brain (serge.weis@kepleruniklinikum.at).

Michael Sonnberger is a senior consultant in neuroradiology at the Department of Neuroradiology of the Neuromed Campus of the Kepler University Hospital, Johannes Kepler University, Linz, Austria. He studied medicine at the University of Innsbruck (Austria) and was trained in radiology/neuroradiology at the University of Regensburg (Germany) and at the State Neuropsychiatric Hospital Wagner-Jauregg, Linz, Austria. His fields of expertise are interventional neuroradiology and stroke (michael.sonnberger@kepleruniklinikum.at).

Andreas Dunzinger is a senior consultant in nuclear medicine at the Department of Nuclear Medicine of the Neuromed Campus of the Kepler University Hospital, Johannes Kepler University, Linz, Austria. He studied medicine at the University of Vienna (Austria). He was trained as a general physician at the Hospital of the Sisters of Mercy, Linz, Austria, and in nuclear medicine at the Medical University of Graz and at the State Neuropsychiatric Hospital Wagner-Jauregg, Linz, Austria. His field of expertise is neuronuclear medicine and neuroendocrinology (andreas.dunzinger@kepleruniklinikum.at).

Eva Voglmayr is a trainee in radiology and neuroradiology at the Department of Neuroradiology of the Neuromed Campus of the Kepler University Hospital, Johannes Kepler University, Linz, Austria. She studied medicine at the University of Vienna. Her field of interest is neurodegeneration (eva.voglmayr@kepleruniklinikum.at).

Martin Aichholzer is deputy head of the Department of Neurosurgery at the Neuromed Campus of the Kepler University Hospital, Johannes Kepler University, Linz, Austria. He studied medicine at the University of Vienna and was trained at the Department of Neurosurgery of the Medical University of Vienna (Austria). His field of expertise is skull base surgery (martin.aichholzer@krpleruniklinikum.at).

Raimund Kleiser is a medical physicist and is the head of the imaging center at the Institute of Neuroradiology at the Kepler University Hospital in Linz. He studied physics in Freiburg im Breisgau (Germany) and supplemented his training with the specialization in medical physics. His focus is on functional imaging, for which he established fMRT measuring equipment in prestigious institutions in Germany, Switzerland, and Austria (Raimund.kleiser@kepleruniklinikum.at).

Peter Strasser is molecular biologist at the PMU University Institute for Medical & Chemical Laboratory Diagnostics of the Paracelsus Medical University in Salzburg, Austria. He studied general biology at the University of Salzburg and specialized in biochemistry and molecular genetics. Dr. Strasser's current focus of interest lies in the genetic background of neurological diseases (p.strasser@salk.at).

Part X

The Brain Diseases: Tumors

Tumors of the Nervous System: General Considerations

51.1 Clinical Signs and Symptoms

The clinical signs always depend on the location of the tumor and might be divided into:

- Elevated intracranial pressure (ICP)
- Focal neurologic deficit
- Seizures (focal and/or secondarily generalized) (Table 51.1)

Symptoms of elevated intracranial pressure include:

- Headache
- Vomiting
- Altered level of consciousness
- Visual obscurations
- Diplopia

Signs of elevated intracranial pressure include:

- Papilledema
- Reduced level of consciousness
- Meningism

Signs and symptoms of focal neurologic dysfunction, based on topography, include:

- Supratentorial
  – Hemiparesis
  – Aphasia
  – Cognitive impairment
  – Visual loss
  – Sensory loss
  – Changes in behavior or personality
- Infratentorial
  – Ataxia
  – Dysarthria
  – Cranial neuropathies
- Spine
  – Spine and radicular pain
  – Paraparesis/paraplegia
  – Sensory loss with sensory level
  – Bowel, bladder, and/or sexual dysfunction

Table 51.1 Tumor-associated epilepsy: association between tumor type and seizure frequency, modified after van Breemen et al. (2007) reproduced with kind permission by Elsevier

Tumor type	Frequency in %
Dysembryoblastic neuroepithelial tumor (DNT)	100
Ganglioglioma	80–90
Low-grade astrocytoma	75
Meningioma	29–60
Glioblastoma	29–49
Metastasis	20–35
Primary CNS lymphoma	10

51.2 Definitions

Definitions of oncologic aspects can be found at the following homepage: http://www.cancer.gov/dictionary?cdrid=45651

51.2.1 Neuro-oncology

Neuro-oncology is the medical specialization directed at the diagnosis and treatment of brain tumors and other tumors of the nervous system.

51.2.2 Tumor

An abnormal mass of tissue that results when cells divide more than they should or do not die when they should. Tumors may be benign (not cancer), or malignant (cancer). Tumor is also called neoplasm.

51.2.3 Neoplasia

Abnormal and uncontrolled cell growth.

51.2.4 Brain Tumor

The growth of abnormal cells in the tissues of the brain. Brain tumors can be benign (not cancer) or malignant (cancer).

51.2.5 Malignant Versus Benign

Benign: Not cancerous. Benign tumors may grow larger but do not spread to other parts of the body. Benign is also called non-malignant.
Malignant: Cancerous. Malignant cells can invade and destroy nearby tissue and spread to other parts of the body.

Malignancy usually refers to lesions with the potential to metastasize. As a matter of fact, metastases of brain tumors are extremely rare, even in the most aggressive neoplasms. However, brain tumors might apt to be lethal despite the absence of histological evidence of malignancy, mainly due to their topographical localization, i.e., diffuse astrocytoma WHO grade II affecting the brain stem.

Criteria for malignancy include:

- Cellularity
  - Nuclear density or number of tumor nuclei per unit area of tumor as seen on the microscopic slide
- Pleomorphism
  - Variability in nuclear size and shape
- Nuclear atypia
  - Atypical nuclei are generally greater than normal in size and have a higher density of nuclear chromatin.
- Mitotic activity
  - Mitoses are usually more numerous in tumors with aggressive behavior. The number of mitoses can be expressed as the mitotic count (number of mitoses per high-power field).
- Anaplasia
  - Feature of malignant cells including:
    o pleomorphism
    o nuclear atypia
    o increased nuclear size
    o higher nuclear:cytoplasmic ratio

51.2.6 Seeding and Metastases

Seeding
- The spread of tumor through existing spaces such as the meninges or along parenchymal surfaces
- Macroscopically:
  - The seeded surface of the brain, spinal cord, or ventricle may appear cloudy or opaque.
  - More extensive seeding expands the subarachnoidal space, which can be studded or filled with a granular or shaggy, exudate-like infiltrate.
  - Seeding is more common in aggressive tumors that originate in the parenchyma, such as medulloblastoma and ependymoma, and generally signifies a poor prognosis.
- Microscopically:
  - Tumor cells tend to spread along the pathways of lesser resistance, particularly in the

loose, acellular subpial and subependymal regions, along fiber tracts such as the corpus callosum, and in the spaces around vessels and neurons.
- Infiltrating neoplastic cells are seen microscopically adjacent to the leptomeninges and ventricles, surrounding the perivascular Virchow–Robin spaces, and enveloping neurons (satellitosis), i.e., "secondary structures" after Scherer.

Metastatic Disease
- Discontinuous spread of a brain tumor to distant sites beyond the central nervous system.
- The spread of tumor cells into the adjacent dura mater or bone is not considered to be a metastatic process.

51.2.7 Various Modalities of Therapy

- **Chemotherapy**
  - Treatment with drugs that kill cancer cells.
- **Radiation therapy**
  - The use of high-energy radiation from x-rays, gamma rays, neutrons, protons, and other sources to kill cancer cells and shrink tumors. Radiation may come from a machine outside the body (external-beam radiation therapy), or it may come from radioactive material placed in the body near cancer cells (internal radiation therapy). Systemic radiation therapy uses a radioactive substance, such as a radiolabeled monoclonal antibody, that travels in the blood to tissues throughout the body. Also called irradiation and radiotherapy.
- **Targeted therapy**
  - A type of treatment that uses drugs or other substances to identify and attack specific types of cancer cells with less harm to normal cells. Some targeted therapies block the action of certain enzymes, proteins, or other molecules involved in the growth and spread of cancer cells. Other types of targeted therapies help the immune system kill cancer cells or deliver toxic substances directly to cancer cells and kill them. Targeted therapy may have fewer side effects than other types of cancer treatment. Most targeted therapies are either small-molecule drugs or monoclonal antibodies.
- **Biological therapy**
  - A type of treatment that uses substances made from living organisms to treat disease. These substances may occur naturally in the body or may be made in the laboratory. Some biological therapies stimulate or suppress the immune system to help the body fight cancer, infection, and other diseases. Other biological therapies attack specific cancer cells, which may help keep them from growing or kill them. They may also lessen certain side effects caused by some cancer treatments. Types of biological therapy include immunotherapy (such as vaccines, cytokines, and some antibodies), gene therapy, and some targeted therapies. Also called biological response modifier therapy, biotherapy, and BRM therapy.
- **Concomitant therapy**
  - Occurring or existing at the same time as something else. In medicine, it may refer to a condition a person has or a medication a person is taking that is not being studied in the clinical trial he or she is taking part in.
- **Adjuvant therapy**
  - Additional cancer treatment given after the primary treatment to lower the risk that the cancer will come back. Adjuvant therapy may include chemotherapy, radiation therapy, hormone therapy, targeted therapy, or biological therapy.

51.2.8 Endpoints on Clinical Trials

The definition for disease endpoints can be found on the following home page: http://www.cancer.gov/dictionary?cdrid=45651

- **Complete remission (CR)**
  - The disappearance of all signs of cancer in response to treatment. This does not always

mean the cancer has been cured. Also called complete response.
- **Partial remission (PR)**
  - A decrease in the size of a tumor, or in the extent of cancer in the body, in response to treatment. Also called partial response.
- **Stable disease**
  - Cancer that is neither decreasing nor increasing in extent or severity.
- **Progressive disease (PD)**
  - Cancer that is growing, spreading, or getting worse.
- **Overall survival (OS)**
  - The length of time from either the date of diagnosis or the start of treatment for a disease, such as cancer, that patients diagnosed with the disease are still alive. In a clinical trial, measuring the overall survival is one way to see how well a new treatment works.
- **Event-free survival (EFS)**
  - In cancer, the length of time after primary treatment for a cancer ends that the patient remains free of certain complications or events that the treatment was intended to prevent or delay. These events may include the return of the cancer or the onset of certain symptoms, such as bone pain from cancer that has spread to the bone. In a clinical trial, measuring the event-free survival is one way to see how well a new treatment works.
- Progression-free survival (PFS)
  - The length of time during and after the treatment of a disease, such as cancer, that a patient lives with the disease but it does not get worse. In a clinical trial, measuring the progression-free survival is one way to see how well a new treatment works.
- Disease-free survival (DFS)–Relapse-free survival (RFS)
  - In cancer, the length of time after primary treatment for a cancer ends that the patient survives without any signs or symptoms of that cancer. In a clinical trial, measuring the disease-free survival is one way to see how well a new treatment works.

51.3 Histologic Tumor Characteristics

51.3.1 Cellularity

- The number and type of cells in a given tissue
  - Nuclear density or number of tumor nuclei per unit area of tumor as seen on the microscopic slide
- Low number, i.e., low cellularity, of tumor cells correlates with low malignancy
- High number, i.e., high cellularity, of tumor cells correlates with high malignancy

51.3.2 Anaplasia

- Tumor cells have undergone retrogression from a more highly differentiated state to a lower level of differentiation.
- Primitive cells with poor cytoplasmic differentiation.
- Nuclear abnormalities include:
  - Pleomorphism
  - Nuclear atypia
  - Increased nuclear size
  - Higher nuclear:cytoplasmic ratio

51.3.3 Metaplasia

- Non-neoplastic, reactive, and reversible change during which a normal cell appears to differentiate into another cell type
- Adaptive change that allows cells to cope with an unfavorable environment

51.3.4 Pleomorphism

- Variability in nuclear size and shape

51.3.5 Mitoses

Atypical mitoses (Fig. 51.1a–d)

51.3 Histologic Tumor Characteristics

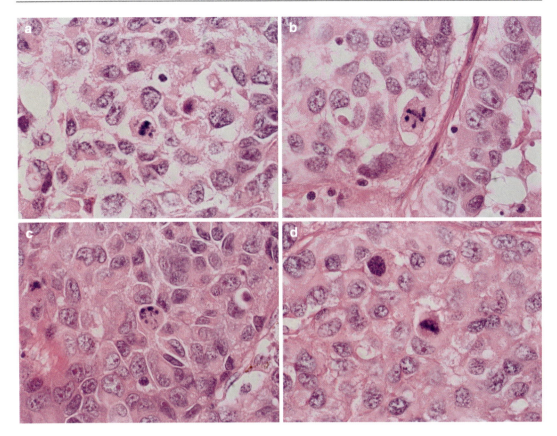

Fig. 51.1 Mitotic figure in brain tumors (a–d)

- Defects of mitosis result in various nuclear abnormalities, namely, micronuclei, binucleation, broken egg appearance, pyknotic nuclei, and increased numbers of and/or abnormal mitotic figures

A recent classification of chromosome segregation errors at mitosis defines

- abnormalities in spindle symmetry
  - such as spindle multipolarity and size asymmetry of anaphase-telophase poles
- in abnormal sister chromatid segregation
  - such as chromosome bridges, chromatid bridges, chromosome lagging, and acentric fragment lagging
- Combinations of these changes result in more complex abnormalities (Tvedten 2009).

51.3.6 Reactive Versus Neoplastic

- Reactive changes occur in response to injury from trauma, infection, vascular disease, and tumor
- The cells that participate in the reactive process are activated and proliferate so that they can stimulate neoplasia histologically
- One of the most difficult diagnostic problems involves the distinction between reactive astrogliosis and low-grade astroglioma.
  - In astrogliosis, the architecture of the nervous system is preserved, while in astroglioma it is effaced by infiltrating neoplastic cells.
  - Reactive astrogliosis is immunohistochemically negative for IDH-1 while low-grade astrogliomas are usually IDH-1 positive.

- Moreover, the amounts of cellularity, pleomorphism, and atypia are less in a reactive process, and mitoses are rarely encountered.

51.3.7 Endothelial Proliferation and Neovascularity
(Fig. 51.2a, b)

- In order to expand, tumors require their own blood supply.
- The individual blood vessels within an area of neovascularity may be larger than those normally found in the nervous system parenchyma.
- They are also tortuous, with a lumen that varies in diameter along its course.
- Endothelial proliferation often occurs in capillaries or in small venules, which become filled with endothelial cells, so that they resemble renal glomeruli.
- Endothelial proliferation and neovascularity are under the influence of tumor angiogenesis factors.
- Endothelial proliferation is an indication of aggressive behavior in tumors of the nervous system. It is commonly found in glioblastoma multiforme, anaplastic astrocytoma, and metastatic tumors.

51.3.8 Necrosis (Fig. 51.2c, d)

Necrosis
- is mediated by:
  - tumor necrosis factors, which are produced by macrophages and other mononuclear elements
  - other cytokines
  - a variety of enzymes liberated by tumor cells which degrade the surrounding normal tissues

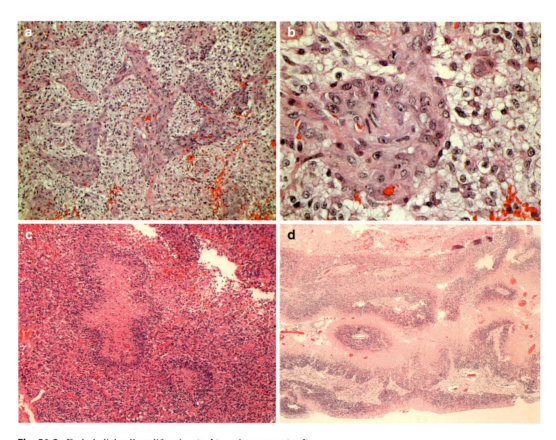

Fig. 51.2 Endothelial cell proliferation (**a**, **b**), and necroses (**c**, **d**)

51.3 Histologic Tumor Characteristics

- Necrosis is generally synonymous with rapid growth.
- Its importance relative to outcome varies with tumor type:
  - In meningiomas, necrosis may reflect a somewhat more aggressive behavior.
  - In astrocytomas, it is regarded as a definite malignant criterion.

Necrosis with Pseudopalisading
- Pseudopalisading is a type of necrosis.
- Non-viable tumor cells are surrounded on one or more sides by rows of neoplastic cells, which assume the appearance of a palisaded or picket fence.
- The pathogenesis of pseudopalisading is unknown.
- Might not reflect a primary organizational behavior of cells of a given tumor type.
- Represent a reaction to external factors occurring within the tumor bed.
- Is a constant feature of glioblastoma multiforme.
- Pseudopalisading may also be seen in other malignant tumors, particularly those of glial origin.

51.3.9 Encapsulation and Invasion

- By definition, when surrounded by a capsule, tumors exhibit indolent growth and relatively benign behavior.
  - Dermoids, epidermoids, and some lipomas are among those benign tumors that are truly encapsulated.
- Meningiomas and nerve sheath tumors are the most common lesions to form a pseudocapsule.
- The majority of CNS tumors are not well circumscribed and are invasive due to the elaboration of tissue-destructive enzymes, such as collagenases and hydrolases, by the tumor cells.
- On the other hand, metastatic tumors with great potential for invasion are paradoxically well demarcated from the surrounding CNS tissue, particularly when they are small.
- Glioblastomas may appear to be well circumscribed grossly, although usually malignant foci can be found histologically outside the boundary between the tumor and normal brain.

51.3.10 Rosettes

A rosette (imitation rose) is an organoid structure resembling a flower that has been cross-sectioned, i.e., a rosette consists of (Wippold and Perry 2006):

- A halo or spoke-wheel arrangement of cells surrounding a central core

The central core may be:

- An empty lumen or
- Space filled with cytoplasmic processes

The cells in the rosette with

- Wedge-shaped cytoplasm
- Apex directed towards the central core
- Peripherally positioned nuclei forming a ring around the halo

Table 51.2 Rosette types and associated tumors

Rosette type	Associated tumors
Homer Wright	• Neuroblastoma • Medulloblastoma • Primitive neuroectodermal tumor • Pineoblastoma
Flexner–Wintersteiner	• Retinoblastoma • Pineoblastoma • Medulloepithelioma
True ependymal	• Ependymoma
Perivascular	• Ependymoma • Medulloblastoma • Primitive neuroectodermal tumor • Central neurocytoma • Glioblastoma • Monomorphous pilomyxoid astrocytoma
Pineocytomatous	• Pineocytoma
Neurocytic	• Central neurocytoma

Many types of rosettes have been described (Table 51.2):

- Homer Wright rosette
- Flexner–Wintersteiner rosette
- True ependymal rosette
- Perivascular pseudorosette
- Pineocytomatous and neurocytic rosettes

Homer Wright rosette is

- formed by a circle of tumor cells from which delicate fibrillary processes converge towards a central point.
- Some of the processes may be argentophilic, like neuronal axons, supporting the idea that Homer Wright rosettes represent neuroblastic differentiation.
- As a diagnostic criterion, these rosettes are not always reliable, since they are frequently few in number and difficult to locate.
- Even when present, Homer Wright rosettes are often abortively formed.
- They are typically observed in primitive neuroectodermal tumors including medulloblastoma, neuroblastoma, and pineoblastoma.

Flexner–Wintersteiner rosette

- A central lumen containing small cytoplasmic extensions of the encircling cells
- Central lumen devoid of fiber-rich neuropil
- Ultrastructural features of primitive photoreceptor cells
- Found in retinoblastoma, pineoblastoma, and medulloepithelioma

True ependymal rosette

- Empty-appearing lumen resembles a tubule lumen.
- Tubule-like structures recapitulate ventricle formation.
- Devoid of fiber-rich neuropil or central cytoplasmic projections.
- Found in ependymoma.

Perivascular rosettes

- are arranged around thin-walled blood vessels that appear to be venous in origin.
- A nuclear free zone is formed between the ring of tumor cells and the vascular channel containing the cytoplasmic processes of tumor cells that attach to the vessel wall.
- Perivascular rosettes are characteristic of ependymomas.

Pineocytomatous and neurocytic rosettes

- Larger than Homer Wright rosettes.
- Irregular in contour.
- Cells reflect neuronal differentiation of the tumor.
- Cells are large, less mitotically active, pale, or less hyperchromatic.

51.3.11 Palisades and Pseudopalisades

Palisades are (Wippold et al. 2006)
- arrangement of elongated nuclei stacked in rows
- found in schwannomas

Verocay bodies
- Stacked arrangements of elongated palisading nuclei alternating with clear zones devoid of nuclei (anuclear zones) containing cell processes

Pseudopalisades
- See Sect. 51.3.8

51.3.12 Desmoplasia

- Consists of an exuberant proliferation of mesenchymal tissue composed of:
  - Fibroblasts
  - Collagen
- Stimulated by:
  - A neoplasm confined to the CNS parenchyma
  - Invasion of tumor cells into normal structures containing mesenchymal elements such as the meninges
- Desmoplasia is a reactive rather than a neoplastic process.

- Histologically, the proliferating mesenchymal tissue appears to be part of the tumor itself.
- A desmoplastic response is common in such tumors as medulloblastoma and ganglioglioma.

51.3.13 Reactive Astrogliosis

- Presence of reactive astrocytes
- With abundant cytoplasm (DD: gemistocytic astrocytes)
- GFAP-immunopositive
- Usually found at the border of the tumor

51.3.14 Microglial Activation

- Presence of reactive microglia
- Ramified to rounded forms
- Immunopositive for IBA1, HLA-DRII

51.3.15 Perivascular Lymphocytic Cuffing

- Presence of lymphocytes in the perivascular spaces
- Predominantly CD3-positive T-lymphocytes
- Rarely found in brain tumors
- Mark the attempt of the immune system to react against tumor growth

51.4 WHO Classification of Tumors of the Central Nervous System

A rough classification of tumors affecting the central nervous system can be given as follows (Louis et al. 2016):

- Diffuse astrocytic and oligodendroglial tumors
- Other astrocytic tumors
- Ependymal tumors
- Other gliomas
- Choroid plexus tumors
- Neuronal and mixed neuronal-glial tumors
- Tumors of the pineal region
- Embryonal tumors
- Tumors of cranial and paraspinal nerves
- Meningiomas
- Mesenchymal, non-meningothelial tumors
- Melanocytic tumors
- Lymphomas
- Histiocytic tumors
- Germ cell tumors
- Tumors of the sellar region
- Familial tumor syndromes
- Metastatic tumors

The detailed World Health Organization (WHO) classification of tumors of the nervous system is given in Table 51.3.

The tumors listed under World Health Organization (WHO) classification of tumors of the nervous system (Louis et al. 2016) as

Table 51.3 The detailed World Health Organization (WHO) classification of tumors of the nervous system listed by increasing grade is given as follows (Louis et al. 2016)

Tumor group	Tumor type	WHO grade
Astrocytic tumors	Subependymal giant cell astrocytoma	I
	Pilocytic astrocytoma	I
	Pilomyxoid astrocytoma	II
	Diffuse astrocytoma	II
	Pleomorphic xanthoastrocytoma	II
	Anaplastic astrocytoma	III
	Glioblastoma	IV
	Giant cell glioblastoma	IV
	Gliosarcoma	IV
	Gliomatosis cerebri	II, IV

(continued)

Table 51.3 (continued)

Tumor group	Tumor type	WHO grade
Oligodendroglial tumors	Oligodendroglioma	II
	Anaplastic Oligodendroglioma	III
Oligo-astrocytic tumors	Oligo-astrocytoma	II
	Anaplastic Oligo-astrocytoma	III
Ependymal tumors	Subependymoma	I
	Myxopapillary ependymoma	I
	Ependymoma	II
	Anaplastic ependymoma	III
Choroid plexus tumors	Choroid plexus papilloma	I
	Atypical choroid plexus papilloma	II
	Choroid plexus carcinoma	III
Other neuroepithelial tumors	Angiocentric glioma	I
	Chordoid glioma of the third ventricle	II
	Astroblastoma	II, III
Neuronal and mixed neuronal-glial tumors	Gangliocytoma	I
	Ganglioglioma	I
	Paraganglioma of the spinal cord	I
	Papillary glioneuronal tumor	I
	Rosette-forming glioneuronal tumor of the fourth ventricle	I
	Desmoplastic infantile astrocytoma/ganglioglioma	I
	Dysembryoplastic neuroepithelial tumor	I
	Central neurocytoma	II
	Extraventricular neurocytoma	II
	Cerebellar liponeurocytoma	II
	Anaplastic ganglioglioma	III
Pineal tumors	Pineocytoma	I
	Pineal parenchymal tumor of intermediate type	II, III
	Papillary tumor of the pineal region	II, III
	Pineoblastoma	IV
Embryonal tumors	Medulloblastoma	IV
	CNS primitive neuroectodermal tumor (PNET)	IV
	Atypical teratoid/rhabdoid tumor (ATRT)	IV
Tumors of the cranial and paraspinal nerves	Schwannoma	I
	Neurofibroma	I
	Perineurioma	I, II, III
	Malignant peripheral nerve sheath tumor (MPNST)	IV
Meningeal tumors	Meningioma	I
	Atypical meningioma	II
	Anaplastic/malignant meningioma	III
Tumors of the sellar region	Craniopharyngioma	I
	Granular cell tumor of the neurohypophysis	I
	Pituicytoma	I
	Spindle cell oncocytoma of the adenohypophysis	I

Table 51.3 (continued)

Tumor group	Tumor type	WHO grade
Germ cell Tumors	Germinoma	
	Embryonal carcinoma	
	Yolk sac tumor	
	Choriocarcinoma	
	Teratoma • Mature • Immature • With malignant transformation	
	Mixed germ cell tumor	
Lymphomas and hematopoietic neoplasms	Maligant lymphomas	
	Plasmacytoma	
	Granulocytic sarcoma	

mesenchymal, non-meningothelial tumors consist of soft tissue tumors and bone tumors. They have their own WHO classification systems which are described in Chaps. 79 and 80.

51.5 Grading Systems for Brain Tumors

51.5.1 WHO Grading System

The grading of brain tumors as given by the WHO is listed in Table 51.4.

Table 51.4 WHO grading system

Grade I	• Tumors with low proliferative potential and • the possibility of cure following surgery
Grade II	• Infiltrative in nature • Despite low level of proliferation, often recur • Tend to progress to higher grades
Grade III	• Lesions with histological evidence of malignancy, including nuclear atypia and brisk mitotic activity • Adjuvant radiation and/or chemotherapy
Grade IV	• Cytologically malignant, mitotically active, necrosis-prone neoplasms associated with • rapid pre- and postoperative disease evolution and fatal outcome

51.5.2 Kernohan et al. (1949)

Grading was introduced to help the clinician with regard to prognosis. A four-tier grading system was first proposed by Kernohan et al. (1949) (Table 51.5).

51.5.3 Ringertz (1950)

A three-tier grading system was proposed by Ringertz (1950).

- Grade I
  - Well differentiated
- Grade II
  - Anaplastic astrocytoma
- Grade III
  - Glioblastoma multiforme

The Ringertz grading system reads as follows:

- Grade 1 = astrocytoma
  - Roughly equivalent to WHO grade II
  - Mild hypercellularity
  - Mild nuclear atypia (nuclear enlargement, hyperchromasia, pleomorphism)
  - Rare mitotic figures
- Grade 2 = anaplastic astrocytoma
  - Roughly equivalent to WHO grade III
  - More cellular than grade 1
  - More nuclear atypia

Table 51.5 Kernohan grading system

	Grade 1	Grade 2	Grade 3	Grade 4
Cell density:	Low	Low to moderate	High	Very high
Cell form:	Uniform	Size irregularities	Polymorphic	Polymorphic, multinucleated giant cells
Cell nucleus:	Monomorphic	Irregularities in size and chromatin content	Polymorphic	Polymorphic, hyperchromatic
Degenerative changes:	Cyst formation is possible	Possible	Present	Present
Mitoses:	None	A few typical	Some atypical	Many atypical
Necroses:	None	None	A few	Widely spread or disseminated
Endothelial proliferation:	None	None	Moderate	Strong
Connective tissue:				Strong proliferation

- More mitotic figures
- Endothelial proliferation (note this is a WHO grade IV feature)
- Grade 3 = glioblastoma
  - Roughly equivalent to WHO grade IV
  - Presence of geographic necrosis ± surrounding pseudopalisading tumor cells

51.5.4 St. Anne/Mayo (Daumas-Duport et al. 1988)

A quite confusing grading system was proposed as a simple and reproducible method by Daumas-Duport et al. (1988) (Table 51.6).
Criteria used:

- Nuclear atypia
- Mitoses
- Endothelial proliferation
- Necrosis

Summing up the number of criteria

- Grade 1—0 criteria
- Grade 2—1 criterion
- Grade 3—2 criteria
- Grade 4—3 or 4 criteria

The weak points in this grading system are:

- Defining a Grade 1 with 0 criteria
- Defining a Grade 4 with the presence of 2 criteria (necrosis, endothelial proliferation)

Table 51.6 Frequency of criteria in various grades

Criteria	Grade 1	Grade 2	Grade 3	Grade 4	Grade 4
Criterion number	0	1	2	3	4
Nuclear atypia	0	100	100	100	100
Mitoses	0	0	92	100	100
Necrosis	0	0	2	48	100
Endothelial proliferation	0	0	6	52	100

51.5.5 Smith Grading for Oligodendroglioma

A grading system for oligodendrogliomas was proposed by Smith et al. (1983).
Criteria used:

- Endothelial proliferation
  - Marked increase in the size and number of endothelial cells within small vessel walls.
  - Coded present or absent
- Necrosis
  - Eosinophilic coagulation necrosis and/or areas of debris filled with macrophages
  - Coded present or absent
- Maximal nuclear/cytoplasmic ratio
  - A ratio approximating that found in the normal oligodendroglial cell was considered low and anything above that high
  - Coded high or low
- Maximal cell density
  - Cell density approximating or just above that found in normal brain white matter

was considered low while sheets of cells, either back to back or with little intervening extracellular neuropil was considered high.
  – Coded high or low
- Pleomorphism
  – Variability in nuclear and cytoplasmic size and shape
  – Coded present or absent

Grading is done as follows:

- Grade A
  – If all five features were judged absent and low.
- Grade B
  – If pleomorphism was present and/or if cell density and nuclear/cytoplasmic ratio were high.
- Grade C
  – Tumors showing pleomorphism, endothelial proliferation, and high nuclear/cytoplasmic ratio and cell density.
- Grade D
  – Tumors in which all five features were coded present and high.

51.6 Frequencies of Brain Tumors

Frequencies of brain tumors as reported by the Central Brain Tumor Registry of the United states (CBTRUS) (Ostrom et al. 2013, 2014, 2015, 2016) are given in the following Tables 51.7, 51.8, and 51.9.

51.7 Molecular Neuropathology: The Hallmarks of Cancer

The hallmarks of cancer as described by Hanahan and Weinberg (2011) are characterized by (Fig. 51.3):

- *Growth signal autonomy:*
  – Normal cells need external signals from growth factors to divide.
  – Cancer cells are not dependent on normal growth factor signaling.
  – Acquired mutations short-circuit growth factor pathways leading to unregulated growth.
- *Evasion of growth inhibitory signals:*
  – Normal cells respond to inhibitory signals to maintain homeostasis (most cells of the body are not actively dividing).

Table 51.7 Distribution (in %) of primary brain and CNS tumors *by histology*

Tumor type	Overall	Malignant	Non-Malignant
Meningioma	36.6	1.5	53.2
Glioblastoma	14.9	46.6	NA
Pituitary tumors	15.9	NIP	23.4
All other	11.5	14.1	6.8
Nerve sheath tumors	8.2	NIP	12.0
Astrocytomas	5.6	17.1	
Lymphoma	1.9	6.1	NA
Ependymal tumors	1.8	3.5	1.1
Oligodendrogliomas	1.5	4.7	NIP
Embryonal tumors	1.0	3.0	NA
Oligo-astrocytic tumors	0.9	2.7	NIP
Craniopharyngioma	0.8	NA	1.2
Germ cell tumors	0.4	0.8	NA
All other			7.4

All primary brain tumors: $n = 368,117$; malignant primary brain tumors: $n = 117,906$; non-malignant primary brain tumors: $n = 250,211$), data from Ostrom et al. (2016) reproduced with kind permission by Oxford University Press. *NA* not applicable, *NIP* no information provided

Table 51.8 Distribution (in %) of primary brain and CNS tumors *by site*

Site	Overall	Malignant	Non-malignant
Meninges	37.0	1.8	53.0
Pituitary	17.0	0.4	24.9
Other brain	9.0	22.5	2.6
Frontal lobe	8.0	23.6	1.2
Cranial nerves	7.0	1.2	9.6
Temporal lobe	6.0	17.4	0.9
Parietal lobe	4.0	10.6	0.5
Spinal cord and cauda equina	3.0	3.0	3.0
Cerebellum	2.0	4.8	1.4
Cerebrum	2.0	4.5	0.4
Brain stem	2.0	3.6	0.5
Occipital lobe	1.0	2.8	0.2
Ventricle	1.0	1.4	1.0
Other nervous system	1.0	1.0	0.5
Pineal	0.0	0.8	0.3
Nasal cavity	0.0	0.6	NIP

All primary brain tumors: $n = 368,117$; malignant primary brain tumors: $n = 117,906$; non-malignant primary brain tumors: $n = 250,211$), data from Ostrom et al. (2016) reproduced with kind permission by Oxford University Press. *NIP* no information provided

Table 51.9 Distribution (in %) of primary brain and CNS *gliomas* by histology subtypes ($N = 99,165$), data from Ostrom et al. (2016) reproduced with kind permission by Oxford University Press

Tumor type	WHO grade	Frequency
Astrocytoma, diffuse	II	8.1
Astrocytoma, anaplastic	III	6.3
Glioblastoma	IV	55.4
Astrocytoma, pilocytic	I	5.1
Oligodendroglioma	II	5.6
Ependymal tumors		6.8
Oligo-astrocytic tumors	II, III	3.2
Malignant gliomas, NOS		7.3
All other gliomas		2.1

- Cancer cells do not respond to growth inhibitory signals.
- Acquired mutations or gene silencing interfere with the inhibitory pathways.
- *Avoiding immune destruction (emerging hallmark):*
  - There is evidence to support the theory of immune surveillance that states the immune system can recognize and eliminate cancer cells.
  - Successful cancer cells may be those which do not stimulate an immune response or can interfere with the immune response so as to avoid immune destruction.
- *Unlimited replicative potential:*
  - Normal cells have an autonomous counting device to define a finite number of cell doublings after which they become senescent. This cellular counting device is the shortening of chromosomal ends, telomeres, that occurs during every round of DNA replication.
  - Cancer cells maintain the length of their telomeres.
  - Altered regulation of telomere maintenance results in unlimited replicative potential.
- *Tumor-promoting inflammation (an enabling characteristic):*
  - Virtually all tumors contain inflammatory immune cells.
  - Inflammation is an immune response that can facilitate the ability of acquiring the core hallmarks of cancer. For example, inflammatory cells can provide growth factors and enzymes that promote angiogenesis and invasion.
  - In addition, inflammatory cells can release oxygen species that are mutagenic.
- *Invasion and metastasis:*
  - Normal cells maintain their location in the body and generally do not migrate.
  - The movement of cancer cells to other parts of the body is a major cause of cancer deaths.
  - Alterations of the genome may affect the activity and/or levels of enzymes involved in invasion or molecules involved in cell–cell or cellular–extracellular adhesion.
- *Angiogenesis (formation of new blood vessels):*
  - Normal cells depend on blood vessels to supply oxygen and nutrients, but the vascular architecture is more or less constant in the adult.
  - Cancer cells induce angiogenesis, the growth of new blood vessels, needed for tumor survival and expansion.
  - Altering the balance between angiogenic inducers and inhibitors can activate the angiogenic switch.

Fig. 51.3 The hallmark of cancer (reproduced from Pecorino (2016) with kind permission by Oxford University Press)

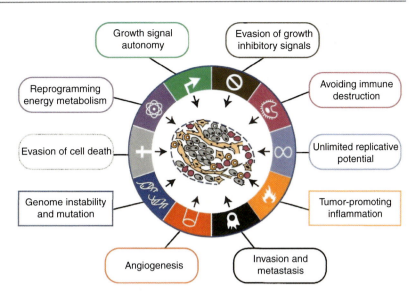

- *Genome instability and mutation (an enabling characteristic):*
  - Acquiring the core hallmarks of cancer usually depends on genomic alterations.
  - Faulty DNA repair pathways can contribute to genomic instability.
- *Evasion of cell death:*
  - Normal cells are removed by apoptosis, often in response to DNA damage.
  - Cancer cells evade apoptotic signals.
- *Reprogramming energy metabolism (emerging hallmark):*
  - Uncontrolled cell division demands increases in fuel and biosynthetic precursors that is obtained by adjusting energy metabolism.
  - Unlike normal cells, cancer cells carry out glycolysis, even in the presence of oxygen. Glycolysis intermediates can be used in biosynthetic pathways.

51.8 Molecular Neuropathology: Cell Cycle

51.8.1 The Cell Cycle in Normal Cells

The term "cell cycle" (or "cell division cycle") refers to a series of highly ordered molecular events that are required for a cell to grow and replicate. One cycle encompasses all steps starting with the formation of a cell by division from a mother cell to its own division to create two new daughter cells.

The cell cycle progresses through several well-defined phases each of which must properly be completed before the next one initiates. This is governed by external signals such as nutrients or growth factors, and in addition, by the action of intracellular sensory mechanisms, the checkpoints, safeguarding the transitions between the phases. Important parameters assessed by the checkpoints include cell size and DNA integrity. The molecular events underlying the management of damaged DNA are detailed later in chapter 51.9 **DNA Damage Response**. Depending on the cellular conditions monitored, it is decided whether to move on to the next step or to reversibly/irreversibly pause the cycle (cell cycle arrest).

In the mammalian cell division cycle, two major phases can be distinguished, *interphase* and *mitosis*, each of which is subdivided into several stages:

- Interphase
  - G1 phase (gap 1)
  - S phase (DNA synthesis)
  - G2 phase (gap 2)
- Mitosis (M phase)
  - Prophase
  - Metaphase

– Anaphase
– Telophase and Cytokinesis

After completing the cycle, a cell may repeat the division process or exit the cycle to move into a "resting" state, the G0 phase. Fully differentiated cells usually remain in G0 throughout their entire life span to carry out their predetermined tasks. Cells can enter G0 (cell cycle arrest) also temporarily at several stages during the cycle when unfavorable conditions or molecular errors are detected by the checkpoints; as soon as the problems are resolved, the cycling process is resumed.

The major checkpoints control the

- G1/S transition (= restriction checkpoint)
- G2/M transition (= DNA replication checkpoint)
- Metaphase/Anaphase transition (= spindle apparatus checkpoint)

At the molecular level, checkpoint activities are executed via protein complex formations involving cyclins and cyclin-dependent kinases (CDKs; the most important are CDK1, CDK2, CDK4, and CDK6). The name "cyclin" refers to the fact that these proteins are synthesized and degraded in a strictly controlled manner during the cell cycle, whereas CDK levels remain quite constant. Thus, the cyclin fluctuations provide an excellent regulatory mechanism in the course of cell division. In general, CDKs are inactive unless they are bound by their respective cyclins; active cyclin/CDK complexes phosphorylate downstream substrates which mediate cell cycle progression.

An additional regulatory tool is provided by CDK inhibitors (CKIs) which bind to cyclin/CDK complexes, thereby blocking CDK activity. Thus, they act as tumor suppressors.

CKIs include members of two protein families:

- the Ink4 family (Inhibitors of kinase 4), inhibiting CDK4- and CDK6 complexes:
  – p15 (p15INK4B; gene: *CDKN2B*)
  – p16 (p16INK4A; gene: *CDKN2A*)
  – p18 (p18INK4C; gene: *CDKN2C*)
  – p19 (p19INK4D; gene: *CDKN2D*)
- the Cip/Kip family (CDK interacting protein/Kinase inhibitory protein), inhibiting CDK1- and CDK2 complexes:
  – p21 (gene: *CDKN1A*)
  – p27 (gene: *CDKN1B*)
  – p57 (gene: *CDKN1C*)

Each checkpoint in the cell cycle depends on specific cyclins (D, E, A, B) and CDKs (details see below) (Fig. 51.4).

The cell division cycle and its regulatory mechanisms in detail:

51.8.1.1 Interphase

The interphase, spanning about 90% of the total time required for a complete cycle, serves the purpose of preparing the cell for division:

- G1 phase:
  – During this phase, the cell has to grow and accumulate organelles before DNA synthesis can start. External signals, mainly growth factors, initiate entry into G1 and promote progression through early G1 stages. Without appropriate growth factor stimulation, however, the cell enters a G0 state where it remains arrested until the required signals are available.
  – In late G1, the first major monitoring mechanism, the *restriction checkpoint*, comes into effect where it is determined whether or not to proceed to S phase. The intracellular checkpoint players involved are D- and E-type cyclins, as well as CDK4, CDK6, and CDK2. Growth factors stimulate the synthesis of cyclin D1 which binds to CDK4 and CDK6. The activated complexes cyclin D1/CDK4, cyclin D1/CDK6, and later in G1, cyclin E/CDK2 phosphorylate pRB (the retinoblastoma protein), thereby stalling its tumor suppressor function. Active pRB binds and inhibits transcription factor E2F which transcribes genes required for G1/S transition. Hence, deactivation of pRB promotes progression into S phase.
  – Notably, E2F also promotes expression of cyclin E; the appearance of the cyclin

Fig. 51.4 Overview of the mammalian cell cycle phases and -checkpoints. G1 checkpoint = restriction checkpoint; G2 checkpoint = DNA replication checkpoint; M checkpoint = spindle apparatus checkpoint. Source: https://commons.wikimedia.org/wiki/File:0332_Cell_Cycle_With_Cyclins_and_Checkpoints.jpg LICENCE NOTICE: OpenStax (https://commons.wikimedia.org/wiki/File:0332_Cell_Cycle_With_Cyclins_and_Checkpoints.jpg), https://creativecommons.org/licenses/by/4.0/legalcode

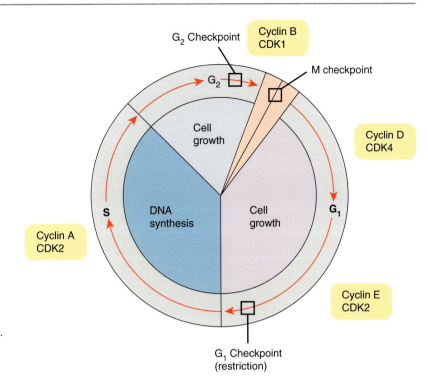

E/CDK2 complex marks a "point of no return": from here, no further growth factor stimulation is needed to drive the cell through the division cycle.
- Another important regulatory molecule, the transcription factor and tumor suppressor protein p53, participates in the cellular management of DNA damage detected during G1 phase.

• S phase:
- During S phase, chromosomal DNA is replicated, resulting in the generation of the respective sister chromatids. At the beginning of S phase, cyclin A appears in the nucleus where it binds to CDK2, and the cyclin A/CDK2 complex initiates DNA synthesis via phosphorylation of proteins involved in the replication machinery. Only after DNA duplication has successfully completed, the cell moves on to G2 Phase.

• G2 phase:
- Basically, G2 serves in preparing the cell for mitosis. The cell continues to grow and synthesizes proteins required for cell division. Near the end of G2, the *DNA replication checkpoint* monitors DNA integrity before G2/M transition is permitted. In the presence of damaged DNA, the cell cycle stalls to enable DNA repair prior to entering mitosis.
- The G2/M transition is triggered by the formation of the cyclin B1/CDK1 complex, also known as the maturation-promoting factor (MPF). Its activity is regulated by two counteracting enzyme types, the Wee1 kinase (inhibitory) and members of the CDC25 phosphatase family (activating). When damaged DNA is detected, another checkpoint kinase (Chk1) comes into play which inactivates CDC25 and consequently MPF, resulting in cell cycle arrest.
- It should be noted that, similar to G1 phase, p53 is also involved in a G2/M arrest in response to DNA damage.

51.8.1.2 Mitosis (M Phase)

In M phase, the cell finally splits into two daughter cells, each receiving identical sets of the previously duplicated chromosomes. In short, a series of cellular events involving major structural rearrangements in the cytoskeleton can be observed during distinct steps in mitosis:

- Prophase:
  - Condensing of the sister chromatids: They become visible in high-resolution light microscopy; each pair is joined at the centromere, a specific DNA sequence to which a protein complex (the kinetochore) is bound.
  - Formation of the spindle apparatus: Two centrosomes, previously duplicated, move to opposite locations within the cell where they become the polar attachment sites for the spindle microtubules. After breakdown of the nuclear envelope in late prophase, the microtubules originating from the two poles connect with the kinetochores of the condensed chromosomes, such that the sister chromatids of each chromosome are linked to opposite poles of the mitotic spindle.
- Metaphase:
  - Planar arrangement of the chromosomes between the spindle poles: The spindle apparatus aligns the chromosomes in the center plane between the poles, establishing a structure called "metaphase plate." At this point, the *spindle apparatus checkpoint* controls the proper alignment of the sister chromatids and the correct attachment of their kinetochores to the spindle microtubules. Unattached kinetochores are recognized as a signal for cycle arrest, and the progression to anaphase is postponed until all connections are established.
- Anaphase:
  - Separation of the chromosomes: The anaphase-promoting complex (cyclosome; APC/C) triggers the degradation of regulatory proteins, including cyclin B, thus rendering MPF inactive. Activity of APC/C also mediates the degradation of cohesins, specific proteins that keep the sister chromatids joined during metaphase plate formation. The disconnected sister chromatids are now referred to as "daughter chromosomes" and are separated by moving towards the opposite centrosomes of the spindle apparatus. Due to forces exerted by microtubules that are not attached to kinetochores, but overlap from opposite centrosomes, the cell becomes elongated which supports chromosome segregation. At the end of anaphase, identical sets of chromosomes have arrived at each spindle pole.
- Telophase/Cytokinesis:
  - Regeneration of nuclear membranes and breakdown of mitotic spindle/cell division.
  - At both poles, new nuclear envelopes are formed around the chromosomes which de-condense, relaxing into chromatin, and the nucleoli reappear. The spindle apparatus breaks down by way of depolymerization of the microtubules.
  - Cytokinesis, the actual division of the cytoplasm after mitosis, begins in late anaphase by forming the so-called cleavage furrow which appears on the cell surface at the equator between the two poles of the elongated cell. The underlying molecular process involves a cytoskeletal structure containing actin and myosin filaments, called the "contractile ring," that assembles beneath the plasma membrane to which it remains attached. When the ring contracts, it pulls the membrane inward until, at full constriction, an intercellular bridge is established. To complete cell division (= abscission process), membrane vesicles are delivered to the region of the intercellular bridge where they fuse with the plasma membrane which ultimately enables the physical separation of the two daughter cells.

51.8.2 The Cell Cycle in Cancer Cells

To a large extent, dysregulation of the cell cycle in cancer cells can be attributed to genetic alterations in proto-oncogenes and/or tumor suppressor genes. Aberrations in the affected genes include somatic or germline mutations, under-/overexpression, and chromosomal instability such as amplifications/deletions (Table 51.10).

Table 51.10 A selection of cell cycle-related genetic anomalies frequently observed in tumor cells

Gene	Protein	Functional type	Biological function(s)	Genetic aberration(s)	Cell cycle checkpoint
RB1	pRB	Tumor suppressor	Proliferation control: inactivates E2F transcription factor	Mutations Deletions	Restriction chpt
P53	p53	Tumor suppressor	DNA damage response: initiates p21 transcription, triggers apoptosis	Mutations Deletions	Restriction chpt DNA replication chpt
CCND1	Cyclin D1	Proto-oncogene	Activates CDK4 and CDK6	Mutations amplification overexpression	Restriction chpt
CDKN2A	p16	Tumor suppressor	Inhibits CDK4-/CDK6 complexes	Mutations Deletions	Restriction chpt
CDKN2B	p15	Tumor suppressor	Inhibits CDK4-/CDK6 complexes	Deletions Mutations	Restriction chpt
CDKN1B	p27	Tumor suppressor	Inhibits cyclin A/E-CDK2 complexes and CDK4 complexes	Mutations	Restriction chpt
CDKN1C	p57	Tumor suppressor	Inhibits cyclin A/E-CDK2 complexes	CDKN1C-promoter methylation	Restriction chpt
CDC25 (A,B,C)	CDC25	Proto-oncogene	Activates CDK1-/CDK2 complexes	Overexpression	Restriction chpt DNA replication chpt

51.9 Molecular Neuropathology: DNA Damage Response

Damage to DNA can be inflicted through several mechanisms which are either of endogenous or exogenous origin. The first category includes DNA replication errors (mismatched bases) or exposure to reactive oxygen species (ROS) which affects mainly mitochondrial DNA. Exogenous damage is caused by external factors such as UV irradiation or mutagenic chemicals.

The types of aberrations range from mutations/base modifications to major structural damage of the double helix.

Frequently encountered chemical modifications of nucleobases are:

- Depurination
- Depyrimidination
- Methylation
- Oxidation

Structural damage of DNA includes (Fig. 51.5):

- Single-Strand breaks (SSBs)
- Double-strand breaks (DSBs)
- Pyrimidine dimers
- Covalent inter- or intrastrand cross-links

51.9.1 Mechanisms of DNA Damage Recognition

It is obvious that efficient cellular DNA damage response (DDR) depends on the reliable detection of aberrant DNA. A variety of sensor proteins recognizes different types of DNA errors and transmits signals to downstream factors involved in DNA repair. Most of these sensor proteins belong to a family referred to as PIKKs (phosphoinositide 3-kinase-related kinases; PI3K-related kinases) and include ATM, ATR, and DNA-PK. Another sensor molecule is PARP1 (poly (ADP-ribose) polymerase 1). Clearly, activation of these proteins represents the most upstream event in DDR cascades.

- ATM (ataxia telangiectasia (A-T) mutated):
  – activated by DSBs via interaction with a cofactor-protein complex (MRN) which

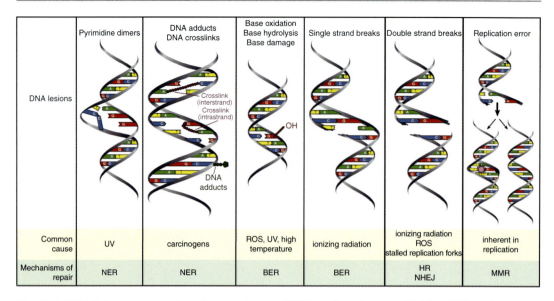

Fig. 51.5 DNA lesions: causes and repair mechanisms. *BER* base excision repair, *HR* homologous recombination, *MMR* mismatch repair, *NER* nucleotide excision repair, *NHEJ* non-homologous end joining, *ROS* reactive oxygen species, *UV* ultraviolet (reprinted from Weeden and Asselin-Labat (2018) with kind permission by Elsevier)

binds to double-stranded DNA ends, thus directing ATM to the site of the lesion; activated ATM phosphorylates downstream effectors such as p53, CHK2 (checkpoint kinase 2), histone H2AX, BRCA1 (breast cancer 1), and many more.
- ATR (ATM- and Rad3-related):
  - recruited to lesions exhibiting ssDNA stretches which are coated with replication protein A (RPA); ssDNA-RPA stretches occur for example at double-strand breaks or are generated at paused replication forks, e.g., as a result of interstrand cross-linking. Thus, ATR is not only sensitive to DSBs but has a wider activity range compared to ATM. A prominent downstream target for phosphorylation by ATR is checkpoint kinase 1, CHK1.
- DNA-PK (DNA-dependent protein kinase):
  - recognizes DSBs in cooperation with factor "Ku," a heterodimer which binds to dsDNA ends, thereby recruiting DNA-PK to dsDNA breaks; Ku is also required for the activation of the DNA-PK catalytic subunit (DNA-PKc). This interaction initiates a repair process known as non-homologous end joining (NHEJ).

- PARP1 (poly(ADP-ribose) polymerase 1):
  - is mainly associated with SSBs, but also recognizes DSBs. PARP1 directly binds to the damaged sites which triggers its activity: unlike the kinases described above, it modifies itself and downstream targets by poly(ADP)ribosylation (PARylation) which is characterized by the attachment of branched ADP-ribose polymers to lysine-, glutamate-, and aspartate side chains in the proteins. Nicotinamide adenine dinucleotide (NAD$^+$) serves as donor molecule for the ADP-ribose monomers.
  - Depending on the DNA lesion detected, PARP1 is involved in the corresponding repair pathways.

51.9.2 Mechanisms of DNA Damage Repair

51.9.2.1 Double-Strand Break Repair (DSBR)

The two pathways available to repair DSBs are:

- homologous recombination (HR) and/or
- non-homologous end joining (NHEJ)

In the presence of a homologous DNA template (sister chromatid), HR is the preferable mechanism due to its largely error-free performance, and it only is observed in S- and G2 phase. On the contrary, NHEJ occurs mainly in G1 and is susceptible to errors since there are no sister chromatids to provide homologous DNA sequences; thus, insertions or deletions are likely to arise during the repair process.

- HR
  - An early step in HR is the phosphorylation of histone H2AX and other downstream proteins of the repair cascade by ATM. In addition, ATR and PARP1 also participate in HR (see above). To initiate the repair mechanism, DNA end resection must occur: DNA-modifying enzymes (endo-, exonucleases) generate 3′-protruding ssDNA strands that are subsequently coated with repair protein A (RPA). Supported by BRCA1, the RAD51 recombinase then binds to RPA-ssDNA which triggers the search for homologous sequences on the sister chromatid. At the site of homology, a loop structure forms, providing a 3′-hydroxyl end as a primer for a DNA polymerase restoring the original sequence.
- NHEJ
  - The major protein complex involved in NHEJ is DNA-PK, recruited by Ku. Upon binding of Ku/DNA-PK to both DNA ends, they become aligned, and DNA-PK phosphorylates downstream repair factors, among them the endonuclease Artemis that is directed to the broken DNA ends. These are then cleaved by Artemis to generate ligatable ends which subsequently become ligated by a complex containing the enzyme ligase IV.

51.9.2.2 Single-Strand Break Repair (SSBR)

Single-strand breaks frequently result from the attack of reactive oxygen species (ROS) or ionizing radiation (IR). PARP1 is the major sensor for SSBs; it attaches to the lesion and there initiates assembly of a protein complex by interaction with XRCC1 (X-ray repair cross complementing 1) which in turn binds repair proteins such as DNA polymerase β, DNA ligase III, and polynucleotide kinase 3′-phosphatase (PNKP). Subsequently, PARP1 is released from the damaged site, and the lesion can be restored by the repair complex.

- Base excision repair (BER)
  - BER may be viewed as a special case in SSBR. Aberrant bases arising from deamination or oxidation are detected, excised, and replaced by the correct complementary bases. In short, a DNA glycosylase recognizes the affected nucleobase and hydrolyzes the N-glycosidic bond between ribose and base, creating an "abasic" site in the DNA. Then, an apurinic/apyrimidinic (AP) endonuclease (Ape1) generates a single-strand break (nick) by cleaving the sugar backbone at this position. The nick is recognized by PARP1 which triggers SSBR as described above.

51.9.2.3 Nucleotide Excision Repair (NER)

In contrast to BER, this repair mechanism is employed upon detection of longer stretches of damaged DNA (between 20 and 30 bases) which result in abnormal structures in the double helix. Two types of repair pathways can be distinguished, global genome NER and transcription-coupled NER. They mainly differ in their mode of damage recognition (Sugasawa 2016), but share a common downstream NER mechanism. Following recognition, the crucial steps are excision of the damaged oligonucleotide, synthesis of a new stretch of complementary DNA and ligation. Repair synthesis requires the activity of TFIIH (TFIIH core complex helicase subunit) which unwinds the affected region; two specific endonucleases cleave 5′ and 3′ of the lesion (ERCC1-XPF complex and XPG, respectively) to remove the damaged strand. The new strand is synthesized by DNA polymerase, and the gaps in the sugar backbone are ligated.

51.9.2.4 Mismatch Repair (MMR)

MMR is a repair mechanism that specifically removes replication errors, including single-base mismatches, but also single- or double base insertions/deletions ("indels"). Evidently, the newly synthesized strand containing the mismatched base(s) must be reliably identified. MSH (MutS homolog) and MLH (MutL homolog) proteins are the key factors in recognition and mismatch repair. MSHs form heterodimers such as MSH2/MSH6 (MutSα) or MSH2/MSH3 (MutSβ) which bind to the mismatched region, triggering interaction with MLH and PCNA (proliferating cell nuclear antigen); the daughter strand is then cleaved around the mismatch, and exonuclease Exo1 excises the wrong base(s). DNA polymerase and ligase finish the repair process.

Common fragile sites (CFSs) are sites on human metaphase chromosomes that are particularly prone to forming cytogenetically defined chromosomal gaps or breaks following the partial inhibition of DNA synthesis (Table 51.11).

Table 51.11 Proteins reported to have a role in CFS stability (Glover et al. 2017)

Protein	Function	Role in CFS expression
DNA replication		
MUS81	Structure-specific endonuclease subunit	M phase replication
EME1	Structure-specific endonuclease subunit	M phase replication
RAD52	Homologous recombination protein	M phase replication
BLM	RecQ helicase	Suppresses inappropriate recombination
TOP1	Type I topoisomerase	Relieves torsional stress downstream of replication and transcriptional machineries
Cell cycle checkpoints		
ATR	Serine/threonine kinase	Cell cycle arrest in response to single-stranded, unreplicated DNA
ATM	Serine/threonine kinase	Cell cycle arrest in response to DNA DSBs
CHK1	Serine/threonine kinase	Cell cycle arrest in response to DNA damage or unreplicated DNA
Claspin	BRCA1 and CHK1 adapter protein	Facilitates the ATR-dependent phosphorylation of BRCA1 and CHK1; replication fork sensor
HUS1	Component of the 9-1-1 cell cycle checkpoint response complex	p53-dependent checkpoint activation and apoptosis
SNM1B	Metallo-β-lactamase superfamily protein	Promotes fork collapse; ATR activation
DNA repair		
RAD51	Recombinase	Homologous recombination
BRCA1	E3 ubiquitin protein ligase	Genome surveillance
FANCD2	Fanconi anemia-linked repair/replication protein	Facilitates replication
DNA-PK	Serine/threonine protein kinase	Non-homologous end joining
Ligase IV	ATP-dependent DNA ligase	Non-homologous end joining
XLF	XRCC4-like factor	Non-homologous end joining
WRN	RecQ helicase	DSB repair
Translesion synthesis		
Pol η	Y family DNA polymerase	DNA synthesis at stalled forks in S phase
Pol κ	Y family DNA polymerase	Replication through repetitive elements
REV3	Polymerase ζ subunit	G2/M phase replication
Structural		
SMC1	Cohesin subunit	Prevents collapse of stalled replications forks

Abbreviations used: *ATR* ataxia telangiectasia and Rad3-related, *BLM* Bloom syndrome protein, *CFS* common fragile site, *DNA-PK* DNA-dependent protein kinase, *DSBs* double-strand breaks, *FANCD2* Fanconi anemia group D2, *SMC1* structural maintenance of chromosomes protein 1, *SNM1B* SNM1 homolog B, *TOP1* DNA topoisomerase 1, *WRN* Werner syndrome ATP-dependent helicase, *XLF* XRCC4-like factor (also known as NHEJ1)

51.10 Molecular Neuro-oncology: Oncogenes

An oncogene is (Table 51.12):

- a gene that is a mutated (changed) form of a gene involved in normal cell growth
  - its protein product is produced in higher quantities
  - its altered product has increased activity
  - "gain-of-function"
- may cause the growth of cancer cells
- Normal gene version of oncogenes are called proto-oncogenes
- Mutations in genes that become oncogenes
  - can be inherited or
  - caused by being exposed to substances in the environment that cause cancer
  - mutation in only one allele is sufficient for an effect (different from tumor suppressor genes)
  - include simple point mutations to major chromosomal rearrangements
- more than 100 oncogenes have been described
- Classification of oncogenes
  - Growth factors
  - Receptors for growth factors
    ○ Receptor tyrosine kinases (RTK)
    ○ G-protein coupled receptors

Table 51.12 Examples of oncogenes activated by amplification in cancer

Cellular oncogene	Location	Protein function	Type of cancer
ABL	9q34.1	Protein tyrosine kinase	• Chronic myeloid leukemia
BCL1	11q13.3	G1/S-specific cyclin D1	• Breast cancer • Squamous cell carcinoma of the head and neck • Bladder cancer
CDK4	12q14	Cyclin-dependent kinase	• Sarcomas
EGFR/ERBB1	7p12	Epidermal growth factor receptor	• Glioblastoma multiforme • Epidermoid carcinoma • Bladder cancer • Breast cancer
ERBB2(NEU)	17q12-q21	Growth factor receptor	• Breast cancer • Ovarian cancer • Stomach cancer • Renal adenocarcinoma • Adenocarcinoma of salivary gland • Colon carcinoma
HSTF1	11q13.3	Fibroblast growth factor	• Breast cancer • Esophageal carcinoma
INT1/WNT1	12q13	Probably growth factor	• Retinoblastoma
INT2	11q13.3	Fibroblast growth factor	• Breast cancer • Esophageal carcinoma • Melanoma • Squamous cell carcinoma of the head and neck
MDM2	12q14.3-q15	p53-binding protein	• Sarcomas
MET	7q31	Hepatocyte growth factor receptor	• Amplified in cell lines from human tumors of nonhematopoietic origin, particularly gastric tumors
MYB	6q22-q23	DNA-binding protein (essential for normal hematopoiesis)	• Leukemias • Colon carcinoma • Melanoma

(continued)

Table 51.12 (continued)

Cellular oncogene	Location	Protein function	Type of cancer
MYC(c-MYC)	8q24.12-q24.13	DNA-binding protein	• Small cell lung cancer • Giant cell carcinoma of lung • Breast cancer • Colon carcinoma • Acute promyelocytic leukemia • Cervical cancer • Gastric adenocarcinoma • Chronic granulocytic leukemia
MYCN (NMYC)	2p24.3	DNA-binding protein	• Neuroblastoma • Small cell lung cancer • Retinoblastoma • Medulloblastoma • Glioblastoma • Rhabdomyosarcoma • Adenocarcinoma of lung • Astrocytoma
MYCL1 (LMYC) MYCLK1	1p32 7p15	DNA-binding protein	• Small cell lung cancer
RAF1 (c-RAF)	3p25	Serine/threonine protein kinase	• Non-small cell lung cancer
HRAS1	11p15.5	GTPase	• Bladder cancer
KRAS2	12p12.1	GTPase	• Adrenocortical tumor • Large cell carcinoma of lung
NRAS	1p13	GTPase	• Breast cancer
REL	2p12-p13	DNA-binding protein	• Non-Hodgkin lymphomas

- Signal transducers
  ○ nonreceptor membrane-associated tyrosine kinases (SRC, ABL, FGR)
  ○ RAS family
  ○ Serine/threonine kinases
- Transcription factors

51.11 Molecular Neuropathology: Tumor Suppressors

A tumor suppressor gene (Table 51.13) is a type of gene that

- makes a protein called a tumor suppressor protein that
  - helps control cell growth
  - stimulate cell death
  - trigger the induction of permanent cell cycle arrest
- Mutations in tumor suppressor genes may lead to cancer

- Also called anti-oncogene
- Negative regulator of oncogenes
- Inactivation of both parental alleles in a single cell (different to oncogenes)
- Inactivating mechanisms include
  - deletions
  - nonsense mutations
  - missense mutations
  - methylation-mediated gene silencing
- "two-hit hypothesis"
  - a germline mutation predisposes the individual to cancer
  - mutations in both alleles are necessary for tumor initiation

p53
- "guardian of the genome": central role in maintaining the integrity of the cell's DNA (Fig. 51.6)
- transcription factor regulating genes involved in:
  - Inhibition of cell cycle
  - DNA repair

51.11 Molecular Neuropathology: Tumor Suppressors

Table 51.13 Examples of tumor suppressor genes

Tumor suppressor gene	Human chromosomal location	Gene function	Human tumors associated with sporadic mutation	Associated cancer syndrome
RB1	13q14	Transcriptional regulator of cell cycle	Retinoblastoma, osteosarcoma	Familial retinoblastoma
Wt1	11p13	Transcriptional regulator	Nephroblastoma	Wilms tumor
p53	17q11	Transcriptional regulator/growth arrest/apoptosis	Sarcomas, breast/brain tumors	Li–Fraumeni
NF1	17q11	Ras-GAP activity	Neurofibromas, sarcomas, gliomas	von Recklinghausen neurofibromatosis
NF2	22q12	ERM protein/cytoskeletal regulator	Schwannomas, meningiomas	Neurofibromatosis type 2
VHL	3p25	Regulates proteolysis	Hemangiomas, renal, pheochromocytoma	von Hippel–Lindau
APC	5q21	Binds/regulates ß-catenin activity	Colon cancer	Familial adenomatous polyposis
INK4a	9p21	p16inka4a cdki for cyclin D-cdk (4/6); p19ARF binds mdm2, stabilizes p53	Melanoma, pancreatic	Familial melanoma
PTC	9q22.3	Receptor for sonic hedgehog	Basal cell carcinoma, medulloblastoma	Gorlin syndrome
BRCA1	17q21	Transcriptional regulator/DNA repair	Breast/ovarian tumors	Familial breast cancer
BRCA2	13q12	Transcriptional regulator/DNA repair	Breast/ovarian tumors	Familial breast cancer
DPC4	18q21.1	Transduces TGF-ß signals	Pancreatic, colon, hamartomas	Juvenile polyposis
FHIT	3p14.2	Nucleoside hydrolase	Lung, stoma, kidney, cervical carcinoma	Familial clear cell renal carcinoma
PTEN	10q23	Dual-specificity phosphatase	Glioblastoma, prostate, breast	Cowden syndrome, BZS, Ldd
TCS2	16	Cell cycle regulator	Renal, brain tumors	Tuberous sclerosis
NKX3.1	8p21	Homeobox protein	Prostate	Familial prostate carcinoma
LKB1	19p13	Serine/threonine kinase	Hamartomas, colorectal, breast	Peutz–Jeghers
E-cadherin	16q22.1	Cell adhesion regulator	Breast, colon, skin, lung carcinoma	Familial gastric cancer
MSH2	2p22	mut S homolog, mismatch repair	Colorectal cancer	HNPCC
MLH1	3p21	mut L homolog, mismatch repair	Colorectal cancer	HNPCC
PMS1	2q31	Mismatch repair	Colorectal cancer	HNPCC
PMS2	7p22	Mismatch repair	Colorectal cancer	HNPCC
MSH6	2p16	Mismatch repair	Colorectal cancer	HNPCC

- Apoptosis
- Angiogenesis
- other roles include:
  - antioxidant responses
  - blocking metabolic reprogramming
  - inhibiting stem cell characteristics
  - blocking metastasis
- 90% of *p53* missense mutations are located in the DNA-binding domain
- p53 protein activity regulators

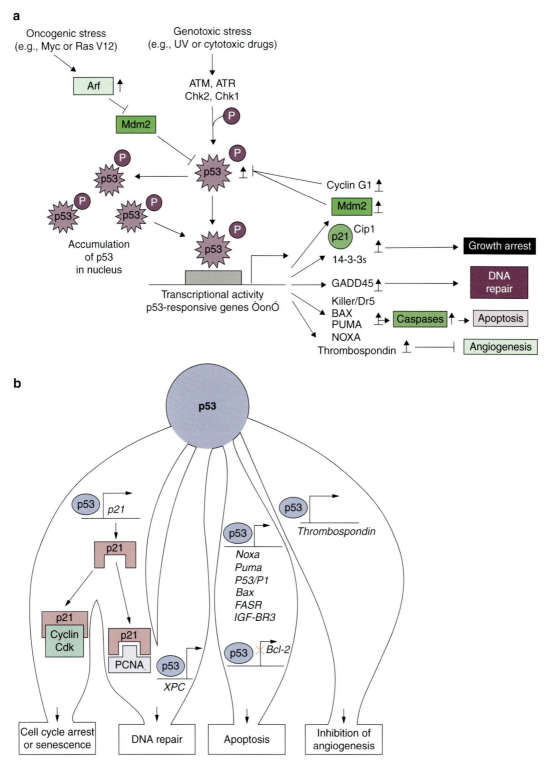

Fig. 51.6 p53 pathway: activation and function of p53 (**a**), downstream effects of p53 (**b**) (**a**: reproduced from Roussel (2013) with kind permission by Wiley; **b**: reproduced from Pecorino (2016) with kind permission by Oxford University Press). For details see text

- MDM2, ligase: degradation
- p21: cell cycle inhibition
- Bax, IGF-BP3: apoptotic response

51.12 Molecular Neuropathology: Cell Death

The many ways cells undergo death include (Tables 51.14, 51.15, and 51.16) (Fig. 51.7):

- Apoptosis
- Autophagy
- Necroptosis
- Ferroptosis
- Pyroptosis
- Parthanatos
- Cyclophilin D (CypD) necrosis
- NETosis

Cell death models are as follows:

- Passive
  - passive necrosis by damage or toxins
- Active
  - Cellular suicide
    - Apoptosis
    - Necroptosis
    - Autophagic cell death
  - Cellular sabotage
    - Generation of ROS
    - Mitotic catastrophe
    - PARP mediated necrosis
    - Ferroptosis

Table 51.14 Proteins involved in various cell death pathways

Cell death modality	Core pathway proteins involved
Apoptosis	• Caspase 8 • Caspase 3 • Caspase 7
Autosis	• Autophagy related (ATG)
Necroptosis	• RIPK3 (receptor-interacting protein kinase) • MLKL (mixed lineage kinase domain-like)
Ferroptosis	• Xc-system (cystin/glutamate antiporter) • GPX4 (glutathione peroxidase) • GSH (reduced glutathione) • LOX (lipoxygenase)
Pyroptosis	• Caspase 1/11 • Gasdermin D
Parthanatos	• PARP-1 (poly-(ADP-ribose)-polymerase) • AIF (apoptosis-inducing factor) • RIPK1 (receptor-interacting protein kinase)
Cyclophilin D (CypD) necrosis	• CypD (cyclophilin D) • mPT (mitochondrial permeability transition pore) • CthD (cathepsin D)
NETosis	• NOX (NADPH oxidase) • mTOR (mechanistic target of rapamycin) • ATG (autophagy related)

51.12.1 Apoptosis

A type of cell death

- in which a series of molecular steps in a cell lead to its death
- This is one method the body uses to get rid of unneeded or abnormal cells
- The process of apoptosis may be blocked in cancer cells
- Also called programmed cell death
- Morphologic features of apoptotic cells
  - cell shrinkage
  - membrane blebbing
  - membrane budding
  - chromatin condensation
- Apoptotic cells are removed during phagocytosis by macrophages
- Caspases (cysteine-rich aspartate proteases), a particular type of proteases, play a central role:
  - cleave intracellular proteins at aspartate residues
  - Caspase cascade
    - one caspase can activate another caspase in a chain reaction
- Inducers of apoptosis include:
  - extracellular signals, i.e., "death factors"
  - internal physical or chemical insults, i.e., DNA damage or oxidative stress

Table 51.15 Main features of PCD subtypes (Kepp et al. 2010), reproduced with kind permission by Wiley

PCD type	Stimuli	Phenotype	Consequences
Apoptosis	• Ligation of death receptors • DNA damage • Reactive oxygen species	• Pyknosis • DNA fragmentation • Plasma membrane blebbing	• Formation of apoptotic bodies • Phagocytosis
Necroptosis	• TNFR1 ligation1 SMAC (second mitochondria-derived activator of caspases) mimetics • TNFR1 ligation1 + caspase inhibition • TRAILR1 ligation1 + caspase inhibition	• Cytoplasmic swelling • Organelle swelling • Disorganized dismantling	• Release of intracellular content • Inflammation
Pyroptosis	• Bacterial infection • Viral infection • Stroke	• Cytoplasmic swelling • DNA fragmentation • Pore formation	• Release of cytokines • Inflammation

Table 51.16 Similarities and differences between apoptosis, necrosis, autophagy, and parthanatos (Fatokun et al. 2014) reproduced with kind permission by Wiley-Blackwell

	Apoptosis	Necrosis	Autophagy	Parthanatos
Variations/subsets in the literature	• Caspase-dependent intrinsic • Caspase-independent intrinsic • Extrinsic apoptosis by death receptors • Extrinsic apoptosis by dependence receptors	• Random or unregulated • Programmed or regulated e.g., necroptosis (some think parthanatos could also be considered a case of regulated necrosis)	• Macroautophagy • Microautophagy • Chaperone-mediated autophagy • Mitophagy	
(Biochemical) signatures mitochondrial	• Caspase activation • Mitochondrial depolarization • MOMP • Irreversible $\Delta\psi m$ dissipation • CYT c release • Release of IMS proteins • Respiratory chain inhibition • BID cleavage • PP2A activation • DAPK1 activation	• Loss of ultrastructure • Swelling	• Degradation	• Depolarization • Irreversible $\Delta\psi m$ dissipation • ATP and NADH depletion • AIF release • CYT c release • Caspase activation (late stage, non-obligatory)
Cytoplasmic	• Shrinkage	• Swelling (including of organelles) • Vacuolation • Organellar disintegration	• Massive vacuolization • Lysosomal degradation • MAP1LC3 lipidation	• PAR polymer accumulation • PAR–AIF interactions (binding) • Condensation • AIF translocation to the nucleus

51.12 Molecular Neuropathology: Cell Death

Table 51.16 (continued)

	Apoptosis	Necrosis	Autophagy	Parthanatos
Nuclear	• PARP cleavage • Chromatin condensation • DNA fragmentation (small-scale, DNA ladder)	• Chromatin digestion • DNA hydrolysis (smear)	• SQSTM1 degradation	• Rapid PARP-1 activation (no cleavage) • PARP-1-mediated PAR synthesis • Chromatin condensation • PAAN activation (putative) • DNA fragmentation (large-scale, ≈50 kb)
Structural (plasma membrane) changes	• Membrane integrity preserved • Formation of apoptotic bodies • Membrane blebbing • Phosphatidylserine externalization	• Loss of integrity • Blebbing • Cell lysis	• Double membrane-bound autophagosomes formed	• Loss of integrity • Phosphatidylserine externalization
Examples of trigger factors and/or conditions	• Death receptor signaling • Dependence receptor signaling • DNA damage • Trophic factor withdrawal • Viral infections	• Excitotoxicity • Ischemia • Stroke • Reactive oxygen/nitrogen species	• Amino acid starvation • Serum starvation • Protein aggregates	• Excitotoxicity • Ischemia • DNA damage • Stroke • Reactive oxygen/nitrogen species
Energy (ATP) requirement	+	−	+	−
(Obligatory) caspase dependence	+	−	−	−
Inflammatory component	−	+	−	−
Major mediator(s)	Caspases (except in b)	• Calpains • CYPD • RIP-1 • RIP-3 (and PARP-1 and AIF, if parthanatos is considered regulated necrosis), etc.	• ATG5 • ATG6 (Beclin-1) • ATG7 • ATG12 • VPS34 • AMBRA-1	• PARP-1 • PAR • AIF
Pharmacological inhibition	Caspase inhibitors, e.g., Z-VAD-fmk (except in b)	• RIP-1 inhibitors, e.g., necrostatin-1 • calpain inhibitors, etc.	• VPS34 inhibitors, e.g., 3-methyladenine and wortmannin	• PARP-1 inhibitors, e.g., DPQ

(continued)

Table 51.16 (continued)

	Apoptosis	Necrosis	Autophagy	Parthanatos
Genetic inhibition (knockout/mutation, RNAi targeting) or inhibition by protein overexpression	• BCL2 overexpression • Inhibition of caspases (3, 8, and 9) • Inhibition of PP2A • CrmA expression	• Inhibition of *RIP-1* or *RIP-3*	• Inhibition of *AMBRA1, ATG5, ATG7, ATG12,* or *BECN1*	• *PARP-1* knockout • AIF downregulation (e.g., in Harlequin mouse)

Abbreviations used: *AIF* apoptosis-inducing factor, *AMBRA1* activating molecule in Beclin-1-regulated autophagy protein 1, *ATG* autophagy, *BCL2* B-cell lymphoma 2, *BECN1* Beclin-1, *CrmA* cytokine response modifier A, *CYPD* cyclophilin D, *CYT* cytochrome, *DAPK1* death-associated protein kinase 1, *DPQ* 3,4-Dihydro-5-[4-(1-piperidinyl)butoxyl]-1(2H)-isoquinolinone, *IMS* intermembrane space, *MAP1LC3* microtubule-associated protein 1 light chain 3, *MOMP* mitochondrial outer membrane permeabilization, *PAAN* parthanatos AIF-associated nuclease, *PAR* poly (ADP-ribose), *PP2A* protein phosphatase 2A, *RIP* receptor

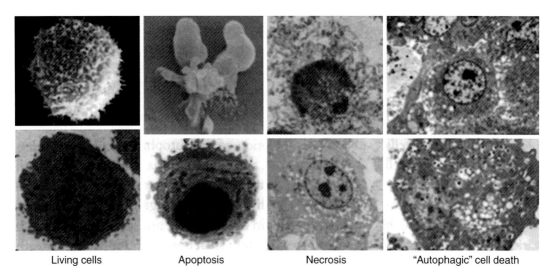

Fig. 51.7 Types of cell death (reproduced from White et al. (2015) with kind permission by Elsevier). For details see text

The extrinsic death receptor pathway (Fig. 51.8a)

- mediated by membrane death receptors
- Death signals, TNF and Fas, activate their death receptors
- Binding causes a change in shape and trimerization of the receptors
- Adaptor proteins (FADD: Fas-associated death domain protein; TRADD:TNF receptor associated death domain protein) recognize the activated receptors and lead to the aggregation of procaspase-8
- Procaspase aggregation leads to caspase-8 activation
- Initiation of
  - A caspase cascade, i.e., executioner caspases (caspase-3, -6, and -7)
  - Proteolysis of target proteins
    ○ nuclear lamins: nuclear shrinkage
    ○ cytoskeletal proteins (actin, intermediate filaments): rearranging cell structure
    ○ specific kinases: cell signaling
    ○ caspase-activated DNase: cleavage of chromatin
  - Apoptosis

- Inhibition of the process by c-Flip via
  - binding to adaptor FADD
  - binding to caspase-8 via a DED
  - inhibiting caspase-8 recruitment and activation

The intrinsic mitochondrial apoptosis pathway (Fig. 51.8b)

- Mediated by mitochondria
- Independent of external stimuli
- Inducers include DNA damage and oxidative stress
- Cell stress triggers the BH3-only protein Bid which binds and activates Bax
- Bax undergoes conformational change, inserts into the outer mitochondrial membrane, and oligomerizes
- The pro-apoptotic members of the Bcl-2 family (e.g., Bax, Bak) act by forming pores in the outer mitochondrial membrane
- The anti-apoptotic members of the Bcl-2 family (e.g., Bcl-2, Mcl-1) bind and sequester pro-apoptotic proteins into apoptosis
- Release of cytochrome c and procaspase-9 into the cytoplasm
- Assembly into a complex called apoptosome
- Caspase aggregation leads to the activation of procaspase-9 and a caspase cascade
- Modulators of the process:
  - inhibitors of apoptosis proteins (IAPs)
  - second mitochondria-derived activator (Smac/DIABLO)

Diseases in which alterations of apoptosis are involved

- Cancer
  - Breast, lung, kidney, ovary and uterus, CNS, gastro-enteric trait, head and neck, melanoma, lymphomas, leukemia
- Neurological disorders
  - Alzheimer, Parkinson, Huntington, amyotrophic lateral sclerosis, stroke
- Cardiovascular disorders
  - Ischemia, heart failure, infectious diseases, bacterial, viral
- Autoimmune diseases
  - Systemic lupus erythematosus, autoimmune lymphoproliferative syndrome, rheumatoid arthritis, thyroiditis

Conditions involving apoptosis

- Physiological conditions
  - Programmed cell destruction in embryonic development for the purpose of sculpting of tissue
  - Physiologic involution such as shedding of the endometrium, regression of the lactating breast
  - Normal destruction of cells accompanied by replacement proliferation such as in the gut epithelium
  - Involution of the thymus in early age
- Pathological conditions
  - Anticancer drug induced cell death in tumors
  - Cytotoxic T-cell induced cell death such as in immune rejection and graft versus host disease
  - Progressive cell death and depletion of CD4+ cells in AIDs
  - Some forms of virus-induced cell death, such as hepatitis B or C
  - Pathologic atrophy of organs and tissues as a result of stimuli removal, e.g., prostatic atrophy after orchidectomy
  - Cell death due to injurious agents like radiation, hypoxia, and mild thermal injury
  - Cell death in degenerative diseases such as Alzheimer disease and Parkinson disease
  - Cell death that occurs in heart diseases such as myocardial infarction

51.12.2 Autophagy

Autophagy is (Fig. 51.9):

- self-degradation pathway.
- lysosome dependent process.
- degrades various cargoes varying from molecules to whole organelles.

Fig. 51.8 Apoptotic pathways: extrinsic pathway (**a**) and intrinsic pathway (**b**) (reproduced from Pecorino (2016) with kind permission by Oxford University Press)

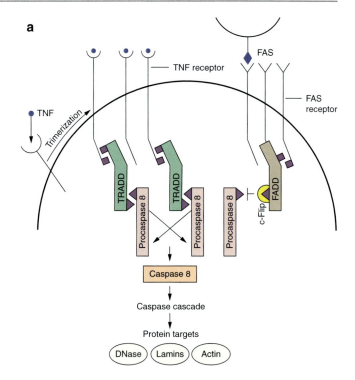
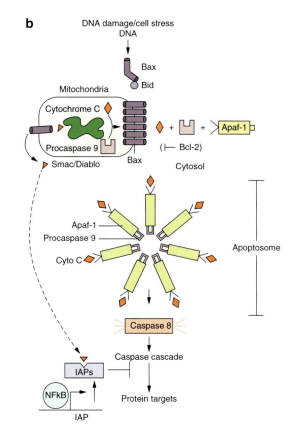

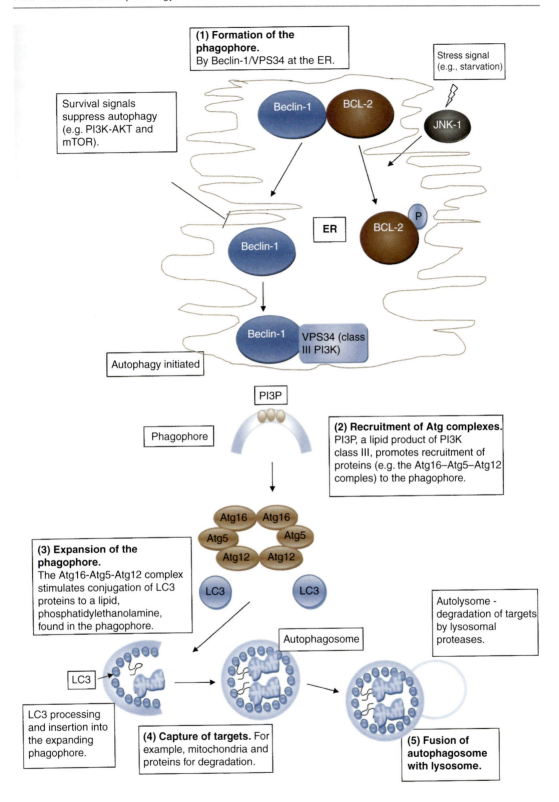

Fig. 51.9 The autophagic process (reproduced from Pelengaris and Khan (2013a) with kind permission by Wiley). For details see text

- an isolation membrane forms in the cytoplasm.
- engulfing cytosolic cargo to create an autophagosome.
- Mature autophagosomes fuse with lysosomes leading to a breakdown of engulfed material, allowing macromolecules to be recycled.

Contradictory effects of autophagy on cancer metastasis

- Anti-metastatic roles
  - Autophagy reduces hypoxia induced tumor necrosis thus precludes inflammatory cells infiltration into tumor, resulting in a reduction on metastasis.
  - Autophagic flux triggers apoptotic cell death in cancer cells at some cases.
  - Autophagy can prevent oncogene-induced cell senescence and accelerate early-stage tumor progression.
  - Autophagic cell death may inhibit cancer metastasis.
  - Autophagy regulates the release of HMGB1 from cancer cells to activate the dendritic cells-mediated anticancer immune responses.
- Pro-metastatic roles
  - Autophagy facilitates the self-adaption of pre-metastatic cells under excessive metabolic and oxidative stress or adverse environments.
  - Detachment of ECM induces autophagy and protects disseminating cancer cells from anoikis.
  - Detachment-induced autophagy also facilitates tumor cells in adverse situations into dormancy.
  - Autophagy is critical for cancer stem cells (CSCs) maintenance and drug resistances; it also sustains the dynamic equilibrium between CSCs and non-CSCs.

51.12.3 Necroptosis

Necroptosis is

- a form of regulated cell death
- induced by ligand binding to
  - TNF family death domain receptors
  - pattern recognizing receptors
  - virus sensors
- The common feature of these receptor systems is the implication of proteins,
  - which contain a receptor interaction protein kinase (RIPK) homology interaction motif (RHIM) mediating recruitment and
  - activation of receptor-interacting protein kinase 3 (RIPK3),
  - which ultimately activates the necroptosis executioner mixed lineage kinase domain-like (MLKL).

51.12.4 Ferroptosis

- results from iron-dependent lipid peroxide accumulation.
- differs from traditional apoptosis and necrosis.
- Ferroptotic cell death is characterized by cytological changes, including cell volume shrinkage and increased mitochondrial membrane density.
- is characterized morphologically by the presence of smaller than normal mitochondria with condensed mitochondrial membrane densities, reduction or vanishing of mitochondria crista, and outer mitochondrial membrane rupture.
- Ferroptosis can be induced by two classes of small-molecule substances known as class 1 (system Xc_ inhibitors) and class 2 ferroptosis inducers [glutathione peroxidase 4 (GPx4) inhibitors].
- In addition to these small-molecule substances, a number of drugs (e.g., sorafenib, artemisinin and its derivatives) can induce ferroptosis.
- Various factors, such as the mevalonate (MVA) and sulfur-transfer pathways, play pivotal roles in the regulation of ferroptosis.

51.12.5 Pyroptosis

Pyroptosis is a

- caspase 1-dependent form of programmed cell death.
- differs in many respects from apoptosis.

- it depends on the activation of caspase-1 or caspase-11 (caspase-5 in humans).
- pyroptosis is an inflammatory type of cell death.
- is triggered by various pathological stimuli, such as stroke, heart attack, or cancer.
- is crucial for controlling microbial infections.
- Pathogens have evolved mechanisms to inhibit pyroptosis, enhancing their ability to persist and cause disease.

51.12.6 Parthanatos

- PAR-mediated cell death
- Poly-ADP-ribose polymerase-1 (PARP-1) has multiple roles
  - from maintaining life to inducing death
- The processes in which PARP-1 is involved include:
  - DNA repair, DNA transcription, mitosis, and caspase-independent cell death

51.12.7 NETosis

- Neutrophil extracellular traps (NETs) are chromatin structures loaded with antimicrobial molecules.
- They can trap and kill various bacterial, fungal and protozoal pathogens, and their release is one of the first lines of defense against pathogens.
- In vivo, NETs are released during a form of pathogen-induced cell death, which was recently named NETosis.
- NETs are associated with severe tissue damage or certain autoimmune diseases.

51.12.8 Caspase-Independent Cell Death

- Pro-apoptotic triggers that cause mitochondrial outer membrane permeabilization (MOMP) also engage cell death even in the absence of caspase activity
- mitochondrial permeabilization is often viewed as a "point-of-no-return"
- shares similarities to apoptosis (namely mitochondrial permeabilization)
- but is distinct morphologically, biochemically, and kinetically

The roles that major known apoptotic participators play in cancer metastasis are given in Table 51.17.

Table 51.17 Roles of the major known apoptotic participators in cancer metastasis (Su et al. 2015) reproduced with kind permission by Springer Nature

Factor	Description	Association with cancer metastasis (representative examples)
Caspases and caspase inhibitors		
Caspase-8	Initiator caspase	Caspase-8 knockout Th-MYCN mice developed advanced neuroblastoma with bone marrow metastasis
Caspase-10	Initiator caspase	Caspase-10 mutations were identified in NSCLC patients with lymph node metastases
Caspase-3	Effector caspase	The caspase-3 protein level negatively correlated with lymph node metastasis in NSCLC patients. Another report described an inverse association between caspase-3 expression and lymph node metastasis in gastric carcinomas, although most of the caspase-3 protein was not activated

(continued)

Table 51.17 (continued)

Factor	Description	Association with cancer metastasis (representative examples)
IAPs (XIAP, survivin, and cIAP1/2)	Caspase inhibitors	Increased levels of the apoptosis inhibitor protein XIAP contributed to the anoikis resistance of circulating human prostate cancer metastatic precursor cells. A recent study showed that intermolecular cooperation between XIAP and survivin stimulated tumor cell invasion and promoted metastasis and that this pathway was independent of the IAP-mediated inhibition of cell death
DAPK	Upstream regulator of caspases-3/6/7	DAPK downregulation or inactivation was observed in several metastatic cancers. In certain cases, DAPK downregulation correlated with metastatic recurrence
Intrinsic apoptotic pathway		
Apaf-1	Key apoptosome component	Apaf-1 gene haploinsufficiency correlated with colorectal carcinoma progression and hepatic metastasis
Bcl-2	Controls mitochondrial membrane permeability	The pulmonary metastatic burden was dramatically augmented in mice inoculated with Bcl-2 transfectants. Elevated nuclear expression of Bcl-2 correlated with increased hepatocellular carcinoma metastasis
Bcl-xL	Controls mitochondrial membrane permeability	Bcl-xL overexpression caused apoptosis resistance and acted as an enhancer of metastasis but not primary tumor growth
Bax	Same as above	Bax expression was markedly decreased in metastatic colorectal cancer cells. Bax inhibitor-1 enhanced cancer metastasis
Maspin	Serine protease inhibitor	Maspin expression was reduced in brain-metastasized breast cancer cells. Decreased expression of maspin restricted the growth and metastasis of colorectal cancer xenografts in mice
Extrinsic apoptotic pathway		
FADD	Key adaptor that transmits death signals mediated by death receptors	Somatic mutations in FADD were observed at a higher frequency in metastatic NSCLC tumors than in the corresponding primary tumors. High FADD expression was associated with regional and distant metastasis in squamous cell carcinoma of the head and neck
FasL and Fas	Key death ligand and its receptor, respectively	Fas-sensitive melanoma clones were highly tumorigenic but were rarely metastatic in wild-type syngeneic mice. However, in FasL-deficient mice, both the incidence and the number of metastases were increased. The ability of osteosarcoma cells to form lung metastases inversely correlated with cell surface Fas expression
sFas and DcR3	Soluble Fas and FasL decoy receptor, respectively	In gastric carcinomas, the serum DcR3 levels closely correlated with the tumor differentiation status and the TNM classification
TRAIL	TNF family death ligand	Mice depleted of NK cells or treated with a TRAIL-blocking antibody exhibited a significant increase in spontaneous liver metastasis

Table 51.17 (continued)

Factor	Description	Association with cancer metastasis (representative examples)
DR4 and DR5	Death receptors for TRAIL	TRAIL receptor deficiency in mice enhanced lymph node metastasis of squamous cell carcinoma without affecting primary tumor development
DcR1, DcR2, and OPG	TRAIL decoy receptors	The expression of decoy receptors in tumor cells served as an alternate mechanism to resist TRAIL-induced apoptosis
Regulators of apoptotic pathways		
JNKs	Dual-role regulators of apoptosis	JNKs induced or inhibited cancer cell apoptosis in a manner that was dependent on the cell type, the stimulus, the duration of JNK activation, and the activity of other pathways. JNKs served dual roles as both suppressors and promoters of cancer metastasis
NF-κB	Transcription factor	Activated NF-κB transactivated many anti-apoptotic genes, including Bcl-2, Bcl-xL, survivin, cIAP-1/2, and c-FLIP, as well as many angiogenesis-related genes. NF-κB activity was closely associated with cancer metastasis
p53 and p63	Transcription factors	p53 upregulated pro-apoptotic genes, such as Fas, DR5, Bax, Bak, and Apaf-1, and repressed anti-apoptotic effectors, such as Bcl-2, Bcl-xL, and survivin. p53 loss or mutation promoted tumor metastasis. The loss of p53 led to invasion and lymph node metastasis of carcinogen-induced colorectal tumors. By interacting with mutant p53, p63 suppressed tumorigenesis and metastasis
TGF-β, TβRI/II, and SMADs	TGF-β pathway genes	The SMAD complex transactivated a series of apoptosis-related genes. TGF-β signals also induced apoptosis via the activation of the ARTS and Daxx-JNK pathways. Prior to tumor initiation and the early stages of progression, TGF-β signaling acted as a tumor suppressor; however, at later stages, it often promoted metastasis
MMPs	Prominent family of proteinases	MMPs played roles in the regulation of ECM turnover, cancer cell migration, cell growth, inflammation, and angiogenesis. They also interfered with the induction of apoptosis in malignant cells via the cleavage of ligands or receptors in the apoptotic pathways

Abbreviations used: *NSCLC* non-small cell lung cancer, *Apaf-1* apoptotic protease-activating factor, *IAPs* cellular inhibitors of apoptosis proteins, *XIAP* X-linked inhibitor of apoptosis, *DAPK* death-associated protein kinase, *FADD* Fas-associated death domain-containing protein, *sFas* soluble Fas, *DcR3* decoy receptor 3, *TRAIL* TNF-related apoptosis-inducing ligand, *DcR1* decoy receptor 1, also referred to as TRAIL-R3, *DcR2* decoy receptor 2, also referred to as TRAIL-R4, *OPG* osteoprotegerin, *DR4* death receptor 4, *TβR I/II* TGF-β receptor I/II, *MMPs* matrix metalloproteinases, *JNK* c-Jun N-terminal kinases

51.13 Molecular Neuropathology: Genomic Instability

Genomic instability is

- not simply the presence of a number of defined mutations
- the result of shortcomings in DNA damage responses (DDR) that greatly increase the rate at which chromosomes and DNA are damaged and that allow cells with such damage to survive and to replicate (Khan 2013)
- result from abnormalities across a range of key cellular processes:
  - cell cycle regulation
  - DNA damage and repair
  - aging
  - telomere function
- comprises several processes:
  - chromosomal instability (CIN)
    ○ gross chromosomal abnormalities
      • deletion and duplication of chromosomes or chromosome parts
      • rearrangements
      • aneuploidy
  - microsatellite instability (MSI)
    ○ alterations in the length of short repetitive sequences—microsatellites

Mutation (Tables 51.18 and 51.19)

- heritable alteration or change in the genetic material
- can be pathogenic
- can arise through exposure to mutagenic agents
- occur spontaneously through errors in the DNA replication and repair

Table 51.18 Main classes, groups, and types of mutation and effects on protein product (Turnpenny and Ellard 2017) reproduced with kind permission by Elsevier

Class	Group	Type	Effect on protein product
Substitution	Synonymous	Silent	Same amino acid
	Nonsynonymous	Missense	Altered amino acid: may after protein function or stability
		Nonsense	Stop codon loss-of-function or expression due to degradation of mRNA
		Splice site	Aberrant splicing: exon skipping or intron retention
		Promoter	Altered gene expression
		Enhancer	Altered gene expression
Deletion	Multiple of 3 (codon)		In-frame deletion of one or more amino acid(s) may affect protein function or stability
	Not multiple of 3	Frameshift	Likely to result in premature termination with loss-of-function or expression
	Large deletion	Partial gene deletion	May result in premature termination with loss-of-function or expression
		Whole gene deletion	Loss of expression
Insertion	Multiple of 3 (codon)		In-frame insertion of one or more amino acid(s) may affect protein function or stability
	Not multiple of 3	Frameshift	Likely to result in premature termination with loss-of-function or expression
	Large insertion	Partial gene duplication	May result in premature termination with loss-of-function or expression
		Whole gene duplication	May have an effect because of increased gene dosage
	Expansion of trinucleotide repeat	Dynamic mutation	Altered gene expression or altered protein stability or function

51.13 Molecular Neuropathology: Genomic Instability

Table 51.19 Some genes that might contribute to the deregulation of the cancer hallmarks

Aberration type	Examples of prominent affected genes
Amplification	• ERBB2 • EGFR • MXCN • MDM2
Frameshift mutation	• APC • RB$_1$ • ATM • NF1
Germline mutation	• BRCA1/2 • TP53 • RB1 • VHL
Missense mutation	• ARID1A • ATM • PIK3CA • IDH1 • KRAS
Nonsense mutation	• CDKN2A • PTEN
Other mutation	• BRAF • PDGFRA • PIK3R1
Splicing mutation	• GATA3 • MEN1 • TSC1
Translocation	• ABL1 • ALK • Bcl2 • MYC

Types of mutations

- Substitution
  - Replacement of a single nucleotide by another
  - Transition: replacement by the same type of nucleotide (C for T)
  - Transversion: substitution of a pyrimidine by a purine
- Deletion
  - Loss of one or more nucleotides
  - Can disrupt the reading frame
- Insertion
  - Addition of one or more nucleotides into a gene
  - Can disrupt the reading frame

Effects of mutations

- Structural effects
  - Synonymous or silent mutations
    - The polypeptide product of the gene is not altered
  - Nonsynonymous mutations
    - Encoded polypeptide is altered
    - Missense mutations: single base-pair substitution results in coding for a different amino acid and the synthesis of an altered protein
    - Nonsense mutation: substitution leads to the generation of one of the stop codons resulting in premature termination of translation of a peptide chain
    - Frameshift mutation: insertion or deletion of nucleotides that are not a multiple of three will disrupt the reading frame
- Mutations in non-coding DNA
  - Occur in promoter sequences, enhancers, or other regulatory regions
  - Effect the level of gene expression
  - Splicing mutations:
    - At highly conserved splice donor (GT) and splice acceptor (AG) sites
    - Result in aberrant splicing
- Functional effects
  - Loss-of-function mutations
    - Result in either reduced activity or complete loss of the gene product
    - Haploinsufficiency: loss-of-function mutations in the heterozygous state in which half normal levels of the gene product result in phenotypic effects
  - Gain-of-function mutation
    - Result in either increased levels of gene expression or the development of a new function of the gene product
  - Dominant-negative mutations
    - A mutant gene in the heterozygous state results in the loss of protein activity or function as a consequence of the mutant gene product interfering with the function of the normal gene product of the corresponding allele

51.14 Molecular Neuropathology: Signal Transduction Pathways

Signal transduction:

- The process by which a cell responds to substances in its environment.
- The binding of a substance to a molecule on the surface of a cell causes signals to be passed from one molecule to another inside the cell.
- These signals can affect many functions of the cell, including cell division and cell death.
- Cells that have permanent changes in signal transduction molecules may develop into cancer.

The following signaling pathways may be distinguished:

- Growth factors
  - Epidermal growth factor (EGF)
  - Transforming growth factor (TGF-α)
  - Platelet-derived growth factor (PDGF-A, PDGF-B)
  - Stem cell Factor (SCF)
  - Insulin-like growth factor 1 (IGF-1)
  - Nerve growth factor (NGF)
  - Glial cell line-derived growth factor (GDNF)
  - Vascular endothelial growth factor (VEGFs)
  - Hepatocyte growth factor (HGF)
  - Tumor necrosis factor (TNFα)
- Protein kinases
- Receptor protein tyrosine kinases
- Mitogen-Activated Protein Kinase (MAPK) signaling
  - *RAS* gene—Ras protein
  - Neurofibromin
  - Downstream signaling of Ras
    ○ BRaf protein—*BRAF* gene
- PI3K-AKT-mTOR signaling (phosphatidylinositol-4,5-biphosphate 3 kinase)-AKT- (mechanistic target of rapamycin)
  - Protein Kinase C (PKC)
  - PTEN
- Hypoxia-Inducible Factor (HIF)
- NF-κB pathways
- Wnt signaling
  - APC (adenomatous polyposis coli)
  - ß-catenin
  - Axin
- Notch signaling
- Hedgehog signaling
- TGFß signaling

PDGFR

- Two isoforms of PDGFR:
  - PDGFR-α and PDGFR-β
  - each isoform is encoded by a separate gene (PDGFR-α: chromosome 4; PDGFR-β: chromosome 5)
- PDGF is a dimeric growth factor composed of homo- or heterodimers of PDGF-A (chromosome 7), which binds only PDGFR-α, and PDGF-β (chromosome 22), which can bind to both PDGFRs, although at higher affinity to PDGFR-β.
- Human astrocytomas have been shown to overexpress both PDGF ligands and their cognate receptors, resulting in paracrine or autocrine growth stimulatory loops.
- Rearrangements and amplification of PDGFs or PDGFRs are rare (amplification in PDGFR-α in ~8% of GBMs)
- Overexpression of PDGFR-α receptor is found in ~24% of human astrocytomas.
- is likely an early induction factor as it is found in all grades.
- Only higher-grade astrocytomas overexpress the ligands, suggestive of autocrine stimulatory loops contributing to tumor progression.
- PDGFR-β overexpression is usually found in higher astrocytoma grades, where it may contribute with other angiogenesis-specific cytokines such as VEGF and angiopoietins to the florid GBM vasculature.

EGFR

- The normal 170 kDa EGFR binds to EGF, transforming growth factor-α (TGF-α), vaccinia virus growth factor, and amphiregulin, resulting in receptor dimerization and activation of downstream signaling pathways.

- This dimerization can form homodimers, or heterodimers with other members of the EGFR family, including ErbB2, ErbB3, and ErbB4.
- Overexpression of EGFR or ErbB1 (chromosome 7p11-p12) is a late event promoting malignant progression to a GBM, with amplification and often accompanying activating mutations.
- Amplification of EGFR is detected in only ~3% of low-grade astrocytomas, ~7% of anaplastic astrocytomas but in 40–50% of GBMs.
- In a large number of GBMs with EGFR gene amplification, mutant forms of EGFR are detected, the most common of which is the truncated 140 kDa EGFRvIII.
  – EGFRvIII results from intragenic deletions in exons 2–7 (801 bases encoding amino acid #6-273) of the extracellular domain of normal EGFR, resulting in a constitutively phosphorylated (activated) mutant EGFRvIII.
  – Aberrations in EGFRvIII turnover and persistent signaling in subcellular locations may be another mechanism how it is more transforming than normal EGFR.
  – GBMs which express EGFRvIII have increased in vitro and in vivo growth advantage in experimental conditions, with some ambiguity as to whether it is a negative survival prognosticator in patients.

p21-Ras
- Three human p21-Ras genes encode for four proteins (Ha, N, K4A, K4B).
- Belong to the important small-G-protein-mediated signaling family.
- Activating mutations (residue 12, 13, 61) of p21-Ras are prevalent in greater than 30% of all human cancers.
- Activation of p21-Ras is regulated by activated receptor protein tyrosine kinases (RPTKs) and its downstream effectors, leading to alterations in cell behavior.
- p21-Ras activation requires
  – post-translational modification to bind to the inner cell membrane
  – where exchange of GDP for GTP can occur by nucleotide exchange factors, such as mSos (mammalian homolog of the Son of sevenless) gene
- Normal inactivation of p21-Ras:GTP to p21-Ras:GDP requires
  – binding of a family of enzymes called Ras-GAPs (GTPase activating protein), among which are p120GAP and neurofibromin (lost in NF-1 tumors)
- In addition to primary activating mutations of p21-Ras, decreased levels of these Ras:GAPs in theory would also lead to elevated levels of active p21-Ras:GTP.
- Activated p21-Ras leads to activation of several downstream signals, which ultimately converge into the nucleus to alter transcription and thereby the cell response.
  – One of these is activation of Raf and subsequent activation of MAPKinase (ERK1,2), leading to its translocation to the nucleus and resultant proliferative signals.
  – Others include activation of PI3-kinase signaling (discussed in greater detail below), PLCγ and PKC.
- Levels of activated p21-Ras are elevated in GBMs likely from aberrant upstream signals generated by overexpressed and mutated receptors such as PDGFR and EGFR.
- Activated p21-Ras is of functional importance in GBM proliferation, angiogenesis, and overall growth.

PI3K-PTEN-AKT (Fig. 51.10)
- PI3-K can be activated either through p21-Ras-dependent or -independent mechanisms, with activation of AKT/PKB and mTOR (mammalian target of rapamycin), which in turn activates a multitude of downstream effector pathways leading to cell survival, proliferation, and cytoskeletal organization.
- PI3-K pathway activation in GBMs is not only from upstream activated RPTKs, but also from loss of its major negative regulator PTEN/MMAC located on chromosome 10q23.
- Aberrations in PI3-kinase signaling have been demonstrated to be of high functional relevance in GBMs, as restoration of normal

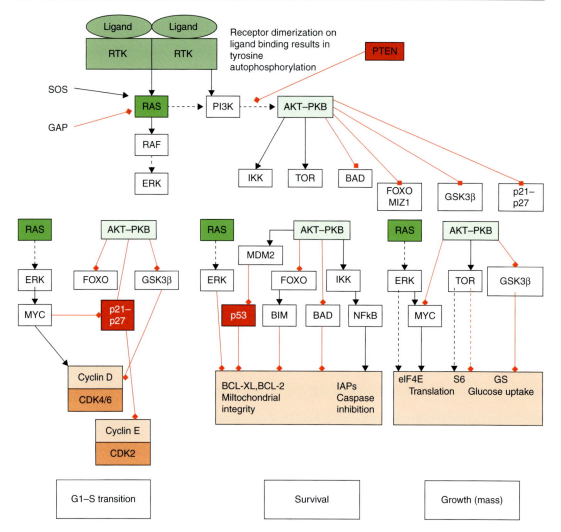

Fig. 51.10 The RAS-PI3K pathway (reproduced from Pelengaris and Khan (2013b) with kind permission by Wiley). For details see text

PTEN activity in human GBM cells leads to G1 cell cycle arrest.
- Loss of PTEN expression, either through mutation, deletion, or gene inactivation, is one of the most common genetic aberrations of GBMs, and is not found in lower-grade astrocytomas.
- PTEN mutations in "Primary GBMs" are somewhat more common (~32%) and are associated with amplifications/mutations of EGFR, compared with mutations in "Secondary GBMs (~4%)."
- The prevalence of loss of PTEN protein expression is higher than the mutational rate and approaches ~70–95% of GBMs, suggesting other mechanisms of PTEN loss such as gene inactivation.
- Activation of AKT/PKB leads to activation of several downstream signaling molecules and pro-survival pathway, i.e., mTOR and its downstream target S6, involved in mRNA translation.

JAK-STAT
- The JAK family of proteins consists of cytoplasmic proteins with four members, JAK1 JAK2, JAK3, and TYK2, which share seven regions of high homology between them known as JAK homology regions (JH1–JH7).

- The C-terminal JH-1 domain encodes the catalytic kinase, with the N-terminal JH3–JH7 implicated in receptor association.
- JAK is recruited to the intracellular domains of certain types of activated receptors, notably the interferon receptors (IFNRs), where it itself is phosphorylated and activated.
- Activated JAKs in turn phosphorylates downstream substrates, notably STATs, which are latent cytoplasmic transcription factors that upon phosphorylation become activated and form homo- or heterodimers.
- Seven STAT proteins have been identified in mammals (STAT1–4, STAT5a, STAT5b, and STAT6)
- These dimers then translocate to the nucleus to regulate gene transcription. In addition to the STATs, JAKs can also recruit other molecules to the receptor, to activate the MAPK or PI3-K pathways.
- One group found Jak1 and STAT3 to be more elevated in low-grade vs high-grade gliomas, while another group found STAT3 was constitutively activated in glioma and medulloblastoma tumors.
- Analysis of these gliomas found activated STAT3 to be mainly localized to endothelial cells, perhaps resulting in inducing transcription of VEGF and thereby playing a role in glioma angiogenesis.

51.14.1 PKC

Protein kinase C (PKC)

- is a large family of phospholipid-dependent serine/threonine kinases
- are involved in a variety of signal transduction pathways
- There are many isozymes of PKC, which differ in their enzymatic properties, tissue expression, and intracellular localization.
- All consist of an N-terminal regulatory domain and a C-terminal kinase domain.
- The inhibitory effect of the regulatory domain can be inhibited by calcium, anionic phospholipid, diacylglycerol (DAG), or tumor-promoting phorbol esters (TPA), depending on the isozyme, hence activating the protein.
- Three classes of PKC isozymes have been described based on their activation by calcium and DAG.
- Conventional PKC isozymes (α, $\beta 1$, $\beta 2$, γ) are dependent on calcium for their activation, while the novel isozymes (δ, ε, η, θ, μ) do not require calcium for their activation. Both classes are activated by DAG, while atypical isozymes (ζ, λ) are neither calcium-dependent, nor activated by DAG. The set of isozymes expressed in a cell varies during development, transformation, differentiation, and senescence.
- PKC is expressed at high levels in the normal developing brain, where it is an important glial mitogen and maturation factor.
- Malignant astrocytoma cell lines and specimens were found to have increased expression of PKC similar to fetal astrocytes, perhaps as a result of de-differentiation.
- In addition, stimulation of aberrant receptors such as EGFR in GBM cells, resulted not only in activation of p21-Ras and PI3-kinase, but also PKC mediated signaling.

51.15 Molecular Neuropathology: Epigenetic Changes

Epigenetics is the study of how age and exposure to environmental factors, such as diet, exercise, drugs, and chemicals, may cause changes in the way genes are switched on and off without changing the actual DNA sequence. These changes can affect a person's risk of disease and may be passed from parents to their children.

Epigenetic regulation of transcription includes:

- Histone modifications
- DNA methylation

Histone modifications

- Post-translational modifications of histone proteins include:
  - acetylation
  - methylation

- phosphorylation
- ubiquitination
- The pattern of these multiple histone modifications helps to specify the components and activity of the transcription regulatory molecular machinery.

DNA methylation

- addition of a methyl group to position 5 of cytosine
- occurs only at cytidine nucleotides which are situated 5′ to guanosine nucleotides (CpGs)
- CpG is under-represented and unequally distributed in the genome
- CpG islands are located in the promoter region of 50% of human genes
- *MGMT* promoter methylation
  - The DNA repair enzyme O6-methylguanine-DNA methyltransferase (MGMT) antagonizes the genotoxic effects of alkylating agents.
  - *MGMT* promoter methylation is the key mechanism of *MGMT* gene silencing and predicts a favorable outcome in patients with glioblastoma who are exposed to alkylating agent chemotherapy.

51.16 Molecular Neuropathology: Telomeres and Telomerase

Telomeres:

- The ends of a chromosome.
- Each time a cell divides, the telomeres lose a small amount of DNA and become shorter.
- Over time, the chromosomes become damaged and the cells die.
- In cancer cells, the telomeres do not get shorter, and may become longer, as the cells divide.
- The shortening of human telomeres has two opposing effects during cancer development.
  - Telomere shortening can exert a tumor-suppressive effect through the proliferation arrest induced by activating the kinases ATM and ATR at unprotected chromosome ends.
  - Loss of telomere protection can lead to telomere crisis, which is a state of extensive genome instability that can promote cancer progression.

Telomerase:

- An enzyme in cells that helps keep them alive by adding DNA to telomeres (the ends of chromosomes).
- Cancer cells usually have more telomerase than most normal cells.
- Common inherited variants near the telomerase-component genes *TERC* and *TERT* are associated both with longer telomere length and increased risk of glioma.
- These mutations facilitate telomere lengthening, thus bypassing a critical mechanism of apoptosis.

51.17 Molecular Neuropathology: Angiogenesis

The process of creation of vessels is divided into the following two steps:

- Vasculogenesis
- Angiogenesis

The following definitions

- Vasculogenesis:
  - In situ differentiation of endothelial precursor cells during development.
- Angiogenesis or neovascularization:
  - Sprouting of capillaries from pre-existing vessels.
- Bone marrow derived vasculogenesis:
  - Mobilization of endothelial precursor cells from bone marrow and their integration and differentiation into sites of adult blood vessel formation.
- Somatic stem cell derived vasculogenesis:
  - Mobilization of precursor cells from differentiated organs and their integration and trans-differentiation into growing blood vessels.

Table 51.20 List of key angiostatic, anti-angiogenic and pro-angiogenic signals, modified after (De Palma et al. 2017), reproduced with kind permission by Springer Nature

Key angiostatic or anti-angiogenic signals	Key pro-angiogenic signals
• Basal lamina • Low VEGFA gradients • Low MMP and cathepsin activity • Angiopoietin (ANGPT1) • Thrombospondin 1(THBS1) • Plasminogen activator inhibitor 1 (PAI1) • Angiostatin • Interferon α (IFN-α) • CXCL9 • CXCL10 • CXCL11 • ECM	• Vascular endothelial growth factor A (VEGFA) • Fibroblast growth factor 2 (FGF2) • CXCL8 • Platelet-derived growth factors (PDGFs) • Placental growth factor (PlGF) • Angiopoietin (ANGPT2) • Interleukin (IL-1ß) • Interleukin 6 (IL-6) • Tumor necrosis factor TNF • BV8 • Matrix metalloproteinases (MMPs) • Cathepsins • Extracellular vesicle EVs • Adipokines • Lactate • Acidosis • ECM

- Vascular morphogenesis:
  – Formation and maturation of functional blood vessels, e.g., interaction of vascular endothelial cells with pericytes and smooth muscle cells.

The hypothesis that tumor growth is angiogenesis-dependent states (Folkman 1971):

- Virtually all tumors would be restricted to a microscopic size in the absence of angiogenesis.
- Tumors would be found to secrete diffusible angiogenic molecules.
- Tumor dormancy due to blocked angiogenesis.
- Antiangiogenesis means the prevention of new capillary sprouts from being recruited into an early tumor implant.
- Discovery of angiogenesis inhibitors.
- Antibody to a tumor angiogenic factor could be an anticancer drug.

A list of key angiostatic, anti-angiogenic and pro-angiogenic signals is given in Table 51.20 while angiogenesis regulators in the tumor microenvironment (TME) are listed in Table 51.21.

51.17.1 Features of Tumor Endothelial Cells

Morphology

- Tumor endothelial cells (ECs) are structurally abnormal (De Palma et al. 2017).
- They generally present excessive fenestrations, uneven surfaces and intra-luminal projections, and loosened intercellular junctions, and can also form multilayered endothelia.
- These features favor vascular leakage and may limit blood flow.

Gene Expression

- The vascular ECs of different tissues and organs show distinct gene expression profiles.
- Tumor ECs may display considerable inter- and intra-tumoral molecular heterogeneity.
- Both gene expression profiling and the use of phage-display peptide libraries identified several tumor-type or stage-specific vascular markers (termed "tumor endothelial markers" or "vascular zip codes") in mouse models of cancer.
- The targeting of such tumor EC-specific markers may facilitate the selective delivery of therapeutic agents to tumor-associated blood vessels (TABVs).

Proliferative Signaling

- Tumor ECs display increased proliferative, migratory and tube-formation capabilities in response to growth factors and cytokines, compared with non-tumor ECs.
- Furthermore, they are resistant to senescence and can grow ex vivo in serum-free conditions.

Table 51.21 Angiogenesis regulators in the tumor microenvironment (TME), modified after (De Palma et al. 2017) data reproduced with kind permission by Elsevier

TME component	Main angiogenesis regulators produced by TME component	Effects of TME component on TABVs
Macrophages	VEGFA, FGF2, CXCL8, CXCL12, PlGF, VEGFC, IL-1β, IL-6, TNF, WNT7B, MMPs, and cathepsins	Pro-angiogenic; induce EC proliferation, migration, and survival, as well as ECM remodeling, to facilitate sprouting angiogenesis
CXCL9, CXCL10, CXCL11, and TNF	Potentially angiostatic under the influence of IFNγ and other	TH1 cytokines
Neutrophils and MDSCs	VEGFA, FGF2, BV8, and MMP9	Pro-angiogenic; the role is well established during early tumor stages or after therapeutic neutralization of VEGFA
Mast cells	FGF2, VEGFA, TNF, CXCL8, chymase, tryptase, and MMP9	Pro-angiogenic during the transition from non-angiogenic to angiogenic tumors
Eosinophils	VEGFA, FGF2, IL-6, CXCL8, and MMP9	Potentially pro-angiogenic, but relevance for tumor angiogenesis unclear
TH2 cells	IL-4	Potentially pro-angiogenic by stimulating the alternative (M2-like) activation of TAMs
TH1 cells	IFNγ	Potentially angiostatic through the induction of CXCL9, CXCL10, and CXCL11 in TAMs or via direct angiostatic or anti-angiogenic effects on ECs
TH17 cells	IL-17	Pro-angiogenic by inducing CAFs to release CSF3, which recruits pro-angiogenic neutrophils
Treg cells	VEGFA	Pro-angiogenic
B-cells	VEGFA, FGF2, MMP9, and IgG	Potentially pro-angiogenic, either directly or via IgG-dependent recruitment and activation of myeloid cells
	Anti-VEGFA or anti-ANGPT2 IgG	Potentially angiostatic through the production of autoantibodies against pro-angiogenic cytokines in the context of immunotherapy
NK cells	VEGFA	Potentially pro-angiogenic, but relevance for tumor angiogenesis unclear
Platelets	VEGFA, PDGFB, FGF2, and CXCL12	Pro-angiogenic
THBS1, PAI1, endostatin, and ANGPT1	Potentially angiostatic	
Pericytes	VEGFA, ANGPT1, and ECM components	Promote EC survival and, possibly, proliferation; they may contribute to stabilization of TABVs
CAFs	VEGFA, PDGFC, FGF2, CXCL12, osteopontin, and CSF3	Pro-angiogenic, both directly and indirectly by recruiting myeloid cells and through ECM production
Adipocytes	Adipokines and free fatty acids	Pro-angiogenic and pro-inflammatory; stimulate peri-tumoral angiogenesis
ECM	Periostin, tenascin-C, fibronectin, osteopontin, and CCN-family proteins	Pro-angiogenic through the storage and concentration of pro-angiogenic factors, and recruitment of pro-angiogenic leukocytes
	THBS1, osteonectin, decorin, proteolytic fragments of type IV and XVIII collagens	Potentially angiostatic
Hypoxia	HIF-inducible genes: VEGFA, CXCL12, and ANGPT2	Pro-angiogenic 2

Table 51.21 (continued)

TME component	Main angiogenesis regulators produced by TME component	Effects of TME component on TABVs
Metabolites	Lactate	
	H+	Pro-angiogenic through increased expression and stabilization of VEGFA mRNA
ROS	Free radicals and non-radical ROS	Potentially pro-angiogenic by enhancing HIF1 transcription and the expression of pro-angiogenic and pro-inflammatory factors; they also generate pro-angiogenic lipid oxidation products
Tumor-derived EVs	Various pro-angiogenic and inflammatory mediators, ECM-remodeling enzymes and mitogenic factors for ECs	Potential pro-angiogenic effects mediated via contacts with, or transfer of their cargo to, ECs; relevance for tumor angiogenesis unclear

Abbreviations used: *ANGPT* angiopoietin, *CAF* cancer-associated fibroblast, *CSF3* colony-stimulating factor 3, *CXCL* CXC-chemokine ligand, *EC* endothelial cell, *ECM* extracellular matrix, *EV* extracellular vesicle, *FGF2* fibroblast growth factor 2, *HIF* hypoxia-inducible factor, *IFNγ* interferon-γ, *IgG* immunoglobulin G, *IL* interleukin, *MDSC* myeloid-derived suppressor cell, *MMP* matrix metalloproteinase, *NK* natural killer, *PAI1* plasminogen activator inhibitor 1, *PDGF* platelet-derived growth factor, *PlGF* placental growth factor, *ROS* reactive oxygen species, *TABV* tumor-associated blood vessel, *TAM* tumor-associated macrophage, *TH* T helper, *THBS1* thrombospondin 1, *TME* tumor microenvironment, *TNF* tumor necrosis factor, *Treg cells* regulatory T-cells, *VEGF* vascular endothelial growth factor

- The upregulation of growth factor and cytokine receptors (for example, vascular endothelial growth factor receptors (VEGFRs)) by tumor ECs may account for such abilities.
- Tumor ECs, but not normal ECs, may express epidermal growth factor receptor (EGFR) and proliferate in response to EGF.
- They also show constitutive activation of PI3K–AKT signaling, which promotes cell survival and resistance to apoptosis.

Metabolism
- Quiescent ECs display relatively high glycolysis rates.
- However, tumor ECs are hyper-glycolytic and largely use aerobic glycolysis to address their energy requirements.

Drug Resistance
- There is evidence for tumor ECs being more resistant than normal ECs to various cytotoxic drugs.
- For example, tumor ECs were shown to acquire resistance to the cytotoxic agent paclitaxel through the upregulation of the ATP-dependent efflux pump, P-glycoprotein 1 (PGY1; also known as ABCB1), which is induced by VEGFA signaling.

Genetic Abnormalities
- Gene and chromosomal abnormalities, including aneuploidy, supernumerary centrosomes, and translocations, have been documented in subpopulations of tumor ECs of both mouse and human origin.
- Tumor ECs may accumulate genetic mutations through several routes.
- They produce substantial amounts of reactive oxygen species (ROS) in response to cycles of anoxia–reoxygenation (oxidative stress), and are directly exposed to ROS released by tumor-infiltrating inflammatory cells and cancer cells.
- Furthermore, hypoxia represses the cellular DNA repair machinery.
- Both processes, coupled to the high proliferation rate of tumor ECs, can be directly mutagenic and also promote genetic instability in tumor.
- Alternatively, genetic alterations in tumor ECs might result from the direct *trans*-differentiation of cancer cells or, possibly, cancer stem cells into ECs.

51.18 Molecular Neuro-oncology: Glioma Invasion and Microenvironment

Invasion
- The beginning or incursion of a disease.
- Local spread of a malignant neoplasm by infiltration or destruction of adjacent tissue; for epithelial neoplasms, invasion signifies infiltration beneath the epithelial basement membrane.
- Entrance of foreign cells into a tissue, such as polymorphonuclear leukocytes in inflammation.

Infiltration
- the diffusion or accumulation of substances or cells not normal to it or in amounts in excess of the normal

A tumor is a product of aberrant genomes interacting with an enabling microenvironment

- a tumor creates its own microenvironment.
- an aberrant microenvironment causes a tumor.

Microenvironment (Fig. 51.11)
- Promoting microenvironment
  - a microenvironment favorable for the growth of a tumor cell
  - wounding of tissue promotes tumor formation
  - causal relationship between tumor growth and angiogenesis
- Suppressive microenvironment
  - embryonic microenvironment can induce tumors to function normally in development.

A review of the molecular mechanisms in glioma cell motility is given by (Armento et al. 2017)

Extracellular Matrix (ECM)
- ECM constitutes 10–20% of brain volume.
- It is produced by the surrounding cells.
- ECM not only has a structural function but also a major role in brain development, cell survival, migration, maturation, differentiation, and tissue homeostasis.
- The main components of the brain ECM are:
  - proteoglycans
  - hyaluronan
  - link-proteins like TN-C
  - others
- Another ECM type in the brain is the basement membrane that covers blood vessels and is part of the perivascular space.
- Deregulated ECM dynamics is a hallmark of cancer.
- The ECM of glioma differs from that of the healthy brain
  - Whereas universal ECM components are expressed uniformly in healthy brains, in

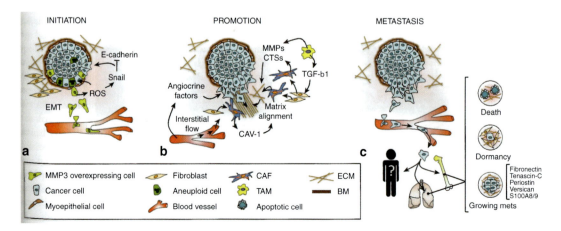

Fig. 51.11 The microenvironment (reproduced from Ghajar et al. (2015) with kind permission by Elsevier). For details see text

high-grade glioma fibrous proteins and laminin are upregulated.
- Besides, the interaction of the ECM component hyaluronan with its receptor CD44, both being overexpressed in glioma cells, is a major requirement for glioma invasion.
- For glioma cells to invade the healthy brain tissue, the intact ECM has to be destroyed and remodeled.
- ECM degrading and remodeling enzymes include several MMPs, A Disintegrin and Metalloproteinase with Thrombospondin Motifs (ADAMTS), the serine protease plasmin, 6-O-sulfatases, heparanases, cathepsins, and urokinase (uPa).

Matrix Metalloproteinases

- MMPs are a family of secreted or membrane-anchored endoproteinases.
  - main function is the degradation and remodeling of the ECM.
- MMP expression in the normal brain is low.
- In glioma, MMPs are overexpressed or activated.
- MMP-2 and MMP-9
  - expression correlates with tumor grade and progression.
  - convert latent pro-migratory transforming growth factor (TGF)-β into its active form, which in turn induces MMP-2 in a feedback loop.
- MMP-9 expression or activity can be regulated by: activation of signal transducer and activator of transcription (STAT)3; epidermal growth factor (EGF); FN; vitronectin (VN); interleukin (IL)-1β; tumor necrosis factor (TNFα); and TGF-β.
- MMP-14 is expressed by surrounding microglia cells. MMP-14 activates MMP-2 by cleaving its pro-peptide
- MMP-3, -7, -12, -13, -16, -19, and -26 are also highly expressed and mostly associated with enhanced glioma invasion.
- MMPs are inhibited by the four tissue inhibitors of metalloproteinases (TIMP), TIMP-1–4.
- High TIMP-1 levels and TIMP-3 silencing are associated with a poor prognosis for glioma patients.

Integrins—The Link Between the ECM and Cells

- Integrins are catalytic inactive heterodimeric transmembrane glycoproteins responsible for cell–ECM interactions.
  - are the link between the ECM and the cytoskeleton and important for signal transduction.
- To date, 24 integrins composed of different combinations of 18 α- and 8 β-subunits have been identified.
- The α/β combination determines ligand specificity. Typical ECM ligands for integrins are laminin, collagen, and FN, which are part of the basement membrane in the brain and are expressed by high-grade gliomas.
- Other integrin ligands are thrombospondin (TSP), osteopontin (OPN), VN, and TN-C, all being overexpressed in gliomas.
- Upon ligand binding, integrins form clusters, leading to activation of the focal adhesion kinase (FAK) and finally to enhanced migration. FAK is active and overexpressed in gliomas, and its expression correlates with the tumor grade.
- Upon integrin clustering, the cytoplasmic domain attaches to cytoskeletal components to form focal adhesion points at the leading edge of migrating cells. This adhesion points give cells a polarity which enable them to move forward. In GBM, integrin β1 is overexpressed and is associated with migration.
- Integrin α9β1 expression correlates with glioma grade and influences MMP-9 expression. Furthermore, integrin α5β1 can stimulate MMP-2 expression upon interaction with angiopoietin.
- In addition, integrin αvβ3 and αvβ5 expression is associated with disease progression. Both can bind to the latency-associated peptide (LAP) of the LAP-TGF-β complex and thereby release active TGF-β.

- In summary, integrins are substantial for glioma cell migration, establishing the link between the brain ECM and the tumor cells.

Chondroitin Sulfate Proteoglycans, Glycoproteins, and Galectins
- chondroitin sulfate proteoglycans (CSPG)
- a class of proteoglycans which are overexpressed in glioma and associated with increased glioma invasion. A subgroup of CSPG, the lecticans, forms tertiary complexes with hyaluronan and TN-R.
- Three of them, versican, BEHAB/brevican, and neurocan, are overexpressed in glioma and enhance glioma motility.
- Invasion-promoting ECM glycoproteins secreted in glioma are:
  - Secreted Protein Acidic and Rich in Cysteine (SPARC)
  - TN-C supporting cell adhesion through integrin binding
  - OPN and VN
  - TSP-1, a multifunctional matrix glycoprotein, is implicated in cell adhesion, migration, invasion, and activation of TGF-β.
- Galectins are soluble lectins with specificity for β-galactoside
  - allow them to bind to proteoglycans and glycoproteins in the brain ECM.
  - In malignant gliomas, galectin-1, -3, and -8 are overexpressed and promote glioma cell migration and invasion by modulating the actin cytoskeleton.

Migration-Associated Changes of the Cytoskeleton
- Cell migration is a multistep process
  - initiated by binding of chemoattractants or pro-migratory factors to cell surface receptors
  - followed by the activation or inactivation of diverse small GTPases and cytoskeleton reorganization

Small GTPases
The most important and well-characterized small GTPases associated with cytoskeletal remodeling are:

- RhoA is responsible for coordination of contractility at the cell body and cell rear
  - RhoA activity correlates with increased glioma cell migration.
- RAC-1 regulates protrusion formation at the leading edge.
  - RAC-1 protein levels correlate with tumor grade in astrocytomas. In addition, RAC-1 is hyperactivated in GBM (100).
- CDC42 modulates cell polarity.
  - Enhanced activity of CDC42 and RAC-1 has been reported in infiltrating glioma cells.

Axonal Guidance Molecules
- Glioma cell movement can also occur along myelinated neuronal axons of white matter tracts.
- A multitude of proteins act as axonal guidance molecules by either attracting or repelling axonal growth cones and modulating neural cell motility during development.
- The most prominent axonal guidance molecules are:
  - Ephrins (Eph)
  - Netrins
  - Slits and their roundabout (Robo) receptors
  - Semaphorins (Sema) and their receptors plexin and neuropilin (NRP)

Ephrins
- Ephrins serve as ligands of ephrin receptors (EphRs), a family of proteins containing nine EphR class A and five EphR class B members.
- Interaction of Eph and EphR regulates cell–cell interaction by forward (Eph to EphR) or reverse (EphR to Eph) signaling.
- Eph regulates cell migration, adhesion, morphology, differentiation, proliferation, and survival through Jun-N-terminal kinase (JNK), STAT3, PKB/AKT, Rho GTPase, and paxillin pathways.
- Eph proteins have a dual role in glioma cell migration:
  - Negative regulation that inhibits migration.

- Positive regulation that promotes migration.
- These proteins might serve as regulators of the "Go or Grow" behavior of GBM.

Netrins
- Netrins are a family of laminin-related proteins.
- Netrin-1, the most prominent representative of the netrin family, is widely expressed in fetal and adult brain tissues.
- Netrin-1 binds to UNC5-family dependence receptor (DR) deleted in colorectal cancer (DCC), or other UNC5 molecules.
- While the absence of netrin-1, DCC/UNC induces apoptosis, the absence of the DRs or enhanced netrin-1 expression is tumorigenic.
- Netrin expression is associated with poor patient prognosis in lower-grade gliomas.
- In GBM cells, elevated netrin expression activates notch signaling, finally resulting in the gain of stemness and enhancement of invasiveness of these cells.

Slit/Robo
- Slit (Slit 1–3) and the Robo receptor family proteins are evolutionarily conserved molecules.
- During normal development, secreted Slit proteins regulate axon guidance and neuronal precursor cell migration by mediating chemo-repulsive signals on cells expressing Robo.
- In glioma, Slit2 and Robo1 provide different patterns.
  - By hypermethylation of its promoter, the expression of Slit is low in most gliomas, whereas the expression of Robo1 is high.
  - Slit2/Robo1 signaling inhibits glioma cell migration and invasion by inactivation of CDC42 signaling.
- In vivo, Slit-2 mitigates infiltration of glioma cells into the healthy brain, indicating that a chemo-repulsive signal transmitted by the interaction of Slit2/Robo1 participates in glioma cell migration or guidance

Semaphorins and Their Receptors
- Semaphorins (Sema) are membrane-anchored and transmembrane proteins.
- Class 3 semaphorins (Sema3) transfer their function through a receptor complex consisting of plexins and neuropilin (NRP)-1 and -2.
- Downstream signaling of Sema involves RhoA, RAC-1, and cofilin, leading to the reorganization of the cytoskeleton.
- In GBM cells, inactivation of RhoA by Sema3F leads to the collapse of the cytoskeleton, whereas inhibition of Sema3F promotes cell motility.
- Similar effects have been observed for Sema3G, and higher expression of Sema3G in GBM patients has been associated with a better prognosis.

The Role of TGF-β in Glioma Cell Motility
- The TGF-β superfamily of cytokines consists of TGF-β 1–3.
- Master regulators of inflammation and cell differentiation.
- Play a key role in tumor progression and metastasis.
- After binding to the TGF-β receptor (TGFβ-R)-I, TGFβ-RII is phosphorylated. This in turn phosphorylates SMAD2/3, which then combines with SMAD4. This complex translocates to the nucleus and regulates gene expression.
- TGF-β is heavily secreted by glioma cells in vitro and in vivo.
  - TGF-β promotes a mesenchymal phenotype in GBM cells, enhancing invasion and migration in vitro, and in an orthotopic mouse model.
  - TGF-β also stimulates the production of reactive oxygen species (ROS) and activates ERK1/2, JNK, and NFκB. NFκB finally upregulates the expression of MMP-9.
  - Other mechanisms of TGF-β influencing the ECM and promoting migration include the upregulation of integrin αvβ3 and the versican isoforms V0/V1.

- TGF-β suppresses phosphatase and tensin homolog (PTEN) in glioma cells through enhanced miR10a/b expression.
- In reaction to radiation treatment, the invasion capability of glioma cells is enhanced and TGF-β is upregulated. This suggests a role for TGF-β in treatment resistance.

EMT-Like Processes
- EMT is a process by which epithelial cells lose their polarity and cell–cell adhesion, resulting in a mesenchymal phenotype characterized by enhanced motility, chemoresistance, and stem-like properties.
- Among the signals that have been shown to induce EMT in glioma are TGF-β, EGF, and Hypoxia-Inducible Factor (HIF).

TWIST
- TWIST1 and TWIST2 are helix-loop-helix TFs involved in EMT during development and cancer progression.
- In glioma, TWIST was found to be a possible prognostic marker, and its expression correlates with tumor grade.
- TWIST overexpression promotes invasion of glioma cells in vitro and in orthotopic glioma xenotransplants in vivo by inducing the expression of EMT-associated genes like MMP-2 and FN-1.

SNAIL, SLUG
- The SNAIL family of transcriptional repressors.
- Consisting of SNAIL/SNAI1 and SLUG/SNAI2.
- Drive invasion and metastasis in various carcinomas.
- SNAIL binds to E-box DNA sequences of genes related to an epithelial phenotype through carboxy-terminal zinc finger domains, thereby suppressing their expression.
- Knockdown of SNAIL in glioma cells by siRNA diminished glioma migration and invasion.
- In GBM, the Rho family GTPase (RND)-3 has been shown to promote the degradation of SNAIL in vitro and in vivo, while downregulation of RND3 strongly induces SNAIL expression and migration.
- SLUG expression was found to correlate with histologic grade and invasive phenotype in glioma, whereas knockdown of SLUG attenuated invasion and prolonged survival in an intracranial mouse model.

ZEB
- The TFs Zinc finger E-box Binding homeobox proteins (ZEB)-1 and -2 bind to E-boxes of DNA sequences, thereby repressing cell polarity-associated genes such as E-cadherin/CDH1, cell adhesion molecules, and stemness-inhibiting miR-200.
- GBM patients, ZEB-1 overexpression correlated with poor overall survival.
- ZEB-1 and PDGFRα were found to be co-expressed in tissue samples from GBM patients, while high expression of both ZEB-1 and activated PDGFRα was identified to significantly coincide with poor survival.
- Protein Tyrosine Phosphatase/Nonreceptor type (PTPN)-1 is a regulator of ZEB-1-induced and PDGFR-induced EMT in glioma.
- The hypoxic marker HIF1α and ZEB-1 were shown to colocalize in hypoxic areas of human GBM.
- ZEB-2 was overexpressed in glioma tissue samples compared to healthy brain tissue, and higher expression of ZEB-2 correlated with glioma pathology grading.

Cadherins
- Cadherins are Ca2+-dependent transmembrane molecules.
- Important role in cell to cell adhesion, recognition, and signaling.
- In tissues of GBM and healthy brain, the expression of E-cadherin is generally only marginal.
- In a minor subset of GBM showing epithelial differentiation, high expression of E-cadherin is observed, correlating with poorer clinical outcome compared to GBM with low or no E-cadherin expression.

- N-cadherin is frequently downregulated in GBM compared to the healthy brain.
- N-cadherin overexpression has been shown to decrease glioma invasion in vitro and in vivo.

51.19 Molecular Neuro-oncology: MicroRNAs

MicroRNAs (miRNAs) are

- small cellular non-coding RNAs of approximately 20 nucleotides in length
- bind to 3′ untranslated regions (UTRs) of target mRNAs
- thereby blocking translation
- mediating degradation of the transcripts
- important modulators of gene expression
- involved in a wide variety of cellular processes

Apart from their crucial function in normal cells, miRNAs were also recognized as important players in tumor development. Cancer cells frequently express dysregulated miRNAs which can be classified in two categories:

- upregulated miRNAs with oncogenic activity (termed oncomiRs)
- downregulated miRNAs with tumor suppressor properties

OncomiRs act by targeting transcripts from tumor suppressor genes; on the other hand, downregulation of the tumor suppressor miRNAs results in their diminished ability to inhibit oncogene expression (loss-of-function). To date, of all known miRNAs only a few have been characterized with respect to their specific function.

51.20 Molecular Neuro-oncology: Stem Cell Hypothesis

Stem Cell (SC)
- A cell from which other types of cells develop (blood cells develop from blood-forming stem cells)
- Involved in the regeneration of tissues during the lifetime of the individual
- May remain dormant until a physiological signal is received (breast stem cells responding to pregnancy hormones)
- Two defining features
  - ability to self-renew
  - ability to give rise to committed progenitors of differentiated cell types of one or more lineages
- Upon cell division
  - one daughter cell maintains characteristics of stem cells
  - the other daughter cell shows characteristics of commitment towards differentiation

Embryonic Stem Cells (ESC)
- unspecialized progeny of cells that reside in the inner cell mass of the fertilized egg

Cancer Stem Cell (CSC)
- subpopulations of cells with stem cell properties that initiate and maintain the cancer phenotype
- ability to
  - self-renewal
  - to give rise to phenotypically diverse cancer cells with limited proliferative potential that make up the rest of the tumor
  - initiate new tumors when transplanted into host animals
- have surface proteins characteristic of the stem cell normally present ion the tissue
- Carcinogenesis hypotheses:
  - self-renewal provides increased opportunities for carcinogenic changes to occur.
  - altered regulation of self-renewal directly underlies carcinogenesis.

Brain Cancer Stem Cells
- display normal neural stem cell markers
- proportion of brain CSCs correlates with prognosis
- fast-growing tumors (GBM) have more brain CSCs than low-growing tumors
- extensively infiltrate brain tissue

- resist radiotherapy and chemotherapy
- thought to represent the ultimate drivers of disease progression
- stem cell associated genes/proteins
  - NESTIN, GFAP, SOX2, A2B5, NANOG, OKT4, CD44, and KLF4
  - CD133
  - CD44
  - CD109
    - a GPI-anchored protein, on a population of perivascular CSCs
    - CD109-expressing CSCs appear to drive the proliferation of adjacent non-stem tumor cells (NSTCs)
  - Prominin-1 (PROM1/Cd133)
    - PROM1 is a single-chain polypeptide of 865 amino acids with 5-TM regions, extracellular N-terminus, and cytoplasmic C-terminus
  - Npm1 (Nucleophosmin/B23)
    - is a non-ribosomal nucleolar protein
    - very abundant 37kDa phosphoprotein
    - mainly localized in the nucleolus
- Perivascular niche-components and soluble factors
  - Notch pathway
  - TGF-beta pathway
  - Nitric oxide (NO) pathway
  - Other pathways
    - Sonic hedgehog (SHH)
    - Wnt
    - Integrin signaling
  - The vascular niche promotes both glioma stem-like cell self-renewal and invasion.
  - Distinct blood vessel properties in each niche modulate niche-specific GSC phenotypes.
  - Perivascular maintenance and invasive GSC subpopulations interconvert.
  - Vascular changes drive GSC plasticity.
  - Increased understanding of the dual role of the vasculature in GSC regulation is a pre-requisite to the development of improved therapies.

Glioma Stem-Like Cells
- are a subset of cells within the bulk tumor that possess self-renewal and multi-lineage differentiation properties similar to somatic stem cells
- These cells also are at the apex of the cellular hierarchy and cause tumor initiation and expansion after chemo-radiation.

Molecular Mechanisms of Self-Renewal
- Wnt signaling pathway (Fig. 51.12):
  - important for regulating pattern formation during development
  - involved in the self-renewal process
  - WNT signaling is inactivated in the absence of WNT ligands
  - Under these conditions, β-catenin forms a complex with Dishevelled, AXIN, APC, and GSK3β.
  - β-Catenin is phosphorylated by GSK3β and then degraded by the proteasome
  - Wnt proteins
    - secreted intercellular signaling molecules
    - act as ligand to trigger a specific signal transduction pathway
  - canonical pathway: ß-catenin dependent
    - Unphosphorylated β-catenin is shuttled into the nucleus, leading to transcriptional activation of WNT signaling-target genes.
  - non-canonical pathway: ß-catenin-independent pathways
    - Non-canonical WNT signaling consists of the planar cell polarity (PCP) and Ca2+ pathways.
    - The PCP signaling pathway has relevance for cell survival and skeletal rearrangement.
    - The nuclear factor of activated T-cell-mediated Ca2+ signaling pathway is concerned with intracellular Ca2+ release and cell fate regulation.
  - mutations
    - inactivate the function of adenomatous polyposis coli (APC)
    - activate ß-catenin
    - rarely alter ligand wnt
- Hedgehog signaling pathway (Fig. 51.13):
  - Important for regulating pattern formation in the embryo.

51.21 Carcinogenic Agents

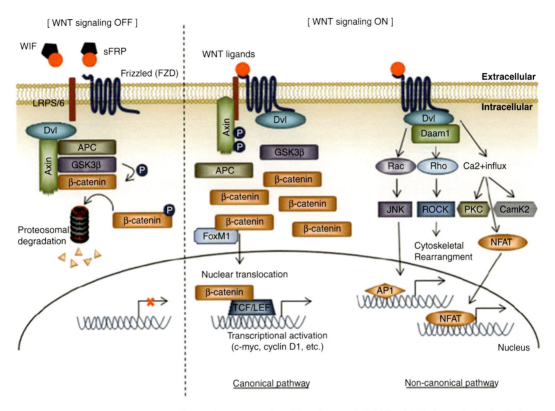

Fig. 51.12 Overview of WNT signaling pathway (reproduced from Lee et al. (2016) with kind permission by Springer Nature). For details see text

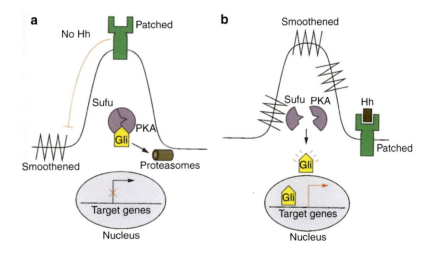

Fig. 51.13 The Hedgehog signaling pathway (reproduced from Pecorino (2016) with kind permission by Oxford University Press). For details see text

- Hh proteins (sonic, desert, and Indian) are secreted intercellular signaling molecules.
- Transmembrane protein Patched and Smoothened are responsible for signal transduction by Hh.
  o *Patched* is a tumor suppressor gene.

51.21 Carcinogenic Agents

Carcinogens are responsible for cancer-causing mutations.

The following classes of carcinogens are distinguished:

- Radiation
  - Ionizing radiation
  - Ultraviolet radiation
- Chemicals
  - Polycyclic aromatic hydrocarbons (PAHs)
  - Aromatic amines
  - Azo dyes
  - Nitrosamines and nitrosamides
  - Hydrazo and azoxy compounds
  - Carbamates
  - Halogenated compounds
  - Natural products
  - Inorganic carcinogens
  - Miscellaneous compounds (alkylating agents, aldehydes, phenolics)
- Infectious pathogens
  - Human papillomavirus (cervical cancer)
  - Kaposi sarcoma-associated herpesvirus (Kaposi sarcoma)
  - Hepatitis B virus (liver cancer)
  - Epstein-Barr virus (EBV) (nasopharyngeal carcinoma)
  - Human T-cell lymphotropic virus type 1 (HTLV-1) (acute T-cell leukemia)
  - *Helicobacter pylori* (gastric cancer)
- Particular endogenous reactions
  - Oxidative perspiration, lipid peroxidation
    - produce reactive oxygen species (ROS)
  - Hydrolysis of the glycosidic bond between a base and deoxyribose

51.22 Common Molecular Changes in Brain Tumors

Frequently encountered molecular changes in brain tumors are listed in Table 51.22.

Table 51.22 Frequently encountered molecular changes in brain tumors

Tumor type	Typical molecular changes
Diffuse astrocytic and oligodendroglial tumors	
Astrocytoma, diffuse, grade II	• *IDH1/2* mutation • *ATRX* mutations/loss of nuclear expression • *TP53* mutations
Astrocytoma, anaplastic grade III	• *IDH1/2* mutation • *ATRX* mutation/loss of nuclear expression • *TP53* mutations
Glioblastoma, grade IV	• *MGMT*-promoter methylation • *H3F3A-K27* mutation • *ATRX* mutation/loss of nuclear expression • *TP53* mutations • *PPM1D* mutation • DNA hypomethylation • *CIMP* • *PDGFRA* amplification • *TERT* promoter mutation • Chromosome 7 • Chromosome 10 loss • *EGFR* amplification • *PTEN* mutation • *CDKN2A* deletion
Oligodendroglioma, grade II	• *IDH1/2* mutation • 1p/19q co-deletion • *CIC* mutation • *TERT* promoter mutation
Oligodendroglioma anaplastic, grade III	• *IDH1/2* mutation • 1p/19q co-deletion • *CIC* mutation • *TERT* promoter mutation

Table 51.22 (continued)

Tumor type	Typical molecular changes
Other astrocytic tumors	
Astrocytoma pilocytic grade I	• *BRAF* fusion • *BRAF*-V600 E • *NF1* • *FGRR1* • *PTPN11* mutations • *NTRK2* fusion
Subependymal giant cell astrocytoma, grade I	• *TSC1* germline mutation • *TSC2* mutation
Pleomorphic xanthoastrocytoma, grade II	• *BRAF*-V600E mutation • *CDKN2A* deletion
Intrinsic pons glioma	• *H3F3A-K27* mutation • *ACVR1* mutation • *IDH1/2* mutation • *ATRX* mutation/loss of nuclear expression • *TP53* mutation • *PPM1D* mutation
Ependymal tumors	
Subependymoma, grade I	• Unknown
Myxopapillary ependymoma, grade I	• Unknown
Ependymoma, grade II	• *RELA* fusions (supratentorial) • *NF2* mutation (spinal) • Various DNA methylation patterns (posterior cerebral fossa)
Ependymoma anaplastic, grade III	• *RELA* fusions (supratentorial) • Various DNA methylation patterns (posterior cerebral fossa)
Other gliomas	
Chordoid glioma of the third ventricle	• Losses of 11q13 and 9p21 • No *EGFR* amplifications • No chromosome 7 gain • No *TP53* mutations • No changes in *CDKN2A*, *CDK4*, *MDM2* • No *IDH1/2* mutations • No *BRAF* V600E mutation
Angiocentric glioma	• Rearrangements at the *MYB* locus on 6q23 • *MYB* fusion with *QKI* or *ESR1* • Loss of chromosomal bands 6q24 to q25 • Copy number gain of two adjacent clones from chromosomal band 11p11.2 containing the PTPRJ gene • Lack of mutations in *IDH1*, *IDH2*, *BRAF* V600
Astroblastoma	• Gains of chromosomes 19 and 20q • Losses of chromosomes 10 and X • Lack of *IDH1* and *IDH2* mutations
Choroid plexus tumors	
Choroid plexus papilloma	• *TP53* mutations are rare • Hyperploidy • *MGMT* promoter methylation
Atypical choroid plexus papilloma	• Similar to choroid plexus papilloma • Higher expression of cell cycle-related genes
Choroid plexus carcinoma	• Complex chromosomal alterations • *TP53* mutations in 50% of cases • Combination of *TP53*-R72 with *MDM2* SNP309 polymorphism found in 90% of cases • Hyper- or hypodiploidy

(continued)

Table 51.22 (continued)

Tumor type	Typical molecular changes
Neuronal and mixed neuronal-glial tumors	
Dysembryoplastic neuroepithelial tumor	• Gains of whole chromosomes 5 and 7 (20–30% of cases) • *BRAF* V600 mutation (30% of cases) • Activation of mTOR signaling • Lack of *TP53*, *IDH1/IDH2*, *H3F3A* K27M mutations
Gangliocytoma	• Genetic data have not been reported
Ganglioglioma	• Chromosomal abnormalities found in 1/3 of cases • Gain of chromosome 7 • Chromosomal imbalances • *BRAF* V600 mutation (20–60% of cases) • MAPK pathway activation: fusion of *BRAF* to *KIAA1549*, *FXR1*, and *MACF1* • Reduced expression of neurodevelopmental genes (e.g., *LDB2*) • No *IDH1/IDH2*, *TP53*, *PTEN* mutations • No *EGFR* or *CDK4* amplification
Anaplastic ganglioglioma	• Loss of *CDKN2A/B* and *DMBT1* • Gain/amplification of CDK4 • *CDKN2A* deletion • *BRAF* V600 mutation (in 50% of cases)
Dysplastic cerebellar gangliocytoma	• 85% of Cowden syndrome • *PTEN* germline mutation • Germline variants of *SDHB* (1p35-36) or *SDHD* (11q23)
Desmoplastic infantile astrocytoma and ganglioglioma	• Large chromosomal alterations are rare • Focal losses at 5q13.3, 10q21.3, and 21q22.11 • Frequent gains at 7q31 including hepatocyte growth factor receptor (*MET*) • Less frequent gains at 4q12 (*KDR*, *KIT*, and *PDGFRA*) and 12q14.3 (*MDM2*) • No *KIAA1549-BRAF* fusion • Rare *BRAF* V600E mutations
Papillary glioneuronal tumor	• Translocation t(9;17) (q31;q24) results in an *SCL44A1-PRKCA* fusion oncogene
Rosette-forming glioneuronal tumor	• *PIK3CA* and *FGFR1* mutations • No *KIAA1549-BRAF* fusion • No *BRAF* V600E, *IDH1/IDH2* mutation • No 1p/19q co-deletion • No mutations in *AKT1*, *AKT2*, *AKT3*, *EGFR*, *GNAQ*, *GNAS*, *KRAS*, *MET*, *NRAS*, *RET*
Diffuse leptomeningeal glioneuronal tumor	• *KIAA1549-BRAF* fusion (75% of cases) • Deletions of chromosomal arm 1p (59% of cases) • 1p/19q co-deletions (18% of cases) • No *BRAF* V600E, *IDH1/IDH2* mutations
Central neurocytoma	• Numerous DNA copy number alterations • *MYCN* gain • Overexpression of genes from the WNT signaling pathway • No 1p/19q co-deletion
Extraventricular neurocytoma	• 1p/19q co-deletion • No *IDH1/IDH2* mutation • No *MGMT* methylation
Cerebellar liponeurocytoma	• *TP53* missense mutations (20% of cases)absence of isochromosome 17q • No mutations in *PTCH*, *CTNNB1*, and *APC* • No mutations in *BRAF*, *IDH1/IDH2*

51.22 Common Molecular Changes in Brain Tumors

Table 51.22 (continued)

Tumor type	Typical molecular changes

Paraganglioma	• Autosomal dominant germline mutations in:
	  – *SDHD* (associated with inherited paraganglioma-1)
	  – *SDHA* and *SDHAF2* (associated with paraganglioma-2)
	  – *SDHC* (associated with paraganglioma-3)
	  – *SDHB* (associated with paraganglioma-4)
	  – *TMEM127* (tumor suppressor)
	  – *MAX* (tumor suppressor)
	  – *VHL* (associated with von Hipple–Lindau disease)
	  – *RET* (associated with multiple endocrine neoplasia type2)
	  – *NF1* (associated with neurofibromatosis type 1)
	• Mutations in: *SDHD*, SDHAF2, *SDHB, SDHC, SDHA, TMEM127*, and *MAX*

Tumors of the pineal gland	
Pineocytoma	• Pseudodiploid or hypotriploid profile • Numerical and structural abnormalities: loss of all or part of chromosome 22, loss or partial deletion of chromosome 11, loss of chromosome 14, gain of chromosomes 5 and 19 • No relationship with *RB1* gene • High-level expression of genes encoding enzymes related to melatonin synthesis (*TPH1*, *ASMT*) and genes involved in retinal phototransduction (OPN4, *RGS16*, *CRB3*)
Pineal parenchymal tumor of intermediate differentiation	• Chromosomal imbalances: 4q gain, 12q gain, 22 loss
Pineoblastoma	• Structural alterations on chromosome 1 • Losses on chromosomes 9, 13, and 16 • No changes in *TP53* and *CDKN1A* • Overexpression of *PRAME*, *CD24*, *POU4F2*, and *HOXD13*
Papillary tumor of the pineal gland	• Imbalances on chromosomes 4 (75% of cases), 9 (87.5% of cases), and 10 (87.5% of cases) • Losses of chromosome 3, 10, 14, and 22 • Gains of whole chromosomes 8, 9, and 12 • No *BRAF* V600E mutation
Embryonal tumors	
Medulloblastoma, WNT-activated	• Somatic mutations in exon 3 of *CTNNB1* (90% of cases) • Mutations in *DDX3X* (50% of cases), *SMARCA4* (26.3% of cases), *KMT2D* (12.5% of cases), *TP53* (12.5% of cases) • Monosomy 6
Medulloblastoma, SHH-activated	• Hedgehog signaling pathway genes altered in 87% of cases • *PTCH1* (9q22) loss-of-function • Structural variations or mutations in *MYCL*, *GLI2*, *PPM1D*, *YAP1*, *PTEN*, *SUFU*, and *MDM4* • Somatic mutations are rare • Point mutations in *TERT* promoter (21–83% of cases), *TP53* (associated with chromothripsis)
Medulloblastoma, non-WNT/non-SHH	• Overexpression of *MYC*, amplification of *MYC* accompanied by *MYC-PVT1* fusion • Mutated genes: *KDM6A* (13% of cases), *SMARCA4* (10.5%), *SNCAIP* (10.4%), *OTX2* (7.7%), *MYCN* (6.3%), *KMT2C* (5.3%), *CDK6* (4.7%), *CTDNEP1* (4.6%), *LRP1B* (4.6%), *KTMT2D* (4%), and *ZMYM3* (3.7%) • *GFI1* and *GFI1B* activated through enhancer hijacking • Copy number alteration on chromosome 17: 17p deletions, 17q gain, combination of these in form of an isodicentric 17q

(continued)

Table 51.22 (continued)

Tumor type	Typical molecular changes
Medulloblastoma, classic	
Desmoplastic/nodular medulloblastoma	• Associated with nevoid basal cell carcinoma syndrome (Gorlin syndrome) • Activation of the SHH pathway • Mutations in: *PTCH1, SMO, SUFU, SHH, GLI2, MYCN* • Rare mutations in: *LDB1, DDX3X, TERT* promoter • Allelic losses on chromosome 9q and 10q
Medulloblastoma with extensive nodularity	• Mutations in SHH pathway genes • Frequent mutations in *SUFU*
Large cell/anaplastic medulloblastoma	• Amplifications of *MYC* and *GLI2* • *TP53* mutations • Chromothripsis (chromosome shattering)
Embryonal tumor with multilayered rosettes, C19MC-altered	• Gains of chromosomes 2, 7q, and 11q • Loss of chromosome 6q • Focal high-level amplicon: upregulated cluster of miRNAs (a polycistron) named C19MC • C19MC amplification in 96% of cases • Fusion of C19MC to the *TTYH1* gene • Increased expression of LIN28A
Atypical teratoid/rhabdoid tumor	• Mutation or loss of the *SMARCB1* locus at 22q11.2 • Mutation in *SMARCA4* (young age, poor prognosis) • Involvement of the Hippo signaling pathway with overexpression of Yap1
Tumors of cranial and peripheral nerves	
Schwannoma	• *NF2* gene • Merlin (schwannomin) protein • Inactivating mutations in 60% of cases
Neurofibroma	• *NF1* gene (17q) • Activation of RAS/MAPK and ALT/mTOR pathways • Losses of chromosomes 19p, 19q, and 22q • Loss of *CDKN2A/CDKN2B* as sign of malignant transformation
Perineurioma	• Monosomy of chromosome 22 • Loss of chromosomes 13, 10, 22q
Malignant peripheral nerve sheath tumor	• Genetic inactivation in *NF1, CDKN2A*, and the PRC2 components *SUZ12* and *EED* • Gene amplifications in *ITGB4, PDGFRA, BIRC5, CCNE2, EGFR, HGF, MET, TERT*, and *CDK4*
Meningiomas	
Meningioma	• NF2 gene mutations • Changes in other genes: *LARGE, MN1, AP1B1, SMARCB1, AKT1, TRAF7, KLF4, SMO, SMARCE1, TERT* promoter, *NDRG2, MEG3, RPS6KB1, EPB41L3* • Loss of chromosome 22q (WHO grade I) • Loss of chromosomes 1p, 6q, 10, 14q, 18q (WHO grades II, III) • Gain of chromosomes 1q, 9p, 12q, 15q, 17q, 20q (WHO grades II, III) • Loss of chromosome 9p (WHO grade III)

Common genetic, epigenetic, and chromosomal aberrations associated with the major glioma entities are listed in Table 51.23.

Predictive molecular biomarkers relevant to gliomas (Reifenberger et al. 2017)

Predictive biomarkers in clinical use

• *MGMT* promoter methylation
  – Prediction of benefit from alkylating chemotherapy in patients with IDH-wild-type gliomas, in particular elderly patients (aged ≥70 years) with glioblastoma
• 1p/19q co-deletion

Table 51.23 Common genetic, epigenetic, and chromosomal aberrations associated with the major glioma entities, modified after Reifenberger et al. (2017), reproduced with kind permission by Springer Nature

Glioma entity	Genetic	Epigenetic	Chromosomal
Diffuse astrocytic and oligodendroglial tumors			
Diffuse astrocytoma, *IDH*-mutant	• *IDH1* mutation • *IDH2* mutation • *TP53* mutation • *ATRX* mutation	• G-CIMP	• Trisomy 7 or 7q gain • LOH 17p
Anaplastic astrocytoma, *IDH*-mutant	• *IDH1* mutation • *IDH2* mutation • *TP53* mutation • *ATRX* mutation	• G-CIMP	• Trisomy 7 or 7q gain • LOH 17p
Oligodendroglioma, *IDH*-mutant and 1p/19q-co-deleted	• *IDH1* mutation • *IDH2* mutation • *TERT* mutation • *CIC* mutation • *FUBP1* mutation	• G-CIMP	• 1p/19q co-deletion
Anaplastic oligodendroglioma, *IDH*-mutant and 1p/19q-co-deleted	• *IDH1* mutation • *IDH2* mutation • *TERT* mutation • *CIC* mutation • *FUBP1* mutation • *TCF12* mutation • *CDKN2A* deletion	• G-CIMP	• 1p/19q co-deletion
Glioblastoma, *IDH*-mutant	• *IDH1* or *IDH2* • *TP53* • *ATRX* mutation • *CDKN2A* homozygous deletion	• G-CIMP	• Trisomy 7 or 7q gain • LOH 17p • 10q deletion
Glioblastoma, *IDH*-wild-type	• *TERT* • *PTEN* • *TP53* • *PIK3CA* • *PIK3R1* • *NF1* • *H3F3A-G34* mutation • *CDKN2A* • *PTEN* homozygous deletion • *EGFR* • *PDGFRA* • *MET* • *CDK4* • *CDK6* • *MDM2* • *MDM4* amplification • *EGFRvIII* rearrangement	• *MGMT* promoter methylation	• Trisomy 7 or 7q gain • monosomy 1 • double minute chromosomes

(continued)

Table 51.23 (continued)

Glioma entity	Genetic	Epigenetic	Chromosomal
Diffuse midline glioma, H3-K27M-mutant	• H3F3A-K27M or HIST1H3B/C-K27M • TP53 • PPMD1 • ACVR1 • FGFR1 mutation • PDGFRA • MYC • MYCN • CDK4 • CDK6 • CCND1-3 • ID2 • MET amplification	• Loss of histone-H3-lysine trimethylation	–
Well-differentiated pediatric diffuse glioma	• MYB or MYBL rearrangement • FGFR1 duplication	–	–
Other (astrocytic) gliomas			
Pilocytic astrocytoma	• BRAF • RAF1 • NTRK2 gene fusions • BRAF-V600E • NF1 • KRAS • FGFR1 • PTPN11 mutation	–	–
Pleomorphic xanthoastrocytoma	• BRAF-V600E mutation • CDKN2A/ • p14ARF homozygous deletion	–	–
Subependymal giant cell astrocytoma	• TSC1 or TSC2 mutation	–	–
Angiocentric glioma	• MYB–QKI gene fusions/rearrangements	–	–
Supratentorial ependymal tumors			
Ependymoma, RELA-fusion positiveII	• C11orf95–RELA fusion	–	• 11q aberrations
EpendymomaII	• YAP1 gene fusions	–	• 11q aberrations
Posterior fossa (PF) ependymal tumors			
Ependymoma PF-AII	–	• PF-A DNA methylation profile with global hypermethylation	• Stable genotype
Ependymoma PF-BII	–	• PF-B DNA methylation profile	• Multiple copy number imbalances (CIN)
Spinal intramedullary ependymal tumors			
Ependymoma	• NF2 mutation	–	• 22q deletion

- Prediction of benefit from upfront radiotherapy and PCV as opposed to radiotherapy alone in patients with anaplastic glioma

Examples of emerging novel predictive biomarkers

- *BRAF* mutation
  - Identification of patients with BRAF-V600-mutant gliomas eligible for BRAF-inhibitor therapy
- *IDH1/IDH2* mutation
  - Identification of patients with IDH-mutant diffuse gliomas eligible for peptide-based vaccination or mutant-IDH inhibitors
- *EGFRvIII* expression
  - Identification of patients with EGFRvIII-positive glioblastomas eligible for EGFRvIII-peptide-based vaccination
  - PCV, procarbazine, CCNU (lomustine), and vincristine
- *EGFR* amplification
  - Identification of patients with EGFR-amplified glioblastomas eligible for treatment with anti-EGFR antibodies
- *FGFR–TACC* fusion
  - Identification of patients with FGFR–TACC-positive glioblastomas eligible for FGFR-inhibitor therapy

51.23 Treatment for Brain Tumors

Treatment recommendations as given by the European Association of Neuro-Oncology (EANO) are shown in Table 51.24.

Agents used in the treatment of brain tumors are shown in Table 51.25.

Table 51.24 Treatment recommendation from the European Association of Neuro-Oncology (EANO), modified after Weller et al. (2017) reproduced with kind permission by Elsevier

Tumor type	First line treatment	Salvage therapies
Diffuse astrocytic and oligodendroglial tumors		
Diffuse astrocytoma, *IDH*-mutant	• Watch-and-wait or • radiotherapy followed by PCV (or temozolomide plus radiotherapy followed by temozolomide)	• Nitrosourea • (or temozolomide rechallenge • or bevacizumab)
Gemistocytic astrocytoma, *IDH*-mutant	• Watch-and-wait or • radiotherapy followed by PCV (or temozolomide plus radiotherapy followed by temozolomide)	• Nitrosourea • (or temozolomide rechallenge • or bevacizumab)
Diffuse astrocytoma, *IDH*-wild-type	• Watch-and-wait (remains controversial) • radiotherapy • radiotherapy followed by PCV, or temozolomide and radiotherapy followed by temozolomide (according to MGMT status [remains controversial])	• Temozolomide • Nitrosourea • (or temozolomide rechallenge) • or bevacizumab
Diffuse astrocytoma, not otherwise specified	• Watch-and-wait • or radiotherapy • followed by PCV (or temozolomide plus radiotherapy followed by temozolomide)	• Nitrosourea • (or temozolomide rechallenge • or bevacizumab)
Anaplastic astrocytoma, *IDH*-mutant	• Radiotherapy • followed by temozolomide	• Nitrosourea • or temozolomide rechallenge • or bevacizumab
Anaplastic astrocytoma, *IDH*-wild-type	• Radiotherapy • or temozolomide plus radiotherapy • followed by temozolomide, according to MGMT status (remains controversial)	• Temozolomide • or nitrosourea • (or temozolomide rechallenge) • or bevacizumab

(continued)

Table 51.24 (continued)

Tumor type	First line treatment	Salvage therapies
Anaplastic astrocytoma, not otherwise specified	• Radiotherapy • followed by temozolomide and radiotherapy • followed by temozolomide, according to MGMT status (remains controversial)	• Nitrosourea • or temozolomide rechallenge • or bevacizumab
Glioblastoma, *IDH*-wild-type (including giant cell glioblastoma, gliosarcoma, and epithelioid glioblastoma)	• Temozolomide • plus radiotherapy • followed by temozolomide for patients aged 70 years or younger • radiotherapy alone (MGMT unmethylated) • or temozolomide plus radiotherapy followed by temozolomide or temozolomide alone (MGMT methylated) for patients older than 70 years	• Nitrosourea • or temozolomide rechallenge • or bevacizumab • radiotherapy for radiotherapy-naive patients
Glioblastoma, *IDH*-mutant	• Radiotherapy • with or without temozolomide • followed by temozolomide	• Nitrosourea or temozolomide rechallenge or bevacizumab
Glioblastoma, not otherwise specified	• Temozolomide • plus radiotherapy • followed by temozolomide for patients aged 70 years or younger • radiotherapy alone (MGMT unmethylated) • or temozolomide plus radiotherapy followed by temozolomide or temozolomide alone (MGMT methylated) for patients older than 70 years	• Nitrosourea or temozolomide rechallenge or bevacizumab • radiotherapy for radiotherapy-naive patients
Diffuse midline glioma, *H3-K27M* mutant	• Radiotherapy or • temozolomide plus radiotherapy • followed by temozolomide	
Oligodendroglioma, *IDH*-mutant and 1p/19q-co-deleted	• Watch-and-wait or • Radiotherapy • followed by PCV	• Temozolomide or • bevacizumab
Oligodendroglioma, not otherwise specified	• Watch-and-wait or • Radiotherapy • followed by PCV	• Temozolomide or • bevacizumab
Anaplastic oligodendroglioma, *IDH*-mutant and 1p/19q-co-deleted	• Radiotherapy • followed by PCV	• Temozolomide or • bevacizumab
Anaplastic oligodendroglioma, not otherwise specified	• Radiotherapy • followed by PCV	• Temozolomide or • bevacizumab
Oligo-astrocytoma, not otherwise specified	• Watch-and-wait or • radiotherapy • followed by PCV	• Temozolomide or • bevacizumab
Anaplastic oligo-astrocytoma, not otherwise specified	• Radiotherapy followed by PCV	• Temozolomide or • bevacizumab
Other astrocytic tumors		
Pilocytic astrocytoma, Pilomyxoid astrocytoma	• Surgery only	• Surgery followed by radiotherapy
Subependymal giant cell astrocytoma	• Surgery only	• Surgery
Pleomorphic xanthoastrocytoma	• Surgery only	• Surgery
Anaplastic pleomorphic xanthoastrocytoma	• Radiotherapy	• Surgery • followed by chemotherapy with temozolomide

Abbreviations used: *IDH* isocitrate dehydrogenase, *PCV* procarbazine, lomustine, and vincristine, *RTOG* Radiation Therapy Oncology Group, *MGMT* O^6-methylguanine DNA methyltransferase, *H3* histone 3

Table 51.25 Agents used in the treatment of brain tumors (Chang and Johnson 2012) reproduced with kind permission by Saunders

Target	Agent
Angiogenesis	
VEGF	• Bevacizumab • Aflibercept
VEGFR	• Cediranib
Notch	
Tumor growth factors	
EGFR	• Cetuximab • Nimotuzumab • Erlotinib • Gefitinib
HGF/SF	
Growth factor effectors	
RAS	• Tipifarnib • Lonafarnib
RAF	• Sorafenib
AKT	• Perifosine
mTOR	• Sirolimus • Temsirolimus • Everolimus
PKC-ß	• Enzastaurin
Signaling pathways	
PDGFR, c-kit, Abl	• Imatinib
EGFR, VEGFR	• Vandetanib
EGFR, HER2	• Lapatinib
PDGFR, VEGFR, c-kit, Flt-3	• Sunitinib
Flt-3, PDGFR, c-kit	• Tandutinib
Raf, VEGFR, PDGFR, c-kit, Flt3	• Sorafenib
VEGFR, c-Met, RET	
VEGFR, PDGFR	• Vatalanib
VEGFR, PDGFR, c-kit	• Pazopanib
Scr family	• Dasatinib
Integrins	
Integrins	• Cilengitide

Selected References

Andrabi SA, Dawson TM, Dawson VL (2008) Mitochondrial and nuclear cross talk in cell death: parthanatos. Ann N Y Acad Sci 1147:233–241. https://doi.org/10.1196/annals.1427.014

Armento A, Ehlers J, Schötterl S, Naumann U (2017) Molecular mechanisms of glioma cell motility. In: De Vleeschouwer S (ed) Glioblastoma. Codon Publications, Brisbane, pp 73–94

Audia A, Conroy S, Glass R, Bhat KPL (2017) The impact of the tumor microenvironment on the properties of glioma stem-like cells. Front Oncol 7:143. https://doi.org/10.3389/fonc.2017.00143

Bencivenga D, Caldarelli I, Stampone E, Mancini FP, Balestrieri ML, Della Ragione F, Borriello A (2017) p27(Kip1) and human cancers: a reappraisal of a still enigmatic protein. Cancer Lett 403:354–365. https://doi.org/10.1016/j.canlet.2017.1006.1031. Epub 2017 July 5.

Bergsbaken T, Fink SL, Cookson BT (2009) Pyroptosis: host cell death and inflammation. Nat Rev Microbiol 7(2):99–109. https://doi.org/10.1038/nrmicro2070

Blackford AN, Jackson SP (2017) ATM, ATR, and DNA-PK: the trinity at the heart of the DNA damage response. Mol Cell 66(6):801–817. https://doi.org/10.1016/j.molcel.2017.1005.1015

Borriello A, Caldarelli I, Bencivenga D, Criscuolo M, Cucciolla V, Tramontano A, Oliva A, Perrotta S, Della Ragione F (2011) p57(Kip2) and cancer: time for a critical appraisal. Mol Cancer Res 9(10):1269–1284. https://doi.org/10.1158/1541-7786.MCR-1211-0220. Epub 2011 Aug 4.

Branzk N, Papayannopoulos V (2013) Molecular mechanisms regulating NETosis in infection and disease. Semin Immunopathol 35(4):513–530. https://doi.org/10.1007/s00281-013-0384-6

Cao JY, Dixon SJ (2016) Mechanisms of ferroptosis. Cell Mol Life Sci 73(11–12):2195–2209. https://doi.org/10.1007/s00018-016-2194-1

Cesselli D, Armento A, Ehlers J, Schotterl S, Naumann U (2017) Molecular mechanisms of glioma cell motility. Int J Mol Sci. https://doi.org/10.3390/ijms19010147; https://doi.org/10.15586/codon.glioblastoma.2017; https://doi.org/10.15586/codon.glioblastoma.2017.ch5

Chang SM, Johnson DR (2012) Biologic therapy for malignant glioma. In: Kaye AH, Laws ER (eds) Brain tumors, 3rd edn. Saunders, pp 102–113

Chen PY, Xu HS, Qin XL, Zong HL, He XG, Cao L (2017) Cancer stem cell markers in glioblastoma—an update. J Neuro-Oncol 21(14):3207–3211. https://doi.org/10.1007/s11060-018-2763-2

Codrici E, Enciu AM, Popescu ID, Mihai S, Tanase C (2016) Glioma stem cells and their microenvironments: providers of challenging therapeutic targets. Stem Cells Int 2016:5728438. https://doi.org/10.1155/2016/5728438

Coly PM, Gandolfo P, Castel H, Morin F (2017) The autophagy machinery: a new player in chemotactic cell migration. Front Neurosci 11:78. https://doi.org/10.3389/fnins.2017.00078

Coon EA, Benarroch EE (2018) DNA damage response: selected review and neurologic implications. Neurology 90(8):367–376. https://doi.org/10.1212/WNL.0000000000004989

Daumas-Duport C, Scheithauer B, O'Fallon J, Kelly P (1988) Grading of astrocytomas. A simple and reproducible method. Cancer 62(10):2152–2165

David KK, Andrabi SA, Dawson TM, Dawson VL (2009) Parthanatos, a messenger of death. Front Biosci (Landmark Edition) 14:1116–1128

De Palma M, Biziato D, Petrova TV (2017) Microenvironmental regulation of tumour angiogenesis. Nat Rev Cancer 17(8):457–474. https://doi.org/10.1038/nrc.2017.51

Dellovade T, Romer JT, Curran T, Rubin LL (2006) The hedgehog pathway and neurological disorders. Annu Rev Neurosci 29:539–563. https://doi.org/10.1146/annurev.neuro.29.051605.112858

Demers M, Wagner DD (2014) NETosis: a new factor in tumor progression and cancer-associated thrombosis. Semin Thromb Hemost 40(3):277–283. https://doi.org/10.1055/s-0034-1370765

Dirks PB (2010) Brain tumor stem cells: the cancer stem cell hypothesis writ large. Mol Oncol 4(5):420–430. https://doi.org/10.1016/j.molonc.2010.08.001

Fatokun AA, Dawson VL, Dawson TM (2014) Parthanatos: mitochondrial-linked mechanisms and therapeutic opportunities. Br J Pharmacol 171(8):2000–2016. https://doi.org/10.1111/bph.12416

Favaloro B, Allocati N, Graziano V, Di Ilio C, De Laurenzi V (2012) Role of apoptosis in disease. Aging 4(5):330–349. https://doi.org/10.18632/aging.100459

Fink SL, Cookson BT (2005) Apoptosis, pyroptosis, and necrosis: mechanistic description of dead and dying eukaryotic cells. Infect Immun 73(4):1907–1916. https://doi.org/10.1128/iai.73.4.1907-1916.2005

Fitzwalter BE, Thorburn A (2015) Recent insights into cell death and autophagy. FEBS J 282(22):4279–4288. https://doi.org/10.1111/febs.13515

Folkman J (1971) Tumor angiogenesis: therapeutic implications. N Engl J Med 285(21):1182–1186. https://doi.org/10.1056/nejm197111182852108

Freese JL, Pino D, Pleasure SJ (2010) Wnt signaling in development and disease. Neurobiol Dis 38(2):148–153. https://doi.org/10.1016/j.nbd.2009.09.003

Gallagher LE, Williamson LE, Chan EY (2016) Advances in autophagy regulatory mechanisms. Cells 5(2):24. https://doi.org/10.3390/cells5020024

Ghajar CM, Correia AL, Bissell MJ (2015) The role of the microenvironment in tumor initiation, progression, and metastasis. In: Mendelsohn J, Gray JW, Howley PM, Israel MA, Thompson CB (eds) The molecular basis of cancer, 4th edn. Elsevier Saunders, pp 239–255

Glover TW, Wilson TE, Arlt MF (2017) Fragile sites in cancer: more than meets the eye. Nat Rev Cancer 17(8):489–501. https://doi.org/10.1038/nrc.2017.52

Goldar S, Khaniani MS, Derakhshan SM, Baradaran B (2015) Molecular mechanisms of apoptosis and roles in cancer development and treatment. Asian Pac J Cancer Prev 16(6):2129–2144

Gordy C, He YW (2012) The crosstalk between autophagy and apoptosis: where does this lead? Protein Cell 3(1):17–27. https://doi.org/10.1007/s13238-011-1127-x

Hale JS, Sinyuk M, Rich JN, Lathia JD (2013) Decoding the cancer stem cell hypothesis in glioblastoma. CNS Oncol 2(4):319–330. https://doi.org/10.2217/cns.13.23

Hanahan D, Weinberg RA (2011) Hallmarks of cancer: the next generation. Cell 144(5):646–674. https://doi.org/10.1016/j.cell.2011.02.013

Heddleston JM, Hitomi M, Venere M, Flavahan WA, Yang K, Kim Y, Minhas S, Rich JN, Hjelmeland AB (2011) Glioma stem cell maintenance: the role of the microenvironment. Curr Pharm Des 17(23):2386–2401

Huang SY, Yang JY (2015) Targeting the Hedgehog pathway in pediatric medulloblastoma. Cancers 7(4):2110–2123. https://doi.org/10.3390/cancers7040880

Iyyathurai J, Decuypere JP, Leybaert L, D'Hondt C, Bultynck G (2016) Connexins: substrates and regulators of autophagy. BMC Cell Biol 17(Suppl 1):20. https://doi.org/10.1186/s12860-016-0093-9

Jia Y, Wang Y, Xie J (2015) The Hedgehog pathway: role in cell differentiation, polarity and proliferation. Arch Toxicol 89(2):179–191. https://doi.org/10.1007/s00204-014-1433-1

Johung T, Monje M (2017) Neuronal activity in the glioma microenvironment. Curr Opin Neurobiol 47:156–161. https://doi.org/10.1016/j.conb.2017.10.009

Kazzaz NM, Sule G, Knight JS (2016) Intercellular interactions as regulators of NETosis. Front Immunol 7:453. https://doi.org/10.3389/fimmu.2016.00453

Kenific CM, Debnath J (2015) Cellular and metabolic functions for autophagy in cancer cells. Trends Cell Biol 25(1):37–45. https://doi.org/10.1016/j.tcb.2014.09.001

Kepp O, Galluzzi L, Zitvogel L, Kroemer G (2010) Pyroptosis—a cell death modality of its kind? Eur J Immunol 40(3):627–630. https://doi.org/10.1002/eji.200940160

Kernohan JW, Mabon RF et al (1949) A simplified classification of the gliomas. Proc Staff Meet Mayo Clin 24(3):71–75

Keulers TG, Schaaf MB, Rouschop KM (2016) Autophagy-dependent secretion: contribution to tumor progression. Front Oncol 6:251. https://doi.org/10.3389/fonc.2016.00251

Khan M (2013) Genetic instability, chromosomes, and repair. In: Pelengaris S, Khan M (eds) The molecular biology of cancer. A bridge from bench to bedside. Wiley-Blackwell, p 620

Kim BW, Kwon DH, Song HK (2016) Structure biology of selective autophagy receptors. BMB Rep 49(2):73–80

Kitao H, Iimori M, Kataoka Y, Wakasa T, Tokunaga E, Saeki H, Oki E, Maehara Y (2018) DNA replication stress and cancer chemotherapy. Cancer Sci 109(2):264–271. https://doi.org/10.1111/cas.13455. Epub 2017 Dec 22.

Koff JL, Ramachandiran S, Bernal-Mizrachi L (2015) A time to kill: targeting apoptosis in cancer. Int J Mol Sci 16(2):2942–2955. https://doi.org/10.3390/ijms16022942

LaRock CN, Cookson BT (2013) Burning down the house: cellular actions during pyroptosis. PLoS Pathog 9(12):e1003793. https://doi.org/10.1371/journal.ppat.1003793

Lee Y, Lee JK, Ahn SH, Lee J, Nam DH (2016) WNT signaling in glioblastoma and therapeutic opportunities. Lab Invest 96(2):137–150. https://doi.org/10.1038/labinvest.2015.140

Liebelt BD, Shingu T, Zhou X, Ren J, Shin SA, Hu J (2016) Glioma stem cells: signaling, microenvironment, and therapy. Stem Cells Int 2016:7849890. https://doi.org/10.1155/2016/7849890

Lin L, Baehrecke EH (2015) Autophagy, cell death, and cancer. Mol Cell Oncol 2(3):e985913. https://doi.org/10.4161/23723556.2014.985913

Liu YC, Lee IC (2018) Biomimetic brain tumor niche regulates glioblastoma cells towards a cancer stem cell phenotype. J Pathol. https://doi.org/10.1002/path.5024; https://doi.org/10.1007/s11060-018-2763-2

Lopez J, Tait SW (2015) Mitochondrial apoptosis: killing cancer using the enemy within. Br J Cancer 112(6):957–962. https://doi.org/10.1038/bjc.2015.85

Louis DN, Ohgaki H, Wiestler OD, Cavenee WK, Ellison DW, Figarella-Branger D, Perry A, Reifenberger G, Von Deimling A (2016) WHO classification of tumours oft he central nervous system, Revised 4th edn. IARC, Lyon

Mancias JD, Kimmelman AC (2016) Mechanisms of selective autophagy in normal physiology and cancer. J Mol Biol 428(9 Pt A):1659–1680. https://doi.org/10.1016/j.jmb.2016.02.027

Manini I, Caponnetto F, Bartolini A, Ius T, Mariuzzi L, Di Loreto C, Beltrami AP (2018) Role of microenvironment in glioma invasion: what we learned from in vitro models. 19(1). https://doi.org/10.3390/ijms19010147

Marechal A, Zou L (2013) DNA damage sensing by the ATM and ATR kinases. Cold Spring Harb Perspect Biol 5(9). (pii): a012716. https://doi.org/10.1101/cshperspect.a012716

Masuda S, Nakazawa D, Shida H, Miyoshi A, Kusunoki Y, Tomaru U, Ishizu A (2016) NETosis markers: quest for specific, objective, and quantitative markers. Clin Chim Acta 459:89–93. https://doi.org/10.1016/j.cca.2016.05.029

Masui K, Kato Y, Sawada T, Mischel PS, Shibata N (2017) Molecular and genetic determinants of glioma cell invasion. Int J Mol Sci 18(12). https://doi.org/10.3390/ijms18122609

Mathiassen SG, De Zio D, Cecconi F (2017) Autophagy and the cell cycle: a complex landscape. Front Oncol 7:51. https://doi.org/10.3389/fonc.2017.00051

Matias D, Predes D, Niemeyer Filho P, Lopes MC, Abreu JG, Lima FRS, Moura Neto V (2017) Microglia-glioblastoma interactions: new role for Wnt signaling. Biochim Biophys Acta 1868(1):333–340. https://doi.org/10.1016/j.bbcan.2017.05.007

McCord M, Mukouyama YS, Gilbert MR, Jackson S (2017) Targeting WNT signaling for multifaceted glioblastoma therapy. Front Cell Neurosci 11:318. https://doi.org/10.3389/fncel.2017.00318

Mondal A, Kumari Singh D, Panda S, Shiras A (2017) Extracellular vesicles as modulators of tumor microenvironment and disease progression in glioma. Front Oncol 7:144. https://doi.org/10.3389/fonc.2017.00144

Murray JM, Carr AM (2018) Integrating DNA damage repair with the cell cycle. Curr Opin Cell Biol 52:120–125. https://doi.org/10.1016/j.ceb.2018.1003.1006

Noelanders R, Vleminckx K (2017) How Wnt signaling builds the brain: bridging development and disease. Neuroscientist 23(3):314–329. https://doi.org/10.1177/1073858416667270

Olsson AK, Cedervall J (2016) NETosis in cancer—platelet-neutrophil crosstalk promotes tumor-associated pathology. Front Immunol 7:373. https://doi.org/10.3389/fimmu.2016.00373

Ortensi B, Setti M, Osti D, Pelicci G (2013) Cancer stem cell contribution to glioblastoma invasiveness. Stem Cell Res Ther 4(1):18. https://doi.org/10.1186/scrt166

Ostrom QT, Gittleman H, Farah P, Ondracek A, Chen Y, Wolinsky Y, Stroup NE, Kruchko C, Barnholtz-Sloan JS (2013) CBTRUS statistical report: primary brain and central nervous system tumors diagnosed in the United States in 2006-2010. Neuro-Oncology 15(Suppl 2):ii1–i56. https://doi.org/10.1093/neuonc/not151

Ostrom QT, Gittleman H, Liao P, Rouse C, Chen Y, Dowling J, Wolinsky Y, Kruchko C, Barnholtz-Sloan J (2014) CBTRUS statistical report: primary brain and central nervous system tumors diagnosed in the United States in 2007-2011. Neuro-Oncology 16(Suppl 4):iv1–i63. https://doi.org/10.1093/neuonc/nou223

Ostrom QT, Gittleman H, Fulop J, Liu M, Blanda R, Kromer C, Wolinsky Y, Kruchko C, Barnholtz-Sloan JS (2015) CBTRUS statistical report: primary brain and central nervous system tumors diagnosed in the United States in 2008-2012. Neuro-Oncology 17(Suppl 4):iv1–iv62. https://doi.org/10.1093/neuonc/nov189

Ostrom QT, Gittleman H, Xu J, Kromer C, Wolinsky Y, Kruchko C, Barnholtz-Sloan JS (2016) CBTRUS statistical report: primary brain and other central nervous system tumors diagnosed in the United States in 2009-2013. Neuro-Oncology 18(Suppl 5):v1–v75. https://doi.org/10.1093/neuonc/now207

Patel SS, Tomar S, Sharma D, Mahindroo N, Udayabanu M (2017) Targeting sonic hedgehog signaling in neurological disorders. Neurosci Biobehav Rev 74(Pt A):76–97. https://doi.org/10.1016/j.neubiorev.2017.01.008

Payne LS, Huang PH (2013) The pathobiology of collagens in glioma. Mol Cancer Res 11(10):1129–1140. https://doi.org/10.1158/1541-7786.mcr-13-0236

Pecorino L (2016) Molecular biology of cancer. Mechanisms, targets, and therapeutics, 4th edn. Oxford University Press

Pelengaris S, Khan M (2013a) Cell death. In: Pelengaris S, Khan M (eds) The molecular biology of cancer. A bridge from bench to bedside, 2nd edn. Wiley-Blackwell, pp 266–294

Pelengaris S, Khan M (2013b) Growth signaling pathways and the new era of targeted treatment of cancer. In: Pelengaris S, Khan M (eds) The molecular biology of cancer. A bridge from bench to bedside, 2nd edn. Wiley-Blackwell, pp 146–187

Pietronigro EC, Della Bianca V, Zenaro E, Constantin G (2017) NETosis in Alzheimer's disease. Front Immunol 8:211. https://doi.org/10.3389/fimmu.2017.00211

Platten M, Ochs K, Lemke D, Opitz C, Wick W (2014) Microenvironmental clues for glioma immunotherapy. Curr Neurol Neurosci Rep 14(4):440. https://doi.org/10.1007/s11910-014-0440-1

Rahman R, Heath R, Grundy R (2009) Cellular immortality in brain tumours: an integration of the cancer stem cell paradigm. Biochim Biophys Acta 1792(4):280–288. https://doi.org/10.1016/j.bbadis.2009.01.011

Rahman M, Deleyrolle L, Vedam-Mai V, Azari H, Abd-El-Barr M, Reynolds BA (2011) The cancer stem cell hypothesis: failures and pitfalls. Neurosurgery 68(2):531–545. ; discussion 545. https://doi.org/10.1227/NEU.0b013e3181ff9eb5

Rao R, Salloum R, Xin M, Lu QR (2016) The G protein Galphas acts as a tumor suppressor in sonic hedgehog signaling-driven tumorigenesis. Cell Cycle (Georgetown, TX) 15(10):1325–1330. https://doi.org/10.1080/15384101.2016.1164371

Reifenberger G, Wirsching HG, Knobbe-Thomsen CB, Weller M (2017) Advances in the molecular genetics of gliomas—implications for classification and therapy. Nat Rev Clin Oncol 14(7):434–452. https://doi.org/10.1038/nrclinonc.2016.204

Remijsen Q, Kuijpers TW, Wirawan E, Lippens S, Vandenabeele P, Vanden Berghe T (2011) Dying for a cause: NETosis, mechanisms behind an antimicrobial cell death modality. Cell Death Differ 18(4):581–588. https://doi.org/10.1038/cdd.2011.1

Ringertz N (1950) Grading of gliomas. Acta Pathol Microbiol Scand 27(1):51–64

Roussel MF (2013) Tumor suppressors. In: Pelengaris S, Khan M (eds) The molecular biology of cancer. A bridge from bench to bedside, 2nd edn. Wiley-Blackwell, pp 239–265

Satyanarayana A, Kaldis P (2009) Mammalian cell-cycle regulation: several Cdks, numerous cyclins and diverse compensatory mechanisms. Oncogene 28(33):2925–2939. https://doi.org/10.1038/onc.2009.2170. Epub 2009 June 29.

Seton-Rogers S (2014) Glioblastoma: cancer stem cell knockout. Nat Rev Cancer 14(7):452–453. https://doi.org/10.1038/nrc3771

Sharma A, Shiras A (2016) Cancer stem cell-vascular endothelial cell interactions in glioblastoma. Biochem Biophys Res Commun 473(3):688–692. https://doi.org/10.1016/j.bbrc.2015.12.022

Silver DJ, Lathia JD (2018) Revealing the glioma cancer stem cell interactome, one niche at a time. J Pathol 244(3):260–264. https://doi.org/10.1002/path.5024

Smith MT, Ludwig CL, Godfrey AD, Armbrustmacher VW (1983) Grading of oligodendrogliomas. Cancer 52(11):2107–2114

Steindler DA (2006) Redefining cellular phenotypy based on embryonic, adult, and cancer stem cell biology. Brain Pathol (Zurich, Switzerland) 16(2):169–180. https://doi.org/10.1111/j.1750-3639.2006.00011.x

Su Z, Yang Z, Xu Y, Chen Y, Yu Q (2015) Apoptosis, autophagy, necroptosis, and cancer metastasis. Mol Cancer 14:48. https://doi.org/10.1186/s12943-015-0321-5

Sugasawa K (2016) Molecular mechanisms of DNA damage recognition for mammalian nucleotide excision repair. DNA Repair (Amst) 44:110–117. https://doi.org/10.1016/j.dnarep.2016.1005.1015. Epub 2016 May 20.

Suwala AK, Hanaford A, Kahlert UD, Maciaczyk J (2016) Clipping the wings of glioblastoma: modulation of WNT as a novel therapeutic strategy. J Neuropathol Exp Neurol 75(5):388–396. https://doi.org/10.1093/jnen/nlw013

Suzuki H, Osawa T, Fujioka Y, Noda NN (2017) Structural biology of the core autophagy machinery. Curr Opin Struct Biol 43:10–17. https://doi.org/10.1016/j.sbi.2016.09.010

Tang C, Chua CL, Ang BT (2007) Insights into the cancer stem cell model of glioma tumorigenesis. Ann Acad Med Singap 36(5):352–357

Thomas TM, Yu JS (2017) Metabolic regulation of glioma stem-like cells in the tumor micro-environment. Cancer Lett 408:174–181. https://doi.org/10.1016/j.canlet.2017.07.014

Turgeon MO, Perry NJS, Poulogiannis G (2018) DNA damage, repair, and cancer metabolism. Front Oncol 8:15. https://doi.org/10.3389/fonc.2018.00015. eCollection 2018.

Turnpenny P, Ellard S (2017) Emery's elements of medical genetics, 15th edn. Elsevier

Tvedten H (2009) Atypical mitoses: morphology and classification. Vet Clin Pathol 38(4):418–420. https://doi.org/10.1111/j.1939-165X.2009.00201.x

van Breemen MS, Wilms EB, Vecht CJ (2007) Epilepsy in patients with brain tumours: epidemiology, mechanisms, and management. Lancet Neurol 6(5):421–430. https://doi.org/10.1016/s1474-4422(07)70103-5

Veeravagu A, Bababeygy SR, Kalani MY, Hou LC, Tse V (2008) The cancer stem cell-vascular niche complex in brain tumor formation. Stem Cells Dev 17(5):859–867. https://doi.org/10.1089/scd.2008.0047

Wang Y, Dawson VL, Dawson TM (2009) Poly(ADP-ribose) signals to mitochondrial AIF: a key event in parthanatos. Exp Neurol 218(2):193–202. https://doi.org/10.1016/j.expneurol.2009.03.020

Wang Z, Wang F, Tang T, Guo C (2012) The role of PARP1 in the DNA damage response and its application in tumor therapy. Front Med 6(2):156–164. https://doi.org/10.1007/s11684-11012-10197-11683. Epub 2012 June 3.

Weeden CE, Asselin-Labat ML (2018) Mechanisms of DNA damage repair in adult stem cells and implications for cancer formation. Biochim Biophys Acta 1864(1):89–101. https://doi.org/10.1016/j.bbadis.2017.1010.1015. Epub 2017 Oct 14.

Weller M, van den Bent M, Tonn JC, Stupp R, Preusser M, Cohen-Jonathan-Moyal E, Henriksson R, Le Rhun E, Balana C, Chinot O, Bendszus M, Reijneveld JC, Dhermain F, French P, Marosi C, Watts C, Oberg I, Pilkington G, Baumert BG, Taphoorn MJB, Hegi M, Westphal M, Reifenberger G, Soffietti R, Wick W (2017) European Association for Neuro-Oncology

(EANO) guideline on the diagnosis and treatment of adult astrocytic and oligodendroglial gliomas. The Lancet Oncology 18(6):e315–e329. https://doi.org/10.1016/s1470-2045(17)30194-8

Wenzel ES, Singh ATK (2018) Cell-cycle checkpoints and aneuploidy on the path to cancer. In Vivo 32(1):1–5. https://doi.org/10.21873/invivo.11197

White E, Green DR, Letai AG (2015) Apoptosis, necrosis, and autophagy. In: Mendelsohn J, Gray JW, Howley PM, Israel MA, Thompson CB (eds) The molecular basis of cancer, 4th edn. Elsevier Saunders, pp 209–227

Williams GH, Stoeber K (2012) The cell cycle and cancer. J Pathol 226(2):352–364. https://doi.org/10.1002/path.3022. Epub 2011 Oct 28.

Wippold FJ 2nd, Perry A (2006) Neuropathology for the neuroradiologist: rosettes and pseudorosettes. AJNR Am J Neuroradiol 27(3):488–492

Wippold FJ 2nd, Lammle M, Anatelli F, Lennerz J, Perry A (2006) Neuropathology for the neuroradiologist: palisades and pseudopalisades. AJNR Am J Neuroradiol 27(10):2037–2041

Wong RS (2011) Apoptosis in cancer: from pathogenesis to treatment. J Exp Clin Cancer Res 30:87. https://doi.org/10.1186/1756-9966-30-87

Xie J, Bartels CM, Barton SW, Gu D (2013) Targeting hedgehog signaling in cancer: research and clinical developments. Onco Targets Ther 6:1425–1435. https://doi.org/10.2147/ott.s34678

Xie Y, Hou W, Song X, Yu Y, Huang J, Sun X, Kang R, Tang D (2016) Ferroptosis: process and function. Cell Death Differ 23(3):369–379. https://doi.org/10.1038/cdd.2015.158

Yin Z, Pascual C, Klionsky DJ (2016) Autophagy: machinery and regulation. Microb Cell (Graz, Austria) 3(12):588–596. https://doi.org/10.15698/mic2016.12.546

Yipp BG, Kubes P (2013) NETosis: how vital is it? Blood 122(16):2784–2794. https://doi.org/10.1182/blood-2013-04-457671

Yu H, Guo P, Xie X, Wang Y, Chen G (2017) Ferroptosis, a new form of cell death, and its relationships with tumourous diseases. J Cell Mol Med 21(4):648–657. https://doi.org/10.1111/jcmm.13008

Zaffagnini G, Martens S (2016) Mechanisms of selective autophagy. J Mol Biol 428(9 Pt A):1714–1724. https://doi.org/10.1016/j.jmb.2016.02.004

Zhang K, Zhang J, Han L, Pu P, Kang C (2012) Wnt/beta-catenin signaling in glioma. J NeuroImmune Pharmacol 7(4):740–749. https://doi.org/10.1007/s11481-012-9359-y

Zuccarini M, Giuliani P, Ziberi S, Carluccio M, Iorio PD, Caciagli F, Ciccarelli R (2018) The role of Wnt signal in glioblastoma development and progression: a possible new pharmacological target for the therapy of this tumor. Genes 9(2). https://doi.org/10.3390/genes9020105

Diffuse Astrocytoma WHO Grade II

Diffuse Astrocytic and Oligodendroglial Tumors

WHO Definition

2016—Diffuse astrocytoma, IDH-mutant: A diffusely infiltrating astrocytoma with a mutation in either the IDH1 or IDH2 gene (von Deimling et al. 2016).

Gemistocytic astrocytoma, IDH-mutant: A variant of IDH-mutant diffuse astrocytoma characterized by the presence of a conspicuous (though variable) proportion of gemistocytic neoplastic astrocytes (gemistocytes) (von Deimling et al. 2016).

Diffuse astrocytoma, IDH-wild-type: A diffusely infiltrating astrocytoma without mutations in the IDH genes (von Deimling et al. 2016).

Diffuse astrocytoma, NOS: A tumor with morphological features of diffuse astrocytoma, but in which IDH mutation status has not been fully assessed (von Deimling et al. 2016).

2007—A diffusely infiltrating astrocytoma that typically affects young adults and is characterized by a high degree of cellular differentiation and slow growth; the tumor occurs throughout the CNS but is preferentially located supratentorially and has an intrinsic tendency for malignant progression to anaplastic astrocytoma and, ultimately, glioblastoma (von Deimling et al. 2007).

2000—An astrocytic neoplasm characterized by a high degree of cellular differentiation, slow growth, a diffuse infiltration of neighboring brain structures. These lesions typically affect young adults and have an intrinsic tendency for malignant progression to anaplastic astrocytoma and, ultimately, glioblastoma (Kleihues et al. 2000).

1993—A generic term applied to diffusely infiltrating tumors composed of well-differentiated astrocytes (Kleihues et al. 1993).

1979—A tumor composed predominantly of astrocytes (Zülch 1979).

WHO Grade
- WHO grade II

52.1 Epidemiology

Incidence
- Incidence rate: 1.4/one million population a year
- Make up 10–15% of all astrocytic tumors

Age Incidence
- Young adults aged 30–40 years
- Mean age: 34 years

Sex Incidence
- Male:Female ratio: 1.18:1

Localization
- Any part of the brain
- Preferentially in the frontal and temporal lobes
- Brain stem and spinal cord
- Rarely the cerebellum

52.2 Neuroimaging Findings

General Imaging Findings
- Homogeneous, primary white matter mass
- May extend into gray matter

CT Non-Contrast-Enhanced
- Homogeneous hypo-/isodense mass

CT Contrast-Enhanced
- No enhancement
- Minimal enhancement may demonstrate malignant progression

MRI-T2 (Fig. 52.1a)
- Homogeneous hyperintense
- Adjacent cortex appears swollen (extended)

MRI-FLAIR (Fig. 52.1b)
- Homogeneous hyperintense

MRI-T1 (Fig. 52.1c)
- Homogeneous hypointense

MRI-T1 Contrast-Enhanced (Fig. 52.1d)
- In general no enhancement but possible
- Enhancement is suspicious of malignant progression

MRI-T2*/SWI
- Calcification and hemorrhages rare

MR-Diffusion Imaging
- No restricted diffusion

MRI-Perfusion (Fig. 52.1e)
- Slight elevation of rCBV
- Lower rCBV compared to astrocytoma WHO grade III or glioblastoma WHO grade IV

MR-Diffusion Tensor Imaging (Fig. 52.1f)
- Difficult to distinguish tumor borders due to the interstitial edema and diffuse brain tissue infiltration of the tumor

MR-Spectroscopy (Fig. 52.1g)
- Elevated choline
- Low NAA
- Myoinositol/choline ratio increased and may demonstrate real extent of tumor

Nuclear Medicine Imaging Findings
- Astrocytomas WHO II show normally hypometabolism in FDG-PET
- Radiotracers like FET (a marker of amino acid uptake, L-system) or FLT (a marker of DNA biosynthesis) may be positive or negative in astrocytomas WHO II
- Some studies suggest a better prognosis for patients with no amino acid uptake in low-grade gliomas than for patients with amino acid uptake
- Results obtained for MET are similar to FET
  - The advantage of FET is that it is taken up in a lesser amount by inflammatory tissue and its longer half-life of 110 min as compared to a relatively short half-life of 20 min of C-11 used in MET
- Dynamic FET-PET enables the measurement of the tracer kinetic

52.3 Neuropathology Findings

Macroscopic Features (Fig. 52.2a–h)
- Gross-anatomical borders are blurred
- Enlargement and distortion of invaded brain structures
- Gray or yellow-whitish color

52.3 Neuropathology Findings

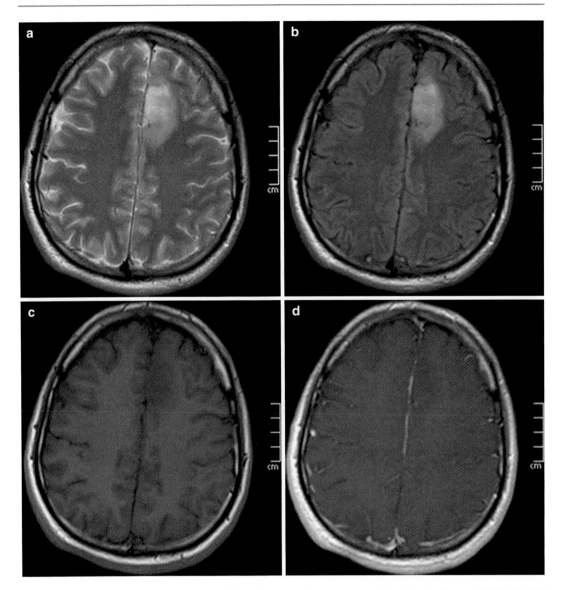

Fig. 52.1 Diffuse left frontal astrocytoma with homogeneous signal intensity in T2 (**a**) and FLAIR (**b**), without enhancement T1 (**c**), T1contrast (**d**). MR-perfusion demonstrates no areas of pathologic elevated rCBV (**e**). DTI (**f**), and spectroscopy (**g**)

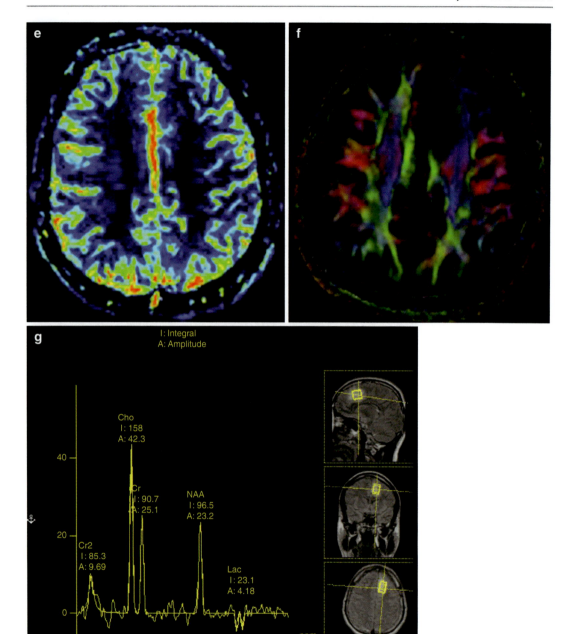

Fig. 52.1 (continued)

- Areas of the tumor tissue might be firm or softened or granular or cystic

Microscopic Features (Fig. 52.3a–d)
- Well-differentiated neoplastic astrocytes
- In a loosely structured tumor matrix
- Neoplastic astrocytes with
  - Round to oval nuclei
  - Vesicular with intermediate-sized masses of chromatin
  - Distinct nucleolus
  - No stainable cytoplasm

52.3 Neuropathology Findings

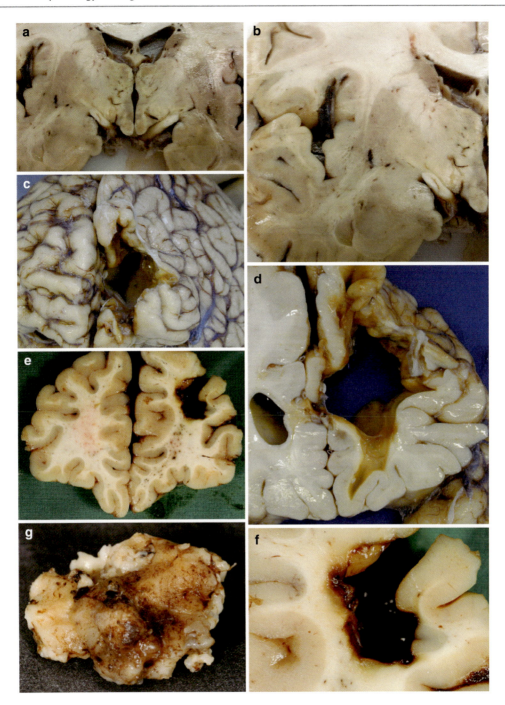

Fig. 52.2 Diffuse astrocytoma (WHO grade II): Autopsy specimen showing diffuse growth of the tumor into and with enlargement of the amygdala extending into the basal ganglia and insula (→) (**a**, **b**). Postoperative appearance of brain tissue displays some hemorrhagic residues at various extensions at the borders of the resection (**c–f**). Surgical specimens of tumor tissue are of gray or yellow-whitish color (**g–j**), with blurred borders (**h**, **j**), enlargement and distortion of invaded structures (**g–j**), invaded hippocampal formation (**j**). Areas of the tumor tissue might be cystic → (**h**)

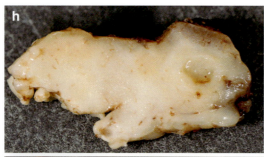
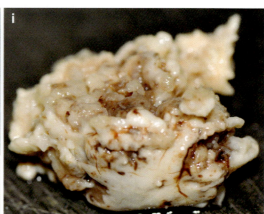
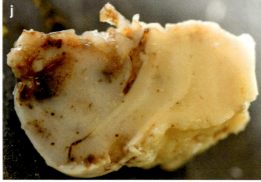

Fig. 52.2 (continued)

- Increase in number and size of neoplastic astrocytes
- Microcysts
- Absent mitotic activity
- Absence of necroses
- Absence of microvascular proliferation

Based on histologic features, besides diffuse astrocytoma, the following type is also distinguished:

- Gemistocytic astrocytoma (Fig. 52.4a–f)
  - Plump, glassy, eosinophilic cell bodies of angular shape
  - Stout, randomly oriented processes form a coarse fibrillary network
  - Eccentric nuclei with nucleoli and densely clumped chromatin
  - Should account for more than 20% of all tumor cells for the diagnosis of gemistocytic astrocytoma
  - Perivascular lymphocytic infiltrates are frequent

In previous editions of the WHO classification system, the following two types of astrocytomas were defined:

- Fibrillary astrocytoma
  - Most frequent variant
  - Composed of fibrillary astrocytes
  - Cell processes form a loose fibrillary matrix
- Protoplasmic astrocytoma
  - Rare variant
  - Protoplasmic astrocytes consist of: Small cell body with a few processes
  - Uniformly round to oval nucleus

Immunophenotype (Fig. 52.5a–h)
- IDH-1 R123H mutation-specific antibody
  - Reactivity seen in 80–90%
  - Expressed in the nucleus
  - Expressed in the cytoplasm
  - Differentiates tumor tissue from surrounding non-neoplastic tissue and/or reactive astrogliosis
  - Full assessment of IDH mutation status in anaplastic astrocytomas involves sequence analysis for IDH1 codon 132 and IDH2 codon 172 mutations in cases that are immunohistochemically negative for the IDH1 R132H-mutation

52.3 Neuropathology Findings

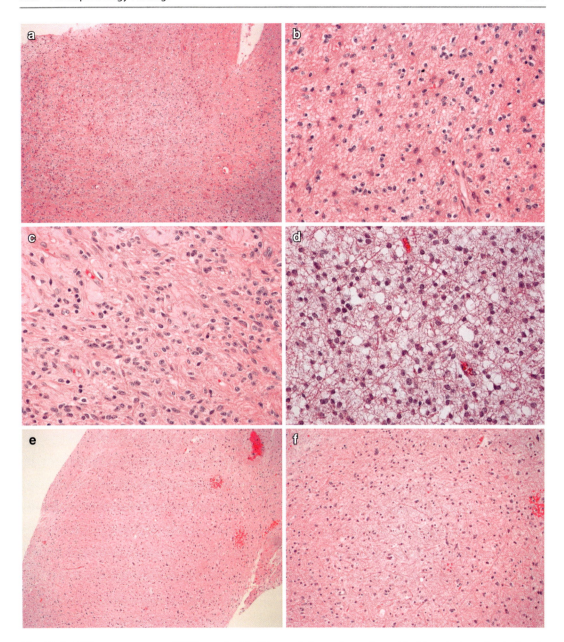

Fig. 52.3 Diffuse astrocytoma (WHO grade II): The tumor is of low to moderate cellularity and composed of well-differentiated neoplastic astrocytes in a loosely structured tumor matrix. The tumor cells have a small cell body, few processes, uniformly round to oval nucleus, distinct nucleolus, vesicular with intermediate-sized masses of chromatin, and no stainable cytoplasm (protoplasmic astrocytes) (**a–h**; stereotactic biopsy: **e–h**). Other tumors are made up of fibrillary astrocytes with cell processes forming a loose fibrillary matrix (**i–l**). Microcystic formation is evident at various degrees (**d**)

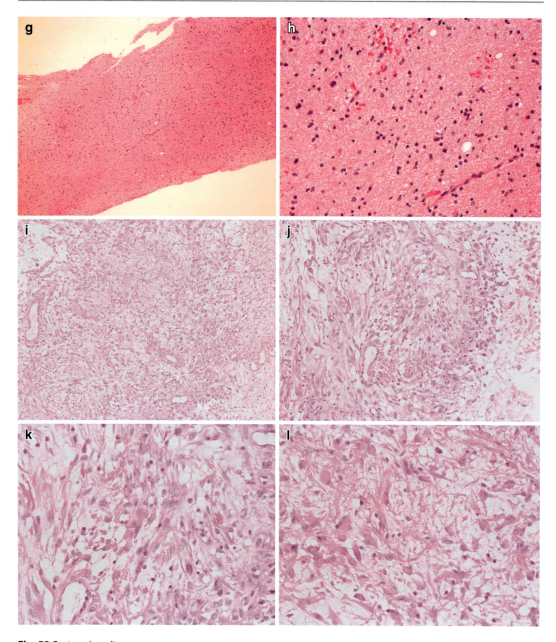

Fig. 52.3 (continued)

- Glial fibrillary acidic protein (GFAP)
  - Expressed at variable degree
  - In the cellular processes
  - Often as a perinuclear rim
  - GFAP-positive fibrillary matrix
- S-100
  - Expressed in the nucleus
  - Expressed in cell processes
- Vimentin
  - Pattern similar to GFAP
  - Seen mainly in the perinuclear region
- ß-Crystallin
  - Same reactivity pattern as S-100

52.3 Neuropathology Findings

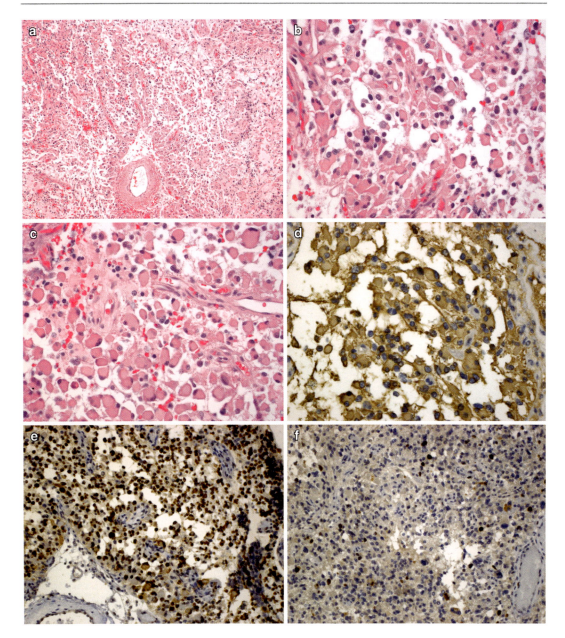

Fig. 52.4 Gemistocytic astrocytoma (WHO grade II): The tumor is composed of cells with flattened eccentric nuclei and massively enlarged cytoplasm (**a–c**). The tumor cells are immunopositive for GFAP (**d**), numerous tumor cells show p53 reactivities (**e**). Low Ki67 proliferation rate (**f**)

- ATRX
  - Loss in the setting of ATRX mutations
  - Retained nuclear reactivity in the nucleus of non-neoplastic vascular endothelial cells
- p53
  - Frequent in gemistocytic astrocytoma
- Bcl-2
  - Frequent in gemistocytic astrocytoma

Proliferation Markers (Fig. 52.5i, j)
- Lack of mitotic activity
- Mean Ki-67 LI around 2.5%, usually less than 4%

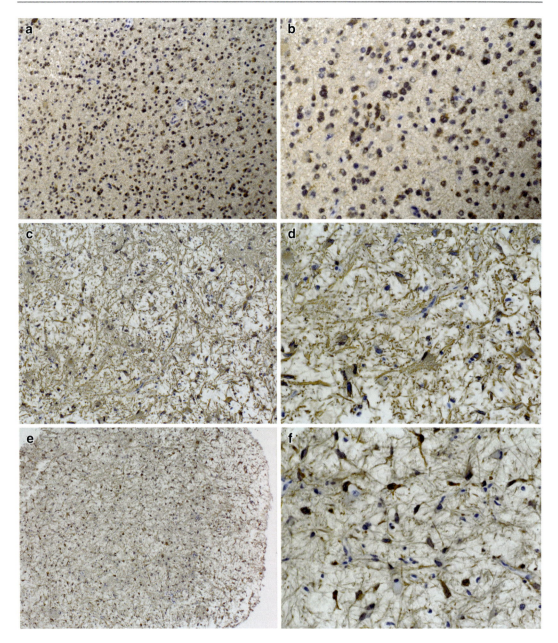

Fig. 52.5 Diffuse astrocytoma (WHO grade II)—Immunophenotype: IDH1 R123H (**a, b**), GFAP (**c, d**), S100 (**e, f**), p53 (**g, h**), Ki-67 (**i, j**)

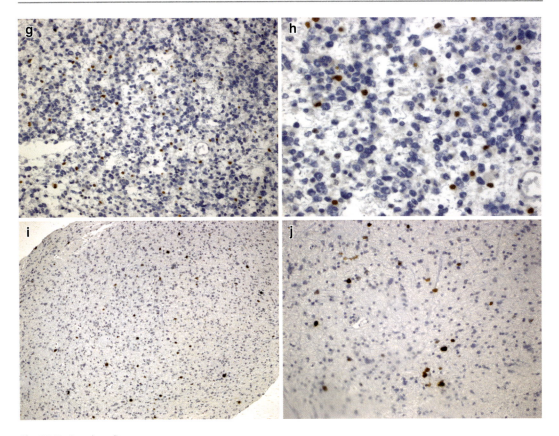

Fig. 52.5 (continued)

Ultrastructural Features
- Presence of glial intermediate filaments (7–11 nm in diameter) in the perikaryon and cell processes
- Limited diagnostic value (especially for delineating reactive astrogliosis)
- Fibrillary and protoplasmic tumor cells
- **Protoplasmic tumor cells**:
  – Resemble non-neoplastic astrocytes
  – Prominent bipolar processes
  – 20 nm microtubules
  – 6–9 nm glial filaments
  – Zonulae adherentes possible
  – Nuclei:
    Irregular or lobulated
    Marginated chromatin
  – Abundant organelles
  – Membrane-bound vesicles
  – Rough endoplasmic reticulum
  – Glial filaments scarce or absent in the perikaryal cytoplasm
- **Fibrillary**:
  – Abundant 6–9 nm glial filaments
  – In perikaryal cytoplasm and processes
  – Cytoplasmic organelles sparse
- **Microcytic tumor**:
  – Cysts as separate, rounded loculi of extracellular space enclosed by basement membrane
- **Gemistocytic**:
  – Flattened eccentric nuclei
  – Massively enlarged cytoplasm
  – Contains diffusely scattered organelles
  – Filled by meshwork of haphazardly oriented, short length of 6–9 nm glial filaments
- **Rosenthal fiber**:
  – Cell process distended by a large mass of similar electron-dense material

- Expanded extracellular space
- Tumor cell processes form tenuous, complex, and loose meshwork

Differential Diagnosis
- Reactive astrogliosis

52.4 Molecular Neuropathology

52.4.1 Pathogenesis

- De novo

52.4.2 Genetics

In line with the pronounced tendency of astrocytoma WHO grade II tumors to progress to higher grade gliomas (anaplastic astrocytoma, WHO grade III, and secondary glioblastoma, WHO grade IV), some of the genetic traits associated with these malignant tumors are already laid out in diffuse astrocytoma. In particular, gains of chromosome 7 and losses of chromosome 17p which occur at high frequencies should be noted (see also Chap. 54: Glioblastoma).

Genes affected in astrocytomas WHO grade II include:

- *IDH1/2* (isocitrate dehydrogenase 1, isocitrate dehydrogenase 2):
- The *IDH1* gene (chromosome locus 2q33.3) and the *IDH2* gene (chromosome locus 15q26.1), encoding the $NADP^+$-dependent enzymes isocitrate dehydrogenase 1 and isocitrate dehydrogenase 2, respectively, are mutated in the majority of WHO grade II astrocytomas. Of particular importance is an *IDH1* point mutation, resulting in a transition of arginine to histidine in the enzyme's catalytic site at amino acid position 132 (R132H). This mutation was found in up to 80% of grade II gliomas as well as in the majority of WHO grade III astrogliomas and secondary glioblastomas; to date, it is regularly analyzed and serves as a specific diagnostic marker in these tumors.
- At a much lower frequency, functional mutations are also reported in the *IDH2* gene; here, the major target is codon 172 which translates into arginine in the wild-type enzyme. R172 represents the analogous residue to R132 in IDH1 and was found to be mutated primarily in patients lacking the typical IDH1 mutation.
- *TP53* (tumor suppressor gene, on chromosome 17p13.1, encoding tumor protein 53):
- In more than 60% of diffuse astrocytomas, monoallelic deletion (loss of heterozygosity; LOH) of the chromosome 17p region harboring *TP53* has been described; moreover, in the majority of cases, mutations in the remaining *TP53* allele ultimately result in a total lack of the functional gene product.
- *PDGFRA* (oncogenic; encoding platelet-derived growth factor receptor, α-peptide):
- In WHO grade II astrocytomas, upregulation of PDGFR-α expression can be observed, although supporting evidence is based on relatively low sample sizes. In addition, elevated PDGFR-α levels are more frequently correlated with higher grade gliomas. Taken together, it therefore remains uncertain to which extent PDGFR-α overexpression contributes to tumorigenesis in diffuse astrocytoma.
- Absence of 1p/19q co-deletion (see Chap. 58—Oligodendroglioma).

52.4.3 Epigenetics

So far, the best studied epigenetic feature associated with grade II astrocytomas is promoter hypermethylation of two tumor suppressor genes, *ARF* and *MGMT*:

- The *ARF* gene codes for the tumor suppressor protein p14ARF which acts as a supporting factor in the TP53 pathway
- The *MGMT* gene encodes the DNA repair enzyme O^6-methylguanine-DNA methyltransferase; by removing the methyl group from mutagenic O^6-methylguanine residues, the enzyme contributes to genome integrity

Promoter hypermethylation results in reduced expression of the tumor suppressor genes and, as a result, in diminished protein function.

52.4.4 Gene Expression

Several genes differentially expressed in astrocytomas WHO grade II—as compared to healthy controls—were identified in recent years:

- Upregulated expression:
  - *CD9*
  - *CSPG2*, also known as *VCAN* (versican)
  - *NTF3* (neurotrophin 3)
  - *EGFR* (epidermal growth factor receptor)
  - *PDGFRA* (platelet-derived growth factor receptor, alpha polypeptide)
  - *TIMP3* (TIMP metallopeptidase inhibitor 3)
- Downregulated expression:
  - *TYRO3* (TYRO3 protein tyrosine kinase)

52.5 Treatment and Prognosis

Treatment
- Surgery with an attempt of total removal
- Chemotherapy (in individual cases after incomplete tumor resection)

Biologic Behavior–Prognosis–Prognostic Factors
- Median survival time: 6–8 years
- Tumor progression might occur after 4–5 years
- Gemistocytic astrocytoma prone to progress to anaplastic astrocytoma and glioblastoma
- No unambiguous parameter predicting occurrence of and speed to malignant progression
  - Favorable parameters include:
    o Young age at diagnosis
    o Gross total resection
    o Presence of epilepsy as a single symptom
    o Presence of microcysts in tumor tissue
    o Loss of ATRX expression in IDH-mutated astrocytomas
  - Non-favorable parameters include:
    o Tumor size (resected volume)
    o Neurologic deficit
    o KI-67 LI of >5%
    o Presence of a significant fraction of gemistocytes
- Changes in various genes, e.g., mutation, deletion, amplification (Table 52.1)

Table 52.1 Molecular predictors for clinical outcome, data from Wang and Bettegowda (2015) reproduced with kind permission by Elsevier

Overall poorer outcomes	Overall better outcomes
IDH1/2 wild-type	*IDH1/2* mutant
• *EGFR/PFGRA/MET* amplification • *PTEN* deletion • *TP53* mutation/deletion • *NF1* mutation/deletion • *CDK4* amplification • *MDM2/4* amplification • *PI3K* mutation • *RB1* mutation • *CDKN2A/B* mutation/deletion • *TERT* mutation	• *TP53* mutation/deletion • *ATRX* mutation/deletion • *RB1* mutation/deletion • *CDK4/6* amplification • *CDKN2A* deletion • *MDM2/4* amplification • *PDGFRA* amplification • *PTEN* mutation/deletion

Selected References

Ajlan A, Recht L (2014) Supratentorial low-grade diffuse astrocytoma: medical management. Semin Oncol 41(4):446–457. https://doi.org/10.1053/j.seminoncol.2014.06.013

Arevalo-Perez J, Peck KK, Young RJ, Holodny AI, Karimi S, Lyo JK (2015) Dynamic contrast-enhanced perfusion MRI and diffusion-weighted imaging in grading of gliomas. J Neuroimaging 25(5):792–798. https://doi.org/10.1111/jon.12239

Ashby LS, Shapiro WR (2004) Low-grade glioma: supratentorial astrocytoma, oligodendroglioma, and oligoastrocytoma in adults. Curr Neurol Neurosci Rep 4(3):211–217

Castillo M, Smith JK, Kwock L (2000) Correlation of myo-inositol levels and grading of cerebral astrocytomas. AJNR Am J Neuroradiol 21(9):1645–1649

Catalaa I, Henry R, Dillon WP, Graves EE, McKnight TR, Lu Y, Vigneron DB, Nelson SJ (2006) Perfusion, diffusion and spectroscopy values in newly diagnosed cerebral gliomas. NMR Biomed 19(4):463–475. https://doi.org/10.1002/nbm.1059

Chawla S, Wang S, Wolf RL, Woo JH, Wang J, O'Rourke DM, Judy KD, Grady MS, Melhem ER, Poptani H (2007) Arterial spin-labeling and MR spectroscopy in the differentiation of gliomas. AJNR Am J Neuroradiol 28(9):1683–1689. https://doi.org/10.3174/ajnr.A0673

von Deimling A, Burger PC, Nakazato Y, Ohgaki H, Kleihues P (2007) Diffuse astrocytoma. In: Louis DN, Ohgaki H, Wiestler OD, Cavenee WK (eds) WHO classification of tumours of the central nervous system. International Agency for Research on Cancer, Lyon, pp 25–29

von Deimling A, Huse JT, Yan H, Brat DJ, Reifenberger G, Ohgaki H, Kleihues P, Berger MS, Weller M, Nakazato Y, Burger PC, Ellison DW, Louis DN (2016) Diffuse astrocytoma, IDH-mutant. In: Louis DN, Ohgaki H, Wiestler OD, Cavenee WK (eds) WHO classification of tumours of the central nervous system, revised 4th edn. IARC, Lyon, pp 18–23

Hakyemez B, Erdogan C, Ercan I, Ergin N, Uysal S, Atahan S (2005) High-grade and low-grade gliomas: differentiation by using perfusion MR imaging. Clin Radiol 60(4):493–502. https://doi.org/10.1016/j.crad.2004.09.009

Hollingworth W, Medina LS, Lenkinski RE, Shibata DK, Bernal B, Zurakowski D, Comstock B, Jarvik JG (2006) A systematic literature review of magnetic resonance spectroscopy for the characterization of brain tumors. AJNR Am J Neuroradiol 27(7):1404–1411

Isaacs H Jr (2016) Perinatal (fetal and neonatal) astrocytoma: a review. Childs Nerv Syst 32(11):2085–2096. https://doi.org/10.1007/s00381-016-3215-y

Kleihues P, Burger PC, Scheithauer BW (1993) Histological typing of tumours of the central nervous system, 2nd edn. Springer-Verlag, Berlin

Kleihues P, Davis RL, Ohgaki H, Burger PC, Westphak MM, Cavenee WK (2000) Diffuse astrocytoma. In: Kleihues P, Cavenee WK (eds) Pathology and genetics of tumours of the nervous system, 3rd edn. IARC, Lyon, pp 22–26

Knizetova P, Darling JL, Bartek J (2008) Vascular endothelial growth factor in astroglioma stem cell biology and response to therapy. J Cell Mol Med 12(1):111–125. https://doi.org/10.1111/j.1582-4934.2007.00153.x

Lee EJ, Lee SK, Agid R, Bae JM, Keller A, Terbrugge K (2008) Preoperative grading of presumptive low-grade astrocytomas on MR imaging: diagnostic value of minimum apparent diffusion coefficient. AJNR Am J Neuroradiol 29(10):1872–1877. https://doi.org/10.3174/ajnr.A1254

Marko NF, Weil RJ (2013) The molecular biology of WHO Grade II gliomas. Neurosurg Focus 34(2):E1. https://doi.org/10.3171/2012.3112.FOCUS12283

Ohgaki H, Kleihues P (2011) Genetic profile of astrocytic and oligodendroglial gliomas. Brain Tumor Pathol 28(3):177–183. https://doi.org/10.1007/s10014-011-0029-1. Epub 2011 Mar 26

Pedersen CL, Romner B (2013) Current treatment of low grade astrocytoma: a review. Clin Neurol Neurosurg 115(1):1–8. https://doi.org/10.1016/j.clineuro.2012.07.002

Rodriguez FJ, Lim KS, Bowers D, Eberhart CG (2013) Pathological and molecular advances in pediatric low-grade astrocytoma. Annu Rev Pathol 8:361–379. https://doi.org/10.1146/annurev-pathol-020712-164009

Rutka JT, Akiyama Y, Lee SP, Ivanchuk S, Tsugu A, Hamel PA (2000) Alterations of the p53 and pRB pathways in human astrocytoma. Brain Tumor Pathol 17(2):65–70

Ryskalin L, Limanaqi F, Biagioni F, Frati A, Esposito V, Calierno MT, Lenzi P, Fornai F (2017) The emerging role of m-TOR up-regulation in brain astrocytoma. Histol Histopathol 32(5):413–431. https://doi.org/10.14670/hh-11-835

Turner DA, Adamson DC (2011) Neuronal-astrocyte metabolic interactions: understanding the transition into abnormal astrocytoma metabolism. J Neuropathol Exp Neurol 70(3):167–176. https://doi.org/10.1097/NEN.0b013e31820e1152

Wang J, Bettegowda C (2015) Genomic discoveries in adult astrocytoma. Curr Opin Genet Dev 30:17–24. https://doi.org/10.1016/j.gde.2014.12.002

Wessels PH, Weber WE, Raven G, Ramaekers FC, Hopman AH, Twijnstra A (2003) Supratentorial grade II astrocytoma: biological features and clinical course. Lancet Neurol 2(7):395–403

Zülch KJ (1979) Histological typing of tumours of the central nervous system. World Health Organization, Geneva

Anaplastic Astrocytoma WHO Grade III

Diffuse Astrocytic and Oligodendroglial Tumors

WHO Definition

2016—Anaplastic astrocytoma, IDH-mutant: A diffusely infiltrating astrocytoma with focal or dispersed anaplasia, significant proliferative activity, and a mutation in either the IDH1 or IDH2 gene (von Deimling et al. 2016).

Anaplastic astrocytoma, IDH-wild-type: A diffusely infiltrating astrocytoma with focal or dispersed anaplasia and significant proliferative activity but without mutations in the IDH genes (von Deimling et al. 2016).

Anaplastic astrocytoma, NOS: A tumor with morphological features of anaplastic astrocytoma, but in which IDH mutation status has not been fully assessed (von Deimling et al. 2016).

2007—A diffusely infiltrating, malignant astrocytoma that primarily affects adults, preferentially located in the cerebral hemispheres, and that is histologically characterized by nuclear atypia, increased cellularity, and significant proliferative activity. The tumor may arise from diffuse astrocytoma WHO grade II or de novo, i.e., without evidence of a less malignant precursor lesion, and has an inherent tendency to undergo progression (Kleihues et al. 2007).

2000—A diffusely infiltrating astrocytoma with focal or dispersed anaplasia, and a marked proliferative potential. Anaplastic astrocytomas arise from low-grade astrocytomas, but are also diagnosed at first biopsy, without indication of a less malignant precursor lesion. They have an intrinsic tendency for malignant progression to glioblastoma (Kleihues et al. 2000).

1993—An astrocytoma with focal or diffuse anaplasia, e.g., increased cellularity, pleomorphism, nuclear atypia, and mitotic activity (Kleihues et al. 1993).

1979—An astrocytoma of one of the recognized subtypes containing areas of anaplasia. It may be difficult focally to distinguish from glioblastoma. However, the prognosis in anaplastic astrocytoma is not as invariably sinister as in the usual glioblastoma. It corresponds histologically to grade III (Zülch 1979).

WHO Grade
- WHO grade III

53.1 Epidemiology

Incidence
- Incidence rate: 0.44 per 100,000
- Make up 6% of all astrocytic tumors

Age Incidence
- Mean age: 45–51 years

Sex Incidence
- Male:Female ratio: 1.6:1

Localization
- Any part of the brain
- Preferentially the cerebral hemispheres
- Brain stem and spinal cord
- Rarely the cerebellum

53.2 Neuroimaging Findings

General Imaging Findings
- Diffuse infiltrating mass, predominantly in the hemispheric white matter

CT Non-Contrast-Enhanced
- Hypodense

CT Contrast-Enhanced
- Variable enhancement

MRI-T2 (Figs. 53.1a and 53.2a)
- Hyperintense inhomogeneous

MRI-FLAIR (Figs. 53.1b and 53.2b)
- Hyperintense inhomogeneous

MRI-T1 (Figs. 53.1c and 53.2c)
- Iso- to hypointense

MRI-T1 Contrast-Enhanced (Figs. 53.1d and 53.2d)
- Variable enhancement

MRI-T2*/SWI
- Calcification and hemorrhages rare

MR-Diffusion Imaging
- No restricted diffusion
- ADC value lower than in glioblastoma

MRI-Perfusion (Figs. 53.1e and 53.2e)
- rCBV elevated

MR-Diffusion Tensor Imaging (Fig. 53.2f)
- Difficult to distinguish tumor borders due to the interstitial edema and diffuse brain infiltration of the tumor

MR-Spectroscopy (Figs. 53.1f and 53.2g)
- NAA decreased
- Choline elevated

Nuclear Medicine Imaging Findings
- Astrocytomas WHO grade III are normally FDG-avid (CAVE: the normal gray matter of the cortex, the striatum, and the thalamus take up FDG due to their normal glucose-based metabolism).
- Radiotracers like FET (a marker of amino acid uptake (L-system)) or FLT (a marker of DNA biosynthesis) have the advantage of nearly no uptake in the healthy brain tissues resulting in a much better tumor-to-background ratio.
- Images can show homogeneous or heterogeneous uptake representing the tumor biology.
- SUV (calculated as ratio of the concentration of the radiotracer corrected by the body weight of the patient) can predict therapeutic outcomes.
- Results obtained for MET are similar to FET.
  - The advantage of FET is that it is taken up in a lesser amount by inflammatory tissue and its longer half-life of 110 min as compared to a relatively short half-life of 20 min of C-11 used in MET.
- Dynamic FET-PET enables the measurement of the tracer kinetic.
- Possibility of non-invasive tumor grading is being discussed (especially in dynamic FET-PET studies).
- Sensitivity of FET-PET for astrocytoma WHO grade III is about 95%.

53.2 Neuroimaging Findings

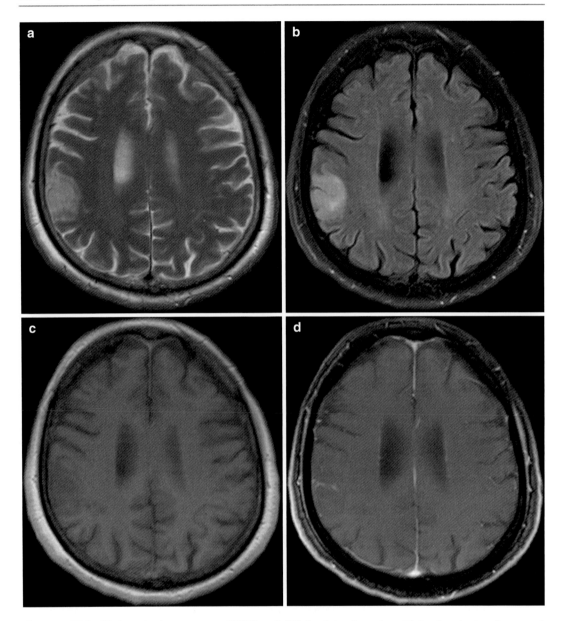

Fig. 53.1 Right sided anaplastic astrocytoma (WHO grade III), involving the cortex with focal moderate enhancement. T2 (**a**), FLAIR (**b**), T1 (**c**), T1 contrast (**d**), rCBV (**e**), and Spectroscopy (**f**)

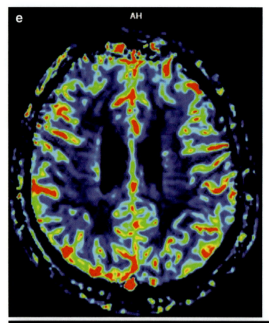
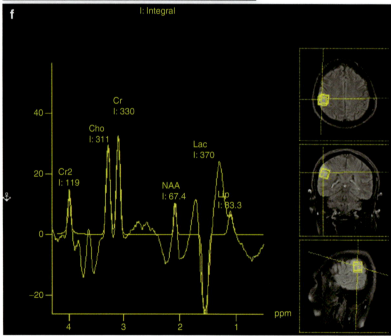

Fig. 53.1 (continued)

53.2 Neuroimaging Findings

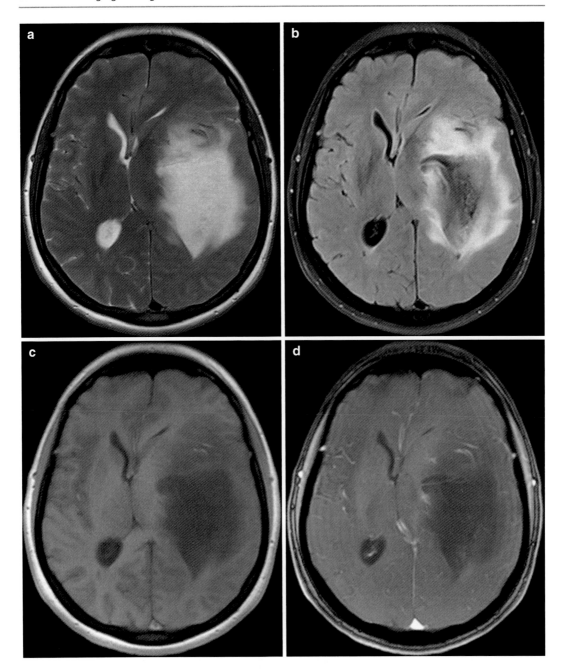

Fig. 53.2 Left hemispheric anaplastic astrocytoma (WHO grade III) with mass effect and inhomogeneous enhancement with increased recurrence risk. T2 (**a**), FLAIR (**b**), T1 (**c**), T1 contrast (**d**), rCBV (**e**), DTI (**f**), and spectroscopy (**g**)

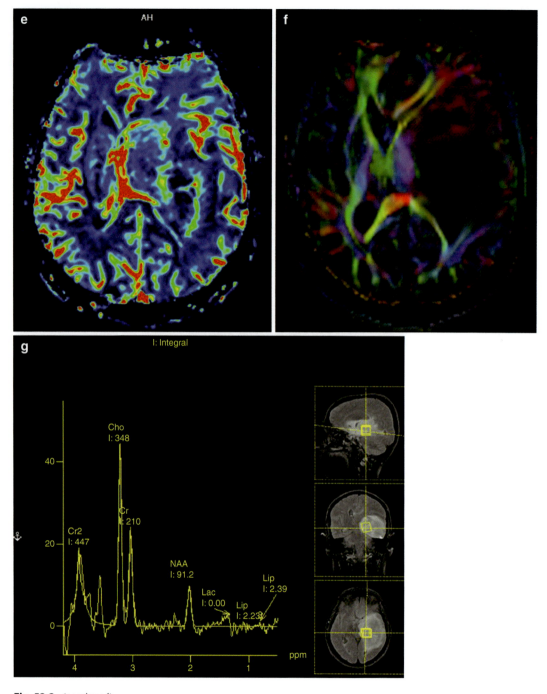

Fig. 53.2 (continued)

53.3 Neuropathology Findings

Macroscopic Features (Fig. 53.3a–f)
- Infiltration of the surrounding brain with tissue destruction
- Areas of granularity, opacity, and soft consistency
- Discernible tumor mass on cut surface

53.3 Neuropathology Findings

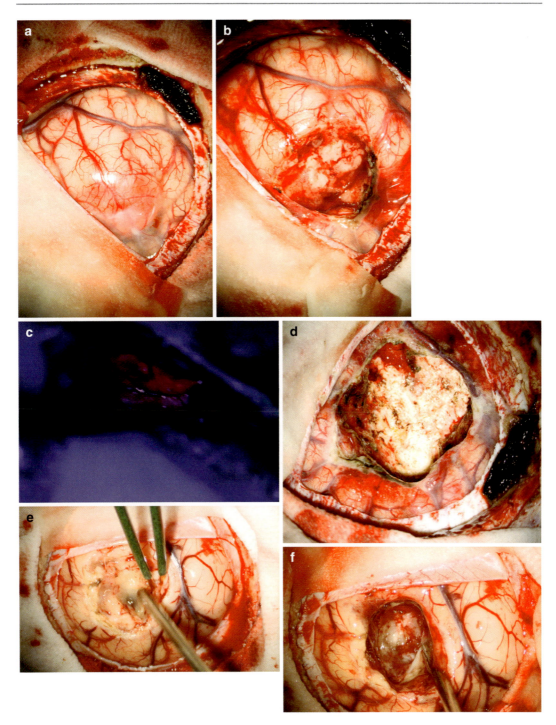

Fig. 53.3 Anaplastic astrocytoma (WHO grade III): Intraoperative appearance: The surface of the brain is protruding and shows variegated color (**a**); whitish color of the exposed tumor (**b**); the tumor displays reddish fluorescence after preoperative administration of ALA (**c**); the resection cavity (**d**); exposure of the tumor tissue with opacity and soft consistency (**e**); and reddish-brownish color (**f**)

Microscopic Features (Fig. 53.4a–i)
- Increased cellularity as compared to astrocytoma WHO grade II
- Distinct nuclear atypia characterized by increased variations of:
  - Nuclear size
  - Shape
  - Chromatin coarsening and dispersion
  - Nucleolar prominence
- Presence of mitotic activity
  - In small biopsy samples, one mitosis is enough for the diagnosis
  - In large tumor tissues, one mitosis is **not** enough for the diagnosis

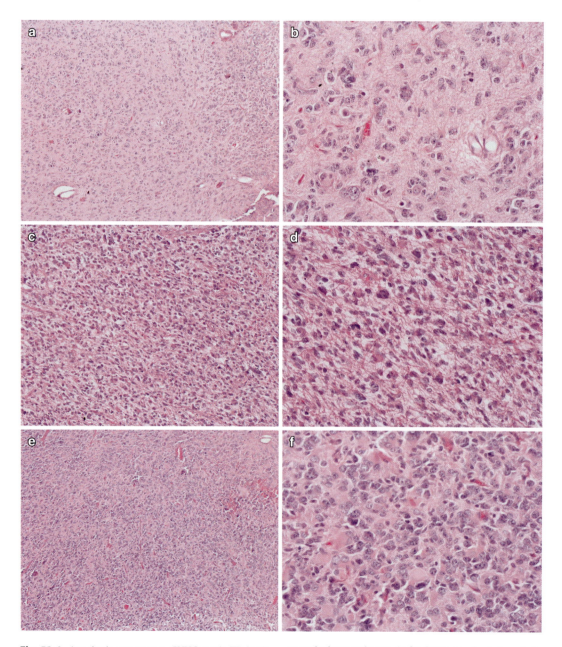

Fig. 53.4 Anaplastic astrocytoma (WHO grade III) is histologically characterized by an increased cellularity of tumor cells with distinct nuclear atypia, increased nuclear size and shape, chromatin coarsening and dispersion as well as nucleolar prominence (**a–h**). Presence of mitotic activity and multinucleated giant cells is noted (**g, h**). Diffuse infiltration of the cerebral cortex by tumor cells (**i–l**) (→ **i**). Note that the pial surface is reached by the tumor (∗) (**i**)

53.3 Neuropathology Findings

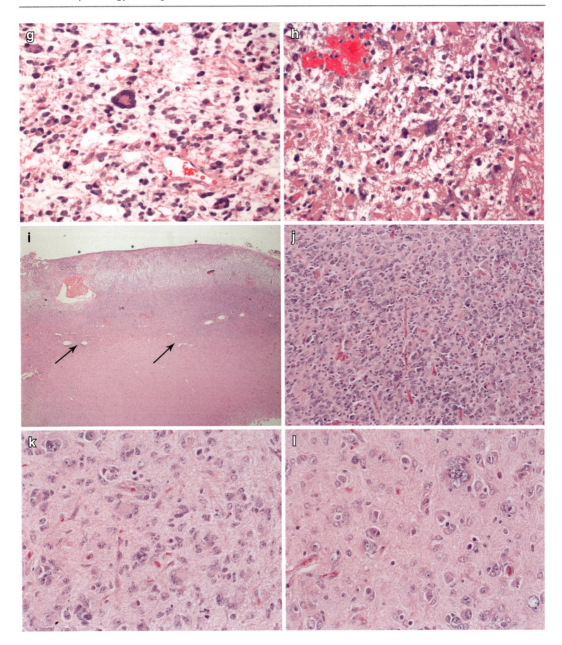

Fig. 53.4 (continued)

- Presence of multinucleated tumor cells possible
- Presence of abnormal mitoses possible
- Absence of microvascular proliferation
- Absence of necroses

Immunophenotype (Fig. 53.5a–j)
- IDH-1 R123H mutation-specific antibody

– Reactivity seen in 44–69%
– Expressed in the nucleus
– Expressed in the cytoplasm
– Differentiates tumor tissue from surrounding non-neoplastic tissue and/or reactive astrogliosis
– Full assessment of IDH mutation status in anaplastic astrocytomas involves sequence analy-

sis for IDH1 codon 132 and IDH2 codon 172 mutations in cases that are immunohistochemically negative for the IDH1 R132H-mutation
- Glial fibrillary acidic protein (GFAP)
  - Expressed at variable degree
  - In the cellular processes
  - Often as a perinuclear rim
  - GFAP-positive fibrillary matrix
- S-100
  - Expressed in the nucleus
  - Expressed in cell processes
- Vimentin
  - Pattern similar to GFAP
  - Seen mainly in the perinuclear region

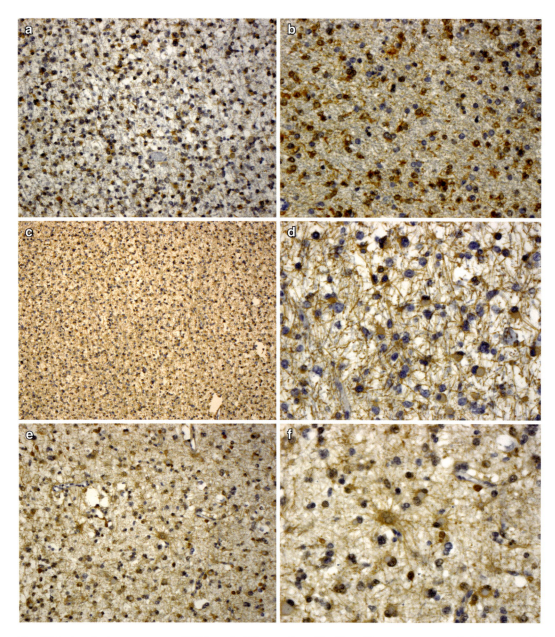

Fig. 53.5 Anaplastic astrocytoma (WHO grade III)—Immunophenotype: IDH1 R123H (**a**, **b**), GFAP (**c**, **d**), S100 (**e**, **f**), p53 (**g**, **h**). Infiltrative zone of cerebral cortex shows NeuN-positive neurons surrounded by tumor cells (**i**, **j**). Moderate Ki-67 proliferation rate (**k**, **l**)

53.3 Neuropathology Findings

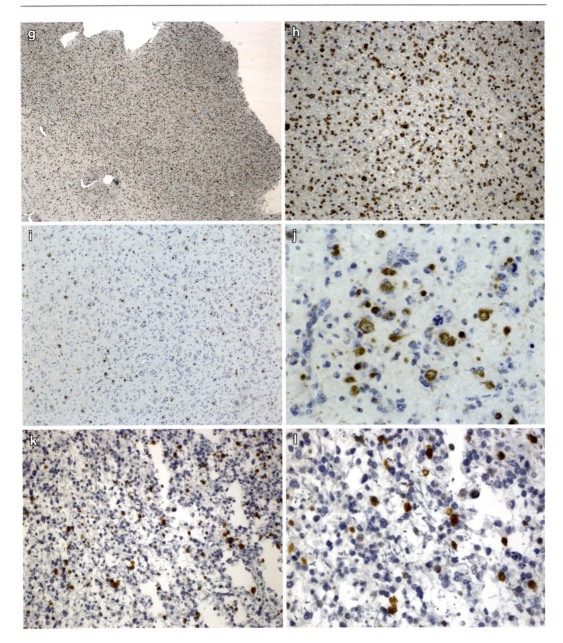

Fig. 53.5 (continued)

- ß-crystallin
  - Same reactivity pattern as S-100
- P53
  - Frequent in gemistocytic astrocytoma
- Bcl-2
  - Frequent in gemistocytic astrocytoma

Proliferation Markers (Fig. 53.5k, l)
- Mitotic activity present
- Ki-67 LI: 5–10%

Ultrastructural Features
- Presence of glial intermediate filaments (7–11 nm in diameter) in the perikaryon and cell processes in variable amount
- Reduced extracellular space
- Large nuclei with irregular outline
- Prominent nucleolus
- Presence of mitotic figures
- Scant perinuclear cytoplasm
- Sparse organelles
- Abundant polyribosomes

Differential Diagnosis
- Astrocytoma WHO grade II
- Glioblastoma WHO grade IV
- The presence of a component morphologically resembling oligodendroglioma is compatible with the diagnosis of AA in the absence of 1p/19q co-deletion

53.4 Molecular Neuropathology

Pathogenesis
- Derived from precursor cells committed to astrocytic differentiation
- Evolution from astrocytoma WHO grade II
- De novo without an identifiable precursor lesion
- Anaplastic astrocytomas frequently evolve from diffuse astrocytomas (WHO grade II) and eventually progress further to secondary glioblastomas (WHO grade IV). Accordingly, the genetic background of anaplastic astrocytomas includes features that are also found in astrocytic tumors of both WHO grades II and IV (see Chaps. 52 and 54).

IDH-wild-type anaplastic astrocytoma

- Uncommon
- accounts for about 20% of all anaplastic astrocytomas
- have the highest incidence of wild-type IDH1 and IDH2 among the WHO grade II and III diffuse glioma variants

Genetic aberrations observed in anaplastic astrocytoma WHO grade III include:

- Point mutation in the *IDH1* (isocitrate dehydrogenase 1) gene (up to 80% of cases)
- Mutations in ATRX (63% of cases)
- Absence of 1p/19q co-deletion
- Gains of chromosome 7
- Losses of chromosome 17p
- Mutations in the tumor suppressor gene *TP53* (tumor protein 53) (82% of cases)
- Loss of heterozygosity (LOH) on chromosomes 6q, 11p, 19q, and 22q

Table 53.1 Changed gene expression between anaplastic astrocytoma and glioblastoma, modified after Rao et al. (2014) reproduced with kind permission by Public Library of Science, open access

Gene symbol	Gene name	Fold change
CDKN3	Cyclin-dependent kinase inhibitor 3	2.0
CHI3L1	Chitinase 3-like 1	5.5
COL4	Collagen, type IV	3.5
DCN	Decorin	2.7
DLL3	Delta-like 3 protein precursor; delta homolog	−4.3
FABP7	Fatty acid binding protein 7	3.1
IGFBP2	Insulin-like growth factor binding protein 2	3.4
IGFBP3	Insulin-like growth factor binding protein 3	2.6
LAMB1	Laminin, beta 1	2.2
LGALS1	Lectin, galactoside-binding, soluble, 1	2.4
LGALS3	Lectin, galactoside-binding, soluble, 3	2.7
PBEF1	Pre-B-cell colony enhancing factor 1	2.1
PLAT	Plasminogen activator, tissue	2.2
PTTG1	Pituitary tumor transforming 1	2.1
TIMP1	Tissue inhibitor of metalloproteinase 1	4.0
TOP2A	Topoisomerase (DNA) II alpha	2.2

- Deletions of the chromosome 9p21 region carrying the tumor suppressor genes
- *CDKN2A* (cyclin-dependent kinase inhibitor 2A)
- *CDKN2B* (cyclin-dependent kinase inhibitor 2B)
- Mutations in the *RB1* gene (retinoblastoma 1) (~25% of cases)
- Mutations in Notch pathway genes (*NOTCH1, NOTCH2, NOTCH4, NOTCH2NL*), including a recurrent *NOTCH1*-A465T mutation (31% of cases)

The extent of changed gene expression between anaplastic astrocytoma and glioblastoma is given in Table 53.1.

53.5 Treatment and Prognosis

Treatment
- Surgery
- Radiotherapy
- Chemotherapy

Biologic Behavior–Prognosis–Prognostic Factors
- Median survival: 4–6 years
- Strong tendency to progress to IDH-mutant glioblastoma within 2 years
- Increasing age is a negative factor
- EGFR-amplification leads to shorter survival
- Anaplastic astrocytoma without IDH mutation
    - Share molecular features with IDH-wild-type glioblastoma
    - Share molecular features with H3 K27M-mutant gliomas if located preferentially in midline locations
    - Tumors in this category are clinically more aggressive than are IDH-mutant anaplastic astrocytomas and may follow a clinical course more similar to that of glioblastoma

Selected References

Barker CA, Chang M, Beal K, Chan TA (2014) Survival of patients treated with radiation therapy for anaplastic astrocytoma. Radiol Oncol 48(4):381–386. https://doi.org/10.2478/raon-2014-0019

Butowski NA, Sneed PK, Chang SM (2006) Diagnosis and treatment of recurrent high-grade astrocytoma. J Clin Oncol 24(8):1273–1280. https://doi.org/10.1200/jco.2005.04.7522

Chow LM, Baker SJ (2012) Capturing the molecular and biological diversity of high-grade astrocytoma in genetically engineered mouse models. Oncotarget 3(1):67–77. https://doi.org/10.18632/oncotarget.425

von Deimling A, Huse JT, Yan H, Brat DJ, Ohgaki H, Kleihues P, Berger MS, Weller M, Burger PC, Ellison DW, Rosenblum MK, Reifenberger G, Paulus W, Wesseling P, Aldape KD, Louis DN (2016) Anaplastic astrocytoma, IDH-mutant. In: Louis DN, Ohgaki H, Wiestler OD, Cavenee WK (eds) WHO classification of tumours of the central nervous system, revised 4th edn. IARC, Lyon, pp 24–27

Grimm SA, Chamberlain MC (2016) Anaplastic astrocytoma. CNS Oncol 5(3):145–157. https://doi.org/10.2217/cns-2016-0002

Grimm SA, Pfiffner TJ (2013) Anaplastic astrocytoma. Curr Treat Options Neurol 15(3):302–315. https://doi.org/10.1007/s11940-013-0228-7

Hollingworth W, Medina LS, Lenkinski RE, Shibata DK, Bernal B, Zurakowski D, Comstock B, Jarvik JG (2006) A systematic literature review of magnetic resonance spectroscopy for the characterization of brain tumors. AJNR Am J Neuroradiol 27(7):1404–1411

Jellison BJ, Field AS, Medow J, Lazar M, Salamat MS, Alexander AL (2004) Diffusion tensor imaging of cerebral white matter: a pictorial review of physics, fiber tract anatomy, and tumor imaging patterns. AJNR Am J Neuroradiol 25(3):356–369

Johnson DR, Galanis E (2014) Medical management of high-grade astrocytoma: current and emerging therapies. Semin Oncol 41(4):511–522. https://doi.org/10.1053/j.seminoncol.2014.06.010

Killela PJ, Pirozzi CJ, Reitman ZJ, Jones S, Rasheed BA, Lipp E, Friedman H, Friedman AH, He Y, McLendon RE, Bigner DD, Yan H (2014) The genetic landscape of anaplastic astrocytoma. Oncotarget 5(6):1452–1457. https://doi.org/10.18632/oncotarget.1505

Kleihues P, Burger PC, Scheithauer BW (1993) Histological typing of tumours of the central nervous system, 2nd edn. Springer-Verlag, Berlin

Kleihues P, Davis RL, Coons SW, Burger PC (2000) Anaplastic astrocytoma. In: Kleihues P, Cavenee WK (eds) Pathology and genetics of tumours of the nervous system, 3rd edn. IARC Press, Lyon, pp 27–28

Kleihues P, Burger PC, Rosenblum MK, Paulus W, Scheithauer BW (2007) Anaplastic astrocytoma. In: Louis DN, Ohgaki H, Wiestler OD, Cavenee WK (eds) WHO classification of tumours of the central nervous system, 4th edn. International Agency for Research on Cancer, Lyon, pp 30–32

Law M, Yang S, Wang H, Babb JS, Johnson G, Cha S, Knopp EA, Zagzag D (2003) Glioma grading: sensitivity, specificity, and predictive values of perfusion MR imaging and proton MR spectroscopic imaging compared with conventional MR imaging. AJNR Am J Neuroradiol 24(10):1989–1998

Lee EJ, Lee SK, Agid R, Bae JM, Keller A, Terbrugge K (2008) Preoperative grading of presumptive low-grade astrocytomas on MR imaging: diagnostic value of minimum apparent diffusion coefficient. AJNR Am J Neuroradiol 29(10):1872–1877. https://doi.org/10.3174/ajnr.A1254

Llaguno SA, Chen J, Kwon CH, Parada LF (2008) Neural and cancer stem cells in tumor suppressor mouse models of malignant astrocytoma. Cold Spring Harb Symp Quant Biol 73:421–426. https://doi.org/10.1101/sqb.2008.73.005

Minniti G, Scaringi C, Arcella A, Lanzetta G, Di Stefano D, Scarpino S, Bozzao A, Pace A, Villani V, Salvati M, Esposito V, Giangaspero F, Enrici RM (2014) IDH1 mutation and MGMT methylation status predict survival in patients with anaplastic astrocytoma treated with temozolomide-based chemoradiotherapy. J Neurooncol 118(2):377–383. https://doi.org/10.1007/s11060-014-1443-0

Nano R, Capelli E, Facoetti A, Benericetti E (2009) Immunobiological and experimental aspects of malignant astrocytoma. Anticancer Res 29(7):2461–2465

Rao SA, Srinivasan S, Patric IR, Hegde AS, Chandramouli BA, Arimappamagan A, Santosh V, Kondaiah P, Rao MR, Somasundaram K (2014) A 16-gene signature distinguishes anaplastic astrocytoma from glioblastoma. PLoS One 9(1):e85200. https://doi.org/10.1371/journal.pone.0085200

Reardon DA, Rich JN, Friedman HS, Bigner DD (2006) Recent advances in the treatment of malignant astrocytoma. J Clin Oncol 24(8):1253–1265. https://doi.org/10.1200/jco.2005.04.5302

Riemenschneider MJ, Reifenberger G (2009) Astrocytic tumors. In: von Deimling A (ed) Gliomas, Recent results in cancer research, vol 171. Springer, Berlin, Heidelberg, pp 3–24

Sarkar C, Jain A, Suri V (2009) Current concepts in the pathology and genetics of gliomas. Indian J Cancer 46(2):108–119

Sathornsumetee S, Rich JN, Reardon DA (2007) Diagnosis and treatment of high-grade astrocytoma. Neurol Clin 25(4):1111–1139, x. https://doi.org/10.1016/j.ncl.2007.07.004

Schiff D (2017) Benefit with adjuvant chemotherapy in anaplastic astrocytoma. Lancet. https://doi.org/10.1016/s0140-6736(17)31477-0

Scoccianti S, Magrini SM, Ricardi U, Detti B, Krengli M, Parisi S, Bertoni F, Sotti G, Cipressi S, Tombolini V, Dall'oglio S, Lioce M, Saieva C, Buglione M, Mantovani C, Rubino G, Muto P, Fusco V, Fariselli L, de Renzis C, Masini L, Santoni R, Pirtoli L, Biti G (2012) Radiotherapy and temozolomide in anaplastic astrocytoma: a retrospective multicenter study by the Central Nervous System Study Group of AIRO (Italian Association of Radiation Oncology). Neuro Oncol 14(6):798–807. https://doi.org/10.1093/neuonc/nos081

See SJ, Gilbert MR (2004) Anaplastic astrocytoma: diagnosis, prognosis, and management. Semin Oncol 31(5):618–634

Shin JY, Diaz AZ (2016) Anaplastic astrocytoma: prognostic factors and survival in 4807 patients with emphasis on receipt and impact of adjuvant therapy. J Neurooncol 129(3):557–565. https://doi.org/10.1007/s11060-016-2210-1

Stupp R, Reni M, Gatta G, Mazza E, Vecht C (2007) Anaplastic astrocytoma in adults. Crit Rev Oncol Hematol 63(1):72–80. https://doi.org/10.1016/j.critrevonc.2007.03.003

Tabatabai G, Stupp R, Wick W, Weller M (2013) Malignant astrocytoma in elderly patients: where do we stand? Curr Opin Neurol 26(6):693–700. https://doi.org/10.1097/wco.0000000000000037

Ushio Y, Tada K, Shiraishi S, Kamiryo T, Shinojima N, Kochi M, Saya H (2003) Correlation of molecular genetic analysis of p53, MDM2, p16, PTEN, and EGFR and survival of patients with anaplastic astrocytoma and glioblastoma. Front Biosci 8:e281–e288

Xue L, Xu Z, Wang K, Wang N, Zhang X, Wang S (2016) Network analysis of microRNAs, transcription factors, target genes and host genes in human anaplastic astrocytoma. Exp Ther Med 12(1):437–444. https://doi.org/10.3892/etm.2016.3272

Zülch KJ (1979) Histological typing of tumours of the central nervous system. World Health Organization, Geneva

Glioblastoma

Diffuse Astrocytic and Oligodendroglial Tumors

WHO Definition

2016 – Glioblastoma, IDH-wildtype: A high-grade glioma with predominantly astrocytic differentiation; featuring nuclear atypia, cellular pleomorphism (in most cases), mitotic activity, and typically a diffuse growth pattern, as well as microvascular proliferation and/or necrosis; and which lacks mutations in the IDH genes (Louis et al. 2016).

Epithelioid glioblastoma: A high-grade diffuse astrocytic tumour variant with a dominant population of closely packed epithelioid cells, some rhabdoid cells, mitotic activity, microvascular proliferation, and necrosis (Ellison et al. 2016).

Glioblastoma, IDH-mutant: A high-grade glioma with predominantly astrocytic differentiation; featuring nuclear atypia, cellular pleomorphism (in most cases), mitotic activity, and typically a diffuse growth pattern, as well as microvascular proliferation and/or necrosis; with a mutation in either the IDH1 or IDH2 gene (Ohgaki et al. 2016).

Glioblastoma, NOS: A high-grade glioma with predominantly astrocytic differentiation; featuring nuclear atypia, cellular pleomorphism (in most cases), mitotic activity, and typically a diffuse growth pattern, as well as microvascular proliferation and/or necrosis; in which IDH mutation status has not been fully assessed (Ohgaki et al. 2016).

2007 - The most frequent primary brain tumor and the most malignant neoplasm with predominant astrocytic differentiation; histopathological features include nuclear atypia, cellular pleomorphism, mitotic activity, vascular thrombosis, microvascular proliferation and necrosis (Kleihues et al. 2007).

2000 - Glioblastoma is the most malignant astrocytic tumour, composed of poorly differentiated neoplastic astrocytes. Histopathological features include cellular polymorphism, nuclear atypia, brisk mitotic activity, vascular thrombosis, microvascular proliferation and necrosis. Glioblastoma typically affects adults and is preferentially located in the cerebral hemispheres. Glioblastomas may develop from diffuse astrocytomas WHO grade II or anaplastic astrocytomas ('secondary glioblastoma'), but more frequently, they manifest after a short clinical history *de novo,* without evidence of a less malignant precursor lesion ('primary glioblastoma') (Kleihues et al. 2000).

1993 - An anaplastic, often cellular brain tumor composed of poorly differentiated, fusiform, round or pleomorphic cells and occasional multinucleated giant cells. Essential for the histological diagnosis is the presence of prominent vascular proliferation and/or necrosis (Kleihues et al. 1993).

1979 - An anaplastic, highly cellular tumour consisting of fusiform cells, small poorly differentiated round cells, or pleomorphic cells alone or in varying combinations. Necrosis, pseudopalissading, fistulous vessels and vascular endothelial proliferation, haemorrhage, and invasive growth are usually prominent features. Some of the cells demonstrate slender glial processes (Zülch 1979).

WHO grade
- WHO grade IV

Glioblastoma or glioblastoma multiforme (GBM) is a highly malignant neuroectodermal tumor composed of densely packed, anaplastic, and highly dedifferentiated tumor cells making the histogenetic typing difficult.

The following two types of GBM are distinguished:

- Primary GBM: de novo manifestation without recognizable precursor lesion
- Secondary GBM: develops slowly from diffuse astrocytoma (WHO grade II) or anaplastic astrocytoma (WHO grade III) → malignant progression

54.1 Epidemiology

Incidence
- the most frequent tumor of the CNS
- represents approximately 20-30% of all primary tumors of the CNS
- represents approximately 50-60% of all gliomas
- 3-4 new cases per 100,000 population per year

Age Incidence
- affects predominantly persons between 40-80 years of age
- mean age: 60-65 years
- In children, 6.5% of primary tumors are GBMs

Sex Incidence
- Male:Female ratio: 2:1 to 3:2
- 50-65% of the affected population are male

Localisation
- All regions of the brain and spinal cord are susceptible
- A preferential involvement of the telencephalon is noted
- The white matter is characteristically involved.
- The following list gives an average incidence of the involved brain regions:
  - temporal 38 %
  - frontal 24 %
  - fronto-parieto-temporal 14 %
  - temporo-parieto-occipital 11 %
  - parietal 9 %
  - occipital 4 %
  - cerebellum 0.2 %
- combined fronto-temporal location is quite typical

54.2 Neuroimaging Findings

General Imaging Findings
- Irregular, heterogeneous, ring enhancing mass of variable size with central necrosis and surrounding vasogenic edema

CT non-contrast-enhanced (Figs. 54.1a and 54.2a)
- Lobulated, irregular tumor, hypo- or isodense
- Hypodense necrosis and hyperdense hemorrhage are common
- Large area of perifocal hypodensity representing edema
- Occasional calcifications

CT contrast-enhanced (Fig. 54.1b)
- Irregular, thick, ring-like enhancement
- Rarely patchy or homogeneous enhancement

MRI - T2 (Fig. 54.2c, d)
- Hyperintense lesion
- Tumor tissue cannot be well differentiated from surrounding edema
- Flow voids representing neovascularity are rare

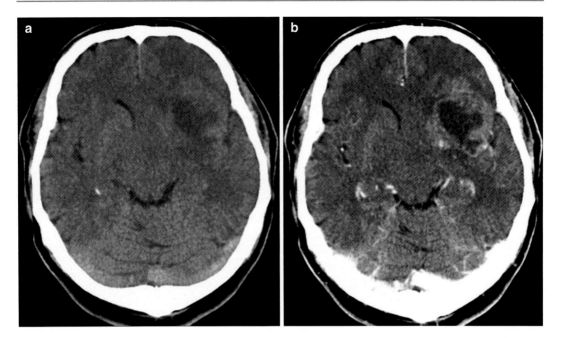

Fig. 54.1 CT-scan. Axial CT showing a left temporal mass with necrotic core (**a**) and irregular peripheral enhancement (**b**)

MRI - FLAIR (Figs. 54.3a, 54.4a, 54.5c, d, 54.6a, and 54.7a, b)
- Irregular, hyperintense mass consisting of tumor tissue, tumor infiltration and large surrounding edema

MRI - T1 (Figs. 54.2b and 54.3b)
- Heterogeneous iso- or hyperintense mass with hypointense core due to necrosis
- Common subacute hemorrhages appear hyperintense

MRI - T1 contrast-enhanced (Figs. 54.2d, 54.3c, 54.4b, 54.5a, b, e, 54.6b, and 54.7c, d)
- Irregular, occasionally nodular, ring-like pattern
- Variations of solid, multifocal enhancement possible

MRI - T2∗/SWI
- Reveals intratumoral hemorrhage

MRI - Diffusion Imaging (Fig. 54.6c)
- No restricted diffusion
- ADC values reduced and lower than in low grade gliomas
- High signal in ADC map is related to surrounding edema

MRI - Perfusion (Fig. 54.3d)
- Elevated rCBV
- Related permeability tends to increase with tumor grade

MRI - Diffusion Tensor Imaging (Fig. 54.6d, e)
- Increased FA – values may help assess tumor grade
- Larger peritumoral abnormalities may indicate high grade glioma

MR - Spectroscopy (Figs. 54.4c and 54.8)
- Elevated peaks of choline, lactate, lipid and myoinositol
- Reduced NAA peak

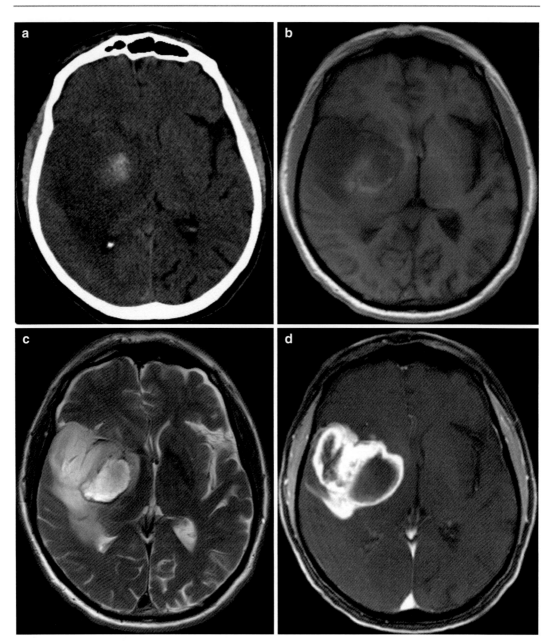

Fig. 54.2 Hemorrhagic GBM: Axial CT shows a right temporal hemorrhage with surrounding mass effect and midline shift (**a**). Subacute bleedings are demonstrated with a slightly hyperintense ring on T1 related to the deposition of methemoglobin (**b**). The dark ring on T2 demonstrates hemosiderin deposits (**c**) at the border of the necrotic core surrounded by solid contrast-enhanced tumor formations (**d**)

54.2 Neuroimaging Findings

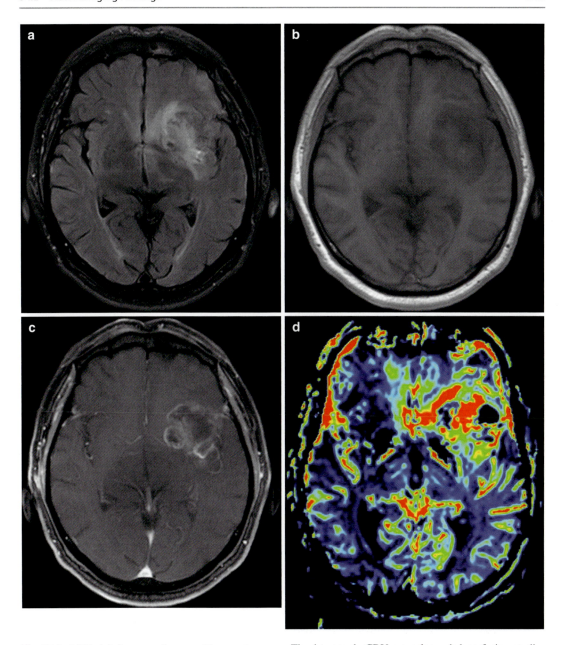

Fig. 54.3 MRI: A left temporal mass with necrotic core and irregular peripheral enhancement. The lesion is hyperintense on FLAIR (**a**), iso- to hypointense on T1 (**b**). The increased rCBV on color-coded perfusion studies correlates with contrast-enhanced tumor areas (**c**, **d**)

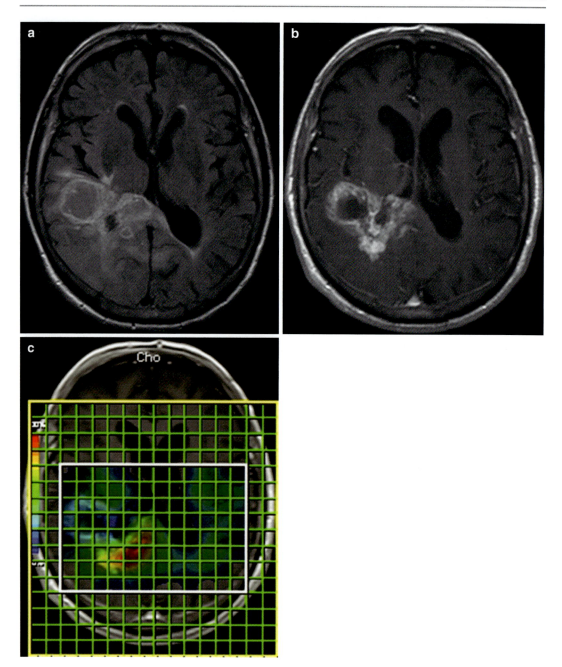

Fig. 54.4 MRI: FLAIR and T1-contrast demonstrate a right hemispheric glioblastoma infiltrating the splenium of the corpus callosum (**a**, **b**). Elevated choline values are shown with MR-Spectroscopy in choline mapping (**c**)

Fig. 54.5 Multifocal GBM: Axial (**a**, **b**) and sagittal (**e**) T1-contrast enhanced images display a case of multifocal glioblastoma connected by a large hyperintensive area due to diffuse tumor infiltration/ edema as seen on FLAIR images (**c**, **d**)

54.2 Neuroimaging Findings

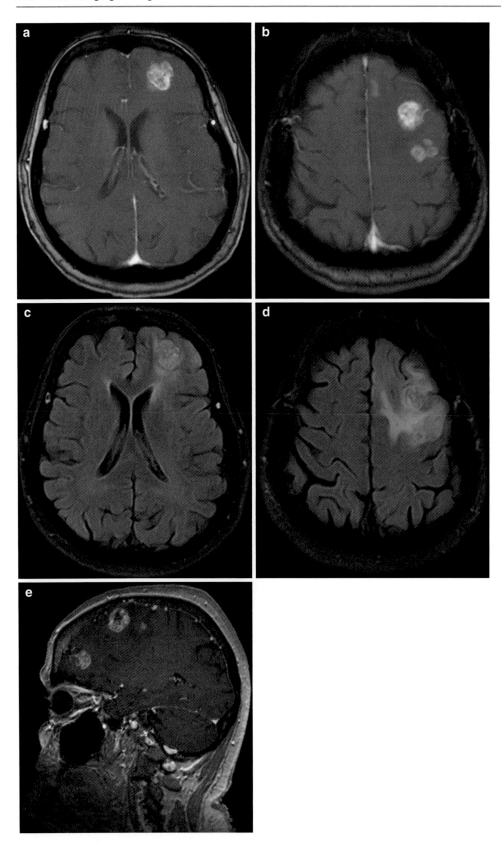

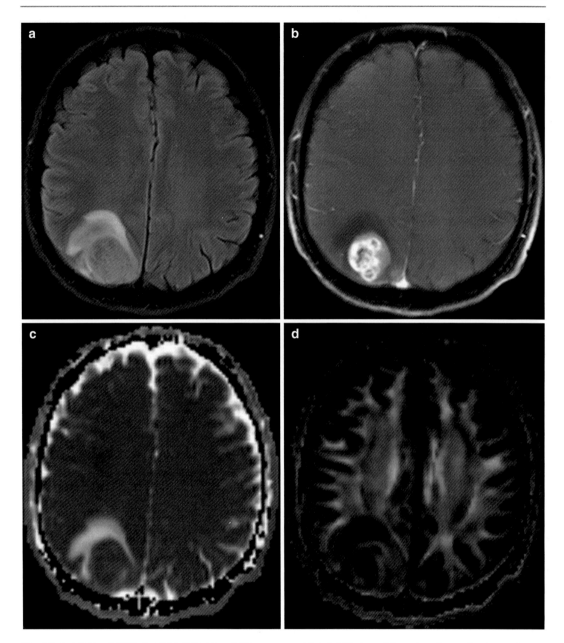

Fig. 54.6 ADC and DTI: Axial FLAIR (**a**) and T1 contrast (**b**) demonstrate a well-defined occipital lobe mass. The low signal intensity on the ADC map (**c**) due to restricted diffusion of the enhancing region inversely correlates with higher cellularity. Elevated FA-values are shown with DTI (**d, e**)

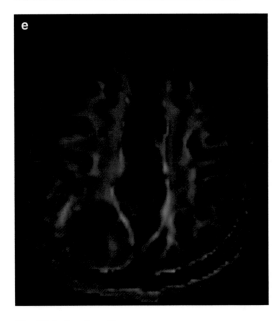

Fig. 54.6 (continued)

Nuclear Medicine Imaging Findings
(Figs. 54.9, 54.10, 54.11, 54.12, and 54.13)
- Historically gliomas were addressed by 201Thallium or 99Technetium-MIBI SPECT
- PET/CT is the modality of choice to:
  - monitor the biological behavior of gliomas
  - identify the most metabolic region to be chosen as the biopsy site
  - determine the gross tumor volume for radiation planning
  - differentiate post-radiogenic pseudo-progression from tumor progression
  - monitor the biological effect during therapy
  - monitor the biological behavior of the tumor after therapy
  - diagnosis of a relapse

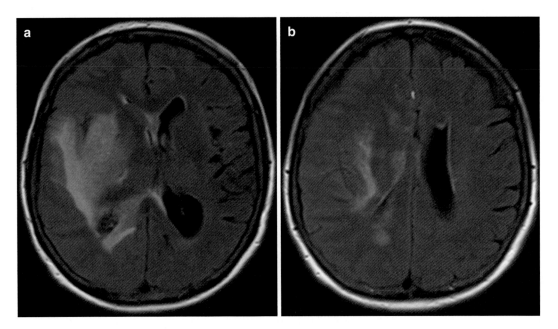

Fig. 54.7 Intraventricular GBM: FLAIR (**a**, **b**) and T1-contrast (**c**, **d**) show an enhancing tumor with a cystic component, peritumoral edema, and intraventricular spreading

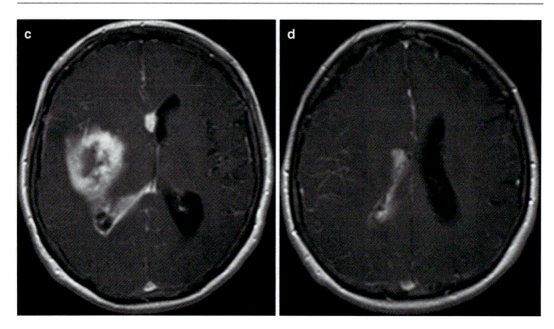

Fig. 54.7 (continued)

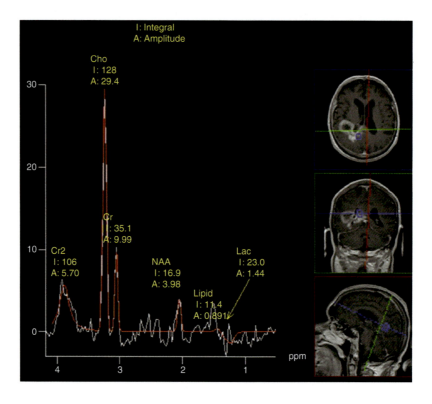

Fig. 54.8 MRS: MR spectroscopy (135 msec) shows an elevation of the choline (Cho) peak and a decreased peak for NAA. At 135 msec the lactate peak is inverted.

54.2 Neuroimaging Findings

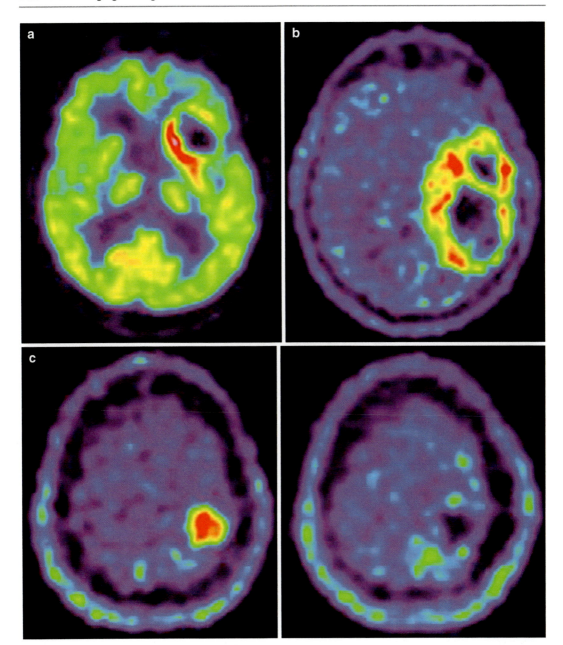

Fig. 54.9 PET-scans: FDG - PET of a glioblastoma left frontal and striatal with central necrosis and the metabolic most active part of the tumor in the striatal area. Note the relatively high uptake in the healthy gray matter (**a**). FET - PET of a huge left hemispheric glioblastoma with two necrotic zones and heterogeneous biological behavior (**b**). FET - PET of a glioblastoma in the left parietal lobe before (left) and after (right) surgery (**c**). MRI, FET - PET (D1) and fused MRI/FET - PET (D2) of a glioblastoma of the splenium of the corpus callosum bulging into the ventricle (**d**), Fusion of MRI and FET-PET (**e**)

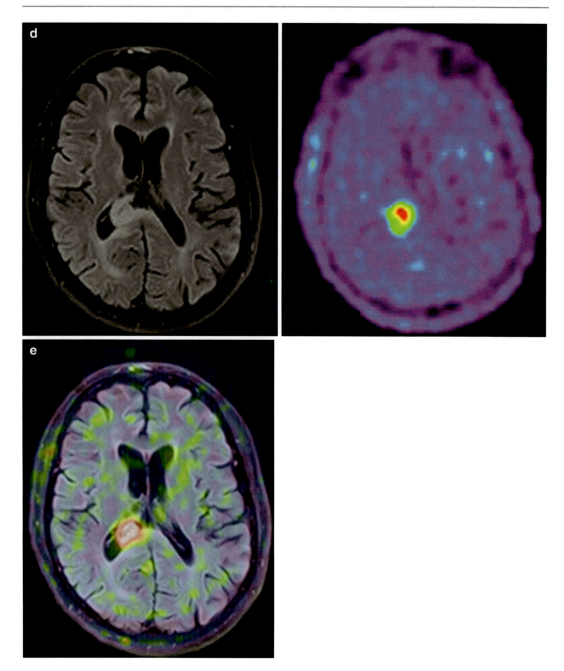

Fig. 54.9 (continued)

- GBMs are normally FDG-avid (CAVE: the normal gray matter of the cortex, the striatum and the thalamus take up FDG due to their normal glucose-based metabolism)
- Results obtained for MET are similar to FET
  - the advantage of FET is that it is taken up in a lesser amount by inflammatory tissue and its longer half-life of 110 minutes as compared to a relatively short half-life of 20 minutes of C-11 used in MET
- Images can show homogeneous or heterogeneous uptake representing the tumour biology
- SUV (calculated as ratio of the concentration of the radiotracer corrected by the body weight of the patient) can predict therapeutic outcomes

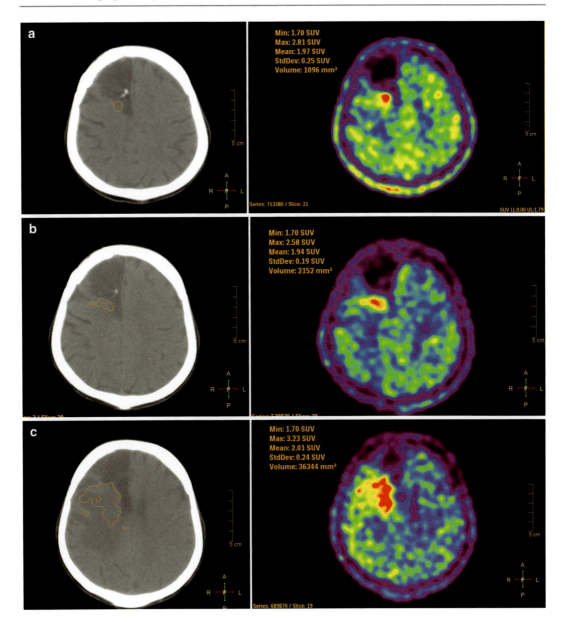

Fig. 54.10 PET-scan. Course of the patient with glioblastoma: shortly after surgery (**a**), 6 months after surgery (**b**), and 1 year after surgery (**c**)

- Results obtained for MET are similar to FET with the advantage of FET to be taken up in a lesser amount in inflammatory tissue and the longer half-life of 110 minutes compared to a relatively short half-life of 20 minutes of C-11 used in MET
- Dynamic FET - PET enables the measurement of the tracer kinetic
- Possibility of non-invasive tumour grading is being discussed (especially in dynamic FET - PET studies)
- Sensitivity of FET - PET for glioblastoma is about 95% (gliomatosis cerebri can be false negative)
- Possible influence of bevacicumab therapy has to be considered
- Hypoxia-PET tracers like 18F-FMISO and perfusion PET tracers like 15O-H_2O are under investigation for their utility in predicting treatment response

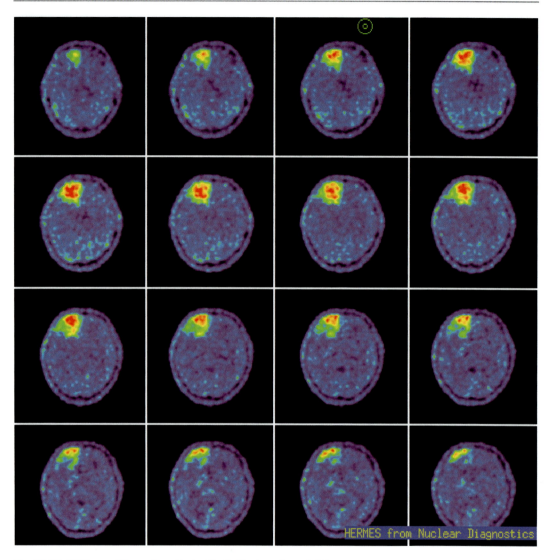

Fig. 54.11 PET scan. Slices of a patient with glioblastoma frontal right.

54.3 Neuropathology Findings

Macroscopic Features (Figs. 54.14a–f and 54.15a–h)
- Intraoperative features:
  - The exposed surface of the brain does not necessarily display broadened gyri and narrowed sulci.
  - While approaching the lesion, the color of the tissue changes into glistening blue-gray.
  - The tumor is very soft, showing areas of necroses as well as thrombosed vessels.
- The tumor shows all in all a variegated appearance.
- Tumors of large size
- Involves several lobes
- Tumors spread to the contralateral hemisphere through the corpus callosum displaying a symmetrical tumor growth into both hemispheres, i.e. butterfly GBM.
- Multiplicity is defined as the widely separated localisation of the tumor in different lobes or even different hemispheres. Multiple locations of tumor growth are rare and are found in 2-5% of cerebral GBM.

54.3 Neuropathology Findings

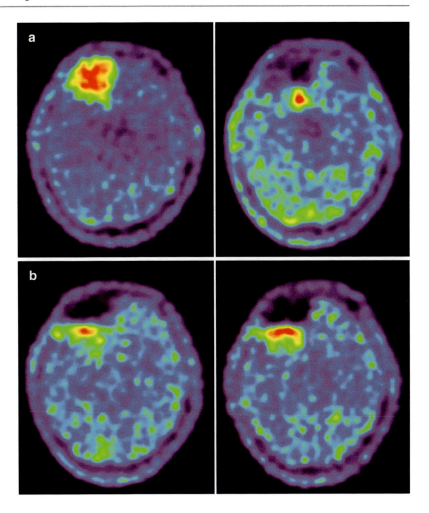

Fig. 54.12 PET scan showing the course of a patient before (**a**) and after resection (**b**) and combined radio-chemotherapy from March to December

- Grossly, the brain shows broadened and flattened gyri.
- An infiltration of the meninges by the tumor is possible and is reflected by the opacity of the leptomeninges and/or its attachment to the dura.
- Invasion of the tumor into the ventricles can be observed.
- The tumor is usually not sharply demarcated presenting with a broad and diffuse zone of infiltration.
- The cut surface characteristically shows a vari-colored appearance ranging from grey, brown, white, yellow to dark red.
- The consistency of the irregular outer zone is often firmer due to astrocytic growth.
- Necroses are found in about 25%. They can be large and make up as much as 80% of the tumor mass.
- The red appearance of certain areas of the tumor is mainly due to diapedesis. These hemorrhagic areas might be large.
- Cysts may be present.

A correlation of neuropathological features with CT findings is shown in Table 54.1.

Microscopic Features (Figs. 54.6a–f, 54.16a–r, 54.17a–d, 54.18a–d, 54.19a, f, and 54.20a–h)

- A high diversity of cell forms is encountered in glioblastoma, thus, the former term of "glioblastoma multiforme".

A high variability of pathological features are found and encompass:

- Anaplastic cells displaying astrocytic features
- Neoplastic oligodendroglia

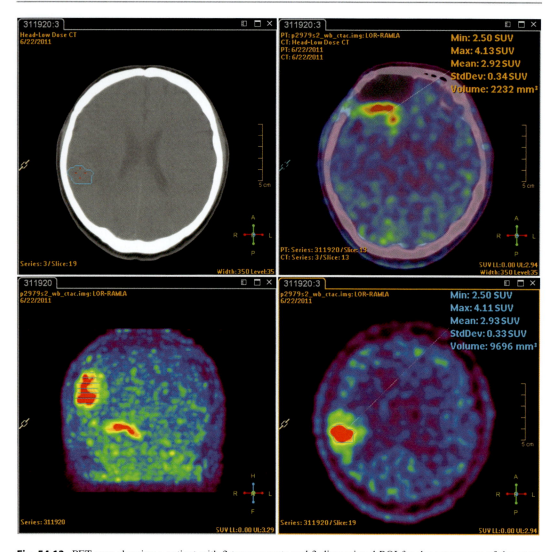

Fig. 54.13 PET scan showing a patient with 2 tumour parts and 3-dimensional ROI for the assessment of the gross tumor volume and the maximum SUV

- High density of small, poorly differentiated cells
- Marked polymorphism of tumor cells including multinucleated giant cells
- Areas showing cells with astrocytic, oligodendroglial, and rarely ependymal differentiation
- Atypical mitoses are often present
- Vascular endothelial cell proliferation
- Typical tumor necroses, i.e. palisading with cells arranged side by side in rows and their processes directed towards a central area of necrosis
- Large areas of necroses

Based on the predominant features, a classification into the following types can be done but is of no clinical significance or prognostic relevance:

- GBM multiforme type or classical type:
  - composed of areas displaying heterogeneous features and anaplastic areas with pleomorphic cells
- Small cell GBM:
  - composed of uniform small, densely packed, and hyperchromatic cells many with perinuclear halo. High number of mitoses can be found.

54.3 Neuropathology Findings

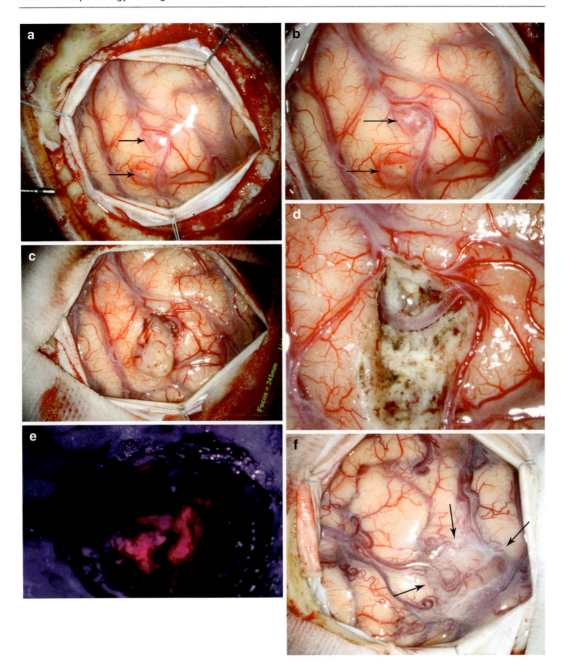

Fig. 54.14 Intraoperative features show straightened vessels (veins) and two suspicious areas characterized by color discoloration (→) (**a**, **b**). After incision of the cortex the tumor becomes evident as a whitish-greyish colored mass (**c**). The tumor bed is shown after removal of the mass (**d**). The tumor lights up in red under fluorescence after ALA administration prior to surgery (**e**). The vessels of the cortical surfaced might appear tortuous (**f**)

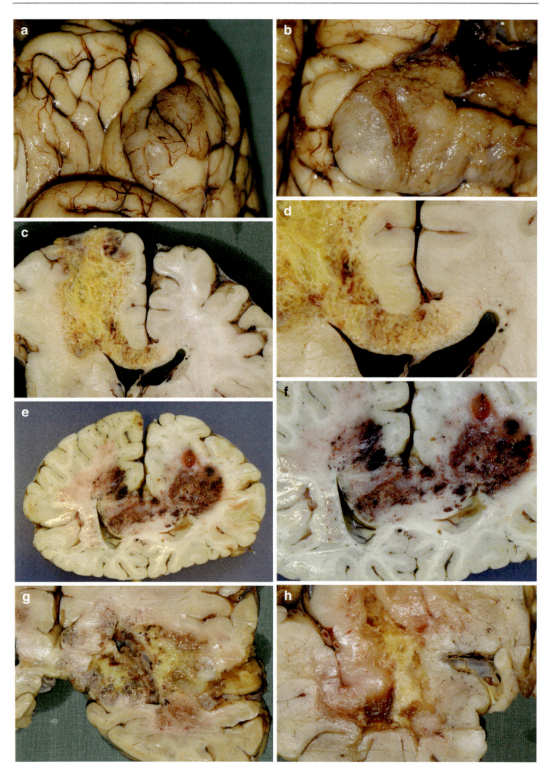

Fig. 54.15 Macroscopic appearance (autopsy material). Tumor involving the left lateral fronto-orbital region (**a**) displayed by roughened irregular surface (**b**). Butterfly GBM originates in the left frontal lobe and crosses the midline via the corpus callosum (**c, d**). Hemorrhagic butterfly GBM (**e, f**). GBM of the temporal lobe displays vari-colored appearance, blurred borders, and central necrosis (**g, h**)

54.3 Neuropathology Findings

Table 54.1 Correlation of neuropathological features with CT findings

Neuropathology features	CT features
central area of necrosis	region of low density
surrounding hypercellular zone	rim with marked contrast enhancement
outer region of peripheral tumor infiltration	perilesional zone of low density

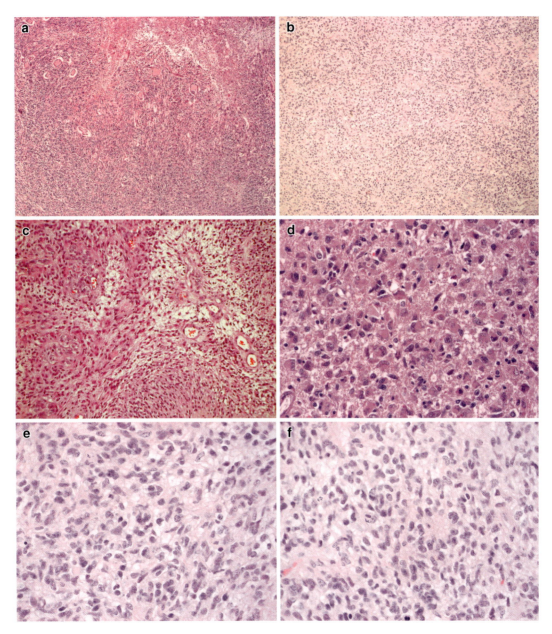

Fig. 54.16 Histologic appearance. GBM composed of high cellular areas (**a**, **b**) paucicellular areas (**c**) with astrocytic-like tumor highly pleomorphic cells (**d**), densely packed round cells (**e**, **f**), cells with oligodendroglia-like appearance (**g**), multinucleated giant cell (**h**), fibrillar appearing astrocytic-like tumor cells (**i**), two mitotic figures (**j**), gemistocytic astrocytes (**k**, **l**), epitheloid-like tumor cells (**m**, **n**), undifferentiated small cells partly grouped in nests, i.e. PNET-like islands (**o**, **p**). GBM with small cell component (**q**, **r**). Stain: H&E

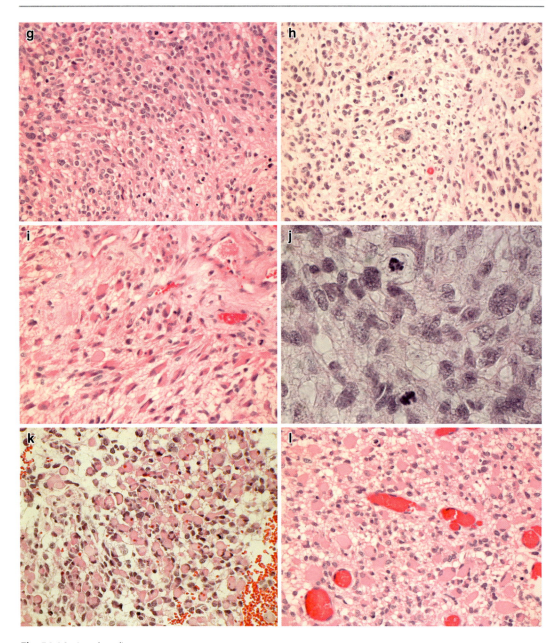

Fig. 54.16 (continued)

54.3 Neuropathology Findings

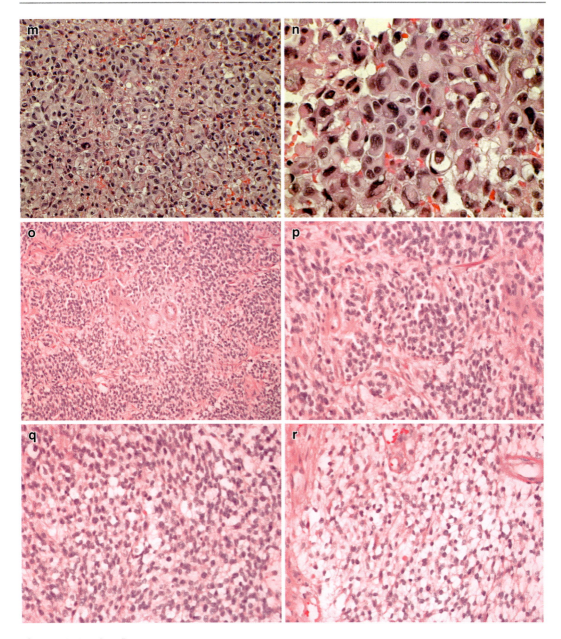

Fig. 54.16 (continued)

- GBM with primitive neuronal component:
  - contain foci with PNET-like tumor cells
- GBM with oligodendroglioma component:
  - contain foci with oligodendroglioma-like tumor cells
- Granular cell glioblastoma:
  - contain large cells with a granular, periodic acid-Schiff (PAS)-positive cytoplasm
- Lipidized GBM:
  - contain tumor cells with foamy cytoplasm
- Adenoid GBM:
  - focal gland-like architecture
- Giant cell glioblastoma (see Chap. 55):
  - numerous giant cells
- Gliosarcoma (see Chap. 55):
  - sarcomatoid areas

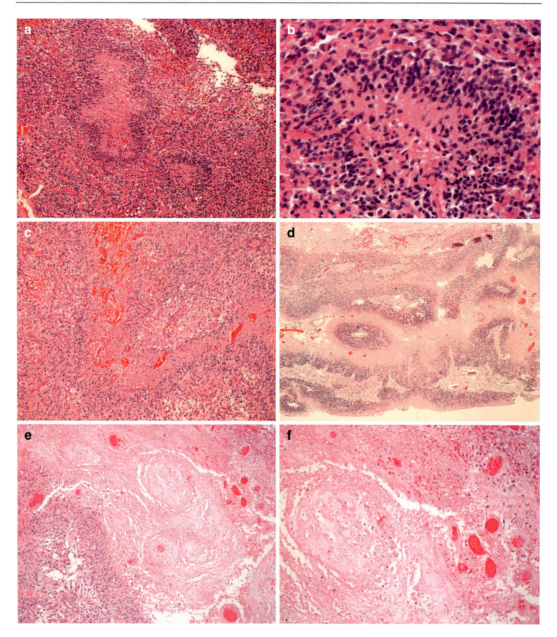

Fig. 54.17 Types of necroses. Distinct types of necroses including pseudopalisading necroses (**a**, **b**), large-sized pseudopalisading necroses (**c**), confluent areas of pseudopalisading necroses (**d**), large areas of tumor necroses (**e**, **f**)

54.3 Neuropathology Findings

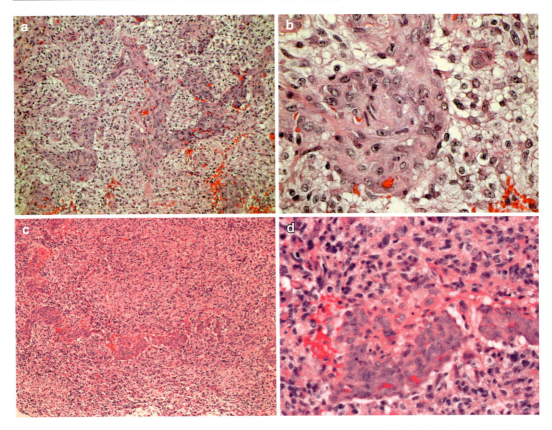

Fig. 54.18 Endothelial proliferation. High number of vessels show endothelial proliferation (**a**), glomeruloid-like vascular endothelial proliferation (**b**), and garland-like vascular endothelial proliferation (**c, d**)

Epitheloid GBM
- relatively uniform population of epithelioid cells showing
  - focal discohesion
  - scant intervening neuropil
  - distinct cell memebrane
  - eosinophilic neoplasm
  - paucity of cytoplasmic processes
  - laterally positioned nucleus
- variations:
  - cytoplasmic filamentous-like balls
  - rhabdoid cells
  - xanthomatous changes
- Zonal necrosis
- Absence of
  - Squamous nests
  - Glandular formation
  - Adenoid features

Rare variants of glioblastoma include the following features: (a) solid cellular trabeculae, (b) papillary pattern, and (c) squamous changes.

Immunophenotype (Figs. 54.12a–d, 54.21a–d, and 54.22a–j)
- IDH-1 R123H mutation-specific antibody
  - Approximately 90% of primary GBM show no IDH-1 mutation visualized with an antibody directed against the R132H mutation.
  - The remaining 10% of GBMs which show the most common IDH-1 R132H mutation are secondary GBMs
- GFAP
  - The astrocytic nature of the tumor cells can be demonstrated in less anaplastic regions by the evidence of GFAP-positivity.

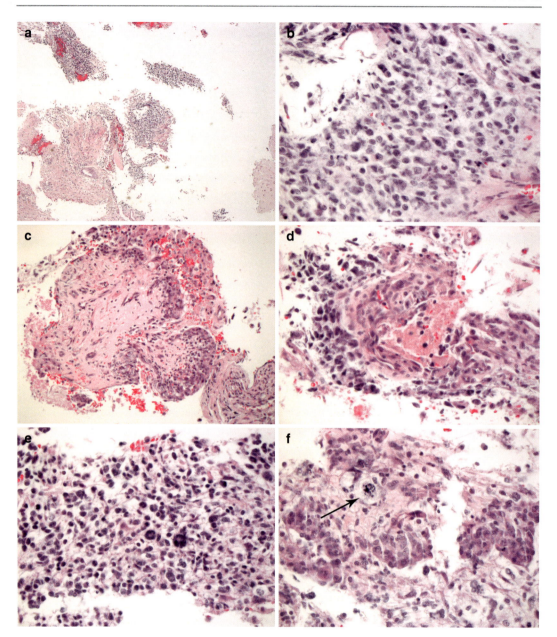

Fig. 54.19 Biopsy material. Biopsy material is often sparse (**a**) which makes the diagnosis difficult. Small areas with tumor cells (**b**), areas with brain tissue and vascular endothelial proliferations (**c**), areas with tumor cells and vascular proliferation (**d**), multinucleated tumor cells (**e**), and tumor tissue containing one mitotic figure (→) (**f**)

54.3 Neuropathology Findings

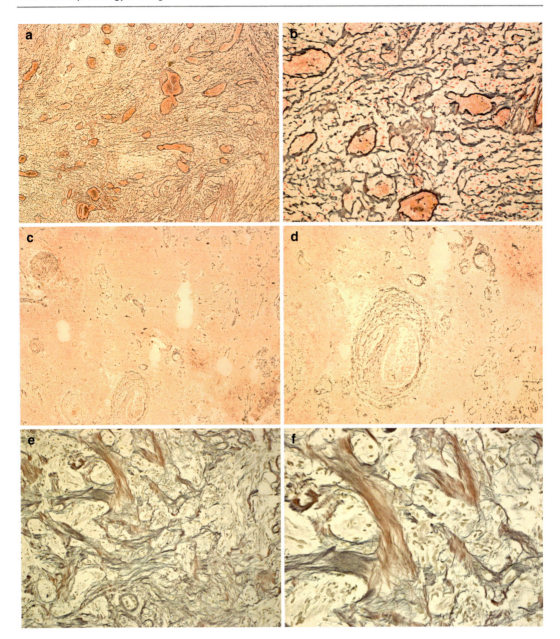

Fig. 54.20 Special stains. Reticulin staining demonstrates areas with large amounts of reticulin fibers abundant around blood vessels (**a-b**, **e-f**) as well as areas with low reticulin fiber production (**c-d**). Elastic fibers are also present in the tumor in varying amounts as demonstrated by the Elastica van Gieson stain (**g-h**)

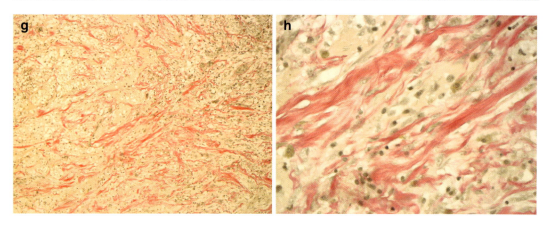

Fig. 54.20 (continued)

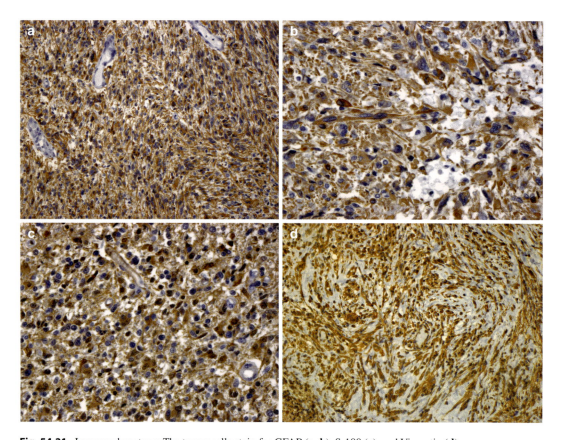

Fig. 54.21 Immunophenotype: The tumor cells stain for GFAP (**a**, **b**), S-100 (**c**), and Vimentin (**d**)

54.3 Neuropathology Findings

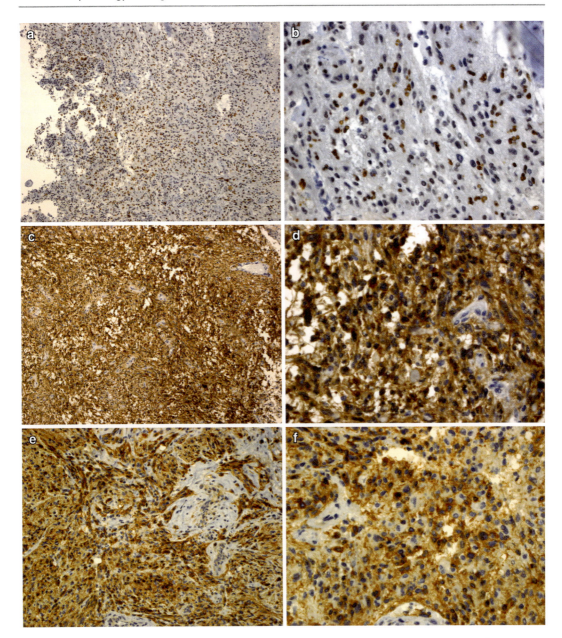

Fig. 54.22 Immunophenotype of pathway-specific markers. p53 staining at low (**a**) and high magnification (**b**), IDH1 R123H (**c, d**), Platelet derived growth factor receptor (PDGFR) (**e, f**), Vascular Epithelial Growth Factor receptor (VEGFR) positive cells (**g, h**), and tumor cells with epithelial growth factor receptor (EGFR) vIII mutation (**i, j**)

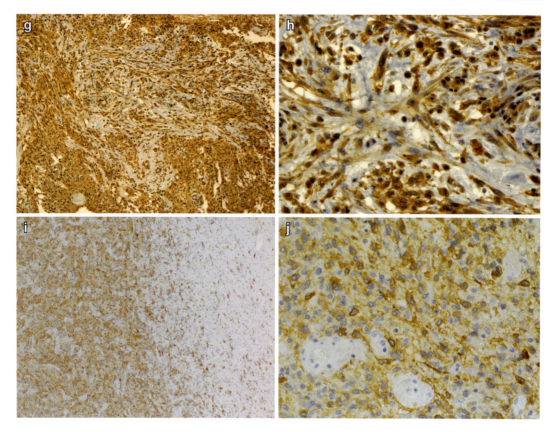

Fig. 54.22 (continued)

– The number of GFAP-positive cells is inversely proportional to the degree of anaplasia.

A list of antibodies with positive or negative immunostaining results are given in Table 54.2.

Proliferation Markers (Fig. 54.23a, b)
- Mitoses and atypical mitoses are frequent
- Labelling indices of cells positive for the various proliferation markers show a high range of variation
- A high index of 3H-Thymidin positive cells is mainly found in the small cell component. If the index is higher than 5%, a fatal outcome has to be expected to occur within one year's time.
- The number of AgNOR per nucleus ranges between 1.6 to 15.5 in GBM.
- Labelling indices of cells positive for the following proliferation markers were reported:
  – BRdU: 1.3 - 38.1 % of cells were labelled
  – Ki-67: 0.8 - 40.0 % of cells were labelled
  – PCNA: 3.3 - 50.0 % of cells were labelled

Table 54.2 Immunophenotype of epitheloid GBM

Positivities	Negativities
• Vimentin	• Melan-A
• S-100	• Desmin
• GFAP	• Myoglobin
• SMARCB1	• Smooth muscle antigen
• SMARCA4	
• Braf V600E mutation specific antibody	
• Some cases express	
– Epithelial markers	
– Cytokeratins	
– EMA	
– Synaptophysin	
– NFP	

- No clear-cut correlation between proliferation index and clinical outcome or survival time.

Ultrastructural Features
- Ultrastructural features of GBM are summarized in Table 54.3.

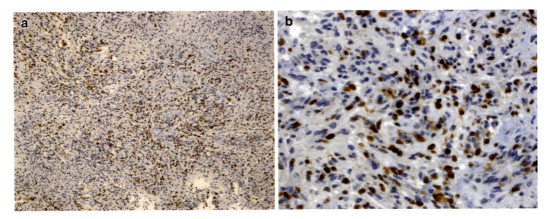

Fig. 54.23 Immunophenotype. Proliferating cells stained with Ki-67 at low (**a**) and high magnification (**b**)

Differential Diagnosis

1. *GBM and Anaplastic Astrocytoma*
   We consider the presence of necroses as the differentiating criterion. The presence of necroses, i.e. either typical tumor necroses with pseudopalisading or large areas of necroses, is the criterion for the diagnosis of glioblastoma. A prominent glomeruloid vascular endothelial proliferation is seen in glioblastoma, while in anaplastic astrocytoma only an incipient vascular proliferation can be noted (Table 54.4).
2. *Metastases*
   The distinction between GBM and metastases might sometimes prove to be difficult (Table 54.5).

54.4 Molecular Neuropathology

54.4.1 Pathogenesis

- *de novo* genesis of highly anaplastic tumor cells (primary glioblastoma).
- anaplastic areas develop rapidly within astrocytomas, oligodendrogliomas or ependymomas and overgrow the primary less anaplastic areas (secondary glioblastoma). This pathogenic mechanism becomes obvious when the clinical history is of long duration with several surgical interventions. With progression of the disease, the grade of anaplasia of the tumors removed is also progressing.

Table 54.3 Ultrastructural features of GBM

Cell component/ characteristics	Features
Cell shape	• considerable degree of pleomorphism • ruffling of the cell surface
Cell size	• considerable degree of pleomorphism,
Cytoplasm	• plications of the cytoplasmic membrane • astroglial cytoplasmic filaments are lacking in more immature tumor cells
Nucleus	• considerable degree of pleomorphism • intranuclear inclusions are common • juxtanuclear membranous stacks
Mitochondria	• marked increase in number • enlarged • presence of atypical cristae

Table 54.4 Differential diagnostic criteria between anaplastic astrocytoma and GBM

Anaplastic Astrocytoma	Glioblastoma multiforme
high cell density	high cell density
marked cellular pleomorphism	marked cellular pleomorphism
moderate to high number of mitoses	high number of mitoses
incipient endothelial cell proliferation, not always present	prominent endothelial cell proliferation, always present
no necroses	typical tumor necroses and/or large areas of necroses

Table 54.5 Some diagnostic clues to differentiate between metastasis and GBM

Glioblastoma multiforme	Metastatic carcinoma
infiltrative behavior	discrete, circumscribed deposition
fibrillary background	collagenous stroma and discrete cell borders
randomly distributed necroses	mostly perivascular necroses
necroses with pseudopalisading	absent
vascular endothelial proliferation	absent
cell features • small cell to gigantocellular • heterogeneous (multiforme) • glial, fibrillary	cell features: • large • homogeneous • epithelial
Immunohistochemistry: • EMA negative • Cytokeratin (usually negative, sometimes positive) • GFAP positive	Immunohistochemistry: • EMA positive • Cytokeratin positive • GFAP usually negative, border possibly positive (reactive astrocytes)

54.4.2 Genetics

Genome-wide analyses revealed that basically three major signalling cascades are affected by genetic aberrations in GBM:

- the TP53 (tumor protein 53) pathway
- the RTK (receptor tyrosine kinase)/RAS/PI3K (phosphoinositide 3-kinase) pathway, both involved in the regulation of cellular growth, apoptosis and proliferation
- the RB1 (retinoblastoma) pathway, controlling the G1 to S phase transition in the cell cycle

54.4.2.1 Pathway-Related Genes

The compilation outlined below contains a selection of pathway-related genes which are commonly altered in GBM, with respect to their properties, chromosomal location, and nature of pathogenic changes (Table 54.6).

IDH1/2 mutations
- In addition to the pathway-related gene alterations, another important genetic trait in GBM are recurrent point mutations in the IDH1 gene, which is located on chromosome 2q33.3 and encodes the cytosolic enzyme isocitrate dehydrogenase 1 (IDH1).
  – Wild-type IDH1 is involved in cytosolic NADPH production, but to date, the role of the mutated gene in gliomagenesis is not yet fully understood.
  – It is important to note that IDH1 is mutated mainly in secondary GBM but only rarely in primary GBM.
  – Interestingly, the point mutations described so far in *IDH1* appear to be restricted to codon 132, corresponding to an arginine residue located in the substrate binding site of the enzyme.
  – The point mutations observed in GBM are all functional, in most cases resulting in an Arg132His substitution.
  – The detection of mutated *IDH1* is therefore used to support discrimination between these two tumor subtypes, possibly also indicating a prognostic potential of *IDH* mutations which, however, needs to be explored in more detail.
- Mutations in the *IDH2* gene at chromosome position 15q26.1, encoding the mitochondrial isoenzyme isocitrate dehydrogenase 2 (*IDH2*), are found at a considerably lower frequency.

54.4.2.2 *TERT* Promoter Mutations

Mutations in the promoter region of the *TERT* gene result in elevated expression levels of the gene product telomerase reverse transcriptase. This enzyme is crucial for maintaining the integrity of chromosomal telomeres in the course of eukaryotic cell division. Thus, enhanced expression of the protein promotes proliferation of the cells. *TERT* promoter mutations were found in the vast majority of adult primary glioblastomas, but rarely in pediatric primary glioblastomas,

54.4 Molecular Neuropathology

Table 54.6 Genes involved in GBM

Genes	Gene characteristics/function
TP 53 pathway	
TP53 (tumor protein p53)	• tumor suppressor gene • located on chromosome 17p13.1 • mutations, deletions
MDM2 (E3 ubiquitin protein ligase)	• oncogene • overexpression inhibits p53 function • located on chromosome 12q14-15 • amplification
CDKN2A: (cyclin-dependent kinase inhibitor 2A)	• encoding tumor suppressors p14ARF and p16INK4A (involved in RB1 pathway; see below) • located on chromosome 9p21 • deletions
RTK (receptor tyrosine kinase)/RAS/PI3K (phosphoinositide 3-kinase) pathway	
RTK: *EGFR* (epidermal growth factor receptor):	• oncogenic properties • chromosome 7p12 • mutations, amplification [gain of chromosome 7, double minutes]
RTK: *PDGFRA* (platelet-derived growth factor receptor; α-peptide)	• oncogenic properties • chromosome 4q12 • amplification
PTEN (phosphatase and tensin homolog)	• tumor suppressor gene • inhibitor in the PI3 kinase pathway (PI3K activates the oncogenic Akt pathway) • chromosome 10q23.3 • mutations, deletion
PIK3CA	• oncogene • encoding the PI3 kinase catalytic subunit α • chromosome 3q26.3 • mutations, amplification
PIK3R1	• oncogene • encoding the PI3 kinase regulatory subunit 1 (α) • chromosome 5q13.1 • mutations
NF1 (neurofibromin 1)	• tumor suppressor gene • negative regulator of the oncogenic Ras pathway • chromosome 17q11.2 • mutations, deletions
RB1 pathway	
RB1 (retinoblastoma 1)	• tumor suppressor gene • chromosome 13q14.2 • mutations, deletions
CDKN2A (cyclin-dependent kinase inhibitor 2A)	• encoding tumor suppressors p16INK4A and p14ARF (involved in TP53 pathway; see above) • chromosome 9p21 • deletions
CDKN2B (cyclin-dependent kinase inhibitor 2B)	• encoding tumor suppressor p15INK4B (inhibits CDK4) • chromosome 9p21 • deletions
CDK4 (cyclin-dependent kinase 4)	• oncogenic properties • chromosome 12q14 • amplification

lower grade astrocytomas and secondary glioblastomas.

54.4.2.3 ATRX Mutations

The *ATRX* gene (α-thalassemia/mental retardation syndrome X-linked), located at Xq21.1 on the long arm of the X chromosome, encodes the nuclear protein ATRX. ATRX is an essential factor participating in telomere stabilization and chromatin remodelling. Loss of ATRX function due to missense mutations in the *ATRX* gene has been observed in a variety of tumors. These *ATRX* mutations are strongly associated with a mechanism known as the ALT (alternative lengthening of telomeres) phenotype which is activated in cancer cells to maintain their replicative potential. *ATRX* mutations are frequently identified in secondary glioblastomas and in *IDH*-mutated astrocytomas.

It should be pointed out that *TERT* promoter mutations and *ATRX* mutations apparently occur mutually exclusive in glioma cells. Moreover, a strong correlation could be established between

- *TERT* promoter mutations and wild-type *IDH1*
- *ATRX*- and *IDH1* mutations

Thus, combined analyses of these molecular markers allow a reliable determination of the GBM subtype.

In summary, genes which are mutated in GBM are involved in the regulation of

- Cell signalling
- Cell proliferation and survival
- Cell cycle
- Apoptosis
- NADPH production

54.4.2.4 Mutation Affecting Oncogenes/Tumor Suppressor Genes

Somatic mutations frequently found to cause activation of oncogenes and/or inactivation of tumor suppressor genes are listed in Table 54.7

Table 54.7 Somatic mutations in oncogenes/tumor suppressor genes in GBM

Gene Name	Gene Symbol	Somatic Mutations (% GBM samples)
Tumor protein p53	TP53	31 - 42
Phosphatase and tensin homolog	PTEN	24 - 37
Neurofibromin 1	NF1	15 - 21
Epidermal growth factor receptor	EGFR	14 - 18
Retinoblastoma 1	RB1	8 - 13
Phosphoinositide-3-kinase, regulatory subunit 1 (alpha)	PIK3R1	7 - 10
Phosphoinositide-3-kinase, catalytic, alpha polypeptide	PIK3CA	7 - 10

(mutation frequencies compiled from Dunn et al. 2012; Bleeker et al. 2012).

54.4.2.5 Chromosomal Aberrations

Apart from somatic mutations, genomic instability resulting in somatic copy number alterations (SCNA's) is a major determining factor in GBM. The most important chromosomal abnormalities are depicted in Table 54.8 (LOH = loss of heterozygosity).

54.4.2.6 Genetic Characteristics of Primary and Secondary Glioblastomas

The differentiation between primary and secondary GBM is reflected by distinct pathogenetic patterns in the two tumor subtypes. Major differences that are consistently observed mainly involve key regulatory genes such as *EGFR*, *PTEN*, *TP53* and most strikingly, *IDH1* (see above). In the following, only the most significant differences are summarized.

Primary GBM:
- A characteristic feature is the amplification of the *EGFR* oncogene accompanied by LOH on chromosome 10q where the tumor-suppressor gene *PTEN* is located

54.4 Molecular Neuropathology

Table 54.8 Chromosomal aberrations in GBM

Chromosomal Abnormality	Genes affected	
	Oncogenes	tumor suppressor genes
Amplification of chromosome region 3q26	PIK3CA	
Amplification of chromosome region 4q12	PDGFRA	
Gain of chromosome 7	EGFR	
Amplification of chromosome region 7p11	EGFR	
Loss of chromosome 9p regions		CDKN2A, CDKN2B
Loss of chromosome 10		PTEN
LOH in chromosome region 10q		PTEN
Amplification of chromosome region 12q14-15	MDM2, CDK4	
LOH in chromosome region 13q		RB1
LOH in chromosome region 17p		TP53
Loss of chromosome region 17q11.2		NF1

- Complete loss of chromosome 10 has been reported
- About one third of primary GBMs display mutated *PTEN* which is not the case in secondary glioblastoma
- *TP53* mutations are found at a significantly lower rate in primary than in secondary GBM
- *EGFR* amplification and mutations in *PTEN* and *TP53* show a preferred correlation pattern, i.e. *EGFR* amplification and *PTEN* mutations are associated with low *TP53* mutation frequencies
- *ERGFRvIII* mutations are seen in about 35% of GBMs.
- Another feature prevailing in adult primary glioblastomas are the TERT promoter mutations resulting in higher cellular levels of the telomerase reverse transcriptase
- TERT promoter mutations were identified in more than 80% of adult primary glioblastomas, but only in ~10% of secondary glioblastomas (Killela et al. 2013)

Secondary GBM:
- In contrast to primary glioblastomas, a high frequency of *TP53* mutations - often occurring together with LOH in chromosome 17p - is detected in secondary GBM.
- The occurrence of high *TP53* mutation rates is largely complemented by a lack of *EGFR* amplification, probably indicating a mutually exclusive relationship.
- A chromosomal aberration associated predominantly with secondary GBM is LOH in chromosome 19q (54%), in contrast to primary GBM (6%).
- *IDH* mutations are highly indicative for secondary GBM but are only sporadically observed in primary glioblastoma.
- *ATRX* mutations have been predominantly detected in secondary glioblastomas (57%) (Watson et al. 2015).

A graphical representation of the molecular alterations occurring in primary GBM as compared to secondary GBM is illustrated below:

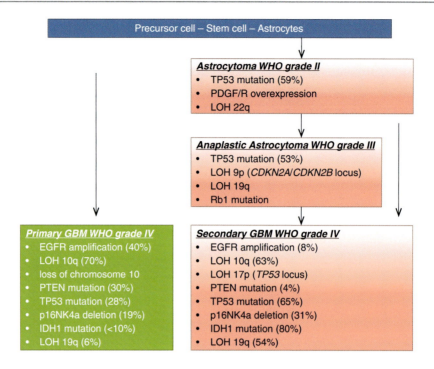

Epitheloid GBM
- *Braf* V600E mutation (50% of cases)
- *H3F3A* K27M mutation
- Absence of IDH1 and IDH2 mutations
- Copy number variations in:
  - *EGFR:* amplification
  - *CDKN2A:* homozygous deletion
  - *PTEN:* loss
- Rare copy number variations in
  - *PDGFRA*
  - *PTEN*
  - *MET*

54.4.2.7 A Novel Molecular Classification of GBM into Four Distinct Subtypes

Based entirely on genomic and gene expression profiling, a new classification model was recently proposed for glioblastoma (Verhaak et al. 2010). This scheme suggests to replace the currently accepted primary and secondary GBM subtypes with four redefined subgroups:

- Proneural
- Neural
- Classical
- Mesenchymal

The essential intention of this approach was to relate the specific molecular signature of each tumor subgroup to the progenitor cell type from which it may have developed, thus providing a basis for better and more specific therapeutic strategies.

Each of the four subtypes was shown to display characteristic features:

- The hallmarks in the ***proneural subtype*** were amplification of *PDGFRA* and high levels of *PDGFRA* expression, frequent *IDH1*- and *TP53* mutations as well as *TP53* LOH, all features which are reminiscent of secondary GBM.
- In the ***neural subtype***, an expression pattern of neuron markers very similar to that in normal tissue was observed, indicating that this subtype is not defined by a specific pathogenetic signature.
- The ***classical subtype*** is characterized mainly by chromosome 7 amplification (*EGFR*) with

corresponding enhanced *EGFR* expression, chromosome 10 loss (*PTEN*) and loss of chromosome 9p regions (*CDKN2A*); no abnormalities were detected in *PDGFRA*, *IDH1*, *TP53* and *NF1*.
- The prevailing feature in the **mesenchymal subtype** was loss of the *NF1* locus on chromosome 17q11.2, correlating with low *NF1* expression levels.

54.4.3 Epigenetics

DNA methylation
- DNA hypermethylation of promoter regions is a frequently observed mechanism in glioblastomas by which tumor suppressor genes (such as for example *TP53*, *PTEN*, or *CDKN2A*) are silenced.
- In recent years, the *MGMT* gene, encoding the DNA repair enzyme O^6-methylguanine-DNA methyltransferase, has received particular attention. Guanine alkylated at its O^6 position represents a mutagenic DNA lesion that is normally repaired by the MGMT enzymatic activity. It transfers the alkyl group from the nucleobase to an active cysteinyl residue in its own sequence.
- In glioblastoma chemotherapy, alkylating drugs like the widely used temozolomide (TMZ) are employed to introduce DNA damage in tumor cells with the intention to trigger apoptosis and cell death. Active MGMT counteracts this mechanism, thus conferring resistance to the treatment.
- Hypermethylation of the *MGMT* promoter, abolishing the transcription of the gene, was demonstrated in a high percentage of GBMs, i.e. in up to 75% of secondary and approximately 35% of primary glioblastomas.
- It is obvious that patients with glioblastoma lacking *MGMT* expression show better responsiveness to TMZ chemotherapy, especially in elderly patients (>65 years), which also has been implicated with improved prognosis.

MicroRNAs
- In GBM, most of the miRNAs surveyed were shown to be overexpressed, and some have been functionally studied, e.g. miR-10b, miR-17, miR-21, miR-93, miR-221 and miR-222.
- The smaller cluster of downregulated miRNAs includes, among others, miR-7, miR-34a, miR-128 and miR-137.
- For a detailed update on miRNAs and their specific targets in glioblastoma, the reader is referred to a systematic review (Moller et al. 2013).

54.4.4 Gene Expression

Microarray-based analyses of differentially expressed genes have lately been used to characterize GBM subtypes correlating with patients' response to treatment and prognosis of survival. Recently, an intensified search for a "consensus" expression profile from several independent GBM data sets produced a limited number of statistically robust marker panels (de Tayrac et al. 2011; Colman et al. 2010; Bredel et al. 2009). Each proposed panel contains only a handful of marker genes which were validated for their potential to support classification of GBM subtypes for predicting clinical outcome.

- In summary, the marker genes included in the panels described above are *POLD2*, *CYCS*, *MYC*, *AKR1C3*, *YME1L1*, *ANXA7*, and *PDCD4* (Bredel et al. 2009); *EDNRB*, *CHAF1B*, *PDLIM4*, and *HJURP* (de Tayrac et al. 2011); *AQP1*, *CHI3L1*, *EMP3*, *GPNMB*, *IGFBP2*, *LGALS3*, *OLIG2*, *PDPN*, and *RTN1* (Colman et al. 2010).
- Genes associated with a better prognosis of survival were *EDNRB*, *OLIG2*, *RTN1*
- Genes associated with worse prognosis include *CHAF1B*, *PDLIM4*, *HJURP*, *AQP1*, *CHI3L1*, *EMP3*, *GPNMB*, *IGFBP2*, *LGALS3*, and *PDPN*.
- Alternatively spliced genes (Table 54.9)

Table 54.9 Alternatively spliced genes in GBM, modified after Marcelino Meliso et al. (2017), reproduced with kind permission by Springer Nature

Gene	Gene ontology terms
Rbfoxl	• Nucleotide binding • Nucleic acid binding • RNA binding • mRNA binding • Protein binding
App	• DNA binding • Binding, • Protein binding • Peptidase activity • Transition metal ion binding • PTB domain binding
Cacna1g	• Ion channel activity • Scaffold protein binding
Cald1	• Protein binding • Cadherin binding involved in cell–cell adhesion
Clta and Cltb	• Structural molecule activity • Protein binding • Peptide binding
Dync1l2	• Microtubule motor activity • Protein binding
Kcnc2	• Voltage-gated potassium channel activity • Ion channel binding
Nf1	• GTPase activator activity • Protein binding
Rtn4	• Protein binding • poly(A) RNA binding • Cadherin binding involved in cell–cell adhesion
Sncb	• Phospholipase inhibitor activity • Calcium ion binding
Tnc	• Syndecan binding
Tpd52l2	• Protein homodimerization and heterodimerization activity • poly(A) RNA binding
Aff2	• G-quadruplex RNA binding
Gnal	• GTPase activity • Signal transducer activity • GTP binding • Metal ion binding
Arpp21	• Nucleic acid binding • Calmodulin binding
Cacna2d3	• Voltage-gated ion channel activity • Calcium channel activity • Metal ion binding
Hist1h3j	• Protein binding • Nucleosomal DNA binding • Histone binding • Protein heterodimerization activity • Cadherin binding involved in cell–cell adhesion
Rgs7	• Signal transducer activity • GTPase activator activity • G-protein beta-subunit binding
Apba2	• Beta-amyloid binding • Protein binding
Map4	• Structural molecule activity • Protein binding • Microtubule binding • poly(A) RNA binding

Table 54.9 (continued)

Gene	Gene ontology terms
Nuf2	• Protein binding
Inpp5f	• Protein binding • Protein homodimerization activity
Top2a	• Magnesium ion binding • DNA binding • Chromatin binding • Protein binding • ATP binding • DNA-dependent ATPase activity • Drug binding • Protein homodimerization and heterodimerization activity • Histone deacetylase binding • poly(A) RNA binding
Ttn	• Protein kinase activity • Calcium ion binding • Protein binding • Calmodulin binding • ATP binding • Structural constituent of muscle • Protein self-association
Neb	• Actin binding • Protein binding • Structural constituent of muscle
Pkd1	• Calcium channel activity • Protein binding • Carbohydrate binding • Ion channel binding
Egf	• Protein tyrosine kinase activity • Ras guanyl-nucleotide exchange factor activity • Epidermal growth factor receptor binding • Calcium ion binding • Protein binding • Growth factor activity • Wnt-protein binding
Adgre5	• Transmembrane signaling receptor activity • G-protein coupled receptor activity • Calcium ion binding • Protein binding
Cbl	• Transcription factor activity • Sequence-specific DNA binding • Signal transducer activity • Calcium ion binding • Protein binding • Zinc ion binding • Ligase activity • Receptor tyrosine kinase binding • Cadherin binding involved in cell–cell adhesion
Rsu1	• Protein binding
Klf6	• Nucleic acid binding • DNA binding • Protein binding • Metal ion binding
Ca12	• Carbonate dehydratase activity • Zinc ion binding
Ghrh	• Growth hormone–releasing hormone activity • Growth hormone-releasing hormone receptor binding

54.5 Treatment and Prognosis

54.5.1 Treatment: State of the Art

State of the art therapy (STUPP scheme) (Stupp et al. 2005, 2006) after the surgical intervention consists of:

- Focal radiation therapy (RT): a total of 60 Gy delivered as 30 sessions with 2 Gy dose for a duration of 6 weeks.
- Temozolomide (TMZ)
  - During RT: 75 mg/m^2 daily (including weekends) for up to 49 days. Administration 1-2 hours before RT or in the morning on days without RT
  - Maintenance: 150-200 mg/m^2 daily for 5 days a week, then 23 days rest. 4 weeks constitute a cycle. 6 cycles are to be administered.
- Antiemetic prophylaxis with metoclopramide or 5HT3 antagonists.
- Pneumocystis carinii pneumonia prophylaxis during continuous TMZ administration only. Pentamide inhalations or trimethroprim/sulfametoxale 3x/week.

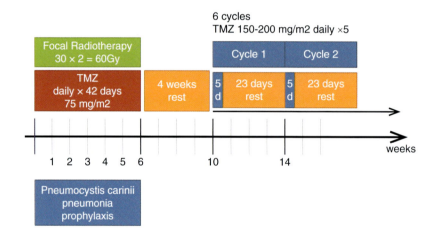

The survival data obtained under the STUPP schema are shown in Table 54.10 and contrasted with historical survival data (Table 54.11).

Recently, the administration of the antiangiogenic agent bevacizumab (Avastin) with radiotherapy-temozolomide for newly diagnosed GBMs was advocated (Chinot et al. 2014; Gilbert et al. 2014). The results were as follows:

- no improvement of overall survival (1-year survival: 72.4% vs 66.3%; 15.7 vs 16.1 months)
- progression-free survival was prolonged (from 6.2-7.3 months to 10.6-10.7 months)

Table 54.10 The survival data obtained under the STUPP schema are reported as follows

Survival	Mean (months)	Range (months)
Overall survival	18	2-92
Progression free survival	16	2-72

Per year survival	Percent	Stupp et al. (2009)
2-year	34	27.2
3-year	24	16.0
4-year	11	12.1
5-year	11	9.8

54.5 Treatment and Prognosis

Table 54.11 Historical survival data

	Median survival (weeks)	1-year survival (%)	2-year survival (%)
Overall survival	30.1	27.1	9.7
Resection	44	38	10
Resection + 50 Gy	50.6	45	18
Biopsy	19	22	8
Biopsy + 50 Gy	33.0	35	13

- maintenance of baseline quality of life and performance status were improved
- higher rate of adverse events

54.5.2 Treatment: Historical Aspects

In order to demonstrate the enormous progress made during the last decade in the treatment of GBM, we present here some historical aspects:

- It should not be denied that between various neurosurgical departments and among neurosurgeons within a neurosurgical unit, there is no clear consensus concerning the treatment of glioblastoma.
- Several treatment schemes have been proposed (Devaux et al. 1993):
  - no treatment after the diagnosis made on stereotactic brain biopsy,
  - partial tumor removal to ameliorate mass effects,
  - radical tumor resection,
  - radical tumor resection + radiation therapy
  - radical tumor resection + radiation therapy + chemotherapy
- The straightforward and accurate application of microsurgical techniques significantly reduced the incidence of morbidity and mortality.
- Patients with glioblastoma, who after tumor resection underwent radiation therapy with a dose of greater than 50 Gy, survived longer than those patients who underwent only radical tumor resection.
- Patients undergoing radical tumor resection and radiation therapy survive longer than those patients who are subjected to stereotactic biopsy and radiotherapy.
- The second important determinant of patient survival is the dose of radiation. Patients receiving a dose lower than 50 Gy either with radical tumor resection or stereotactic biopsy have a significant shorter survival time than those receiving a radiation dose greater than 50 Gy. In daily practice, a radiation dose of 60 Gy is usually administered.
- In general, no significant prolongation of the survival time after adjuvant chemotherapy supplementing radical tumor resection and radiotherapy was noted. In selected cases, adjuvant chemotherapy can be considered. Inclusion criteria for adjuvant chemotherapy are: Karnofsky Performance Scale score higher than 60% as well as normal hematopoetic, renal, and liver functions.
- In terms of median survival time, 12-months survival time, and 24 months survival time, the following data were reported:

Biologic Behavior – Prognosis - Prognostic factors

- The prognosis of GBM is poor.
- Glioblastoma is a tumor of rapid growth which is also reflected by the short clinical history (average 2-3 months; no case longer than 6 months). The aggressiveness of the tumor is due to the small cell component of the tumor.
- Due to the infiltrating growth behavior, complete tumor resection is not always possible. GBM is therefore characterized by a high rate of recurrency.
- The untreated tumors lead to death within a few months (see Treatment).
- In general, metastases are rare. However, metastases along the cerebrospinal fluid spaces within the cranial cavity or spinal canal can be observed. In old studies using autopsy material, metastases within the nervous system have been described in 12 % of the cases.

- Metastases outside the brain and CSF spaces are found in extremely rare occasions.
- Prognostic factors include among others:
  - Age of the patient
  - Karnofsky Performance score
  - Amount of resected tumor tissue
  - MGMT methylation status (methylated promotor ➔ better response to TMZ ➔ better overall survival)
  - IDH-1 mutation status (mutation ➔ better overall survival)
  - Polymorphisms in genes including *EGFR*, *TP53*, Carcinogen-metabolizing gene, immune function (e.g. Interleukin-4), DNA repair, Telomerase hTERT
  - microRNA expression

Selected References

Aldape K, Zadeh G, Mansouri S, Reifenberger G, von Deimling A (2015) Glioblastoma: pathology, molecular mechanisms and markers. Acta Neuropathol 129(6):829–848. https://doi.org/10.1007/s00401-015-1432-1

Alfardus H, McIntyre A, Smith S (2017) MicroRNA regulation of glycolytic metabolism in glioblastoma. BioMed Res Int 2017:9157370. https://doi.org/10.1155/2017/9157370

Anil R, Colen RR (2016) Imaging genomics in glioblastoma multiforme: a predictive tool for patients prognosis, survival, and outcome. Magn Reson Imaging Clin N Am 24(4):731–740. https://doi.org/10.1016/j.mric.2016.07.002

Areeb Z, Stylli SS, Koldej R, Ritchie DS, Siegal T, Morokoff AP, Kaye AH, Luwor RB (2015) MicroRNA as potential biomarkers in glioblastoma. J Neurooncol 125(2):237–248. https://doi.org/10.1007/s11060-015-1912-0

Auffinger B, Spencer D, Pytel P, Ahmed AU, Lesniak MS (2015) The role of glioma stem cells in chemotherapy resistance and glioblastoma multiforme recurrence. Expert Rev Neurother 15(7):741–752. https://doi.org/10.1586/14737175.2015.1051968

Bleeker FE, Molenaar RJ, Leenstra S (2012) Recent advances in the molecular understanding of glioblastoma. J Neurooncol 108(1):11–27. https://doi.org/10.1007/s11060-11011-10793-11060. Epub 12012 Jan 11020.

Bredel M, Scholtens DM, Harsh GR, Bredel C, Chandler JP, Renfrow JJ, Yadav AK, Vogel H, Scheck AC, Tibshirani R, Sikic BI (2009) A network model of a cooperative genetic landscape in brain tumors. JAMA 302(3):261–275. https://doi.org/10.1001/jama.2009.1997

Chinot OL, Wick W, Mason W, Henriksson R, Saran F, Nishikawa R, Carpentier AF, Hoang-Xuan K, Kavan P, Cernea D, Brandes AA, Hilton M, Abrey L, Cloughesy T (2014) Bevacizumab plus radiotherapy-temozolomide for newly diagnosed glioblastoma. N Engl J Med 370(8):709–722. https://doi.org/10.1056/NEJMoa1308345

Colman H, Zhang L, Sulman EP, McDonald JM, Shooshtari NL, Rivera A, Popoff S, Nutt CL, Louis DN, Cairncross JG, Gilbert MR, Phillips HS, Mehta MP, Chakravarti A, Pelloski CE, Bhat K, Feuerstein BG, Jenkins RB, Aldape K (2010) A multigene predictor of outcome in glioblastoma. Neuro Oncol 12(1):49–57. https://doi.org/10.1093/neuonc/nop1007. Epub 2009 Oct 1020

Corso CD, Bindra RS, Mehta MP (2017) The role of radiation in treating glioblastoma: here to stay. J Neurooncol 134(3):479–485. https://doi.org/10.1007/s11060-016-2348-x

Crespo I, Vital AL, Gonzalez-Tablas M, Patino Mdel C, Otero A, Lopes MC, de Oliveira C, Domingues P, Orfao A, Tabernero MD (2015) Molecular and genomic alterations in glioblastoma multiforme. Am J Pathol 185(7):1820–1833. https://doi.org/10.1016/j.ajpath.2015.02.023

de Tayrac M, Aubry M, Saikali S, Etcheverry A, Surbled C, Guenot F, Galibert MD, Hamlat A, Lesimple T, Quillien V, Menei P, Mosser J (2011) A 4-gene signature associated with clinical outcome in high-grade gliomas. Clin Cancer Res 17(2):317–327. https://doi.org/10.1158/1078-0432.CCR-1110-1126. Epub 2011 Jan 1111

Delgado-Lopez PD, Corrales-Garcia EM (2016) Survival in glioblastoma: a review on the impact of treatment modalities. Clin Transl Oncol 18(11):1062–1071. https://doi.org/10.1007/s12094-016-1497-x

Devaux BC, O'Fallon JR, Kelly PJ (1993) Resection, biopsy, and survival in malignant glial neoplasms. A retrospective study of clinical parameters, therapy, and outcome. J Neurosurg 78(5):767–775. https://doi.org/10.3171/jns.1993.78.5.0767

Di Costanzo A, Scarabino T, Trojsi F, Giannatempo GM, Popolizio T, Catapano D, Bonavita S, Maggialetti N, Tosetti M, Salvolini U, d'Angelo VA, Tedeschi G (2006a) Multiparametric 3T MR approach to the assessment of cerebral gliomas: tumor extent and malignancy. Neuroradiology 48(9):622–631. https://doi.org/10.1007/s00234-006-0102-3

Di Costanzo A, Trojsi F, Giannatempo GM, Vuolo L, Popolizio T, Catapano D, Bonavita S, d'Angelo VA, Tedeschi G, Scarabino T (2006b) Spectroscopic, diffusion and perfusion magnetic resonance imaging at 3.0 Tesla in the delineation of glioblastomas: preliminary results. J Exp Clin Cancer Res 25(3):383–390

Diaz RJ, Ali S, Qadir MG, De La Fuente MI, Ivan ME, Komotar RJ (2017) The role of bevacizumab in the treatment of glioblastoma. J Neurooncol 133(3):455–467. https://doi.org/10.1007/s11060-017-2477-x

Dunn GP, Rinne ML, Wykosky J, Genovese G, Quayle SN, Dunn IF, Agarwalla PK, Chheda MG, Campos B,

Selected References

Wang A, Brennan C, Ligon KL, Furnari F, Cavenee WK, Depinho RA, Chin L, Hahn WC (2012) Emerging insights into the molecular and cellular basis of glioblastoma. Genes Dev 26(8):756–784. https://doi.org/10.1101/gad.187922.187112

Ellison DW, Kleinschmidt-DeMasters BK, Park S-H (2016) Epithelioid glioblastoma. In: Louis DN, Ohgaki H, Wiestler OD, Cavenee WK (eds) WHO classification of tumours of the central nervous system, revised 4th ed. IARC, Lyon, pp 50–51

Franceschi E, Minichillo S, Brandes AA (2017) Pharmacotherapy of glioblastoma: established treatments and emerging concepts. CNS drugs 31(8):675–684. https://doi.org/10.1007/s40263-017-0454-8

Gilbert MR, Dignam JJ, Armstrong TS, Wefel JS, Blumenthal DT, Vogelbaum MA, Colman H, Chakravarti A, Pugh S, Won M, Jeraj R, Brown PD, Jaeckle KA, Schiff D, Stieber VW, Brachman DG, Werner-Wasik M, Tremont-Lukats IW, Sulman EP, Aldape KD, Curran WJ Jr, Mehta MP (2014) A randomized trial of bevacizumab for newly diagnosed glioblastoma. N Engl J Med 370(8):699–708. https://doi.org/10.1056/NEJMoa1308573

Ho IAW, Shim WSN (2017) Contribution of the microenvironmental niche to glioblastoma heterogeneity. Biomed Res Int 2017:9634172. https://doi.org/10.1155/2017/9634172

Killela PJ, Reitman ZJ, Jiao Y, Bettegowda C, Agrawal N, Diaz LA Jr, Friedman AH, Friedman H, Gallia GL, Giovanella BC, Grollman AP, He TC, He Y, Hruban RH, Jallo GI, Mandahl N, Meeker AK, Mertens F, Netto GJ, Rasheed BA, Riggins GJ, Rosenquist TA, Schiffman M, Shih IM, Theodorescu D, Torbenson MS, Velculescu VE, Wang TL, Wentzensen N, Wood LD, Zhang M, McLendon RE, Bigner DD, Kinzler KW, Vogelstein B, Papadopoulos N, Yan H (2013) TERT promoter mutations occur frequently in gliomas and a subset of tumors derived from cells with low rates of self-renewal. Proc Natl Acad Sci U S A 110(15):6021–6026. https://doi.org/10.1073/pnas.1303607110

Kleihues P, Burger PC, Aldape KD, Brat DJ, Biernat W, Bigner DD, Nakazato Y, Plate KH, Giangaspero F, von Deimling A, Ohgaki H, Cavenee WK (2007) Glioblastoma. In: Louis DN, Ohgaki H, Wiestler OD, Cavenee WK (eds) WHO classification of tumours of the central nervous system, 4th edn. International Agency for Research on Cancer, Lyon, pp 33–46

Kleihues P, Burger PC, Collins VP, Newcomb EW, Ohgaki H, Cavenee WK (2000) Glioblastoma. In: Kleihues P, Cavenee WK (eds) Pathology and genetics of tumours of the nervous system, 3rd edn. IARC Press, Lyon, pp 29–39

Kleihues P, Burger PC, Scheithauer BW (1993) Histological typing of tumours of the central nervous system, 2nd edn. Springer, Berlin

Lakin N, Rulach R, Nowicki S, Kurian KM (2017) Current advances in checkpoint inhibitors: lessons from non-central nervous system cancers and potential for glioblastoma. Front Oncol 7:141. https://doi.org/10.3389/fonc.2017.00141

Law M, Yang S, Wang H, Babb JS, Johnson G, Cha S, Knopp EA, Zagzag D (2003) Glioma grading: sensitivity, specificity, and predictive values of perfusion MR imaging and proton MR spectroscopic imaging compared with conventional MR imaging. AJNR Am J Neuroradiol 24(10):1989–1998

Louis DN, Suvá ML, Burger PC, Perry A, Kleihues P, Aldape KD, Brat DJ, Biernat W, Bigner DD, Nakazato Y, Plate KH, Giangaspero F, Ohgaki H, Cavenee WK, Wick W, Barnholtz-Sloan J, Rosenblum MK, Hegi M, Stupp R, Hawkins C, Verhaak RGW, Ellison DW, von Deimling A (2016) Glioblastoma, IDH-wildtype. In: Louis DN, Ohgaki H, Wiestler OD, Cavenee WK (eds) WHO classification of tumours of the central nervous system, revised 4th edn. IARC, Lyon, pp 28–45

Marcelino Meliso F, Hubert CG, Favoretto Galante PA, Penalva LO (2017) RNA processing as an alternative route to attack glioblastoma. Human genetics. 136(9):1129–1141. https://doi.org/10.1007/s00439-017-1819-2

Maxwell R, Jackson CM, Lim M (2017) Clinical trials investigating immune checkpoint blockade in glioblastoma. Curr Treat Options Oncol 18(8):51. https://doi.org/10.1007/s11864-017-0492-y

Miranda A, Blanco-Prieto M, Sousa J, Pais A, Vitorino C (2017) Breaching barriers in glioblastoma. Part I: molecular pathways and novel treatment approaches. Int J Pharm 531(1):372–388. https://doi.org/10.1016/j.ijpharm.2017.07.056

Moller HG, Rasmussen AP, Andersen HH, Johnsen KB, Henriksen M, Duroux M (2013) A systematic review of microRNA in glioblastoma multiforme: micromodulators in the mesenchymal mode of migration and invasion. Mol Neurobiol 47(1):131–144. https://doi.org/10.1007/s12035-12012-18349-12037. Epub 12012 Oct 12032

Ohgaki H, Kleihues P, von Deimling A, Louis DN, Reifenberger G, Yan H, Weller M (2016) Glioblastoma, IDH-mutant. In: Louis DN, Ohgaki H, Wiestler OD, Cavenee WK (eds) WHO classification of tumours of the central nervous system, revised 4th edn. IARC, Lyon, pp 52–56

Paldino MJ, Barboriak D, Desjardins A, Friedman HS, Vredenburgh JJ (2009) Repeatability of quantitative parameters derived from diffusion tensor imaging in patients with glioblastoma multiforme. J Magn Reson Imaging 29(5):1199–1205. https://doi.org/10.1002/jmri.21732

Sahebjam S, Sharabi A, Lim M, Kesarwani P, Chinnaiyan P (2017) Immunotherapy and radiation in glioblastoma. J Neurooncol 134(3):531–539. https://doi.org/10.1007/s11060-017-2413-0

Shea A, Harish V, Afzal Z, Chijioke J, Kedir H, Dusmatova S, Roy A, Ramalinga M, Harris B, Blancato J, Verma M, Kumar D (2016) MicroRNAs in glioblastoma multiforme pathogenesis and therapeutics. Cancer Med 5(8):1917–1946. https://doi.org/10.1002/cam4.775

Shiroishi MS, Boxerman JL, Pope WB (2015) Physiologic MRI for assessment of response to therapy and prognosis in glioblastoma. Neuro Oncol 18(4):467–478. https://doi.org/10.1093/neuonc/nov179

Stavrovskaya AA, Shushanov SS, Rybalkina EY (2016) Problems of glioblastoma multiforme drug resistance. Biochem Biokhim 81(2):91–100. https://doi.org/10.1134/s0006297916020036

Stupp R, Mason WP, van den Bent MJ, Weller M, Fisher B, Taphoorn MJ, Belanger K, Brandes AA, Marosi C, Bogdahn U, Curschmann J, Janzer RC, Ludwin SK, Gorlia T, Allgeier A, Lacombe D, Cairncross JG, Eisenhauer E, Mirimanoff RO, European Organisation for Research and Treatment of Cancer Brain Tumor and Radiotherapy Groups, National Cancer Institute of Canada Clinical Trials Group (2005) Radiotherapy plus concomitant and adjuvant temozolomide for glioblastoma. N Engl J Med 352(10):987–996.

Stupp R, Hegi ME, van den Bent MJ, Mason WP, Weller M, Mirimanoff RO, Cairncross JG, European Organisation for Research and Treatment of Cancer Brain Tumor and Radiotherapy Groups, National Cancer Institute of Canada Clinical Trials Group (2006) Changing paradigms—an update on the multidisciplinary management of malignant glioma. Oncologist 11(2):165–180.

Tipping M, Eickhoff J, Ian Robins H (2017) Clinical outcomes in recurrent glioblastoma with bevacizumab therapy: an analysis of the literature. J Clin Neurosci 44:101–106. https://doi.org/10.1016/j.jocn.2017.06.070

Touat M, Duran-Pena A, Alentorn A, Lacroix L, Massard C, Idbaih A (2015) Emerging circulating biomarkers in glioblastoma: promises and challenges. Expert Rev Mol Diagn 15(10):1311–1323. https://doi.org/10.1586/14737159.2015.1087315

Verhaak RG, Hoadley KA, Purdom E, Wang V, Qi Y, Wilkerson MD, Miller CR, Ding L, Golub T, Mesirov JP, Alexe G, Lawrence M, O'Kelly M, Tamayo P, Weir BA, Gabrie S, Winckler W, Gupta S, Jakkula L, Feiler HS, Hodgson JG, James CD, Sarkaria JN, Brennan C, Kahn A, Spellman PT, Wilson RK, Speed TP, Gray JW, Meyerson M, Getz G, Perou CM, Hayes DN (2010) An integrated genomic analysis identifies clinically relevant subtypes of glioblastoma characterized by abnormalities in PDGFRA, IDH1, EGFR and NF1. Cancer Cell 17(1):98

Watson LA, Goldberg H, Berube NG (2015) Emerging roles of ATRX in cancer. Epigenomics 7(8):1365–1378. https://doi.org/10.2217/epi.1315.1382. Epub 2015 Dec 1368

Zülch KJ (1979) Histological typing of tumours of the central nervous system. World Health Organization, Geneva

Gliosarcoma WHO Grade IV-Giant Cell Glioblastoma WHO Grade IV

Diffuse Astrocytic and Oligodendroglial Tumors

55.1 Gliosarcoma WHO Grade IV

WHO Definition
2016: A variant of IDH-wild-type glioblastoma, characterized by a biphasic tissue pattern with alternating areas displaying glial and mesenchymal differentiation (Burger et al. 2016).

2007: A glioblastoma variant characterized by a biphasic tissue pattern with alternating areas displaying glial and mesenchymal differentiation (Kleihues et al. 2007b).

2000: A glioblastoma variant characterized by a biphasic tissue pattern with alternating areas displaying glial and mesenchymal differentiation (Ohgaki et al. 2000a).

1993: A glioblastoma admixed with a sarcomatous component (Kleihues et al. 1993).

1979: Glioblastoma with sarcomatous component [mixed glioblastoma and sarcoma]: This tumor consists of a glioblastoma as described above with a sarcomatous component within the tumor. The sarcomatous component, which originates from a malignant transformation of the hyperplastic vascular elements, may predominate in some cases (Zülch 1979).

WHO Grade
- WHO grade IV

55.1.1 Epidemiology

Incidence
- 2–8% of all glioblastomas

Age Incidence
- Mean age: 52 years
- Age range: 40–60 years

Sex Incidence
- Male:Female ratio: 1.3:1

Localization
- Cerebral hemispheres
- Rarely posterior fossa and spinal cord
- Multifocal occurrence possible

55.1.2 Neuroimaging Findings

General Imaging Findings
- Infiltrating, well-demarcated mass, often with cystic components, and heterogeneous enhancement

- Can infiltrate dura or skull
- Often not to distinguish from glioblastoma multiforme

CT Non-Contrast-Enhanced
- Heterogeneous hypodense
- Demonstrates dural or skull involvement

CT Contrast-Enhanced
- Inhomogeneous, strong, peripheral enhancement

MRI-T2 (Fig. 55.1a)
- Heterogeneous hyperintense
- Prominent surrounding edema
- Cysts and necrosis are common

MRI-FLAIR (Fig. 55.1b)
- Heterogeneous due to cysts and necrosis with edema

MRI-T1 (Fig. 55.1c)
- Heterogeneous hypointense

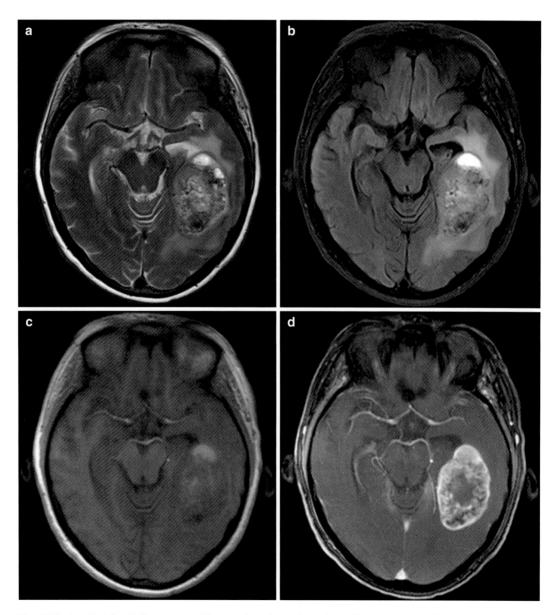

Fig. 55.1 A well-defined gliosarcoma with necrosis and cyst formations. The strong enhancing wall of the tumor is attached to the dura of the left tentorium. T2 (**a**), FLAIR (**b**), T1 (**c**), T1 (**d**, **e**), rCBV (**f**)

55.1 Gliosarcoma WHO Grade IV

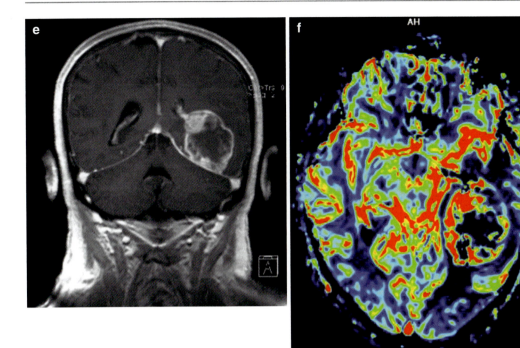

Fig. 55.1 (continued)

MRI-T1 Contrast-Enhanced (Figs. 55.1d, e)
- Strong heterogeneous peripheral enhancement
- Enhancement of the dura indicates dura involvement

MRI-T2*/SWI
- Hemorrhage may be seen

MR-Diffusion Imaging
- Restricted diffusion in solid components described

MRI-Perfusion (Fig. 55.1f)
- Elevated rCBV

MR-Spectroscopy
- NAA decreased
- Cho increased
- Lactate and lipid peaks

Nuclear Medicine Imaging Findings
- Gliosarcomas are normally FDG-avid (CAVE: the normal gray matter of the cortex, the striatum, and the thalamus take up FDG due to their normal glucose-based metabolism).
- FDG-PET can be used to assess the damage to healthy brain tissue.
- Radiotracers like FET (a marker of amino acid uptake (L-system)) or FLT (a marker of DNA biosynthesis) have the advantage of nearly no uptake in the healthy brain tissues resulting in a much better tumor-to-background ratio.
- Images can show homogeneous or heterogeneous uptake representing the tumor biology.
- SUV (calculated as ratio of the concentration of the radiotracer corrected by the body weight or body surface of the patient) can predict therapeutic outcomes.
- Results obtained for MET are similar to FET with the advantage of FET to be taken up in a lesser amount in inflammatory tissue and the longer half-life of 110 min compared to a relatively short half-life of 20 min of C-11 used in MET.
- Dynamic FET-PET enables the measurement of the tracer kinetic.

- Possibility of non-invasive tumor grading is being discussed (especially in dynamic FET-PET studies).
- Sensitivity of FET-PET for gliosarcomas is about 95%.
- Possible influence of bevacizumab therapy has to be considered.
- Hypoxia tracers are under investigation especially for radiotherapy planning.

55.1.3 Neuropathology Findings

Macroscopic Features (Fig. 55.2a–h)
- Firm, well-circumscribed mass

Microscopic Features (Fig. 55.3a–h)
- Biphasic tissue pattern composed of:
  - A mixture of gliomatous and sarcomatous tissues
- Gliomatous component
  - Anaplastic astrocytic tumor cells like in glioblastoma
- Sarcomatous component
  - Signs of malignant transformation with
    - Nuclear atypia, mitotic activity, and necroses
  - Shows pattern of fibrosarcoma with
    - Densely packed long bundles of spindle cells
- Epithelial differentiation
  - With carcinomatous features
    - Gland-like formations
    - Adenoid formations
    - Squamous metaplasia
- Mesenchymal differentiation possible with formation of:
  - Cartilage
  - Bone
  - Osteoid-chondral tissue
  - Smooth and striated muscle
- Special stains reveal:
  - Collagen in the mesenchymal part (trichrome stain)
  - Connective tissue fibers in the sarcomatous part (reticulin stain)

Immunophenotype (Fig. 55.4a–f)
- GFAP-positivity in the glial part
- GFAP-negativity of the malignant mesenchymal part
- P53 positivities in the gliomatous and the sarcomatous parts

Proliferation Markers (Fig. 55.4g, h)
- High mitotical activity
- Ki-67 LI high

Ultrastructural Features
- Considerable degree of pleomorphism in cell shape and size
- Ruffling of the cell surface
- Plications of the cytoplasmic membrane
- Astroglial cytoplasmic filaments are lacking in more immature tumor cells
- Intranuclear inclusions are common
- Mitochondria increased in number, enlarged with atypical cristae
- Sarcomatous component

Differential Diagnosis
- Glioblastoma with florid fibroblastic proliferation

55.1.4 Molecular Neuropathology

Pathogenesis
- Obsolete: collision tumor of a separate astrocytic and sarcomatous component
- Sarcomatous component results from advanced glioma dedifferentiation with
  - Subsequent loss of *GFAP* expression
  - Acquisition of a sarcomatous phenotype
  - Expression of *TP53* in both tumor components
  - Identical *PTEN* and *TP53* mutations in both components
  - *P16* deletion in both components
  - *MDM2* and *CDK4* co-amplification in both components

55.1 Gliosarcoma WHO Grade IV

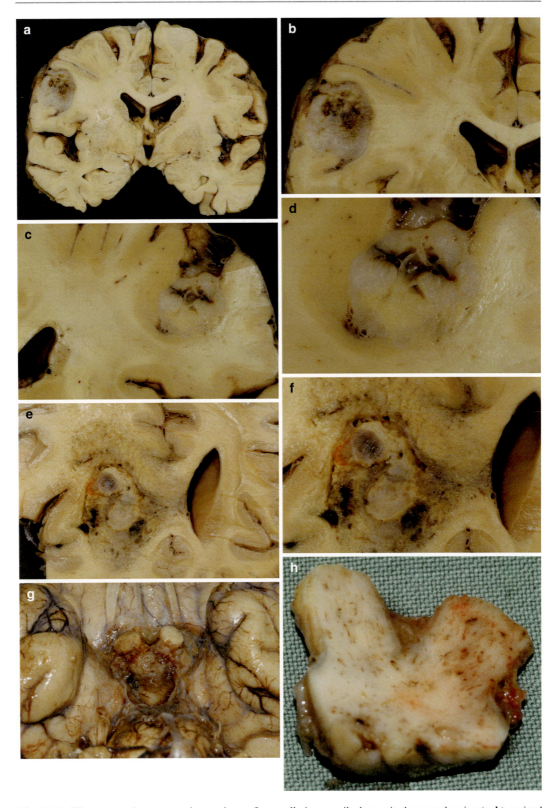

Fig. 55.2 Gliosarcoma: Autopsy specimens show a firm, well-circumscribed mass in the central region (**a**, **b**), parietal lobe (**c**, **d**), caudate nucleus and corpus callosum (**e**, **f**), and the optic chiasm (**g**, **h**)

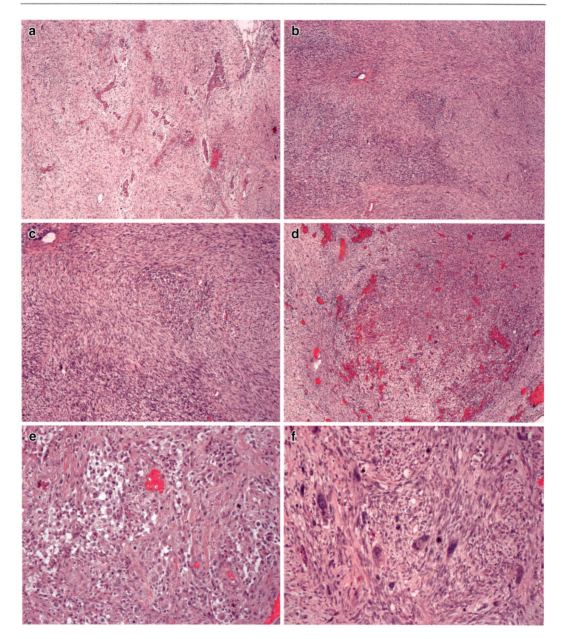

Fig. 55.3 Gliosarcoma: Highly cellular tumor presenting a biphasic tissue pattern composed of a mixture of gliomatous and sarcomatous tissues (**a–g**). The gliomatous component consists of anaplastic astrocytic tumor cells like in glioblastoma, whereas the sarcomatous component shows signs of malignant transformation with nuclear atypia (**f, g**), and mitotic activity. Densely packed long bundles of spindle cells are evident. Conspicuous reticulin network is located between the tumor cells (**h**)

55.1 Gliosarcoma WHO Grade IV

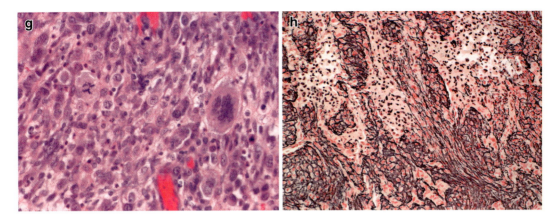

Fig. 55.3 (continued)

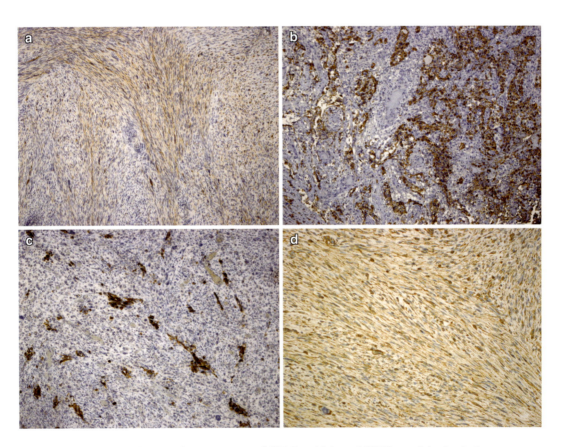

Fig. 55.4 Gliosarcoma—Immunophenotype: areas of GFAP-positivity and GFAP-negativity (**a–c**); the sarcomatous component is vimentin positive (**d–f**); high Ki67 proliferation rate (**g, h**)

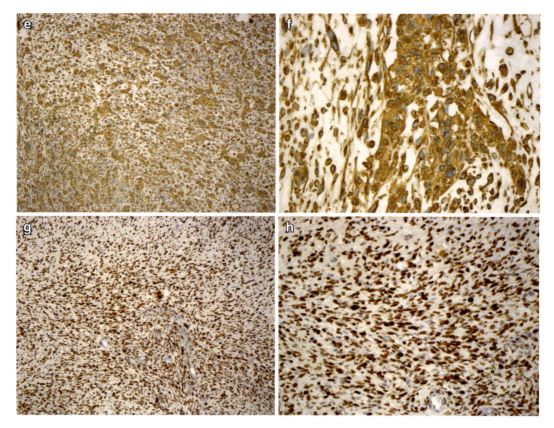

Fig. 55.4 (continued)

Genetics, Epigenetics, Gene Expression
- *TP53* mutations in 23%
- *PTEN* mutations in 38%
- *P16* deletion in 37%
- *MDM2* amplification in 5%
- *EGFR* amplification in 0%

55.1.5 Treatment and Prognosis

Treatment
- Surgery
- Radiotherapy
- Chemotherapy

Biologic Behavior–Prognosis–Prognostic Factors
- Poor prognosis
- Somewhat more favorable than glioblastoma

55.2 Giant Cell Glioblastoma WHO Grade IV

WHO Definition

2016: A rare histological variant of IDH-wild-type glioblastoma, histologically characterized by bizarre, multinucleated giant cells and an occasionally abundant reticulum network (Ohgaki et al. 2016).

2007: A histological variant of glioblastoma with a predominance of bizarre, multinucleated giant cells, an occasionally abundant stromal reticulin network, and high frequency of *TP53* mutations (Kleihues et al. 2007a).

2000: A histological variant of glioblastoma with a predominance of bizarre, multi-nucleated giant cells, on occasionally abundant stromal reticulin network, and a high frequency of *TP53* mutations (Ohgaki et al. 2000b).

1993: A glioblastoma with a marked predominance of bizarre, multinucleated giant cells and, on occasion, an abundant stromal reticulin network. GFAP expression may be highly variable (Kleihues et al. 1993).

1979: A glioblastoma with a predominance of bizarre ("monstrous") giant cells, with many nuclei, frequently showing an abundant reticulin network in its stroma (Zülch 1979).

WHO Grade
- WHO grade IV

55.2.1 Epidemiology

Incidence
- Rare
- 1% of all brain tumors
- 5% of glioblastomas

Age Incidence
- Mean age: 41 years

Sex Incidence
- Male:female ratio: 1:1

Localization
- Subcortically in the
  - Temporal lobe
  - Parietal lobe

55.2.2 Neuroimaging Findings

General Imaging Findings
- Giant cell glioblastoma indistinguishable from glioblastoma multiforme (see Chap. 54).

Nuclear Medicine Imaging Findings
- Giant cell glioblastomas are normally FDG-avid (CAVE: the normal gray matter of the cortex, the striatum, and the thalamus take up FDG due to their normal glucose-based metabolism).
- Radiotracers like FET (a marker of amino acid uptake (L-system)) or FLT (a marker of DNA biosynthesis) have the advantage of nearly no uptake in the healthy brain tissues resulting in a much better tumor-to-background ratio.
- Images can show homogeneous or heterogeneous uptake representing the tumor biology.
- SUV (calculated as ratio of the concentration of the radiotracer corrected by the body weight of the patient) can predict therapeutic outcomes.
- Results obtained for MET are similar to FET with the advantage of FET to be taken up in a lesser amount in inflammatory tissue and the longer half-life of 110 min compared to a relatively short half-life of 20 min of C-11 used in MET.
- Dynamic FET-PET enables the measurement of the tracer kinetic.
- Possibility of non-invasive tumor grading is being discussed (especially in dynamic FET-PET studies).
- Sensitivity of FET-PET for giant cell glioblastomas is about 95%.
- Possible influence of bevacizumab therapy has to be considered.
- Hypoxia tracers are under investigation especially for radiotherapy planning.

55.2.3 Neuropathology Findings

Macroscopic Features
- Tumors of large size
- Involving several lobes
- Grossly, the brain shows broadened and flattened gyri
- The tumor is usually not sharply demarcated presenting with a broad and diffuse zone of infiltration
- The cut surface characteristically shows a vari-colored appearance ranging from gray, brown, white, yellow to dark red
- The consistency of the irregular outer zone is often firmer due to astrocytic growth
- Necroses are found

Microscopic Features (Fig. 55.5a–f)
- Numerous multinucleated giant cells
  - With bizarre appearance
  - Diameter exceeds 500 μm
  - Heavily lipidized
  - Number of nuclei from a few to more than 20
- Small fusiform cells
- Reticulin network
- Atypical mitoses frequent
- Necroses (geographic or pseudopalisading) present
- Microvascular proliferation rare

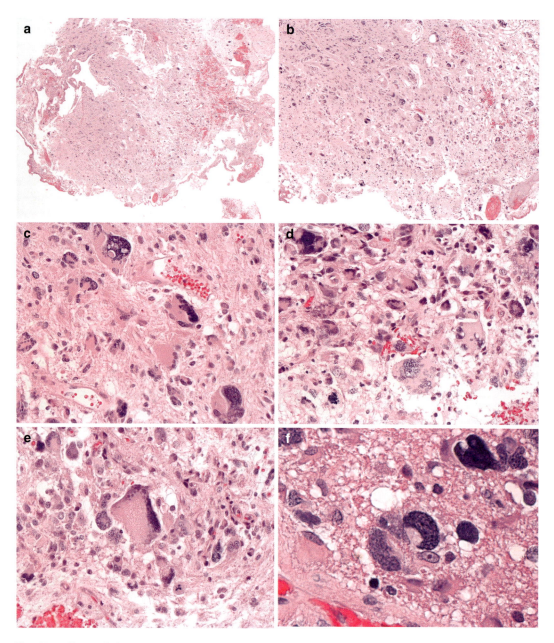

Fig. 55.5 Giant cell GBM: Moderately cellular tumor containing numerous multinucleated giant cells with bizarre appearances (**a–f**)

55.2 Giant Cell Glioblastoma WHO Grade IV

Immunophenotype (Fig. 55.6a–d)
- Giant cells positive for
  - S-100
  - Vimentin
  - Class III ß-tubulin
  - P53
  - EGFR
- Highly variable GFAP expression
- AURKB expression
- Negativity for neuronal markers

Proliferation Markers (Fig. 55.6e, f)
- High as in glioblastoma

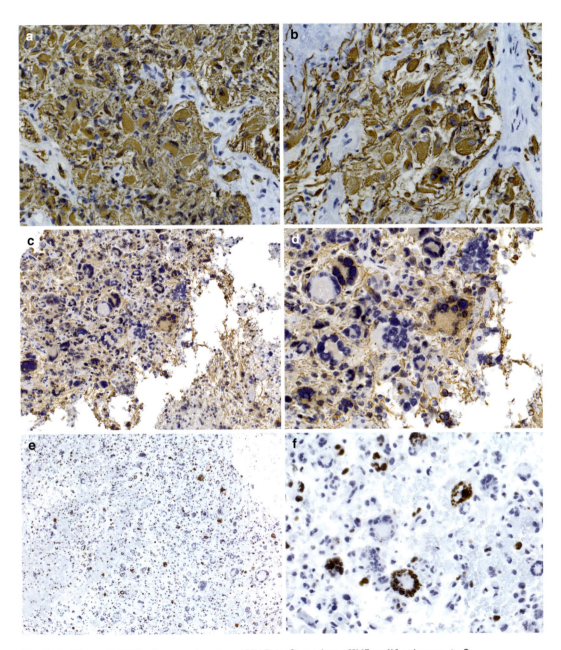

Fig. 55.6 Giant cell GBM—Immunophenotype: GFAP (**a–d**); moderate Ki67 proliferation rate (**e, f**)

Ultrastructural Features
- Considerable degree of pleomorphism in cell shape and size
- Extremely large tumor cells
- Ruffling of the cell surface
- Plications of the cytoplasmic membrane
- Astroglial cytoplasmic filaments are lacking in more immature tumor cells
- Intranuclear inclusions are common
- Mitochondria increased in number, enlarged with atypical cristae

Differential Diagnosis
- GBM

55.2.4 Molecular Neuropathology

Pathogenesis
- De novo after short preoperative history without clinical or radiologic evidence of a less malignant precursor lesion

Genetics, Epigenetics, Gene Expression
- *TP53* mutation 75–90%
- *PTEN* mutations 33%
- *EGFR* amplification/overexpression rare
- *P16* homozygous deletion
- Hybrid position with glioblastoma

55.2.5 Treatment and Prognosis

Treatment
- Surgery
- Radiotherapy
- Chemotherapy

Biologic Behavior–Prognosis–Prognostic Factors
- Poor prognosis
- Lesser infiltrative behavior than glioblastoma

Selected References

Burger PC, Giangaspero F, Ohgaki H, Biernat W (2016) Gliosarcoma. In: Louis DN, Ohgaki H, Wiestler OD, Cavenee WK (eds) WHO classification of tumours of the central nervous system, revised 4th edn. IARC, Lyon, pp 48–49

Han SJ, Yang I, Tihan T, Chang SM, Parsa AT (2010a) Secondary gliosarcoma: a review of clinical features and pathological diagnosis. J Neurosurg 112(1):26–32. https://doi.org/10.3171/2009.3.jns081081

Han SJ, Yang I, Tihan T, Prados MD, Parsa AT (2010b) Primary gliosarcoma: key clinical and pathologic distinctions from glioblastoma with implications as a unique oncologic entity. J Neurooncol 96(3):313–320. https://doi.org/10.1007/s11060-009-9973-6

Karremann M, Butenhoff S, Rausche U, Pietsch T, Wolff JE, Kramm CM (2009) Pediatric giant cell glioblastoma: new insights into a rare tumor entity. Neuro Oncol 11(3):323–329. https://doi.org/10.1215/15228517-2008-099

Kleihues P, Burger PC, Scheithauer BW (1993) Histological typing of tumours of the central nervous system, 2nd edn. Springer-Verlag, Berlin

Kleihues P, Burger PC, Aldape KD, Brat DJ, Biernat W, Bigner DD, Nakazato Y, Plate KH, Giangaspero F, von Deimling A, Ohgaki H, Cavenee WK (2007a) Glioblastoma. In: Louis DN, Ohgaki H, Wiestler OD, Cavenee WK (eds) WHO classification of tumours of the central nervous system, 4th edn. International Agency for Research on Cancer, Lyon, pp 33–46

Kleihues P, Burger PC, Aldape KD, Brat DJ, Biernat W, Bigner DD, Nakazato Y, Plate KH, Giangaspero F, von Deimling A, Ohgaki H, Cavenee WK (2007b) Gliosarcoma. In: Louis DN, Ohgaki H, Wiestler OD, Cavenee WK (eds) WHO classification of tumours of the central nervous system, 4th edn. International Agency for Research on Cancer, Lyon, pp 48–49

Kozak KR, Moody JS (2009) Giant cell glioblastoma: a glioblastoma subtype with distinct epidemiology and superior prognosis. Neuro Oncol 11(6):833–841. https://doi.org/10.1215/15228517-2008-123

Lohkamp LN, Schinz M, Gehlhaar C, Guse K, Thomale UW, Vajkoczy P, Heppner FL, Koch A (2016) MGMT promoter methylation and BRAF V600E mutations are helpful markers to discriminate pleomorphic xanthoastrocytoma from giant cell glioblastoma. PLoS One 11(6):e0156422. https://doi.org/10.1371/journal.pone.0156422

Mallya V, Siraj F, Singh A, Sharma KC (2015) Giant cell glioblastoma with calcification and long-term survival. Indian J Cancer 52(4):704–705. https://doi.org/10.4103/0019-509x.178417

McAleer MF, Brown PD (2015) Therapeutic management of gliosarcoma in the temozolomide era. CNS Oncol 4(3):171–178. https://doi.org/10.2217/cns.14.61

Oh T, Rutkowski MJ, Safaee M, Sun MZ, Sayegh ET, Bloch O, Tihan T, Parsa AT (2014) Survival outcomes of giant cell glioblastoma: institutional experience in the management of 20 patients. J Clin Neurosci 21(12):2129–2134. https://doi.org/10.1016/j.jocn.2014.04.011

Oh JE, Ohta T, Nonoguchi N, Satomi K, Capper D, Pierscianek D, Sure U, Vital A, Paulus W, Mittelbronn M, Antonelli M, Kleihues P, Giangaspero F, Ohgaki

H (2016) Genetic alterations in gliosarcoma and giant cell glioblastoma. Brain Pathol 26(4):517–522. https://doi.org/10.1111/bpa.12328

Ohgaki H, Biernat W, Reis R, Hegi M, Kleihues P (2000a) Gliosarcoma. In: Kleihues P, Cavenee WK (eds) Pathology and genetics of tumours of the nervous system, 3rd edn. IARC Press, Lyon, pp 42–44

Ohgaki H, Peraud A, Nakazato Y, Watanabe K, von Deimling A (2000b) Giant cell glioblastoma. In: Kleihues P, Cavenee WK (eds) Pathology and genetics of tumours of the nervous system, 3rd edn. IARC Press, Lyon, pp 40–41

Ohgaki H, Kleihues P, Plate KH, Nakazato Y, Bigner DD (2016) Giant cell glioblastoma. In: Louis DN, Ohgaki H, Wiestler OD, Cavenee WK (eds) WHO classification of tumours of the central nervous system, revised 4th edn. IARC, Lyon, pp 46–47

Okami N, Kawamata T, Kubo O, Yamane F, Kawamura H, Hori T (2002) Infantile gliosarcoma: a case and a review of the literature. Childs Nerv Syst 18(6–7):351–355. https://doi.org/10.1007/s00381-002-0602-3

Sampaio L, Linhares P, Fonseca J (2017) Detailed magnetic resonance imaging features of a case series of primary gliosarcoma. Neuroradiol J 30(6):546–553. https://doi.org/10.1177/1971400917715879

Schuss P, Ulrich CT, Harter PN, Tews DS, Seifert V, Franz K (2011) Gliosarcoma with bone infiltration and extracranial growth: case report and review of literature. J Neurooncol 103(3):765–770. https://doi.org/10.1007/s11060-010-0437-9

Valle-Folgueral JM, Mascarenhas L, Costa JA, Vieira F, Soares-Fernandes J, Beleza P, Alegria C (2008) Giant cell glioblastoma: review of the literature and illustrated case. Neurocirugia (Astur) 19(4):343–349

Winkler PA, Buttner A, Tomezzoli A, Weis S (2000) Histologically repeatedly confirmed gliosarcoma with long survival: review of the literature and report of a case. Acta Neurochir 142(1):91–95

Zipp L, Schwartz KM, Hewer E, Yu Y, Stippich C, Slopis JM (2012) Magnetic resonance imaging and computed tomography findings in pediatric giant cell glioblastoma. Clin Neuroradiol 22(4):359–363. https://doi.org/10.1007/s00062-012-0130-9

Zülch KJ (1979) Histological typing of tumours of the central nervous system. World Health Organization, Geneva

Gliomatosis Cerebri

WHO Definition

2016—Gliomatosis cerebri was deleted as a tumor entity. Instead it was defined to be a growth pattern under the topics "diffuse astrocytoma, IDH-wild-type," "anaplastic astrocytoma, IDH-wild-type," and "glioblastoma, IDH-wild-type." Like other diffuse gliomas, diffuse astrocytoma can manifest at initial clinical presentation with a gliomatosis cerebri pattern of extensive involvement of CNS, with the affected area ranging from most of one cerebral hemisphere (three lobes or more) to both cerebral hemispheres with additional involvement of the deep gray matter structures, brain stem, cerebellum, and spinal cord (von Deimling et al. 2016b; von Deimling et al. 2016a; Louis et al. 2016).

2007—A diffuse glioma (usually astrocytic) growth pattern consisting of exceptionally extensive infiltration of a large region of the central nervous system, with involvement of at least three cerebral lobes, usually with bilateral involvement of the cerebral hemispheres and/or deep gray matter, and frequent extension to the brain stem, cerebellum, and even the spinal cord. Gliomatosis cerebri most commonly displays an astrocytic phenotype although oligodendroglioma and mixed oligo-astrocytoma can also present within the gliomatosis cerebri growth pattern (Fuller and Kros 2007).

2000—Gliomatosis cerebri is a diffuse glial tumor infiltrating the brain extensively, involving more than two lobes, frequently bilaterally and often extending to infratentorial structures and even to the spinal cord (Lantos and Bruner 2000).

1993—Diffuse neoplastic glial cell infiltration of the brain involving several cerebral lobes and, on occasion, infratentorial structures and the spinal cord (Kleihues et al. 1993).

1979—A rare entity consisting in an extremely diffuse involvement of one or both cerebral hemispheres by glial cells which have undergone neoplastic transformation, with variable degrees of differentiation. It may contain foci of glioblastoma (Zülch 1979).

56.1 Epidemiology

Incidence
- Rare

Age Incidence
- All ages possible
- Mean age: 40–50 years

Sex Incidence
- Male:Female ratio: 1:1

Localization
- Any region of the central nervous system
- Most commonly the cerebral hemispheres (75%)
- Bilateral involvement in 77% of the cases

56.2 Neuroimaging Findings

General Imaging Findings
- Diffuse infiltrating
- Involved structures appear extended
- Almost no mass effect

CT Non-Contrast-Enhanced (Fig. 56.1i)
- Slight hypodense
- Loss of white and gray matter differentiation
- Can appear normal

CT Contrast-Enhanced
- Usually no enhancement

MRI-T2 (Figs. 56.1a and 56.2a)
- Homogeneous hyperintense

MRI-FLAIR (Figs. 56.1b and 56.2b)
- Homogeneous hyperintense
- Gives best impression of tumor extent

MRI-T1 (Figs. 56.1c and 56.2c)
- Iso- to hypointense

MRI-T1 Contrast-Enhanced (Figs. 56.1d and 56.2d)
- No enhancement typical
- In some cases focal enhancement—suspicious of malignant progression

MRI-T2∗/SWI
- No hemorrhage

MR-Diffusion Imaging (Figs. 56.1e, f and 56.2e)
- No restricted diffusion.

MRI-Perfusion (Figs. 56.1g and 56.2f)
- rCBV low (absence of de novo vascularization)

MR-Diffusion Tensor Imaging
- Fiber tracks seem to be preserved.

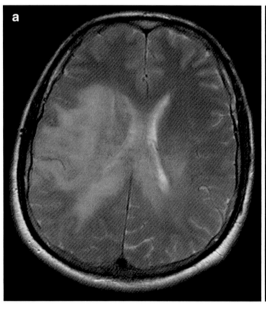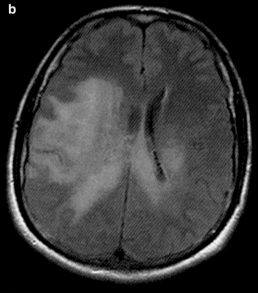

Fig. 56.1 A right-sided diffuse infiltrating mass with extension across the splenium, which is hyperintense in T2 (**a**) and FLAIR (**b**), hypointense in T1 (**c**), without contrast enhancement in T1 contrast (**d**). DWI and ADC do not reveal any restricted diffusion (**e, f**) or elevation of rCBV in MR-perfusion (**g**). In MR-spectroscopy, the typical elevation of the myoinositol peak (=ins) is seen (**h**). CT (**i**)

56.2 Neuroimaging Findings

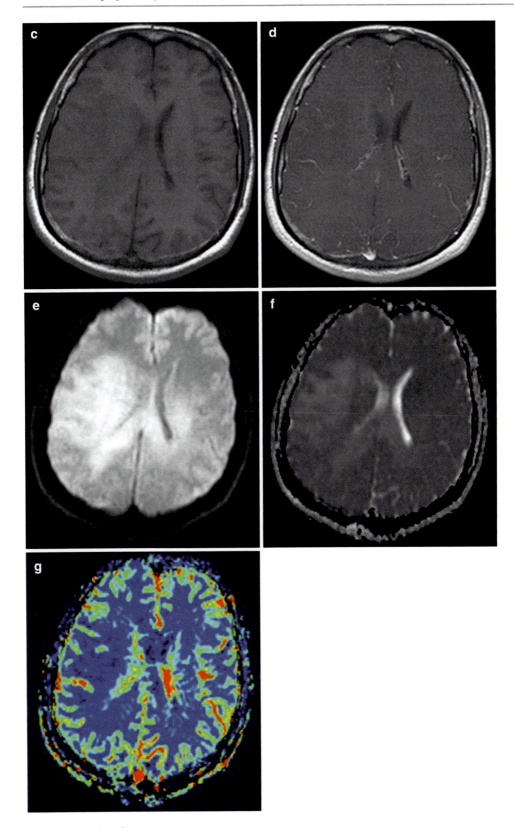

Fig. 56.1 (continued)

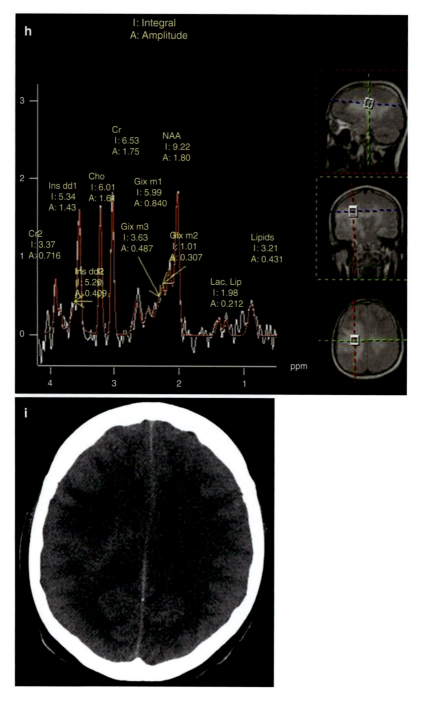

Fig. 56.1 (continued)

56.5 Treatment and Prognosis

MR-Spectroscopy (Fig. 56.1h)
- Myoinositol elevated
- NAA decreased
- Choline increased

Nuclear Medicine Imaging Findings
- Gliomatosis shows inhomogeneous uptake with often only slight uptake in large regions representing the inhomogeneous proliferation of malignant tumor cells.
- Due to the normal uptake behavior of the residual neuronal cells, FET uptake can be only faint in regions with less malignant transformed cells.
- In regions with accumulation of malignant cells, FET uptake is increased.

56.3 Neuropathology Findings

Macroscopic Features
- Swollen firm lesion
- Blurred distinction between gray and white matter

Microscopic Features
- Proliferation of small glial cells with elongated fusiform nuclei.
- Astrocytic features of tumor cells.
  - Large cells with irregular pleomorphic nuclei
- Infiltrated white matter shows signs of demyelination with preserved neurons and axons.
- Features of oligodendroglioma.
- Absence of microvascular proliferation and necrosis.
- Gliomatosis cerebri might show areas of tumor manifestation corresponding to
  - Diffuse astrocytoma, WHO grade II (see Chap. 52)
  - Anaplastic astrocytoma, WHO grade III (see Chap. 53)
  - Glioblastoma, WHO grade IV (see Chap. 54)

Immunophenotype
- GFAP-positivity variable
- S-100-positivity variable
- MAP 2
- CD44 (hyaluronic acid receptor)
- Matrix metalloproteinases
- Fibroblast growth factor receptor 1 (FGFR1)

Proliferation Markers
- Ki-67-LI ranges between 1 and 30% depending on the grade of the tumor

Ultrastructural Features
- See ultrastructural features of astrocytoma grade II, anaplastic astrocytoma WHO grade III, and glioblastoma WHO grade IV

Differential Diagnosis
- Astrocytic tumors grade II, III, and IV
- Oligodendrogliomas grade II, III
- Oligo-astrocytomas grade II, III

56.4 Molecular Neuropathology

Pathogenesis
- Two hypotheses:
- Subtype of glioma with unusual infiltrative capacity
- Simultaneous neoplastic transformation at different regional sites ("field cancerization")
- Monoclonal origin of gliomatosis cerebri with widespread tumor infiltration

Genes
- Not well investigated
- *TP53* mutations (see Chaps. 52 and 54)
- *IDH1* R132H mutation
- *Alpha-internexin* (INA)
- *MGMT* promoter methylation
- *PTEN* mutation

56.5 Treatment and Prognosis

Treatment
- Biopsy for establishing the diagnosis
- Resection usually impossible because of diffuse spread
- Radiation
- Chemotherapy with
  - Temozolamide
  - PCV (procarbazine, carmustine, vincristine)

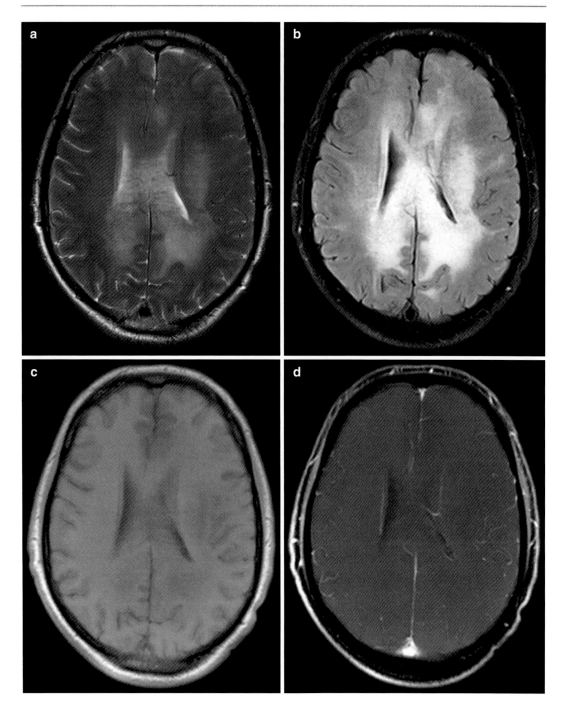

Fig. 56.2 A bi-hemispheric gliomatosis cerebri T2 (**a**), FLAIR (**b**), T1 (**c**), T1 contrast-enhanced (**d**), ADC (**e**) and rCBV (**f**)

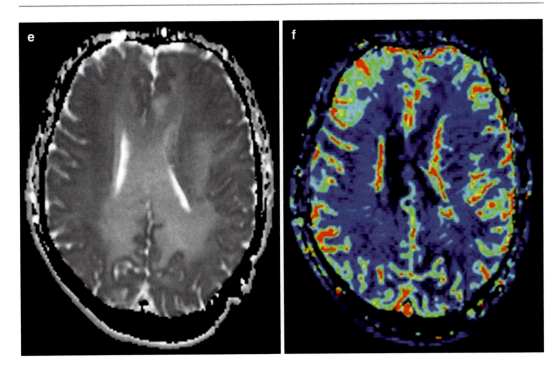

Fig. 56.2 (continued)

Biologic Behavior–Prognosis–Prognostic Factors

- Median survival: 11–38 months
- Median survival depends on:
  - Age at onset (<42 years)
  - Karnofsky performance status at time of clinical presentation (>80)
  - WHO grade of the tumor
  - Histologic subtype
  - Ki67
  - MGMT promoter methylation status

Selected References

Akai H, Mori H, Aoki S, Masutani Y, Kawahara N, Shibahara J, Ohtomo K (2005) Diffusion tensor tractography of gliomatosis cerebri: fiber tracking through the tumor. J Comput Assist Tomogr 29(1):127–129

Boisselier B, De Carli E, Rousseau A (2017) Molecular alterations in pediatric gliomatosis cerebri are similar to those in less invasive forms of pediatric diffuse glioma. J Neurooncol 133(1):217–219. https://doi.org/10.1007/s11060-017-2432-x

Broniscer A (2016) Gliomatosis cerebri in children shares molecular characteristics with other pediatric gliomas. J Neuro-Oncol 131(2):299–307. https://doi.org/10.1007/s00401-015-1532-y

Chen S, Tanaka S, Giannini C, Morris J, Yan ES, Buckner J, Lachance DH, Parney IF (2013) Gliomatosis cerebri: clinical characteristics, management, and outcomes. J Neuro-Oncol 112(2):267–275. https://doi.org/10.1007/s11060-013-1058-x

D'Urso OF, D'Urso PI, Marsigliante S, Storelli C, Luzi G, Gianfreda CD, Montinaro A, Distante A, Ciappetta P (2009) Correlative analysis of gene expression profile and prognosis in patients with gliomatosis cerebri. Cancer 115(16):3749–3757. https://doi.org/10.1002/cncr.24435

Freund M, Hahnel S, Sommer C, Martmann M, Kiessling M, Tronnier V, Sartor K (2001) CT and MRI findings in gliomatosis cerebri: a neuroradiologic and neuropathologic review of diffuse infiltrating brain neoplasms. Eur Radiol 11(2):309–316. https://doi.org/10.1007/s003300000653

Fuller GN, Kros JM (2007) Gliomatosis cerebri. In: Louis DN, Ohgaki H, Wiestier OD, Cavenee WK (eds) WHO classification of tumours of the central nervous system, 4th edn. International Agency for Research on Cancer, Lyon, pp 50–2

Guzman-de-Villoria JA, Sanchez-Gonzalez J, Munoz L, Reig S, Benito C, Garcia-Barreno P, Desco M (2007) 1H MR spectroscopy in the assessment of gliomatosis cerebri. AJR Am J Roentgenol 188(3):710–714. https://doi.org/10.2214/ajr.06.0055

Herrlinger U (2012) Gliomatosis cerebri. Handb Clin Neurol 105:507–515. https://doi.org/10.1016/b978-0-444-53502-3.00005-7

Herrlinger U, Jones DTW, Glas M, Hattingen E, Gramatzki D, Stuplich M, Felsberg J, Bahr O, Gielen GH, Simon M, Wiewrodt D, Schabet M, Hovestadt V, Capper D, Steinbach JP, von Deimling A, Lichter P, Pfister SM, Weller M, Reifenberger G (2016) Gliomatosis cerebri: no evidence for a separate brain tumor entity. Acta Neuropathol 131(2):309–319. https://doi.org/10.1007/s00401-015-1495-z

Kararizou E, Likomanos D, Gkiatas K, Markou I, Triantafyllou N, Kararizos G (2006) Magnetic resonance spectroscopy: a noninvasive diagnosis of gliomatosis cerebri. Magn Reson Imaging 24(2):205–207. https://doi.org/10.1016/j.mri.2005.10.032

Kleihues P, Burger PC, Scheithauer BW (1993) Histological typing of tumours of the central nervous system, 2nd edn. Springer, Berlin

Lantos PL, Bruner JM (2000) Gliomatosis cerebri. In: Kleihues P, Cavenee WK (eds) Pathology and genetics of tumours of the nervous system, 3rd edn. IARC Press, Lyon, pp 92–93

Louis DN, Suvá ML, Burger PC, Perry A, Kleihues P, Aldape KD, Brat DJ, Biernat W, Bigner DD, Nakazato Y, Plate KH, Giangaspero F, Ohgaki H, Cavenee WK, Wick W, Barnholtz-Sloan J, Rosenblum MK, Hegi M, Stupp R, Hawkins C, Verhaak RGW, Ellison DW, von Deimling A (2016) Glioblastoma, IDH-wildtype. In: Louis DN, Ohgaki H, Wiestler OD, Cavenee WK (eds) WHO classification of tumours of the central nervous system, Revised 4th edn. IARC, Lyon, pp 28–45

Maharaj MM, Phan K, Xu J, Fairhall J, Reddy R, Rao PJV (2017) Gliomatosis cerebri: prognosis based on current molecular markers. J Clin Neurosci 43:1–5. https://doi.org/10.1016/j.jocn.2017.04.043

Mohana-Borges AV, Imbesi SG, Dietrich R, Alksne J, Amjadi DK (2004) Role of proton magnetic resonance spectroscopy in the diagnosis of gliomatosis cerebri: a unique pattern of normal choline but elevated Myo-inositol metabolite levels. J Comput Assist Tomogr 28(1):103–105

Rajz GG, Nass D, Talianski E, Pfeffer R, Spiegelmann R, Cohen ZR (2012) Presentation patterns and outcome of gliomatosis cerebri. Oncol Lett 3(1):209–213. https://doi.org/10.3892/ol.2011.445

Ruda R, Bertero L, Sanson M (2014) Gliomatosis cerebri: a review. Curr Treat Options Neurol 16(2):273. https://doi.org/10.1007/s11940-013-0273-2

Uysal E, Erturk M, Yildirim H, Karatag O, Can M, Tanik C, Basak M (2005) Multivoxel magnetic resonance spectroscopy in gliomatosis cerebri. Acta Radiol 46(6):621–624

von Deimling A, Huse JT, Yan H, Brat DJ, Ohgaki H, Kleihues P, Berger MS, Weller M, Burger PC, Ellison DW, Rosenblum MK, Reifenberger G, Paulus W, Wesseling P, Aldape KD, Louis DN (2016a) Anaplastic astrocytoma, IDH-mutant. In: Louis DN, Ohgaki H, Wiestler OD, Cavenee WK (eds) WHO classification of tumours of the central nervous system, Revised 4th edn. IARC, Lyon, pp 24–27

von Deimling A, Huse JT, Yan H, Brat DJ, Reifenberger G, Ohgaki H, Kleihues P, Berger MS, Weller M, Nakazato Y, Burger PC, Ellison DW, Louis DN (2016b) Diffuse astrocytoma, IDH-mutant. In: Louis DN, Ohgaki H, Wiestler OD, Cavenee WK (eds) WHO classification of tumours of the central nervous system, Revised 4th edn. IARC, Lyon, pp 18–23

Ware ML, Hirose Y, Scheithauer BW, Yeh RF, Mayo MC, Smith JS, Chang S, Cha S, Tihan T, Feuerstein BG (2007) Genetic aberrations in gliomatosis cerebri. Neurosurgery 60(1):150–158, discussion 158. https://doi.org/10.1227/01.neu.0000249203.73849.5d

Yu A, Li K, Li H (2006) Value of diagnosis and differential diagnosis of MRI and MR spectroscopy in gliomatosis cerebri. Eur J Radiol 59(2):216–221. https://doi.org/10.1016/j.ejrad.2006.03.001

Zülch KJ (1979) Histological typing of tumours of the central nervous system. World Health Organization, Geneva

Pilocytic Astrocytoma WHO Grade I

Other Astrocytic Tumors

WHO Definition

2016—An astrocytoma classically characterized by a biphasic pattern with variable proportions of compacted bipolar cells with Rosenthal fibers and loose-textured multipolar cells with microcysts and occasional granular bodies (Collins et al. 2016).

2007—A relatively circumscribed, slowly growing, often cystic astrocytoma occurring in children and young adults, histologically characterized by a biphasic pattern with varying proportions of compacted bipolar cells associated with Rosenthal fibers and loose-texture multipolar cells associated with microcysts and eosinophilic granular bodies/hyaline droplets (Scheithauer et al. 2007).

2000—A generally circumscribed, slowly growing, often cystic astrocytoma occurring in children and young adults, histologically characterized by a biphasic pattern with varying proportion of compacted bipolar cells with Rosenthal fibers and loose-textured multipolar cells with microcysts and granular bodies (Burger et al. 2000).

1993—A circumscribed astrocytoma composed, at least in part, of bipolar fusiform or "piloid" cells with dense fibrillation. Tumor cells tend to form compact parallel bundles. Particularly common is a biphasic pattern in which pilocytic areas are intimately associated with a loosely structured microcystic component consisting of protoplasmic, poorly fibrillated neoplastic astrocytes (Kleihues et al. 1993).

1979—An astrocytoma composed predominantly of fusiform cells which possess unusually long wavy fibrillary processes. Stellate astrocytes are also frequently found (Zülch 1979).

WHO Grade
- WHO grade I

57.1 Epidemiology

Incidence
- 0.4 per 100,000 persons per year
- 5–6% of all gliomas

Age Incidence
- Children: First two decades of life
- Adults:
  - mean age 25 years
  - rare in patients older than 50 years

Sex Incidence
- Male:Female ratio 1:1

Localization
- Throughout the neuraxis
- Optic nerve
- Optic chiasm/hypothalamus
- Thalamus
- Basal ganglia
- Cerebellum
- Brain stem
- Spinal cord
- Children:
  - Cerebellum (67%)
  - Hypothalamus/optic pathway
  - Thalamus/basal ganglia

57.2 Neuroimaging Findings

General Imaging Findings
- Predominant cystic mass with enhancing mural nodule
- Moderate to absent edema

CT Non-Contrast-Enhanced
- Hypodense cyst, solid tumor hypo- to isodense
- Calcifications possible

CT Contrast-Enhanced
- Solid components enhanced

MRI-T2/FLAIR (Figs. 57.1a, b and 57.2a, b)
- Solid components hyperintense to brain
- Cyst hyperintense to CSF

MRI-T1 (Figs. 57.1c and 57.2c)
- Solid component iso- to hypointense to parenchyma
- Cyst iso- to hyperintense to CSF

MRI-T1 Contrast-Enhanced (Figs. 57.1d and 57.2d, e)
- Solid components show strong heterogeneous enhancement
- Cyst wall may enhance

MRI-T2∗/SWI
- Calcifications possible
- Hemorrhage uncommon

MR-Diffusion Imaging (Fig. 57.2f)
- No restricted diffusion

MRI-Perfusion
- Slight elevation of rCBV in solid component

MR-Spectroscopy
- Choline elevated
- Lactate elevated
- NAA low
- Looks like a high-grade glioma, despite the benign character of the tumor

Nuclear Medicine Imaging Findings (Fig. 57.3)
- Pilocytic astrocytomas show a typically high FDG and amino acid uptake although the reason for this uptake is not fully clear.
- Hypometabolic pilocytic astrocytomas do occur.

57.3 Neuropathology Findings

Macroscopic Features (Figs. 57.4a–d and 57.5)
- Soft, gray discrete mass
- Cyst formation intratumoral and paratumoral
- Syrinx formation in the spinal cord
- Calcification possible
- Hemosiderin deposits possible

Microscopic Features (Fig. 57.6a–r)
- Low to moderate cellularity.
- Heterogeneity of histologic features.
- Biphasic pattern:
  - Loose-textured multipolar cells (protoplasmic astrocytes) with microcysts and granular bodies/hyaline droplets
  - Compacted bipolar cells with Rosenthal fibers

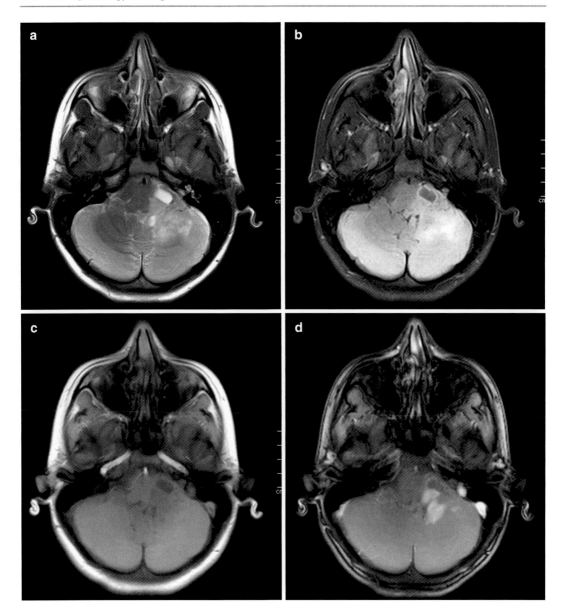

Fig. 57.1 Pilocytic astrocytoma in the most common location—the cerebellum T2 (**a**), FLAIR (**b**), T1 (**c**), T1 contrast (**d**)

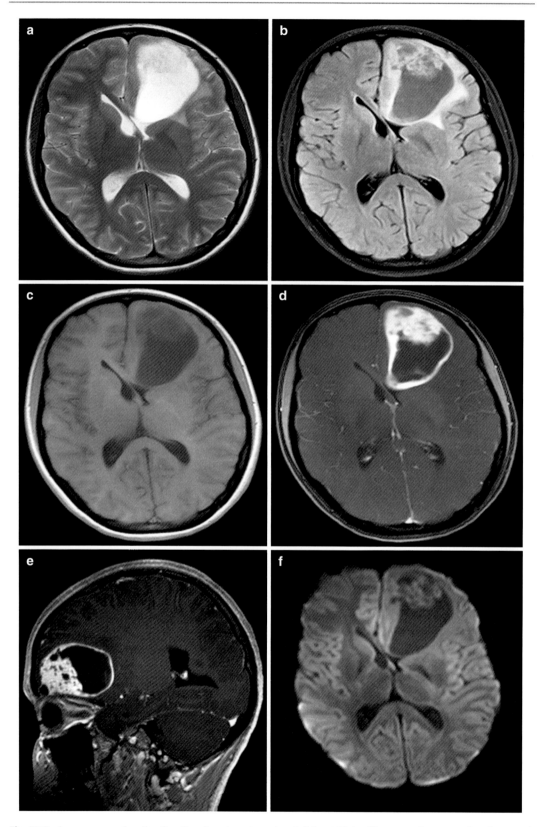

Fig. 57.2 An uncommon location for pilocytic astrocytoma, i.e., left frontal lobe. The tumor shows an enhancing mural nodule, as well as enhancement of the cyst wall and moderate edema. T2 (**a**), FLAIR (**b**), T1 (**c**), T1 c (**d, e**), DWI (**f**)

57.3 Neuropathology Findings

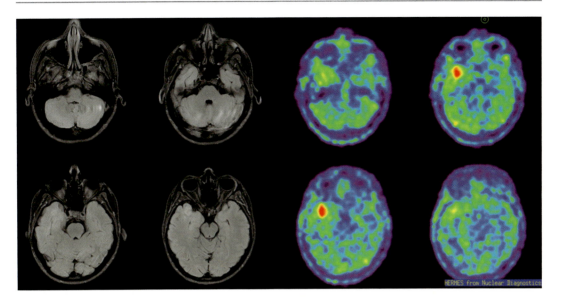

Fig. 57.3 FET-PET/CT slices of a pilocytic astrocytoma temporal right with correlating MRI (FLAIR)

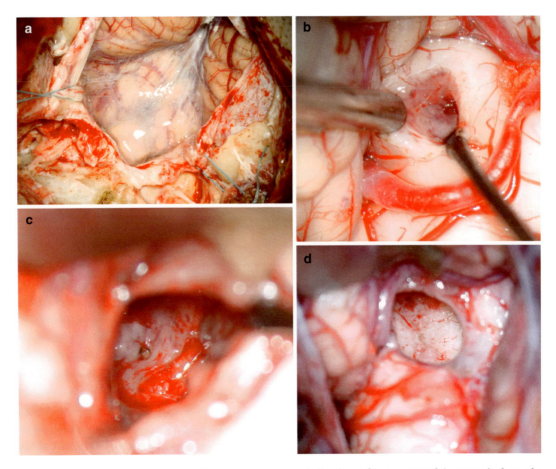

Fig. 57.4 Intraoperative appearance of pilocytic astrocytoma (WHO grade I). Translucent leptomeninges and view of the cerebellar hemispheres (**a**), transsection of the cerebellar tissue (**b**), exposure of the tumor in form of a soft, gray discrete mass (**c**, **d**)

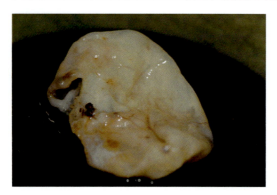

Fig. 57.5 Resected membranous cyst formation

- Protoplasmic astrocytes:
  - Round to oval nuclei
  - Small cell body
  - Short, cobweb-like processes poor in fibrils
- Cyst formation:
  - Common feature
  - Single or multiple
  - Cyst content contains factors stimulating vascular proliferation
- Rosenthal fibers:
  - Elongated nuclei
    Intracytoplasmic corkscrew-shaped, eosinophilic and hyaline masses (fibers) (GFAP-positivity)
- Eosinophilic granular bodies (EGB):
  - Globular aggregates within astrocytic processes
  - Eosinophilic
  - PAS-positive
- Tumor cell alignment in pallisades.
- Trapped neurons.
- Oligodendroglioma-like cells:
  - Arranged in sheets
  - Dispersed within the parenchyma
- No well-defined borders towards the surrounding brain tissue:
  - Infiltration zone extends between millimeters to centimeters.

- No aggressive overrunning of brain tissue by tumor.
- Mitoses are rare.
- Highly vascularized tumor.
- Not indicative as signs of malignancy are:
  - Hyalinized and glomeruloid vascular proliferation
  - Infarct-like, non-palisading necrosis
  - Infiltration of the leptomeninges
- Regressive changes include:
  - Hyalizined, ectatic vessels (DD cavernous angioma)
  - Previous hemorrhage (hemosiderin)
  - Calcification
  - Lymphocytic infiltrates

Immunophenotype (Fig. 57.7a–h)
- Lack of tumor-specific markers
- Rosenthal fibers
  - GFAP
- Eosinophilic granular bodies
  - α-1 antichymotrypsin
  - α-1 antitrypsin
- IDH1 R123H negative

Proliferation Markers (Fig. 57.7i, j)
- Mitoses are rare.
- Ki-67 LI: low.

Ultrastructural Features
- Rosenthal fibers:
  - Within astrocytic process
  - Amorphous, electron-dense elements surrounded by intermediate glial filaments

Differential Diagnosis
- Diffuse astrocytoma WHO grade II
- Oligodendroglioma WHO grade II
- Ganglion cell tumor (ganglioblastoma, ganglioneuroma)

57.3 Neuropathology Findings

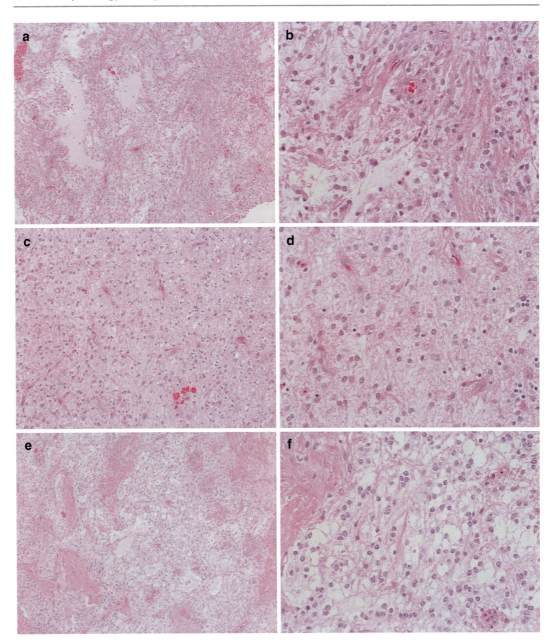

Fig. 57.6 Pilocytic astrocytoma (WHO grade I): Tumor of low to moderate cellularity (**a–j**) showing heterogeneity of histologic features with a biphasic pattern which consists of loose-textured multipolar cells (protoplasmic astrocytes) (**a–d**). Oligodendroglioma-like cells are arranged in sheets and dispersed within the parenchyma (**e, f**). Microcysts of various size (**g, h**). Rosenthal fibers consist of elongated nuclei and are discernible as intracytoplasmic corkscrew-shaped, eosinophilic and hyaline masses (fibers) (**i–l**) which are (GFAP-positivity, Fig. 56.7b). Eosinophilic granular bodies (EGB) are eosinophilic PAS-positive globular aggregates within astrocytic processes (**m, n**). Regressive changes are represented by strongly hyalinized, partly ectatic vessels (**o–r**) and a few hemosiderinophages (**q, r**)

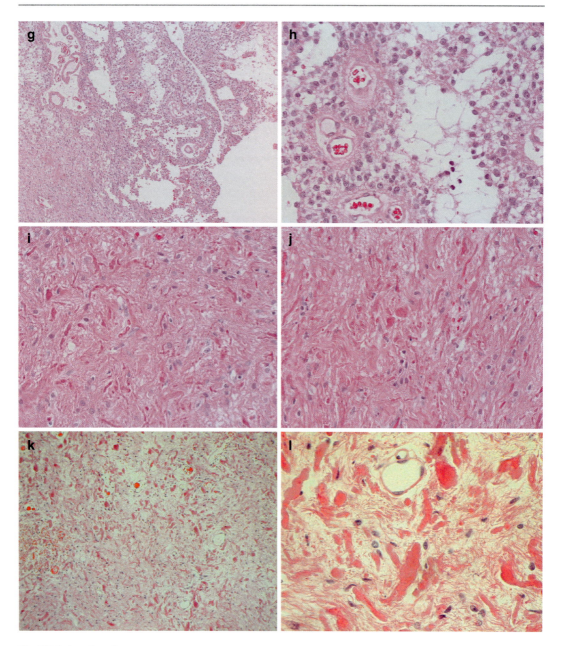

Fig. 57.6 (continued)

57.3 Neuropathology Findings

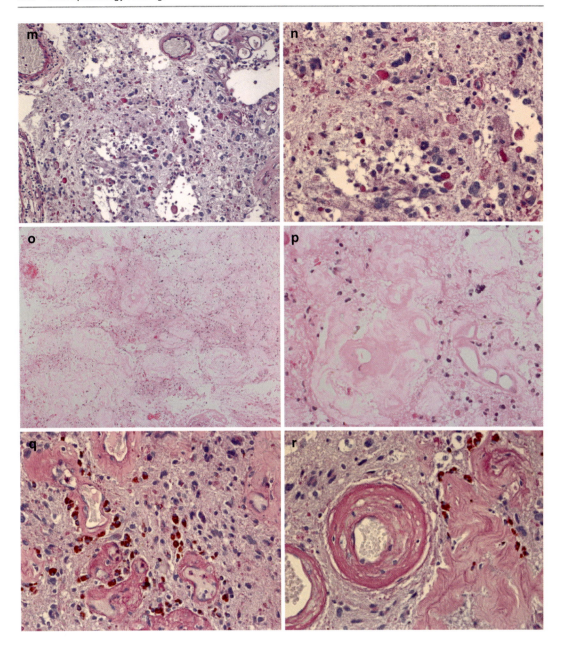

Fig. 57.6 (continued)

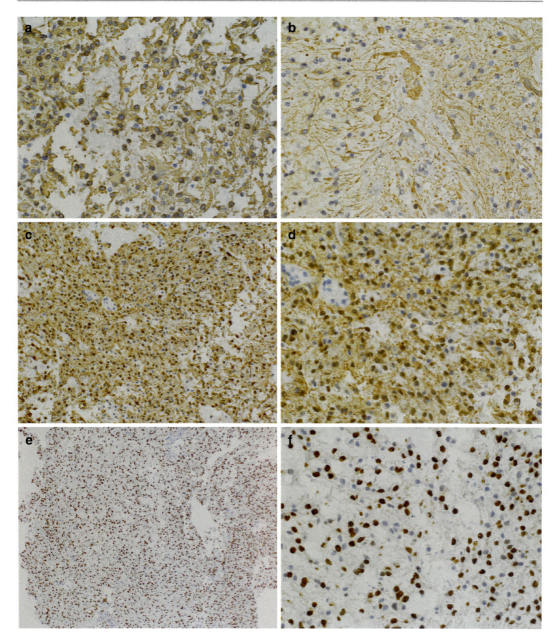

Fig. 57.7 Pilocytic astrocytoma (WHO grade I)—Immunophenotype: Tumor cells (**a**) and Rosenthal fibers (**b**) are positive for GFAP, S-100 (**c, d**), Olig2 (**e, f**), ATRX (**g, h**). Low Ki-67 proliferation rate (**i, j**)

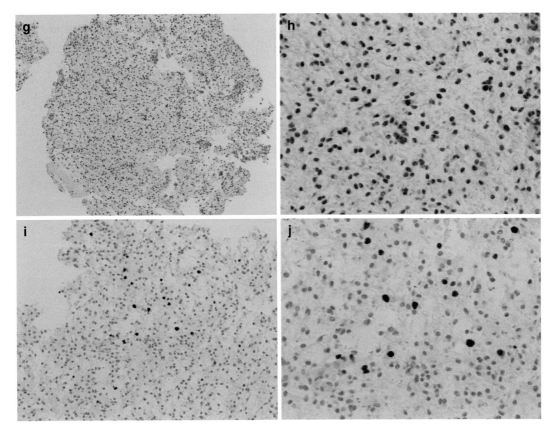

Fig. 57.7 (continued)

57.4 Molecular Neuropathology

57.4.1 Pathogenesis

- Derive from piloid cells
  - Similar to cells found around chronic lesions of the hypothalamus, cerebellum, spinal cord, or glial stromal cells of the pineal gland

57.4.2 Genetics

Patients suffering from neurofibromatosis type 1 (NF1), a hereditary tumor syndrome (Chap. 70), frequently develop pilocytic astrocytoma. About one-third of pilocytic astrocytomas are observed in NF1 patients, whereas the sporadic types of this tumor are NF1 independent.

- *NF1-associated pilocytic astrocytoma*
- Neurofibromin, encoded by the *NF1* gene on chromosome 17q11.2, functions as a tumor suppressor by inhibiting oncogenic Ras (= *Ra*t *sarcoma*) signaling. In neurofibromatosis type 1 and in NF1-associated pilocytic astrocytoma, *NF1* gene deletions and mutations result in loss of functional neurofibromin.
- *NF1-independent pilocytic astrocytoma*
  - In sporadic pilocytic astrocytoma, typical genetic aberrations (>60%) are duplications at chromosome region 7q34, affecting the *BRAF* gene (v-raf murine sarcoma viral oncogene homolog B). These duplications create in-frame fusions of *BRAF* with the upstream *KIAA1549* gene. The resulting aberrant fusion proteins contain the BRAF kinase domain and were shown to exhibit constitutive BRAF kinase activity which in

turn activates the oncogenic MAPK (mitogen-activated protein kinase) signaling pathway.
- Oncogenic BRAF activation not only occurs via gene duplication but may also be the result of mutations occurring around codon 600:
    ○ a T > A mutation at nucleotide position 1799, creating the replacement of the wild-type valine 600 by a glutamate residue in the protein (referred to as the BRAF^{V600E} mutation)
    ○ two different 3 bp-insertions, both resulting in an additional threonine residue at amino acid position 599.
- These activating mutations occur at a much lower frequency than the *KIAA1549/BRAF* fusions (~9%).
- Similar to the *BRAF* fusions, albeit less common, are fusions on chromosome 3p25 between the *SRGAP3* (SLIT-ROBO Rho GTPase-activating protein 3) gene and the *RAF1* (v-raf-1 murine leukemia viral oncogene homolog 1) gene. RAF1 is a positive regulator of the oncogenic MAPK signaling pathway; in *SRGAP3/RAF1* fusions, the auto-inhibitory region of RAF1 is lost, leading to a constitutive activation of the MAPK pathway (Table 57.1).

Table 57.1 Summary of mutations in pilocytic astrocytoma, modified after Collins et al. (2015)

MAPK pathway aberration	Diagnostic utility
KIAA1549:BRAF	• Highly recurrent in PA • Extremely rare in other entities
Other *BRAF/RAF1* fusions	• Recurrent in PA • Extremely rare in other entities
BRAF V600E	• Recurrent in supratentorial PA • Common in ganglioglioma, pleomorphic xanthoastrocytoma, dysembryoplastic neuroepithelial tumor
KRAS	• Rare in PA • Frequency not fully established in other entities
FGFR1 mutation	• Recurrent in midline PA • Frequency not fully established in other entities
FGFR1-ITD/ fusion	• Rare in PA • Observed in other low-grade gliomas
NTRK fusions	• Recurrent in PA • Observed in other low-grade gliomas and infant high-grade gliomas
NF1	• Typically germline • Closely associated with optic pathway PA

Reproduced with kind permission by Springer Nature

57.4.3 Epigenetics

- To date, epigenomic investigations in pilocytic astrocytoma are still sparse. One study on microRNA (miR) expression (Birks et al. 2011) revealed
    - overexpression of *miR-29a, miR-34a, miR-138, miR-299–5p, miR-432*, and
    - underexpression of *miR-93, miR-106b, miR-129, miR-135a, miR-135b*
- Somatic mitochondrial mutations, mostly single nucleotide exchanges, were recently reported in pilocytic astrocytoma. Some of the mutations resided in coding regions, causing amino acid alterations. The affected gene products were identified as proteins involved in electron transport/oxidative phosphorylation (Lueth et al. 2009).

57.5 Treatment and Prognosis

Treatment
- Surgery

Biologic Behavior–Prognosis–Prognostic Factors
- Slowly growing tumor.
- Rarely spontaneous regression.
- Usually long-term survival.

- Metastases along the neuraxis are possible usually with the primary affection of the hypothalamus.
- No sign of aggressive behavior.
- Maintain for a long time (years to decades) grade I status.
- Regressive changes rather than anaplasia.
- No prognostic significance for:
  - Increased cellularity
  - Nuclear abnormalities
  - Occasional mitoses
- Anaplastic (atypical, malignant) pilocytic astrocytoma grade III:
  - Multiple mitoses per single high-power field
  - Endothelial proliferation
  - Palisading necroses

Selected References

Bian SX, McAleer MF, Vats TS, Mahajan A, Grosshans DR (2013) Pilocytic astrocytoma with leptomeningeal dissemination. Child's Nerv Syst 29(3):441–450. https://doi.org/10.1007/s00381-012-1970-y

Bikowska-Opalach B, Szlufik S, Grajkowska W, Jozwiak J (2014) Pilocytic astrocytoma: a review of genetic and molecular factors, diagnostic and prognostic markers. Histol Histopathol 29(10):1235–1248. https://doi.org/10.14670/hh-29.1235

Birks DK, Barton VN, Donson AM, Handler MH, Vibhakar R, Foreman NK (2011) Survey of MicroRNA expression in pediatric brain tumors. Pediatr Blood Cancer 56(2):211–216. https://doi.org/10.1002/pbc22723. Epub 22010 Nov 22723

Burger PC, Scheithauer BW, Paulus W, Szymas J, Giannini C, Kleihues P (2000) Pilocytic astrocytoma. In: Kleihues P, Cavenee WK (eds) Pathology and genetics of tumours of the nervous system, 3rd edn. IARC Press, Lyon, pp 45–51

Chourmouzi D, Papadopoulou E, Konstantinidis M, Syrris V, Kouskouras K, Haritanti A, Karkavelas G, Drevelegas A (2014) Manifestations of pilocytic astrocytoma: a pictorial review. Insights Imaging 5(3):387–402. https://doi.org/10.1007/s13244-014-0328-2

Collins VP, Jones DT, Giannini C (2015) Pilocytic astrocytoma: pathology, molecular mechanisms and markers. Acta Neuropathol 129(6):775–788. https://doi.org/10.1007/s00401-015-1410-7

Collins VP, Tihan T, VandenBerg SR, Burger PC, Hawkins C, Jones D, Giannini C, Rodriguez F, Figarella-Branger D (2016) Pilocytic astrocytoma. In: Louis DN, Ohgaki H, Wiestler OD, Cavenee WK (eds) WHO classification of tumours of the central nervous system, Revised 4th edn. IARC, Lyon, pp 80–88

Gaudino S, Martucci M, Russo R, Visconti E, Gangemi E, D'Argento F, Verdolotti T, Lauriola L, Colosimo C (2017) MR imaging of brain pilocytic astrocytoma: beyond the stereotype of benign astrocytoma. Child's Nerv Syst 33(1):35–54. https://doi.org/10.1007/s00381-016-3262-4

Jones DT, Gronych J, Lichter P, Witt O, Pfister SM (2012) MAPK pathway activation in pilocytic astrocytoma. Cell Mol Life Sci 69(11):1799–1811. https://doi.org/10.1007/s00018-011-0898-9

Kleihues P, Burger PC, Scheithauer BW (1993) Histological typing of tumours of the central nervous system, 2nd edn. Springer, Berlin

Koeller KK, Rushing EJ (2004) From the archives of the AFIP: pilocytic astrocytoma: radiologic-pathologic correlation. Radiographics 24(6):1693–1708. https://doi.org/10.1148/rg.246045146

Lueth M, Wronski L, Giese A, Kirschner-Schwabe R, Pietsch T, von Deimling A, Henze G, Kurtz A, Driever PH (2009) Somatic mitochondrial mutations in pilocytic astrocytoma. Cancer Genet Cytogenet 192(1):30–35. https://doi.org/10.1016/j.cancergencyto.2009.03.002

Marko NF, Weil RJ (2012) The molecular biology of WHO grade I astrocytomas. Neuro Oncol 14(12):1424–1431. https://doi.org/10.1093/neuonc/nos1257. Epub 2012 Oct 1422

Matyja E, Grajkowska W, Stepien K, Naganska E (2016) Heterogeneity of histopathological presentation of pilocytic astrocytoma—diagnostic pitfalls. A review. Folia Neuropathol 54(3):197–211

Pfister S, Witt O (2009) Pediatric Gliomas. In: von Deimling A (ed) Gliomas. Recent results in cancer research, vol 171. Springer, Berlin, pp 67–81

Reis GF, Tihan T (2015) Therapeutic targets in pilocytic astrocytoma based on genetic analysis. Semin Pediatr Neurol 22(1):23–27. https://doi.org/10.1016/j.spen.2014.12.001

Sadighi Z, Slopis J (2013) Pilocytic astrocytoma: a disease with evolving molecular heterogeneity. J Child Neurol 28(5):625–632. https://doi.org/10.1177/0883073813476141

Scheithauer BW, Hawkins C, Tihan T, VandenBerg SR, Burger PC (2007) Pilocytic astrocytoma. In: Louis DN, Ohgaki H, Wiestler OD, Cavenee WK (eds) WHO classification of tumours of the central nervous system. International Agency for Research on Cancer, Lyon, pp 14–21

Sexton-Oates A, Dodgshun A, Hovestadt V, Jones DT, Ashley DM, Sullivan M, MacGregor D, Saffery R (2018) Methylation profiling of paediatric pilocytic astrocytoma reveals variants specifically associated with tumour location and predictive of recurrence. Mol Oncol 12(8):1219–1232. https://doi.org/10.1002/1878-0261.12062

Trifiletti DM, Peach MS, Xu Z, Kersh R, Showalter TN, Sheehan JP (2017) Evaluation of outcomes after stereotactic radiosurgery for pilocytic astrocytoma. J Neuro-Oncol 134(2):297–302. https://doi.org/10.1007/s11060-017-2521-x

Xia J, Yin B, Liu L, Lu Y, Geng D, Tian W (2016) Imaging features of pilocytic astrocytoma in cerebral ventricles. Clin Neuroradiol 26(3):341–346. https://doi.org/10.1007/s00062-015-0370-6

Ye JM, Ye MJ, Kranz S, Lo P (2014) A 10 year retrospective study of surgical outcomes of adult intracranial pilocytic astrocytoma. J Clin Neurosci 21(12):2160–2164. https://doi.org/10.1016/j.jocn.2014.04.015

Zülch KJ (1979) Histological typing of tumours of the central nervous system. World Health Organization, Geneva

58
Oligodendroglioma WHO Grade II- Anaplastic Oligodendroglioma WHO Grade III

Diffuse Astrocytic and Oligodendroglial Tumors

58.1 Oligodendroglioma WHO Grade II

WHO Definition
2016—Oligodendroglioma, IDH-mutant, and 1p/19q co-deleted: A diffusely infiltrating, slow-growing glioma with IDH1 or IDH2 mutation and co-deletion of chromosomal arms 1p and 19q (Reifenberger et al. 2016b).

Oligodendroglioma, NOS: A diffusely infiltrating glioma with classic oligodendroglial histology, in which molecular testing for combined IDH mutation and 1p/19q co-deletion could not be completed or was inconclusive (Reifenberger et al. 2016b).

2007—A diffusely infiltrating, well-differentiated glioma of adults, typically located in the cerebral hemispheres, composed of neoplastic cells morphologically resembling oligodendroglia and often harboring deletions of chromosomal arms 1p and 19q (Reifenberger et al. 2007b).

2000—A well-differentiated, diffusely infiltrating tumor of adults, typically located in the cerebral hemispheres and composed predominantly of cells morphologically resembling oligodendroglia (Reifenberger et al. 2000b).

1993—A tumor composed predominantly of neoplastic oligodendrocytes (Kleihues et al. 1993).

1979—A tumor composed predominantly of oligodendroglial cells (Zülch 1979).

WHO Grade
- WHO grade II

58.1.1 Epidemiology

Incidence
- 0.27–0.35 per 100.000 persons
- 2.5% of all primary brain tumors
- 5–6% of all gliomas

Age Incidence
- Adults
- Mean age: 40–45 years
- Rare in children

Sex Incidence
- Male:Female ratio: 1.1:1

Localization
- Cortex and white matter of the cerebral hemispheres
- Frontal lobe in 50–65% of all cases
- Parietal and occipital lobes
- Involvement of more than one cerebral lobe
- Bilateral tumor spread possible
- Rarely in the posterior fossa, basal ganglia, brain stem, and spinal cord

58.1.2 Neuroimaging Findings

General Imaging Findings
- Well-defined infiltrative mass, involved cortex appears enlarged; calcifications common

CT Non-Contrast-Enhanced
- Hypo- to isodense
- Detects calcifications

CT Contrast-Enhanced
- In half of cases strong enhancement

MRI-T2/FLAIR (Figs. 58.1a, b and 58.2a, b)
- Heterogeneous, hyperintense (calcifications and cysts)
- Peritumoral edema rare

MRI-T1 (Figs. 58.1c and 58.2c)
- Hypo- to isointense

MRI-T1 Contrast-Enhanced (Figs. 58.1d and 58.2d)
- Heterogeneous, variable enhancement in 50% of cases

MRI-T2*/SWI
- Strong signal reduction (blooming) due to calcifications
- Hemorrhages uncommon

MR-Diffusion Imaging
- No restricted diffusion

MRI-Perfusion (Fig. 58.1e)
- Elevation of rCBV

MR-Spectroscopy (Fig. 58.1f)
- Choline elevated
- NAA reduced

Nuclear Medicine Imaging Findings (Figs. 58.3, 58.4, 58.5, 58.6, 58.7, 58.8, 58.9, and 58.10)
- FDG shows often hypometabolism in oligodendrogliomas WHO grade II.
- Radiotracers like FET (a marker of amino acid uptake (L-system)) or FLT (a marker of DNA biosynthesis) have the advantage of nearly no uptake in the healthy brain tissues. They may be positive or negative in oligodendrogliomas WHO grade II.
- Some studies suggest a better prognosis for patients with no amino acid uptake in low-grade gliomas than for patients with amino acid uptake.
- Images can show homogeneous or heterogeneous uptake representing the tumor biology.
- Results obtained for MET are similar to FET with the advantage of FET to be taken up in a lesser amount in inflammatory tissue and the longer half-life of 110 min compared to a relatively short half-life of 20 min of C-11 used in MET.
- Hypoxia tracers are under investigation for radiotherapy planning.

58.1.3 Neuropathology Findings

Macroscopic Features
- Well-defined masses
- Soft to gelatinous (mucoid degeneration)
- Grayish-pink color
- Infiltration of the leptomeninges possible
- Frequent calcifications
- Possible intratumoral cystic degeneration and/or hemorrhages

Microscopic Features (Fig. 58.11a–h)
- Monomorphic cells with
- Round nuclei
- Perinuclear halo only seen on paraffin sections (honeycomb appearance)
- Moderate cellularity
- Minigemistocytes or microgemistocytes
  – Somewhat larger cells with often eccentric cytoplasm
  – Positive for GFAP
- Sometimes tumor cells have signet ring appearance

58.1 Oligodendroglioma WHO Grade II

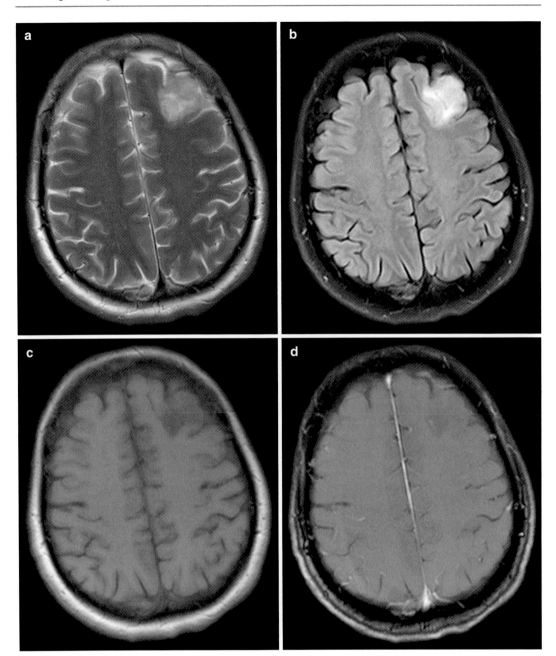

Fig. 58.1 Scans of a left frontal oligodendroglioma (WHO grade II), involving the cortex in T2 (**a**), FLAIR (**b**), T1 (**c**), T1 contrast (**d**), normal rCBV (**e**), and slight elevation of choline in MR-spectroscopy (**f**)

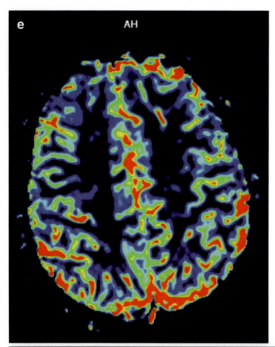

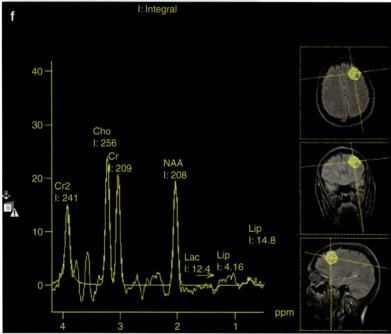

Fig. 58.1 (continued)

58.1 Oligodendroglioma WHO Grade II

- Microcalcifications
  - Associated with blood vessels
  - Within the tumor tissue
  - In the invaded brain tissue
- Mucoid/cystic degeneration
- Dense network of branching capillaries
  - Chicken-wire pattern
- Tumor cells form secondary structures like
  - Perineuronal satellitosis
  - Perivascular aggregates
  - Subpial accumulations
- Absent or low mitotic activity

Immunophenotype (Fig. 58.12a–d)
- Specific and sensitive marker not available
- IDH-1 R123H mutation-specific antibody
  - Reactivity seen in 67–82%
  - Expressed in the nucleus
  - Expressed in the cytoplasm
  - Differentiates tumor tissue from surrounding non-neoplastic tissue and/or reactive astrogliosis
- ATRX
- Expression of
  - S-100

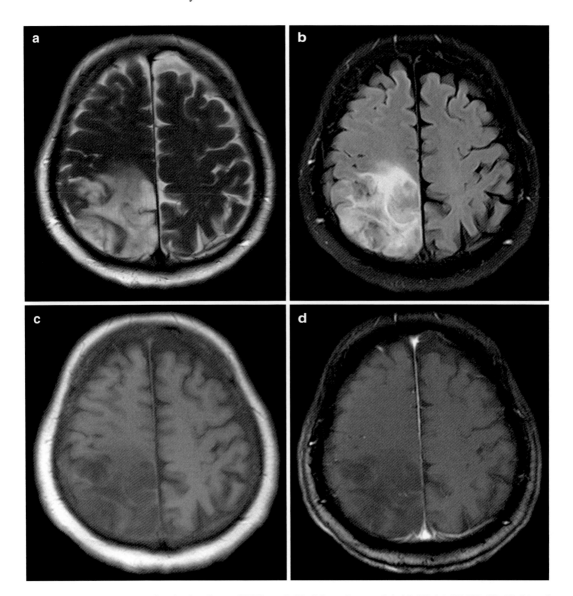

Fig. 58.2 Inhomogeneous oligodendroglioma (WHO grade II) right parieto-occipital in T2 (**a**), FLAIR (**b**), T1 (**c**) and T1gd (**d**)

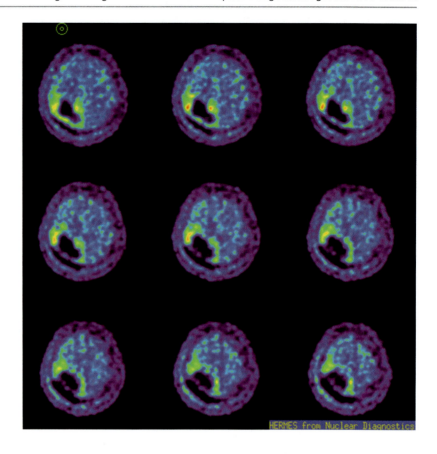

Fig. 58.3 FET-PET of an oligodendroglioma (WHO grade II) (right parietal) after resection with remaining viable tumor tissue (slices)

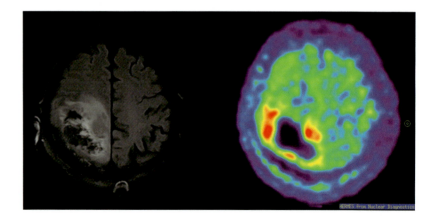

Fig. 58.4 FET-PET of an oligodendroglioma (WHO grade II) (right parietal) after resection in combination with postoperative MRI

- CD57
- γ-enolase
- MAP 2
- Expression of transcription factors OLIG-1, OLIG-2, SOX10
- GFAP expressed in minigemistocytes or intermingled reactive astrocytes
- Lack of nuclear p53 staining
- Synaptophysin expression mainly in the residual neuropil at infiltrating borders
- Oligodendroglioma-associated markers
  - NOGO-A
  - Alpha-internexin
- Loss of nuclear CIC or FUBP1 expression

58.1 Oligodendroglioma WHO Grade II

Fig. 58.5 FET-PET of an oligodendroglioma (WHO grade II) with focal increased proliferation left frontal before and after resection

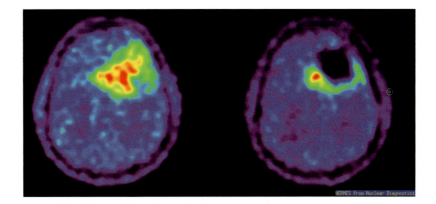

Fig. 58.6 FET-PET of an oligodendroglioma (WHO grade II) with focal increased proliferation after resection with remaining viable tumor tissue (slices)

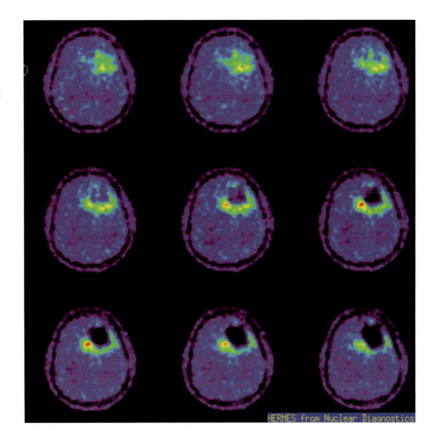

Proliferation Markers (Fig. 58.12e, f)
- Absent or low mitotic activity
- Ki-67 LI below 5%

Ultrastructural Features
- Similarities to normal oligodendrocytes, i.e.,
- Abundant, electron-lucent perikaryal cytoplasm
- Regular, rounded nuclei
- Fine granular nuclear chromatin
- Prominent nucleolus
- Cytoplasm with
  - Scant ribosomes
  - Scant endoplasmic reticulum
  - Numerous mitochondria
    Of abnormal large size
    Deranged architecture
    Skein-like appearance, i.e., fusiform membranous bodies

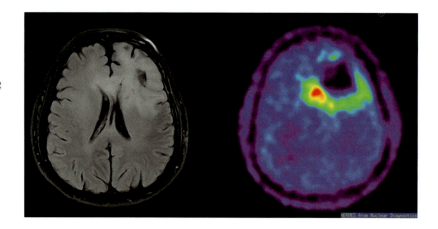

Fig. 58.7 FET-PET of an oligodendroglioma (WHO grade II) with focal increased proliferation after resection with remaining viable tumor tissue in combination with MRI

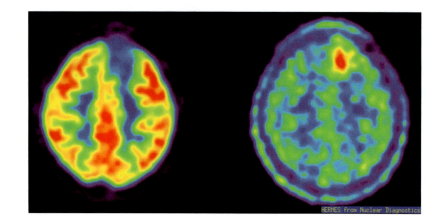

Fig. 58.8 FDG-PET (left) and FET-PET (right) of an oligodendroglioma (WHO grade II) demonstrating reduced FDG metabolism in contrast to increased FET uptake

- Absence of junctional attachments between tumor cells
- Cell processes
  - Electron-lucent, interdigitating
  - Contain 20 nm microtubules
  - Lamellar organization with parallel bundles
  - Form spirals, i.e., concentric membrane structures

Differential Diagnosis
- Reactive lesions
- Neoplastic lesions
  - Clear cell ependymoma (pseudorosettes, EMA immunoreactivity)
  - Neurocytoma (immunohistochemistry for synaptophysin)
  - Dysembryoplastic neuroepithelial tumor
  - Pilocytic astrocytoma
  - Clear cell meningioma (EMA immunoreactivity, abundant diastase-sensitive PAS-positive material)
  - Metastatic clear cell carcinomas (immunoreactivities for EMA and cytokeratins)

58.1.4 Molecular Neuropathology

58.1.4.1 Pathogenesis
- De novo
- From oligodendrocytes or other glial precursor cells

58.1.4.2 Genetics
- The most commonly detected genomic aberration in oligodendrogliomas is a heterozygous loss (LOH) of the short arm of chromosome 1 associated with LOH of the long arm of chromosome 19 (1p/19q co-deletion). The vast majority of oligodendro-

58.1 Oligodendroglioma WHO Grade II

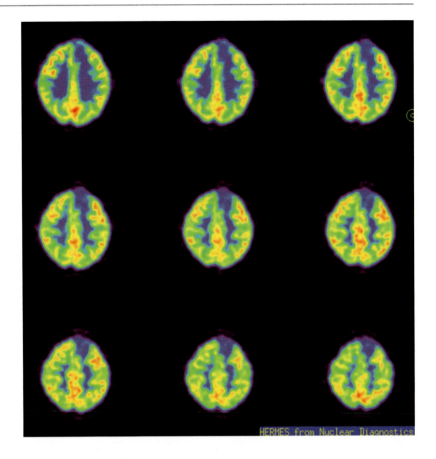

Fig. 58.9 FDG-PET slices of an FDG-negative oligodendroglioma (WHO grade II)

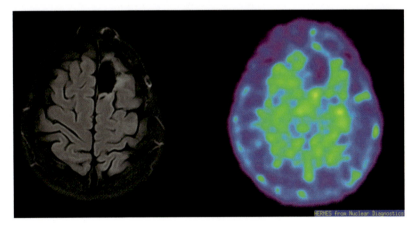

Fig. 58.10 FET-PET and MRI after successful resection of an oligodendroglioma (WHO grade II) left frontal

gliomas exhibit this genetic anomaly, with incidences of up to 90% reported for WHO grade II and somewhat lower for WHO grade III tumors (50–70%). Moreover, the 1p/19q co-deletion apparently occurs mutually exclusive of the TP53 mutations and chromosome 17p losses which are more common in astrocytic tumors (see Chaps. 52–54). Thus, the 1p/19q co-deletion represents a genetic hallmark in oligodendrogliomas.

- Mutations in the *IDH1*- and *IDH2* genes (encoding isocitrate dehydrogenase 1 and −2, respectively) are another characteristic feature in oligodendrogliomas. IDH1 localizes to the

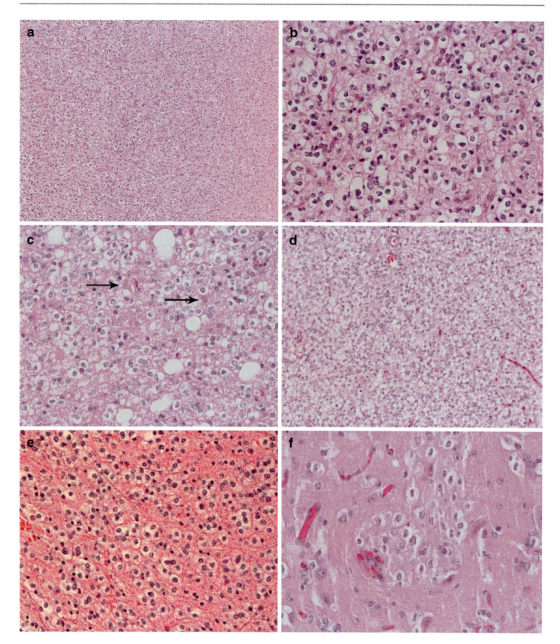

Fig. 58.11 Oligodendroglioma (WHO grade II): Moderately cellular tumor composed of monomorphic cells with round nuclei, perinuclear halo only seen on paraffin sections (honeycomb appearance) (**a–f**). Minigemistocytes or microgemistocytes are somewhat larger cells with often eccentric cytoplasm (arrow) (**c**); cystic degeneration (**c**), dense network of branching capillaries (chicken-wire pattern) (**b**). Diffuse infiltration of the upper layers of the cerebral cortex; the tumor cells reach the pial surface (**g, h**)

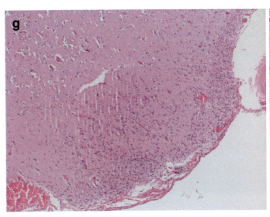
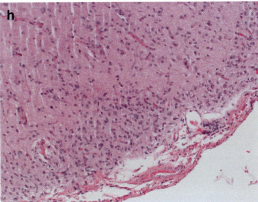

Fig. 58.11 (continued)

cytosol and IDH2 to the mitochondrion, and both enzymes are NADP⁺ dependent. The most frequently observed mutation in IDH1 (>70%) is an arginine to histidine exchange at amino acid position 132 (R132H) in the substrate-binding site of the enzyme. In IDH2, the homologous site was found to be mutated (R172K), however, in only a small fraction of the tumors (Yan et al. 2009).

- Similarly, IDH1/2 mutations were described in astrocytomas WHO grades II and III and in secondary glioblastomas (see Chaps. 52–54); in oligodendrogliomas they appear to be strongly associated with the 1p/19q co-deletion.
- Novel genetic anomalies have recently been correlated with oligodendrogliomas:
- Point mutations in the *CIC* (capicua transcriptional repressor) gene, located at chromosome 19q13.2; its gene product acts as a transcriptional repressor downstream of the receptor tyrosine kinase (RTK) pathway. Interestingly, *CIC* mutations occur in the majority (~70%) of oligodendrogliomas exhibiting the 1p/19q co-deletion plus IDH mutations.
- Point mutations in the *FUBP1* (far upstream element-binding protein 1) gene on chromosome 1p31.1; FUBP1 is a transcriptional regulator of the c-*Myc* oncogene. Most of the *FUBP1* mutations (>70%) are found in oligodendrogliomas that also carry *CIC* mutations.

58.1.4.3 Epigenetics

Several genes were shown to be affected by promoter hypermethylation, resulting in reduced expression levels:

- the *MGMT* gene, encoding the DNA repair enzyme O⁶-methylguanine-DNA methyltransferase
- *CDKN2A* (cyclin-dependent kinase inhibitor 2A) and *CDKN2B* (cyclin-dependent kinase inhibitor 2B)
- *RB1* (retinoblastoma 1)
- *DAPK1* (death-associated protein kinase 1)
- *ESR1* (estrogen receptor 1)

58.1.4.4 Gene Expression

Commonly observed in oligodendrogliomas are elevated expression levels of:

- *PDGFA* (platelet-derived growth factor, alpha polypeptide)
- *PDGFB* (platelet-derived growth factor, beta polypeptide)
- *PDGFR* (platelet-derived growth factor receptor, alpha polypeptide)
- *PDGFR* (platelet-derived growth factor receptor, beta polypeptide)

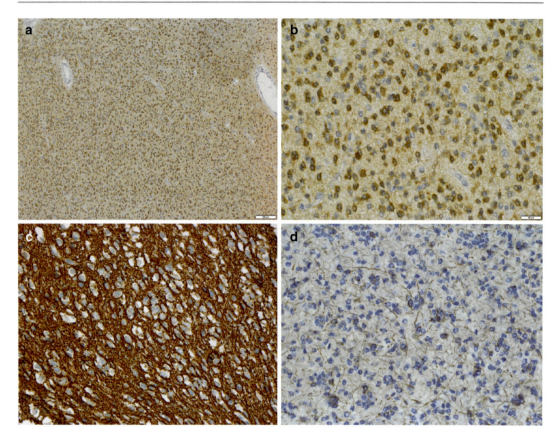

Fig. 58.12 Oligodendroglioma (WHO grade II)—Immunophenotype: IDH1 R123H (**a**, **b**); GFAP (**c**, **d**); low Ki-67 proliferation rate (**e**, **f**)

58.1.5 Treatment and Prognosis

Treatment
- Surgery

Biologic Behavior–Prognosis–Prognostic Factors
- Slowly growing tumors.
- Mean survival 11.6 years.
- Factors accounting for favorable outcome:
  - Young age
  - Frontal localization
  - Postoperative Karnofsky score
  - Lack of contrast enhancement
  - Macroscopically complete surgical removal
  - KI-67 LI less than 5%
  - Loss of 1p or combined 1p/19q loss
- Recurrence with malignant progression is common with longer progression-free intervals.

58.2 Anaplastic Oligodendroglioma WHO Grade III

WHO Definition
2016—Anaplastic oligodendroglioma, IDH-mutant, and 1p/19q co-deleted: An IDH-mutant and 1p/19q co-deleted oligodendroglioma with focal or diffuse histological features of anaplasia (in particular, pathological microvascular proliferation and/or brisk mitotic activity) (Reifenberger et al. 2016a).

Anaplastic oligodendroglioma, NOS: A diffusely infiltrating anaplastic glioma with classic oligodendroglial histology, in which molecular testing for combined IDH mutation and 1p/19q co-deletion could not be completed or was inconclusive (Reifenberger et al. 2016a).

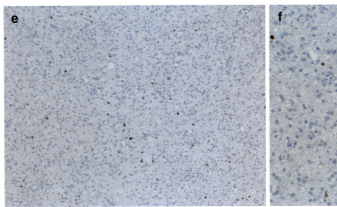
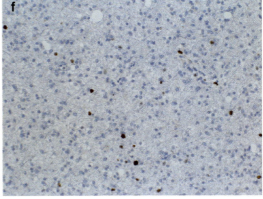

Fig. 58.12 (continued)

2007—An oligodendroglioma with focal or diffuse histological features of malignancy and a less favorable prognosis (Reifenberger et al. 2007a).

2000—An oligodendroglioma with focal or diffuse histological features of malignancy and a less favorable prognosis (Reifenberger et al. 2000a).

1993—An oligodendroglioma with focal or diffuse anaplasia, e.g., high cellularity, nuclear polymorphism, and brisk mitotic activity (Kleihues et al. 1993).

1979—An oligodendroglioma with areas of anaplasia (Zülch 1979).

WHO Grade
- WHO grade III

58.2.1 Epidemiology

Incidence
- Incidence: 0.07–0.18 per 100,000 population.
- 1.2% of all primary tumors.
- 20–35% of oligodendrogliomas are anaplastic oligodendrogliomas.

Age Incidence
- Adults
- Mean age: 45–50 years

Sex Incidence
- Male:Female ratio: 1.1:1

Localization
- Frontal lobe
- Temporal lobe

58.2.2 Neuroimaging Findings

General Imaging Findings
- Similar to oligodendroglioma WHO grade II; cysts, hemorrhages. and peritumoral edema are more common than in oligodendrogliomas WHO grade II

CT Non-Contrast-Enhanced (Fig. 58.13e)
- Hypo- to isointense
- Calcifications

CT Contrast-Enhanced
- Variable enhancement, more intense than low-grade tumors

MRI-T2/FLAIR (Fig. 58.13a, b)
- Heterogeneous hyperintense due to calcifications, cysts. and hemorrhages.
- Adjacent cortex appears expanded.

MRI-T1 (Fig. 58.13c)
- Hypo- to isointense

MRI-T1 Contrast-Enhanced (Fig. 58.13d)
- Enhancement more often and intense than in WHO grade II tumors

MRI-T2*/SWI
- Strong signal reduction (blooming) due to calcifications

MR-Diffusion Imaging
- No diffusion restriction

MRI-Perfusion
- Elevation of rCBV

MR-Spectroscopy (Fig. 58.13f)
- Choline elevated
- NAA reduced

Nuclear Medicine Imaging Findings
- FDG can show hypermetabolism in anaplastic oligodendrogliomas WHO grade III.

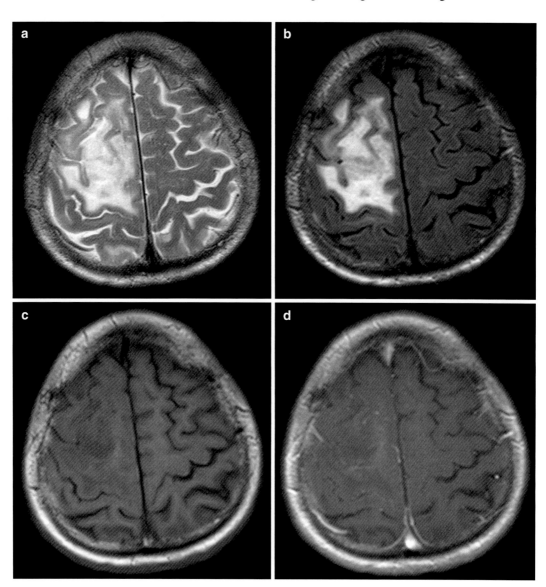

Fig. 58.13 Anaplastic oligodendroglioma (WHO grade III) in T2 (**a**), FLAIR (**b**), T1 (**c**), without contrast enhancement in T1 contrast (**d**). CT reveals an intratumoral calcification (**e**). MR-spectroscopy demonstrates a more elevated choline peak as compared to oligoastrocytoma WHO grade II (**f**)

58.2 Anaplastic Oligodendroglioma WHO Grade III

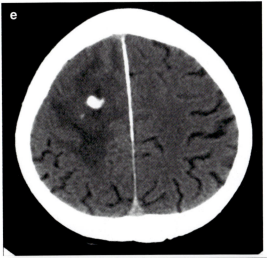

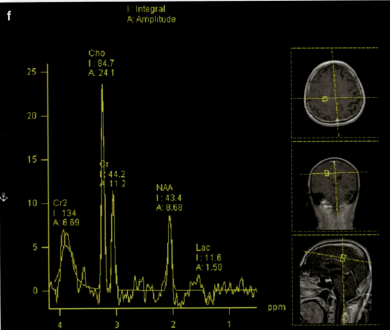

Fig. 58.13 (continued)

- Amino acid uptake is normally positive in anaplastic oligodendrogliomas WHO III with a higher uptake than in oligodendrogliomas WHO grade II.
- Images can show homogeneous or heterogeneous uptake representing the tumor biology.
- Results obtained for MET are similar to FET:
  - the advantage of FET is that it is taken up in a lesser amount by inflammatory tissue and its longer half-life of 110 min as compared to a relatively short half-life of 20 min of C-11 used in MET.
- Hypoxia tracers are under investigation for radiotherapy planning.

58.2.3 Neuropathology Findings

Macroscopic Features (Fig. 58.14a, b)
- Well-defined masses.
- Soft to gelatinous (mucoid degeneration).
- Grayish-pink color.
- Infiltration of the leptomeninges possible.
- Frequent calcifications.
- Possible intratumoral cystic degeneration and/or hemorrhages.
- Areas of necrosis might be seen.

Microscopic Features (Fig. 58.15a–j)
- Cellular
- Diffusely infiltrating
- Tumor cells are reminiscent of oligodendrocytes with:
  - Round hyperchromatic nuclei
  - Perinuclear halo
  - Scant cellular processes
- Tumor cells with
  - marked cellular and nuclear pleomorphism
  - multinucleated giant cells
  - spindle cell appearance
- Gliofibrillary oligodendrocytes
- Minigemistocytes
- Microcalcifications
- Dense network of branching capillaries (chicken-wire pattern) still preserved
  - With microvascular proliferation
- Necroses
  - Not indicative of shorter survival!

Immunophenotype (Fig. 58.16a–f)
- IDH-1 R123H mutation-specific antibody
- Reactivity seen in 49–89%
- Expressed in the nucleus
- Expressed in the cytoplasm
- Differentiates tumor tissue from surrounding non-neoplastic tissue and/or reactive astrogliosis
- GFAP partly positive
- Olig 2-positive
- Loss of nuclear CIC or FUBP1 expression
- ATRX

Proliferation Markers (Fig. 58.16g, h)
- High mitotic activity

Ultrastructural Features
- See Sect. 58.1

Differential Diagnosis
- Anaplastic astrocytoma (WHO grade III)
- Anaplastic oligo-astrocytoma (WHO grade III)
- Glioblastoma (WHO grade IV)
- Neurocytoma (central or extraventricular)
- Ependymoma

58.2.4 Molecular Neuropathology

58.2.4.1 Pathogensis
- De novo
- Progression from oligodendroglioma WHO grade II in 6–7 years

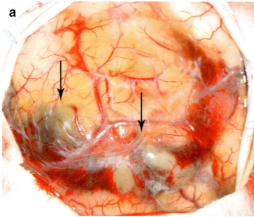

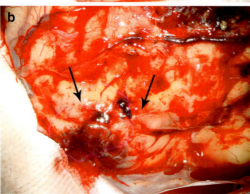

Fig. 58.14 Anaplastic oligodendroglioma (WHO grade III): Intraoperative appearance: the surface of the brain is extended and discolored (yellowish-brownish) (arrow) (**a**); the yellowish colored tumor is exposed after incisure of the brain surface (arrow) (**b**)

58.2 Anaplastic Oligodendroglioma WHO Grade III

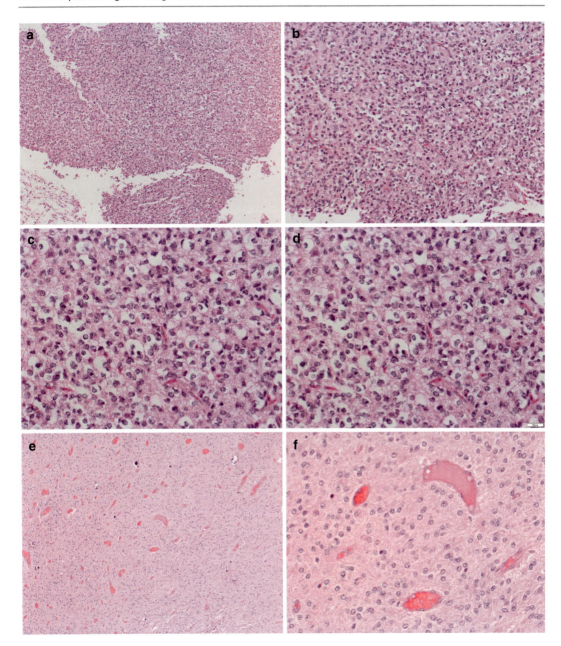

Fig. 58.15 Anaplastic oligodendroglioma (WHO grade III): Moderate to highly cellular, diffusely infiltrating tumor. The tumor cells are reminiscent of oligodendrocytes with round hyperchromatic nuclei, perinuclear halo, and scant cellular processes. The tumor cells show marked cellular and nuclear pleomorphism and sometimes a spindle cell appearance (**a–d**); dense network of branching capillaries (chicken-wire pattern) (**e, f**); calcifications are often present (**g, h**); areas of necrosis (**i, j**)

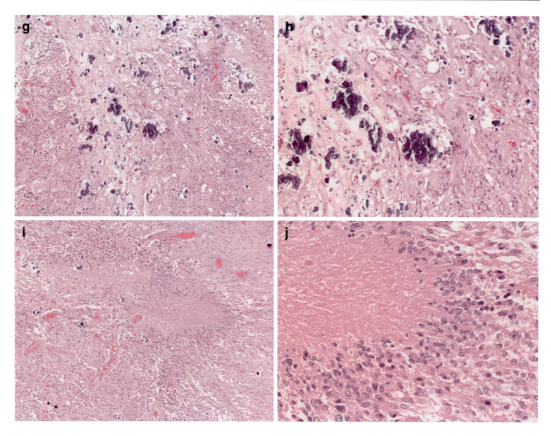

Fig. 58.15 (continued)

58.2.4.2 Genetics

- The most commonly detected genomic aberration in oligodendrogliomas is a heterozygous loss (LOH) of the short arm of chromosome 1 associated with LOH of the long arm of chromosome 19 (1p/19q co-deletion). The vast majority of oligodendrogliomas exhibit this genetic anomaly, with incidences of up to 90% reported for WHO grade II and somewhat lower for WHO grade III tumors (50–70%). Moreover, the 1p/19q co-deletion apparently occurs mutually exclusive of the TP53 mutations and chromosome 17p losses which are more common in astrocytic tumors (see Chaps. 52–54). Thus, the 1p/19q co-deletion represents a genetic hallmark in oligodendrogliomas.
- Mutations in the *IDH1*- and *IDH2* genes (encoding isocitrate dehydrogenase 1 and −2, respectively) are another characteristic feature in oligodendrogliomas. IDH1 localizes to the cytosol and IDH2 to the mitochondrion, and both enzymes are $NADP^+$-dependent. The most frequently observed mutation in IDH1 (>70%) is an arginine to histidine exchange at amino acid position 132 (R132H) in the substrate-binding site of the enzyme. In IDH2, the homologous site was found to be mutated (R172), however, in only a small fraction of the tumors (Yan et al. 2009).
- Similarly, IDH1/2 mutations were described in astrocytomas grade II and III and in secondary glioblastomas (see Chaps. 52–54); in oligodendrogliomas they appear to be strongly associated with the 1p/19q co-deletion.
- Novel genetic anomalies have recently been correlated with oligodendrogliomas:
- Point mutations in the *CIC* (capicua transcriptional repressor) gene, located at chromosome 19q13.2; its gene product acts as a transcrip-

58.2 Anaplastic Oligodendroglioma WHO Grade III

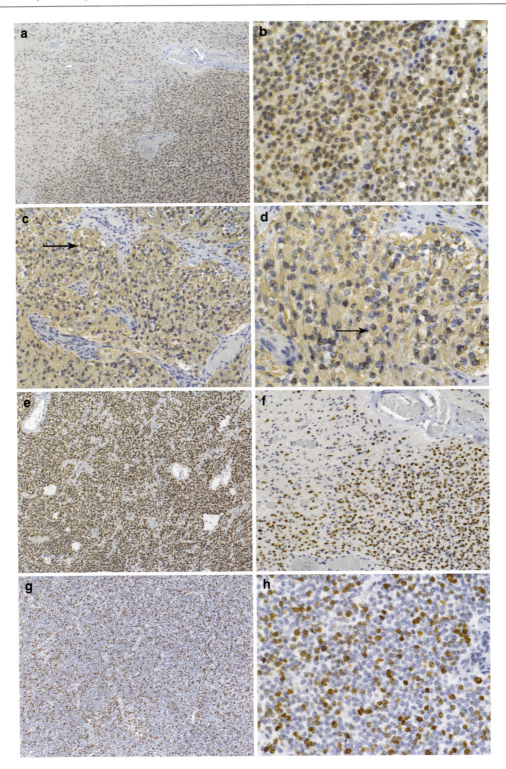

Fig. 58.16 Anaplastic oligodendroglioma (WHO grade III)—Immunophenotype: IDH1 R123H (**a**, **b**); GFAP-positive minigemistocytes (arrow) (**c**, **d**); Olig2 (**e**, **f**); moderate Ki-67 proliferation rate (**g**, **h**)

tional repressor downstream of the receptor tyrosine kinase (RTK) pathway. Interestingly, *CIC* mutations occur in the majority (~70%) of oligodendrogliomas exhibiting the 1p/19q co-deletion plus IDH mutations.
- Point mutations in the *FUBP1* (far upstream element-binding protein 1) gene on chromosome 1p31.1; FUBP1 is a transcriptional regulator of the c-*Myc* oncogene. Most of the *FUBP1* mutations (>70%) are found in oligodendrogliomas that also carry *CIC* mutations.

58.2.4.3 Epigenetics
Several genes were shown to be affected by promoter hypermethylation, resulting in reduced expression levels:

- *MGMT* gene, encoding the DNA repair enzyme O^6-methylguanine-DNA methyltransferase
- *CDKN2A* (cyclin-dependent kinase inhibitor 2A) and *CDKN2B* (cyclin-dependent kinase inhibitor 2B)
- *RB1* (retinoblastoma 1)
- *DAPK1* (death-associated protein kinase 1)
- *ESR1* (estrogen receptor 1)

58.2.4.4 Gene Expression
Commonly observed in oligodendrogliomas are elevated expression levels of:

- *PDGFA* (platelet-derived growth factor, alpha polypeptide)
- *PDGFB* (platelet-derived growth factor, beta polypeptide)
- *PDGFR* (platelet-derived growth factor receptor, alpha polypeptide), and
- *PDGFR* (platelet-derived growth factor receptor, beta polypeptide)

58.2.5 Treatment and Prognosis

Treatment
- Surgery
- Radiotherapy
- Chemotherapy
  - PCV regimen: procarbazine, CCNU, vincristine

Biologic Behavior–Prognosis–Prognostic Factors
- Median survival time 4–5 years
- Longer survival and longer progression-free intervals in patients with 1p/19q loss
- Possibly better prognosis with
  - CDKN2A deletion
  - PTEN mutation
  - chromosome 10 loss
- Patient age
- Factors for poor prognosis:
  - Ring enhancement

Selected References

Aldape K, Burger PC, Perry A (2007) Clinicopathologic aspects of 1p/19q loss and the diagnosis of oligodendroglioma. Arch Pathol Lab Med 131(2):242–251. https://doi.org/10.1043/1543-2165(2007)131[242:caoqla]2.0.co;2

Alentorn A, Sanson M, Idbaih A (2012) Oligodendrogliomas: new insights from the genetics and perspectives. Curr Opin Oncol 24(6):687–693. https://doi.org/10.1097/CCO.0b013e328357f4ea

Cahill DP, Louis DN, Cairncross JG (2015) Molecular background of oligodendroglioma: 1p/19q, IDH, TERT, CIC and FUBP1. CNS Oncol 4(5):287–294. https://doi.org/10.2217/cns.15.32

Cairncross G, Jenkins R (2008) Gliomas with 1p/19q codeletion: a.k.a. oligodendroglioma. Cancer J 14(6):352–357. https://doi.org/10.1097/PPO.0b013e31818d8178

Ellis TL, Stieber VW, Austin RC (2003) Oligodendroglioma. Curr Treat Options in Oncol 4(6):479–490

Engelhard HH, Stelea A, Cochran EJ (2002) Oligodendroglioma: pathology and molecular biology. Surg Neurol 58(2):111–117, discussion 117

Harris BT, Hattab EM (2013) Molecular pathology of the central nervous system. In: Cheng L, Eble JN (eds) Molecular surgical pathology. Springer, New York, pp 357–405

Hartmann C, von Deimling A (2009) Molecular pathology of oligodendroglial tumors. In: von Deimling A (ed) Gliomas. Recent results in cancer research, vol 171. Springer, Berlin, pp 25–49

Kleihues P, Burger PC, Scheithauer BW (1993) Histological typing of tumours of the central nervous system, 2nd edn. Springer, Berlin

Koeller KK, Rushing EJ (2005) From the archives of the AFIP: oligodendroglioma and its variants: radiologic-pathologic correlation. Radiographics 25(6):1669–1688. https://doi.org/10.1148/rg.256055137

Lwin Z, Gan HK, Mason WP (2009) Low-grade oligodendroglioma: current treatments and future hopes. Expert Rev Anticancer Ther 9(11):1651–1661. https://doi.org/10.1586/era.09.127

Selected References

Marko NF, Weil RJ (2013) The molecular biology of WHO Grade II gliomas. Neurosurg Focus 34(2):E1. https://doi.org/10.3171/2012.3112.FOCUS12283

Matthews S, Succar P, Jelinek H, McParland B, Buckland M, McLachlan CS (2012) Diagnosis of oligodendroglioma: molecular and classical histological assessment in the twenty-first century. Asia Pac J Clin Oncol 8(3):213–216. https://doi.org/10.1111/j.1743-7563.2012.01527.x

Reifenberger G, Collins VP, Hartmann C, Hawkins C, Kros JM, Cairncross JG, Yokoo H, Yip S, Louis DN (2016a) Anaplastic oligodendroglioma, IDH-mutant and 1p/19q-codeleted. In: Louis DN, Ohgaki H, Wiestler OD, Cavenee WK (eds) WHO classification of tumours of the central nervous system, Revised 4th edn. IARC, Lyon, pp 70–74

Reifenberger G, Collins VP, Hartmann C, Hawkins C, Kros JM, Cairncross JG, Yokoo H, Yip S, Louis DN (2016b) Oligodendroglioma, IDH-mutant and 1p/19q-codeleted. In: Louis DN, Ohgaki H, Wiestler OD, Cavenee WK (eds) WHO classification of tumours of the central nervous system, Revised 4th edn. IARC, Lyon, pp 60–69

Reifenberger G, Kros JM, Burger PC, Louis DN, Collins VP (2000a) Anaplastic oligoastrocytoma. In: Kleihues P, Cavenee WK (eds) Pathology and genetics of tumours of the nervous system, 3rd edn. IARC Press, Lyon, pp 68–69

Reifenberger G, Kros JM, Burger PC, Louis DN, Collins VP (2000b) Oligodendroglioma. In: Kleihues P, Cavenee WK (eds) Pathology and genetics of tumours of the nervous system, 3rd edn. IARC Press, Lyon, pp 56–61

Reifenberger G, Kros JM, Louis DN, Collins VP (2007a) Anaplastic oligodendroglioma. In: Louis DN, Ohgaki H, Wiestler OD, Cavenee WK (eds) WHO classification of tumours of the central nervous system, 4th edn. International Agency for Research on Cancer, Lyon, pp 60–62

Reifenberger G, Kros JM, Louis DN, Collins VP (2007b) Oligodendroglioma. In: Louis DN, Ohgaki H, Wiestler OD, Cavenee WK (eds) WHO classification of tumours of the central nervous system, 4th edn. International Agency for Research on Cancer, Lyon, pp 54–59

Reifenberger G, Louis DN (2003) Oligodendroglioma: toward molecular definitions in diagnostic neuro-oncology. J Neuropathol Exp Neurol 62(2):111–126

Simonetti G, Gaviani P, Botturi A, Innocenti A, Lamperti E, Silvani A (2015) Clinical management of grade III oligodendroglioma. Cancer Manag Res 7:213–223. https://doi.org/10.2147/cmar.s56975

Smits M (2016) Imaging of oligodendroglioma. Br J Radiol 89(1060):20150857. https://doi.org/10.1259/bjr.20150857

Ueki K (2005) Oligodendroglioma: impact of molecular biology on its definition, diagnosis and management. Neuropathology 25(3):247–253

van den Bent MJ (2007) Anaplastic oligodendroglioma and oligoastrocytoma. Neurol Clin 25(4):1089–1109. https://doi.org/10.1016/j.ncl.2007.07.013. ix-x.

Van Den Bent MJ, Bromberg JE, Buckner J (2016) Low-grade and anaplastic oligodendroglioma. Handb Clin Neurol 134:361–380. https://doi.org/10.1016/b978-0-12-802997-8.00022-0

Van den Bent MJ, Reni M, Gatta G, Vecht C (2008) Oligodendroglioma. Crit Rev Oncol Hematol 66(3):262–272. https://doi.org/10.1016/j.critrevonc.2007.11.007

van den Bent MJ, Smits M, Kros JM, Chang SM (2017) Diffuse infiltrating oligodendroglioma and astrocytoma. J Clin Oncol 35(21):2394–2401. https://doi.org/10.1200/jco.2017.72.6737

Wesseling P, van den Bent M, Perry A (2015) Oligodendroglioma: pathology, molecular mechanisms and markers. Acta Neuropathol 129(6):809–827. https://doi.org/10.1007/s00401-015-1424-1

Xu M, See SJ, Ng WH, Arul E, Back MF, Yeo TT, Lim CC (2005) Comparison of magnetic resonance spectroscopy and perfusion-weighted imaging in presurgical grading of oligodendroglial tumors. Neurosurgery 56(5):919–926, discussion 919–926

Yan H, Parsons DW, Jin G, McLendon R, Rasheed BA, Yuan W, Kos I, Batinic-Haberle I, Jones S, Riggins GJ, Friedman H, Friedman A, Reardon D, Herndon J, Kinzler KW, Velculescu VE, Vogelstein B, Bigner DD (2009) IDH1 and IDH2 mutations in gliomas. N Engl J Med 360(8):765–773. https://doi.org/10.1056/NEJMoa0808710

Zülch KJ (1979) Histological typing of tumours of the central nervous system. World Health Organization, Geneva

59 Oligo-astrocytoma WHO Grade II-Anaplastic Oligo-astrocytoma WHO Grade III

Diffuse Astrocytic and Oligodendroglial Tumors

59.1 Oligo-astrocytoma WHO Grade II

WHO Definition
2016—Oligo-astrocytoma, NOS: A diffusely infiltrating, slow-growing glioma composed of a conspicuous mixture of two distinct neoplastic cell types morphologically resembling tumor cells with either oligodendroglial or astrocytic features, and in which molecular testing could not be completed or was inconclusive (Reifenberger et al. 2016).

2007—A diffusely infiltrating glioma composed of a conspicuous mixture of two distinct neoplastic cell types morphologically resembling the tumor cells in oligodendrogliomas and diffuse astrocytoma of WHO grade II (von Deimling et al. 2007b).

2000—A tumor composed of a conspicuous mixture of two distinct neoplastic cell types morphologically resembling the tumor cells in oligodendroglioma and diffuse astrocytoma of WHO grade II (Reifenberger et al. 2000b).

1993—A tumor with a conspicuous mixture of neoplastic oligodendrocytes and astrocytes, either diffusely intermingled or separated into distinct areas (Kleihues et al. 1993).

1979—A tumor in which there is a conspicuous mixture of oligodendroglial cells and astrocytes. These elements may be either separated into distinct areas or intermingled. Histologically, the tumor corresponds to grade II (Zülch 1979).

WHO Grade
- WHO grade II

59.1.1 Epidemiology

Incidence
- Annual incidence: 0.1 per 100.000
- 9–19% of supratentorial low-grade gliomas

Age Incidence
- Mean age: 35–45 years

Sex Incidence
- Male:Female ratio: 1.3:1

Localization
- Cerebral hemispheres
- Rarely brain stem

59.1.2 Neuroimaging Findings

General Imaging Findings
- No imaging features to differentiate oligo-astrocytomas from pure oligodendrogliomas, characteristics of both correlate within tumor grade.

CT Non-Contrast-Enhanced
- Heterogeneous, hypodense

CT Contrast-Enhanced
- Variable enhancement

MRI-T2/FLAIR (Fig. 59.1a, b)
- Heterogeneous, hyperintense

MRI-T1 (Fig. 59.1c)
- Hypointense

MRI-T1 Contrast-Enhanced (Fig. 59.1d)
- Variable enhancement

MRI-T2∗/SWI
- Reveals calcifications

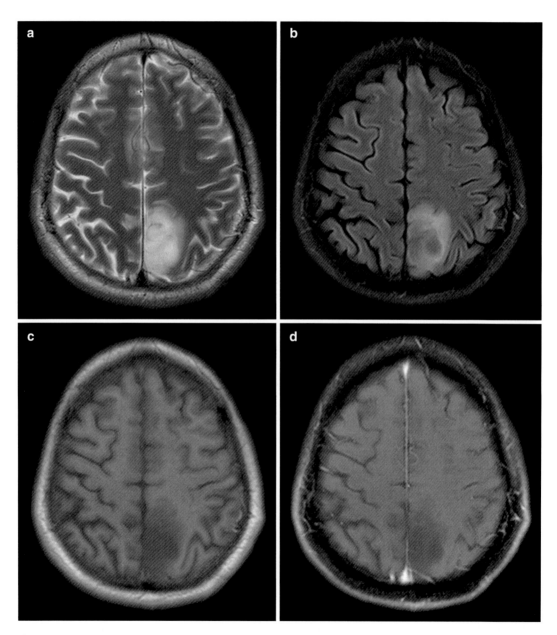

Fig. 59.1 Oligo-astrocytoma (WHO grade II) left occipital in T2 (**a**), FLAIR (**b**), T1 (**c**), T1 contrast without enhancement (**d**), normal rCBV (**e**), and slight elevation of choline in MR-spectroscopy (**f**)

59.1 Oligo-astrocytoma WHO Grade II

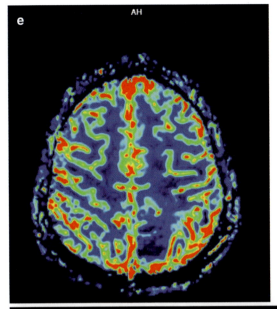

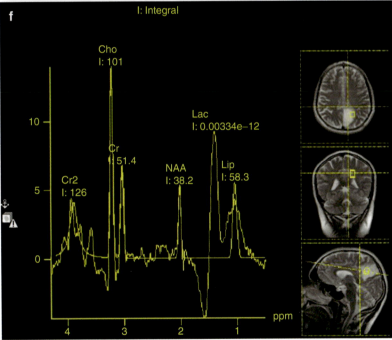

Fig. 59.1 (continued)

MR-Diffusion Imaging
- No restricted diffusion

MRI-Perfusion (Fig. 59.1e)
- High rCBV

MR-Spectroscopy (Fig. 59.1f)
- NAA decreased
- Choline increased

Nuclear Medicine Imaging Findings (Fig. 59.2, 59.3, and 59.4)
- FDG shows often hypometabolism in oligo-astrocytomas WHO grade II.
- Radiotracers like FET (a marker of amino acid uptake (L-system)) or FLT (a marker of DNA biosynthesis) have the advantage of nearly no uptake in the healthy brain tissues. They may be positive or negative in oligo-astrocytomas WHO grade II.
- Some studies suggest a better prognosis for patients with no amino acid uptake in low-grade gliomas than for patients with amino acid uptake.
- Images can show homogeneous or heterogeneous uptake representing the tumor biology.
- Results obtained for MET are similar to FET:
  - the advantage of FET is that it is taken up in a lesser amount by inflammatory tissue and its longer half-life of 110 min as compared to a relatively short half-life of 20 min of C-11 used in MET
- Hypoxia tracers are under investigation for radiotherapy planning.

59.1.3 Neuropathology Findings

Macroscopic Features
- Gross-anatomical borders are blurred.
- Enlargement and distortion of invaded structures.
- Gray or yellow-whitish color.
- Areas of the tumor tissue might be firm, softened, granular, or cystic.

Microscopic Features (Fig. 59.5a–f)
- Moderate cellularity.
- Presence of neoplastic glial cells with astrocytic or oligodendroglial phenotypes:
  - Biphasic (compact) variant with juxtaposition of distinct areas of oligodendroglial and astrocytic differentiation

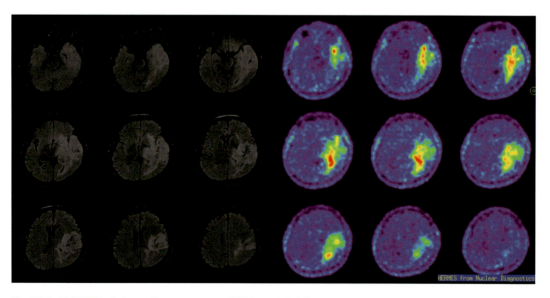

Fig. 59.2 FET-PET of a large oligo-astrocytoma WHO grade II left temporal and parietal with inhomogeneous uptake representing inhomogeneous tumor biology

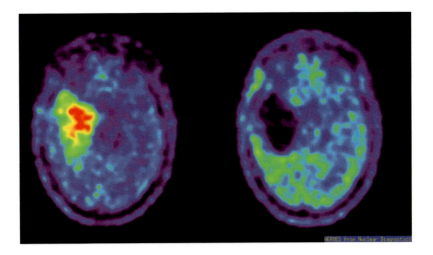

Fig. 59.3 FET-PET before and after successful resection of an oligo-astrocytoma WHO grade II right temporal

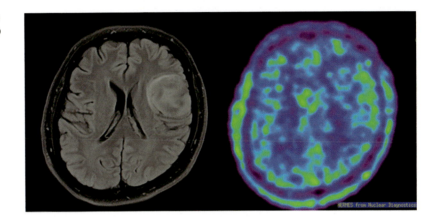

Fig. 59.4 FET negative oligo-astrocytoma WHO grade II left frontal

- Intermingled (diffuse) variant with intimate mixture of oligodendroglial and astrocytic tumor cells
- Astrocytic tumor component is fibrillary, protoplasmatic, or gemistocytic.
- Microcalcifications.
- Microcysts.
- Absence of necroses.
- Absence of microvascular proliferation.

Immunophenotype (Fig. 59.6a–d)
- IDH-1 R123H mutation-specific antibody
  - Reactivity seen in 50–100%
  - Expressed in the nucleus
  - Expressed in the cytoplasm
  - Differentiates tumor tissue from surrounding non-neoplastic tissue and/or reactive astrogliosis
- Glial fibrillary acidic protein (GFAP)
  - expressed at variable degree
  - in the cellular processes
  - often as a perinuclear rim
  - GFAP-positive fibrillary matrix
- S-100
  - Expressed in the nucleus
  - Expressed in cell processes
- Vimentin
  - Pattern similar to GFAP
  - Seen mainly in the perinuclear region

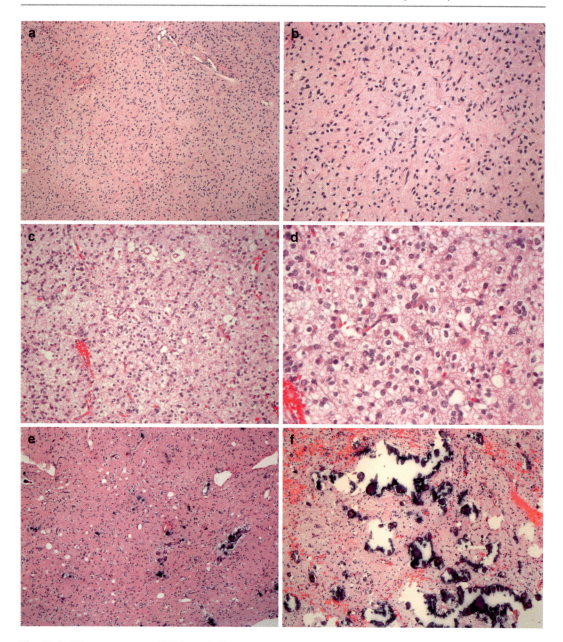

Fig. 59.5 Oligo-astrocytoma (WHO grade II): Moderately cellular tumor with areas of neoplastic glial cells with astrocytic (**a, b**) or oligodendroglial phenotypes (**c, d**). Microcalcifications (**e, f**)

59.1 Oligo-astrocytoma WHO Grade II

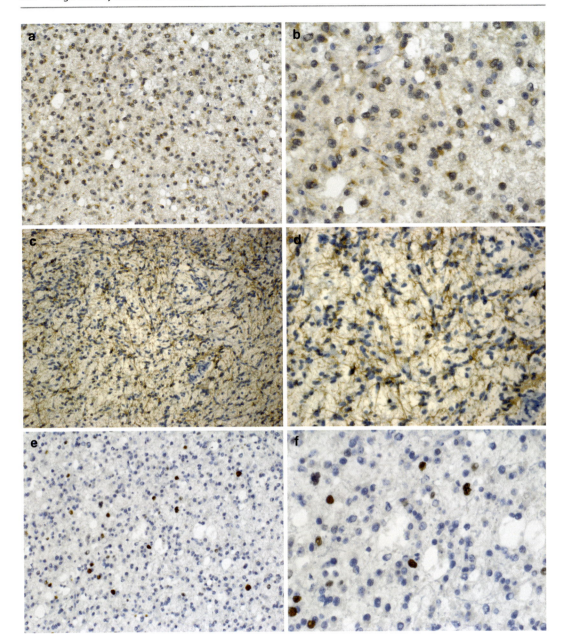

Fig. 59.6 Oligo-astrocytoma (WHO grade II)—Immunophenotype: IDH1 R123H (**a**, **b**); GFAP (**c**, **d**); low Ki-67 proliferation rate (**e**, **f**)

Proliferation Markers (Fig. 59.6e, f)
- No or low mitotic activity
- Ki-67 LI: up to 6%

Ultrastructural Features
- Mixture of features seen in astrocytomas and oligodendrogliomas (Chaps. 52 and 58)

Differential Diagnosis
- Oligodendroglioma

59.1.4 Molecular Neuropathology

Pathogenesis
- De novo

Genes
- Similar to oligodendrogliomas, albeit at a lower frequency, heterozygous chromosome 1p/19q co-deletions have been described in oligo-astrocytomas (30–50% of the cases). Notably, 19q deletion without 1p loss is often observed in these tumors.
- Several genetic aberrations which are reminiscent of astrocytic tumors can be detected in about 30% of cases, e.g.:
  - Mutations in the tumor suppressor gene *TP53*
  - Loss of heterozygosity (LOH) of chromosome 17p
  - Anomalies of chromosome 10
  - Amplification of the *EGFR* (epidermal growth factor receptor) gene

59.1.5 Treatment and Prognosis

Treatment
- Surgery

Biologic Behavior–Prognosis–Prognostic Factors
- Median survival: 6.3 years
- 5-year survival rate: 58%
- 10-year survival rate: 32%
- Factors associated with longer survival include:
  - Young age at operation
  - Gross total tumor removal
  - Postoperative radiation therapy
  - Low Ki-67 indices
  - Combined loss of 1p and 19q (60 months progression-free survival with presence of 1p/19q loss compared to 30 months without loss)

59.2 Anaplastic Oligo-astrocytoma WHO Grade III

WHO Definition
2016—Anaplastic oligo-astrocytoma, NOS: An oligo-astrocytoma, NOS, with focal or diffuse histological features of anaplasia, including increased cellularity, nuclear atypia, pleomorphism, and brisk mitotic activity (Reifenberger et al. 2016).

2007—An oligo-astrocytoma with histological features of malignancy, such as increased cellularity, nuclear atypia, pleomorphism, and increased mitotic activity (von Deimling et al. 2007a).

2000—An oligo-astrocytoma with histological features of malignancy, such as increased cellularity, nuclear atypia, pleomorphism, and increased mitotic activity (Reifenberger et al. 2000a).

1993—An oligo-astrocytoma with histological evidence of anaplasia, e.g., increased cellularity, nuclear atypia, and brisk mitotic activity. Vascular proliferation and focal necrosis may be seen (Kleihues et al. 1993).

WHO Grade
- WHO grade III

59.2 Anaplastic Oligo-astrocytoma WHO Grade III

59.2.1 Epidemiology

Incidence
- 1–4% of gliomas

Age Incidence
- Mean age: 44 years

Sex Incidence
- Male:Female ratio: 1.15:1

Localization
- Cerebral hemisphere
  - Frontal lobe
  - Temporal lobe

59.2.2 Neuroimaging Findings

General Imaging Findings
- No imaging features to differentiate oligo-astrocytomas from pure oligodendrogliomas.
- Characteristics of both correlate within tumor grade.
- Similar to anaplastic oligodendroglioma WHO grade III.
- Cysts, hemorrhages, and peritumoral edema are more common than in oligo-astrocytoma WHO grade II.

CT Non-Contrast-Enhanced
- Hypo- to isointense
- Calcifications

CT Contrast-Enhanced
- Variable enhancement

MRI-T2/FLAIR (Figs. 59.7a, b and 59.8a, b)
- Heterogeneous hyperintense due to calcifications, cysts, and hemorrhages.
- Adjacent cortex appears expanded.

MRI-T1 (Figs. 59.7c and 59.8c)
- Hypo- to isointense

MRI-T1 Contrast-Enhanced (Figs. 59.7d and 59.8d)
- Enhancement more often than in WHO grade II tumors

MRI-T2∗/SWI
- Strong signal reduction (blooming) due to calcifications

MR-Diffusion Imaging
- No diffusion restriction

MRI-Perfusion (Fig. 59.7e)
- Elevation of rCBV

MR-Spectroscopy (Fig. 59.7f)
- Choline elevated
- NAA reduced

Nuclear Medicine Imaging Findings (Figs. 59.9, 59.10, and 59.11)
- FDG can show hypermetabolism in oligo-astrocytomas WHO grade III.
- Amino acid uptake is normally positive in oligo-astrocytomas WHO grade III with a higher uptake than in oligodendrogliomas WHO II.
- Images can show homogeneous or heterogeneous uptake representing the tumor biology.
- Results obtained for MET are similar to FET:
  - the advantage of FET is that it is taken up in a lesser amount by inflammatory tissue and its longer half-life of 110 min as compared to a relatively short half-life of 20 min of C-11 used in MET.
- Hypoxia tracers are under investigation for radiotherapy planning.

59.2.3 Neuropathology Findings

Macroscopic Features (Fig. 59.12a–f)
- Infiltration of the surrounding brain with tissue destruction
- Areas of granularity, opacity, and soft consistency
- Discernible tumor mass on cut surface

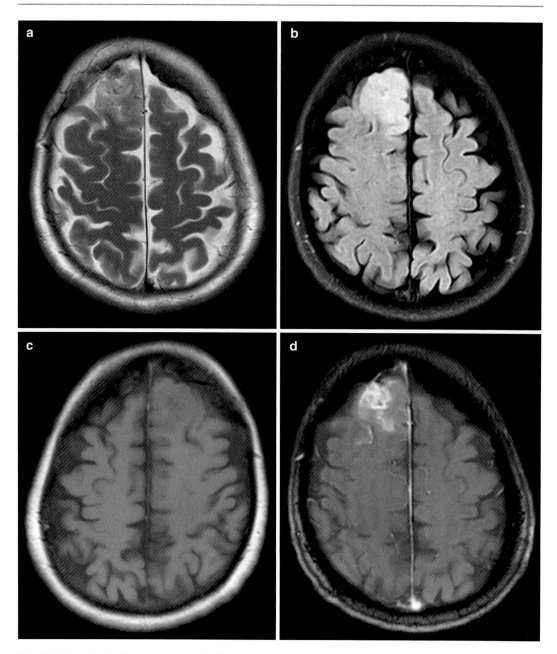

Fig. 59.7 Anaplastic oligo-astrocytoma WHO grade III left frontal, predominantly cortical in T2 (**a**), FLAIR (**b**), T1 (**c**), and irregular enhancement in T1 contrast (**d**), with elevated rCBV (**e**) and massive increase of choline (**f**)

59.2 Anaplastic Oligo-astrocytoma WHO Grade III

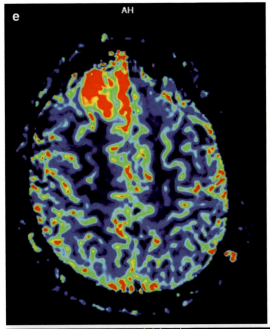

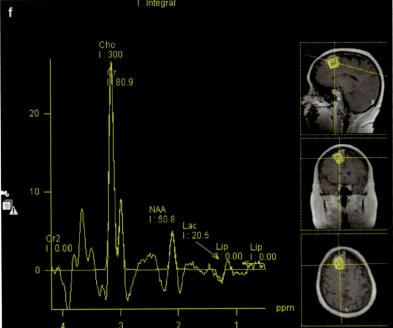

Fig. 59.7 (continued)

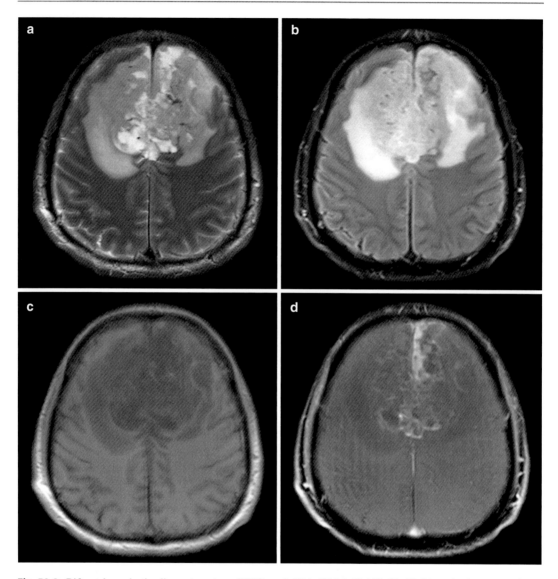

Fig. 59.8 Bifrontal anaplastic oligo-astrocytoma WHO grade III in T2 (**a**), FLAIR (**b**), T1 (**c**), and enhancement in T1 contrast (**d**)

Microscopic Features (Fig. 59.13a–h)
- Increased cellularity as compared to oligo-astrocytoma WHO grade II.
- Distinct nuclear atypia characterized by increased variations of:
  - Nuclear size
  - Shape
  - Chromatin coarsening and dispersion
  - Nucleolar prominence
- Cellular pleomorphism.
- High mitotic activity.
- Necroses: tumors with necroses should be classified as "glioblastoma with oligodendroglial component."

Immunophenotype (Fig. 59.14a–h)
- IDH-1 R123H mutation-specific antibody
  - Reactivity seen in 49–100%
  - Expressed in the nucleus
  - Expressed in the cytoplasm

59.2 Anaplastic Oligo-astrocytoma WHO Grade III

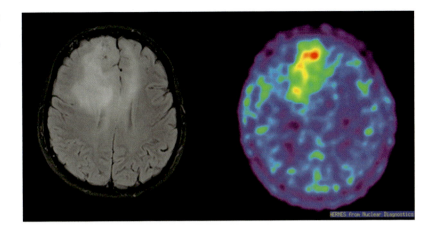

Fig. 59.9 FET-PET and MRI of an anaplastic oligo-astrocytoma WHO grade III right frontal demonstrating inhomogeneous biological behavior and presenting the most malignant area in the front, thereby guiding biopsy

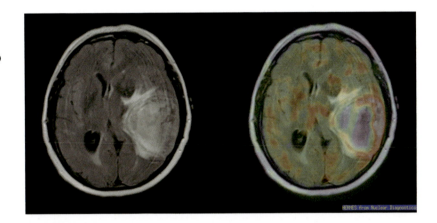

Fig. 59.10 MRI and fused FET-PET/MRI of an extended anaplastic oligo-astrocytoma WHO grade III of the left hemisphere with a large central necrosis

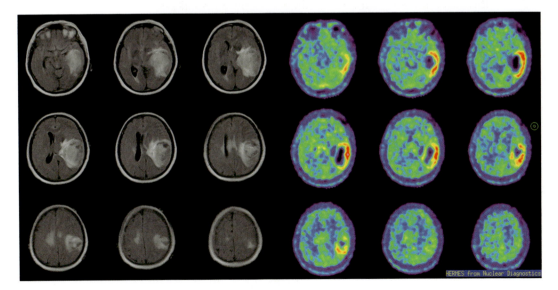

Fig. 59.11 MRI and FET-PET slices of an extended anaplastic oligo-astrocytoma WHO grade III of the left hemisphere with a large central necrosis

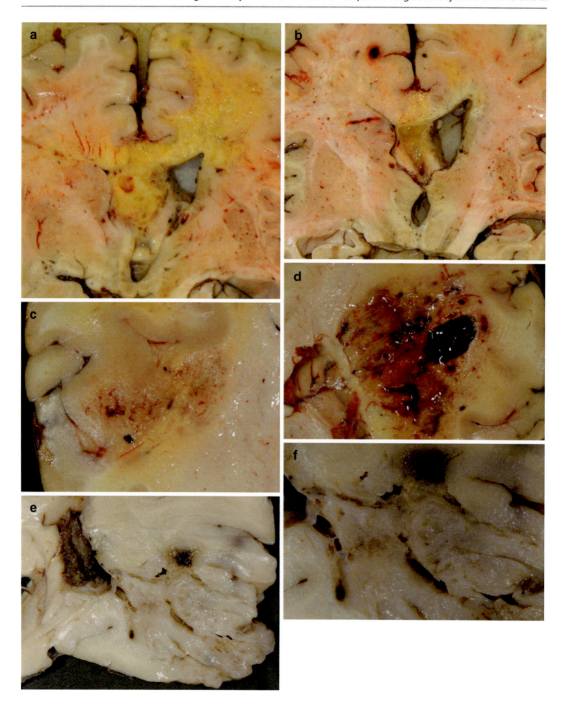

Fig. 59.12 Anaplastic oligo-astrocytoma (WHO grade III): Autopsy specimen with tumor manifestation infiltrating the parietal lobe and corpus callosum (**a, b**), occipital lobe (**c**) with hemorrhagic component (**d**), and the temporal lobe (**e, f**)

59.2 Anaplastic Oligo-astrocytoma WHO Grade III

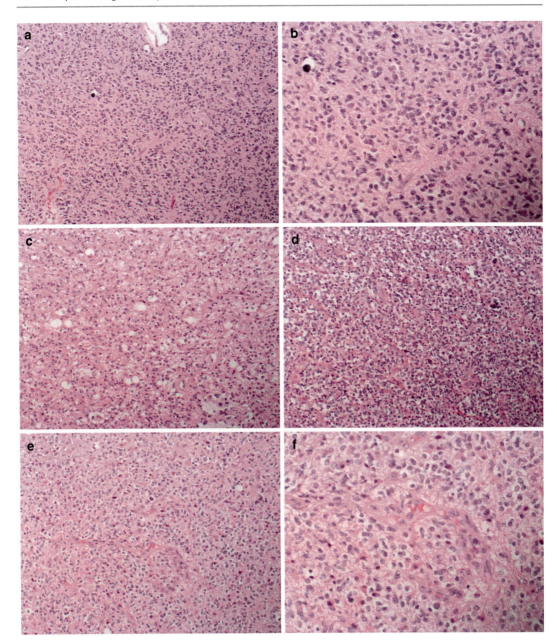

Fig. 59.13 Anaplastic oligo-astrocytoma (WHO grade III): Tumor with increased cellularity with areas of neoplastic glial cells with astrocytic (**a**, **b**), intermediate (**c**, **d**), or oligodendroglial phenotypes (**e**, **f**); areas with high cellular pleomorphism (**g**, **h**)

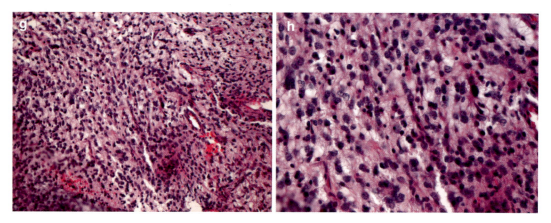

Fig. 59.13 (continued)

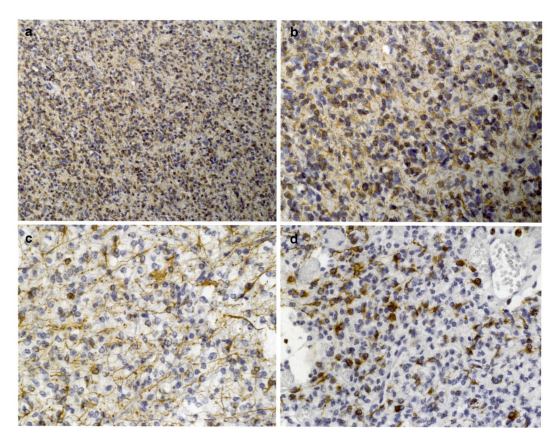

Fig. 59.14 Anaplastic oligo-astrocytoma (WHO grade III): Immunophenotype: GFAP (**a–d**); S100 (**e, f**); p53 (**g, h**); high Ki-67 proliferation rate (**i, j**)

59.2 Anaplastic Oligo-astrocytoma WHO Grade III

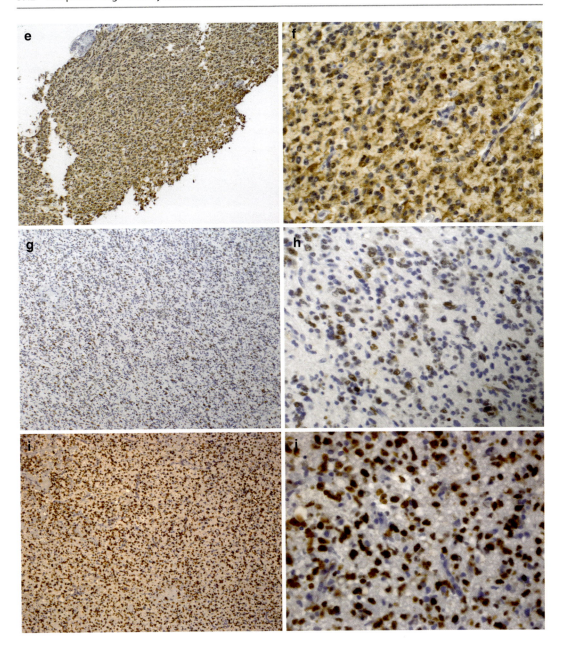

Fig. 59.14 (continued)

- Differentiates tumor tissue from surrounding non-neoplastic tissue and/or reactive astrogliosis
- Glial fibrillary acidic protein (GFAP)
  - expressed at variable degree
  - in the cellular processes
  - often as a perinuclear rim
  - GFAP-positive fibrillary matrix
- S-100
  - Expressed in the nucleus
  - Expressed in cell processes
- Vimentin
  - Pattern similar to GFAP
  - Seen mainly in the perinuclear region

Proliferation Markers (Fig. 59.14i, j)
- High mitotic activity
- Ki-67 LI: >5%

Ultrastructural Features
- Mixture of features seen in anaplastic astrocytomas and oligodendrogliomas (Chaps. 53 and 58)

Differential Diagnosis
- Anaplastic oligodendroglioma
- Anaplastic astrocytoma
- Glioblastoma

59.2.4 Molecular Neuropathology

Pathogenesis
- De novo
- Malignant progression from oligo-astrocytoma WHO grade II

Genes
- Similar to oligodendrogliomas, albeit at a lower frequency, heterozygous chromosome 1p/19q co-deletions have been described in oligo-astrocytomas (30–50% of the cases). Notably, 19q deletion without 1p loss is often observed in these tumors.
- Several genetic aberrations which are reminiscent of astrocytic tumors can be detected in about 30% of cases, e.g.:
  - Mutations in the tumor suppressor gene *TP53*
  - Loss of heterozygosity (LOH) of chromosome 17p
  - Anomalies of chromosome 10
  - Amplification of the *EGFR* (epidermal growth factor receptor) gene

59.2.5 Treatment and Prognosis

Treatment
- Surgery
- Radiation therapy
- Chemotherapy (PCV)

Biologic Behavior–Prognosis–Prognostic Factors
- Median survival time: 2.8 years
- 5-year survival rate: 36%
- 10-year survival rate: 9%
- Prognostic markers:
  - Necroses (glioblastoma with oligodendroglial component)
  - 1p status

Selected References

Alentorn A, Sanson M, Idbaih A (2012) Oligodendrogliomas: new insights from the genetics and perspectives. Curr Opin Oncol 24(6):687–693. https://doi.org/10.1097/CCO.1090b1013e328357f32 8354ea

Bai HX, Zou Y, Lee AM, Tang X, Zhang P, Yang L (2016) Does morphological assessment have a role in classifying oligoastrocytoma as 'oligodendroglial' versus 'astrocytic'? Histopathology 68(7):1114–1115. https://doi.org/10.1111/his.12891

Barresi V, Lionti S, Valori L, Gallina G, Caffo M, Rossi S (2017) Dual-genotype diffuse low-grade glioma: is it really time to abandon oligoastrocytoma as a distinct entity? J Neuropathol Exp Neurol 76(5):342–346. https://doi.org/10.1093/jnen/nlx024

Ducray F, del Rio MS, Carpentier C, Psimaras D, Idbaih A, Dehais C, Kaloshi G, Mokhtari K, Taillibert S, Laigle-Donadey F, Omuro A, Sanson M, Delattre JY, Hoang-Xuan K (2011) Up-front temozolomide in elderly patients with anaplastic oligodendroglioma and oligoastrocytoma. J Neuro-Oncol 101(3):457–462. https://doi.org/10.1007/s11060-010-0264-z

Selected References

Harris BT, Hattab EM (2013) Molecular pathology of the central nervous system. In: Cheng L, Eble JN (eds) Molecular surgical pathology. Springer, New York, pp 357–405

Hartmann C, von Deimling A (2009) Molecular pathology of oligodendroglial tumors. In: von Deimling A (ed) Gliomas. Recent results in cancer research, vol 171. Springer, Berlin, pp 25–49

Huse JT, Diamond EL, Wang L, Rosenblum MK (2015) Mixed glioma with molecular features of composite oligodendroglioma and astrocytoma: a true "oligoastrocytoma"? Acta Neuropathol 129(1):151–153. https://doi.org/10.1007/s00401-014-1359-y

Kleihues P, Burger PC, Scheithauer BW (1993) Histological typing of tumours of the central nervous system, 2nd edn. Springer, Berlin

Koeller KK, Rushing EJ (2005) From the archives of the AFIP: oligodendroglioma and its variants: radiologic-pathologic correlation. Radiographics 25(6):1669–1688. https://doi.org/10.1148/rg.256055137

Marko NF, Weil RJ (2013) The molecular biology of WHO Grade II gliomas. Neurosurg Focus 34(2):E1. https://doi.org/10.3171/2012.3112.FOCUS12283

Naugle DK, Duncan TD, Grice GP (2004) Oligoastrocytoma. Radiographics 24(2):598–600. https://doi.org/10.1148/rg.242035069

Reifenberger G, Collins VP, Hartmann C, Hawkins C, Kros JM, Cairncross JG, Yokoo H, Yip S, Louis DN (2016) Oligoastrocytoma, NOS. In: Louis DN, Ohgaki H, Wiestler OD, Cavenee WK (eds) WHO classification of tumours of the central nervous system, Revised 4th edn. International Agency for Research on Cancer, Lyon, pp 75–77

Reifenberger G, Kros JM, Burger PC, Louis DN, Collins VP (2000a) Anaplastic oligoastrocytoma. In: Kleihues P, Cavenee WK (eds) Pathology and genetics of tumours of the nervous system, 3rd edn. IARC Press, Lyon, pp 68–69

Reifenberger G, Kros JM, Burger PC, Louis DN, Collins VP (2000b) Oligoastrocytoma. In: Kleihues P, Cavenee WK (eds) Pathology and genetics of tumours of the nervous system, 3rd edn. IARC Press, Lyon, pp 65–67

Sahm F, Lass U, Herold-Mende C, von Deimling A, Hartmann C, Mueller W (2013) Analysis of CIC-associated CpG island methylation in oligoastrocytoma. Neuropathol Appl Neurobiol 39(7):831–836. https://doi.org/10.1111/nan.12045

Sahm F, Reuss D, Koelsche C, Capper D, Schittenhelm J, Heim S, Jones DT, Pfister SM, Herold-Mende C, Wick W, Mueller W, Hartmann C, Paulus W, von Deimling A (2014) Farewell to oligoastrocytoma: in situ molecular genetics favor classification as either oligodendroglioma or astrocytoma. Acta Neuropathol 128(4):551–559. https://doi.org/10.1007/s00401-014-1326-7

von Deimling A, Reifenberger G, Kros JM, Louis DN, Collins VP (2007a) Anaplastic oligoastrocytoma. In: Louis DN, Ohgaki H, Wiestler OD, Cavenee WK (eds) WHO classification of tumours of the central nervous system, 4th edn. International Agency for Research on Cancer, Lyon, pp 66–67

von Deimling A, Reifenberger G, Kros JM, Louis DN, Collins VP (2007b) Oligoastrocytoma. In: Louis DN, Ohgaki H, Wiestler OD, Cavenee WK (eds) WHO classification of tumours of the central nervous system, 4th edn. International Agency for Research on Cancer, Lyon, pp 63–65

Zülch KJ (1979) Histological typing of tumours of the central nervous system. World Health Organization, Geneva

Ependymal Tumors

60.1 General Aspects

Based on histopathologic criteria, the following types of ependymal tumors are distinguished:

Subependymoma	WHO grade I
Myxopapillary ependymoma	WHO grade I
Ependymoma	WHO grade II
Anaplastic ependymoma	WHO grade III

60.1.1 Clinical Signs and Symptoms

- Subependymoma in the ventricular system
  - Ventricular obstruction
  - Raised intracranial pressure
- Spinal cord
  - Motor or sensory deficits
- Myxopapillary ependymoma
  - Back pain often of long duration
- Ependymoma
  - Localization-dependent
  - Hydrocephalus
  - Increased intracranial pressure (headache, nausea, vomiting, dizziness)
  - Cerebellar ataxia
  - Visual disturbance
  - Paresis

60.1.2 Nuclear Medicine Imaging Findings

- Overall, only few studies are available dealing with ependymomas.
- FDG shows often hypometabolism in ependymoma WHO II.
- FDG can show hypermetabolism in ependymoma WHO III.
- Radiotracers like FET (a marker of amino acid uptake (L-system)) or FLT (a marker of DNA biosynthesis) may be positive or negative in ependymomas WHO II.
- Amino acid uptake is normally positive in ependymomas WHO III with a higher uptake than in ependymomas WHO II.
- Some studies suggest a better prognosis for patients with no amino acid uptake than for patients with amino acid uptake.

60.1.3 Molecular Neuropathology

Depending on their location in the brain, human ependymomas display specific genetic signatures, allowing a distinct categorization into three major anatomical subgroups: supratentorial region, infratentorial region (posterior fossa), and spinal cord. Both supratentorial as well as infratentorial ependymomas can be further subclassified:

Supratentorial ependymomas

- The majority of the tumors exhibit a chromosomal rearrangement within region 11q12.1–q13.3 where an open reading frame, *C11orf95*, is fused to *RELA*, a proto-oncogene involved in NF-κB signaling. *C11orf95-RELA* fusions occur in ~70% of supratentorial ependymomas and are more common in children than in adults.
- In the remaining *C11orf95-RELA*-negative cases, *YAP1-MAMLD1* fusions are observed. *YAP1* encodes a protein that participates in the hippo signaling pathway which regulates organ size by mediating cell proliferation, renewal, and apoptosis. The *MAMLD1* gene product acts as a transcriptional activator. This tumor type is more common in younger children.

Infratentorial ependymomas fall into two genetic subclasses based on epigenetic features, namely the extent of CpG island methylation which is referred to as the CpG island methylator phenotype (CIMP).

- The posterior fossa group A (PFA) is characterized by high levels of CpG island methylation and therefore classified as CIMP-positive (CIMP+). It is associated with younger age and poor prognosis.
- In contrast, the posterior fossa group B (PFB) is classified as CIMP-negative (CIMP−) and correlates with older age and better prognosis.

Spinal cord ependymomas are

- Often associated with frequent mutations in the *NF2* gene which actually is a well-established genetic hallmark in neurofibromatosis type 2 (Chap. 71).
- Spinal cord ependymomas are more common in adults than in children and associated with a better prognosis.
- More common in adults than in children.

Genetic characteristics, neuropathology types, age at disease onset and outcome in RELA fusion-positive ependymomas are given in Table 60.1.

Involved genes from various pathways include (Pajtler et al. 2015b):

- Apoptosis
- Embryonal development

Table 60.1 Ependymoma, RELA fusion-positive

Compartment	Group	Genetic characteristics	Dominant pathology	Age at presentation	Outcome
Supratentorial	ST-EPN-*RELA*	*RELA* fusion gene	Classic/anaplastic	Infancy to adulthood	Poor
	ST-EPN-*YAP1*	*YAP1* fusion gene	Classic/anaplastic	Infancy to childhood	Good
	ST-SE	Balanced genome	Subependymoma	Adulthood	Good
Posterior fossa	PF-EPN-A	Balanced genome	Classic/anaplastic	Infancy	Poor
	PF-EPN-B	Genome-wide polyploidy	Classic/anaplastic	Childhood to adulthood	Good
	PF-SE	Balanced genome	Subependymoma	Adulthood	Good
Spinal	SP-EPN	*NF2* mutation	Classic/anaplastic	Childhood to adulthood	Good
	SP-MPE	Genome-wide polyploidy	Myxopapillary	Adulthood	Good
	SP-SE	6q deletion	Subependymoma	Adulthood	Good

Modified after Pajtler et al. (2015a), Pajtler et al. (2015b) reproduced with kind permission from Elsevier and Springer Nature

- Cell cycle
- Cell migration
- Tissue morphogenesis
- cAMP metabolism
- Dopamine signaling
- Ion homeostasis
- Cell adhesion
- Chemotaxis
- Extracellular matrix
- Carbohydrate metabolism
- Calcium signaling
- Synapse organization
- Neuron development
- Aminoglycan metabolism
- Fatty acid metabolism
- Mast cell, leukocytes
- Hypoxia
- CNS development
- Axon extension
- Cell growth
- Stem cell differentiation
- Forebrain development
- Angiogenesis
- Epithelial cell proliferation
- Blood coagulation
- Chemokine signaling
- Cytokine secretion
- Chromatid segregation
- Signal transduction pathways
    - STAT
    - Protein kinases
    - MAPK
    - ERK1/2
    - SMAD
    - BMP
    - WNT
    - VEGF
    - PDGF
    - Insulin
    - Rho GTPase

Pathogenesis–Ependymoma
- Radial glia as a possible cell of origin

Pathogenesis–Anaplastic Ependymoma
- De novo
- Progression from low-grade ependymomamo

Pathogenesis–Myxopapillary Ependymoma
- Ependymal glial cells of the filum terminale

Pathogenesis–Subependymoma
- De novo from
    - subependymal glial precursor cells
    - astrocytes of the subependymal plate
    - ependymal cells
    - mixture of astrocytes and ependymal cells
- Rare familial cases

60.2 Ependymoma WHO Grade II

WHO Definition
2016—Ependymoma: A circumscribed glioma composed of uniform small cells with round nuclei in a fibrillary matrix and characterized by perivascular anucleate zones (pseudorosettes) with ependymal rosettes also found in about one quarter of cases (Ellison et al. 2016c).

Papillary ependymoma: A rare histological variant of ependymoma characterized by well-formed papillae (Ellison et al. 2016c).

Clear cell ependymoma: A histological variant of ependymoma characterized by an oligodendrocyte-like appearance, with perinuclear haloes due to cytoplasmic clearing (Ellison et al. 2016c).

Tanycytic ependymoma: A histological variant of ependymoma characterized by arrangement of tumor cells in fascicles of variable width and cell density and by elongated cells with spindle-shaped nuclei (Ellison et al. 2016c).

Ependymoma, RELA fusion-positive: A supratentorial ependymoma characterized by a RELA fusion gene (Ellison et al. 2016a).

2007—A generally slowly growing tumor of children and young adults, originating from the wall of the ventricles or from the spinal canal and composed of neoplastic ependymal cells (McLendon et al. 2007b).

2000—A slowly growing tumor of children and young adult, originating from the wall of the cerebral ventricles or from the spinal canal and composed of neoplastic ependymal cells (Wiestler et al. 2000b).

1993—A tumor composed predominantly of neoplastic ependymal cells (Kleihues et al. 1993).

1979—A tumor composed predominantly of uniform ependymal cells forming rosettes, canals and perivascular pseudorosettes (Zülch 1979).

WHO Grade
- WHO grade II

60.2.1 Epidemiology

Incidence
- 0.20 per 100,000 persons
- 2–9% of all neuroepithelial tumors
- 6–12% of all intracranial tumors

Age Incidence
- All age groups
- Children: infratentorial ependymomas mean age 6.4 years
- Adults: spinal ependymomas age 30–40 years

Sex Incidence
- Male:Female ratio 1:1

Localization
- Any site along the ventricular system and spinal cord
- Decreasing frequency:
  - Fourth ventricle
  - Spinal cord
  - Lateral ventricle
  - Third ventricle
- Spinal cord:
  - Cervical segment
  - Cervico-thoracic segment
- Supratentorial parenchymal ependymomas
- Extraneural ependymomas in
  - Ovaries
  - Broad ligament
  - Soft tissues
  - Mediastinum
  - Sacro-coccygeal region

60.2.2 Neuroimaging Findings

General Imaging Findings
- Heterogeneous, soft tumor with contrast enhancement, in two-third located on the fourth ventricle, growing through the foramina of Magendie and Luschka

CT Non-Contrast-Enhanced
- Heterogeneous hypo- to isodense
- Cysts and calcifications (50%) common
- Associated hydrocephalus

CT Contrast-Enhanced
- Variable enhancement

MRI-T2 (Fig. 60.1a)
- Heterogeneous hyperintense

MRI-FLAIR (Fig. 60.1b)
- Heterogeneous hyperintense

MRI-T1 (Fig. 60.1c)
- Solid component iso- to hypointense

MRI-T2∗/SWI
- Calcification and hemorrhages hypointense

MRI-T1 Contrast-Enhanced (Fig. 60.1d)
- Variable enhancement

MR-Diffusion Imaging
- No restricted diffusion
- ADC value significantly higher, compared to medulloblastoma

MRI-Perfusion
- High rCBV

MR-Spectroscopy
- NAA decreased
- Cho increased
- Lactate elevated
- Similar to PNET and astrocytoma

60.2 Ependymoma WHO Grade II

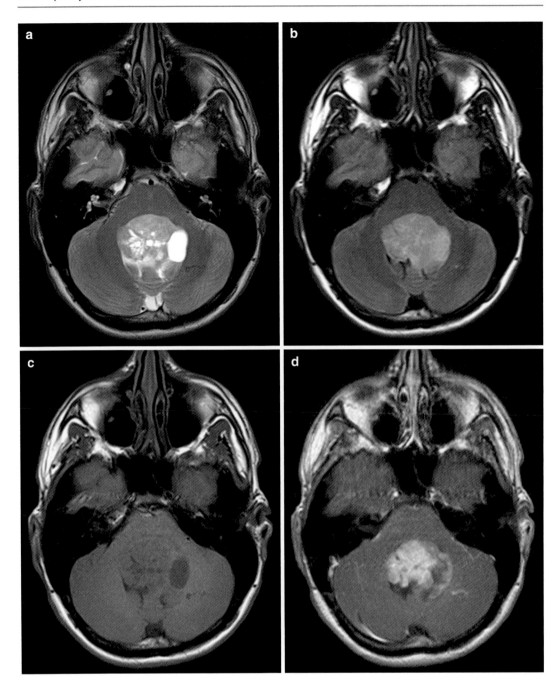

Fig. 60.1 Ependymoma (WHO grade I), typically located at the fourth ventricle in T2 (**a**), FLAIR (**b**), T1 (**c**), and T1gd with strong enhancement (**d**)

60.2.3 Neuropathology Findings

Macroscopic Features (Figs. 60.2a–h and 60.3a, b)
- Soft tan masses
- Well demarcated
- "Plastic ependymoma"
  - Fills the fourth ventricle
  - Merges out of the foramina of Luschka or Magendie
  - Surrounds the brain stem by subarachnoidal growth

Microscopic Features (Fig. 60.4a–n)
- Moderately cellular tumor
- Monomorphic nuclear morphology with

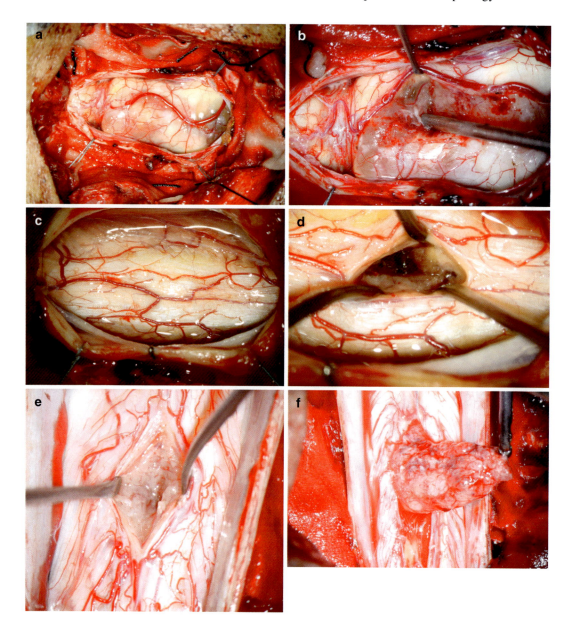

Fig. 60.2 Ependymoma (WHO grade I): Intraoperative appearances of ependymoma (**a–h**). Bulging of spinal cord tissue with reddish-yellowish discoloration (**a, c**), after splitting of the spinal cord (**b, d**). Exposed tumor tissue is of grayish color (**e–h**)

60.2 Ependymoma WHO Grade II

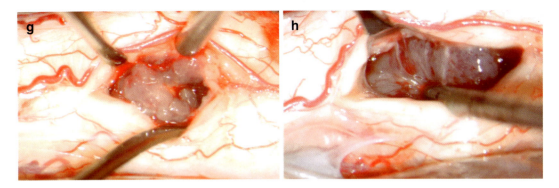

Fig. 60.2 (continued)

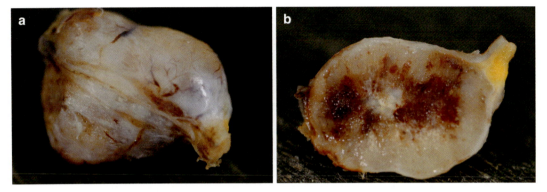

Fig. 60.3 Ependymoma (WHO grade I): Gross-anatomical surgical specimen presenting as a well-demarcated soft tan mass with brownish color and reddish confluent microhemorrhages (**a**, **b**)

- Round to oval nuclei
- "Salt and pepper" speckling of the chromatin
- Perivascular pseudorosettes
  - Tumor cells arranged radially around blood vessels with perivascular anuclear zones of GFAP-rich fibrillary processes
- Ependymal rosettes
  - Columnar cells arranged around a central lumen
- Regressive changes:
  - Myxoid degeneration
  - Hemorrhages
  - Calcification
  - Cartilage or bone formation
- Hyalinization of vessel walls
- Sharp tumor/parenchyma interface

The following ependymoma variants are considered:

- Papillary ependymoma
  - Formation of linear, epithelial-like surfaces
  - Well-formed papillae
- Clear cell ependymoma
  - Clear perinuclear halos (oligodendroglia-like)
  - Preferentially located in the supratentorial compartment
- Tanycytic ependymoma
  - Arrangement of tumor cells in fascicles
  - Spindly, bipolar cells resembling tanycytes
  - Commonly affecting the spinal cord
- Cellular ependymoma (deleted in the new WHO classification)
  - Conspicuous cellularity without increased mitotic activity
  - Common in extraventricular locations

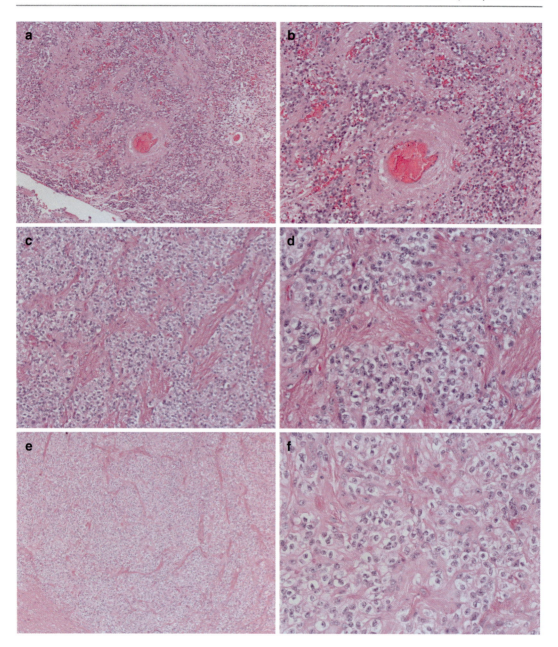

Fig. 60.4 Ependymoma (WHO grade I): a moderately cellular tumor (**a–n**). The tumor cells show monomorphic nuclear morphology with round to oval nuclei and "salt and pepper" speckling of the chromatin (**a–n**). Perivascular pseudorosettes are present (**a, b**), i.e., tumor cells are arranged radially around blood vessels with perivascular anuclear zones of GFAP-rich fibrillary processes. Ependymal rosettes are made up of columnar cells arranged around a central lumen (**i, j**). Regressive changes consist of myxoid degeneration (**k, l**). Hyalinization of vessel walls (**m, n**)

60.2 Ependymoma WHO Grade II

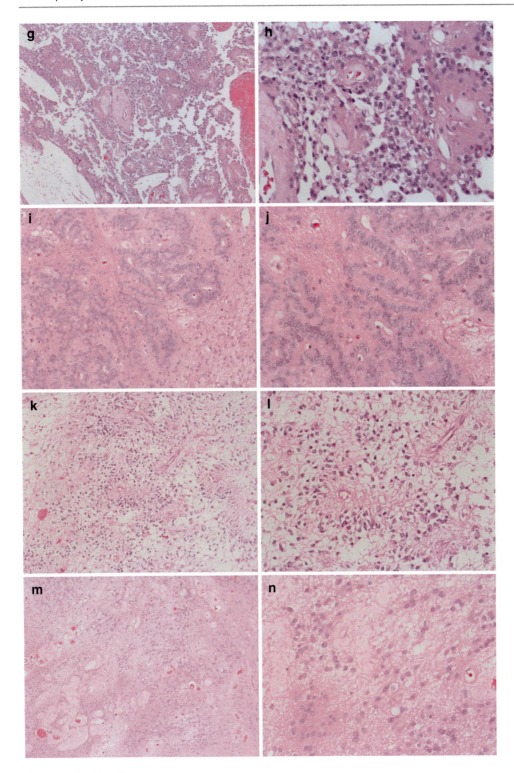

Fig. 60.4 (continued)

Immunophenotype (Fig. 60.5a–h)

IHC-positivities	IHC-negativities
• GFAP • Vimentin • S-100 • EMA dot-like reactivities • Alarin • Nestin	• Neuronal markers • IDH-1

Proliferation Markers
- Mitoses: rare or absent
- Ki-67 LI: <4% (longer survival)
- Ki-67 LI: >5% (shorter survival time)

Ultrastructural Features
- Show characteristics of ependymal cells with
  - Cilia in a 9 + 2 arrangement

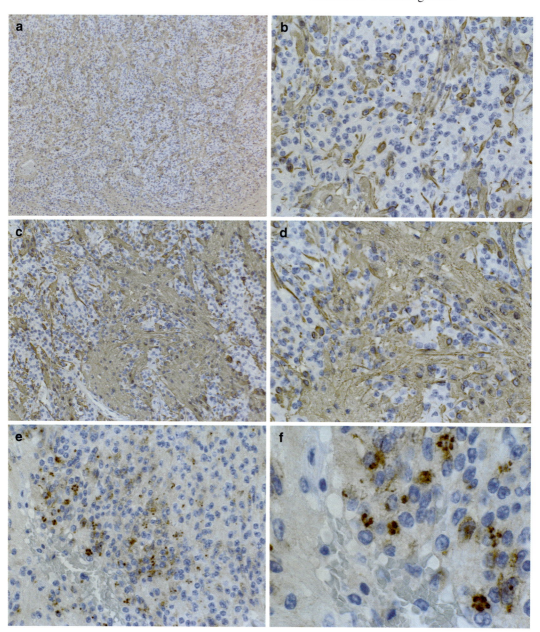

Fig. 60.5 Ependymoma (WHO grade I)—Immunophenotype: tumor cells reactive positively with GFAP (**a–d**), EMA dots (**e, f**), some tumor cells stain with the pancytokeratin AE1/AE3 antibody (**g, h**)

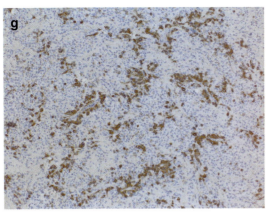 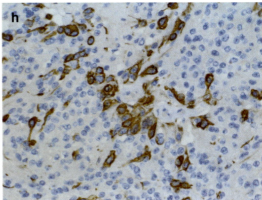

Fig. 60.5 (continued)

- Blepharoplasts
- Microvilli at the luminal surface
- Zonulae adherentes

Differential Diagnosis
- Intraspinal
  - Diffuse astrocytoma
  - Pilocytic astrocytoma
  - Schwannomas
  - Meningioma
  - Hemangioblastoma
- Intracranial
  - Oligodendroglioma
  - Neurocytoma
  - Medulloblastoma
- Papillary ependymoma
  - Choroid plexus papilloma
  - Metastatic carcinoma
- Clear cell ependymoma
  - Oligodendroglioma
  - Central neurocytoma
  - Clear cell carcinoma
  - Hemangioblastoma

60.2.4 Treatment and Prognosis

Treatment
- Surgery

Biologic Behavior–Prognosis–Prognostic Factors
- Factor with worse prognosis:
  - Age (children: tumor often located in the posterior fossa)
  - Localization:
    ○ posterior fossa worser than supratentorial
    ○ cerebral lesions worser than spinal lesions
  - Cerebrospinal dissemination
- Ki-67 LI:
  - <4% (longer survival)
  - >5% (shorter survival)

60.3 Anaplastic Ependymoma WHO Grade III

WHO Definition

2016—A circumscribed glioma composed of uniform small cells with round nuclei in a fibrillary matrix and characterized by perivascular anucleate zones (pseudorosettes), ependymal rosettes in about one quarter of cases, a high nuclear-to-cytoplasmic ratio, and a high mitotic count (Ellison et al. 2016b).

2007—A malignant glioma of ependymal differentiation with accelerated growth and unfavorable clinical outcome, particularly in children; histologically characterized by high mitotic activity, often accompanied by microvascular proliferation and pseudopalisading necrosis (McLendon et al. 2007a).

2000—A malignant glioma of ependymal origin with accelerated growth and unfavorable clinical outcome, particularly in children. Anaplastic ependymomas exhibit high mitotic activity, often accompanied by microvascular proliferation and pseudopalisading necrosis (Wiestler et al. 2000a).

1993—An ependymal tumor with histological evidence of anaplasia, e.g., high cellularity, variable nuclear atypia, marked mitotic activity, and often prominent vascular proliferation (Kleihues et al. 1993).

1979—An ependymoma containing areas of anaplasia, or a tumor resembling a glioblastoma or medulloblastoma in which features indicative of ependymal differentiation can be recognized (Zülch 1979).

WHO Grade
- WHO grade III

60.3.1 Epidemiology

Incidence
- 0.20 per 100,000 persons

Age Incidence
- Childhood

Sex Incidence
- Male:Female ratio 1:1

Localization
- Any site along the ventricular system and spinal cord
- Decreasing frequency:
  - Fourth ventricle
  - Spinal cord
  - Lateral ventricle
  - Third ventricle
- Spinal cord:
  - Cervical segment
  - Cervico-thoracic segment
- Supratentorial parenchymal ependymomas
- Extraneural ependymomas in
  - Ovaries
  - Broad ligament
  - Soft tissues
  - Mediastinum
  - Sacro-coccygeal region

60.3.2 Neuroimaging Findings

General Imaging Findings (Fig. 60.6)
- Imaging features are similar to grade II ependymomas

60.3.3 Neuropathology Findings

Macroscopic Features
- Soft tan masses
- Well demarcated
- Invasion of neighboring tissue
- Possible hemorrhages
- Possible necrotic areas

Microscopic Features (Fig. 60.7a–l)
- Increased cellularity.
- Brisk mitotic activity.
- Microvascular proliferation.
- Geographic tumor necroses are not a diagnostic feature of malignancy in the absence of vascular proliferation.
- Perivascular pseudorosettes.

Immunophenotype (Fig. 60.8a–f)

IHC-positivities	IHC-negativities
• GFAP • Vimentin • S-100 • EMA dot-like reactivities • Alarin • Nestin	• Neuronal markers • IDH-1

Proliferation Markers (Fig. 60.8g, h)
- Brisk mitotic activity
  - ≥10 mitoses per 10 high-power field
- KI-67 LI: variably high

Ultrastructural Features
- Show characteristics of ependymal cells with
  - Cilia in a 9 + 2 arrangement
  - Blepharoplasts
  - Microvilli at the luminal surface
  - Zonulae adherentes

60.3 Anaplastic Ependymoma WHO Grade III

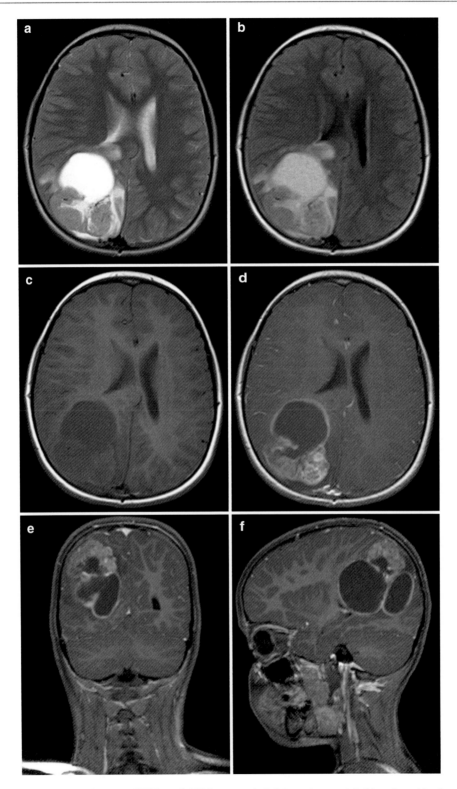

Fig. 60.6 Anaplastic ependymoma (WHO grade III) in an atypical right parieto-occipital location with a large cyst in T2 (**a**), FLAIR (**b**), T1 (**c**), and heterogeneous enhancement in T1gd (**d, e, f**)

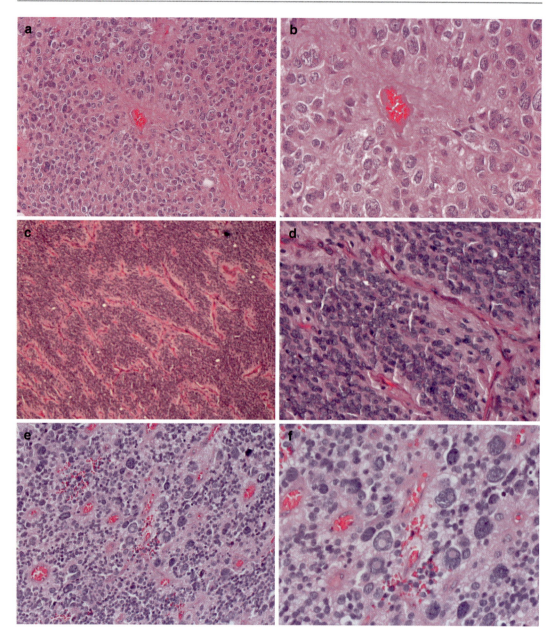

Fig. 60.7 Anaplastic ependymoma (WHO grade III) characterized by increased cellularity, brisk mitotic activity, cellular pleomorphism, and perivascular pseudorosettes (**a–l**)

60.3 Anaplastic Ependymoma WHO Grade III

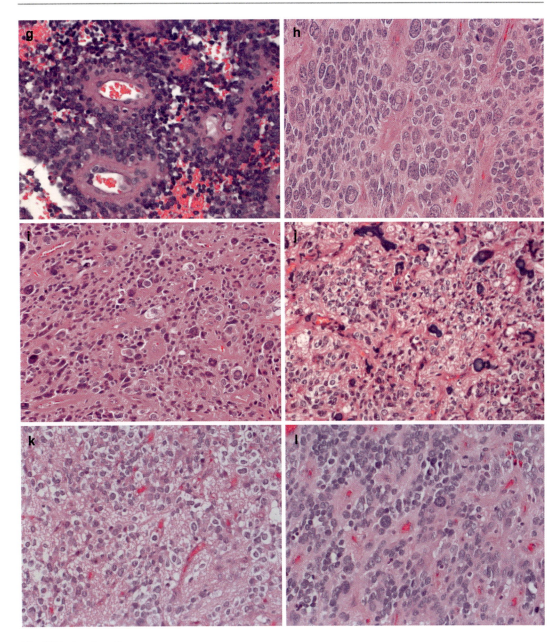

Fig. 60.7 (continued)

Differential Diagnosis
- Intraspinal
  - Diffuse astrocytoma
  - Pilocytic astrocytoma
  - Schwannomas
  - Meningioma
  - Hemangioblastoma
- Intracranial
  - Oligodendroglioma
  - Neurocytoma
  - Medulloblastoma
  - Glioblastoma
  - Choroid plexus carcinoma
  - Ependymoblastoma
  - Atypical teratoid/rhabdoid tumor

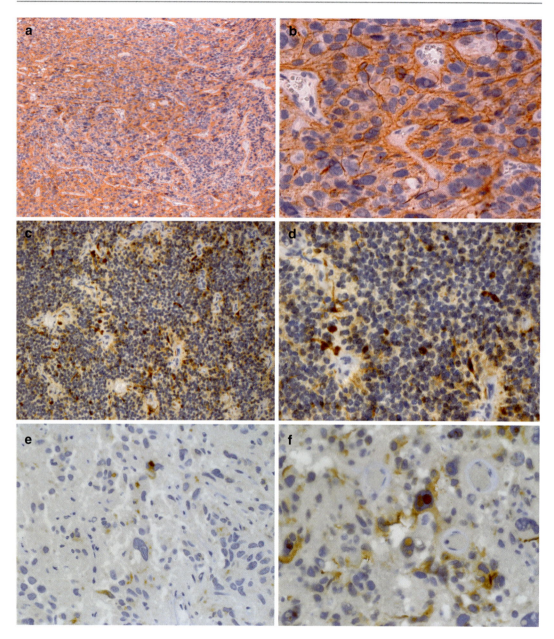

Fig. 60.8 Anaplastic ependymoma (WHO grade III)—Immunophenotype: tumor cells are partly positive for GFAP (**a**, **b**), S-100 (**c**, **d**), EMA dots (**e**, **f**), moderate Ki-67 proliferation rate (**g**, **h**)

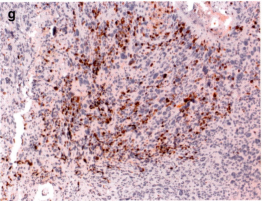 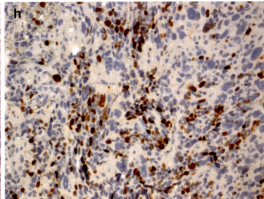

Fig. 60.8 (continued)

60.3.4 Treatment and Prognosis

Treatment
- Surgery
- Radiation
- Chemotherapy

Biologic Behavior–Prognosis–Prognostic Factors
- Predictive factors of bad prognosis
  - High cell density + brisk mitotic activity
  - High cell density + vascular proliferation and/or cytologic atypia
  - Extent of resection (spinal tumors)
  - P53

60.4 Myxopapillary Ependymoma (WHO Grade I)

WHO Definition
2016—A glial tumor arising almost exclusively in the region of the conus medullaris, cauda equina, and filum terminale, and histologically characterized by elongated, fibrillary processes arranged in radial patterns around vascularized, mucoid, fibrovascular cores (McLendon et al. 2016a).

2007—A slowly growing ependymal glioma with preferential manifestation in young adults and almost exclusive location in the region of the conus medullaris, cauda equina, and filum terminale of the spinal cord; typically characterized histologically by tumor cells arranged in a papillary manner around vascularized myxoid stromal cores (McLendon et al. 2007c).

2000—Myxopapillary ependymomas are slowly growing gliomas with preferential manifestation in young adults and are almost exclusively located in the conus-cauda-filum terminale region of the spinal cord. They are histologically characterized by tumor cells arranged in a papillary manner around vascularized mucoid stromal cores (Wiestler et al. 2000c).

1993—A variant of ependymoma that occurs almost exclusively in the region of the cauda equina and originates from the filum terminale. It is histologically characterized by cuboidal to elongated tumor cells arranged in a perivascular papillary pattern around central cores of mucinous or hyalinized perivascular stroma (Kleihues et al. 1993).

1979—A tumor that occurs virtually exclusively in the region of the cauda equina and originates from the filum terminale or the conus medullaris. It is composed of ependymal cells often arranged in a perivascular papillary manner around central cores of acellular hyaline connective tissue. The stroma is highly vascular, and hemorrhages are frequent. Mucin is often demonstrable in the cytoplasm of the tumor cells. Material with a similar staining reaction in the stroma may be so prominent that the architecture is blurred. It corresponds histologically to grade I, rarely II (Zülch 1979).

WHO Grade
- WHO grade I

60.4.1 Epidemiology

Incidence
- 9–13% of ependymal tumors
- 0.05 (females)—0.08% (males) per 100.000

Age Incidence
- Mean age: 36 years

Sex Incidence
- Male:Female ratio: 2.2:1

Localization
- Conus medullaris–cauda equina–filum teminale
- Rarely nerve roots
- Rare erosion of the adjacent bone
- Rarely cervical-thoracic spine, fourth ventricle, lateral ventricle, brain
- Subcutaneous sacro-coccygeal or presacral region

60.4.2 Neuroimaging Findings

General Imaging Findings
- Lobulated, solid, enhancing mass at filum terminale

CT Non-Contrast-Enhanced
- Isodense
- Scalloping of spinal canal/adjacent bone possible

CT Contrast-Enhanced
- Homogeneous enhancement

MRI-T2 (Fig. 60.9a, d)
- Homogenous, hyperintense mass
- Hypointense signal (hemosiderin) in case of hemorrhage

MRI-T1 (Fig. 60.9b)
- Isointense

MRI-T1 Contrast-Enhanced (Fig. 60.9c, e)
- Strong enhancement

60.4.3 Neuropathology Findings

Macroscopic Features
- Lobulated
- Soft
- Greyish
- Encapsulated
- No gross infiltration

Microscopic Features (Fig. 60.10a–h)
- Cuboidal to elongated tumor cells.
- Radially arranged in a papillary way around vascularized stromal cores.
- Minimal or no papillary regions may be encountered.
- Fascicles of elongated cells.
- Myxoid matrix:
  - Alcian-blue positive
  - Between tumor cells and blood vessels
  - Microcysts

Immunophenotype (Fig. 60.10i–n)

IHC-positivity	IHC-negativity
• GFAP • S-100 • Vimentin • Alarin	– Cytokeratins – IDH1

Proliferation Markers (Fig. 60.10o, p)
- Mitotic activity low
- Ki-67 LI: <3%

60.4 Myxopapillary Ependymoma (WHO Grade I)

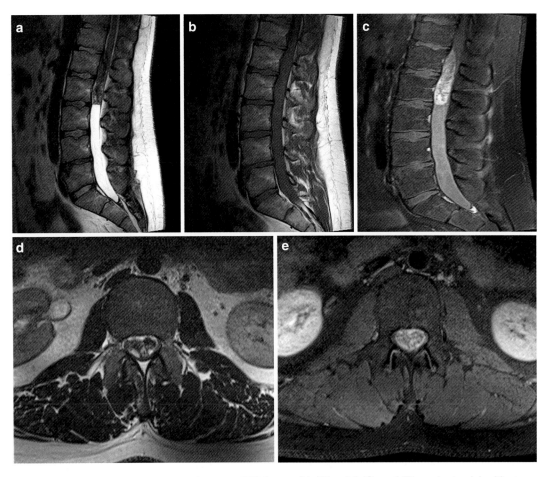

Fig. 60.9 Spinal myxopapillary ependymoma (WHO grade I), typically located in the conus medullaris and filum terminale t2 sag(**a**), T1 sag(**b**), T1 contrast, fat sat sag(**c**), T2 axial (**d**), and T1 contrast axial with strong enhancement (**e**)

Ultrastructural Features
- junctions of zonula adherens type
- cytoplasmic thickening
- wide spaces containing amorphous material or loose filaments
- cilia
- abundant basement membrane structures
- aggregation of microtubules within endoplasmic reticulum

Differential Diagnosis
- Chordoma
- Myxoid chondrosarcoma
- Paraganglioma
- Mesothelioma
- Papillary adenocarcinoma

60.4.4 Treatment and Prognosis

Treatment
- Surgery

Biologic Behavior–Prognosis–Prognostic Factors
- good prognosis
- late recurrence with incomplete resection
- metastases with incomplete resection
- subarachnoid dissemination

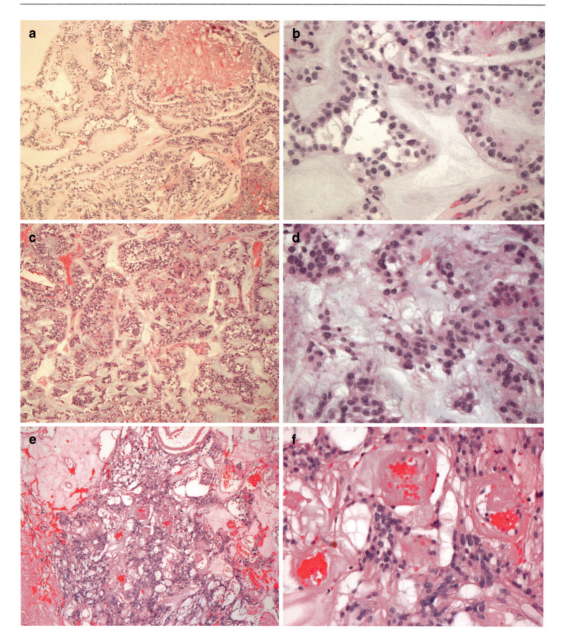

Fig. 60.10 Myxopapillary ependymoma (WHO grade I) is made up of cuboidal to elongated tumor cells which are radially arranged in a papillary way around vascularized stromal cores (**a–f**). The myxoid matrix is located between tumor cells and blood vessels and stain Alcian-blue positive (**g, h**). Immunophenotype: tumor cells are positive for GFAP (**i–l**), s-100 (**m**), EMA dots (**n**). Low Ki-67 proliferation rate (**o, p**)

60.4 Myxopapillary Ependymoma (WHO Grade I)

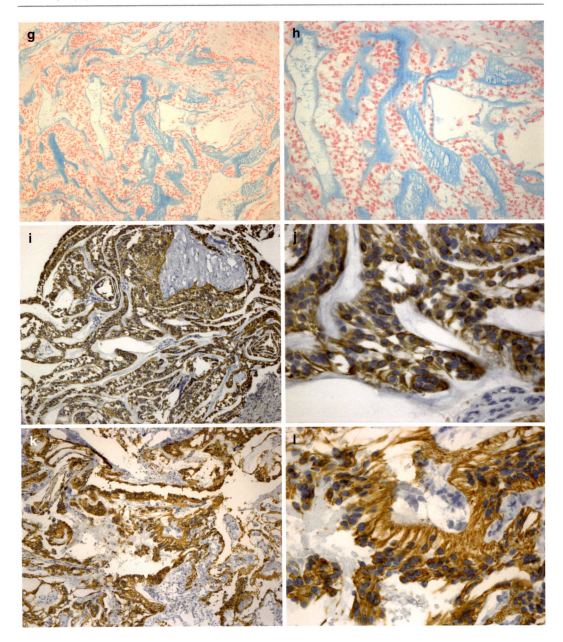

Fig. 60.10 (continued)

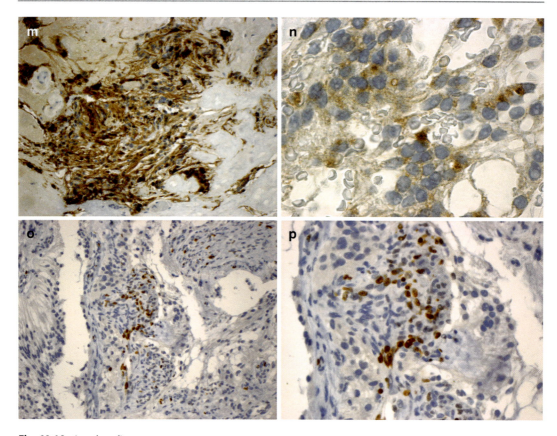

Fig. 60.10 (continued)

60.5 Subependymoma (WHO Grade I)

WHO Definition

2016—A slow-growing, exophytic, intraventricular glial neoplasm characterized by clusters of bland to mildly pleomorphic, mitotically inactive cells embedded in an abundant fibrillary matrix with frequent microcystic change (McLendon et al. 2016b).

2007—A slowly growing, benign neoplasm, typically attached to a ventricular wall, composed of glial tumor cell clusters embedded in an abundant fibrillary matrix with frequent microcystic change (McLendon et al. 2007d).

2000—A slowly growing, benign neoplasm, typically attached to a ventricular wall, composed of glial tumor cells clusters embedded in an abundant fibrillary matrix with frequent microcystic change (Wiestler and Schiffer 2000).

1993—A nodular tumor composed of nests of ependymal cells in a dense glial fibrillary matrix (Kleihues et al. 1993).

1979—A tumor composed of nests of uniform ependymal cells in a stroma of dense acellular glial fibers. These glial fibers could be produced either by admixed astrocytes or by the ependymal cells themselves (Zülch 1979).

WHO Grade
- WHO grade I

60.5 Subependymoma (WHO Grade I)

60.5.1 Epidemiology

Incidence
- Low
- 8% of ependymal tumors

Age Incidence
- All ages
- Frequently in middle-aged and elderly patients

Sex Incidence
- Male:Female ratio: 2.3:1

Localization
- Fourth ventricle (50% of cases)
- Lateral ventricle (30% of cases)
- Third ventricle
- Septum pellucidum
- Spinal cord
  - Cervical level
  - Cervico-thoracic level

60.5.2 Neuroimaging Findings

General Imaging Findings
- Lobulated, well-defined, solid mass, typically in the foramen Magendie of the fourth ventricle

CT Non-Contrast-Enhanced
- Iso- to hypodense
- Calcifications less common than in ependymoma

CT Contrast-Enhanced
- None to mild enhancement

MRI-T1
- Homogenous hypo- to isointense

MRI-T2 (Fig. 60.11a, b)
- Homogenous, hyperintense mass
- Edema at adjacent parenchyma is absent

MRI-Flair (Fig. 60.11c)
- Hyperintense

MRI-T2*
- In case of calcifications, hypointense

MRI-T1 Contrast-Enhanced (Fig. 60.11d)
- None to mild enhancement

MR-Diffusion Imaging
- No diffusion restriction
- ADC value elevated

MR-Spectroscopy
- Slightly decreased NAA

60.5.3 Neuropathology Findings

Macroscopic Features (Fig. 60.12a–f)
- Firm nodules
- Variable size
- Bulge into the ventricular system
- Well demarcated

Microscopic Features (Fig. 60.13a–l)
- Clusters of isomorph nuclei embedded in a dense fibrillar matrix of glial cell processes.
- Nuclei resemble subependymal glia.
- Ependymal rosettes:
  - Orientation of cell processes around vessels
- Admixed histological features of both subependymoma and ependymoma.
- Small cysts.
- Calcifications possible.
- Hemorrhages possible.
- Prominent tumor vasculature with microvascular proliferation.
- Mitoses: rare or absent.

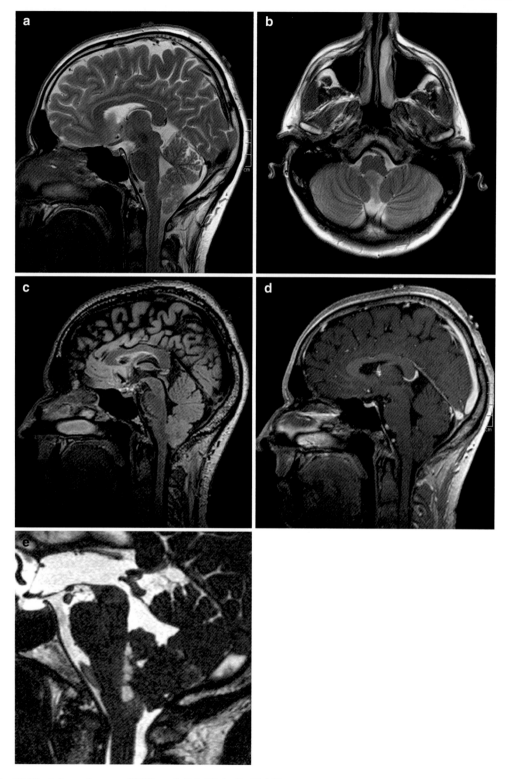

Fig. 60.11 Subependymoma (WHO grade I) in T2 (**a**, **b**), FLAIR (**c**), T1 contrast without enhancement (**d**), and in 3D CISS (**e**)

60.5 Subependymoma (WHO Grade I)

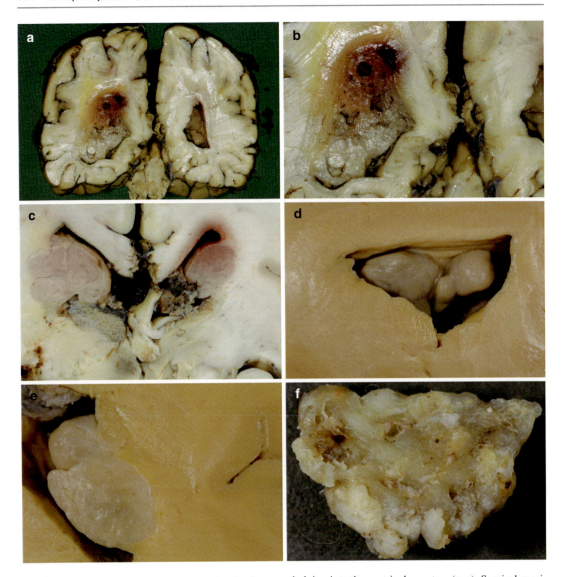

Fig. 60.12 Subependymoma (WHO grade I). Gross-anatomical autopsy specimen shows well-demarcated firm nodules of variable size and whitish-grayish color bulging into the ventricular system (**a–e**). Surgical specimen of whitish-grayish color (**f**)

Immunophenotype (Fig. 60.14a–l)
- GFAP variable extent
- Alarin
- NCAM and neuron-specific enolase

Proliferation Markers (Fig. 60.14m, n)
- Mitoses: rare or absent
- Ki-67 LI: <1%

Ultrastructural Features
- Typical ependymal characteristics:
  - Cilia formation
  - Microvilli
  - Abundant intermediate filaments

Differential Diagnosis
- Ependymoma
- Astrocytoma
- Pilocytic astrocytoma
- Central neurocytoma

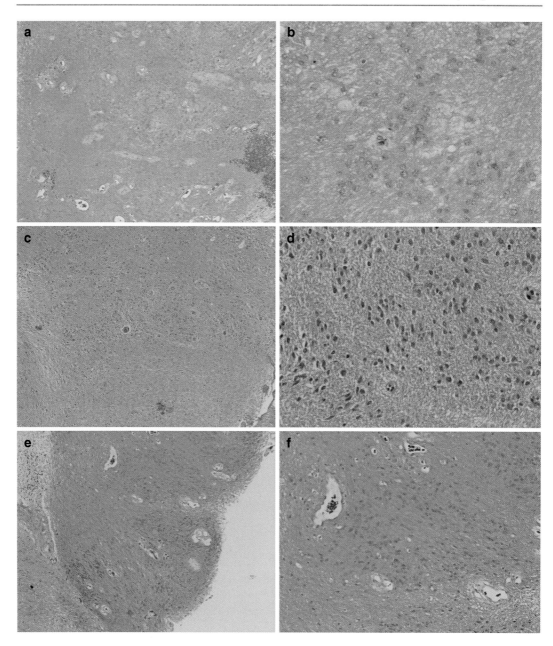

Fig. 60.13 Subependymoma (WHO grade I): Histologically, the tumor is characterized by clusters of isomorph nuclei embedded in a dense fibrillar matrix of glial cell processes (**a–h**). Ependymal rosettes show orientation of cell processes around vessels (**e, f**). Cyst formation is possible (**g, h**). Prominent vessel with wall hyalinization (**h–j**). Alcian-blue positive matrix (**k, l**)

60.5 Subependymoma (WHO Grade I)

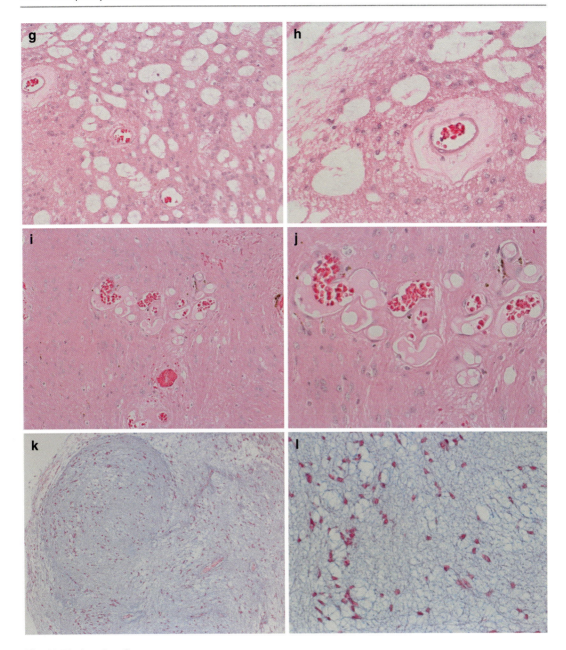

Fig. 60.13 (continued)

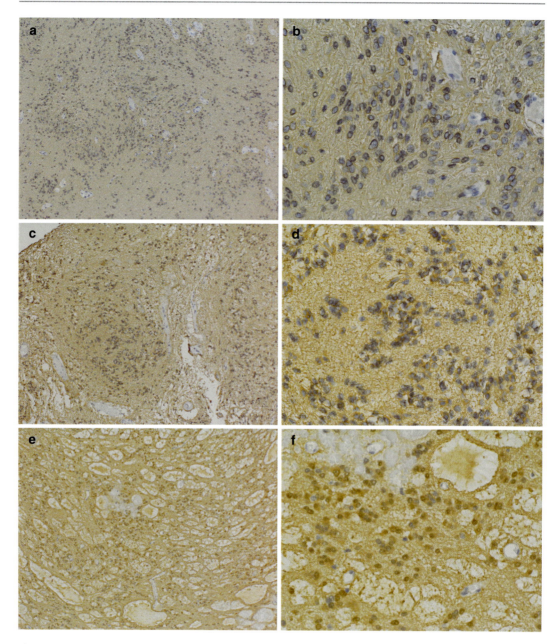

Fig. 60.14 Subependymoma (WHO grade I)—Immunophenotype: Tumor cells are positive for GFAP (**a–d**), S-100 (**e, f**), few cells express Olig 2 (**g, h**), few cells are ATRX-positive (**i, j**), EMA dots (**k, l**). Low Ki-67 proliferation rate (**m, n**)

60.5 Subependymoma (WHO Grade I)

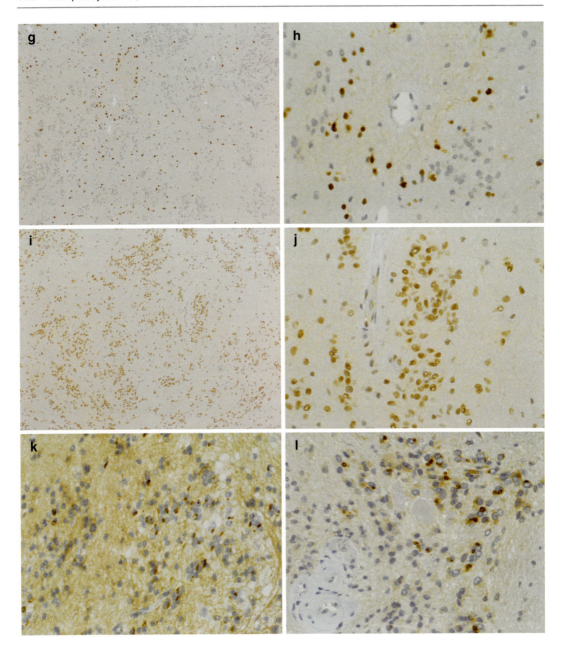

Fig. 60.14 (continued)

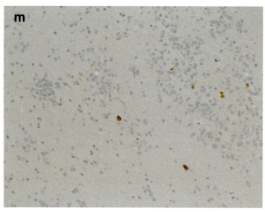 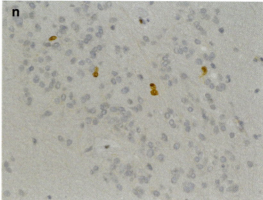

Fig. 60.14 (continued)

60.5.4 Treatment and Prognosis

Treatment
- Surgery

Biologic Behavior–Prognosis–Prognostic Factors
- good prognosis
- recurrence after incomplete resection

Selected References

Chiechi MV, Smirniotopoulos JG, Jones RV (1995) Intracranial subependymomas: CT and MR imaging features in 24 cases. AJR Am J Roentgenol 165(5):1245–1250. https://doi.org/10.2214/ajr.165.5.7572512

Dorfer C, Tonn J, Rutka JT (2016) Ependymoma: a heterogeneous tumor of uncertain origin and limited therapeutic options. Handb Clin Neurol 134:417–431. https://doi.org/10.1016/b978-0-12-802997-8.00025-6

Ellison DW, Korshunov A, Witt H (2016a) Ependymoma, RELA fusion-positive. In: Louis DN, Ohgaki H, Wiestler OD, Cavenee WK (eds) WHO classification of tumours of the central nervous system, Revised 4th edn. IARC, Lyon, p 112

Ellison DW, McLendon R, Wiestler OD, Kros JM, Korshunov A, Ng H-K, Witt H, Hirose T (2016b) Anaplastic ependymoma. In: Louis DN, Ohgaki H, Wiestler OD, Cavenee WK (eds) WHO classification of tumours of the central nervous system, Revised 4th edn. IARC, Lyon, pp 113–114

Ellison DW, McLendon R, Wiestler OD, Kros JM, Korshunov A, Ng H-K, Witt H, Hirose T (2016c) Ependymoma. In: Louis DN, Ohgaki H, Wiestler OD, Cavenee WK (eds) WHO classification of tumours of the central nervous system, Revised 4th edn. IARC, Lyon, pp 106–111

Gilbert MR, Ruda R, Soffietti R (2010) Ependymomas in adults. Curr Neurol Neurosci Rep 10(3):240–247. https://doi.org/10.1007/s11910-010-0109-3

Gupta K, Salunke P (2017) Understanding ependymoma oncogenesis: an update on recent molecular advances and current perspectives. Mol Neurobiol 54(1):15–21. https://doi.org/10.1007/s12035-015-9646-8

Jain A, Amin AG, Jain P, Burger P, Jallo GI, Lim M, Bettegowda C (2012) Subependymoma: clinical features and surgical outcomes. Neurol Res 34(7):677–684. https://doi.org/10.1179/1743132812y.0000000064

Kahan H, Sklar EM, Post MJ, Bruce JH (1996) MR characteristics of histopathologic subtypes of spinal ependymoma. AJNR Am J Neuroradiol 17(1):143–150

Khatua S, Ramaswamy V, Bouffet E (2017) Current therapy and the evolving molecular landscape of paediatric ependymoma. Eur J Cancer 1990(70):34–41. https://doi.org/10.1016/j.ejca.2016.10.013

Kilday JP, Rahman R, Dyer S, Ridley L, Lowe J, Coyle B, Grundy R (2009) Pediatric ependymoma: biological perspectives. Mol Cancer Res 7(6):765–786. https://doi.org/10.1158/1541-7786.mcr-08-0584

Kim JH, Huang Y, Griffin AS, Rajappa P, Greenfield JP (2013) Ependymoma in children: molecular considerations and therapeutic insights. Clin Transl Oncol 15(10):759–765. https://doi.org/10.1007/s12094-013-1041-1

Kleihues P, Burger PC, Scheithauer BW (1993) Histological typing of tumours of the central nervous system, 2nd edn. Springer, Berlin

Koeller KK, Rosenblum RS, Morrison AL (2000) Neoplasms of the spinal cord and filum terminale: radiologic-pathologic correlation. Radiographics 20(6):1721–1749. https://doi.org/10.1148/radiographics.20.6.g00nv151721

Selected References

Mack SC, Taylor MD (2009) The genetic and epigenetic basis of ependymoma. Childs Nerv Syst 25(10):1195–1201. https://doi.org/10.1007/s00381-009-0928-1

McLendon R, Schiffer D, Rosenblum MK, Wiestler OD (2016a) Myxopapillary ependymoma. In: Louis DN, Ohgaki H, Wiestler OD, Cavenee WK (eds) WHO classification of tumours of the central nervous system, Revised 4th edn. IARC, Lyon, pp 104–105

McLendon R, Schiffer D, Rosenblum MK, Wiestler OD, Rushing EJ, Hirose T, Santi M (2016b) Subependymoma. In: Louis DN, Ohgaki H, Wiestler OD, Cavenee WK (eds) WHO classification of tumours of the central nervous system, Revised 4th edn. IARC, Lyon, pp 102–103

McLendon R, Wiestler OD, Kros JM, Korshunov A, Ng H-K (2007a) Anaplastic ependymoma. In: Louis DN, Ohgaki H, Wiestler OD, Cavenee WK (eds) WHO classification of tumours of the central nervous system, 4th edn. International Agency for Research on Cancer, Lyon, pp 79–80

McLendon R, Wiestler OD, Kros JM, Korshunov A, Ng H-K (2007b) Ependymoma. In: Louis DN, Ohgaki H, Wiestler OD, Cavenee WK (eds) WHO classification of tumours of the central nervous system, 4th edn. International Agency for Research on Cancer, Lyon, pp 74–78

McLendon RE, Rosenblum MK, Schiffer D, Wiestler OD (2007c) Myxopapillary ependymoma. In: Louis DN, Ohgaki H, Wiestler OD, Cavenee WK (eds) WHO classification of tumours of the central nervous system, 4th edn. International Agency for Research on Cancer, Lyon, pp 72–73

McLendon RE, Schiffer D, Rosenblum MK, Wiestler OD (2007d) Subependymoma. In: Louis DN, Ohgaki H, Wiestler OD, Cavenee WK (eds) WHO classification of tumours of the central nervous system, 4th edn. International Agency for Research on Cancer, Lyon, pp 70–71

Merchant TE, Pollack IF, Loeffler JS (2010) Brain tumors across the age spectrum: biology, therapy, and late effects. Semin Radiat Oncol 20(1):58–66. https://doi.org/10.1016/j.semradonc.2009.09.005

Pajtler KW, Pfister SM, Kool M (2015a) Molecular dissection of ependymomas. Oncoscience 2(10):827–828. https://doi.org/10.18632/oncoscience.202

Pajtler KW, Witt H, Sill M, Jones DT, Hovestadt V, Kratochwil F, Wani K, Tatevossian R, Punchihewa C, Johann P, Reimand J, Warnatz HJ, Ryzhova M, Mack S, Ramaswamy V, Capper D, Schweizer L, Sieber L, Wittmann A, Huang Z, van Sluis P, Volckmann R, Koster J, Versteeg R, Fults D, Toledano H, Avigad S, Hoffman LM, Donson AM, Foreman N, Hewer E, Zitterbart K, Gilbert M, Armstrong TS, Gupta N, Allen JC, Karajannis MA, Zagzag D, Hasselblatt M, Kulozik AE, Witt O, Collins VP, von Hoff K, Rutkowski S, Pietsch T, Bader G, Yaspo ML, von Deimling A, Lichter P, Taylor MD, Gilbertson R, Ellison DW, Aldape K, Korshunov A, Kool M, Pfister SM (2015b) Molecular classification of ependymal tumors across All CNS compartments, histopathological grades, and age groups. Cancer Cell 27(5):728–743. https://doi.org/10.1016/j.ccell.2015.04.002

Pfister S, Hartmann C, Korshunov A (2009) Histology and molecular pathology of pediatric brain tumors. J Child Neurol 24(11):1375–1386. https://doi.org/10.1177/0883073809339213

Ragel BT, Osborn AG, Whang K, Townsend JJ, Jensen RL, Couldwell WT (2006) Subependymomas: an analysis of clinical and imaging features. Neurosurgery 58(5):881–890; . discussion 881-890. https://doi.org/10.1227/01.neu.0000209928.04532.09

Rumboldt Z, Camacho DL, Lake D, Welsh CT, Castillo M (2006) Apparent diffusion coefficients for differentiation of cerebellar tumors in children. AJNR Am J Neuroradiol 27(6):1362–1369

Tamburrini G, D'Ercole M, Pettorini BL, Caldarelli M, Massimi L, Di Rocco C (2009) Survival following treatment for intracranial ependymoma: a review. Childs Nerv Syst 25(10):1303–1312. https://doi.org/10.1007/s00381-009-0874-y

Wiestler OD, Schiffer D (2000) Subependymoma. In: Kleihues P, Cavenee WK (eds) Pathology and genetics of tumours of the nervous system, 3rd edn. IARC Press, Lyon, pp 80–81

Wiestler OD, Schiffer D, Coons SW, Prayson RA, Rosenblum MK (2000a) Anaplastic ependymoma. In: Kleihues P, Cavenee WK (eds) Pathology and genetics of tumours of the nervous system, 3rd edn. IARC Press, Lyon, pp 76–77

Wiestler OD, Schiffer D, Coons SW, Prayson RA, Rosenblum MK (2000b) Ependymoma. In: Kleihues P, Cavenee WK (eds) Pathology and genetics of tumours of the nervous system, 3rd edn. IARC Press, Lyon, pp 72–76

Wiestler OD, Schiffer D, Coons SW, Prayson RA, Rosenblum MK (2000c) Myxopapillary ependymoma. In: Kleihues P, Cavenee WK (eds) Pathology and genetics of tumours of the nervous system, 3rd edn. IARC Press, Lyon, pp 78–79

Witt H, Korshunov A, Pfister SM, Milde T (2012) Molecular approaches to ependymoma: the next step(s). Curr Opin Neurol 25(6):745–750. https://doi.org/10.1097/WCO.0b013e328359cdf5

Yao Y, Mack SC, Taylor MD (2011) Molecular genetics of ependymoma. Chin J Cancer 30(10):669–681. https://doi.org/10.5732/cjc.011.10129

Yuh EL, Barkovich AJ, Gupta N (2009) Imaging of ependymomas: MRI and CT. Childs Nerv Syst 25(10):1203–1213. https://doi.org/10.1007/s00381-009-0878-7

Zacharoulis S, Moreno L (2009) Ependymoma: an update. J Child Neurol 24(11):1431–1438. https://doi.org/10.1177/0883073809339212

Zülch KJ (1979) Histological typing of tumours of the central nervous system. World Health Organization, Geneva

Choroid Plexus Tumors

61.1 General Aspects

Choroid plexus tumors: Intraventricular, papillary neoplasm derived from choroid plexus epithelium (Paulus and Brandner 2007).

The following tumors affecting the choroid plexus are distinguished:

• Choroid plexus papilloma	WHO grade I
• Atypical choroid plexus papilloma	WHO grade II
• Choroid plexus carcinoma	WHO grade III

61.1.1 Epidemiology

Incidence
- Annual incidence: 0.3 per 1,000,000 population per year
- 0.3–0.6% of all brain tumors

Age Incidence
- Median age:
  - Lateral and third ventricle: 1.5 years
  - Fourth ventricle: 22 years
  - Cerebellopontine angle: 35.5 years
- Patients under 15 years of age: 2–4%
- Patients under 1 year of age: 10–20%

Sex Incidence
- Male:Female ratio: 1.2:1
  - Lateral ventricle 1:1
  - Fourth ventricle: 3:2

Localization
- Lateral ventricles (50%)
- Fourth ventricle (40%)
- Third ventricle (5%)
- Cerebellopontine angle (rare)
- Involvement of 2 or 3 ventricles (5%)

61.1.2 Nuclear Medicine Imaging Findings

- Rare reports deal with the imaging of choroid plexus papilloma in Tc-99 m brain perfusion scans. These findings have no current clinical impact.
- Overall, only few studies are available dealing with choroid plexus carcinomas.
- FDG can show hypermetabolism in choroid plexus carcinomas.
- Amino acid uptake is described to be positive in choroid plexus carcinomas.
- Hypoxia tracers are under investigation for radiotherapy planning.

61.1.3 Differential Diagnosis

- Normal choroid plexus
- Metastatic carcinomas
  - Choroid plexus tumor positive for:
    o Inward rectifier potassium channel Kir7.1 (74% of cases)
    o Stanniocalcin-1 (83% of cases)
    o Excitatory amino acid transporter-1 (EAAT1) (66%)
  - Metastatic carcinoma positive for:
    o HEA125
    o BerEP4
    o Carcinoembryonic antigen (CEA)
- Atypical teratoid/rhabdoid tumor (AT/RT)
  - Loss of INI immunoreativity in AT/RT

61.1.4 Molecular Neuropathology

Pathogenesis
- unknown

Genes
- Different genetic pathways between choroid plexus papilloma and carcinoma
- Choroid plexus papilloma
  - Gains on chromosomes 7, 9, 12, 15, 17, 18
- Choroid plexus carcinoma
  - Loss of heterozygosity on chromosomes 1p, 1q, 3p, 5q, 9q, 10q, 13q, 18q, 22q

61.1.5 Treatment and Prognosis

Treatment
- Surgery
- Controversial
  - Radiotherapy
  - Chemotherapy

Biologic Behavior–Prognosis–Prognostic Factors
- Choroid plexus papilloma:
  - 5-year survival rate: 100%
  - 5-year local control: 100% with gross total resection, 68% after subtotal resection
  - 1-year survival rate: 90%
  - 5-year survival rate: 81%
  - 10-year survival rate: 77%
  - Malignant progression is rare
- Choroid plexus carcinoma:
  - 1-year survival rate: 71%
  - 5-year survival rate: 41%
  - 10-year survival rate: 35%
- Poor prognosis, recurrence and/or fatal outcome correlated with:
  - Mitoses
  - Necrosis
  - Brain invasion
  - Lack of immunoreactivity for transthyretin
  - Decreased expression of S-100 protein

61.2 Choroid Plexus Papilloma WHO Grade I

WHO Definition
2016—A benign ventricular papillary neoplasm derived from choroid plexus epithelium, with very low or absent mitotic activity (Paulus et al. 2016c).

2007—Choroid plexus tumors: Intraventricular, papillary neoplasm derived from choroid plexus epithelium (Paulus and Brandner 2007).

Choroid plexus papilloma: Delicate fibrovascular connective tissue fronds are covered by a single layer of uniform cuboidal to columnar epithelial cells with round or oval, basally situated monomorphic nuclei (Paulus and Brandner 2007).

2000—Choroid plexus tumors: Intraventricular, papillary neoplasms derived from choroid plexus epithelium (Aguzzi et al. 2000).

Choroid plexus papilloma: This benign, papillary tumor is composed of delicate fibrovascular connective tissue fronds covered by a single layer of uniform cuboidal to columnar epithelial cells with round or oval, basally situated monomorphic nuclei. Conspicuous mitotic activity, brain invasion, and necroses are absent (Aguzzi et al. 2000).

1993—An epithelial tumor of the choroid plexus of the central ventricles. It is composed of a simple or pseudostratified layer of cuboidal to columnar cells resting upon a basement membrane overlying papillary, vascularized connective tissue cores (Kleihues et al. 1993).

1979—A papillary tumor composed of usually a single layer of low columnar or cuboidal cells which lie upon a basement membrane covering a delicate vascular connective tissue core. Sometimes, they are heavily calcified (Zülch 1979).

WHO Grade
- WHO grade I

61.2.1 Neuroimaging Findings

General Imaging Findings
- Well-delineated, lobulated, intraventricular mass with strong enhancement
- Rarely invasion into adjacent parenchyma

CT Non-Contrast-Enhanced
- Iso- to hyperdense
- Calcifications common
- May cause hydrocephalus (obstructive or CSF overproduction)

CT Contrast-Enhanced
- Strong enhancement

MRI-T2/FLAIR (Fig. 61.1a, b)
- Iso- to hyperintense
- Flow voids demonstrate vascularity

MRI-T1 (Fig. 61.1c)
- Iso- to hypointense

MRI-T1 Contrast-Enhanced (Figs. 61.1d, e and 61.2a–c)
- Strong homogeneous enhancement

MRI-T2∗/SWI
- Calcifications and hemorrhage common

MR-Diffusion Imaging
- No restricted diffusion

MRI-Perfusion (Fig. 61.2d)
- CBV increased

MR-Spectroscopy (Fig. 61.2e)
- NAA decreased
- Choline elevated
- Lactate elevated in case of necrosis
- Myoinositol elevated

61.2.2 Neuropathology Findings

Macroscopic Features (Fig. 61.3a–d)
- Circumscribed cauliflower-like mass
- Adheres to ventricular wall
- Well delineated from the brain tissue
- Cyst formation possible
- Hemorrhages possible

Microscopic Features (Fig. 61.4a–f)
- Single layer of cuboidal or columnar epithelial cells with
  - Round to oval nuclei
  - Basally situated monomorphic nuclei
- Underlying delicate fibrovascular connective tissue
- Unusual but possible features:
  - Brain invasion
  - High cellularity
  - Nuclear pleomorphism

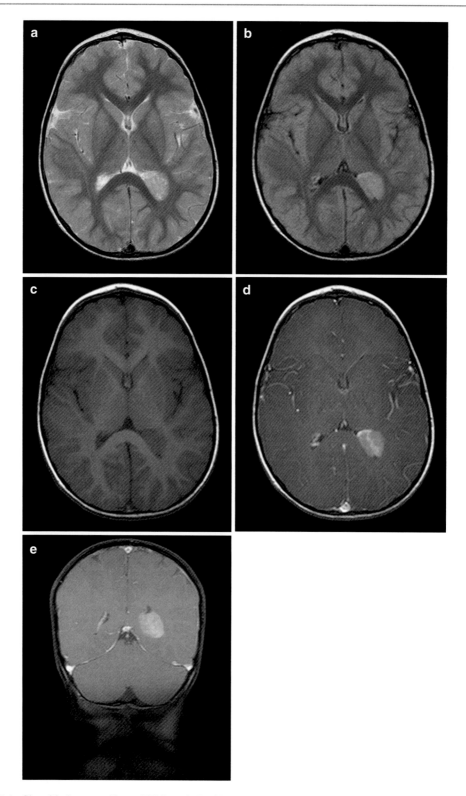

Fig. 61.1 Choroid plexus papilloma WHO grade I with cystic components, located in the posterior horn of the left ventricle in T2 (**a**), FLAIR (**b**), T1 (**c**), and T1 contrast with enhancement (**d**, **e**)

61.2 Choroid Plexus Papilloma WHO Grade I

- Necroses
- Focal blurring of the papillary pattern
- Unusual histologic features include:
  - Oncocytic change
  - Mucinous degeneration
  - Melanization
- Tubular glandular architecture
- Xanthomatous change of connective tissue
- Angioma-like blood vessels
- Formation of bone, cartilage, or adipose tissue

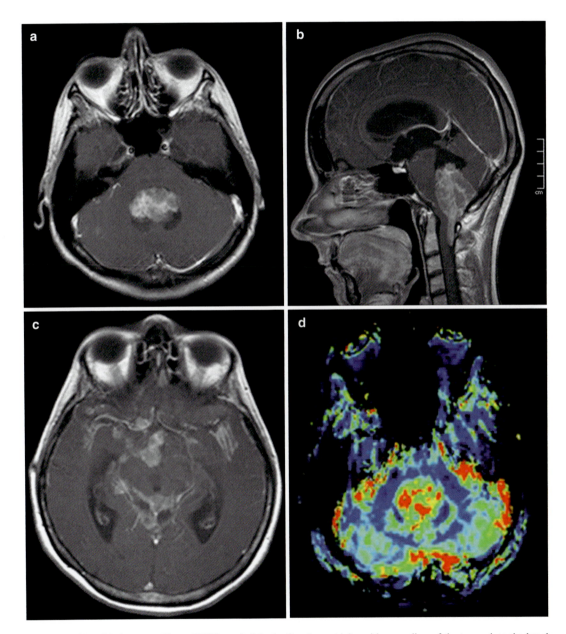

Fig. 61.2 Choroid plexus papilloma WHO grade I in the fourth ventricle, with spreading of the tumor into the basal subarachnoidal space T1 contrast (**a–c**), increased CBV (**d**), and mild elevation of choline in MR-spectroscopy (**e**)

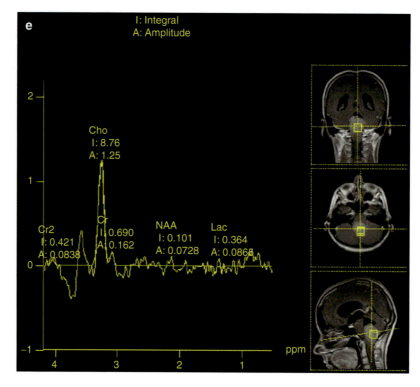

Fig. 61.2 (continued)

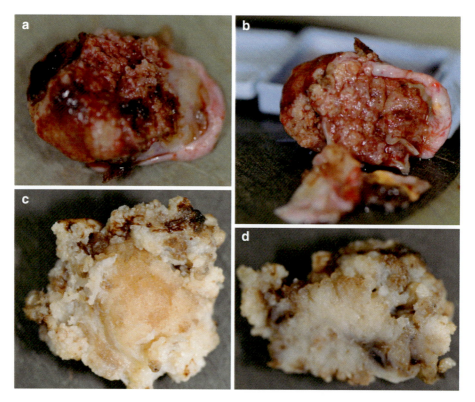

Fig. 61.3 Choroid plexus papilloma WHO grade I: Surgical specimen showing a circumscribed cauliflower-like mass (**a–d**)

61.2 Choroid Plexus Papilloma WHO Grade I

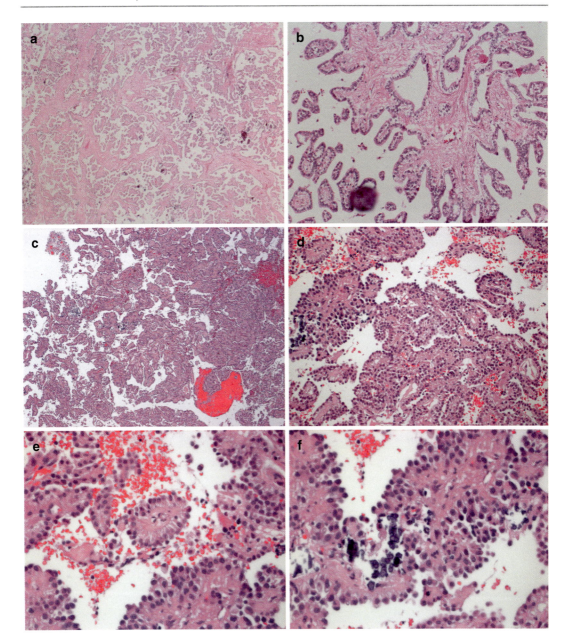

Fig. 61.4 Choroid plexus papilloma WHO grade I: A moderately cellular papillary tumor made up of single layers of cuboidal or columnar epithelial cells with round to oval nuclei and basally situated monomorphic nuclei resting on an underlying delicate fibrovascular connective tissue (**a–f**). Immunophenotype: Tumor cells are positive for pre-albumin (**g, f**), S-100 (**i, j**), pancytokeratin AE1/AE3 (**k, l**). Few cells are positive for GFAP (**m, n**) and synaptophysin (**o, p**)

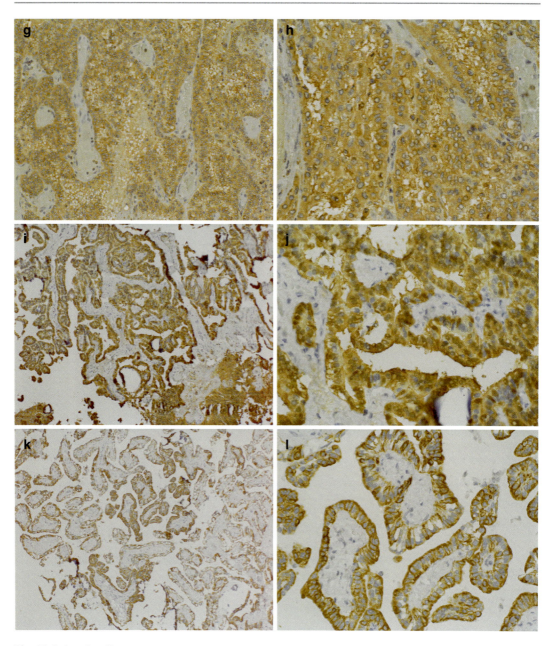

Fig. 61.4 (continued)

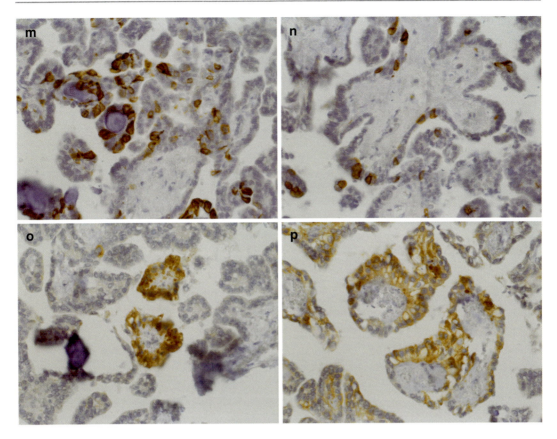

Fig. 61.4 (continued)

Immunophenotype (Fig. 61.4g–p)

IHC-positivity	IHC-negativity
• Cytokeratins (CK7-positive, CK20-negative) • Vimentin • Transthyretin (pre-albumin) (70% of cases) • Podoplanin • S-100 (55–90% of cases) • GFAP (25–55% of cases) • Inward rectifier potassium channel Kir7.1 (74% of cases) • Stanniocalcin-1 (83% of cases) • Excitatory amino acid transporter-1 (EAAT1) (66%) • Alarin • Synaptophysin	• Epithelial membrane antigen (EMA)

Proliferation Markers
- Low mitotic activity
- Ki-67 LI:
  - mean: 1.9%
  - range: 0.2–6%

Ultrastructural Features
- Interdigitating cell membranes
- Tight junctions
- Microvilli
- Apical cilia
- Basement membrane at the abluminal pole

61.3 Atypical Choroid Plexus Papilloma (WHO Grade II)

WHO Definition
2016—A choroid plexus papilloma that has increased mitotic activity but does not fulfill the criteria for choroid plexus carcinoma (Paulus et al. 2016a).

2007—Choroid plexus tumors: Intraventricular, papillary neoplasm derived from choroid plexus epithelium with increased mitotic activity (Paulus and Brandner 2007).

Atypical choroid plexus papilloma: Atypical CPP is defined as CPP with increased mitotic activity (Paulus and Brandner 2007).

2000—Tumors where the distinction between choroid plexus tumors and choroid plexus carcinomas is not always clear-cut (Aguzzi et al. 2000).

WHO Grade
- WHO grade II

61.3.1 Neuroimaging Findings

- Indistinguishable from choroid plexus papilloma WHO grade I or choroid plexus carcinoma

61.3.2 Neuropathology Findings

Macroscopic Features
- Circumscribed cauliflower-like mass
- Adheres to ventricular wall
- Well delineated from the brain tissue
- Cyst formation possible
- Hemorrhages possible

Microscopic Features (Fig. 61.5a–h)
- Single layer of cuboidal or columnar epithelial cells with
  - Round to oval nuclei
  - Basally situated monomorphic nuclei
- Underlying delicate fibrovascular connective tissue
- Increased mitotic activity (2 or more mitoses per 10 randomly selected high-power field)
- Two of the following features might be present:
  - Increased cellularity
  - Nuclear pleomorphism
  - Blurring of the papillary pattern resulting in solid growth
  - Areas of necroses

Immunophenotype (Fig. 61.5i–p)

IHC-positivities	IHC-negativities
• Cytokeratins (CK7-positive, CK20-negative) • Vimentin • Transthyretin (pre-albumin) (70% of cases) • Podoplanin • S-100 (55–90% of cases) • GFAP (25–55% of cases) • Inward rectifier potassium channel Kir7.1 (74% of cases) • Stanniocalcin-1 (83% of cases) • Excitatory amino acid transporter-1 (EAAT1) (66%) • Alarin • Synaptophysin	• Epithelial membrane antigen (EMA)

Proliferation Markers (Fig. 61.5q, r)
- Moderate mitotic activity

61.4 Choroid Plexus Carcinoma WHO Grade III

WHO Definition

2016—A frankly malignant epithelial neoplasm most commonly occurring in the lateral ventricles of children, showing at least four of the following five histological features: frequent mitoses, increased cellular density, nuclear pleomorphism, blurring of the papillary pattern with poorly structured sheets of tumor cells, and necrotic areas (Paulus et al. 2016b).

2007—Intraventricular, papillary neoplasm derived from choroid plexus epithelium with frank signs of malignancy (Paulus and Brandner 2007).

2000—Choroid plexus tumors: Intraventricular, papillary neoplasms derived from choroid plexus epithelium (Aguzzi et al. 2000).

Choroid plexus carcinoma: This solid tumor shows frank signs of malignancy, including nuclear pleomorphism, frequent mitoses, high nucleus: cytoplasm ratios, increased cellu-

61.4 Choroid Plexus Carcinoma WHO Grade III

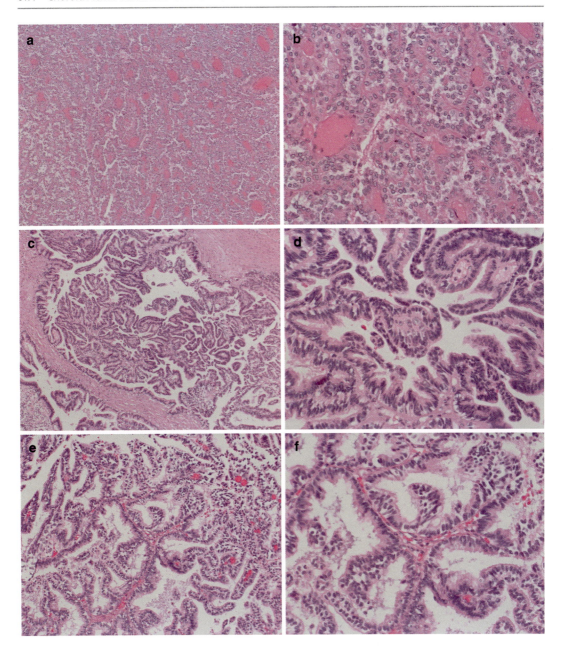

Fig. 61.5 Atypical choroid plexus papilloma (WHO grade II): The tumor consists of single layers of cuboidal or columnar epithelial cells with round to oval nuclei and basally situated monomorphic nuclei (**a–h**). Increased cellularity, nuclear pleomorphism and blurring of the papillary pattern resulting in solid growth characterize atypical choroid plexus papilloma (**a–h**). Immunophenotype: Tumor cells are positive for vimentin (**i, j**), pancytokeratin (**k, l**). Few cells show positivities for GFAP (**m, n**) and synaptophysin (**o, p**). Moderate Ki-67 proliferation rate (**q, r**)

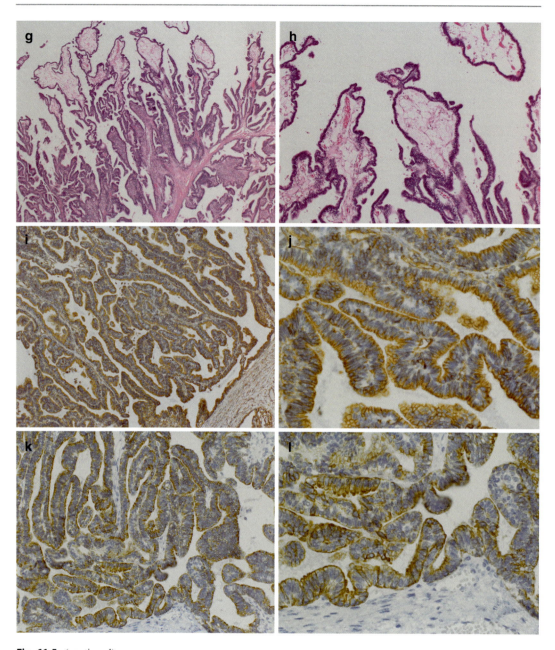

Fig. 61.5 (continued)

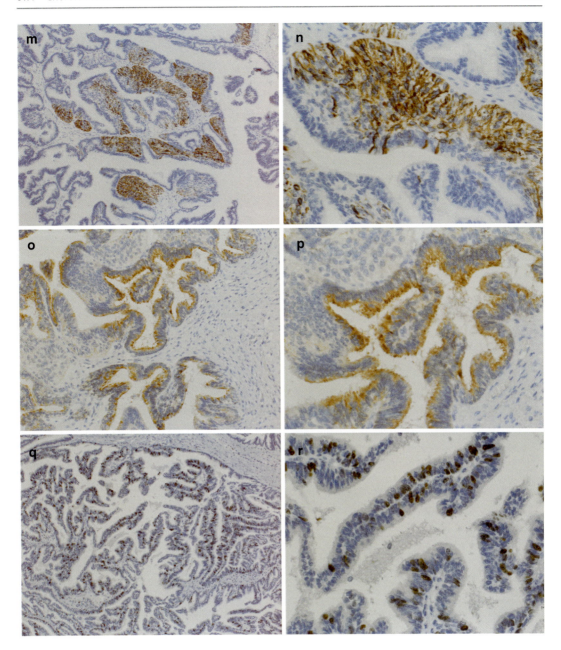

Fig. 61.5 (continued)

lar density, blurring of the papillary pattern with poorly structured sheets of tumor cells, necrotic areas, and often brain invasion (Aguzzi et al. 2000).

1993—A choroid plexus tumor with histological evidence of anaplasia, e.g., increased mitotic activity, nuclear atypia, loss of papillary differentiation with transition to patternless cellular sheets and necrosis (Kleihues et al. 1993).

1979—A choroid plexus papilloma with areas of anaplasia (Zülch 1979).

WHO Grade
- WHO grade III

61.4.1 Neuroimaging Findings

General Imaging Findings
- Intraventricular, lobulated mass with inhomogeneous enhancement and frequent invasion into adjacent parenchyma

CT Non-Contrast-Enhanced (Fig. 61.7a)
- Iso- to hyperdense
- Calcifications common
- May cause hydrocephalus

CT Contrast-Enhanced
- Heterogeneous enhancement

MRI-T2/FLAIR (Figs. 61.6a, b and 61.7b, c)
- Mixed signal of tumor
- Hyperintense peritumoral edema

MRI-T1 (Figs. 61.6c and 61.7d)
- Iso- to hypointense

MRI-T1 Contrast-Enhanced (Figs. 61.6d–f and 61.7e, f)
- Heterogeneous enhancement (versus homogenous in choroid plexus papilloma)

MRI-T2∗/SWI
- Calcifications and hemorrhage common

MR-Diffusion Imaging
- No restricted diffusion

MRI-Perfusion
- CBV increased

MR-Spectroscopy (Fig. 61.6g)
- NAA decreased
- Choline elevated
- Lactate in case of necrosis
- Myoinositol elevated

61.4.2 Neuropathology Findings

Macroscopic Features
- Circumscribed cauliflower-like mass
- Adheres to ventricular wall
- Well delineated from the brain tissue
- Cyst formation possible
- Hemorrhages possible

Microscopic Features (Fig. 61.8a–c)
- Signs of malignancy (at least four of the five):
  - Frequent mitoses (>5 per 10 high-power field)
  - Increased cellular density
  - Nuclear polymorphism
  - Blurring of the papillary pattern with poorly structured sheets of tumor
  - Areas of necroses

Immunophenotype

Positivity	Negativity
- Cytokeratins (CK7-positive, CK20-negative) - Transthyretin (pre-albumin) (less frequent) - S-100 (less frequent) - GFAP (20% of cases) - Alarin	- Epithelial membrane antigen (EMA)

Proliferation Markers (Fig. 61.8d)
- Ki-67 LI:
  - mean: 13.8%
  - range: 7–60%

61.4.3 Molecular Neuropathology

- Preserved expression of
  - *SMARCB1*
  - *SMARCA4*
- Complex chromosomal alterations
- Cytogenetics:
  - Hyperploidy
  - Hypoploidy
- *PT53* mutations (50% of cases)
  - *TP53*-R72 variant and MDM2 SNP309 polymorphism (90% of cases) → reduced *TP53* activity

61.4 Choroid Plexus Carcinoma WHO Grade III

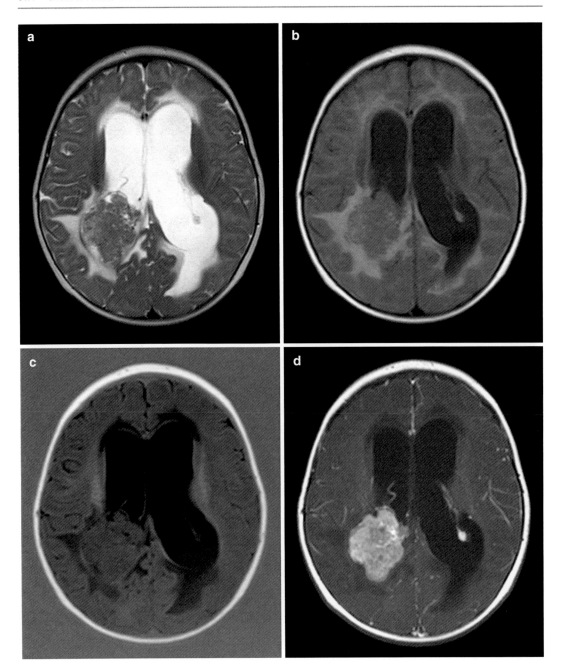

Fig. 61.6 Choroid plexus carcinoma (WHO grade III) in the posterior cornu of the right ventricle T2 (**a**), FLAIR (**b**), T1 (**c**), T1 contrast with strong enhancement (**d, e, f**), and obvious elevation of choline in MR-spectroscopy (**g**)

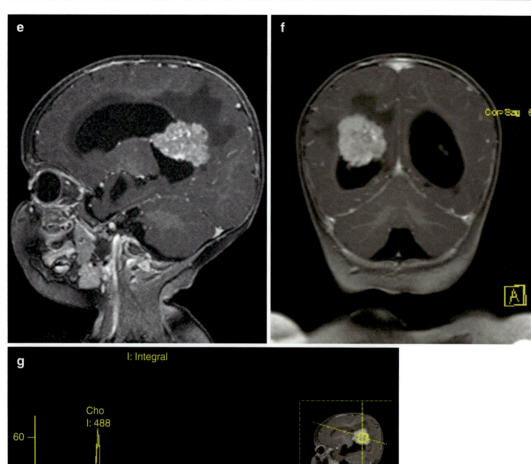

Fig. 61.6 (continued)

61.4 Choroid Plexus Carcinoma WHO Grade III

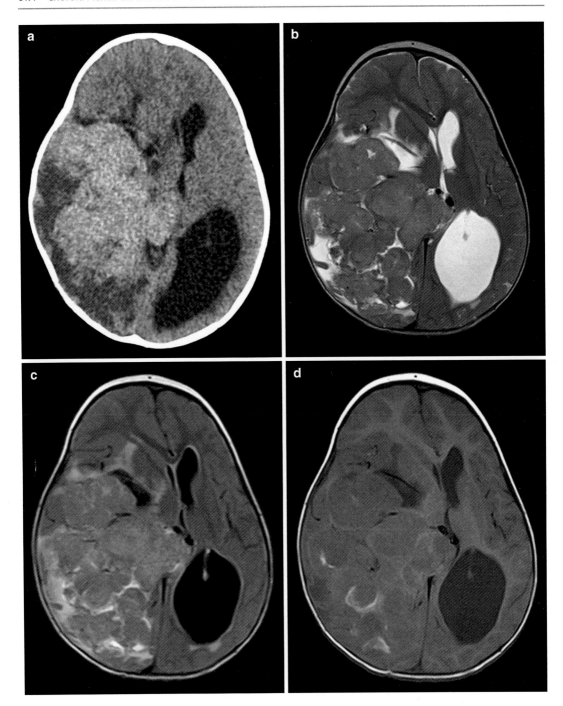

Fig. 61.7 Choroid plexus carcinoma (WHO grade III): CT (**a**), T2 (**b**), FLAIR (**c**), T1 (**d**), T1 contrast (**e, f**)

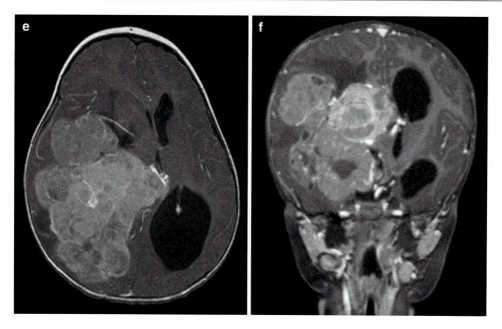

Fig. 61.7 (continued)

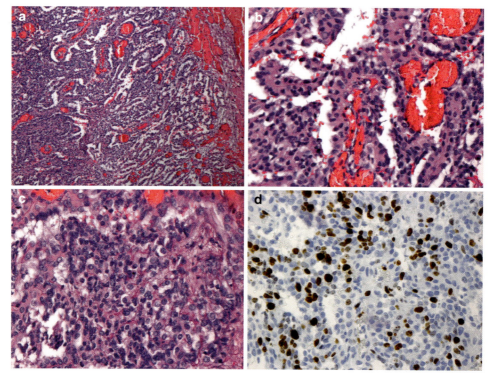

Fig. 61.8 Choroid plexus carcinoma (WHO grade III) characterized by blurring of the papillary pattern with poorly structured sheets of tumor (**a–c**), increased cellular density (**a–c**), nuclear polymorphism (**b**, **c**), frequent mitoses, and moderate to high Ki67 proliferation rate (**d**)

Selected References

Aguzzi A, Brandner S, Paulus W (2000) Choroid plexus tumours. In: Kleihues P, Cavenee WK (eds) Pathology and genetics of tumours of the nervous system, 3rd edn. IARC Press, Lyon, pp 84–85

Gopal P, Parker JR, Debski R, Parker JC Jr (2008) Choroid plexus carcinoma. Arch Pathol Lab Med 132(8):1350–1354. https://doi.org/10.1043/1543-2165(2008)132[1350:cpc]2.0.co;2

Guermazi A, De Kerviler E, Zagdanski AM, Frija J (2000) Diagnostic imaging of choroid plexus disease. Clin Radiol 55(7):503–516. https://doi.org/10.1053/crad.1999.0476

Jaiswal AK, Jaiswal S, Sahu RN, Das KB, Jain VK, Behari S (2009) Choroid plexus papilloma in children: diagnostic and surgical considerations. J Pediatr Neurosci 4(1):10–16. https://doi.org/10.4103/1817-1745.49100

Kamaly-Asl ID, Shams N, Taylor MD (2006) Genetics of choroid plexus tumors. Neurosurg Focus 20(1):E10

Kaur C, Rathnasamy G, Ling EA (2016) The choroid plexus in healthy and diseased brain. J Neuropathol Exp Neurol 75(3):198–213. https://doi.org/10.1093/jnen/nlv030

Kleihues P, Burger PC, Scheithauer BW (1993) Histological typing of tumours of the central nervous system, 2nd edn. Springer-Verlag, Berlin

Koeller KK, Sandberg GD (2002) From the archives of the AFIP. Cerebral intraventricular neoplasms: radiologic-pathologic correlation. Radiographics 22(6):1473–1505. https://doi.org/10.1148/rg.226025118

Naeini RM, Yoo JH, Hunter JV (2009) Spectrum of choroid plexus lesions in children. AJR Am J Roentgenol 192(1):32–40. https://doi.org/10.2214/ajr.08.1128

Paulus W, Brandner S (2007) Choroid plexus tumours. In: Louis DN, Ohgaki H, Wiestler OD, Cavenee WK (eds) WHO classification of tumours of the central nervous system, 4th edn. International Agency for Research on Cancer, Lyon, pp 82–85

Paulus W, Brandner S, Hawkins C, Tihan T (2016a) Atypical choroid plexus papilloma. In: Louis DN, Ohgaki H, Wiestler OD, Cavenee WK (eds) WHO classification of tumours of the central nervous system, Revised 4th edn. IARC, Lyon, pp 126–127

Paulus W, Brandner S, Hawkins C, Tihan T (2016b) Choroid plexus carcinoma. In: Louis DN, Ohgaki H, Wiestler OD, Cavenee WK (eds) WHO classification of tumours of the central nervous system, Revised 4th edn. IARC, Lyon, pp 128–129

Paulus W, Brandner S, Hawkins C, Tihan T (2016c) Choroid plexus papilloma. In: Louis DN, Ohgaki H, Wiestler OD, Cavenee WK (eds) WHO classification of tumours of the central nervous system, Revised 4th edn. IARC, Lyon, pp 124–126

Safaee M, Oh MC, Bloch O, Sun MZ, Kaur G, Auguste KI, Tihan T, Parsa AT (2013) Choroid plexus papillomas: advances in molecular biology and understanding of tumorigenesis. Neuro-Oncology 15(3):255–267. https://doi.org/10.1093/neuonc/nos289

Spector R, Keep RF, Robert Snodgrass S, Smith QR, Johanson CE (2015) A balanced view of choroid plexus structure and function: focus on adult humans. Exp Neurol 267:78–86. https://doi.org/10.1016/j.expneurol.2015.02.032

Wolburg H, Paulus W (2010) Choroid plexus: biology and pathology. Acta Neuropathol 119(1):75–88. https://doi.org/10.1007/s00401-009-0627-8

Zülch KJ (1979) Histological typing of tumours of the central nervous system. World Health Organization, Geneva

62. Dysembryoplastic Neuroepithelial Tumor (DNT)

Neuronal and Mixed Neuronal-Glial Tumors

WHO Definition

2016—A benign glioneural neoplasm typically located in the temporal lobe of children or young adults with early-onset epilepsy; predominantly with a cortical location and a multinodular architecture; and with a histological hallmark of a specific glioneuronal element characterized by columns made up of bundles of axons oriented perpendicularly to the cortical surface (Pietsch et al. 2016).

2007—Benign, usually supratentorial glial-neuronal neoplasms, occurring in children or young adults, characterized by a predominantly cortical location and by drug-resistant partial seizures; typically exhibiting a complex columnar and multinodular architecture and often associated with cortical dysplasia (Daumas-Duport et al. 2007).

2000—Benign, usually supratentorial, glial-neuronal neoplasms characterized by a predominantly cortical location and occurrence in children and young adults with a long-standing history of partial seizures. Dysembryoplastic neuroepithelial tumors typically exhibit a multinodular architecture and may be associated with cortical dysplasia (Daumas-Duport et al. 2000).

1993—A benign, supratentorial mixed glial-neuronal neoplasm characterized by its intracortical location, multinodular architecture, and heterogeneous cellular composition. Cortical dysplasia may also be present (Kleihues et al. 1993).

WHO Grade
- WHO grade I

62.1 Epidemiology

Incidence
- Among all neuroepithelial tumors:
  - 1.2% in patients under 20 years of age
  - 0.2% in patients over 20 years of age
- In epilepsy surgery material:
  - 13.5% in children
  - 12% in adults

Age Incidence
- 3 weeks to 38 years.
- First seizure occurs before the age of 20 in 90% of cases.

Sex Incidence
- Male:Female: 1.5:1

Localization
- Supratentorial cortex
- Predilection for the temporal lobe (50% of cases)

- Other regions include:
  - Caudate nucleus
  - Lateral ventricle
  - Septum pellucidum
  - Trigonoseptal region
  - Midbrain
  - Tectum
  - Cerebellum
  - Brain stem

62.2 Neuroimaging Findings

General Imaging Features
Well-delineated, bubbly mass, cortical-subcortical location, without surrounding edema.

CT Non-contrast-Enhanced
- Hypodense, triangular mass
- Calcification possible

CT Contrast-Enhanced
- No enhancement in most of the cases
- Nodular enhancement possible

MRI-T2 (Figs. 62.1a, b and 62.2a)
- Hyperintense
- Multicystic appearance

MRI-FLAIR (Figs. 62.1c and 62.2b)
- Hypo- to isointense with hyperintense rim along tumor border

MRI-T1 (Fig. 62.2c)
- Hypointense

MRI-T1 Contrast-Enhanced (Figs. 62.1d and 62.2d)
- Usually no enhancement
- Nodular enhancement possible

MRI-T2*/SWI
- Reveals possible calcification
- Almost no hemorrhage

MR-Diffusion Imaging
- No restricted diffusion

MRI-Perfusion
- rCBV decreased

MR-Spectroscopy (Fig. 62.2e)
- NAA reduced

Nuclear Medicine Imaging Findings
- FDG usually presents hypometabolism.
- Amino acid PET presents usually with increased uptake.

62.3 Neuropathology Findings

Macroscopic Features
- Variable size (millimeters to centimeters)
- Single or multiple firm nodules
- Viscous consistency
- Exophytic growth possible

Microscopic Features (Fig. 62.3a–l)
- "Specific glioneuronal element":
  - Columns oriented perpendicular to the cortical surface,
  - Formed by bundles of axons lined by small oligodendroglia-like cells,
  - Neurons float in a pale eosinophilic matrix,
  - Scattered stellate, GFAP-positive astrocytes,
  - Variation from columnar to alveolar or compact structure,
- Histological forms have no clinical or therapeutic relevance:
  - Simple form
    - Consists of the unique glioneuronal element
  - Complex form
    - Consists of the unique glioneuronal element
    - Glial nodules are present
    - Presence of astrocytic, oligodendrocytic, and neuronal components

62.3 Neuropathology Findings

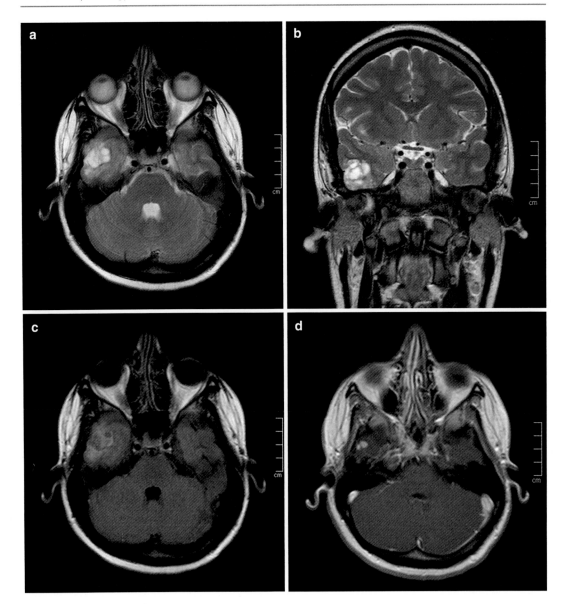

Fig. 62.1 Classic multicystic appearance of a right temporal DNT in T2 axial (**a**) and coronal (**b**), FLAIR (**c**). Nodular enhancement in T1 contrast is rare (**d**)

- Glial components have variable appearances:
  - Form typical nodules
  - Show diffuse growth pattern
  - Resemble diffuse gliomas
  - May show nuclear atypia
  - Rare mitoses
- Microvascular network
  - Vary from poor to exuberant
  - Glomerular formations possible
  - Hyperplastic endothelial cells
  - Vascular calcifications
- Cortical dysplasia
  - Disorganization of the cortex is observed in 80% of the cases

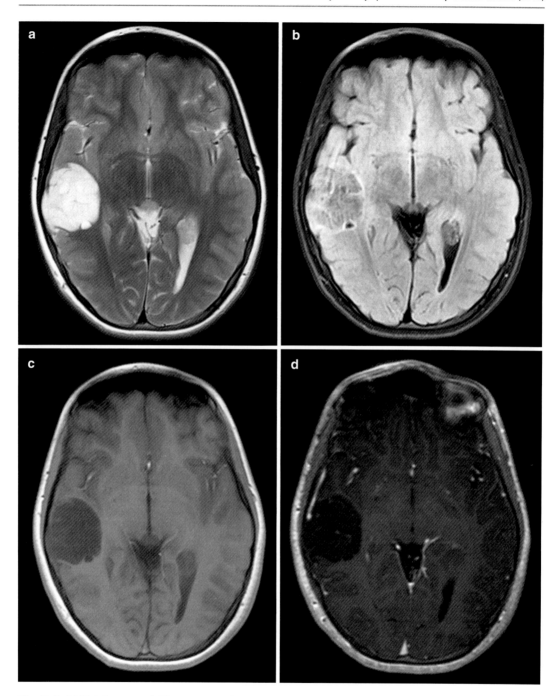

Fig. 62.2 DNT right temporal, T2 (**a**), FLAIR (**b**), T1 (**c**), T1 contrast (**d**), and spectroscopy (**e**)

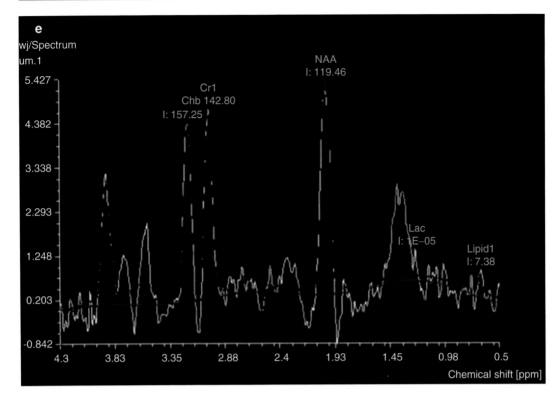

Fig. 62.2 (continued)

Immunophenotype (Fig. 62.4a–n)
- GFAP for the astrocytic component
- NeuN for floating neurons

Proliferation Markers
- Ki-67-LI: 0–8%

Ultrastructural Features
- Glial/oligodendroglial features
  - Pericellular lamination
  - Intermediate filaments
- Neuronal features
  - Dense core granules
  - Synapses

Differential Diagnosis
- Low-grade diffuse gliomas
- Oligodendroglioma
- Ganglioglioma
- Extraventricular neurocytoma
- Rosette-forming glioneuronal tumor of the fourth ventricle

62.4 Molecular Neuropathology

Pathogenesis
- Malformative origin
  - Presence of focal cortical dysplasia
  - Ectopic neurons in the white matter
- Otherwise unknown

Genes
- No 1p/19q co-deletions
- No deletions on 17q
- No *TP53* gene mutations

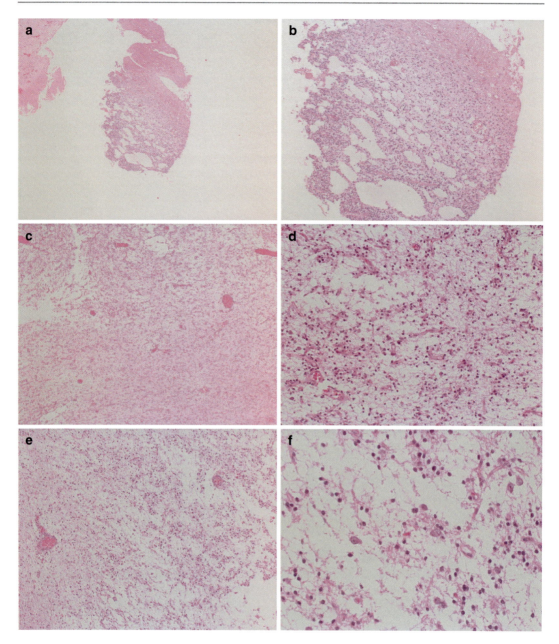

Fig. 62.3 Tumor showing a "nodule" composed of columns oriented perpendicular to the cortical surface (**a–d**), formed by bundles of axons lined by small oligodendroglia-like cells (**e–g**). Neurons float in a pale eosinophilic matrix (**f, h–l**; **k, l**: Cresyl violet stain)

62.4 Molecular Neuropathology

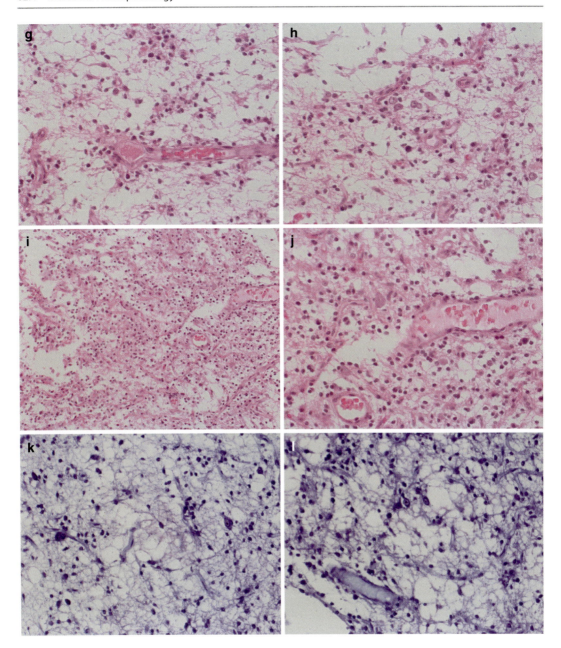

Fig. 62.3 (continued)

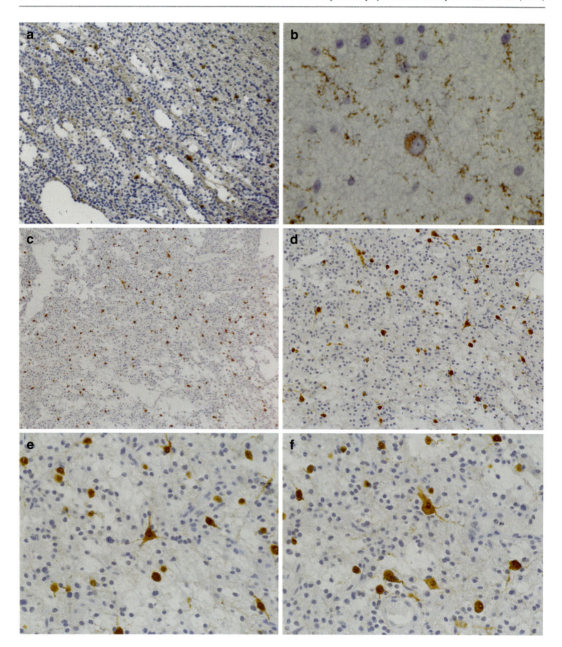

Fig. 62.4 Immunophenotype: Floating neurons are positive for NeuN (**a–f**), matrix positive for synaptophysin (**g, h**), axons positive for neurofilament (**i**), glial cells express Olig2 (**j**). Network of GFAP-positive processes (**k, l**) and scattered stellate, GFAP-positive astrocytes (**m, n**)

62.4 Molecular Neuropathology

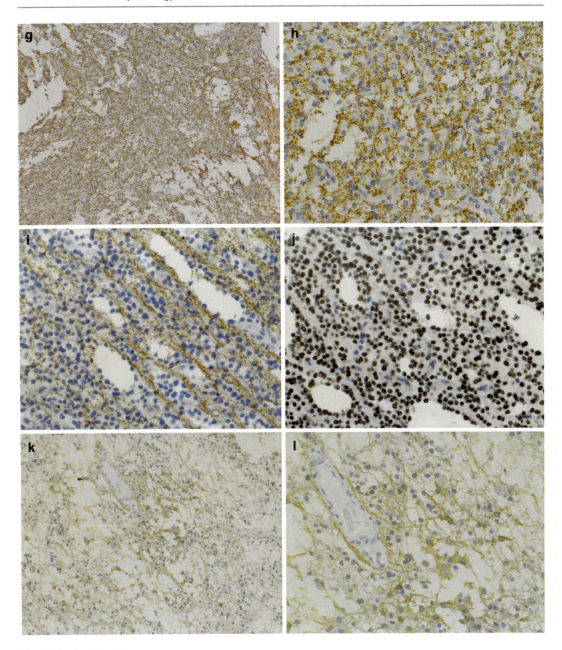

Fig. 62.4 (continued)

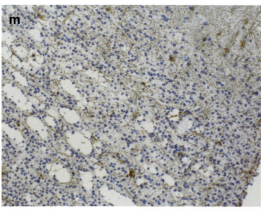 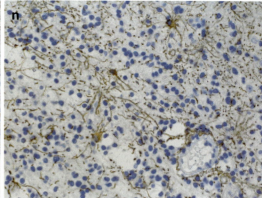

Fig. 62.4 (continued)

62.5 Treatment and Prognosis

Treatment
- surgery

Biologic Behavior–Prognosis–Prognostic Factors
- benign tumor
- no recurrence (even after partial resection)
- risk factors for recurrent seizures:
  – longer preoperative history of seizures
  – residual tumor
  – presence of cortical dysplasia adjacent to DNT

Selected References

Adamek D, Korzeniowska A, Morga R, Lopatka P, Jelenska-Szygula I, Danilewicz B (2001) Dysembryoplastic neuroepithelial tumour (DNT). Is the mechanism of seizures related to glutamate? An immunohistochemical study. Folia neuropathologica/Association of Polish Neuropathologists and Medical Research Centre. Pol Acad Sci 39(2):111–117

Alexander H, Tannenburg A, Walker DG, Coyne T (2015) Progressive dysembryoplastic neuroepithelial tumour. J Clin Neurosci 22(1):221–224. https://doi.org/10.1016/j.jocn.2014.07.022

Bodi I, Selway R, Bannister P, Doey L, Mullatti N, Elwes R, Honavar M (2012) Diffuse form of dysembryoplastic neuroepithelial tumour: the histological and immunohistochemical features of a distinct entity showing transition to dysembryoplastic neuroepithelial tumour and ganglioglioma. Neuropathol Appl Neurobiol 38(5):411–425. https://doi.org/10.1111/j.1365-2990.2011.01225.x

Bulakbasi N, Kocaoglu M, Sanal TH, Tayfun C (2007) Dysembryoplastic neuroepithelial tumors: proton MR spectroscopy, diffusion and perfusion characteristics. Neuroradiology 49(10):805–812. https://doi.org/10.1007/s00234-007-0263-8

Chang EF, Christie C, Sullivan JE, Garcia PA, Tihan T, Gupta N, Berger MS, Barbaro NM (2010) Seizure control outcomes after resection of dysembryoplastic neuroepithelial tumor in 50 patients. J Neurosurg Pediatr 5(1):123–130. https://doi.org/10.3171/2009.8.peds09368

Daumas-Duport C, Scheithauer BW, Chodkiewicz JP, Laws ER Jr, Vedrenne C (1988) Dysembryoplastic neuroepithelial tumor: a surgically curable tumor of young patients with intractable partial seizures. Report of thirty-nine cases. Neurosurgery 23(5):545–556

Daumas-Duport C, Pietsch T, Lantos PL (2000) Dysembryoplastic neuroepithelial tumour. In: Kleihues P, Cavenee WK (eds) Pathology and genetics of tumours of the nervous system, 3rd edn. IARC Press, Lyon, pp 103–106

Daumas-Duport C, Pietsch T, Hawkins C, Shankar SK (2007) Dysembryoplastic neuroepithelial tumour. In: Louis DN, Ohgaki H, Wiestler OD, Cavenee WK (eds) WHO classification of tumours of the central nervous system, 4th edn. International Agency for Research on Cancer, Lyon, pp 99–102

Eye PG, Davidson L, Malafronte PJ, Cantrell S, Theeler BJ (2017) PIK3CA mutation in a mixed dysembryoplastic neuroepithelial tumor and rosette forming glioneuronal tumor, a case report and literature review. J Neurol Sci 373:280–284. https://doi.org/10.1016/j.jns.2016.11.003

Heiland DH, Staszewski O, Hirsch M, Masalha W, Franco P, Grauvogel J, Capper D, Schrimpf D, Urbach H, Weyerbrock A (2016) Malignant transformation of a dysembryoplastic neuroepithelial tumor (DNET) characterized by genome-wide methylation analysis.

Selected References

J Neuropathol Exp Neurol 75(4):358–365. https://doi.org/10.1093/jnen/nlw007

Honavar M, Janota I, Polkey CE (1999) Histological heterogeneity of dysembryoplastic neuroepithelial tumour: identification and differential diagnosis in a series of 74 cases. Histopathology 34(4):342–356

Jensen RL, Caamano E, Jensen EM, Couldwell WT (2006) Development of contrast enhancement after long-term observation of a dysembryoplastic neuroepithelial tumor. J Neurooncol 78(1):59–62. https://doi.org/10.1007/s11060-005-9054-4

Kleihues P, Burger PC, Scheithauer BW (1993) Histological typing of tumours of the central nervous system, 2nd edn. Springer, Berlin

Komori T, Arai N (2013) Dysembryoplastic neuroepithelial tumor, a pure glial tumor? Immunohistochemical and morphometric studies. Neuropathology 33(4):459–468. https://doi.org/10.1111/neup.12033

Kuchelmeister K, Demirel T, Schlorer E, Bergmann M, Gullotta F (1995) Dysembryoplastic neuroepithelial tumour of the cerebellum. Acta Neuropathol 89(4):385–390

Lee DY, Chung CK, Hwang YS, Choe G, Chi JG, Kim HJ, Cho BK (2000) Dysembryoplastic neuroepithelial tumor: radiological findings (including PET, SPECT, and MRS) and surgical strategy. J Neurooncol 47(2):167–174

Lee MC, Kang JY, Seol MB, Kim HS, Woo JY, Lee JS, Jung S, Kim JH, Woo YJ, Kim MK, Kim HI, Kim SU (2006) Clinical features and epileptogenesis of dysembryoplastic neuroepithelial tumor. Childs Nerv Syst 22(12):1611–1618. https://doi.org/10.1007/s00381-006-0162-z

Mano Y, Kumabe T, Shibahara I, Saito R, Sonoda Y, Watanabe M, Tominaga T (2013) Dynamic changes in magnetic resonance imaging appearance of dysembryoplastic neuroepithelial tumor with or without malignant transformation. J Neurosurg Pediatr 11(5):518–525. https://doi.org/10.3171/2013.1.peds11449

Markonis A, Mazioti A, Wozniak G, Lavdas E, Vassiou K, Fezoulidis I (2012) Perfusion sensitive contrast-enhanced magnetic resonance imaging of dysembryoplastic neuroepithelial tumour: a new neuroimaging finding. Neurol Neurochir Pol 46(2):184–188

Parmar HA, Hawkins C, Ozelame R, Chuang S, Rutka J, Blaser S (2007) Fluid-attenuated inversion recovery ring sign as a marker of dysembryoplastic neuroepithelial tumors. J Comput Assist Tomogr 31(3):348–353. https://doi.org/10.1097/01.rct.0000243453.33610.9d

Paudel K, Borofsky S, Jones RV, Levy LM (2013) Dysembryoplastic neuroepithelial tumor with atypical presentation: MRI and diffusion tensor characteristics. J Radiol Case Rep 7(11):7–14. https://doi.org/10.3941/jrcr.v7i11.1559

Pietsch T, Hawkins C, Varlet P, Blümcke I, Hirose T (2016) Dysembryoplastic neuroepithelial tumour. In: Louis DN, Ohgaki H, Wiestler OD, Cavenee WK (eds) WHO classification of tumours of the central nervous system, Revised 4th edn. IARC, Lyon, pp 132–135

Preuss M, Nestler U, Zuhlke CJ, Kuchelmeister K, Neubauer BA, Jodicke A (2010) Progressive biological behavior of a dysembryoplastic neuroepithelial tumor. Pediatr Neurosurg 46(4):294–298. https://doi.org/10.1159/000320729

Sharma MC, Jain D, Gupta A, Sarkar C, Suri V, Garg A, Gaikwad SB, Chandra PS (2009) Dysembryoplastic neuroepithelial tumor: a clinicopathological study of 32 cases. Neurosurg Rev 32(2):161–169; discussion 169–170. https://doi.org/10.1007/s10143-008-0181-1

Shinohara Y, Kinoshita T, Kinoshita F, Moroi J, Yoshida Y, Nakazato Y (2009) F-18 FDG-PET imaging of dysembryoplastic neuroepithelial tumor-like astrocytoma. Clin Nucl Med 34(10):700–702. https://doi.org/10.1097/RLU.0b013e3181b53666

Sontowska I, Matyja E, Malejczyk J, Grajkowska W (2017) Dysembryoplastic neuroepithelial tumour: insight into the pathology and pathogenesis. Folia neuropathologica/Association of Polish Neuropathologists and Medical Research Centre. Pol Acad Sci 55(1):1–13. https://doi.org/10.5114/fn.2017.66708

Stanescu Cosson R, Varlet P, Beuvon F, Daumas Duport C, Devaux B, Chassoux F, Fredy D, Meder JF (2001) Dysembryoplastic neuroepithelial tumors: CT, MR findings and imaging follow-up: a study of 53 cases. J Neuroradiol 28(4):230–240

Tatke M, Sharma A, Malhotra V (1998) Dysembryoplastic neuroepithelial tumour. Childs Nerv Syst 14(7):293–296. https://doi.org/10.1007/s003810050229

Vaquero J, Saldana C, Coca S, Zurita M (2012) Complex form variant of dysembryoplastic neuroepithelial tumor of the cerebellum. Case Rep Pathol 2012:718651. https://doi.org/10.1155/2012/718651

Xu J, Du J, Shan Y (2014) Manifestation and treatment of intraventricular dysembryoplastic neuroepithelial tumor. Chin Med J 127(7):1390

Zhang JG, Hu WZ, Zhao RJ, Kong LF (2014) Dysembryoplastic neuroepithelial tumor: a clinical, neuroradiological, and pathological study of 15 cases. J Child Neurol 29(11):1441–1447. https://doi.org/10.1177/0883073813490831

63

Desmoplastic (Infantile) Astrocytoma/Ganglioglioma (DIA/DIG)

Neuronal and Mixed Neuronal-Glial Tumors

WHO Definition

2016—A benign glioneuronal tumor composed of a prominent desmoplastic stroma with a neuroepithelial population restricted either to neoplastic astrocytes—desmoplastic infantile astrocytoma (DIA)—or to astrocytes together with a variable mature neuronal component—desmoplastic infantile ganglioglioma (DIG)—sometimes with aggregates of poorly differentiated cells (Brat et al. 2016).

2007—Large cystic tumor of infants that involve superficial cerebral cortex and leptomeninges, often attached to dura, with a generally good prognosis following surgical resection; histologically composed of a prominent desmoplastic stroma with a neuroepithelial population, mainly restricted to neoplastic astrocytes (desmoplastic infantile astrocytoma, DIA) or to astrocytes together with a variable neuronal component (desmoplastic infantile ganglioglioma, DIG), in addition to aggregates of poorly differentiated cells, which are present in both (Brat et al. 2007).

2000—Large cystic tumours of infants that involve superficial cerebral cortex and leptomeninges, often attached to dura, with a generally good prognosis following surgical resection. They consist histologically of a prominent desmoplastic stroma with a neuroepithelial population, mainly restricted to neoplastic astrocytes (desmoplastic infantile astrocytoma, DIA) or to astrocytes together with a variable neuronal component (desmoplastic infantile ganglioglioma, DIG), in addition to aggregates of poorly differentiated cells, which are present in both (Taratuto et al. 2000).

1993—A mixed neuronal-glial neoplasm of infancy with a distinct desmoplastic component. It is characterized by a dense fibrous stroma containing an admixture of neuroepithelial cells displaying astrocytic and neuronal differentiation (Kleihues et al. 1993).

WHO Grade
- WHO grade I

63.1 Epidemiology

Incidence
- Rare tumors of childhood
- 0.3% of CNS tumors
- 1.25% of childhood brain tumors
- 16% of intracranial tumors of infancy

Age Incidence
- 1–24 months
- Non-infantile cases: 5–25 years
- Rare cases: 60 years and older

Sex Incidence
- Male:Female ratio: 1.5:1

Localization
- Supratentorial region
- Preferential lobe involvement
  - Frontal
  - Parietal
- Other lobe involvement
  - Temporal
  - Occipital

63.2 Neuroimaging Findings

General Imaging Findings
Large, heterogeneous, supratentorial located, rare tumor, containing a solid nodule (cortical located, contacts dura) and cystic components.
Associated with cortical dysplasia.

CT Non-contrast-Enhanced
- Mixed cystic (hypodense) and solid (hyperdense) components
- Calcifications common

CT Contrast-Enhanced
- Enhancement of solid component

MRI-T2/FLAIR (Fig. 63.1a)
- Cysts hyperintense
- Nodule isointense

MRI-T1
- Cysts hypo- to isointense
- Solid component isointense

MRI-T1 Contrast-Enhanced (Fig. 63.1b–d)
- Intense enhancement of solid component

MRI-T2*/SWI
- Calcifications common

MR-Spectroscopy
- NAA low
- Choline elevated

Nuclear Medicine Imaging Findings
- Few studies are available.
- FDG usually presents hypometabolism.
- Amino acid PET presents usually with increased uptake.

63.3 Neuropathology Findings

Macroscopic Features
- Large tumors
- Can reach a size of 13 cm
- Extracerebral solid superficial part involving the leptomeninges and superficial cortex and attached to the dura mater
- Firm or rubbery consistency
- Gray or white color
- Uni- or multiloculated cysts filled with clear or xanthochromic fluid

Microscopic Features (Fig. 63.2a–j)
- Three distinctive components:
  - Desmoplastic leptomeningeal component
  - Poorly differentiated neuroepithelial component
  - Cortical component
- Desmoplastic leptomeningeal component:
  - Mixture of fibroblast-like, spindle-shaped cells
  - Pleomorphic neoplastic neuroepithelial cells
    - With eosinophilic cytoplasm
    - Arranged in fascicles or in a storiform or whorled pattern
- Poorly differentiated neuroepithelial component:
  - Predominant astrocytic tumor component associated with neoplastic neurons
  - Neoplastic neurons show features of atypical ganglion cells to small polygonal cells
  - Poorly differentiated neuroepithelial cells
    - Small, round, deeply basophilic nuclei and minimal cytoplasm
- Cortical component:
  - Devoid of desmoplasia
  - Multinodular neoplastic component
  - Microcystic nodules

Immunophenotype (Fig. 63.3a–h)
- Fibroblast-like cells
  - Vimentin

63.3 Neuropathology Findings

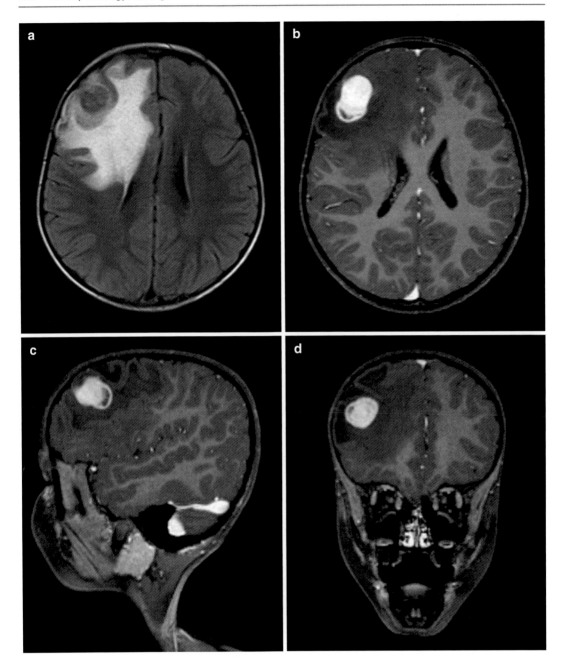

Fig. 63.1 Frontal desmoplastic astrocytoma in FLAIR (**a**), T1 contrast ax, sag, cor (**b–d**)

- Neuroepithelial component
  - GFAP (astrocytes)
  - Neuronal markers (synaptophysin, neurofilament) (neoplastic neuronal cells)
- Fibrillar network
  - Collagen Type IV

- No reactivity for
  - Epithelial markers (AE1/AE3, EMA)

Proliferation Markers
- Mitotic activity: rare
- Ki67-LI: 0.5–5%

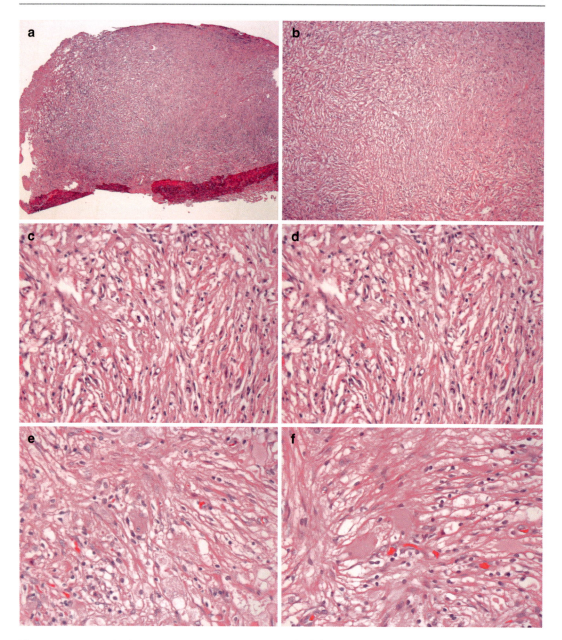

Fig. 63.2 Desmoplastic astrocytoma/ganglioglioma. Moderately cellular tumor (**a**, **b**) composed of a mixture of fibroblast-like, spindle-shaped cells (**c**, **d**); pleomorphic neoplastic neuroepithelial cells with eosinophilic cytoplasm are arranged in fascicles or in a storiform or whorled pattern (**d**, **e**); neoplastic neurons show features of atypical ganglion cells to small polygonal cells (**f**). Focus of accumulation of lymphocytes (**g**, **h**). Intense network of reticulin fibers (**i**, **j**)

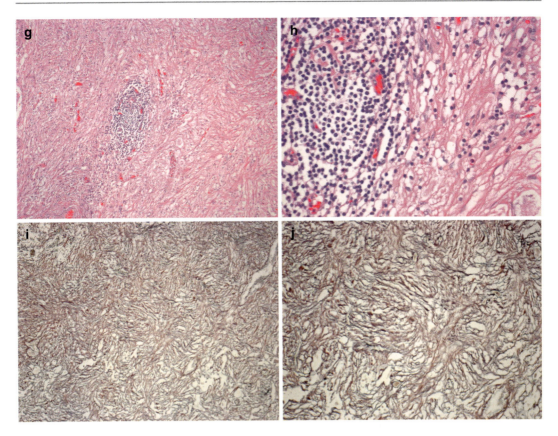

Fig. 63.2 (continued)

Ultrastructural Features
- Astrocytic cells
  - Intermediate filaments arranged in bundles
  - Scattered cisternae of rough endoplasmic reticulum
  - Mitochondria
  - Basal lamina surrounds tumor cells
- Fibroblasts
  - Contain granular endoplasmic reticulum
  - Well-developed Golgi complexes
- Neuronal cells
  - Contain dense core secretory granules
  - Small processes with neurofilaments

Differential Diagnosis
- Neuroepithelial tumors with fibrosis
- Pleomorphic xanthoastrocytoma
- "Gliofibromas"
- Ganglion cell tumor
- Fibroblastic meningioma
- Fibrohistiocytic tumors

63.4 Molecular Neuropathology

Pathogenesis
- Possible embryonal neoplasms programmed to progressive maturation
- Originating from a specialized subpial astrocyte that forms a limiting basal lamina

Genes
- Genetic alterations involve 1p, 3p, 3q, 5q, 7q, 9p, 11q, 14q, 17p, 21q, and 22q
- No *TP53* mutations

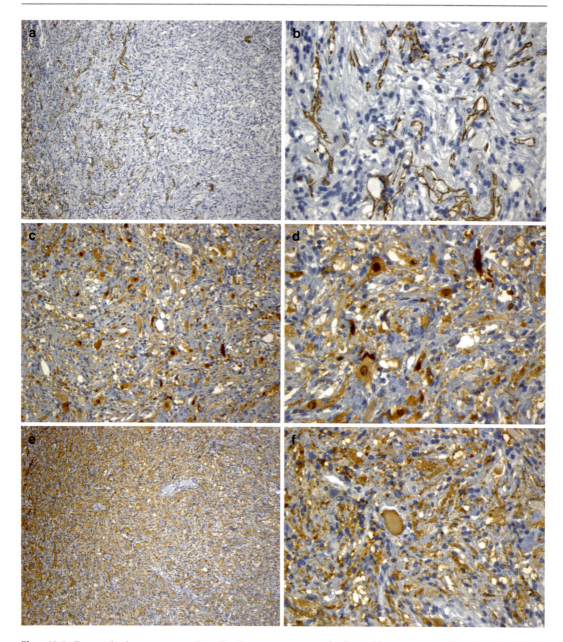

Fig. 63.3 Desmoplastic astrocytoma/ganglioglioma—Immunophenotype: GFAP-positive cytoplasmatic processes (**a**, **b**); S-100-positive astroglial cells (**c**, **d**); synaptophysin-positive neuroepithelial cells (**e**, **f**); CD34-positive neuroglial cells (**g**, **h**)

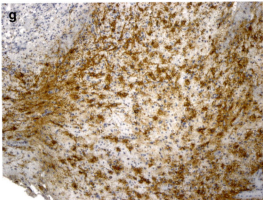
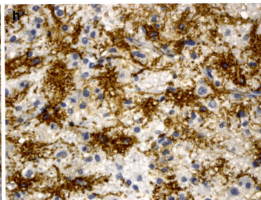

Fig. 63.3 (continued)

63.5 Treatment and Prognosis

Treatment
- Surgical excision

Biologic Behavior–Prognosis–Prognostic Factors
- Benign tumor
- Curation possible after total gross resection
- Recurrence slow even with subtotal gross resection or biopsy alone
- Rare metastasis through the CSF

Selected References

Bader A, Heran M, Dunham C, Steinbok P (2015) Radiological features of infantile glioblastoma and desmoplastic infantile tumors: British Columbia's Children's Hospital experience. J Neurosurg Pediatr 16(2):119–125. https://doi.org/10.3171/2014.10.peds13634

Balaji R, Ramachandran K (2009) Imaging of desmoplastic infantile ganglioglioma: a spectroscopic viewpoint. Childs Nerv Syst 25(4):497–501. https://doi.org/10.1007/s00381-008-0786-2

Bianchi F, Tamburrini G, Massimi L, Caldarelli M (2016) Supratentorial tumors typical of the infantile age: desmoplastic infantile ganglioglioma (DIG) and astrocytoma (DIA). A review. Childs Nerv Syst 32(10):1833–1838. https://doi.org/10.1007/s00381-016-3149-4

Brat DJ, VandenBerg SR, Figarella-Branger D, Taratuto AL (2007) Desmoplastic infantile astrocytoma and ganglioglioma. In: Louis DN, Ohgaki H, Wiestler OD, Cavenee WK (eds) WHO classification of tumours of the central nervous system, 4th edn. International Agency for Research on Cancer, Lyon, pp 96–98

Brat DJ, VandenBerg SR, Figarella-Branger D, Reuss DE (2016) Desmoplastic infantile astrocytoma and ganglioglioma. In: Louis DN, Ohgaki H, Wiestler OD, Cavenee WK (eds) WHO classification of tumours of the central nervous system, Revised 4th edn. IARC, Lyon, pp 144–146

Cerda-Nicolas M, Lopez-Gines C, Gil-Benso R, Donat J, Fernandez-Delgado R, Pellin A, Lopez-Guerrero JA, Roldan P, Barbera J (2006) Desmoplastic infantile ganglioglioma. Morphological, immunohistochemical and genetic features. Histopathology 48(5):617–621. https://doi.org/10.1111/j.1365-2559.2005.02275.x

Ho CY, Gener M, Bonnin J, Kralik SF (2016) Diffusion, perfusion, and histopathologic characteristics of desmoplastic infantile ganglioglioma. J Radiol Case Rep 10(7):1–13. https://doi.org/10.3941/jrcr.v10i7.2715

Hummel TR, Miles L, Mangano FT, Jones BV, Geller JI (2012) Clinical heterogeneity of desmoplastic infantile ganglioglioma: a case series and literature review. J Pediatr Hematol Oncol 34(6):e232–e236. https://doi.org/10.1097/MPH.0b013e3182580330

Iwami K (2007) Desmoplastic infantile ganglioglioma. Childs Nerv Syst 23(6):619–620; author reply 621. https://doi.org/10.1007/s00381-007-0352-3

Kesavadas C, Sonwalker H, Thomas B, Gupta AK, Radhakrishnan VV (2005) Atypical MRI appearance of desmoplastic infantile ganglioglioma. Pediatr Radiol 35(10):1024–1026. https://doi.org/10.1007/s00247-005-1497-4

Khaddage A, Chambonniere ML, Morrison AL, Allard D, Dumollard JM, Pasquier B, Peoc'h M (2004) Desmoplastic infantile ganglioglioma: a rare tumor with an unusual presentation. Ann Diagn Pathol 8(5):280–283

Kleihues P, Burger PC, Scheithauer BW (1993) Histological typing of tumours of the central nervous system, 2nd edn. Springer, Berlin

Loh JK, Lieu AS, Chai CY, Howng SL (2011) Malignant transformation of a desmoplastic infantile ganglioglioma. Pediatr Neurol 45(2):135–137. https://doi.org/10.1016/j.pediatrneurol.2011.04.001

Lonnrot K, Terho M, Kahara V, Haapasalo H, Helen P (2007) Desmoplastic infantile ganglioglioma: novel aspects in clinical presentation and genetics. Surg Neurol 68(3):304–308; discussion 308. https://doi.org/10.1016/j.surneu.2006.11.043

Nikas I, Anagnostara A, Theophanopoulou M, Stefanaki K, Michail A, Hadjigeorgi C (2004) Desmoplastic infantile ganglioglioma: MRI and histological findings case report. Neuroradiology 46(12):1039–1043. https://doi.org/10.1007/s00234-004-1283-2

Tamburrini G, Colosimo C Jr, Giangaspero F, Riccardi R, Di Rocco C (2003) Desmoplastic infantile ganglioglioma. Childs Nerv Syst 19(5–6):292–297. https://doi.org/10.1007/s00381-003-0743-z

Taratuto AL, VandenBerg SR, Rorke LB (2000) Desmoplastic infantile astrocytoma and ganglioglioma. In: Kleihues P, Cavenee WK (eds) Pathology and genetics of tumours of the nervous system, 3rd edn. IARC Press, Lyon, pp 99–102

Trehan G, Bruge H, Vinchon M, Khalil C, Ruchoux MM, Dhellemmes P, Ares GS (2004) MR imaging in the diagnosis of desmoplastic infantile tumor: retrospective study of six cases. AJNR Am J Neuroradiol 25(6):1028–1033

Ganglioglioma/Gangliocytoma

Neuronal and Mixed Neuronal-Glial Tumors

64

WHO Definition
2016—Gangliocytoma: A rare, well-differentiated, slow-growing neuroepithelial neoplasm composed of irregular clusters of mostly mature neoplastic ganglion cells, often with dysplastic features (Capper et al. 2016).

Ganglioglioma: A well-differentiated, slow-growing glioneuronal neoplasm composed of dysplastic ganglion cells (i.e., large cells with dysmorphic neuronal features, without the architectural arrangement or cytological characteristic of cortical neurons) in combination with neoplastic glial cells (Becker et al. 2016b).

2007—Well-differentiated, slowly growing neuroepithelial tumors, composed of neoplastic, mature ganglion cells, alone (gangliocytoma) or in combination with neoplastic glial cells (ganglioglioma); the most frequent entity observed in patients with long-term epilepsy (Becker et al. 2007).

2000—Well-differentiated, slowly growing neuroepithelial tumors composed of neoplastic, mature ganglion cells, either alone (gangliocytoma), or in combination with neoplastic glial cells (ganglioglioma) (Nelson et al. 2000).

1993—A tumor composed predominantly of neoplastic though mature ganglion cells with a minor component of supportive, non-neoplastic glial cells (Kleihues et al. 1993).

1979—Gangliocytoma: A tumor composed predominantly of mature ganglion cells, associated with glial elements that are presumed to be non-neoplastic. A striking mesenchymal stroma may be present. They are often calcified and cystic (Zülch 1979).

Ganglioneuroblastoma: The composition of this tumor involves a complete spectrum of cells from immature neuroblasts to mature ganglion cells. The very similar tumor recognized as "differentiating neuroblastoma" is predominantly neuroblastic but includes foci of ganglion cells. It corresponds histologically to grade III (Zülch 1979).

Neuroblastoma: A cerebral tumor composed predominantly of small, darkly staining, poorly differentiated cells with slender cytoplasmic processes, and a tendency to form Homer Wright rosettes ("pseudorosettes") (Zülch 1979).

64.1 Ganglioglioma

WHO Definition
2016—A well-differentiated, slow-growing glioneuronal neoplasm composed of dysplastic ganglion cells (i.e., large cells with dysmorphic neuronal features, without the architectural arrangement or cytological characteristic of cortical neurons) in combination with neoplastic glial cells (Becker et al. 2016b).

2007—Well-differentiated, slowly growing neuroepithelial tumors, composed of neoplastic, mature ganglion cells, alone (gangliocytoma) or in combination with neoplastic glial cells (ganglioglioma); the most frequent entity observed in patients with long-term epilepsy (Becker et al. 2007).

2000—Well-differentiated, slowly growing neuroepithelial tumors composed of neoplastic, mature ganglion cells, either alone (gangliocytoma), or in combination with neoplastic glial cells (ganglioglioma) (Nelson et al. 2000).

1993—A benign tumor composed of neoplastic astrocytes (rarely oligodendrocytes) and ganglion cells (Kleihues et al. 1993).

1979—A tumor composed of mature ganglion cells and neoplastic glial cells (Zülch 1979).

WHO Grade
- WHO grade I

64.1.1 Epidemiology

Incidence
- 0.4–1.3% of all brain tumors

Age Incidence
- 2 months–70 years
- Median age: 8.5–25 years
- 50% become manifest before the age of 15 years
- 50% become manifest before the age of 30 years
- very rare in elderly subjects

Sex Incidence
- Male:Female: 1.1:1.9–1

Localization
- Any part of the central nervous system
- Predominance for the temporal lobe especially in the hippocampus (70% of the cases)
- They are also encountered in:
  – Hypothalamus
  – Intra- and parasellar region
  – Pineal gland
  – Cerebellum
  – Lower brain stem
  – Medulla oblongata
  – Spinal cord

64.1.2 Neuroimaging Findings

General Imaging Findings
- Well-demarcated supratentorial lesion, containing solid and cystic components
- Often associated with cortical dysplasia

CT Non-contrast-Enhanced (Fig. 64.2a)
- Mixed cystic components or solid
- Calcifications common

CT Contrast-Enhanced
- None to homogeneous enhancement

MRI-T2/FLAIR (Figs. 64.1a, b and 64.2b–d)
- Hyperintense

MRI-T1 (Figs. 64.1c and 64.2e)
- Hypo- to isointense

MRI-T1 Contrast-Enhanced (Figs. 64.1d and 64.2f)
- None to homogeneous enhancement

MRI-T2*/SWI
- Calcifications common

MR-Diffusion Imaging (Fig. 64.1f)
- No restricted diffusion

MRI-Perfusion (Figs. 64.1e and 64.2g)
- Normal to slight elevation of rCBV in solid components

MR-Spectroscopy
- Choline elevated

Nuclear Medicine Imaging Findings
- Few studies are available dealing with gangliogliomas and gangliocytomas.
- FDG usually presents hypometabolism.

64.1 Ganglioglioma

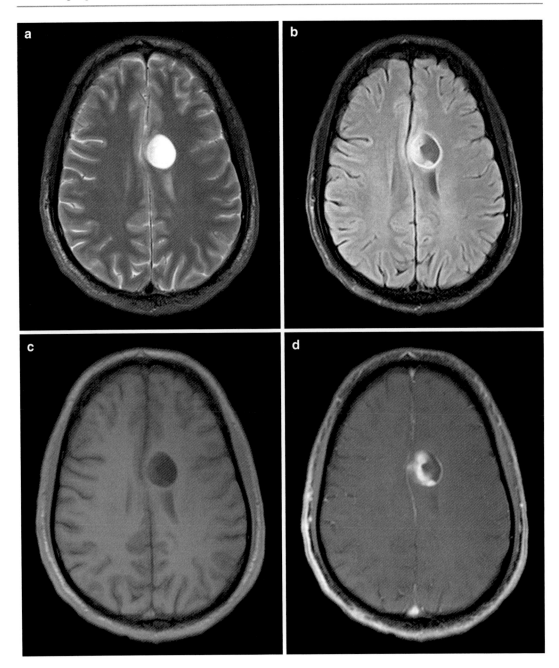

Fig. 64.1 Left parasagittal ganglioglioma WHO grade I in T2 (**a**), FLAIR (**b**), T1 (**c**), T1 contrast (**d**), rCBV (**e**), and DWI (**f**)

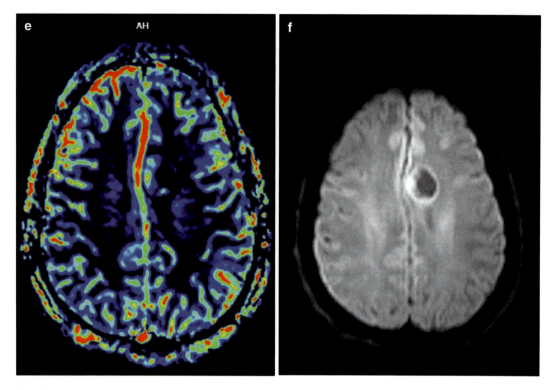

Fig. 64.1 (continued)

- FDG-PET can be used to assess the damage to healthy brain tissue.
- Amino acid PET presents usually with increased uptake.

64.1.3 Neuropathology Findings

Macroscopic Features
- nodular
- firm
- sharply delineated
- encapsulation possible
- white-rough
- cyst formation possible
- calcification frequent
- bleeding rare
- necrosis rare

Microscopic Features (Fig. 64.3a–h)
- Neoplastic neurons
  - contain Nissl substance
  - bi- or multinucleated
  - eosinophilic cytoplasmic vacuolization
  - synapse formation
  - neurofibrils not obligatory
  - myelin sheaths not obligatory
- Neoplastic astrocytes
  - Fibrillary or pilocytic astrocytes.
  - Rosenthal fibers might be present.
  - Responsible for tumor growth.
- Oligodendrocytes
- Lymphocytic infiltrates
  - B-cells

Immunophenotype (Fig. 64.4a–r)
- immunopositive for:
  - CD34
  - synaptophysin
  - neurofilament
  - calcineurin
  - thyrosine hydroxylase
  - GFAP

Proliferation Markers (Fig. 64.4s, t)
- none to very low number of positive cells

64.1 Ganglioglioma

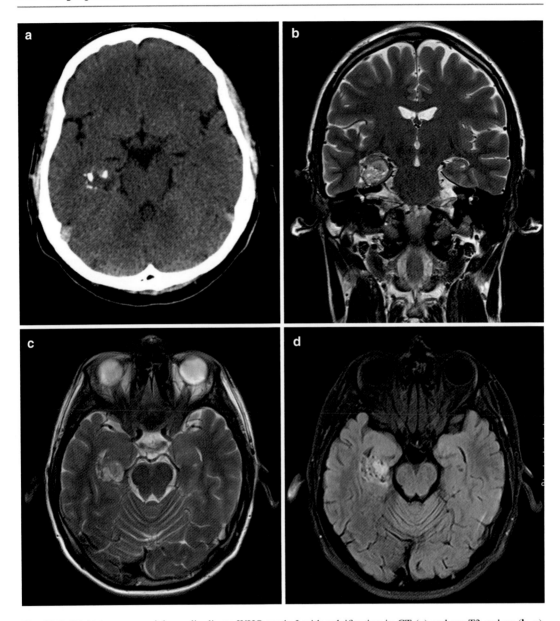

Fig. 64.2 Right temporomesial ganglioglioma WHO grade I with calcification in CT (**a**) and cor T2 and ax (**b**, **c**), FLAIR (**d**), T1 (**e**), T1 contrast (**f**), rCBV (**g**)

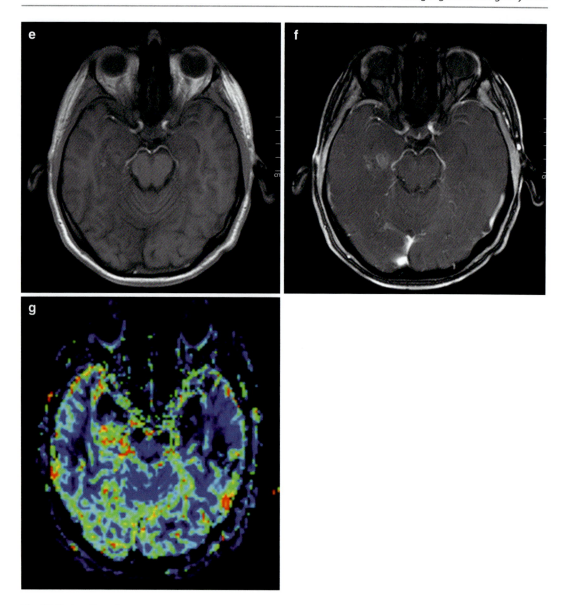

Fig. 64.2 (continued)

Differential Diagnosis
- Astroglioma
- Malformation

64.1.4 Molecular Neuropathology

Pathogenesis
- Unresolved
- Origin from dysplastic, malformative glioneuronal precursor lesion

Molecular Neuropathology
- Gain of chromosome 7.
- Loss of chromosome 9q.
- Deletion of *CDKN2A*.
- Polymorphisms in intron 4 and exon 41 in *TSC2* gene.
- *BRAF* V600E mutation in approximately 25%.
- *IDH* mutation or combined loss of chromosomal arms 1p and 19q exclude a diagnosis of a ganglioglioma.

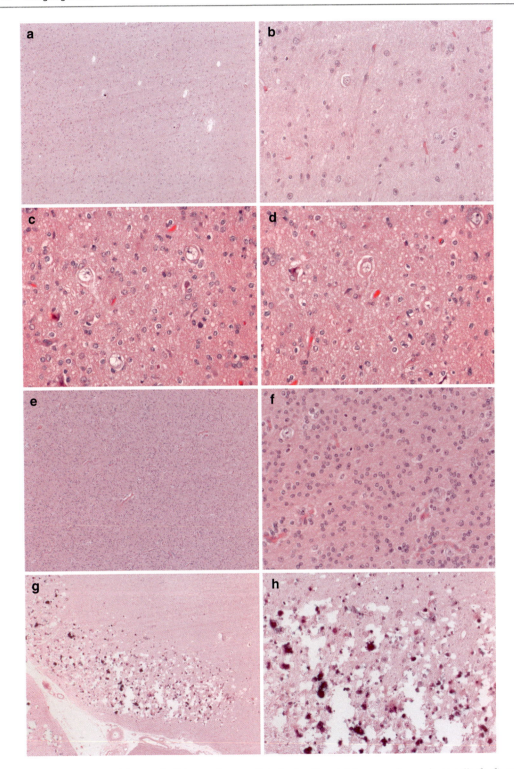

Fig. 64.3 Ganglioglioma: Tumor of mild to moderate cellularity (**a–d**) containing conspicuous large cells (**b–d**), and mainly composed of astroglial cells (**e, f**). Calcifications might be present (**g, h**)

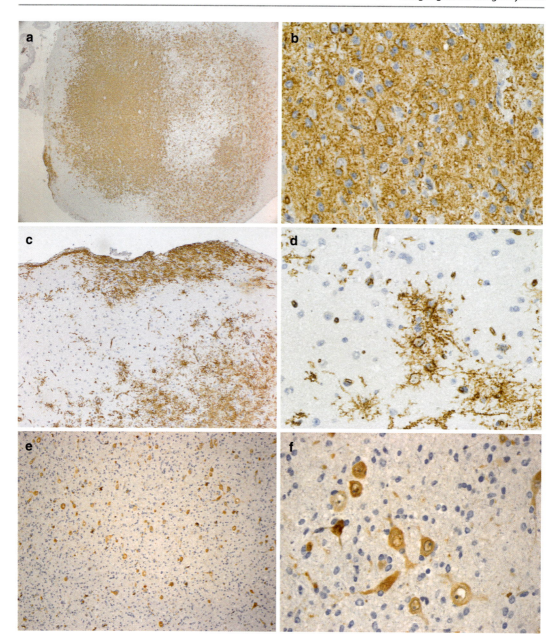

Fig. 64.4 Ganglioglioma—Immunophenotype: Bush-like CD34-positive cells represent the hallmark of the tumor (**a–d**); the large cells are identified as neurons by NeuN staining (**e–h**), neurofilament (**i, j**) and MAP2 (**k, l**). Moderate reactive astrogliosis (**m, n**: GFAP; **o, p**: Vimentin). Mild reactive microgliosis (**q, r**: HLA-DRII). Low ki67 proliferation rate (**s, t**)

64.1 Ganglioglioma

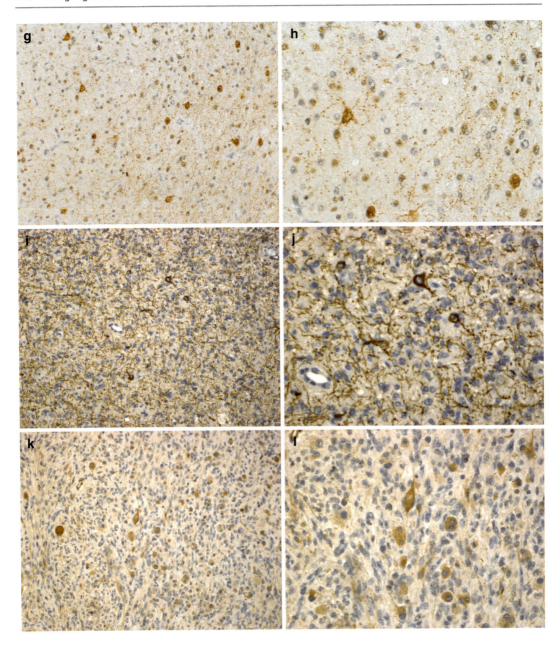

Fig. 64.4 (continued)

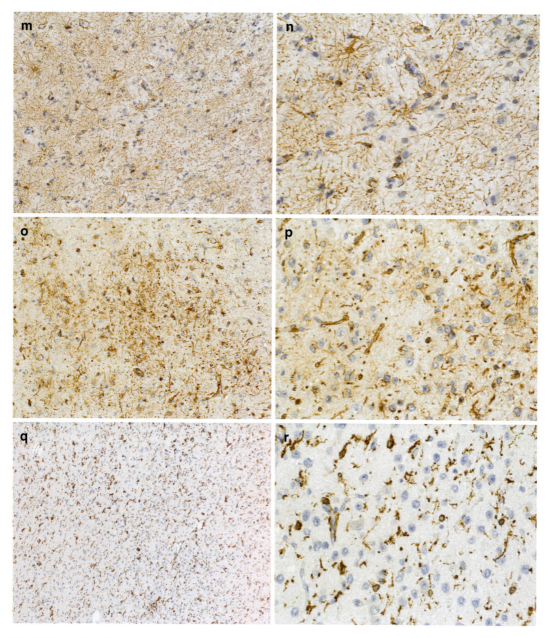

Fig. 64.4 (continued)

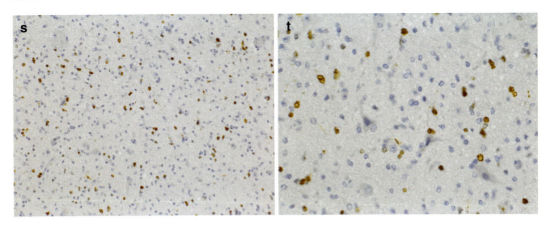

Fig. 64.4 (continued)

64.1.5 Treatment and Prognosis

Treatment
- Surgery

Biologic Behavior–Prognosis–Prognostic Factors
- benign tumor
- good prognosis
- recurrence
  - After long-lasting interval.
  - 94% of cases with 7.5 year recurrence-free survival.
  - Recurrent tumor does not necessarily show higher anaplasia.

64.2 Anaplastic Ganglioglioma

WHO Definition
2016—A glioneuronal tumor composed of dysplastic ganglion cells and an anaplastic glial component with elevated mitotic activity (Becker et al. 2016a).
  2007—In anaplastic gangliogliomas, malignant change almost invariably involves the glial component (Becker et al. 2007).
  2000—Malignant change in anaplastic gangliogliomas invariably involves the glial component (Nelson et al. 2000).
  1993—A rare variant of ganglioglioma in which the glial component shows distinct features of anaplasia, e.g., excessive atypia, increased mitotic activity, vascular proliferation, and necrosis (Kleihues et al. 1993).
  1979—A gangliocytoma or a ganglioglioma showing areas of anaplasia. The tumor correspond histologically to grades III or IV (Zülch 1979).

WHO Grade
- WHO grade III

64.2.1 Epidemiology

Incidence
- rare

Age Incidence
- children

Sex Incidence
- unknown

Localization
- Any part of the central nervous system
- Predominance for the temporal lobe

64.2.2 Neuroimaging Findings

General Imaging Features
- Nonspecific imaging characteristics
- Diffuse, poorly delineated mass with heterogeneous enhancement

CT Non-contrast-Enhanced
- Heterogeneous mass

CT Contrast-Enhanced
- Irregular enhancement

MRI-T1
- Isointense or hypointense

MRI-T2/FLAIR
- Hyperintense

MRI-T1 Contrast-Enhanced
- Irregular enhancement

MRI-Perfusion
- Elevated rCBV

MR-Spectroscopy
- Distinct choline peaks

Nuclear Medicine Imaging Findings
- increased amino acid-tracer uptake

64.2.3 Neuropathology Findings

Macroscopic Features
- nodular
- firm
- sharply delineated
- encapsulation possible
- white-rough
- cyst formation possible
- calcification frequent
- bleeding rare
- necrosis rare

Microscopic Features
- Neoplastic astrocytes
  - Fibrillary or pilocytic astrocytes.
  - Rosenthal fibers might be present.
  - Responsible for tumor growth.
  - Increased cellularity.
  - Increased pleomorphism.
  - Increased number of mitoses.
- Vascular proliferation
- Necrosis
- Neoplastic neurons
  - contain Nissl substance
  - bi- or multinucleated
  - eosinophilic cytoplasmic vacuolization
  - synapse formation
  - neurofibrils not obligatory
  - myelin sheaths not obligatory

Immunophenotype
- immunopositive for:
  - CD34
  - Synaptophysin
  - Neurofilament
  - Calcineurin
  - Thyrosine hydroxylase
  - GFAP

Proliferation Markers
- Few mitoses
- Moderate Ki67 LI

Differential Diagnosis
- Astrocytoma
- Anaplastic astrocytoma

64.2.4 Molecular Neuropathology

Pathogenesis
- Unresolved
- Origin from dysplastic, malformative glioneuronal precursor lesion
- Malignant progression from ganglioglioma WHO grade II

Molecular Neuropathology
- Loss of *CDKN2A/B* and *DMBT1*
- Gain/amplification of *CDK4*
- *BRAF V600E* mutation in approximately 50%

64.2.5 Treatment and Prognosis

Treatment
- Surgery
- Chemotherapy
- Radiotherapy

Biologic Behavior–Prognosis–Prognostic Factors
- reduced 5-year overall and progression-free survival rate
- increased recurrence rate

Selected References

Becker AJ, Wiestler OD, Figarella-Branger D, Blümcke I (2007) Ganglioglioma and gangliocytoma. In: Louis DN, Ohgaki H, Wiestler OD, Cavenee WK (eds) WHO classification of tumours of the central nervous system, 4th edn. International Agency for Research on Cancer, Lyon, pp 103–105

Becker AJ, Wiestler OD, Figarella-Branger D, Blümcke I, Capper D (2016a) Anaplastic ganglioglioma. In: Louis DN, Ohgaki H, Wiestler OD, Cavenee WK (eds) WHO classification of tumours of the central nervous system, Revised 4th edn. IARC, Lyon, p 141

Becker AJ, Wiestler OD, Figarella-Branger D, Blümcke I, Capper D (2016b) Ganglioglioma. In: Louis DN, Ohgaki H, Wiestler OD, Cavenee WK (eds) WHO classification of tumours of the central nervous system, Revised 4th edn. IARC, Lyon, pp 138–141

Capper D, Becker AJ, Giannini C, Figarella-Branger D, Huse JT, Rosenblum MK, Blümcke I, Wiestler OD (2016) Gangliocytoma. In: Louis DN, Ohgaki H, Wiestler OD, Cavenee WK (eds) WHO classification of tumours of the central nervous system, Revised 4th edn. IARC, Lyon, pp 136–137

Dapaah A, Biswas S, Srikandarajah N, Crooks D, Das K, Farah JO (2017) Serial imaging and management of ganglioglioma with unusual presentation and meningeal spread. Acta Neurochir (Wien) 159(3):481–483. https://doi.org/10.1007/s00701-016-3017-8

Drapalo K, Jozwiak J (2018) Parkin, PINK1 and DJ1 as possible modulators of mTOR pathway in ganglioglioma. Int J Neurosci 128(2):167–174. https://doi.org/10.1080/00207454.2017.1366906

Kleihues P, Burger PC, Scheithauer BW (1993) Histological typing of tumours of the central nervous system, 2nd edn. Springer, Berlin

Lee S, Yun TJ, Kang KM, Rhim JH, Park CK, Kim TM, Park SH, Kim IH, Choi SH (2016) Application of diffusion-weighted imaging and dynamic susceptibility contrast perfusion-weighted imaging for ganglioglioma in adults: comparison study with oligodendroglioma. J Neuroradiol 43(5):331–338. https://doi.org/10.1016/j.neurad.2016.06.001

Lucas JT Jr, Huang AJ, Mott RT, Lesser GJ, Tatter SB, Chan MD (2015) Anaplastic ganglioglioma: a report of three cases and review of the literature. J Neurooncol 123(1):171–177. https://doi.org/10.1007/s11060-015-1781-6

Ludemann W, Banan R, Hartmann C, Bertalanffy H, Di Rocco C (2017) Pediatric intracranial primary anaplastic ganglioglioma. Childs Nerv Syst 33(2):227–231. https://doi.org/10.1007/s00381-016-3302-0

Majumdar A, Ahmad F, Sheikh T, Bhagat R, Pathak P, Joshi SD, Seth P, Tandon V, Tripathi M, Saratchandra P, Sarkar C, Sen E (2017) miR-217-casein kinase-2 cross talk regulates ERK activation in ganglioglioma. J Mol Med (Berl) 95(11):1215–1226. https://doi.org/10.1007/s00109-017-1571-z

Nelson JS, Bruner JM, Wiestler OD, VandenBerg SR (2000) Ganglioglioma and gangliocytoma. In: Kleihues P, Cavenee WK (eds) Pathology and genetics of tumours of the nervous system, 3rd edn. IARC Press, Lyon, pp 96–98

Provenzale JM, Ali U, Barboriak DP, Kallmes DF, Delong DM, McLendon RE (2000) Comparison of patient age with MR imaging features of gangliogliomas. AJR Am J Roentgenol 174(3):859–862. https://doi.org/10.2214/ajr.174.3.1740859

Zanello M, Pages M, Tauziede-Espariat A, Saffroy R, Puget S, Lacroix L, Dezamis E, Devaux B, Chretien F, Andreiuolo F, Sainte-Rose C, Zerah M, Dhermain F, Dumont S, Louvel G, Meder JF, Grill J, Dufour C, Pallud J, Varlet P (2016) Clinical, imaging, histopathological and molecular characterization of anaplastic ganglioglioma. J Neuropathol Exp Neurol 75(10):971–980. https://doi.org/10.1093/jnen/nlw074

Zülch KJ (1979) Histological typing of tumours of the central nervous system. World Health Organization, Geneva

65

Neurocytoma: Central—Extraventricular

Neuronal and Mixed Neuronal-Glial Tumors

WHO Definition

2016—Central neurocytoma: An uncommon intraventricular neoplasm composed of uniform round cells with a neural immunophenotype and low proliferation index (Figarella-Branger et al. 2016a).

Extraventricular neurocytoma: A tumor composed of small uniform cells that demonstrate neuronal differentiation but are not IDH-mutant, and that presents throughout the CNS, without apparent association with the ventricular system (Figarella-Branger et al. 2016b).

2007—A neoplasm composed of uniform round cells with neuronal differentiation, typically located in the lateral ventricles in the region of the foramen of Monro (central neurocytoma) or brain parenchyma (extraventricular neurocytoma); affecting mostly young adults, and with a favorable prognosis (Figarella-Branger et al. 2007).

2000—A neoplasm composed of uniform round cells with neuronal differentiation, typically located in the lateral ventricles in the region of the foramen of Monro. It affects mostly young adults and has a favorable prognosis (Figarella-Branger et al. 2000).

1993—An intraventricular tumor composed of uniform round cells with immunohistochemical and ultrastructural features of neuronal differentiation (Kleihues et al. 1993).

WHO Grade
- WHO grade II

65.1 Epidemiology

Incidence
- 0.25–0.5% of all intracranial tumors

Age Incidence
- 8 days to 67 years
- Mean age: 29 years

Sex Incidence
- Male:Female ratio 1:1

Localization
- Central neurocytoma:
  – Intracerebral ventricles:
    o lateral ventricles, anterior part (50% of the cases)
    o third ventricle
- Extraventricular neurocytoma:
  – Tumor arising within the central nervous system
  – Cerebral hemispheres (71% of cases)
  – Frontal lobe (30% of cases)
  – Spinal cord (14% of cases)

65.2 Neuroimaging Findings

General Imaging Findings
Well-defined, intraventricular (frontal horn or body of lateral ventricle), lobulated, bubbly mass, typically broad based to the septum pellucidum.

CT Non-Contrast-Enhanced (Fig. 65.1a)
- Mixed iso- to hyperdense.
- Calcifications common.

- Obstructive hydrocephalus commonly caused by compression of foramina of Monro.
- Hemorrhage is rare.

CT Contrast-Enhanced (Fig. 65.1b)
- Heterogeneous enhancement

MRI-T2 (Fig. 65.1c)
- Heterogeneous hyperintense
- Prominent flow voids

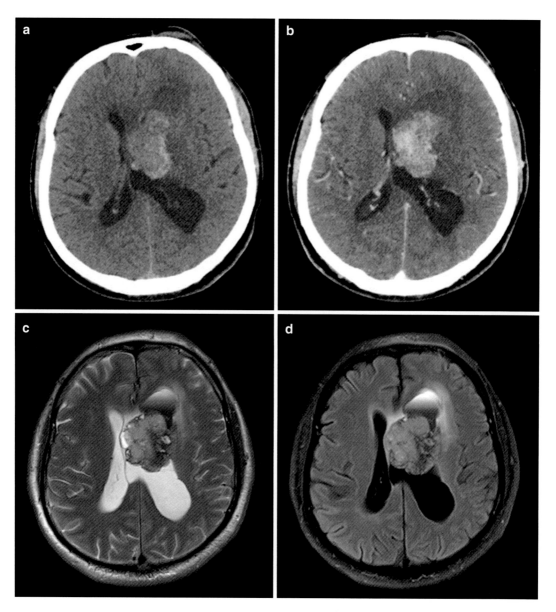

Fig. 65.1 Classic central neurocytoma, intraventricularly located and attached to the septum pellucidum CT (**a**), CT contrast (**b**), T2 (**c**), FLAIR (**d**), T1 (**e**), T1 contrast ax/sag/cor (**f–h**)

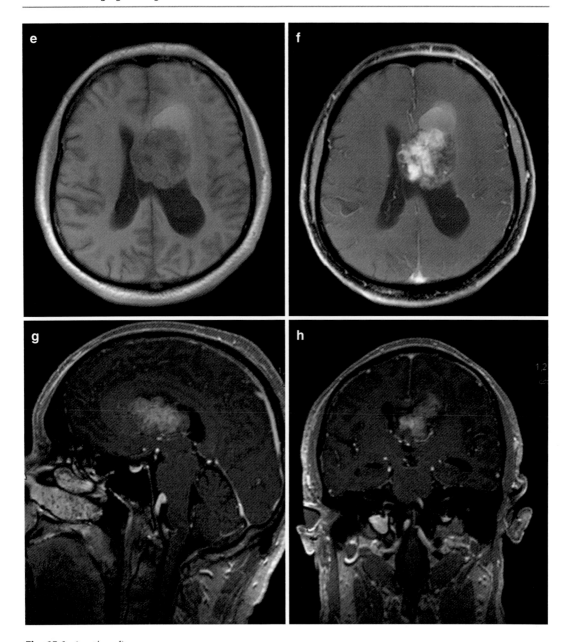

Fig. 65.1 (continued)

MRI-FLAIR (Fig. 65.1d)
- Heterogeneous hyperintense

MRI-T1 (Fig. 65.1e)
- Heterogeneous iso- to hypointense

MRI-T1 Contrast-Enhanced (Fig. 65.1f–h)
- Heterogeneous enhancement

MRI-T2∗/SWI
- Demonstrates calcifications in up to 70% of cases.
- Hemorrhage is rare.

MR-Diffusion Imaging
- ADC decreased

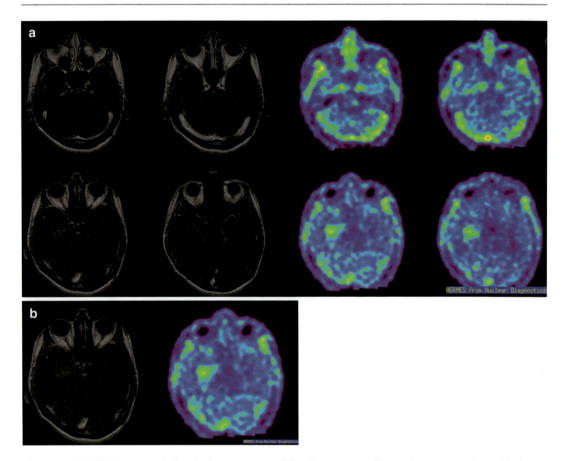

Fig. 65.2 FET-PET hypermetabolism in the temporo-mesial region corresponding to the contrast-enhanced lesion on the MR scan (**a**, **b**)

MR-Spectroscopy
- NAA decreased
- Slight elevation of choline
- Glycine peak at 1.5 ppm

Nuclear Medicine Imaging Findings (Fig. 65.2a, b)
- Only few studies deal with neurocytomas.
- Uptake in brain perfusion SPECT (historically) and Tl-201 (historically).
- Uptake in FDG (depending on the degree of dedifferentiation).
- Better delineation in amino acid PET.

65.3 Neuropathology Findings

Macroscopic Features
- Grayish color
- Friable
- Calcifications
- Hemorrhages
- Attachment to the septum pellucidum

Microscopic Features (Fig. 65.3a–f)
- Previously classified as:
  - Ependymoma of the foramen of Monro
  - Intraventricular oligodendroglioma

65.3 Neuropathology Findings

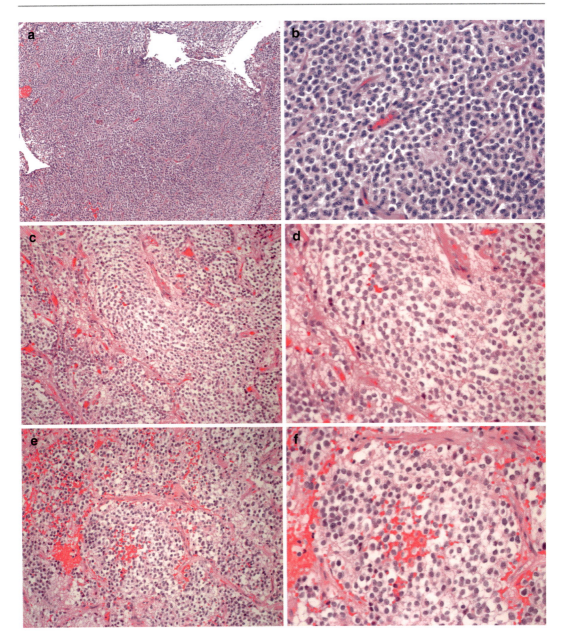

Fig. 65.3 Histological features of central neurocytoma on H&E stained sections (**a–f**). Uniform round cells showing features of neuronal differentiation with a round to oval nucleus, fine speckled chromatin, and occasional nucleolus. Fibrillary areas mimic neuropil

- Uniform round cells showing features of neuronal differentiation (by immunohistochemistry and ultrastructure).
  - Round to oval nucleus with fine speckled chromatin and occasional nucleolus
- Fibrillary areas mimicking neuropil.
- Various architectural patterns include:
  - Oligodendroglioma-like honeycomb appearance
  - Large fibrillary areas mimicking irregular rosettes
  - Cells arranged in straight lines
  - Perivascular pseudorosettes
- Calcifications are frequent (50% of the cases).
- Rare features include:
  - Homer Wright rosettes
  - Ganglioid cells
- Anaplastic features (WHO grade III) include:
  - Brisk mitotic activity
  - Microvascular proliferation
  - Necrosis

Immunophenotype (Fig. 65.4a–d)

Positivity	Negativity
• Synaptophysin (neuropil and perivascular nuclei-free cuffs) • NeuN • Class III ß-tubulin • MAP • Anti-Hu • Olig2	• Neurofilament • Chromogranin A • Alpha-internexin • IDH1 R123H

Proliferation Markers (Fig. 65.4e, f)
- Ki-67 LI: <2%
- Ki-67 LI: >2–3% indicative of atypical neurocytoma

Ultrastructural Features
- Regular round nuclei with fine chromatin.
- Cytoplasm contains mitochondria, Golgi apparatus, cisternae of rough endoplasmatic reticulum.
- Cell processes with microtubules, dense core, and clear vesicles.
- Synapses are well-formed or abnormal.

Differential Diagnosis
- Oligodendroglioma
- Ependymoma
- Pineocytoma
- Dysembryoplastic neuroepithelial tumor

65.4 Molecular Neuropathology

Pathogenesis
- Derivation from neuroglial precursor cells with
  - the potential of dual differentiation
  - originating from the subependymal plate of the lateral ventricles or from circumventricular organs

Molecular Neuropathology
- Central neurocytoma
  - cell of origin unknown
  - derived from neuroglial precursor cells with potentiality of dual differentiation
  - originated from the subependymal plate of the lateral ventricles
  - originated from circumventricular organs
- Extraventricular neurocytoma
  - Mislocated neuronal progenitor cells in brain parenchyma
- Gains on chromosomes 7, 2p, 10q, 18q, 13q
- No *EGFR* amplification
- *TP53* and *MYC* mutations absent or rare
- *WNT* signaling pathway
- 1p/19q deletion
  - None in central neurocytoma
  - Deletion found in extraventricular neurocytoma

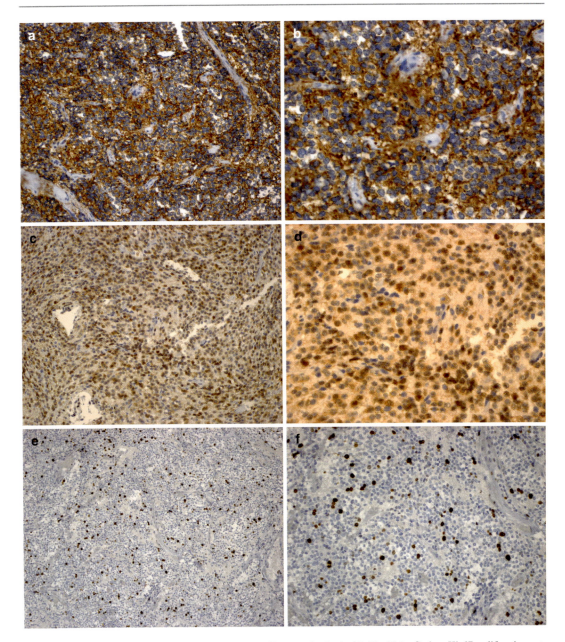

Fig. 65.4 Immunophenotype of central neurocytoma: Synaptophysin (**a**, **b**), NeuN (**c**, **d**), low Ki-67 proliferation rate (**e**, **f**)

65.5 Treatment and Prognosis

Treatment
- Surgery
- Radiotherapy

Biologic Behavior–Prognosis–Prognostic Factors
- Benign tumor
- Prognostic factor: extent of resection.
- Ki-67 LI >2 or 3% indicates shorter recurrence-free intervals.
- Local recurrence common.
- Rare craniospinal dissemination.

Selected References

Bonney PA, Boettcher LB, Krysiak RS 3rd, Fung KM, Sughrue ME (2015) Histology and molecular aspects of central neurocytoma. Neurosurg Clin N Am 26(1):21–29. https://doi.org/10.1016/j.nec.2014.09.001

Bui TT, Lagman C, Chung LK, Tenn S, Lee P, Chin RK, Kaprealian T, Yang I (2017) Systematic analysis of clinical outcomes following stereotactic radiosurgery for central neurocytoma. Brain Tumor Res Treat 5(1):10–15. https://doi.org/10.14791/btrt.2017.5.1.10

Choudhari KA, Kaliaperumal C, Jain A, Sarkar C, Soo MY, Rades D, Singh J (2009) Central neurocytoma: a multi-disciplinary review. Br J Neurosurg 23(6):585–595. https://doi.org/10.3109/02688690903254350

Chuang MT, Lin WC, Tsai HY, Liu GC, Hu SW, Chiang IC (2005) 3-T proton magnetic resonance spectroscopy of central neurocytoma: 3 case reports and review of the literature. J Comput Assist Tomogr 29(5):683–688

Figarella-Branger D, Söylemezoglu F, Kleihues P, Hassoun J (2000) Central neurocytoma. In: Kleihues P, Cavenee WK (eds) Pathology and genetics of tumours of the nervous system, 3rd edn. IARC Press, Lyon, pp 107–109

Figarella-Branger D, Söylemezoglu F, Burger PC (2007) Central neurocytoma and extraventricular neurocytoma. In: Louis DN, Ohgaki H, Wiestler OD, Cavenee WK (eds) WHO classification of tumours of the central nervous system, 4th edn. International Agency for Research on Cancer, Lyon, pp 106–109

Figarella-Branger D, Söylemezoglu F, Burger PC, Park S-H, Honavar M (2016a) Central neurocytoma. In: Louis DN, Ohgaki H, Wiestler OD, Cavenee WK (eds) WHO classification of tumours of the central nervous system, Revised 4th edn. IARC, Lyon, pp 156–158

Figarella-Branger D, Söylemezoglu F, Burger PC, Park S-H, Honavar M (2016b) Extraventricular neurocytoma. In: Louis DN, Ohgaki H, Wiestler OD, Cavenee WK (eds) WHO classification of tumours of the central nervous system, Revised 4th edn. IARC, Lyon, pp 159–160

Karki B, Tamrakar K, Kai XY, Kui WY, Wei ZW (2012) Extraventricular neurocytoma. JNMA J Nepal Med Assoc 52(188):181–187

Kleihues P, Burger PC, Scheithauer BW (1993) Histological typing of tumours of the central nervous system, 2nd edn. Springer, Berlin

Lee SJ, Bui TT, Chen CH, Lagman C, Chung LK, Sidhu S, Seo DJ, Yong WH, Siegal TL, Kim M, Yang I (2016) Central neurocytoma: a review of clinical management and histopathologic features. Brain Tumor Res Treat 4(2):49–57. https://doi.org/10.14791/btrt.2016.4.2.49

Patel DM, Schmidt RF, Liu JK (2013) Update on the diagnosis, pathogenesis, and treatment strategies for central neurocytoma. J Clin Neurosci 20(9):1193–1199. https://doi.org/10.1016/j.jocn.2013.01.001

Sharma MC, Deb P, Sharma S, Sarkar C (2006) Neurocytoma: a comprehensive review. Neurosurg Rev 29(4):270–285; discussion 285. https://doi.org/10.1007/s10143-006-0030-z

Shin HY, Kim JW, Paek SH, Kim DG (2015) The characteristics of neuronal stem cells of central neurocytoma. Neurosurg Clin N Am 26(1):31–36. https://doi.org/10.1016/j.nec.2014.09.009

Yang I, Ung N, Chung LK, Nagasawa DT, Thill K, Park J, Tenn S (2015) Clinical manifestations of central neurocytoma. Neurosurg Clin N Am 26(1):5–10. https://doi.org/10.1016/j.nec.2014.09.011

Rosette-Forming Glioneuronal Tumor (RGNT)

Neuronal and Mixed Neuronal-Glial Tumors

WHO Definition
2016—A neoplasm composed of two distinct histological components: one containing uniform neurocytes forming rosettes and/or perivascular pseudorosettes and the other being astrocytic in nature and resembling pilocytic astrocytoma (Hainfellner et al. 2016).

2007—A rare, slowly growing neoplasm of the fourth ventricular region, preferentially affecting young adults and composed of two distinct histological components, one with uniform neurocytes forming rosettes and/or perivascular pseudorosettes, the other being astrocytic in nature and resembling pilocytic astrocytoma (Hainfellner et al. 2007).

WHO Grade
- WHO grade I

66.1 Epidemiology

Incidence
- rare

Age Incidence
- Age range: 12–59 years
- Mean age: 33 years

Sex Incidence
- Male:Female ratio: 1:1.3

Localization
- Midline
- Fourth ventricle and/or aqueduct
- Brain stem
- Cerebellum
- Pineal gland
- Optic chiasm
- Septum pellucidum
- Spinal cord

66.2 Neuroimaging Findings

General Imaging Findings
- Well-demarcated heterogeneous mass, typically at the top of the fourth ventricle located.
- Cases with associated NF 1 are reported.

CT non-contrast-enhanced
- Hypodense, multicystic
- Calcifications and hemorrhage common

CT contrast-enhanced
- None to inhomogeneous enhancement

MRI-T2 (Fig. 66.1a, e)
- Hyperintense
- Blood-fluid levels possible

MRI-Flair (Fig. 66.1b, f)
- Hyperintense

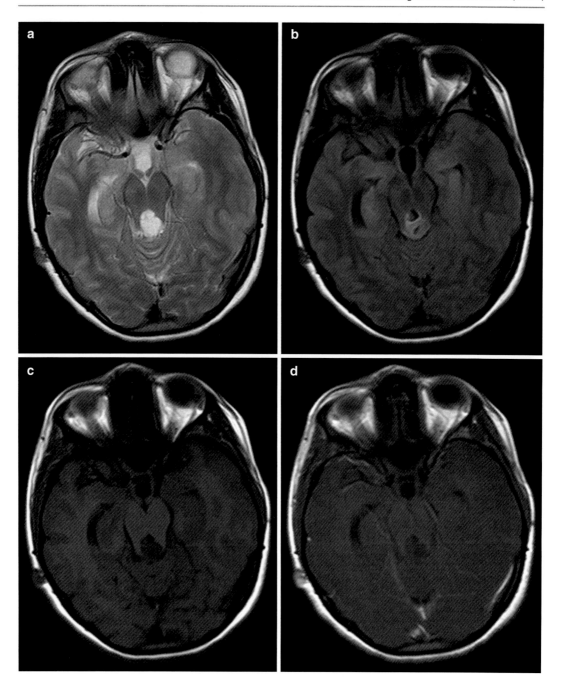

Fig. 66.1 Well-defined rosette-forming glioneural tumor, typically located at the top of the fourth ventricle without contrast enhancement. T2 ax (**a**), Flair (**b**), T1 (**c**), T1 contrast (**d**), T2 sag (**e**), Flair sag (**f**), T1 contrast sag (**g**), MR-spectroscopy 135 (**h**), MR-perfusion CBV (**i**)

66.2 Neuroimaging Findings

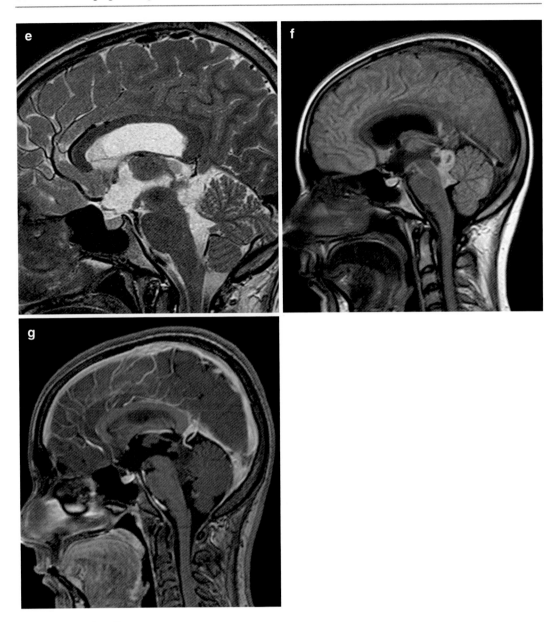

Fig. 66.1 (continued)

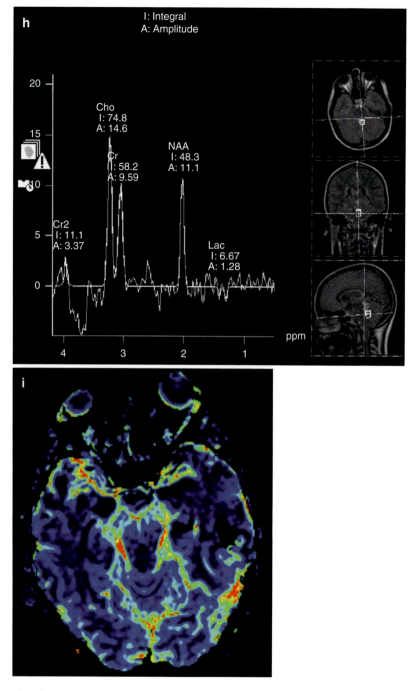

Fig. 66.1 (continued)

MRI-T1 (Fig. 66.1c)
- Hypointense

MRI-T1 Contrast-Enhanced (Fig. 66.1d, g)
- None to inhomogeneous enhancement

MRI-T2∗/SWI
- Calcifications and hemorrhage common

MR-Diffusion Imaging
- No restricted diffusion or hypointense

MRI-Perfusion (Fig. 66.1i)
- No elevation of rCBV

MR-Spectroscopy (Fig. 66.1h)
- NAA decreased
- Slight elevation of choline

Nuclear Medicine Imaging Findings
- No data available

66.3 Neuropathology Findings

Macroscopic Features
- Whitish-brown color

Microscopic Features (Fig. 66.2a–l)
- Characterized by biphasic architecture:
  – Neurocytic
  – Glial
- Neurocytic component:
  – Uniform population of neurocytes forming neurocytic rosettes and/or perivascular pseudorosettes
  – Neurocytic tumor cells:
    ○ Spherical nuclei with fine granular chromatin
    ○ Inconspicuous nuclei
    ○ Scant cytoplasm
    ○ Delicate cytoplasmic processes
  – Neurocytic rosettes:
    ○ ring-like arrays of neurocytic nuclei around delicate eosinophilic neuropil cores
  – Perivascular pseudorosettes:
    ○ delicate cell processes radiating towards vessels
- Glial component
  – Astrocytic tumor cells:
    ○ Spindle to stellate shape
    ○ Elongate to oval nuclei
    ○ Moderate dense chromatin
  – Loosely textured fibrillary background formed by cytoplasmic processes
  – Oligodendroglia-like cells with perinuclear halo
- Well demarcated with some infiltration of the brain parenchyma
- Resembles pilocytic astrocytoma
- Features also encountered:
  – Rosenthal fibers
  – Eosinophilic granular bodies
  – Microcalcifications
  – Hemosiderin deposits
- Absence of mitoses and necrosis
- Vessels may be:
  – Thin-walled
  – Dilated
  – Hyalinized
  – Thrombosed
  – Glomeruloid

Immunophenotype (Fig. 66.3a–h)
- Positivity for
  – Synaptophysin (center of neurocytic rosette, neuropil of perivascular pseudorosettes)
  – MAP-2 (cytoplasm and processes of neurocytic tumor cells)
  – Neuron-specific enolase (NSE) (cytoplasm and processes of neurocytic tumor cells)
  – GFAP (glial component)
  – S-100 (glial component)

Proliferation Markers (Fig. 66.3i, j)
- Absence of mitoses
- Ki-67 LI <3%

Ultrastructural Features
- Astrocytic cells:
  – Dense bundles of glial filaments

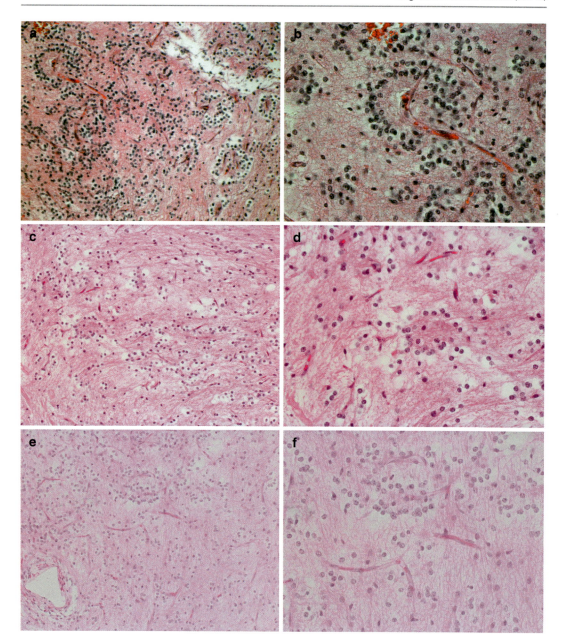

Fig. 66.2 The neurocytic component is made up of a uniform population of neurocytes forming neurocytic rosettes and/or perivascular pseudorosettes (**a–f**). The neurocytic tumor cells have spherical nuclei with fine granular chromatin, inconspicuous nuclei, scant cytoplasm, and delicate cytoplasmic processes (**a–h**). Some tumor cells resemble oligodendrocytes with empty cytoplasm (**g, h**). The glial component is made up of astrocytic tumor cells of spindle to stellate shape with elongate to oval nuclei and moderate dense chromatin (**g–l**). A loosely textured fibrillary background is formed by cytoplasmic processes (**i–l**). (Case contributed by Ognian Kalev, MD, Division of Neuropathology, Neuromed Campus, Kepler University Hospital, Linz, Austria)

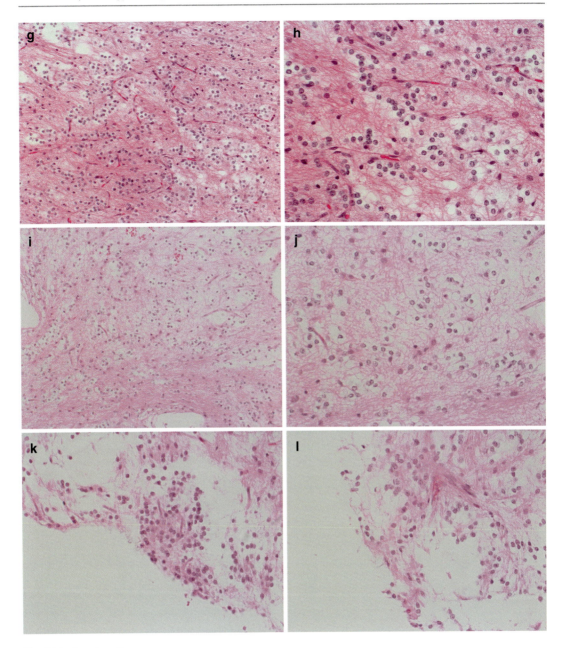

Fig. 66.2 (continued)

- Neurocytic cells:
  - Spherical nuclei
  - Delicate chromatin
  - Cytoplasm with
    o Free ribosomes
    o Rough endoplasmatic reticulum
    o Prominent Golgi apparatus
    o Mitochondria
  - Cytoplasmic processes with
    o Aligned microtubules
    o Dense core vesicles
  - Presynaptic specialization and mature synaptic terminals

Differential Diagnosis
- Astrocytoma WHO grade II

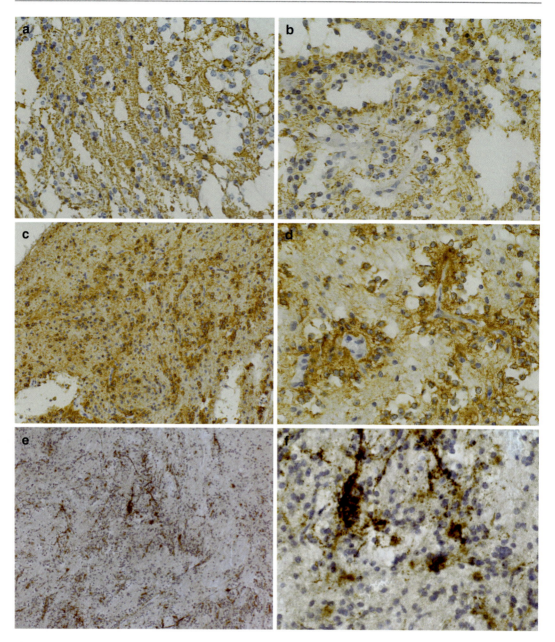

Fig. 66.3 Immunophenotype of rosette-forming glioneural tumor: Astroglial component stains for GFAP (**a, b**), neurocytic component stains for MAP2abc (**c, d**), and synaptophysin (**e, f**). Rosettes are well visualized with Olig2 (**g, h**). Proliferation is very low (Ki-67: **i, j**)

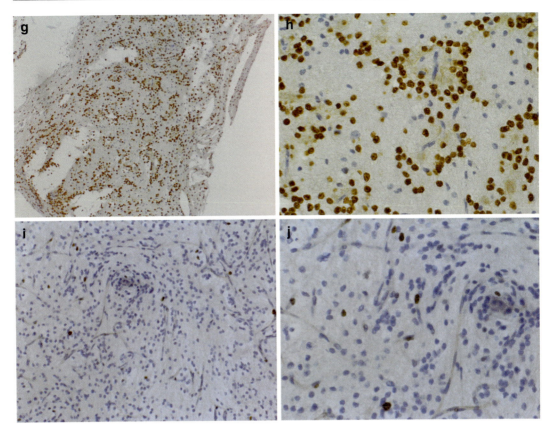

Fig. 66.3 (continued)

- Pilocytic astrocytoma WHO grade I
- Oligodendroglioma WHO grade II

66.4 Molecular Neuropathology

Pathogenesis
  Originates from

- brain tissue surrounding the infratentorial ventricular system
- subependymal plate, i.e., remnants of periventricular germinal matrix

Genes
- Mutations in
  - *PIK3CA*
  - *FGFR1*
- No mutations in
  - *BRAF* V600E
- No fusions in
  - *KIAA1549-BRAF*
- No SNP mutations in
  - *AKT1, AKT2, AKT3, EGFR, GNAQ, GNAS, KRAS, MET, NRAS, RET*
- Possible association with
  - Chiari type I malformation
  - Neurofibromatosis type I

66.5 Treatment and Prognosis

Treatment
- Surgical excision

Biologic Behavior–Prognosis–Prognostic Factors
- Benign tumor
- Favorable prognosis
- Postoperative disabling deficits possible

Selected References

Alnaami I, Aronyk K, Lu JQ, Johnson ES, O'Kelly C (2013) Rosette-forming glioneuronal tumors in the posterior third ventricle. Can J Neurol Sci 40(6):885–888

Bidinotto LT, Scapulatempo-Neto C, Mackay A, de Almeida GC, Scheithauer BW, Berardinelli GN, Torrieri R, Clara CA, Feltrin LT, Viana-Pereira M, Varella-Garcia M, Jones C, Reis RM (2015) Molecular profiling of a rare rosette-forming glioneuronal tumor arising in the spinal cord. PLoS One 10(9):e0137690. https://doi.org/10.1371/journal.pone.0137690

Chakraborti S, Mahadevan A, Govindan A, Bhateja A, Dwarakanath S, Aravinda HR, Phalguni AA, Santosh V, Yasha TC, Rout P, Sampath S, Shankar SK (2012) Rosette-forming glioneuronal tumor—evidence of stem cell origin with biphenotypic differentiation. Virchows Arch 461(5):581–588. https://doi.org/10.1007/s00428-012-1313-0

Dunham C (2015) Uncommon pediatric tumors of the posterior fossa: pathologic and molecular features. Childs Nerv Syst 31(10):1729–1737. https://doi.org/10.1007/s00381-015-2735-1

Eastin M, Shah KJ, Newell KL, Chamoun R (2016) Rosette-forming glioneuronal tumor of the thalamus. Clin Neuropathol 35(5):326–328. https://doi.org/10.5414/np300886

Ellezam B, Theeler BJ, Luthra R, Adesina AM, Aldape KD, Gilbert MR (2012) Recurrent PIK3CA mutations in rosette-forming glioneuronal tumor. Acta Neuropathol 123(2):285–287. https://doi.org/10.1007/s00401-011-0886-z

Eye PG, Davidson L, Malafronte PJ, Cantrell S, Theeler BJ (2017) PIK3CA mutation in a mixed dysembryoplastic neuroepithelial tumor and rosette forming glioneuronal tumor, a case report and literature review. J Neurol Sci 373:280–284. https://doi.org/10.1016/j.jns.2016.11.003

Gao L, Han F, Jin Y, Xiong J, Lv Y, Yao Z, Zhang J (2018) Imaging features of rosette-forming glioneuronal tumours. Clin Radiol 73(3):275–282. https://doi.org/10.1016/j.crad.2017.10.011

Gessi M, Lambert SR, Lauriola L, Waha A, Collins VP, Pietsch T (2012) Absence of KIAA1549-BRAF fusion in rosette-forming glioneuronal tumors of the fourth ventricle (RGNT). J Neurooncol 110(1):21–25. https://doi.org/10.1007/s11060-012-0940-2

Gessi M, Moneim YA, Hammes J, Goschzik T, Scholz M, Denkhaus D, Waha A, Pietsch T (2014) FGFR1 mutations in Rosette-forming glioneuronal tumors of the fourth ventricle. J Neuropathol Exp Neurol 73(6):580–584. https://doi.org/10.1097/nen.0000000000000080

Hainfellner JA, Scheithauer BW, Giangaspero F, Rosenblum MK (2007) Rosette-forming glioneuronal tumour. In: Louis DN, Ohgaki H, Wiestler OD, Cavenee WK (eds) WHO classification of tumours of the central nervous system, 4th edn. International Agency for Research on Cancer, Lyon, pp 115–116

Hainfellner JA, Giangaspero F, Rosenblum MK, Gessi M, Preusser M (2016) Rosette-forming glioneuronal tumour. In: Louis DN, Ohgaki H, Wiestler OD, Cavenee WK (eds) WHO classification of tumours of the central nervous system, Revised 4th edn. IARC, Lyon, pp 150–151

Hakan T, Aker FV (2016) Rosette-forming glioneuronal tumour of the fourth ventricle: case report and review of the literature. Folia neuropathologica/Association of Polish Neuropathologists and Medical Research Centre. Pol Acad Sci 54(1):80–87

Hsu C, Kwan G, Lau Q, Bhuta S (2012) Rosette-forming glioneuronal tumour: imaging features, histopathological correlation and a comprehensive review of literature. Br J Neurosurg 26(5):668–673. https://doi.org/10.3109/02688697.2012.655808

Joseph V, Wells A, Kuo YH, Halcrow S, Brophy B, Scott G, Manavis J, Swift J, Blumbergs PC (2009) The 'rosette-forming glioneuronal tumor' of the fourth ventricle. Neuropathology 29(3):309–314. https://doi.org/10.1111/j.1440-1789.2008.00953.x

Kitamura Y, Komori T, Shibuya M, Ohara K, Saito Y, Hayashi S, Sasaki A, Nakagawa E, Tomio R, Kakita A, Nakatsukasa M, Yoshida K, Sasaki H (2018) Comprehensive genetic characterization of rosette-forming glioneuronal tumors: independent component analysis by tissue microdissection. Brain Pathol 28(1):87–93. https://doi.org/10.1111/bpa.12468

Komori T, Scheithauer BW, Hirose T (2002) A rosette-forming glioneuronal tumor of the fourth ventricle: infratentorial form of dysembryoplastic neuroepithelial tumor? Am J Surg Pathol 26(5):582–591

Lin FY, Bergstrom K, Person R, Bavle A, Ballester LY, Scollon S, Raesz-Martinez R, Jea A, Birchansky S, Wheeler DA, Berg SL, Chintagumpala MM, Adesina AM, Eng C, Roy A, Plon SE, Parsons DW (2016) Integrated tumor and germline whole-exome sequencing identifies mutations in MAPK and PI3K pathway genes in an adolescent with rosette-forming glioneuronal tumor of the fourth ventricle. Cold Spring Harb Mol Case Stud 2(5):a001057. https://doi.org/10.1101/mcs.a001057

Matsumura N, Wang Y, Nakazato Y (2014) Coexpression of glial and neuronal markers in the neurocytic rosettes of rosette-forming glioneuronal tumors. Brain Tumor Pathol 31(1):17–22. https://doi.org/10.1007/s10014-012-0133-x

Medhi G, Prasad C, Saini J, Pendharkar H, Bhat MD, Pandey P, Muthane Y (2016) Imaging features of rosette-forming glioneuronal tumours (RGNTs): a Series of seven cases. Eur Radiol 26(1):262–270. https://doi.org/10.1007/s00330-015-3808-y

Pradhan R, Mondal S, Pal S, Chatterjee S, Banerjee A, Bhattacharyya D (2017) Rosette-forming glioneuronal tumor of the fourth ventricle. Neurol India 65(5):1176–1177. https://doi.org/10.4103/neuroindia.NI_862_16

Selected References

Preusser M, Dietrich W, Czech T, Prayer D, Budka H, Hainfellner JA (2003) Rosette-forming glioneuronal tumor of the fourth ventricle. Acta Neuropathol 106(5):506–508. https://doi.org/10.1007/s00401-003-0758-2

Sharma S (2017) Rosette-forming glioneuronal tumor arising from the spinal cord. World Neurosurg 105:1001. https://doi.org/10.1016/j.wneu.2017.01.016

Smith AB, Smirniotopoulos JG, Horkanyne-Szakaly I (2013) From the radiologic pathology archives: intraventricular neoplasms: radiologic-pathologic correlation. Radiographics 33(1):21–43. https://doi.org/10.1148/rg.331125192

Yin B, Liu L, Chen XR, Li K, Geng DY (2012) Rosette-forming glioneuronal tumor of the fourth ventricle. J Neuroradiol 39(2):129–130. https://doi.org/10.1016/j.neurad.2011.02.004

Pineal Parenchymal Tumors

Tumors of the Pineal Region

67.1 General Aspects

The following tumors affecting the pineal region are distinguished:

- Pineocytoma (WHO grade I)
- Pineal parenchymal tumor of intermediate differentiation (WHO grades II and III)
- Pineoblastoma (WHO grade IV)
- Papillary tumor of the pineal region

67.1.1 Epidemiology

Incidence
- 1% of all intracranial neoplasms
- Pineocytoma: 14–60% of the cases
- Pineal parenchymal tumor of intermediate differentiation: 20% of the cases
- Pineoblastoma: 40% of cases

Age Incidence
- All ages can be affected.
- Mean age: 38 years.

Sex Incidence
- Male:Female ratio: 1:1

Localization
- Pineal region
- Compresses adjacent structures
  - Cerebral aqueduct
  - Brain stem
  - Cerebellum

67.1.2 Nuclear Medicine Imaging Findings

- Pineoblastoma was described to be FET-positive.

67.1.3 Differential Diagnosis

- Primitive neuroectodermal tumor (PNET)
- Metastatic carcinoma

67.1.4 Molecular Neuropathology

Pathogenesis
- Originate from pineocytes or their precursor cells
  - Morphologic similarities.
  - Similar immunoprofile.
  - Similar genetic features.
  - Pineal tumors mimic the developmental stages of the human pineal gland/retina.

Genes
- Pineocytoma
  - Monosomy or loss of chromosome 22
  - Deletions on the distal region of 12q
  - Deletion or loss of chromosome 11

- Expression of enzymes related to melatonin synthesis (*TPH1, HIOMT*) and retinal phototransduction (*OPN4, RGS16, CRB3*)
- Pineal parenchymal tumor of intermediate differentiation
  - Chromosomal imbalances as gains in 4q, 12q, and losses on 22
  - Expression of genes: *PRAME, CD24, POU4F2, HOXD13*
- Pineoblastoma
  - Monosomy 22
  - Chromosomal imbalances on 1q12-qter, 5p13.2-14, 5q21-qter, 6p-12-pter, 14q21-qter
  - No changes in *TP53, Waf/p21*
  - Expression of genes: *PITX2, POU4F2, HOXD13, Hist1H3D, Hist1H4E, DSG1, TERT*

67.2 Pineocytoma

WHO Definition

2016—A well-differentiated pineal parenchymal neoplasm composed of uniform cells forming large pineocytomatous rosettes and/or of pleomorphic cells showing gangliocytic differentiation (Nakazato et al. 2016).

2007—A rare, slowly growing, grossly demarcated pineal parenchymal neoplasm occurring mainly in adults and composed of relatively small, uniform, mature-appearing pineocytes often forming large pineocytomatous rosettes (Nakazato et al. 2007c).

2000—A slow-growing pineal parenchymal neoplasm with predominant manifestation in young adults, composed of small, uniform, mature cells resembling pineocytes with occasional large pineocytomatous rosettes (Mena et al. 2000c).

1993—A rare, differentiated tumor composed of neoplastic pineal parenchymal cells (Kleihues et al. 1993).

1979—A uncommon tumor composed of pineal cells. Their polar processes often radiate towards the vascular stroma (specific silver impregnations for pineal parenchymal cells may demonstrate the typical cell processes with club-like expansions at their tips, as described by Rio-Hortega) (Zülch 1979).

WHO Grade
- WHO grade I

67.2.1 Neuroimaging Findings

General Imaging Findings
- Round, well-delineated, enhancing pineal mass with no invasion, but compression of adjacent structures, hydrocephalus is rare.

CT non-contrast-enhanced (Fig. 67.1a)
- Iso- to hypodense
- Peripheral calcifications

CT contrast-enhanced (Fig. 67.1b)
- Heterogeneous enhancement

MRI-T2 (Fig. 67.1c, d)
- Hyperintense
- Fluid levels possible

MRI-FLAIR (Fig. 67.1e)
- Hyperintense

MRI-T1 (Fig. 67.1f)
- Iso- to hypointense

MRI-T1 Contrast-Enhanced (Fig. 67.1g, h)
- Homogeneous enhancement

MRI-T2∗/SWI
- Blooming due to peripheral calcifications.
- Hemorrhages are rare.

67.2 Pineocytoma

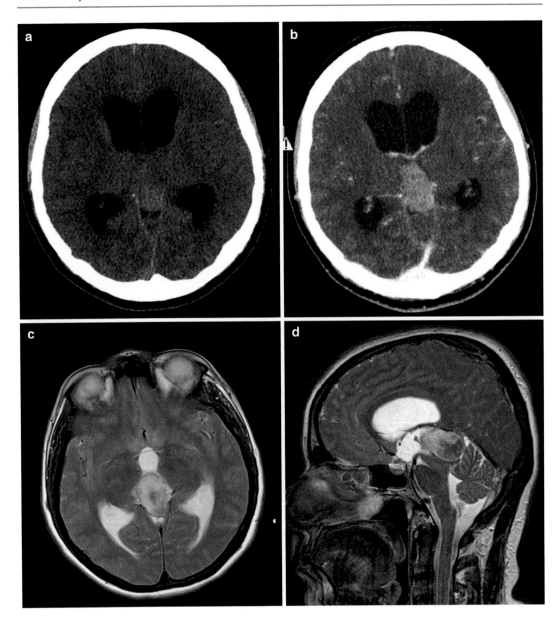

Fig. 67.1 Pineocytoma WHO grade I with peripheral, punctual calcification in CT native (**a**) and homogeneous enhancement in CT contrast (**b**). This is a rare case of hydrocephalus caused by the extension of the tumor in T2 ax/sag (**c**, **d**), FLAIR (**e**), T1 (**f**), T1 contrast ax/sag (**g**, **h**), and 3D CISS (**i**). FET-PET showing hypermetabolism (**j**)

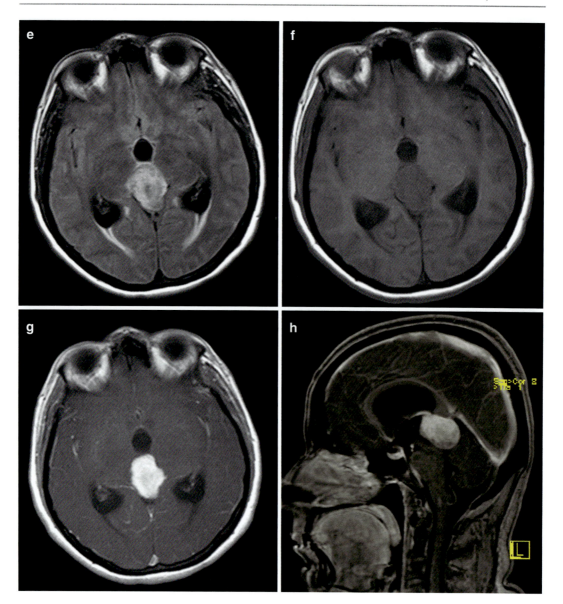

Fig. 67.1 (continued)

67.2 Pineocytoma

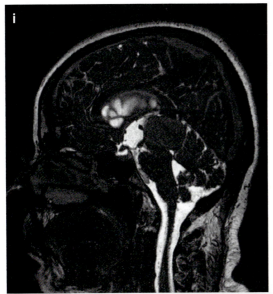

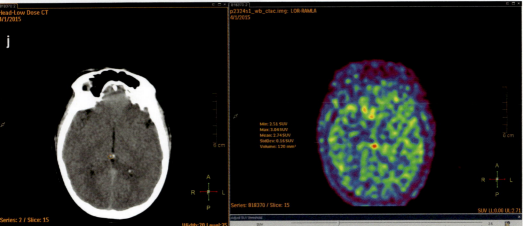

Fig. 67.1 (continued)

Nuclear Medicine Imaging Features (Fig. 67.1j)
- FGD-PET hypermetabolism

67.2.2 Neuropathology Findings

Macroscopic Features
- Well-circumscribed lesion
- Gray-tan color
- Homogeneous or granular cut surface
- Cyst formation possible
- Hemorrhages possible

Microscopic Features (Fig. 67.2a–d)
- Moderate cellularity
- Small, uniform, mature cells resembling pineocytes
  - Round-to-oval nuclei
  - Inconspicuous nucleoli
  - Fine chromatin
  - Moderate, homogeneous eosinophilic cytoplasm
  - Short processes ending in club-shaped expansions
- Tissue growth in sheets or ill-defined lobules

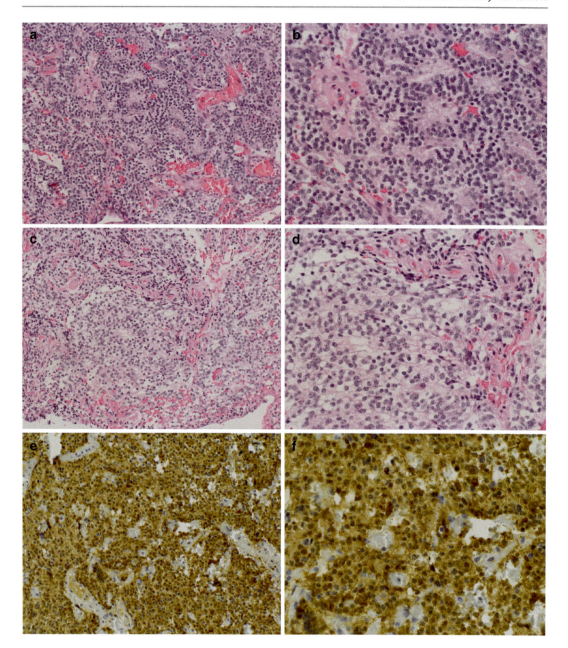

Fig. 67.2 Pineocytoma is characterized by moderate cellularity of mall, uniform, mature cells resembling pineocytes with round-to-oval nuclei, inconspicuous nucleoli, fine chromatin, moderate, homogeneous eosinophilic cytoplasm, and short processes ending in club-shaped expansions (**a–d**). Presence of pineocytomatous rosettes with abundant, delicate cell processes (**a, b**). Tissue growth in sheets or ill-defined lobules (**c, d**). Delicate network of vascular channels (**a–d**). Immunophenotype: positive for PDG9.5 (**e, f**), synaptophysin (**g, h**), chromogranin A (**i, j**), and neurofilament (**k, l**). Fine fibrillar network of GFAP-positive (**m, n**) and S-100-positive (**o, p**) astrocytic processes and cell bodies. Low Ki67 proliferation rate (**q, r**)

67.2 Pineocytoma

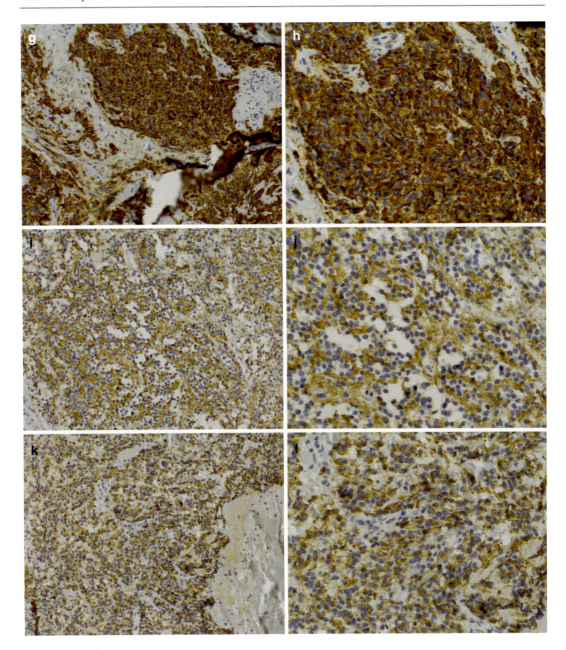

Fig. 67.2 (continued)

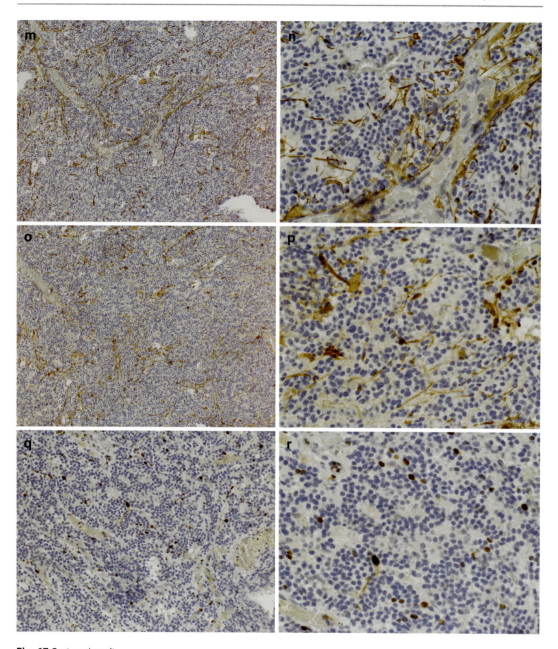

Fig. 67.2 (continued)

67.3 Pineal Parenchymal Tumor of Intermediate Differentiation

- Presence of pineocytomatous rosettes
  - Abundant, delicate cell processes
- Absence of mitoses
- Presence of large giant cells and/or multinucleated giant cells possible
- Delicate network of vascular channels

Immunophenotype (Fig. 67.2e–p)
- Positivity for:
  - Synaptophysin
  - Neuron-specific enolase
  - Neurofilament protein
  - Class III β-tubulin
  - Tau-protein
  - PGP 9.5
  - Chromogranin
  - Serotonin
  - Retinal S-antigen
  - Rhodopsin

Proliferation Markers (Fig. 67.2q, r)
- Mitoses absent to rare
- Ki-67 LI: low

Ultrastructural Features
- Clear and dark cells joined by zonulae adherentes
- Tapering processes ending in bulbous terminals

67.2.3 Treatment and Prognosis

Treatment
- Surgery

Biologic Behavior–Prognosis–Prognostic Factors
- 5-Year survival: 86–100%
- No potential for metastases

67.3 Pineal Parenchymal Tumor of Intermediate Differentiation

WHO Definition
2016—A tumor of the pineal gland that is intermediate in malignancy between pineocytoma and pineoblastoma and is composed of diffuse sheets or large lobules of monomorphic round cells that appear more differentiated than those observed in pineoblastomas (Jouvet et al. 2016a).

2007—A pineal parenchymal neoplasm of intermediate-grade malignancy, affecting all ages and composed of diffuse sheets or large lobules of uniform cells with mild to moderate nuclear atypia and low- to moderate-level mitotic activity. Without justification, the few rare tumors showing coexistent patterns of both pineocytoma and pineoblastoma have occasionally been included in this category (Nakazato et al. 2007a).

2000—Pineal parenchymal tumors with intermediate differentiation are monomorphous tumors characterized by moderately high cellularity, mild nuclear atypia, occasional mitosis, and the absence of large pineocytomatous rosettes (Mena et al. 2000a).

WHO Grade
- WHO grades II or III

67.3.1 Neuropathology Findings

Macroscopic Findings
- Well-circumscribed lesion
- Gray-tan color
- Homogeneous or granular cut surface
- Cyst formation possible
- Hemorrhages possible

Microscopic Features (Fig. 67.3a–f)
- Diffuse or lobulated tumor
- Moderate high cellularity
- Mild to moderate nuclear atypia
- Low to moderate mitotic activity

Immunophenotype
- Positivity for:
  - Synaptophysin
  - Neuron-specific enolase
  - Neurofilament protein
  - Class III β-tubulin
  - Tau-protein
  - PGP 9.5
  - Chromogranin

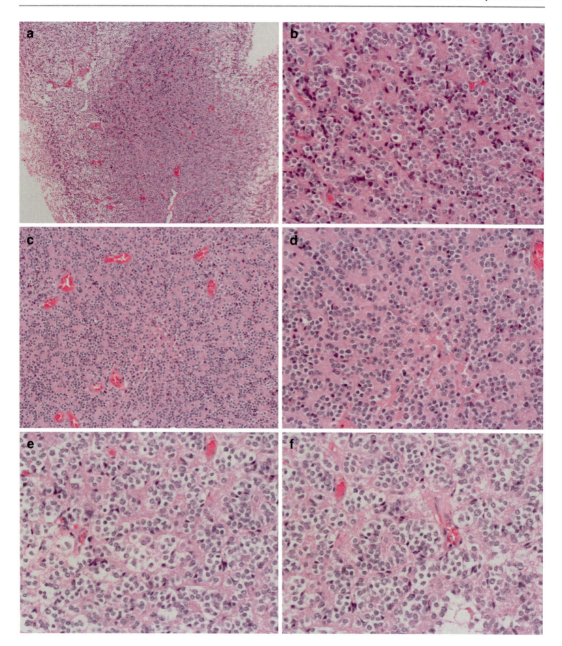

Fig. 67.3 Pineal parenchymal tumor of intermediate differentiation (PPTID) is characterized by a diffuse tumor cell growth of moderate to high cellularity. The tumor cells show mild to moderate nuclear atypia and low to moderate mitotic activity (**a–f**). Some tumor cells have clear cytoplasm appearance (**a–f**)

- Serotonin
- Retinal S-antigen
- Rhodopsin

Proliferation Markers
- Mitoses per 10 high-power field: 0–6
- Ki-67 LI: 3–10%

67.3.2 Treatment and Prognosis

Treatment
- Surgery

Biologic Behavior–Prognosis–Prognostic Factors
- 5-Year survival: 39–74%
- Rare intra- or extraneural metastases
- Prognostic factors include
  - Morphological subtype
  - Grade (II or III)
  - Presence or absence of necrosis
  - Mitotic index
  - Neurofilament protein immunostaining

67.4 Pineoblastoma

WHO Definition
2016—A poorly differentiated, highly cellular, malignant embryonal neoplasm arising in the pineal gland (Jouvet et al. 2016b).
2007—A highly malignant primitive embryonal tumor of the pineal gland, preferentially affecting children, frequently associated with CSF dissemination, and composed of dense, patternless sheets of small cells with round to somewhat irregular nuclei and scant cytoplasm (Nakazato et al. 2007b).
2000—A highly malignant, primitive embryonal tumor of the pineal gland with preferential manifestation in children, composed of patternless sheets of densely packed small cells with round-to-irregular nuclei and scant cytoplasm (Mena et al. 2000b).
1993—A rare, malignant embryonal tumor assumed to originate from precursor cells of the pineal gland (Kleihues et al. 1993).
1979—A rare, highly cellular pineal tumor consisting of small, poorly differentiated cells, whose cytological features and architecture resemble those of medulloblastoma. This tumor corresponds to grade IV (Zülch 1979).

WHO Grade
- WHO grade IV

67.4.1 Neuroimaging Findings

General Imaging Findings
Large, polylobulated mass in pineal region with solid and cystic components, invasion into corpus callosum, midbrain, and thalamus. CSF dissemination is common. Consecutive hydrocephalus.

CT non-contrast-enhanced
- Mixed, cystic, and solid mass with peripheral calcification

CT contrast-enhanced
- Inhomogeneous enhancement

MRI-T2/FLAIR (Fig. 67.4a, b)
- Mixed iso- to hyperintense
- Slight surrounding edema

MRI-T1 (Fig. 67.4c)
- Mixed iso- to hypointense

MRI-T1 Contrast-Enhanced (Fig. 67.4d–f)
- Strong, inhomogeneous enhancement

MRI-T2∗/SWI
- Intratumoral hemorrhages are common.
- Peripheral calcifications.

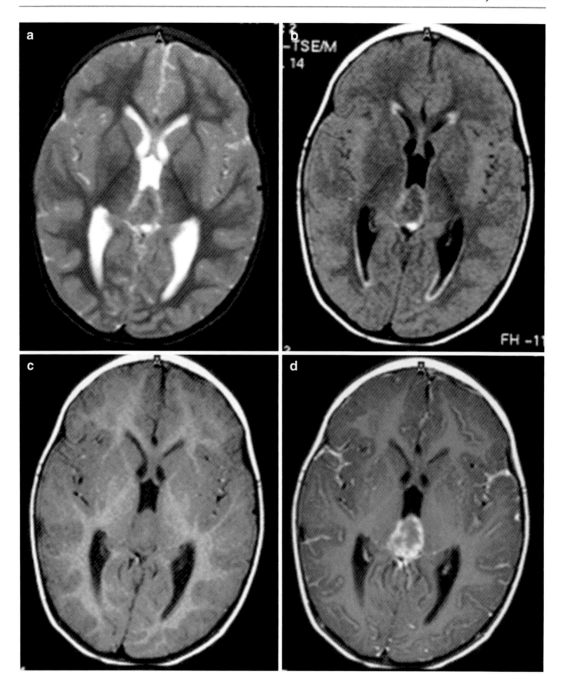

Fig. 67.4 Pineoblastoma in the pineal region in T2 (**a**), FLAIR (**b**), T1 (**c**), with meningeal spreading in T1 contrast ax/sag (**d–f**)

67.4 Pineoblastoma

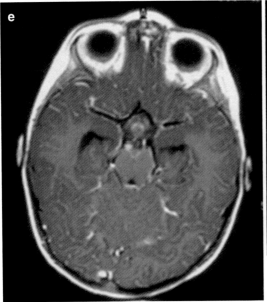
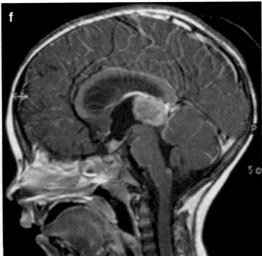

Fig. 67.4 (continued)

MR-Diffusion Imaging
- Restricted diffusion

MRI-Perfusion
- Elevated rCBV

67.4.2 Neuropathology Findings

Macroscopic Features
- Poorly circumscribed lesion
- Gray-tan color
- Cyst formation possible
- Hemorrhages possible
- Infiltration of surrounding tissue and/or leptomeninges

Microscopic Features (Fig. 67.5a–d)
- High cellularity.
- Patternless sheets of small cells with:
  - Round-to-irregular, hyperchromatic nuclei
  - Scant cytoplasm
  - High nuclear-cytoplasmic ratio
- Absence of pineocytomatous rosettes.
- Homer-Wright or Flexner-Wintersteiner rosettes may be present.
- Diffuse tumor cell growth.
- Variable but high mitotic activity.
- Presence of necroses.

Immunophenotype (Fig. 67.5e–h)
- Positivity for:
  - Synaptophysin
  - Neuron-specific enolase
  - Neurofilament protein
  - Class III β-tubulin
  - Tau-protein
  - PGP 9.5
  - Chromogranin
  - Serotonin
  - Retinal S-antigen
  - Rhodopsin

Proliferation Markers (Fig. 67.5i, j)
- KI-67 LI: high

67.4.3 Treatment and Prognosis

Treatment
- Surgery
- Radiotherapy

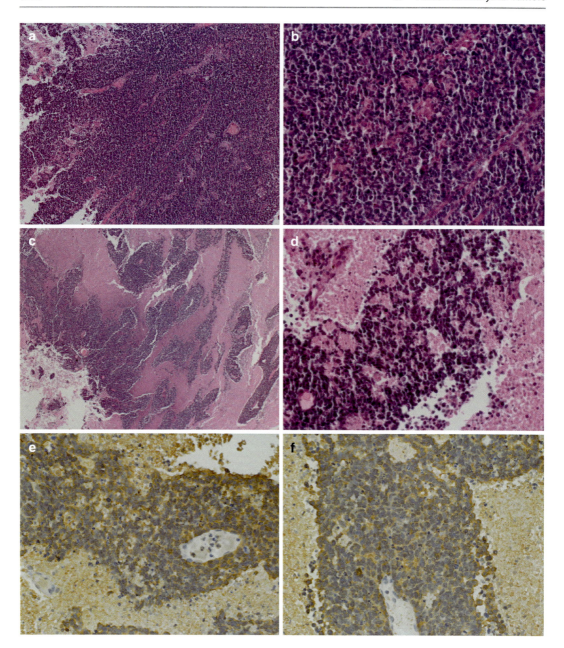

Fig. 67.5 Pineoblastoma is characterized by a high cellularity of patternless sheets of small cells with round-to-irregular, hyperchromatic nuclei, scant cytoplasm, high nuclear-cytoplasmic ratio, and variable but high mitotic activity (**a–d**). Absence of pineocytomatous rosettes; Homer-Wright or Flexner-Wintersteiner rosettes may be present (**d**). Immunophenotype: positive for PGP9.5 (**e, f**), synaptophysin (**g, h**). Fine fibrillar network of GFAP-positive (**i, j**) astrocytic processes and cell bodies

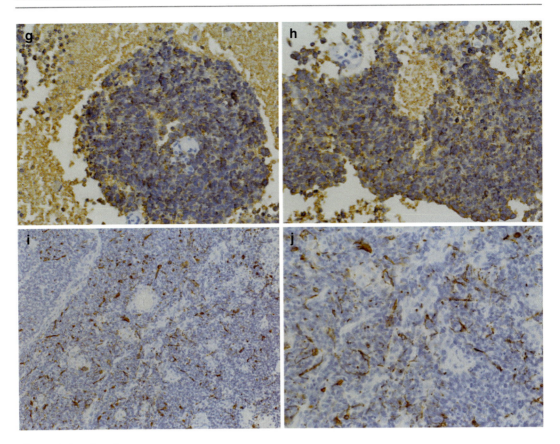

Fig. 67.5 (continued)

Biologic Behavior–Prognosis–Prognostic Factors

- Aggressive tumor
- Prognostic factors:
  - Extent of disease at time of diagnosis
  - Extent of resection
  - Extent of radiotherapy
- Survival rates:
  - 1-Year: 88%
  - 2-Year: 78%
  - 5-Year: 58%
- Metastases:
  - Craniospinal
  - Extracranial
  - Are common cause of death

Selected References

Brown AE, Leibundgut K, Niggli FK, Betts DR (2006) Cytogenetics of pineoblastoma: four new cases and a literature review. Cancer Genet Cytogenet 170(2):175–179. https://doi.org/10.1016/j.cancergencyto.2006.06.009

Chiechi MV, Smirniotopoulos JG, Mena H (1995) Pineal parenchymal tumors: CT and MR features. J Comput Assist Tomogr 19(4):509–517

Clark AJ, Ivan ME, Sughrue ME, Yang I, Aranda D, Han SJ, Kane AJ, Parsa AT (2010) Tumor control after surgery and radiotherapy for pineocytoma. J Neurosurg 113(2):319–324. https://doi.org/10.3171/2009.12.jns091683

Clark AJ, Sughrue ME, Aranda D, Parsa AT (2011) Contemporary management of pineocytoma. Neurosurg Clin N Am 22(3):403–407,. ix. https://doi.org/10.1016/j.nec.2011.05.004

Deiana G, Mottolese C, Hermier M, Louis-Tisserand G, Berthezene Y (2015) Imagery of pineal tumors. Neurochirurgie 61(2–3):113–122. https://doi.org/10.1016/j.neuchi.2014.10.111

Farnia B, Allen PK, Brown PD, Khatua S, Levine NB, Li J, Penas-Prado M, Mahajan A, Ghia AJ (2014) Clinical outcomes and patterns of failure in pineoblastoma: a 30-year, single-institution retrospective review. World Neurosurg 82(6):1232–1241. https://doi.org/10.1016/j.wneu.2014.07.010

Fevre-Montange M, Jouvet A, Privat K, Korf HW, Champier J, Reboul A, Aguera M, Mottolese C (1998) Immunohistochemical, ultrastructural, biochemical and in vitro studies of a pineocytoma. Acta Neuropathol 95(5):532–539

Galluzzi P, de Jong MC, Sirin S, Maeder P, Piu P, Cerase A, Monti L, Brisse HJ, Castelijns JA, de Graaf P, Goericke SL (2016) MRI-based assessment of the pineal gland in a large population of children aged 0-5 years and comparison with pineoblastoma: part I, the solid gland. Neuroradiology 58(7):705–712. https://doi.org/10.1007/s00234-016-1684-z

Ganti SR, Hilal SK, Stein BM, Silver AJ, Mawad M, Sane P (1986) CT of pineal region tumors. AJR Am J Roentgenol 146(3):451–458. https://doi.org/10.2214/ajr.146.3.451

Gasparetto EL, Cruz LC Jr, Doring TM, Araujo B, Dantas MA, Chimelli L, Domingues RC (2008) Diffusion-weighted MR images and pineoblastoma: diagnosis and follow-up. Arq Neuropsiquiatr 66(1):64–68

Gempt J, Ringel F, Oexle K, Delbridge C, Forschler A, Schlegel J, Meyer B, Schmidt-Graf F (2012) Familial pineocytoma. Acta Neurochir 154(8):1413–1416. https://doi.org/10.1007/s00701-012-1402-5

Gomez C, Wu J, Pope W, Vinters H, Desalles A, Selch M (2011) Pineocytoma with diffuse dissemination to the leptomeninges. Rare Tumors 3(4):e53. https://doi.org/10.4081/rt.2011.e53

Jackson AS, Plowman PN (2004) Pineal parenchymal tumours: I. Pineocytoma: a tumour responsive to platinum-based chemotherapy. Clin Oncol (R Coll Radiol) 16(4):238–243

Jouvet A, Nakazato Y, Vasiljevic A (2016a) Pineal parenchymal tumour of intermediate differentiation. In: Louis DN, Ohgaki H, Wiestler OD, Cavenee WK (eds) WHO classification of tumours of the central nervous system, Revised 4 edn. IARC, Lyon, pp 173–175

Jouvet A, Vasiljevic A, Nakazato Y, Tanaka S (2016b) Pineoblastoma. In: Louis DN, Ohgaki H, Wiestler OD, Cavenee WK (eds) WHO classification of tumours of the central nervous system, Revised 4 edn. IARC, Lyon, pp 176–179

Kleihues P, Burger PC, Scheithauer BW (1993) Histological typing of tumours of the central nervous system, 2nd edn. Springer, New York

de Kock L, Sabbaghian N, Druker H, Weber E, Hamel N, Miller S, Choong CS, Gottardo NG, Kees UR, Rednam SP, van Hest LP, Jongmans MC, Jhangiani S, Lupski JR, Zacharin M, Bouron-Dal Soglio D, Huang A, Priest JR, Perry A, Mueller S, Albrecht S, Malkin D, Grundy RG, Foulkes WD (2014) Germ-line and somatic DICER1 mutations in pineoblastoma. Acta Neuropathol 128(4):583–595. https://doi.org/10.1007/s00401-014-1318-7

Korogi Y, Takahashi M, Ushio Y (2001) MRI of pineal region tumors. J Neurooncol 54(3):251–261

Li MH, Bouffet E, Hawkins CE, Squire JA, Huang A (2005) Molecular genetics of supratentorial primitive neuroectodermal tumors and pineoblastoma. Neurosurg Focus 19(5):E3

Mena H, Nakazato Y, Jouvet A, Scheithauer BW (2000a) Pineal parenchymal tumour of intermediate differentiation. In: Kleihues P, Cavenee WK (eds) Pathology and genetics of tumours of the nervous system, 3rd edn. IARC Press, Lyon, p 121

Mena H, Nakazato Y, Jouvet A, Scheithauer BW (2000b) Pineoblastoma. In: Kleihues P, Cavenee WK (eds) Pathology and genetics of tumours of the nervous system, 3rd edn. IARC Press, Lyon, pp 116–118

Mena H, Nakazato Y, Jouvet A, Scheithauer BW (2000c) Pineocytoma. In: Kleihues P, Cavenee WK (eds) Pathology and genetics of tumours of the nervous system, 3rd edn. IARC Press, Lyon, pp 118–120

Miller S, Rogers HA, Lyon P, Rand V, Adamowicz-Brice M, Clifford SC, Hayden JT, Dyer S, Pfister S, Korshunov A, Brundler MA, Lowe J, Coyle B, Grundy RG (2011) Genome-wide molecular characterization of central nervous system primitive neuroectodermal tumor and pineoblastoma. Neuro Oncol 13(8):866–879. https://doi.org/10.1093/neuonc/nor070

Nakamura M, Saeki N, Iwadate Y, Sunami K, Osato K, Yamaura A (2000) Neuroradiological characteristics of pineocytoma and pineoblastoma. Neuroradiology 42(7):509–514

Nakazato Y, Jouvet A, Scheithauer BW (2007a) Pineal parenchymal tumour of intermediate differentiation. In: Louis DN, Ohgaki H, Wiestler OD, Cavenee WK (eds) WHO classification of tumours of the central nervous system, 4th edn. International Agency for Research on Cancer, Lyon, pp 124–125

Nakazato Y, Jouvet A, Scheithauer BW (2007b) Pineoblastoma. In: Louis DN, Ohgaki H, Wiestler OD, Cavenee WK (eds) WHO classification of tumours of the central nervous system, 4th edn. International Agency for Research on Cancer, Lyon, pp 126–127

Nakazato Y, Jouvet A, Scheithauer BW (2007c) Pineocytoma. In: Louis DN, Ohgaki H, Wiestler OD, Cavenee WK (eds) WHO classification of tumours of the central nervous system, 4th edn. International Agency for Research on Cancer, Lyon, pp 122–123

Nakazato Y, Jouvet A, Vasiljevic A (2016) Pineocytoma. In: Louis DN, Ohgaki H, Wiestler OD, Cavenee WK (eds) WHO classification of tumours of the central nervous system, Revised 4 edn. IARC, Lyon, pp 170–172

Parikh KA, Venable GT, Orr BA, Choudhri AF, Boop FA, Gajjar AJ, Klimo P Jr (2017) Pineoblastoma-the experience at St. Jude Children's Research Hospital.

Neurosurgery 81(1):120–128. https://doi.org/10.1093/neuros/nyx005

Serrano J, Infante JR, Rayo JI, Dominguez L, Garcia-Bernardo L, Duran C, Sanchez R (2009) In-111 pentetreotide in recurrent pineocytoma. Clin Nucl Med 34(2):117–118. https://doi.org/10.1097/RLU.0b013e318192c359

Sirin S, de Jong MC, Galluzzi P, Maeder P, Brisse HJ, Castelijns JA, de Graaf P, Goericke SL (2016) MRI-based assessment of the pineal gland in a large population of children aged 0-5 years and comparison with pineoblastoma: part II, the cystic gland. Neuroradiology 58(7):713–721. https://doi.org/10.1007/s00234-016-1683-0

Tate MC, Rutkowski MJ, Parsa AT (2011) Contemporary management of pineoblastoma. Neurosurg Clin N Am 22(3):409–412,. ix. https://doi.org/10.1016/j.nec.2011.05.001

Tate M, Sughrue ME, Rutkowski MJ, Kane AJ, Aranda D, McClinton L, McClinton L, Barani IJ, Parsa AT (2012) The long-term postsurgical prognosis of patients with pineoblastoma. Cancer 118(1):173–179. https://doi.org/10.1002/cncr.26300

Tsunoda S, Sakaki T, Tsujimoto M, Yabuno T, Tsuzuki T, Nakamura M, Hiramatsu K, Morimoto T, Boku E, Iwanaga H et al (1995) Clinicopathological study on pineocytoma. Brain Tumor Pathol 12(1):31–37

Zülch KJ (1979) Histological typing of tumours of the central nervous system. World Health Organization, Geneva

Medulloblastoma

Embryonal Tumors

WHO Definition 2016—Medulloblastoma: An embryonal neuroepithelial tumor arising in the cerebellum or dorsal brain stem, presenting mainly in childhood and consisting of densely packed small round undifferentiated cells with mild to moderate nuclear pleomorphism and a high mitotic count (Ellison et al. 2016c).

Medulloblastoma, NOS: The diagnosis of medulloblastoma, NOS, is appropriate when an embryonal neural tumor is located in the fourth ventricle or cerebellum and the nature of biopsied tissue prevents classification of the tumor in one of the genetically or histologically defined categories (Ellison et al. 2016c).

Medulloblastomas, Histologically Defined:
- **Medulloblastoma, classic**: An embryonal neuroepithelial tumor arising in the cerebellum or dorsal brain stem, consisting of densely packed small round undifferentiated cells with mild to moderate nuclear pleomorphism and a high mitotic count (Ellison et al. 2016a).
- **Desmoplastic/nodular medulloblastoma**: An embryonal neural tumor arising in the cerebellum and characterized by nodular, reticulin-free zones and intervening densely packed, poorly differentiated cells that produce an intercellular network of reticulin-positive collagen fibers (Pietsch et al. 2016).
- **Medulloblastoma with extensive nodularity**: An embryonal tumor of the cerebellum characterized by many large reticulin-free nodules of neurocytic cells against a neuropil-like matrix and by narrow internodular strands of poorly differentiated tumor cells in a desmoplastic matrix (Giangaspero et al. 2016).
- **Large cell/anaplastic medulloblastoma**: An embryonal neural tumor of the cerebellum or dorsal brain stem characterized by undifferentiated cells with marked nuclear pleomorphism, prominent nucleoli, cell wrapping, and high mitotic and apoptotic counts (Ellison et al. 2016d).

Medulloblastomas, Genetically Defined
- **Medulloblastoma, WNT-activated**: An embryonal tumor of the cerebellum/fourth ventricle composed of small uniform cells with round or oval nuclei that demonstrate activation of the WNT signaling pathway (Ellison et al. 2016e).
- **Medulloblastoma, SHH-activated— Medulloblastoma, SHH-activated and TP53-mutant**: An embryonal tumor of the cerebellum with evidence of SHH pathway activation and either germline or somatic TP53 mutation (Eberhart et al. 2016).
- **Medulloblastoma, SHH-activated, and TP53-wild-type**: An embryonal tumor of the cerebellum with molecular evidence of SHH pathway activation and an intact TP53 locus (Eberhart et al. 2016).
- **Medulloblastoma, non-WNT/non-SHH**: An embryonal tumor of the cerebellum consisting

of poorly differentiated cells and excluded from the WNT-activated and SHH-activated groups by molecular testing (Ellison et al. 2016b).

2007—A malignant, invasive embryonal tumor of the cerebellum with preferential manifestation in children, predominantly neuronal differentiation, and an inherent tendency to metastasize via CSF pathways (Giangaspero et al. 2007).

2000—A malignant, invasive embryonal tumor of the cerebellum with preferential manifestation in children, predominantly neuronal differentiation, and an inherent tendency to metastasize via CSF pathways (Giangaspero et al. 2000).

1993—A malignant embryonal childhood tumor located in the cerebellum and composed of densely packed cells with round to oval, or carrot-shaped nuclei and scanty cytoplasm (Kleihues et al. 1993).

1979—A tumor composed of small, poorly differentiated cells with ill-defined cytoplasmic processes and a tendency to form Homer Wright rosettes ("pseudorosettes"). Differentiation into glial or neuronal elements has been observed in some examples (Zülch 1979).

Desmoplastic Medulloblastoma
A tumor with the cellular features of a medulloblastoma, but demonstrating in addition an abundant network of reticulin fibers in its stroma (Zülch 1979).

WHO Grade
- WHO grade IV

68.1 Epidemiology

Incidence
- 0.5–0.8/100,000 in children younger than 19 years of age
- 10% of neuroectodermal tumors
- 16% of all pediatric brain tumors

Age Incidence
- 2/3 become manifest before the age of 15 years

Sex Incidence
- 65% male sex
- Male:Female ratio: 2:1

Localization
- Posterior cranial fossa
- Caudal parts of cerebellar vermis
- Start to proliferate
- Most often from posterior velum medullare
- Rarely from anterior velum medullare, cerebellar hemispheres, pons, or mesencephalon

68.2 Neuroimaging Findings

General Imaging Findings
- Classic medulloblastoma appear well-defined, round, typically arising from the roof of the fourth ventricle, in older children from the cerebellar hemisphere; consecutive hydrocephalus; exclude CSF dissemination of entire neuroaxis.

CT non-contrast-enhanced (Fig. 68.2a)
- Hyperdense
- Calcifications rare

CT contrast-enhanced
- Heterogeneous enhancement

MRI-T2 (Figs. 68.1a, 68.2b, and 68.3a)
- Isointense

MRI-FLAIR (Figs. 68.1b, 68.2c, and 68.3b)
- Hyperintense (helps to distinguish tumor from CSF)

MRI-T1 (Figs. 68.1c, 68.2d, and 68.3c)
- Hypointense

MRI-T1 Contrast-Enhanced (Figs. 68.1d, 68.2e, and 68.3d, e)
- Heterogeneous enhancement
- In case of CSF dissemination: superficial enhancement of brain surface

68.2 Neuroimaging Findings

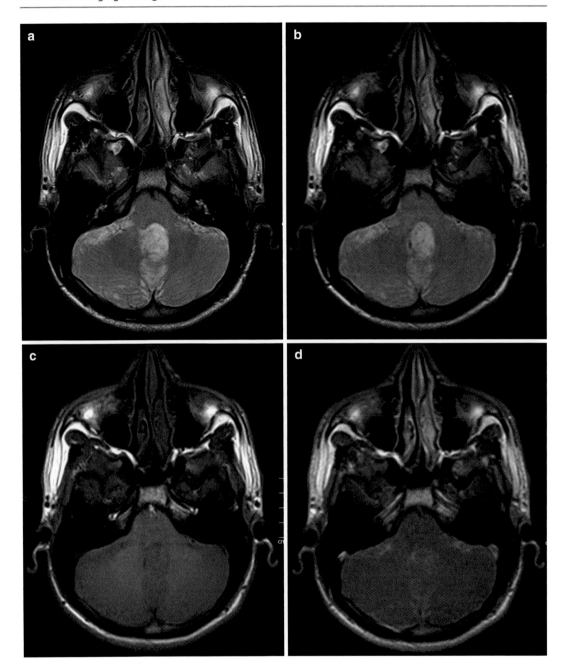

Fig. 68.1 Medulloblastoma in a 6-year-old child located at the roof of the fourth ventricle in T2 (**a**), FLAIR (**b**), T1 (**c**), with CSF dissemination in T1 contrast (**d**)

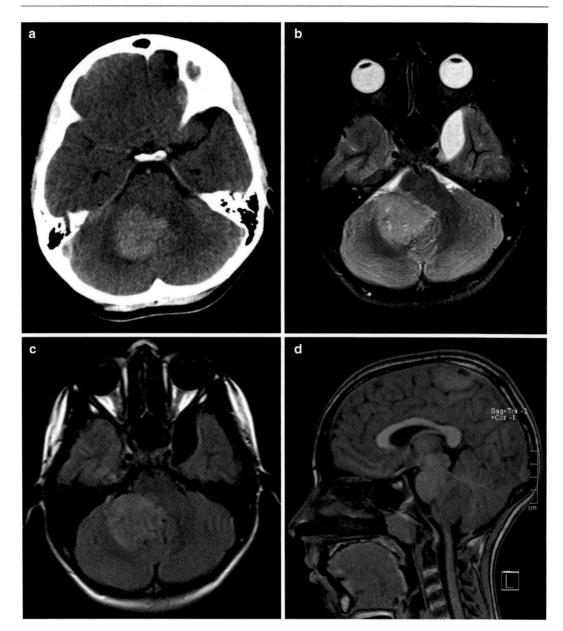

Fig. 68.2 Right-sided medulloblastoma, hyperdense in CT (**a**), hyperintense in STIR and FLAIR (**b**, **c**), hypointense in T1 (**d**), and irregular enhancement in T1 contrast (**e**)

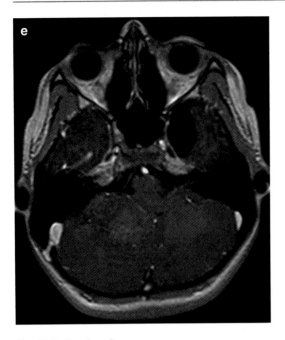

Fig. 68.2 (continued)

MRI-T2∗/SWI
- Calcifications and hemorrhages rare

MR-Diffusion Imaging
- Restricted diffusion
- ADC values lower than in ependymomas

MRI-Perfusion (Fig. 68.3f)
- Elevated rCBV

MR-Spectroscopy
- NAA significantly decreased
- Choline increased
- Lactate peaks

Nuclear Medicine Imaging Findings
- Overall only few studies are available dealing with medulloblastomas.
- FDG can show hypermetabolism.
- Amino acid PET is usually positive in medulloblastoma.
- Hypoxia tracers are under investigation for radiotherapy planning.
- Due to the positive somatostatin receptor status of medulloblastomas, imaging methods like SSR-scan or SSR-PET can be used to differentiate them from gliomas.
- Due to the positive somatostatin receptor status Y-90 labeled compounds have been used for treatment.

68.3 Neuropathology Findings

Macroscopic Features (Fig. 68.4a–d)
- Grayish white
- No sharp borders
- Soft
- Seldomly necroses or hemorrhages or cyst formation
- Infiltrative growth into the leptomeninges → metastases along the CSF way
- Can fill the lumen of the fourth ventricle, growth into the cerebral aqueduct
- Growth through the lateral apertures, through the median aperture into the cerebellomedullary cistern
- Obstruction of ventricles and liquor → hydrocephalus internus

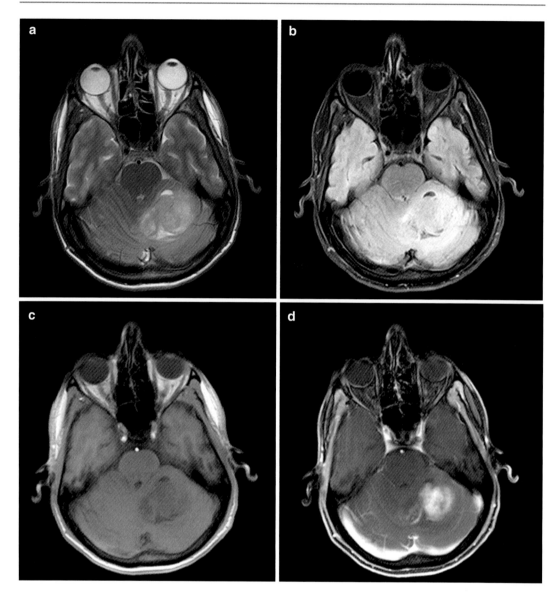

Fig. 68.3 Left cerebellar medulloblastoma of a 33-year-old man in T2 (**a**), Flair (**b**), T1 (**c**), T1 contrast ax/cor (**d**, **e**), and elevated CBV (**f**)

68.3 Neuropathology Findings

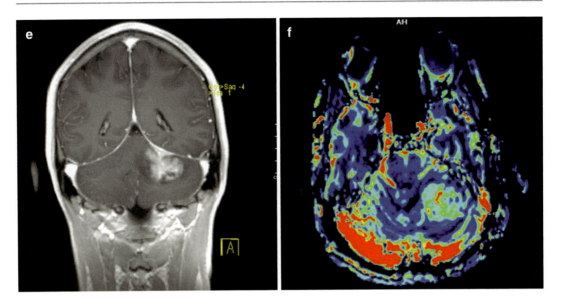

Fig. 68.3 (continued)

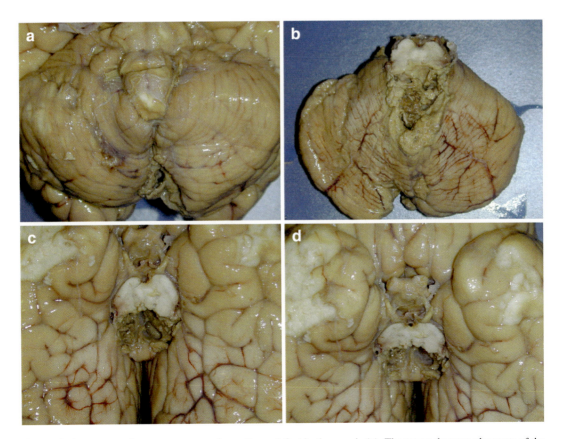

Fig. 68.4 Autopsy specimen post-surgery shows tissue defect in the vermis (**a**). The tumor destroys also parts of the pons (**b**) and lower mesencephalon (**c, d**)

Microscopic Features (Figs. 68.5, 68.6, and 68.7)

- Based on the histological appearance, the following types are distinguished:
- Classic medulloblastoma
- Desmoplastic/nodular medulloblastoma
- Medulloblastoma with extensive nodularity (MBEN)
- Anaplastic medulloblastoma
- Large cell medulloblastoma
- Variants:
    - MB with myogenic differentiation: medullomyoblastoma
    - MB with melanocytic differentiation: melanocytic medulloblastoma

The histological appearance of medulloblastoma is as follows:

- High cell density.
- Cellular polymorphism.
- Densely packed, small, round cells, carotte-shaped.
- Scant cytoplasm, chromatin-rich nucleus.
- Many mitoses.
- Homer Wright pseudorosettes.
- Seldom features: necroses, endothelial proliferation.
- Small cell can contain melanin.
- Connective tissue proliferation when leptomeningeal infiltration:
    - Classic medulloblastoma with leptomeningeal infiltration
    - Desmoplastic medulloblastoma (8–15% of all medulloblastomas)
- Classic medulloblastoma (Fig. 68.5a–l)
    - Highly cellular, patternless tumor
    - Small- to medium-sized nuclei
    - Unapparent nucleoli
    - Nuclear molding
    - Minimal cytoplasm
    - Necrosis
    - Karyorrhexis

- **Desmoplastic/nodular medulloblastoma** (Fig. 68.6a–f)
    - Reticulin-free nodules (pale islands) with low proliferative tumor cells
    - Reticulin-rich internodular tumor with high cellularity and proliferation
- **Medulloblastoma with extensive nodularity**
    - High degree of desmoplasia with predominant reticulin-free pale areas in the form of an expanded lobular architecture
- **Anaplastic medulloblastoma** (Fig. 68.7a–f)
    - High nuclear pleomorphism
    - Nuclear molding
    - Cell–cell wrapping
    - Atypical tumor cell forms
    - High mitotic activity
    - Apoptosis
- **Large cell medulloblastoma**
    - Large tumor cells with vesicular nuclei, prominent nucleoli, and abundant cytoplasm
    - Abundant mitoses and apoptotic figures
- **MB with myogenic differentiation**
    - Old nomenclature: medullomyoblastoma
    - Scattered rhabdomyoblasts or skeletal muscle cells with pink cytoplasm and striations
- **MB with melanocytic differentiation**
    - Old nomenclature: Melanocytic medulloblastoma
    - Presence of melanin-containing tumor cells as undifferentiated or epithelial-like cells, forming tubules, papillae, or cell clusters

Immunophenotype (Fig. 68.8a–r) (Table 68.1)

- expression of glial filament GFAP (84% of cases)
- neurofilaments
- synaptophysin
- NSE
- CD56
- GAB1 (sonic hedgehog pathway tumor)

68.3 Neuropathology Findings

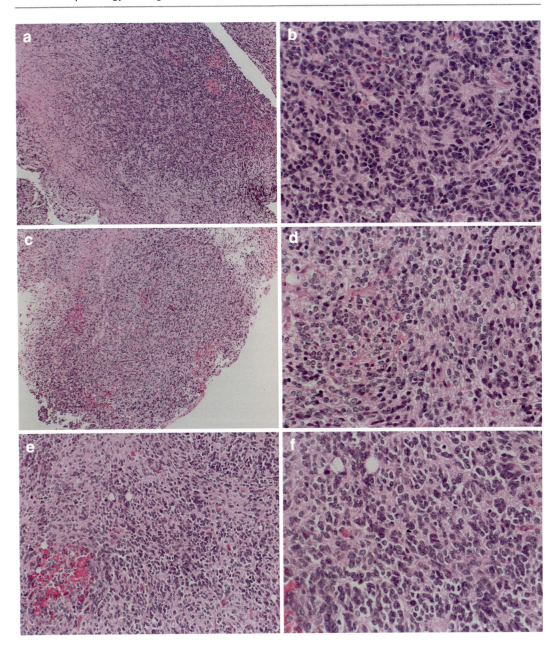

Fig. 68.5 Medulloblastoma is a highly cellular, patternless tumor. The tumor cells have small- to medium-sized nuclei, unapparent nucleoli, nuclear molding, and minimal cytoplasm (**a–j**). The reticulin network is scant (**k, l**)

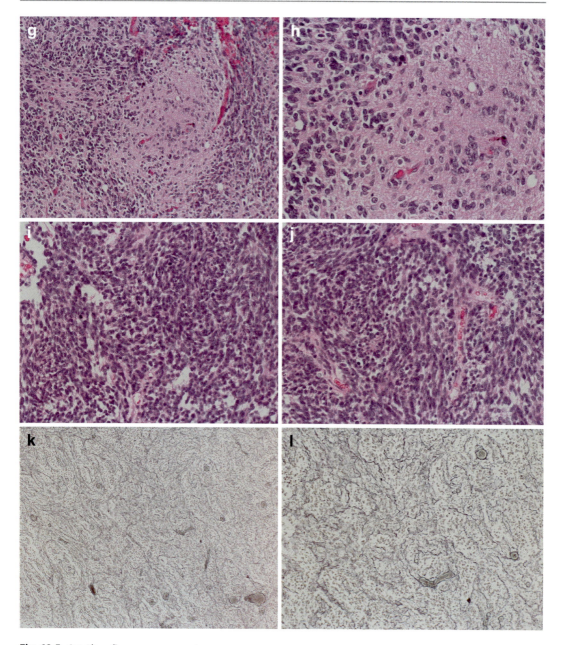

Fig. 68.5 (continued)

68.3 Neuropathology Findings

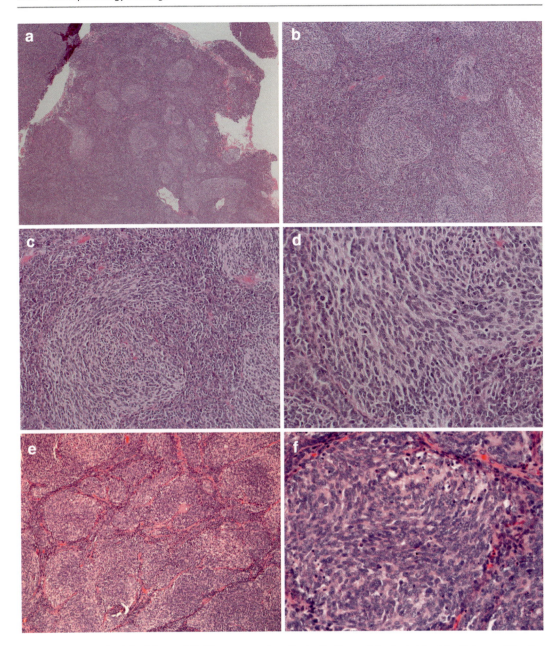

Fig. 68.6 Desmoplastic/nodular medulloblastoma consists of reticulin-free nodules (pale islands) with low proliferative tumor cells and reticulin-rich internodular tumor with high cellularity and proliferation (**a–j**)

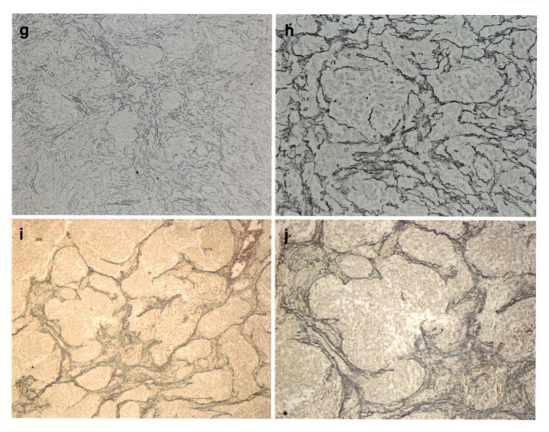

Fig. 68.6 (continued)

- MB with myogenic differentiation
  - Desmin
  - SMA
- MB with melanotic differentiation
  - S-100 protein
- YAP1
- p75
- β-catenin

Proliferation Markers (Fig. 68.8q, r)
- Frequent mitoses
- Ki-67 LI: high
- CAVE: mitoses and proliferating cells might be encountered in low density

Ultrastructural Features
- Neuroblastic differentiation as rosettes or pale islands
  - Cells with neurite-like cytoplasmic processes
  - Adhesion plaques
  - Microtubules arranged in parallel arrays
  - Dense core vesicles
  - Abundant intermediate filaments
- Formation of axons and axosomatic synapses
- MB with myogenic differentiation
  - Thick and thin filaments arranged in sarcomeres and Z-band material
- MB with melanotic differentiation
  - Occulocutaneous melanin with distinct melanosomes

Differential Diagnosis
- Anaplastic astrocytoma
- Ependymoma
- Pineoblastoma
- Atypical teratoid/rhabdoid tumor
- Metastatic carcinoma (small cell carcinoma)

68.3 Neuropathology Findings

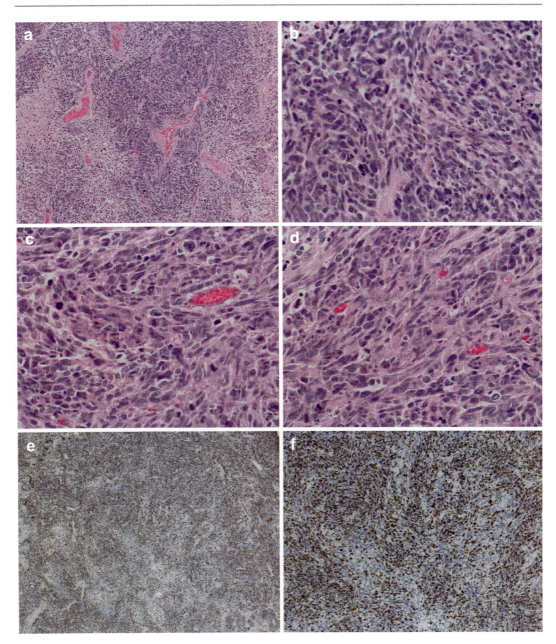

Fig. 68.7 Anaplastic medulloblastoma is characterized by tumor cells with high nuclear pleomorphism, nuclear molding, cell–cell wrapping, atypical tumor cell forms, and high mitotic activity (**a–d**). High Ki-67 proliferation index (**e, f**)

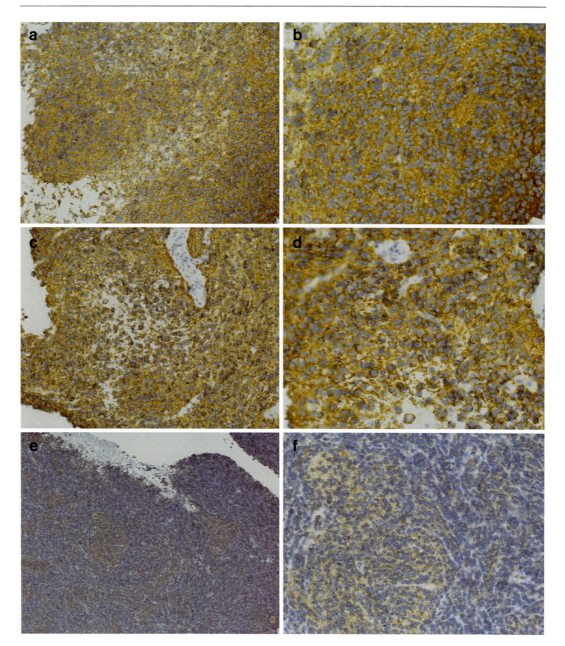

Fig. 68.8 Immunophenotype: tumor cells are positive for synaptophysin (**a**, **b**), CD56 (**c**, **d**). β-catenin (**e–h**) positive tumor cells are found in WNT-activated, SHH-activated, and non-WNT/non-SHH activated medulloblastomas. YAP1 (**i–l**)-positive tumor cells are found in WNT-activated, SHH-activated. GAB1 (p75) (**m**, **n**)-positive tumor cells are found in SHH-activated. A few entrapped GFAP-positive astrocytes are seen (**o**, **p**). High Ki-67 proliferation rate (**q**, **r**)

68.3 Neuropathology Findings

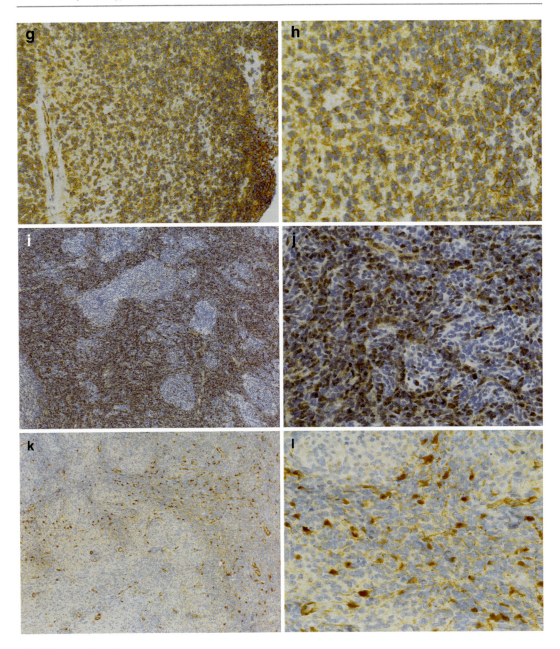

Fig. 68.8 (continued)

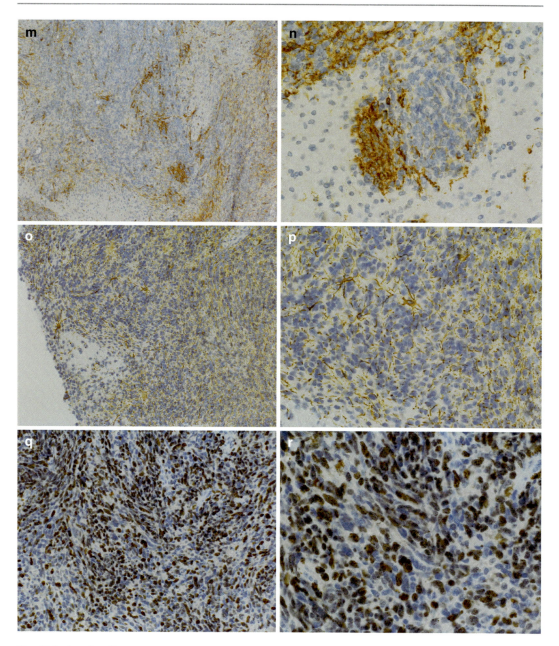

Fig. 68.8 (continued)

Table 68.1 Immunophenotype of genetically defined medulloblastomas; modified after Ellison et al. (2011) data reproduced with kind permission by Springer Nature

	β-catenin	YAP1	GAB1-p75	Filamin-A
WNT-activated	+ (n, c)	+ (n, c)	−	+ (c)
SHH-activated	+ (c)	+ (n, c)	+ (c)	+ (c)
Non-WNT/non-SHH	+ (c)	−	−	−

68.4 Molecular Neuropathology

68.4.1 Pathogenesis

- Derivation from undifferentiated, proliferating embryonal cells
  - Originate from the external granular layer of the cerebellum
    - Precursor neurons controlled by sonic Hedgehog
  - Derived from subependymal matrix cells residing throughout the embryonal central nervous system (PNET concept)

68.4.2 Molecular Classification of Medulloblastomas

Formerly, medulloblastoma was considered as a single tumor entity. In recent years, however, based largely on transcriptome analyses, medulloblastoma was recognized as a heterogeneous disease which falls into four molecular categories: Wnt, Shh, Group 3, and Group 4. The first two groups were termed after the major signaling cascades that are dysregulated in these tumors, i.e., the Wnt ("wingless")- and Shh (Sonic hedgehog) pathway, respectively. Groups 3 and 4 are defined as non-WNT/non-SHH entities with different but distinct transcriptional patterns.

- **Wnt (wingless) group**
  This tumor subtype accounts for ~10% of medulloblastoma cases, typically affects children over 3 years of age and is correlated with very favorable prognosis. Characteristic genetic features include:
  - Mutations
    - Activating somatic mutations in the *CTNNB1* gene, located at chromosome 3p21; it encodes β-catenin which is a key component of the Wnt signaling pathway. Activation and overexpression of β-catenin promotes its translocation from the cytoplasm to the nucleus where it participates in oncogenic transcriptional events.
    - Germline mutations of the tumor suppressor gene *APC* (adenomatous polyposis coli), located at chromosome region 5q21-q22; functional APC protein acts as an inhibitor of the Wnt pathway by negatively regulating β-catenin.
    - Heterozygous mutations in the *TP53* tumor suppressor gene on chromosome 17p13.1
    - Mutations in *DDX3X*
    - Mutations in *SMARCA4*
  - Chromosomal aberrations
    - Monosomy of chromosome 6: partial deletion or complete loss of chromosome 6 is observed in up to 90% of Wnt medulloblastomas; this aberration is virtually absent in the other tumor groups.

- **Shh (Sonic hedgehog) group**
  The Shh group represents ~30% of medulloblastoma cases. Strikingly, the age distribution of Shh tumors shows two peaks of high incidence, one in infants (0–3 years) and one in adults (>16 years); in children, much lower frequencies are observed. The prognosis ranges from good (infants) to intermediate (adults).
  The major genetic abnormalities found in Shh medulloblastomas are summarized below.
  - Mutations and somatic copy number variations (SCNVs)
    - Germline and somatic mutations in the tumor suppressor gene *PTCH1* which is located at chromosome 9q22.3 and encodes the sonic hedgehog receptor patched-1.
    - Germ line and somatic mutations in the tumor suppressor gene *SUFU* encoding the suppressor of fused homolog, a negative regulator in the Shh pathway. The gene is located at chromosome 10q24.32.

- Amplification of the *MYCN* oncogene (v-myc avian myelocytomatosis viral oncogene neuroblastoma-derived homolog) at chromosome 2p24.3.
- Somatic amplification of the Shh-associated oncogenes *GLI1* (chromosome 12q13.2-q13.3; encoding the transcriptional activator GLI family zinc finger 1) and *GLI2* (chromosome 2q14; encoding the transcriptional activator GLI family zinc finger 2).
- Activating somatic mutations in the *SMO* gene, located at chromosome 7q32.3 and encoding the protein Smoothened. Since Smoothened activates GLI1 and GLI2, this results in enhanced Shh signaling.
- Mutations in *DDX3X* or *KMT2D*.
- Amplification of *MYCN*.
– Chromosomal aberrations
- The most frequent observation is loss of chromosome 9q. This chromosomal aberration appears to exclusively occur in Shh medulloblastomas, thereby affecting the tumor suppressor gene *PTCH1* which is located at 9q22.
- Other genetic imbalances include loss of chromosome 10q and 14q and gain of chromosomes 3q and 9p.
– SHH-activated medulloblastomas tend to have similar transcriptome, methylome, and microRNA profiles.

- **Group 3**
Group 3 medulloblastoma (~25%) typically represent a pediatric tumor type which is not observed in adults; it shows a higher incidence in males and has the poorest prognosis of all four tumor subtypes.
– Somatic copy number variations (SCNVs)
- Enhanced *MYC* (v-myc avian myelocytomatosis viral oncogene homolog) amplification is a characteristic feature of this subgroup. *MYC* maps to chromosome 8q24.21 and is classified as a potent proto-oncogene.
– Chromosomal aberrations
- Apart from gain of chromosome 1q and loss of chromosome 10q, the presence of an isochromosome 17q (i17q) has been observed in about 25% of Group 3 medulloblastoma. This chromosomal anomaly results from loss of the entire short arm 17p which is replaced by a copy of 17q. Thus, affected cells harbor one wild-type chromosome 17 and one isochromosome 17q. It should be noted that loss of one copy of 17p also results in the heterozygous deletion of the *TP53* tumor suppressor gene, located at chromosome region 17p13.1.

- **Group 4**
With a frequency of >30%, Group 4 medulloblastoma represents the most common tumor subtype. The high male:female ratio of up to 3:1 is a distinctive feature of this group. Patients have an intermediate prognosis, with a more favorable tendency in children than in adults.
– Somatic copy number variations (SCNVs)
- Sporadically, amplification of the proto-oncogene *MYCN* occurs, whereas *MYC* amplification, typically seen in Group 3 tumors, is almost never observed. In this respect, Group 4 resembles the Shh tumor subgroup.
– Chromosomal aberrations
- The major cytogenetic aberration is the presence of isochromosome 17q which is found in 66% of the tumors.
- Loss of one copy of the X chromosome is another prominent cytogenetic defect that is observed in 80% of female Group 4 medulloblastoma patients. This finding is conspicuously correlated with the above-mentioned gender distribution in this tumor subgroup; its clinical relevance, however, is presently unclear.

The correspondence of histological subtypes with molecular subtypes is shown in Table 68.2, while various characteristics of molecular subgroups are given in Table 68.3.

68.5 Treatment and Prognosis

Table 68.2 The correspondence of histological subtypes with molecular subtypes

Histology	Genetic profile
Classic	• WNT-activated • SHH-activated, *TP53*-mutant • SHH-activated, *TP53*-wild-type • Non-WNT/non-SHH group 3 • Non-WNT/non-SHH group 4
Large cell/ Anaplastic	• WNT-activated • SHH-activated, *TP53*-mutant • SHH-activated, *TP53*-wild-type • Non-WNT/non-SHH group 3 • Non-WNT/non-SHH group 4
Desmoplastic/ nodular	• SHH-activated, *TP53*-mutant • SHH-activated, *TP53*-wild-type
Extensive nodularity	• SHH-activated, *TP53*-wild-type

68.4.3 Epigenetics

68.4.3.1 Affected Genes Involved in Chromatin Modification

Several genes known to contribute to chromatin modification have been found to be mutated in medulloblastoma. Among those are genes that encode factors modulating chromatin structure and post-translational modification of histones.

- In Groups 3 and 4 medulloblastomas, mutations in the *KDM6A* gene have been reported. *KDM6A* is located at chromosome Xp11.2 and codes for the lysine (K)-specific demethylase 6A which is responsible for the demethylation of lysine-27 in histone H3 (H3K27). The protein's activity is an important factor driving cell differentiation.
- Enhanced expression of the *EZH2* gene at chromosome 17q35-q36 (enhancer of zeste 2 polycomb repressive complex 2 subunit) was detected in Groups 3 and 4 tumors. EZH2 is a methyltransferase that methylates H3K27; thus, by counteracting KDM6A function, it is involved in the repression of cell differentiation. The oncogenic activity of EZH2 has already been recognized in a variety of tumor types.
- Mutations in the *SMARCA4* gene (SWI/SNF related, matrix associated, actin-dependent regulator of chromatin, subfamily a, member 4), located at chromosome 19p13.2. The gene product is involved in transcriptional activation by remodeling chromatin structure.

68.5 Treatment and Prognosis

Treatment
- Surgery
- Sensitive towards chemotherapy and radiotherapy
- Craniospinal radiotherapy

Biologic Behavior–Prognosis–Prognostic Factors
- Highly malignant tumor
- High recurrence rate, even after total resection (40–70%)
- Metastasizes in 30% along the CSF ways, ventricles, spinal and extracranial after shunt operations
- 5-year survival rate = 37%
- Genetic type (Table 68.4)
  – WNT-Group
    ○ Better prognosis
  – SHH-Group
    ○ Intermediate prognosis
  – SHH-activated and TP53-mutant
    ○ Very poor prognosis
  – Group 3
    ○ Worst prognosis
    ○ Metastases possible or present at time of diagnosis
- Poor prognosis due to
  – incomplete tumor resection
  – spread
    ○ cerebrospinal fluid
    ○ spinal
    ○ systemic

Table 68.3 Characteristics of molecular subgroups, modified after Coluccia et al. (2016), data reproduced with kind permission by Springer Nature

	WNT	SHH TP53 wild-type	SHH TP53 mutant	Non-WNT/non-SHH	Non-WNT/non-SHH
Group	1	2	2	3	4
prevalence (%)	10	~30	~30	~25	>30
Age	• Childhood • Teens	• Infants • Adults	• Childhood	• Infants • Children	• Infants • Children • Adults
Gender (M:F)	1:2	1:1	1:1	2:1	3:1
Typical localization	Midline/fourth ventricle	Adults: cerebral hemisphere Pediatric: vermis/midline	vermis/midline	Midline/fourth ventricle	Midline/fourth ventricle
Histology	• Classic • Rarely Large cell/Anaplastic	• Desmoplastic/nodular	• LC/A	• Classic • LC/A	• Classic
Metastasis	Low	Low	Low	High	High
Recurrence	Rare	Local	Local	Metastasis	Metastasis
Prognosis	Best	Intermediate		Poor	Intermediate
5-year OA (%)	95	75		50	75
Driver genes	• CTNNB1 (90%) • DDX3X (50%) • SMARCA4 (26%) • TP53 (12%)	• TERT (83%) • PTCH1 (45%) • SMO (14%) • SUFU (8%) • MYCN (8%) • GLI2 (5%) • MLL2 • BCOR1 • LDB1 • GABRG1	• TP53	• GFI1/GFI1B (30%) • MYC (15%) • PVT1 (12%) • OTX2 (10%) • MLL2 • SMARCA4 • CHD7	• KDM6A (13%) • SNCAIP (10%) • MYCN (6%) • GFI1/GFI1B (8%) • OTX2 • DDX31 • CHD7 • CDK6 • MLL2 • MLL3 • ZMYM3
Chromosome	• chr 6 loss	• gain: chr 3q, 9p • loss: chr 9q, 10q, 14q, 17o		• Isochromosome 17q • gain: chr 1q, 7, 18q • loss: chr 5q, 10q, 16q, 17p	• Isochromosome 17q chr X loss • gain: chr 7, 18q • loss: chr 17p, 8, 10,11

68.5 Treatment and Prognosis

Genes with germline mutation	• APC	• PTCH1 • SUFU	• TP53	
Cells of origin	• Lower rhombic lip progenitors • Dorsal brain stem progenitors	• Cerebellar external granule cell layer or cochlear nuclei neuron precursors • Neural stem cells of subventricular zone	• Cerebellar external granule cell layer or cochlear nuclei neuron precursors • Neural stem cells of subventricular zone	• Neuron precursor cells of external granule cell layer • Prominin 1+/lineage neural stem cells	Upper rhombic lip progenitors

Table 68.4 Prognosis based on genetic and histologic type, after Ellison et al. (2016c)

Genetic profile	Histology	Prognosis
WNT-activated	Classic	Low risk tumor
	Large cell/anaplastic	Uncertain clinicopathological significance
SHH-activated TP53 mutant	Classic	Uncommon high risk tumor
	Large cell/anaplastic	High risk tumor
	Desmoplastic/nodular	Uncertain clinicopathological significance
SHH-activated TP53 wild-type	Classic	Standard risk tumor
	Large cell/anaplastic	Uncertain clinicopathological significance
	Desmoplastic/nodular	Low risk tumor
	Extensive nodularity	Low risk tumor
Non-WNT/non-SHH, group 3	Classic	Standard risk tumor
	Large cell/anaplastic	High risk tumor
Non-WNT/non-SHH, group 4	Classic	Standard risk tumor
	Large cell/anaplastic	Uncertain clinicopathological significance

- Poor quality of life associated with therapy-related side effects
  - Long-term physical impairment
  - Endocrine impairment
  - Intellectual and cognitive impairment
- At risk for secondary malignancies

Selected References

Archer TC, Mahoney EL, Pomeroy SL (2017) Medulloblastoma: molecular classification-based personal therapeutics. Neurotherapeutics 14(2):265–273. https://doi.org/10.1007/s13311-017-0526-y

Archer TC, Pomeroy SL (2012) Medulloblastoma biology in the post-genomic era. Future Oncol 8(12):1597–1604. https://doi.org/10.2217/fon.12.151

Aref D, Croul S (2013) Medulloblastoma: recurrence and metastasis. CNS Oncol 2(4):377–385. https://doi.org/10.2217/cns.13.30

Bartlett F, Kortmann R, Saran F (2013) Medulloblastoma. Clin Oncol (R Coll Radiol) 25(1):36–45. https://doi.org/10.1016/j.clon.2012.09.008

Bihannic L, Ayrault O (2016) Insights into cerebellar development and medulloblastoma. Bull Cancer 103(1):30–40. https://doi.org/10.1016/j.bulcan.2015.11.002

Coluccia D, Figuereido C, Isik S, Smith C, Rutka JT (2016) Medulloblastoma: tumor biology and relevance to treatment and prognosis paradigm. Curr Neurol Neurosci Rep 16(5):43. https://doi.org/10.1007/s11910-016-0644-7

Eberhart CG, Giangaspero F, Ellison DW, Haapasalo H, Pietsch T, Wiestler OD, Pfister S (2016) Medullolastoma, SHH-activated. In: Louis DN, Ohgaki H, Wiestler OD, Cavenee WK (eds) WHO classification of tumours of the central nervous system, Revised 4th edn. IARC, Lyon, pp 190–192

Ellison DW, Dalton J, Kocak M, Nicholson SL, Fraga C, Neale G, Kenney AM, Brat DJ, Perry A, Yong WH, Taylor RE, Bailey S, Clifford SC, Gilbertson RJ (2011) Medulloblastoma: clinicopathological correlates of SHH, WNT, and non-SHH/WNT molecular subgroups. Acta Neuropathol 121(3):381–396. https://doi.org/10.1007/s00401-011-0800-8

Ellison DW, Eberhart CG, Giangaspero F, Haapasalo H, Pietsch T, Wiestler OD, Pfister S (2016a) Medulloblastoma, classic. In: Louis DN, Ohgaki H, Wiestler OD, Cavenee WK (eds) WHO classification of tumours of the central nervous system, Revised 4th edn. IARC, Lyon, p 194

Ellison DW, Eberhart CG, Pfister S (2016b) Medulloblastoma, non-WNT/non-SHH. In: Louis DN, Ohgaki H, Wiestler OD, Cavenee WK (eds) WHO classification of tumours of the central nervous system, Revised 4th edn. IARC, Lyon, p 193

Ellison DW, Eberhart CG, Pietsch T, Pfister S (2016c) Medulloblastoma. In: Louis DN, Ohgaki H, Wiestler OD, Cavenee WK (eds) WHO classification of tumours of the central nervous system, Revised 4th edn. IARC, Lyon, pp 184–188

Ellison DW, Giangaspero F, Eberhart CG, Haapasalo H, Pietsch T, Wiestler OD, Pfister S (2016d) Large cell/anaplastic medulloblastoma. In: Louis DN, Ohgaki H, Wiestler OD, Cavenee WK (eds) WHO classification of tumours of the central nervous system, Revised 4th edn. IARC, Lyon, p 200

Ellison DW, Giangaspero F, Eberhart CG, Haapasalo H, Pietsch T, Wiestler OD, Pfister S (2016e) Medulloblastoma, WNT-activated. In: Louis DN, Ohgaki H, Wiestler OD, Cavenee WK (eds) WHO classification of tumours of the central nervous system, Revised 4th edn. IARC, Lyon, pp 188–189

Eran A, Ozturk A, Aygun N, Izbudak I (2010) Medulloblastoma: atypical CT and MRI findings in children. Pediatr Radiol 40(7):1254–1262. https://doi.org/10.1007/s00247-009-1429-9

Selected References

Gerber NU, Mynarek M, von Hoff K, Friedrich C, Resch A, Rutkowski S (2014) Recent developments and current concepts in medulloblastoma. Cancer Treat Rev 40(3):356–365. https://doi.org/10.1016/j.ctrv.2013.11.010

Giangaspero F, Bigner SH, Kleihues P, Pietsch T, Trojanowski JQ (2000) Medulloblastoma. In: Kleihues P, Cavenee WK (eds) Pathology and genetics of tumours of the nervous system, 3rd edn. IARC Press, Lyon, pp 129–137

Giangaspero F, Eberhart CG, Haapasalo H, Pietsch T, Wiestler OD, Ellison DW (2007) Medulloblastoma. In: Louis DN, Ohgaki H, Wiestler OD, Cavenee WK (eds) WHO classification of tumours of the central nervous system, 4th edn. International Agency for Research on Cancer, Lyon, pp 132–140

Giangaspero F, Ellison DW, Eberhart CG, Haapasalo H, Pietsch T, Wiestler OD, Pfister S (2016) Medulloblastoma with extensive nodularity. In: Louis DN, Ohgaki H, Wiestler OD, Cavenee WK (eds) WHO classification of tumours of the central nervous system, Revised 4th edn. IARC, Lyon, pp 198–199

Gopalakrishnan V, Tao RH, Dobson T, Brugmann W, Khatua S (2015) Medulloblastoma development: tumor biology informs treatment decisions. CNS Oncol 4(2):79–89. https://doi.org/10.2217/cns.14.58

Gupta T, Shirsat N, Jalali R (2015) Molecular subgrouping of medulloblastoma: impact upon research and clinical practice. Curr Pediatr Rev 11(2):106–119

Harris BT, Hattab EM (2013) Molecular pathology of the central nervous system. In: Cheng L, Eble JN (eds) Molecular surgical pathology. Springer Science+Business Media, New York, pp 357–405

Huang SY, Yang JY (2015) Targeting the hedgehog pathway in pediatric medulloblastoma. Cancers (Basel) 7(4):2110–2123. https://doi.org/10.3390/cancers7040880

Kijima N, Kanemura Y (2016) Molecular classification of medulloblastoma. Neurol Med Chir 56(11):687–697. https://doi.org/10.2176/nmc.ra.2016-0016

Kim W, Choy W, Dye J, Nagasawa D, Safaee M, Fong B, Yang I (2011) The tumor biology and molecular characteristics of medulloblastoma identifying prognostic factors associated with survival outcomes and prognosis. J Clin Neurosci 18(7):886–890. https://doi.org/10.1016/j.jocn.2011.01.001

Kleihues P, Burger PC, Scheithauer BW (1993) Histological typing of tumours of the central nervous system, 2nd edn. Springer, Berlin

Koeller KK, Rushing EJ (2003) From the archives of the AFIP: medulloblastoma: a comprehensive review with radiologic-pathologic correlation. Radiographics 23(6):1613–1637. https://doi.org/10.1148/rg.236035168

Li KK, Lau KM, Ng HK (2013a) Signaling pathway and molecular subgroups of medulloblastoma. Int J Clin Exp Pathol 6(7):1211–1222. Print 2013

Li KK, Lau KM, Ng HK (2013b) Signaling pathway and molecular subgroups of medulloblastoma. Int J Clin Exp Pathol 6(7):1211–1222

Martirosian V, Chen TC, Lin M, Neman J (2016) Medulloblastoma initiation and spread: where neurodevelopment, microenvironment and cancer cross pathways. J Neurosci Res 94(12):1511–1519. https://doi.org/10.1002/jnr.23917

Northcott PA, Dubuc AM, Pfister S, Taylor MD (2012a) Molecular subgroups of medulloblastoma. Expert Rev Neurother 12(7):871–884. https://doi.org/10.1586/ern.12.66

Northcott PA, Jones DT, Kool M, Robinson GW, Gilbertson RJ, Cho YJ, Pomeroy SL, Korshunov A, Lichter P, Taylor MD, Pfister SM (2012b) Medullomics: the end of the beginning. Nat Rev Cancer 12(12):818–834. https://doi.org/10.1038/nrc3410

Northcott PA, Korshunov A, Pfister SM, Taylor MD (2012c) The clinical implications of medulloblastoma subgroups. Nat Rev Neurol 8(6):340–351. https://doi.org/10.1038/nrneurol.2012.78

Pietsch T, Ellison DW, Haapasalo H, Giangaspero F, Wiestler OD, Pfister S, Eberhart CG (2016) Desmoplastic/nodular medulloblastoma. In: Louis DN, Ohgaki H, Wiestler OD, Cavenee WK (eds) WHO classification of tumours of the central nervous system, Revised 4th edn. IARC, Lyon, pp 195–197

Ramaswamy V, Taylor MD (2017) Medulloblastoma: from myth to molecular. J Clin Oncol 35(21):2355–2363. https://doi.org/10.1200/jco.2017.72.7842

Remke M, Ramaswamy V, Taylor MD (2013) Medulloblastoma molecular dissection: the way toward targeted therapy. Curr Opin Oncol 25(6):674–681. https://doi.org/10.1097/cco.0000000000000008

Roussel MF, Robinson GW (2013) Role of MYC in medulloblastoma. Cold Spring Harb Perspect Med 3(11):a014308. https://doi.org/10.1101/cshperspect.a014308

Rumboldt Z, Camacho DL, Lake D, Welsh CT, Castillo M (2006) Apparent diffusion coefficients for differentiation of cerebellar tumors in children. AJNR Am J Neuroradiol 27(6):1362–1369

Sabia A, Anger WH Jr (2015) Chemotherapy for children with medulloblastoma. Cancer Nurs 38(6):490–492. https://doi.org/10.1097/ncc.0000000000000296

Samkari A, White J, Packer R (2015a) SHH inhibitors for the treatment of medulloblastoma. Expert Rev Neurother 15(7):763–770. https://doi.org/10.1586/14737175.2015.1052796

Samkari A, White JC, Packer RJ (2015b) Medulloblastoma: toward biologically based management. Semin Pediatr Neurol 22(1):6–13. https://doi.org/10.1016/j.spen.2014.12.010

Schroeder K, Gururangan S (2014) Molecular variants and mutations in medulloblastoma. Pharmacogenomics Pers Med 7:43–51. https://doi.org/10.2147/pgpm.s38698

Skowron P, Ramaswamy V, Taylor MD (2015) Genetic and molecular alterations across medulloblastoma subgroups. J Mol Med (Berlin, Germany) 93(10):1075–1084. https://doi.org/10.1007/s00109-015-1333-8

Srinivasan VM, Ghali MG, North RY, Boghani Z, Hansen D, Lam S (2016) Modern management of medulloblastoma: molecular classification, outcomes, and the role of surgery. Surg Neurol Int 7(Suppl 44):S1135–s1141. https://doi.org/10.4103/2152-7806.196922

Taylor MD, Northcott PA, Korshunov A, Remke M, Cho YJ, Clifford SC, Eberhart CG, Parsons DW, Rutkowski S, Gajjar A, Ellison DW, Lichter P, Gilbertson RJ, Pomeroy SL, Kool M, Pfister SM (2012) Molecular subgroups of medulloblastoma: the current consensus. Acta Neuropathol 123(4):465–472. https://doi.org/10.1007/s00401-00011-00922-z. Epub 02011 Dec 00402

Vidal DO, Marques MM, Lopes LF, Reis RM (2013) The role of microRNAs in medulloblastoma. Pediatr Hematol Oncol 30(5):367–378. https://doi.org/10.3109/08880018.2013.783890

Vriend J, Marzban H (2017) The ubiquitin-proteasome system and chromosome 17 in cerebellar granule cells and medulloblastoma subgroups. Cell Mol Life Sci: CMLS 74(3):449–467. https://doi.org/10.1007/s00018-016-2354-3

Yeom KW, Mobley BC, Lober RM, Andre JB, Partap S, Vogel H, Barnes PD (2013) Distinctive MRI features of pediatric medulloblastoma subtypes. AJR Am J Roentgenol 200(4):895–903. https://doi.org/10.2214/ajr.12.9249

Zülch KJ (1979) Histological typing of tumours of the central nervous system. World Health Organization, Geneva

Embryonal Tumors: Other CNS Embryonal Tumors

Tumors of Neuroepithelial Tissue: Embryonal Tumors

69.1 General Aspects

The classification of embryonal tumors led over the last decades to various, partly contradictory and non-conclusive systems. The classification of these tumors still remains in flow and will change based on the acquisition of new molecular insight.

Currently, four major tumor categories should be distinguished as follows:

- Medulloblastoma.
- Embryonal tumor with multilayered rosettes (ETMR), C19MC-altered
- Embryonal tumor with multilayered rosettes, NOS
- Other CNS embryonal tumors
  – Medulloepithelioma
  – CNS neuroblastoma
  – CNS ganglioneuroblastoma
  – CNS embryonal tumor (NOS)
- Atypical teratoid/rhabdoid tumor (AT/RT)
- CNS embryonal tumor with rhabdoid features

A glimpse into a further molecular classification of "Other CNS embryonal tumors" is given by Sturm et al. (2016) as follows:

- CNS neuroblastoma with *FOXR2* activation (CNS NB-*FOXR2*)
- CNS Ewing sarcoma family tumor with *CIC* alteration (CNS EFT-*CIC*)
- CNS high-grade neuroepithelial tumor with *MN1* alteration (CNS HGNET-*MN1*)
- CNS high-grade neuroepithelial tumor with *BCOR* alterations (CNS HGNET-*BCOR*)

WHO Definition
2016—Embryonal tumor with multilayered rosettes, C19MC-altered: An aggressive CNS embryonal tumor with multilayered rosettes and alterations (including amplification and fusions) in the C19MC locus at 19q13.42 (Korshunov et al. 2016).

Embryonal tumor with multilayered rosettes, NOS: An aggressive CNS embryonal tumor with multilayered rosettes, in which copy number at the 19q13 C19MC locus either shows no alteration or has not been tested (Korshunov et al. 2016).

Other CNS embryonal tumors: A group of rare, poorly differentiated embryonal neoplasms of neuroectodermal origin that lack the specific histopathological features or molecular alterations that define other CNS tumors (McLendon et al. 2016).

Medulloepithelioma: A CNS embryonal tumor with a prominent pseudostratified neuroepithelium that resembles the embryonic neural tube in addition to poorly differentiated neuroepithelial cells (McLendon et al. 2016).

CNS neuroblastoma: A CNS embryonal tumor characterized by poorly differentiated neuroepithelial cells, groups of neurocytic cells, and a variable neuropil-rich stroma (McLendon et al. 2016).

CNS ganglioneuroblastoma: A CNS embryonal tumor characterized by poorly differentiated neuroepithelial cells and groups of neurocytic and ganglion cells (McLendon et al. 2016).

CNS embryonal tumor, NOS: A rare poorly differentiated embryonal neoplasm of neuroectodermal origin that lacks the specific histopathological features or molecular alterations that define other CNS tumors (McLendon et al. 2016).

2007—A heterogeneous group of tumors occurring predominantly in children and adolescents. They may arise in the cerebral hemispheres, brain stem, or spinal cord, and are composed of undifferentiated cells which may display divergent differentiation along neuronal, astrocytic, and ependymal lines. CNS/supratentorial PNET is an embryonal tumor composed of undifferentiated or poorly differentiated neuroepithelial cells. Tumors with only neuronal differentiation are termed cerebral neuroblastomas or, if ganglion cells are also present, cerebral ganglioneuroblastomas. Tumors that recreate features of neural tube formation are termed medulloepitheliomas. Tumors with ependymoblastic rosettes are termed ependymoblastomas. Features common to all CNS PNET variants include early-onset and aggressive clinical behavior (McLendon et al. 2007).

2000—Medulloepithelioma: A rare, malignant embryonal brain tumor affecting young children, histologically characterized by papillary, tubular, or trabecular arrangements of neoplastic neuroepithelium mimicking the embryonic neural tube (Becker et al. 2000).

Ependymoblastoma: A rare, malignant, embryonal brain tumor manifesting in neonates and young children, histologically characterized by distinctive multilayered rosettes (Becker and Cruz-Sanchez 2000).

1993—Neuroblastoma
A rare, malignant embryonal tumor composed of neuroblasts or cells with limited neuronal differentiation (Kleihues et al. 1993).

1993—Ganglioneuroblastoma
A neuroblastoma with focally advanced neuronal differentiation, including mature ganglion cells (Kleihues et al. 1993).

69.2 CNS Embryonal Tumor, NOS

WHO Definition
2016—CNS embryonal tumor, NOS: A rare poorly differentiated embryonal neoplasm of neuroectodermal origin that lacks the specific histopathological features or molecular alterations that define other CNS tumors (McLendon et al. 2016).

2007—An embryonal tumor composed of undifferentiated or poorly differentiated neuroepithelial cells which have the capacity for, or display, divergent differentiation along neuronal, astrocytic, muscular, or melanocytic lines. Tumors with only neuronal differentiation are termed cerebral neuroblastoma or, if ganglion cells are also present, ganglioneuroblastomas (McLendon et al. 2007).

2000—An embryonal tumor in the cerebrum or suprasellar region composed of undifferentiated or poorly differentiated neuroepithelial cells which have the capacity for or display divergent differentiation along neuronal, astrocytic, ependymal, muscular, or melanocytic lines. Tumors with a distinct neuronal differentiation are termed *cerebral neuroblastoma* or, if ganglion cells are also present, ganglioneuroblastoma (Rorke et al. 2000).

1993—Small cell, malignant tumors of childhood with predominant location in the cerebellum and a noted capacity for divergent differentiation, including neuronal, astrocytic, ependymal, muscular, and melanotic (Kleihues et al. 1993).

WHO Grade
- WHO grade IV

69.2 CNS Embryonal Tumor, NOS

69.2.1 Epidemiology

Incidence
- Rare
- 1% of pediatric CNS neuroepithelial tumors

Age Incidence
- Young age
  - Mean age: 5.5 years
  - Range: 4 weeks to 20 years

Sex Incidence
- Male:Female ratio: 1.2:1

Localization
- Cerebrum
- Spinal cord
- Suprasellar region

69.2.2 Neuroimaging Findings

General Imaging Findings
- Large heterogeneous, enhancing mass with variable morphology, exclude CSF spreading.

CT non-contrast-enhanced
- Heterogeneous, iso- to hypodense
- Hemorrhages, necrosis, and calcifications are common

CT contrast-enhanced
- Heterogeneous enhancement

MRI-T2 (Fig. 69.1a)
- Heterogeneous
- Solid iso- to slight hyperintense components
- Hyperintense cysts

MRI-FLAIR (Fig. 69.1b)
- Hyperintense solid components
- Moderate peritumoral edema

MRI-T1 (Fig. 69.1c)
- Iso- to hypointense

MRI-T1 Contrast-Enhanced (Fig. 69.1d)
- Heterogeneous enhancement

MRI-T2∗/SWI
- Common calcifications and hemorrhages appear hypointense

MR-Diffusion Imaging
- Restricted diffusion

MRI-Perfusion (Fig. 69.1e)
- Elevated rCBV

MR-Spectroscopy (Fig. 69.1f, g)
- NAA strongly reduced
- Choline elevated
- Lipid and lactate peaks

Nuclear Medicine Imaging Findings
- FDG can show hypermetabolism (although hypometabolism has been described).
- Usually positive in FET-PET.
- Hypoxia tracers are under investigation for radiotherapy planning.
- Due to the positive somatostatin receptor status of PNETs, imaging methods like SSR-scan or SSR-PET can be used to differentiate them from gliomas

69.2.3 Neuropathology Findings

Macroscopic Features (Fig. 69.2a–d)
- Soft to firm mass
- Variable size
- Variably well demarcated from brain tissue
- Pinkish-red to purple color
- Cyst formation possible
- Hemorrhages possible

Microscopic Features (Fig. 69.3a–f)
- Poorly differentiated cells with
  - Round regular nuclei
  - High nuclear: cytoplasmic ratio
- Some cells might show neuronal differentiation
  - Elongated nuclei with vesicular chromatin
  - Processes
  - Nissl substance

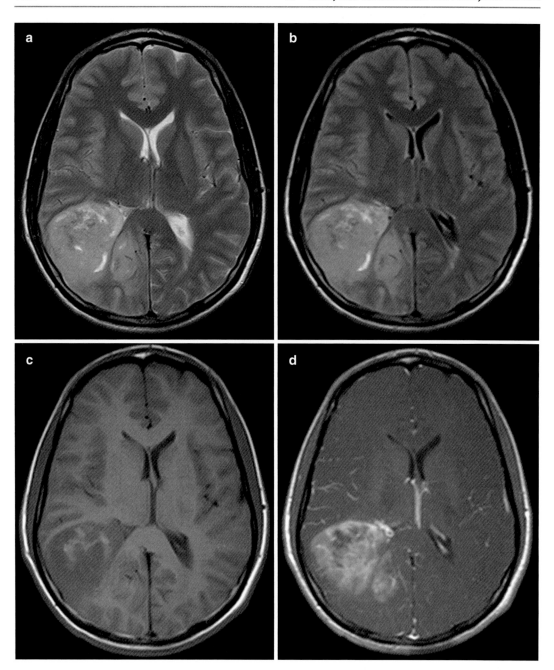

Fig. 69.1 CNS embryonal tumor with heterogeneous signal in T2(**a**) and FLAIR (**b**); T1 (**c**) reflects intratumoral hemorrhage with methemoglobin, irregular enhancement in T1 contrast (**d**) and elevated CBV (**e**), malignant tumor-specific MR-spectroscopy (**f**, **g**)

69.2 CNS Embryonal Tumor, NOS 1633

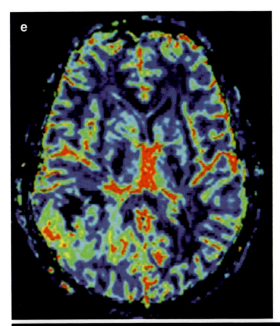

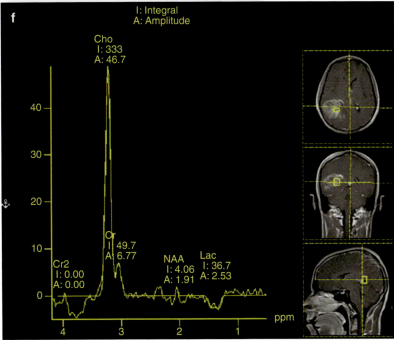

Fig. 69.1 (continued)

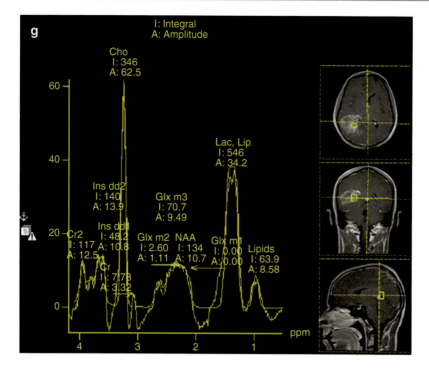

Fig. 69.1 (continued)

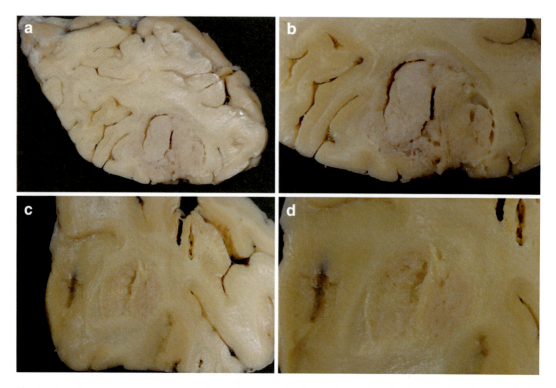

Fig. 69.2 Autopsy specimen of a CNS embryonal tumor presenting as a large, soft to firm mass of grayish-white color which is quite well demarcated from brain tissue (**a–d**). Infiltration into the leptomeningeal spaces (**a, b**) and necrosis (**b, d**) formation are conspicuous

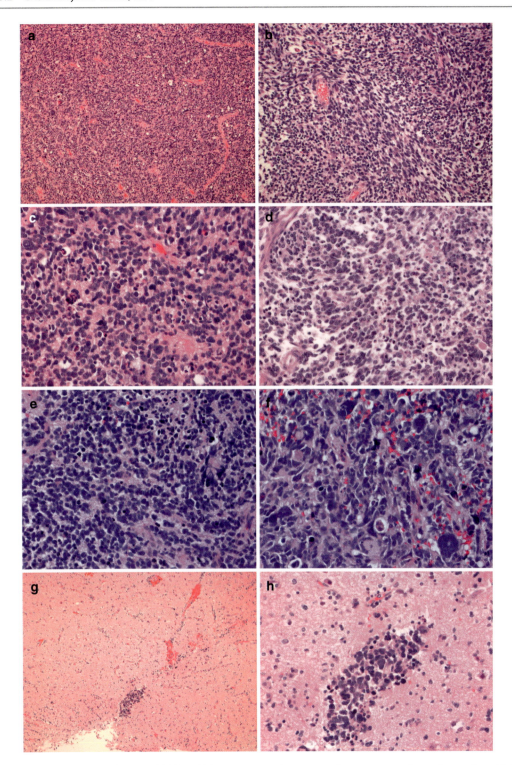

Fig. 69.3 CNS embryonal tumor: highly cellular tumor with partly papillary, tubular, or trabecular arrangements of tumor cells. The tumor cells are of columnar to cuboidal shape with oval to piloid nuclei, perpendicular to the inner and outer surfaces, coarse chromatin, and multiple nucleoli (**a–f**). A focus of tumor cells solitarily located within the brain tissue (**g, h**)

- Fibrous stroma
- Homer Wright rosettes
- Arrangement of tumor cells in parallel streams and palisades
- Calcifications

Immunophenotype (Fig. 69.4a–h)
- Positive for:
  - Synaptophysin
  - Class III β-tubulin
  - Neurofilament
  - S-100
  - NSE

Proliferation Markers
- High mitotic activity
- KI-67 LI: range: 0–80%

Ultrastructural Features
- Poorly differentiated tumor cell
  - Sparse cytoplasmic organelles
  - Presence of dense core vesicles

Differential Diagnosis
- Peripheral primitive neuroectodermal tumor (Ewing sarcoma)
- High-grade astrocytoma with PNET-like component
- Medulloblastoma
- Anaplastic ependymoma
- Anaplastic oligodendroglioma
- Metastatic small cell carcinoma
- Neurocytoma
- Olfactory neuroblastoma

69.2.4 Molecular Neuropathology

Pathogenesis
- Origin from primitive neuroepithelial cells

69.2.5 Treatment and Prognosis

Treatment
- Surgical removal
- Chemotherapy
- Radiotherapy

Biologic Behavior–Prognosis–Prognostic Factors
- Poor prognosis especially in children under age 2

69.3 Embryonal Tumors with Multilayered Rosettes, C19MC-Altered

WHO Definition
2016—Embryonal tumor with multilayered rosettes, C19MC-altered: An aggressive CNS embryonal tumor with multilayered rosettes and alterations (including amplification and fusions) in the C19MC locus at 19q13.42 (Korshunov et al. 2016).

WHO Grade
- WHO grade IV

69.3.1 Epidemiology

Incidence
- Rare

Age Incidence
- Children aged <4 years

Sex Incidence
- Male:Female ratio: 1:1

Localization
- Supratentorial
  - Cerebral hemispheres (70% of cases)
    - Frontal lobes
    - Parieto-occipital
- Infratentorial (30% of cases)
  - Cerebellum
  - Brain stem

69.3.2 Neuropathology Findings

Macroscopic Features
- Well delineated
- Grayish-pink

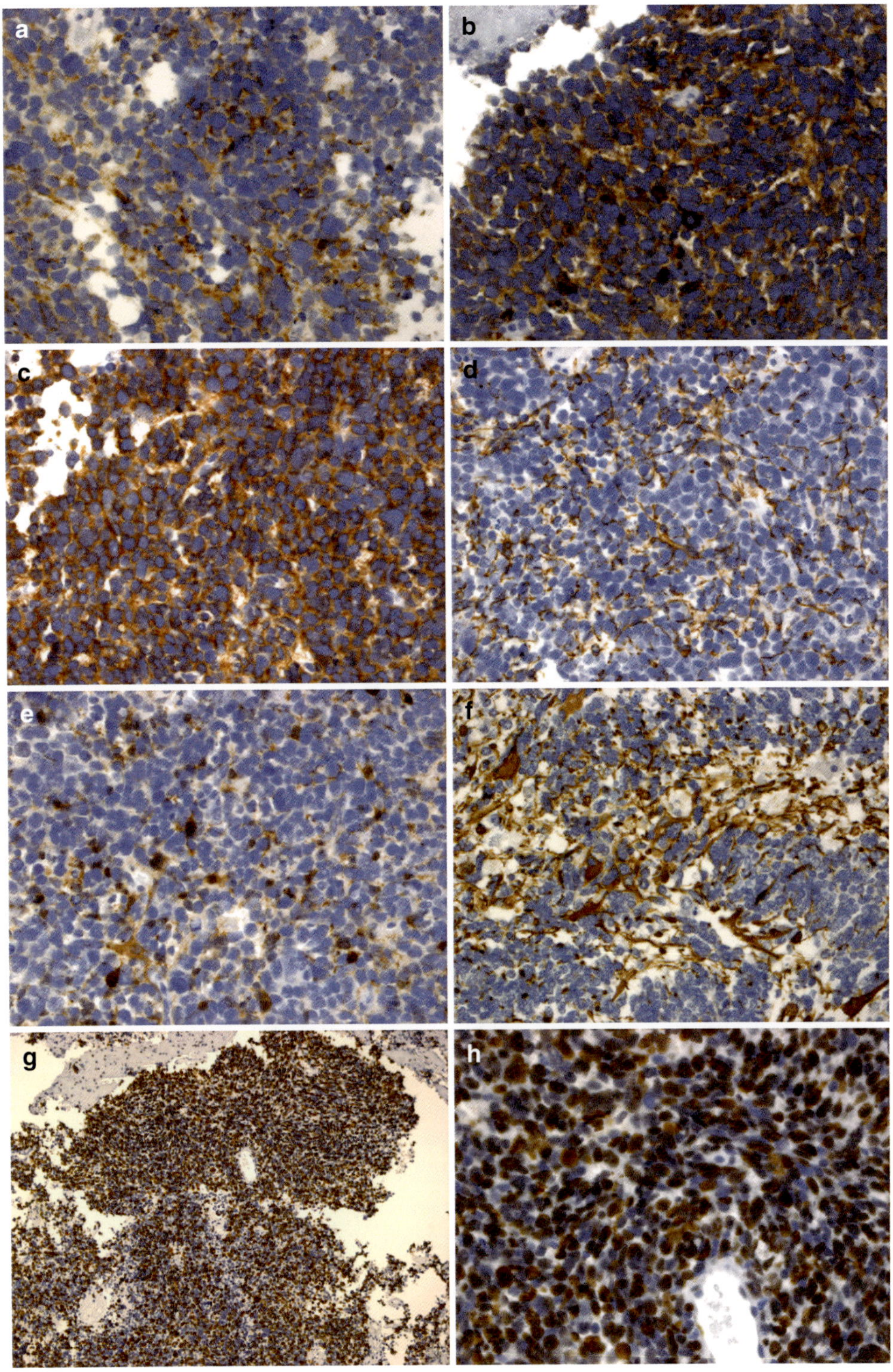

Fig. 69.4 CNS embryonal tumor—Immunophenotype: the tumor cells are positive for neuronal markers synaptophysin (**a**), neuron-specific enolase (NSE) (**b**), microtubule-associated protein (MAP) (**c**). Glial cell elements stain for GFAP (**d**), S-100 (**e**), and vimentin (**f**). High Ki-67 proliferation index (**g**, **h**)

- Possible changes
  - Necrosis
  - Hemorrhage
  - Calcifications
  - Cysts

Microscopic Features

The general histologic characterization of embryonal tumors with multilayered rosettes is as follows:
- Biphasic pattern
  - Cellular areas
    - Small, blue, round cells typical of primitive blast cells
    - Numerous mitoses
    - Apoptosis
  - Paucicellular, neuropil-rich areas
    - Contain same blast cells
    - Large, more differentiated neuronal cells
- Numerous, multilayered rosettes
  - Cells with marked anaplastic nuclear features
  - Mitosis
  - Apoptosis
- Ependymoblastoma pattern
  - Poorly differentiated cells
  - Numerous multilayered rosettes
  - Lack of
    - neuropil-like matrix
    - ganglion cell elements
- Medulloepithelioma pattern
  - Papillary, tubular, and trabecular arrangements of neoplastic pseudostratified epithelium

Ultrastructural Features
- Large nuclei
- Scant cytoplasm
- Few organelles
- Rosette-forming cells show
  - Junctional complexes
  - Abortive cilia
  - Basal bodies at an apical site

Immunophenotype
- A list of antibodies with positive or negative immunostaining results is given in Table 69.1.

Table 69.1 Immunophenotype of embryonal tumors with multilayered rosettes, C19MC-altered

Positivity	Negativity

• Neuroepithelial component
  – Nestin
  – Vimentin
  – Cytokeratins
  – EMA
  – CD99
• Neuropil-like areas
  – Synaptophysin
  – Neurofilament
  – NeuN
	• Neuroepithelial component
	  – Neuronal markers
	  – Glial markers

Proliferation Markers
- High
- Ki-67 LI: 20–80%

Differential Diagnosis
- Peripheral primitive neuroectodermal tumor (Ewing sarcoma)
- High-grade astrocytoma with PNET-like component
- Medulloblastoma
- Anaplastic ependymoma
- Anaplastic oligodendroglioma
- Metastatic small cell carcinoma
- Neurocytoma
- Olfactory neuroblastoma

69.3.3 Molecular Neuropathology

Pathogenesis
- Primitive cell population in the subventricular zone

Molecular Findings
- Gains of chromosomes
  - 2, 7q, 11q
- Loss of chromosomes
  - 6q
- Molecular marker
  - Amplicon at 19q13.42
    - Cluster of microRNA, C19MC
    - Upregulated in tumor

69.3.4 Treatment and Prognosis

Treatment
- Surgery
- Chemotherapy
- Radiotherapy

Biologic Behavior–Prognosis–Prognostic Factors
- Poor
- Rapid growth
- Aggressive clinical course
- Survival time: 12 months
- Local tumor regrowth
- Widespread tumor dissemination

69.4 Medulloepithelioma

WHO Definition

2016—A CNS embryonal tumor with a prominent pseudostratified neuroepithelium that resembles the embryonic neural tube in addition to poorly differentiated neuroepithelial cells (McLendon et al. 2016).

2007—A rare, malignant embryonal brain tumor affecting young children, histologically characterized by papillary, tubular, or trabecular arrangements of neoplastic neuroepithelium mimicking the embryonic neural tube (McLendon et al. 2007).

2000—A rare, malignant embryonal brain tumor affecting young children, histologically characterized by papillary, tubular, or trabecular arrangements of neoplastic neuroepithelium mimicking the embryonic neural tube (Becker et al. 2000).

1993—A very rare, malignant, embryonal tumor resembling primitive medullary epithelium of the neural tube.

69.4.1 Epidemiology

Incidence
- Rare

Age Incidence
- Young age
  - Mean age: 45 months.
  - Range: 5 months to 23 years

Sex Incidence
- Male:Female ratio: 1:1

Localization
- Supra- and infratentorial compartments
- Cerebral hemispheres
  - Periventricular
  - Frequency: temporal, parietal, occipital, frontal lobes
- Intraventricular
- Sellar/parasellar region
- Cauda equina
- Intraorbital and optic nerve

69.4.2 Neuropathology Findings

Macroscopic Features
- Large tumors
- Well demarcated from brain tissue
- Soft to firm mass
- Grayish-pink color
- Infiltration into the leptomeningeal spaces
- Necrosis formation possible
- Hemorrhages possible

Microscopic Features
- Mimic embryonal neural tube
- Papillary, tubular, or trabecular arrangements of tumor cells in the form of a pseudostratified epithelium
- Various lines of differentiation: neural, glial, and mesenchymal
- No cilia or blepharoplasts on the luminal marginal surface
- PAS and collagen type IV positive external limiting membrane on the outer epithelial surface
- Tumor cells
  - Columnar to cuboidal shape
  - Oval to piloid nuclei, perpendicular to the inner and outer surfaces
  - Coarse chromatin
  - Multiple nucleoli

- Abundant mitoses
- Calcifications

Immunophenotype
- Positive for:
  - Nestin (basal areas)
  - Vimentin
  - Synaptophysin
  - NSE
  - MAP
  - GFAP
  - Rarely:
    - Neurofilament
    - Cytokeratins
    - EMA
    - Basic fibroblast growth factor
    - Insulin-like growth factor 1

Proliferation Markers
- High mitotic activity
- KI-67 LI: range: 0–80%

Ultrastructural Features
- Poorly differentiated tumor cells
  - Sparse cytoplasmic organelles
  - Absence of cilia and microvilli
- Neuroepitheliomatous areas
  - Primitive lateral zonulae adherentes
  - Basal lamina on the outer surface of epithelial cells
- Luminal side
  - Amorphous surface coating

Differential Diagnosis
- Peripheral primitive neuroectodermal tumor (Ewing sarcoma)
- High-grade astrocytoma with PNET-like component
- Medulloblastoma
- Anaplastic ependymoma
- Anaplastic oligodendroglioma
- Metastatic small cell carcinoma
- Neurocytoma
- Olfactory neuroblastoma

69.4.3 Molecular Neuropathology

Pathogenesis
- Derivation from a primitive cell population in the subependymal region

69.4.4 Treatment and Prognosis

Treatment
- Surgical removal
- Radiation therapy

Biologic Behavior–Prognosis–Prognostic Factors
- Rapid growing tumor
- Poor prognosis
- Cerebrospinal fluid dissemination
- Death within 1 year after diagnosis

Selected References

Alelu-Paz R, Ropero S (2013) New gene signatures for pediatric brain tumors: a step forward in the understanding of molecular basis of CNS PNET. Transl Pediatr 2(1):3–4. https://doi.org/10.3978/j.issn.2224-4336.2012.10.02

Becker LE, Cruz-Sanchez FF (2000) Ependymoblastom. In: Kleihues P, Cavenee WK (eds) Pathology and genetics of tumours of the nervous system, 3rd edn. IARC Press, Lyon, pp 127–128

Becker LE, Sharma MC, Rorke LB (2000) Medulloepithelioma. In: Kleihues P, Cavenee WK (eds) Pathology and genetics of tumours of the nervous system, 3rd edn. IARC Press, Lyon, pp 124–126

Kleihues P, Burger PC, Scheithauer BW (1993) Histological typing of tumours of the central nervous system, 2nd edn. Springer, Berlin

Korshunov A, McLendon R, Judkins AR, Pfister S, Eberhart CG, Fuller GN, Sarkar C, Ng H-K, Huang A, Kool M, Wesseling P (2016) Embryonal tumour with multilayered rosettes, C19MC-altered. In: Louis DN, Ohgaki H, Wiestler OD, Cavenee WK (eds) WHO classification of tumours of the central nervous system, Revised 4th edn. IARC, Lyon, pp 201–205

Massimino M, Gandola L, Biassoni V, Spreafico F, Schiavello E, Poggi G, Pecori E, Vajna De Pava M, Modena P, Antonelli M, Giangaspero F (2013) Evolving of therapeutic strategies for CNS-

PNET. Pediatr Blood Cancer 60(12):2031–2035. https://doi.org/10.1002/pbc.24540

McLendon R, Judkins AR, Eberhart CG, Fuller GN, Sarkar C, Ng H-K (2007) Central nervous system primitive neuroectodermal tumours. In: Louis DN, Ohgaki H, Wiestler OD, Cavenee WK (eds) WHO classification of tumours of the central nervous system, 4th edn. International Agency for Research on Cancer, Lyon, pp 141–146

McLendon R, Judkins AR, Eberhart CG, Fuller GN, Sarkar C, Ng H-K, Huang A, Kool M, Pfister S (2016) Other CNS embryonal tumours. In: Louis DN, Ohgaki H, Wiestler OD, Cavenee WK (eds) WHO classification of tumours of the central nervous system, Revised 4th edn. IARC, Lyon, pp 206–208

Rogers HA, Miller S, Lowe J, Brundler MA, Coyle B, Grundy RG (2009) An investigation of WNT pathway activation and association with survival in central nervous system primitive neuroectodermal tumours (CNS PNET). Br J Cancer 100(8):1292–1302. https://doi.org/10.1038/sj.bjc.6604979

Rorke LB, Hart MN, McLendon RE (2000) Supratentorial primitive neuroectodermal tumour (PNET). In: Kleihues P, Cavenee WK (eds) Pathology and genetics of tumours of the nervous system, 3rd edn. IARC Press, Lyon, pp 141–144

Sturm D, Orr BA, Toprak UH, Hovestadt V, Jones DT, Capper D, Sill M, Buchhalter I, Northcott PA, Leis I, Ryzhova M, Koelsche C, Pfaff E, Allen SJ, Balasubramanian G, Worst BC, Pajtler KW, Brabetz S, Johann PD, Sahm F, Reimand J, Mackay A, Carvalho DM, Remke M, Phillips JJ, Perry A, Cowdrey C, Drissi R, Fouladi M, Giangaspero F, Lastowska M, Grajkowska W, Scheurlen W, Pietsch T, Hagel C, Gojo J, Lotsch D, Berger W, Slavc I, Haberler C, Jouvet A, Holm S, Hofer S, Prinz M, Keohane C, Fried I, Mawrin C, Scheie D, Mobley BC, Schniederjan MJ, Santi M, Buccoliero AM, Dahiya S, Kramm CM, von Bueren AO, von Hoff K, Rutkowski S, Herold-Mende C, Fruhwald MC, Milde T, Hasselblatt M, Wesseling P, Rossler J, Schuller U, Ebinger M, Schittenhelm J, Frank S, Grobholz R, Vajtai I, Hans V, Schneppenheim R, Zitterbart K, Collins VP, Aronica E, Varlet P, Puget S, Dufour C, Grill J, Figarella-Branger D, Wolter M, Schuhmann MU, Shalaby T, Grotzer M, van Meter T, Monoranu CM, Felsberg J, Reifenberger G, Snuderl M, Forrester LA, Koster J, Versteeg R, Volckmann R, van Sluis P, Wolf S, Mikkelsen T, Gajjar A, Aldape K, Moore AS, Taylor MD, Jones C, Jabado N, Karajannis MA, Eils R, Schlesner M, Lichter P, von Deimling A, Pfister SM, Ellison DW, Korshunov A, Kool M (2016) New brain tumor entities emerge from molecular classification of CNS-PNETs. Cell 164(5):1060–1072. https://doi.org/10.1016/j.cell.2016.01.015

von Bueren AO (2012) CNS PNET molecular subgroups with distinct clinical features. Lancet Oncol 13(8):753–754. https://doi.org/10.1016/s1470-2045(12)70260-7

Embryonal Tumors: Atypical Teratoid/Rhabdoid Tumor (ATRT)

Embryonal Tumors

WHO Definition

2016—A malignant CNS embryonal tumor composed predominantly of poorly differentiated elements and frequently including rhabdoid cells, with inactivation of SMARCB1 (INI1) or (extremely rarely) SMARCA4 (BRG1) (Judkins et al. 2016).

2007—A highly malignant CNS tumor predominantly manifesting in young children, typically containing rhabdoid cells, often with primitive neuroectodermal cells and with divergent differentiation along epithelial, mesenchymal, neuronal, or glial lines; associated with inactivation of the *INI1/hSNF5* gene in virtually all cases (Judkins et al. 2007).

2000—A malignant embryonal CNS tumor manifesting in children and composed of rhabdoid cells, with or without fields resembling a classical primitive neuroectodermal tumor (PNET), epithelial tissue, and neoplastic mesenchyme (Rorke and Biegel 2000).

WHO grade
- WHO grade IV

70.1 Epidemiology

Incidence
- 1–2% of pediatric tumors
- 10% of CNS tumors in infants

Age Incidence
- Mean age: 2 years
- Usually under the age of 3 years

Sex Incidence
- Male:Female ratio: 1.8:1

Localization
- Cerebral hemispheres
- Ventricular system
- Suprasellar region or pineal gland
- Cerebellar hemispheres
- Brain stem
- Spinal cord

70.2 Neuroimaging Findings

General Imaging Findings
- Heterogeneous mass with cysts, calcifications, and necroses. Hydrocephalus is frequent.

CT non-contrast-enhanced
- Heterogeneous, hyperdense to isodense
- Calcifications possible

CT contrast-enhanced
- Heterogeneous enhancement

MRI-T2 (Fig. 70.1a)
- Heterogeneous
- Hyperintense cysts

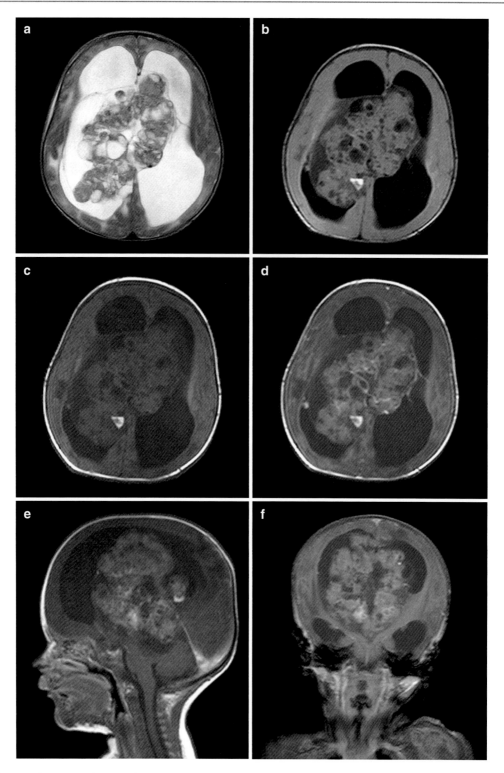

Fig. 70.1 Large central ATRT with heterogeneous signal in T2 (**a**) and FLAIR (**b**); T1 (**c**) and T1 contrast (**d–f**) causing a hydrocephalus

MRI-FLAIR (Fig. 70.1b)
- Heterogeneous
- Minimal to moderate peritumoral edema

MRI-T1 (Fig. 70.1c)
- Heterogeneous

MRI-T1 contrast-enhanced (Fig. 70.1d–f)
- Strong heterogeneous enhancement
- CSF and leptomeningeal dissemination

MRI-T2∗/SWI
- Hypointense calcifications and hemorrhages are common.

MR-Diffusion Imaging
- Restricted diffusion

MRI-Perfusion
- Elevated rCBV

MR-Spectroscopy
- NAA and Cr strongly reduced, Cho elevated, lipid and lactate peaks

Nuclear Medicine Imaging Findings
- FDG can show hypermetabolism.
- FDG-PET can be used to assess the damage to healthy brain tissue.
- Amino acid tracers are usually positive.
- Hypoxia tracers are under investigation for radiotherapy planning.

70.3 Neuropathology Findings

Macroscopic Features (Fig. 70.2a–d)
- Soft to firm in consistency
- Pinkish-red to tan-white
- Demarcated from surrounding parenchyma
- Necrotic foci
- Hemorrhages

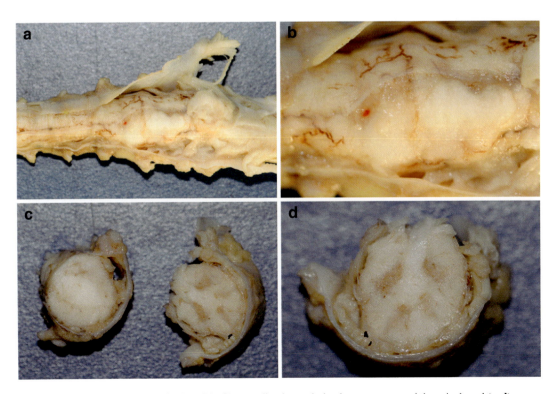

Fig. 70.2 ATRT involving the spinal cord (**a**, **b**) extending beneath the dura mater around the spinal cord (**c**, **d**)

Microscopic Features (Fig. 70.3a–f)
- Cells with classic rhabdoid features:
  - eccentrically placed nucleus with vesicular chromatin
  - prominent eosinophilic nucleoli
  - abundant cytoplasm with eosinophilic globular inclusions
  - well-defined cell borders
- Variable components make up the tumor:
  - Small cell embryonal
  - Primitive neuroectodermal
  - Mesenchymal
  - Epithelial

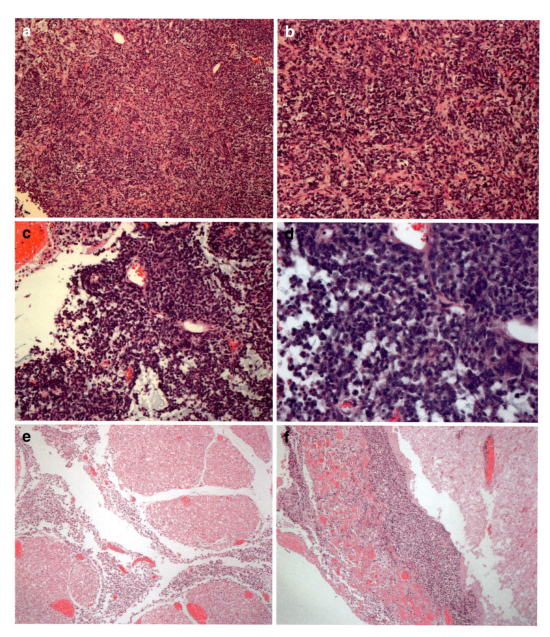

Fig. 70.3 Highly cellular tumor (**a–d**). The tumor cells display classic rhabdoid features with an eccentrically placed nucleus, vesicular chromatin, prominent eosinophilic nucleoli, abundant cytoplasm, and well-defined cell borders. Infiltration of tumor cells into the nerve root area (**e, f**)

70.3 Neuropathology Findings

Immunophenotype (Fig. 70.4a–h)
- Absence of INI1 expression (diagnostic hallmark) (98% of cases)
- Polyphenotypic differentiation along neuroectodermal, epithelial, and mesenchymal lines

A list of antibodies with positive or negative immunostaining results is given in Table 70.1.

Proliferation Markers (Figs. 70.4i, j)
- High mitotic activity
- Ki-67 LI: 50–100%

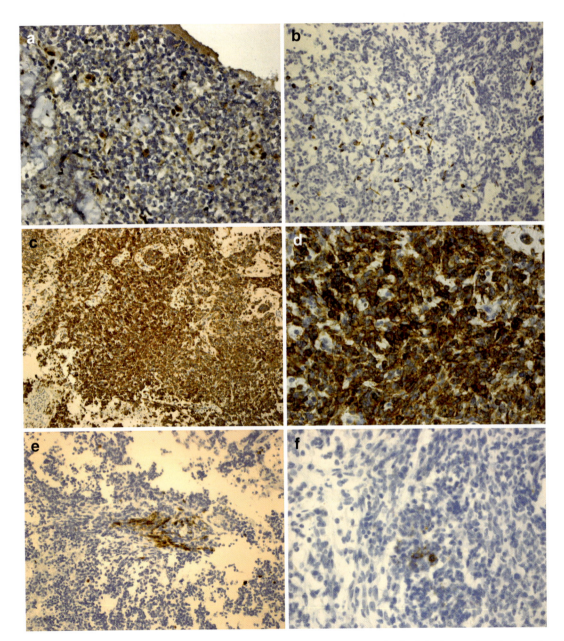

Fig. 70.4 The tumor cells are characteristically negative of INI (**a**), a few cells express GFAP (**b**), numerous cells are positive for MAP 2 (**c**, **d**). Rare reactivities for S100 (**e**) and synaptophysin (**f**). Only the vessels stain for actin (**g**, **h**). The tumor is highly proliferative (Ki67) (**i**, **j**)

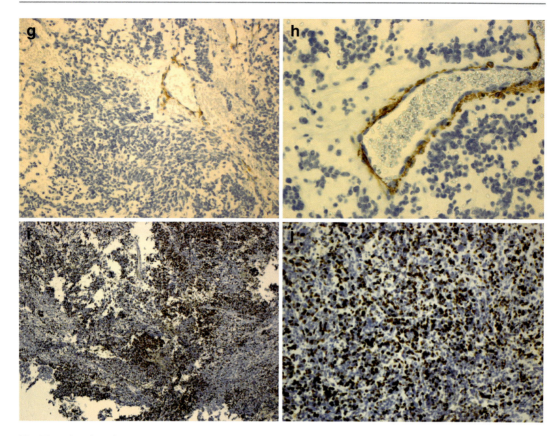

Fig. 70.4 (continued)

Table 70.1 Immunophenotype of atypical teratoid/rhabdoid tumor (ATRT)

Positivity	Negativity
• EMA (95% of cases) • SMA (75% of cases) • Vimentin • GFAP • Neurofilament • Synaptophysin • Keratins	• INI *(diagnostic hallmark!)* • Germ cell markers

Ultrastructural Features
- whorled bundles of intermediate filaments

Differential Diagnosis
- Primitive neuroectodermal tumor (PNET)
- Glioblastoma (GBM)
- Medulloblastoma
- Metastatic carcinoma

70.4 Molecular Neuropathology

Pathogenesis
- Derivation from pluripotent fetal cells

Molecular Findings
- Mutation or loss of INI1 (hSNF5/SMARCB1) locus on chromosome 22q11.2
- Hallmark of AT/RT
- INI1 protein
  - Component of the SWI/SNF complex
  - Alters chromatin structure in an ATP-dependent manner
  - Acts in part via the p16-Rb-E2F and p53-dependent pathways
- Inactivation of SMARCA4 (BRG1)
- Three epigenetic subgroups (Table 70.2):
  - TYR
  - SHH
  - MYC

Table 70.2 Three epigenetic subgroups with distinct enhancer landscapes, modified after Johann et al. (2016) data reproduced with kind permission by Elsevier

	TYR	SHH	MYC
Localization	• Supratentorial 23.4% • Infratentorial 76.6%	• Supratentorial 54.1% • Infratentorial 45.9%	• Supratentorial 61.1% • Infratentorial 38.9%
Gender distribution	• F: 53.9% • M: 46.1%	• F: 41% • M: 59%	• F: 44% • M: 56%
Type of SMARCB1 deletion	• 22q loss: 77% • No aberration: 11% • Focal deletion: 10% • Focal aberration: 2%	• 22q loss: 20% • No aberration: 47% • Focal deletion: 10% • Focal aberration: 23%	• 22q loss: 7% • No aberration: 3% • Focal deletion: 45% • Focal aberration: 45%
Upregulated pathways or drug targets	• Melanogenesis • EZH2 • DNMTs • CCND1 • VEGFA • ERBB2	• SHH pathway • EZH2 • DNMTs • CDK6	• MYC • HOX genes • EZH2 • DNMTs • ERBB2
Methylation	• Hypermethylation • No PMDS	• Hypermethylation • Few PMDs	• Hypomethylation • Many PMDs
Subgroup specific enhancers	• TR • MITF • CCND1	• GLI2 • PTCH2	• MYC • HOXC
Enrichment of transcription factors	• OTX2 • LMX1A	• GLI2 • FOXK1	• MYC • REST
Network analyses	• Feedback loop between OTX2 and MITF	• Important transcription factor targets: SOX11, MN1, GLI2	• Important transcription factor targets: MYC, RARG, PLXND1

70.5 Treatment and Prognosis

Treatment
- Surgery
- Radiotherapy

Biologic Behavior–Prognosis–Prognostic Factors
- Highly aggressive tumor
- Poor prognosis
- Mean survival: 11 months
- Range of survival: 3–24 months
- Age > 3 years associated with longer survival

Selected References

Arslanoglu A, Aygun N, Tekhtani D, Aronson L, Cohen K, Burger PC, Yousem DM (2004) Imaging findings of CNS atypical teratoid/rhabdoid tumors. AJNR Am J Neuroradiol 25(3):476–480

Au Yong KJ, Jaremko JL, Jans L, Bhargava R, Coleman LT, Mehta V, Ditchfield MR (2013) How specific is the MRI appearance of supratentorial atypical teratoid rhabdoid tumors? Pediatr Radiol 43(3):347–354. https://doi.org/10.1007/s00247-012-2530-z

Bruggers CS, Moore K (2014) Magnetic resonance imaging spectroscopy in pediatric atypical teratoid rhabdoid tumors of the brain. J Pediatr Hematol Oncol 36(6):e341–e345. https://doi.org/10.1097/mph.0000000000000041

Chakravadhanula M, Hampton CN, Chodavadia P, Ozols V, Zhou L, Catchpoole D, Xu J, Erdreich-Epstein A, Bhardwaj RD (2015) Wnt pathway in atypical teratoid rhabdoid tumors. Neuro Oncol 17(4):526–535. https://doi.org/10.1093/neuonc/nou229

Dunham C (2010) Pediatric brain tumors: a histologic and genetic update on commonly encountered entities. Semin Diagn Pathol 27(3):147–159

Ginn KF, Gajjar A (2012) Atypical teratoid rhabdoid tumor: current therapy and future directions. Front Oncol 2:114. https://doi.org/10.3389/fonc.2012.00114

Han L, Qiu Y, Xie C, Zhang J, Lv X, Xiong W, Wang W, Zhang X, Wu P (2011) Atypical teratoid/rhabdoid tumors in adult patients: CT and MR imaging features. AJNR Am J Neuroradiol 32(1):103–108. https://doi.org/10.3174/ajnr.A2361

Jeibmann A, Schulz J, Eikmeier K, Johann PD, Thiel K, Tegeder I, Ambree O, Fruhwald MC, Pfister SM, Kool M, Paulus W, Hasselblatt M (2017) SMAD dependent signaling plays a detrimental role in a fly model of SMARCB1-deficiency and the biology of atypical teratoid/rhabdoid tumors. J Neurooncol 131(3):477–484. https://doi.org/10.1007/s11060-016-2326-3

Johann PD, Erkek S, Zapatka M, Kerl K, Buchhalter I, Hovestadt V, Jones DT, Sturm D, Hermann C, Segura Wang M, Korshunov A, Rhyzova M, Grobner S, Brabetz S, Chavez L, Bens S, Groschel S, Kratochwil F, Wittmann A, Sieber L, Georg C, Wolf S, Beck K, Oyen F, Capper D, van Sluis P, Volckmann R, Koster J, Versteeg R, von Deimling A, Milde T, Witt O, Kulozik AE, Ebinger M, Shalaby T, Grotzer M, Sumerauer D, Zamecnik J, Mora J, Jabado N, Taylor MD, Huang A, Aronica E, Bertoni A, Radlwimmer B, Pietsch T, Schuller U, Schneppenheim R, Northcott PA, Korbel JO, Siebert R, Fruhwald MC, Lichter P, Eils R, Gajjar A, Hasselblatt M, Pfister SM, Kool M (2016) Atypical teratoid/rhabdoid tumors are comprised of three epigenetic subgroups with distinct enhancer landscapes. Cancer Cell 29(3):379–393. https://doi.org/10.1016/j.ccell.2016.02.001

Judkins AR, Eberhart CG, Wesseling P (2007) Atypical teratoid/rhabdoid tumour. In: Louis DN, Ohgaki H, Wiestler OD, Cavenee WK (eds) WHO classification of tumours of the central nervous system, 4th edn. International Agency for Research on Cancer, Lyon, pp 147–149

Judkins AR, Eberhart CG, Wesseling P, Hasselblatt M (2016) Atypical teratoid/rhabdoid tumour. In: Louis DN, Ohgaki H, Wiestler OD, Cavenee WK (eds) WHO classification of tumours of the central nervous system, Revised 4th edn. IARC, Lyon, pp 209–212

Meyers SP, Khademian ZP, Biegel JA, Chuang SH, Korones DN, Zimmerman RA (2006) Primary intracranial atypical teratoid/rhabdoid tumors of infancy and childhood: MRI features and patient outcomes. AJNR Am J Neuroradiol 27(5):962–971

Pacheco MC, Dolan M, Bendel A (2017) Ewing sarcoma and atypical teratoid rhabdoid tumor: a FISH and immunohistochemical comparison. Pediatr Dev Pathol 20(5):381–386. https://doi.org/10.1177/1093526617698599

Perreault S, Lober RM, Carret AS, Zhang G, Hershon L, Decarie JC, Vogel H, Yeom KW, Fisher PG, Partap S (2014) Surveillance imaging in children with malignant CNS tumors: low yield of spine MRI. J Neurooncol 116(3):617–623. https://doi.org/10.1007/s11060-013-1347-4

Rorke LB, Biegel JA (2000) Atypical teratoid/rhabdoid tumour. In: Kleihues P, Cavenee WK (eds) Pathology and genetics of tumours of the nervous system, 3rd edn. IARC Press, Lyon, pp 145–148

Schrey D, Carceller Lechon F, Malietzis G, Moreno L, Dufour C, Chi S, Lafay-Cousin L, von Hoff K, Athanasiou T, Marshall LV, Zacharoulis S (2016) Multimodal therapy in children and adolescents with newly diagnosed atypical teratoid rhabdoid tumor: individual pooled data analysis and review of the literature. J Neurooncol 126(1):81–90. https://doi.org/10.1007/s11060-015-1904-0

Sredni ST, Halpern AL, Hamm CA, Bonaldo Mde F, Tomita T (2013) Histone deacetylases expression in atypical teratoid rhabdoid tumors. Childs Nerv Syst 29(1):5–9. https://doi.org/10.1007/s00381-012-1965-8

Torchia J, Golbourn B, Feng S, Ho KC, Sin-Chan P, Vasiljevic A, Norman JD, Guilhamon P, Garzia L, Agamez NR, Lu M, Chan TS, Picard D, de Antonellis P, Khuong-Quang DA, Planello AC, Zeller C, Barsyte-Lovejoy D, Lafay-Cousin L, Letourneau L, Bourgey M, Yu M, Gendoo DM, Dzamba M, Barszczyk M, Medina T, Riemenschneider AN, Morrissy AS, Ra YS, Ramaswamy V, Remke M, Dunham CP, Yip S, Ng HK, Lu JQ, Mehta V, Albrecht S, Pimentel J, Chan JA, Somers GR, Faria CC, Roque L, Fouladi M, Hoffman LM, Moore AS, Wang Y, Choi SA, Hansford JR, Catchpoole D, Birks DK, Foreman NK, Strother D, Klekner A, Bognar L, Garami M, Hauser P, Hortobagyi T, Wilson B, Hukin J, Carret AS, Van Meter TE, Hwang EI, Gajjar A, Chiou SH, Nakamura H, Toledano H, Fried I, Fults D, Wataya T, Fryer C, Eisenstat DD, Scheinemann K, Fleming AJ, Johnston DL, Michaud J, Zelcer S, Hammond R, Afzal S, Ramsay DA, Sirachainan N, Hongeng S, Larbcharoensub N, Grundy RG, Lulla RR, Fangusaro JR, Druker H, Bartels U, Grant R, Malkin D, McGlade CJ, Nicolaides T, Tihan T, Phillips J, Majewski J, Montpetit A, Bourque G, Bader GD, Reddy AT, Gillespie GY, Warmuth-Metz M, Rutkowski S, Tabori U, Lupien M, Brudno M, Schuller U, Pietsch T, Judkins AR, Hawkins CE, Bouffet E, Kim SK, Dirks PB, Taylor MD, Erdreich-Epstein A, Arrowsmith CH, De Carvalho DD, Rutka JT, Jabado N, Huang A (2016) Integrated (epi)-genomic analyses identify subgroup-specific therapeutic targets in CNS rhabdoid tumors. Cancer Cell 30(6):891–908. https://doi.org/10.1016/j.ccell.2016.11.003

Verma V, Johnson CP, Bennion NR, Bhirud AR, Li S, McComb RD, Lin C (2015) Atypical teratoid rhabdoid tumor: long-term survival after chemoradiotherapy. Childs Nerv Syst 31(8):1393–1399. https://doi.org/10.1007/s00381-015-2723-5

Tumors of the Peripheral Nervous System

Tumors of Cranial and Paraspinal Nerves

71.1 General Aspects

71.1.1 Clinical Signs and Symptoms

- Incidental finding
- Radicular pain
- Signs of nerve root or spinal cord compression
- Eighth cranial nerve: hearing loss, tinnitus, disequilibrium
- Cranial nerve palsy
- Present as mass in neurofibromas, painless
- Multiple masses as hallmark of NF1 associated with pigmented cutaneous macules (café-au-lait spots) and freckling
- Progressively enlarging mass with or without neurologic symptoms in cases of malignant peripheral nerve sheath tumor

71.1.2 Classification of Tumors of the Peripheral Nervous System

Tumors affecting the peripheral nervous system are of variegated nature (Table 71.1).

Table 71.1 Tumors of the peripheral nervous system

Schwannoma	• Conventional schwannoma • Cellular schwannoma • Plexiform schwannoma • Melanotic schwannoma
Neurofibroma	• Plexiform neurofibroma • Circumscribed neurofibroma
Perineurioma	• Intraneural perineurioma • Soft tissue perineurioma
Malignant peripheral nerve sheath tumor (MPNST)	• Epithelioid MPNST • MPNST with divergent mesenchymal and/or epithelial differentiation • Melanotic MPNST • Melanotic psammomatous
Miscellaneous benign tumors	• Nerve sheath myxoma and neurothekeoma • Granular cell tumor • Ganglioneuroma
Non-neurogenic tumors	• Peripheral nerve and ectopic meningioma • Paraganglioma of nerve root • Lipoma • Vascular tumors of nerve • Hemangioblastoma of nerve • Adrenal adenoma of spinal nerve root
Hemopoietic neoplasms	• Lymphoma • Leukemia
Hyperplastic lesions	• Neuroma • Localized hypertrophic neuropathy
Hamartoma and choristoma	• Lipofibromatous hamartoma of nerve • Neuromuscular choristoma

71.1.3 Nuclear Medicine Imaging Findings

In general, the resolution limit of the camera system has to be taken into account examining small structures.

Schwannoma (Figs. 71.1 and 71.2)
- Reports state the possibility of detecting schwannomas with SSR-scintigraphy but these findings are not consistent.
- Few reports state a visibility in I123-MIBG scan of atypical schwannoma.
- Malignant schwannomas can be visualized by FDG-PET while MIBI scans are reported to be negative. We detected FET-positive schwannomas.

Neurofibroma
- FDG-PET has been used to differentiate neurofibroma from malignant peripheral nerve sheath tumors.

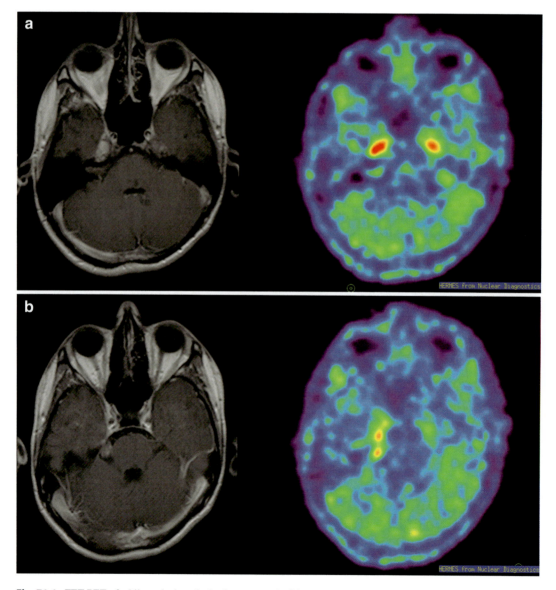

Fig. 71.1 FET-PET of a bilateral trigeminal schwannoma (**a**, **b**)

71.1 General Aspects

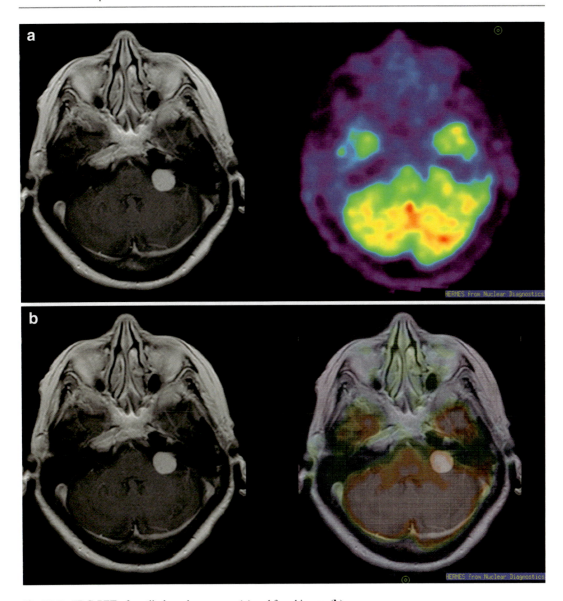

Fig. 71.2 FDG-PET of vestibular schwannoma (**a**) and fused image (**b**)

- Uptake of the following tracers has been described: Tc99m-diphosphonates, Tc99m-DMSA, Tc99m-pertechnetate, Tc99m(In111)-DTPA.

Perineurioma
- No literature available.

Malignant Peripheral Nerve Sheath Tumor (MPNST)
- MPNST have been described as FDG-positive.

Neurofibromatosis I
- Tc99m-diphosphonates are taken up in neurofibromas, plexiform neuromas, and neurofibrosarcomas (especially in soft tissue).
- Tc99m-DMSA is taken up in neurofibromas and neurofibrosarcomas.
- Tc99m-pertechnetate has been described in neurofibromas and plexiform neurofibromas.
- Ga67-citrate is taken up in neurofibrosarcomas.
- Pheochromocytomas can be visualized by FDG, F-DOPA, MIBG-scintigraphy, SSR-scintigraphy, and PET.

71.2 Schwannoma

WHO Definition
2016—A benign, typically encapsulated nerve sheath tumor composed entirely of well-differentiated Schwann cells, with loss of merlin (the NF2 gene product) expression in conventional forms (Antonescu et al. 2016a).

2007—A benign nerve sheath tumor that is typically encapsulated and composed entirely of well-differentiated Schwann cells. Multiple schwannomas are associated with neurofibromatosis type 2 or schwannomatosis (Scheithauer et al. 2007c).

2000—A usually encapsulated benign tumor composed of differentiated neoplastic Schwann cells (Woodruff et al. 2000c).

1993—An encapsulated and sometimes cystic tumor composed of spindle-shaped neoplastic Schwann cells (Kleihues et al. 1993).

1979—Neurilemmoma [Schwannoma, Neurinoma]: A tumor composed of spindle-shaped cells considered to be Schwann cells (Zülch 1979).

WHO Grade
- WHO grade I

71.2.1 Epidemiology

Incidence
- 8% of intracranial tumors
- 85% of cerebellopontine angle tumors
- 29% of spinal nerve root tumors

Age Incidence
- 4th–6th decade

Sex Incidence
- Male:Female ratio: 1:1

Localization
- Skin and subcutaneous tissue
- Eighth cranial nerve in the cerebellopontine angle
- Intraspinal sensory nerve roots
- Rare: spinal intramedullary, cerebrum, intraventricular, visceral, osseous

71.2.2 Neuroimaging Findings

71.2.2.1 Schwannoma of Cranial Nerves

General Imaging Findings
- Strongly contrast-enhancing extra-axial mass, well-defined, along a cranial nerve (except olfactory and optic nerves).

CT non-contrast-enhanced (Fig. 71.3a)
- Iso- to mildly hyperdense
- Enlargement of bony foramina

CT contrast-enhanced
- Strong, homogeneous enhancement

MRI-T2 (Figs. 71.3b and 71.4a)
- Heterogeneous hyperintense

MRI-FLAIR (Fig. 71.4b)
- Heterogeneous hyperintense
- Edema of adjacent brain stem possible
- Hyperintensity in cochlea in case of vestibular schwannoma

MRI-T1 (Fig. 71.4c)
- Isointense

MRI-T1 Contrast-Enhanced (Figs. 71.3c and 71.4d, e)
- Strong, variable enhancement.
- Dural tails are rare.

MRI-T2∗/SWI
- Microhemorrhages possible

MR-CISS (Figs. 71.3d and 71.4f)
- Hypointense tumor surrounded by hyperintense CSF

MR-Diffusion Imaging
- No restricted diffusion

MRI-Perfusion
- Slightly elevated rCBV, significantly lower than in meningioma

71.2 Schwannoma

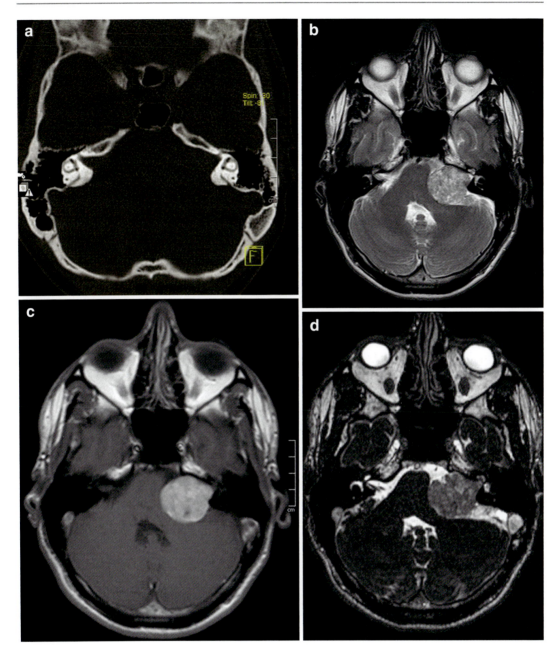

Fig. 71.3 Acoustic schwannoma left with enlargement of internal acoustic meatus in bony CT (**a**), T2 (**b**), T1 contrast (**c**), CISS (**d**)

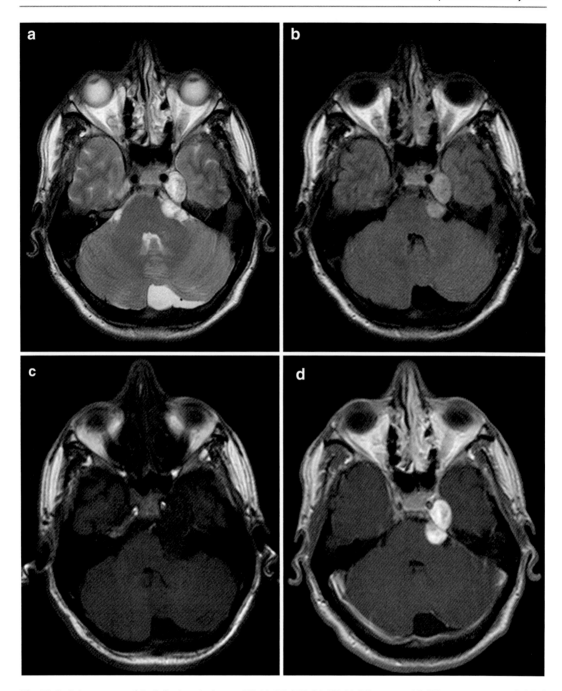

Fig. 71.4 Schwannoma of the left trigeminal nerve T2 (**a**), FLAIR (**b**), T1 (**c**), T1 contrast (**d**), T1 contrast cor (**e**), CISS (**f**)

71.2 Schwannoma

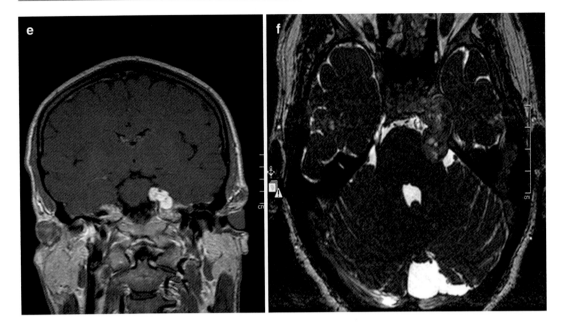

Fig. 71.4 (continued)

71.2.2.2 Parenchymal Schwannoma

General Imaging Findings
- Well-demarcated mass consisting of cyst with mural nodule and ring enhancement, very rare

CT non-contrast-enhanced
- Hypodense cystic component, isodense solid portion
- Calcifications possible

CT contrast-enhanced
- Strong, homogeneous enhancement of solid portion

MRI-T2
- Iso- to hyperintense solid portion
- Cysts strongly hyperintense

MRI-FLAIR
- Hyperintense surrounding edema rare

MRI-T1
- Isointense

MRI-T1 Contrast-Enhanced
- Strong enhancement of mural nodule

MRI-T2*/SWI
- Microhemorrhages and calcifications common

MR-Diffusion Imaging
- No restricted diffusion

MRI-Perfusion
- Slightly elevated rCBV in nodule

71.2.3 Neuropathology Findings

Macroscopic Features (Figs. 71.5 and 71.6)
- Globoid masses (up to 10 cm).
- Usually encapsulated.
- Light tan glistening tissue.
- Bright yellow patches.
- With or without cysts.
- With or without hemorrhages.
- Nerve of origin can be identified.

Microscopic Features (Fig. 71.7)
- The following types of schwannoma are histologically distinguished:
- Conventional schwannoma
- Cellular schwannoma
- Plexiform schwannoma

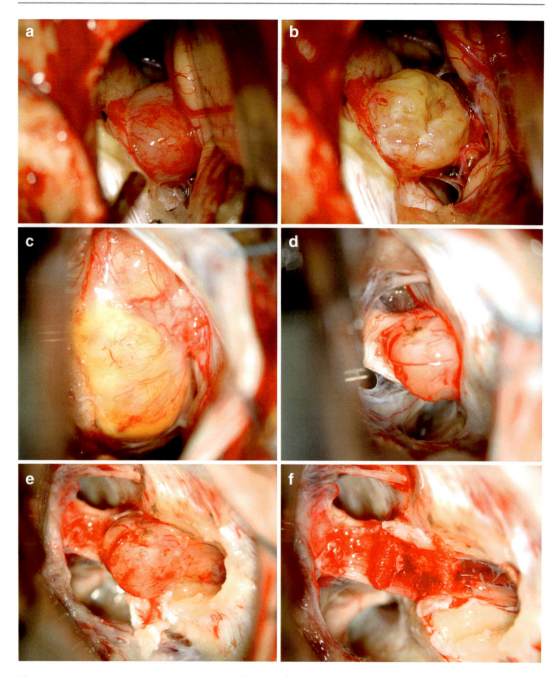

Fig. 71.5 Intraoperative images of schwannoma. Tumor is located at the external meatus. Yellowish color and firm consistency of the tumor (**a–c**). Removal of the mastoid bone in order to expose the tumor in its complete length before removal (**d–f**)

71.2 Schwannoma

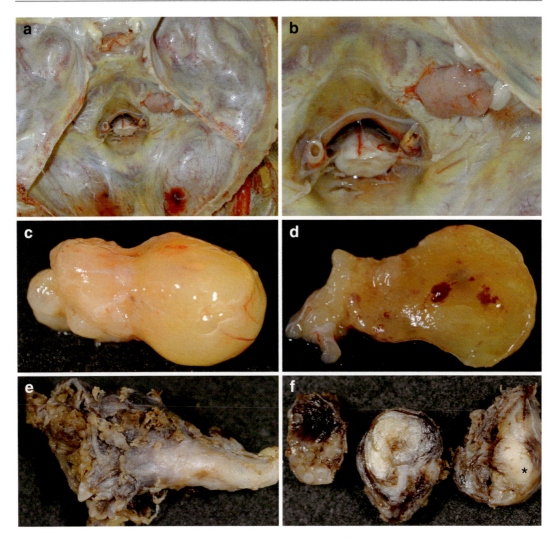

Fig. 71.6 Schwannoma located at the sphenoid ridge (incidental autopsy finding) (**a**, **b**). Surgical specimens of schwannoma (**c–f**) with varying color and consistency (**c**, **d**) yellowish color, soft consistency, hemorrhages at the cut surface, brownish color, hard consistency (**e**, **f**). Some nerve fascicles are still recognizable (∗) (**f**)

- Melanotic schwannoma
- Ancient schwannoma

Conventional Schwannoma
- Composed of neoplastic Schwann cells
  - With moderate quantities of eosinophilic cytoplasm
  - Without discernible cell borders
- Antoni A pattern
  - Areas of compact elongated cells with nuclear palisading (Verocay bodies)
- Antoni B pattern
  - Areas of less cellularity, loose textured cells with indistinct processes and variable lipidization
- Thick-walled and hyalinized vessels

Cellular Schwannoma
- Is defined as a hypercellular schwannoma
- Fascicular growth of cells
- Occasional nuclear hyperchromasia and atypia

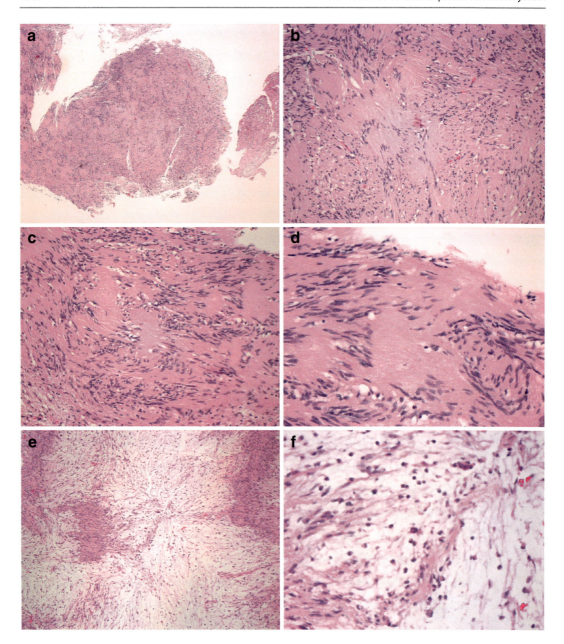

Fig. 71.7 Schwannoma with compact Antoni A areas with Verocay bodies (**a–d**), loose Antoni B areas (**e, f**), Verocay body (**g, h**), areas with lipidization (**i, j**), vessels with hyalinization are often seen (**k, l**), melancytic schwannoma (**m, n**), angiomatous schwannoma (**o–r**) with CD34-positive endothelial cells (**r**); the tumor cells are S-100-positive (**s, t**)

71.2 Schwannoma

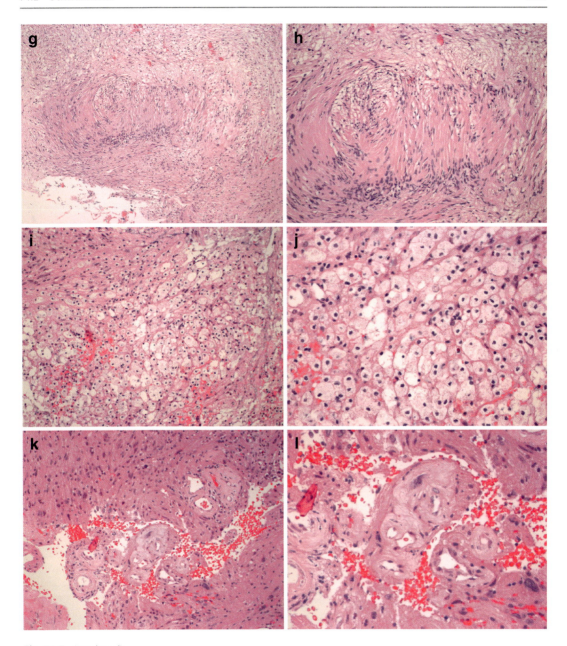

Fig. 71.7 (continued)

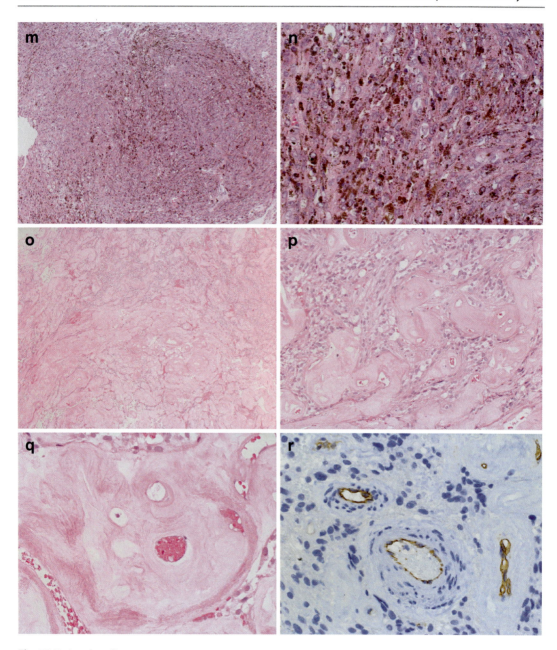

Fig. 71.7 (continued)

71.2 Schwannoma

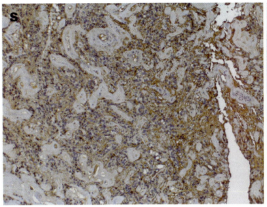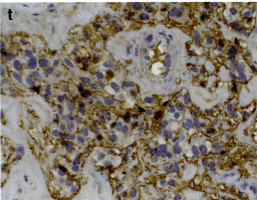

Fig. 71.7 (continued)

- Low-level mitotic activity <4/10 HPF
- Composed predominantly of Antoni A tissue
- Devoid of well-formed Verocay bodies
- Commonly in paravertebral sites
- Pericellular reticulin pattern

Plexiform Schwannoma

- schwannoma growing in plexiform or multinodular manner
- either conventional or cellular type
- mainly affects the skin or subcutaneous tissue
- low association with NF2, no NF1

Melanotic Schwannoma

- pigmented tumor composed of cells with the immunophenotype of Schwann cells.
- contain melanosomes.
- react with melanoma markers (HMB45).
- psammomatous and non-psammomatous variant.
- affect spinal nerves and paraspinal ganglia (non-psammomatous).
- affect autonomic nerves of viscera (psammomatous).
- 50% of patients with psammomatous tumors have Carney complex (autosomal dominant disease with lentiginous facial pigmentation, cardiac myxoma, and endocrine overactivity, i.e., Cushing syndrome associated with multinodular adrenal hyperplasia and acromegaly).
- 10% show malignant course.

Ancient Schwannoma

- Nuclear pleomorphism
  - Bizarre forms with cytoplasmic-nuclear inclusions.
- Occasional mitotic figures

Immunophenotype (Fig. 71.8a–f)

- S-100: strong expression
- Leu-7
- Calretinin
- GFAP focal expression
- Collagen IV stains basal lamina of cell processes
- p53: low levels
- Neurofilament protein-positive axons rarely
- Merlin: loss of expression

Proliferation Markers (Fig. 71.8g, h)

- Cellular schwannomas
  - PCNA: 5.6%
  - Ki-67: 6%

Ultrastructural Features

- Convoluted, moderately thin cytoplasmic processes
- Devoid of pinocytotic vesicles
- Lined by basal lamina
- Stromal long-spacing collagen (Luse body)
- True melanosomes in melanotic schwannomas

Differential Diagnosis

- Cellular schwannoma vs. malignant peripheral nerve sheath tumor
- Schwannoma vs. meningioma

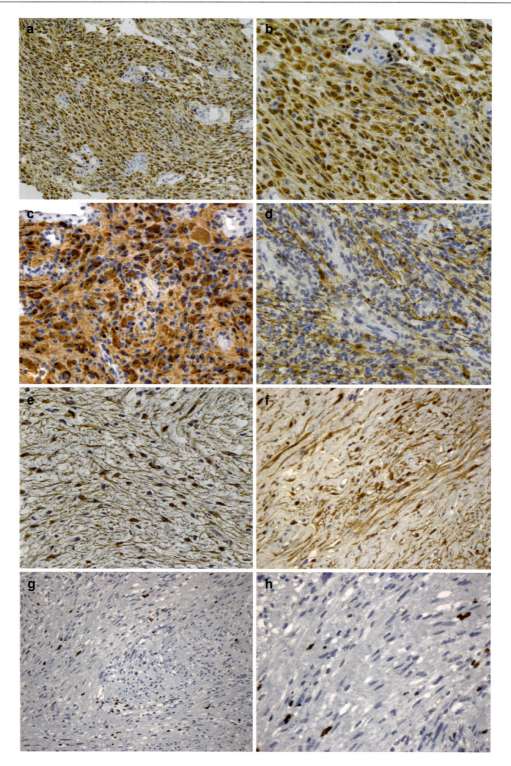

Fig. 71.8 Immunophenotype: schwannoma tumor cells stain immunopositive for S100 (**a–f**). Proliferation is very low (Ki67) (**g, h**)

71.2.4 Molecular Neuropathology

- *NF2* gene
  - Encodes merlin protein
  - Inactivating mutations in 60%
  - Small frameshift mutations resulting in truncated protein products
  - Loss of the remaining wild-type allele on chromosome 22q
  - Loss of merlin expression
- Other genetic changes
  - Loss of chromosome 1p
  - Gain of 9q34
  - Gain of 17q
  - Loss of *PRKAR1A* region on 17q

71.2.5 Treatment and Prognosis

Treatment
- Surgical excision
- Radiosurgery (one treatment session with LINAC or gamma knife or cyberknife)
- Radiotherapy (several sessions of fractionated therapy with LINAC/cyberknife)

Biologic Behavior-Prognosis-Prognostic Factors
- Benign
- Slowly growing
- Infrequently recur
- Rare malignant transformation

Cellular Schwannoma
- Benign, rare recurrences, no metastases, no malignant fatal course

71.3 Neurofibroma

WHO Definition
2016—A benign, well-demarcated, intraneural, or diffusely infiltrative extraneural nerve sheath tumor consisting of neoplastic, well-differentiated Schwann cells intermixed with non-neoplastic elements including perineurial-like cells, fibroblasts, mast cells, a variably myxoid to collagenous matrix, and residual axons or ganglion cells (Perry et al. 2016).

2007—A well-demarcated intraneural or diffusely infiltrative extraneural tumor consisting of a mixture of cell types, including Schwann cells, perineurial-like cells, and fibroblasts; multiple and plexiform neurofibromas are typically associated with neurofibromatosis type 1 (Scheithauer et al. 2007b).

2000—A well-demarcated intraneural or diffusely infiltrative extraneural tumor consisting of a mixture of cell types including Schwann cells, perineurial-like cells, and fibroblasts. Multiple neurofibromas are typically associated with neurofibromatosis 1 (NF1) (Woodruff et al. 2000b).

1993—A demarcated or, particularly in dermal and subcutaneous tissue, diffuse tumor composed of Schwann cells, fibroblasts, and perineurial cells. The lesion varies in cellularity as well as in its content of collagen and mucosubstances (Kleihues et al. 1993).

1979—A localized or diffuse tumor consisting in a mixture of Schwann cells and fibroblasts with loosely arranged collagen fibers and mucoid material, forming an intersecting pattern of wavy fascicles in which neurites may be demonstrable. Antoni A and B patterns are not seen (Zülch 1979).

WHO Grade
- WHO grade I

71.3.1 Epidemiology

Incidence
- Frequent as sporadic solitary nodules
- Less frequent as solitary, multiple, or numerous lesions in NF1

Age Incidence
- All ages

Sex Incidence
- Male:Female ratio: 1:1

Localization
- Cutaneous nodule
- Diffuse but localized involvement of skin and subcutaneous tissue (diffuse cutaneous neurofibroma)
- Extensive to massive involvement of soft tissue (localized gigantism) and "elephantiasis neuromatosa"
- Circumscribed mass in a peripheral nerve
- Plexiform enlargement of a plexus or major nerve trunk

71.3.2 Neuroimaging Findings

General Imaging Findings
- Solitary nodule or diffuse infiltrating plexiform tumor

CT non-contrast-enhanced
- Hypodense
- Plexiform neurofibromas with enlargement of orbital fissure

CT contrast-enhanced
- Strong or moderate, homogeneous enhancement

MRI-T2 (Fig. 71.9a, b)
- Hyperintense

MRI-FLAIR
- Hyperintense

MRI-T1 (Fig. 71.9c, d)
- Isointense

MRI-T1 Contrast-Enhanced (Fig. 71.9e, f)
- Strong, heterogeneous enhancement

MRI-T2*/SWI
- Microhemorrhages possible

MR-Diffusion Imaging
- No restricted diffusion

71.3.3 Neuropathology Findings

Macroscopic Features (Figs. 71.10 and 71.11)
- Nodular
- Circumscribed
- Diffuse involving skin and subcutaneous tissue
- Firm, glistening, gray-tan
- Multinodular tangles ("bag of worms") in plexiform neurofibroma

Microscopic Features (Fig. 71.12a–j)
- Composed of
  - Schwann cells with ovoid to thin curved to elongate nuclei and scant cytoplasm
  - Fibroblasts in a matrix of collagen fibers
- Alcian blue-positive, myxoid material
- Numerous atypical nuclei (atypical neurofibroma)
- Significantly increased cellularity (cellular neurofibroma)
- Rare mitotic figures
- Great variation in stromal collagen formation
- Blood vessels generally lack hyalinization

Ancient Neurofibroma
- Degenerative nuclear atypia

Atypical Neurofibroma
- High cellularity
- Scattered mitotic figures
- Monomorphic cytology
- Fascicular growth
- Cytological atypia
- DD: low-grade malignant peripheral nerve sheath tumor

Plexiform Neurofibroma
- Involvement of multiple fascicles.
- Fascicles are expanded by tumor cells and collagen.
- Residual bundled nerve fibers.

Immunophenotype (Fig. 71.13a–h)
- S-100 invariably seen
- Collagen type IV less consistent
- Limited EMA-positive cells
- Glut-1-positive
- Claudin +

71.3 Neurofibroma

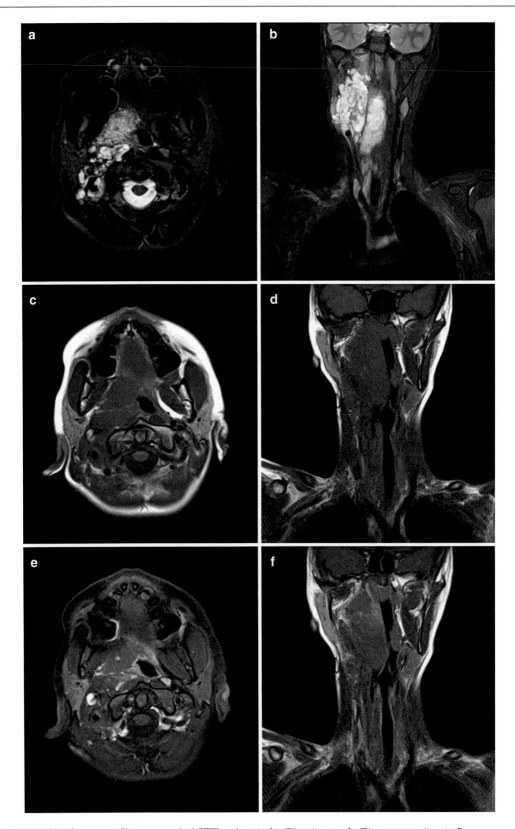

Fig. 71.9 Plexiform neurofibroma: cervical STIR ax/cor (a, b), T1 ax/cor (c, d), T1 contrast ax/cor (e, f)

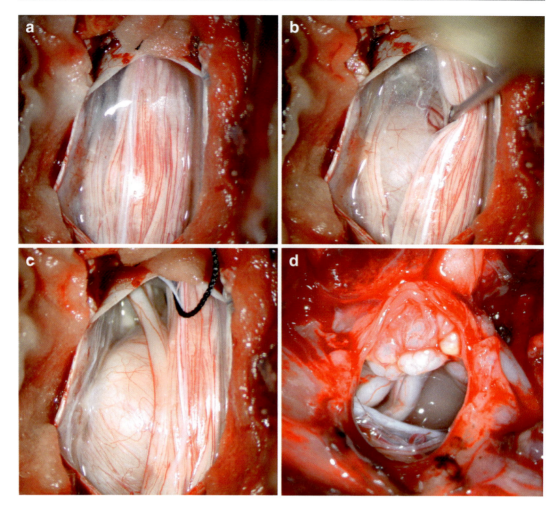

Fig. 71.10 Intraoperative images of a neurofibroma affecting spinal roots (**a**) the dura mater is opened, the arachnoidea is glistening, parts of the cauda equina are seen, the cauda equina is retracted and the tumor visible (**b**, **c**). Note the nerve which rests upon the tumor (**c**). Another example displaying multinodular tangles ("bag of worms") in plexiform neurofibroma (**d**)

Proliferation Markers
- Low

Ultrastructural Features
- Schwann cells either associated or unassociated with axons
- Perineurial-like cells with long, very thin cell processes, numerous pinocytotic vesicles, and interrupted basement membrane

Differential Diagnosis
- Fibroma
- Fibrosarcoma low grade

71.3.4 Molecular Neuropathology

- See below neurofibromatoses

71.3 Neurofibroma

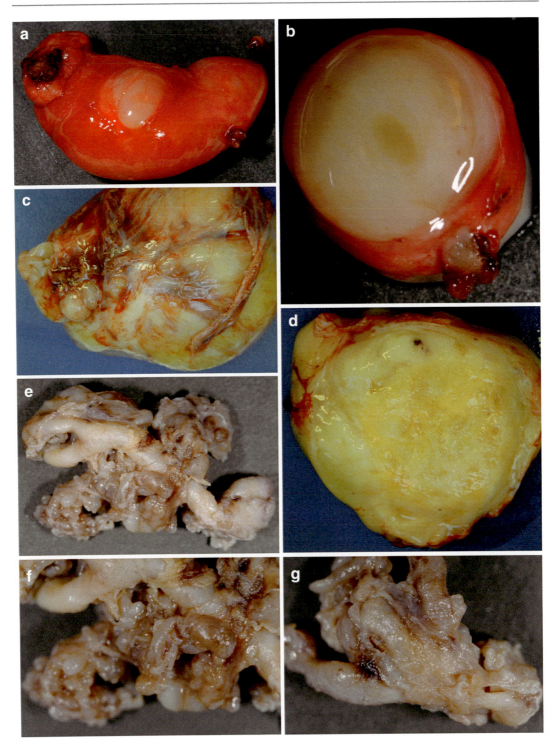

Fig. 71.11 Gross-anatomical appearance of neurofibroma (**a–j**). Firm consistency, yellowish-whitish color (**a–d**), multinodular tangles ("bag of worms") in plexiform neurofibroma (**e–j**), cut surface of the tumor (**j**)

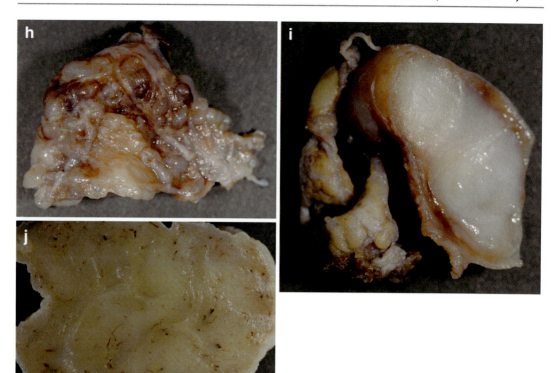

Fig. 71.11 (continued)

71.3.5 Treatment and Prognosis

Treatment
- Surgical excision

Biologic Behavior–Prognosis–Prognostic Factors
- Generally benign behavior.
- Patients are likely to have neurofibromatosis type I.
- Considered to be a precursor lesion for malignant peripheral nerve sheath tumor.
- Malignant transformation occurs in about 5% of the case.

71.4 Perineurioma

Perineurioma was first introduced as a neoplasm in the 2000 WHO Classification of Tumours of the Central Nervous System. Previously, perineuriomas were considered to be a form of hypertrophic neuropathy.

WHO Definition
2016—A tumor composed entirely of neoplastic perineurial cells (Antonescu et al. 2016b).

2007—A tumor composed entirely of neoplastic perineurial cells. Intraneural perineuriomas are benign and consist of proliferating perineurial cells within endoneurium, forming characteristic pseudo-onion bulbs. Soft tissue perineuriomas are typically not associated with nerve and are usually benign (Scheithauer et al. 2007d).

2000—A benign tumor composed entirely of neoplastic perineurial cells. Intraneural perineuriomas exhibit proliferating perineurial cells throughout the endoneurium, with formation of characteristic pseudo-onion bulbs. Soft tissue perineuriomas are unassociated with nerve (Scheithauer et al. 2000).

WHO Grade
- WHO grade I

71.4 Perineurioma

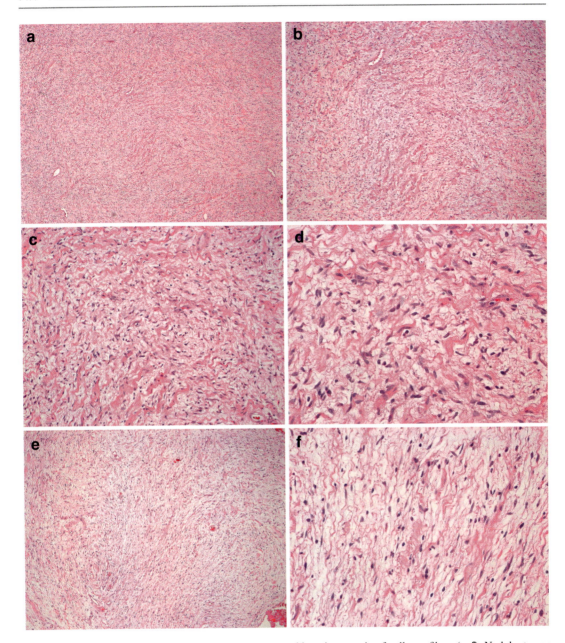

Fig. 71.12 Neurofibroma (**a–j**). Tumor of moderate cellularity composed of cells with ovoid to thin curved to elongate nuclei and scant cytoplasm as well as of fibroblasts in a matrix of collagen fibers (**a–f**). Nodular tumor formation is possible (**g–j**)

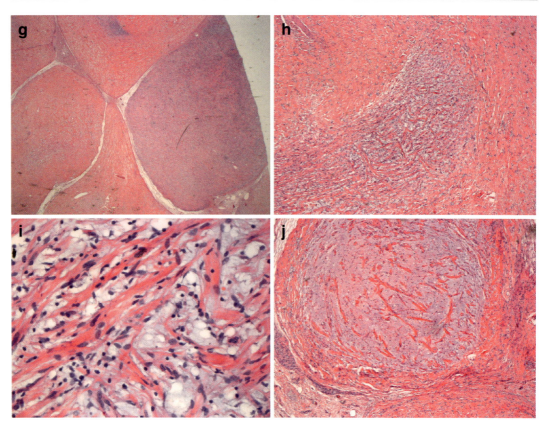

Fig. 71.12 (continued)

71.4.1 Epidemiology

Incidence
- Rare
- 1% of nerve sheath and soft tissue tumors

Age Incidence
- Adolescence
- Early adulthood

Sex Incidence
- No sex predilection

Localization
- Peripheral nerves
  - Extremities
  - Cranial nerves rare
- Soft tissue
  - Not associated with nerve

71.4.2 Neuroimaging Findings

General Imaging Findings
- Similar to schwannomas

CT non-contrast-enhanced
- Iso- to mildly hypodense

CT contrast-enhanced
- Mild enhancement

MRI-T2
- Heterogeneous hyperintense

MRI-FLAIR
- Heterogeneous hyperintense

MRI-T1
- Hypointense

71.4 Perineurioma

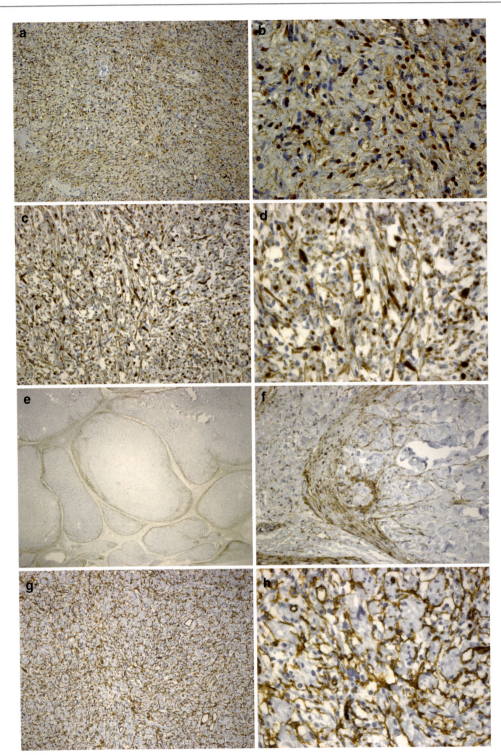

Fig. 71.13 Immunophenotype: Neurofibromas are immunopositive for S-100 (**a–d**). The nodules are surrounded by EMA-positive cells (**e, f**). Some neurofibromas may contain a large number of small vessels (CD34 immunostain) (**g, h**)

MRI-T1 Contrast-Enhanced
- Slight enhancement

71.4.3 Neuropathology Findings

Macroscopic Features
- Segmental, tubular enlargement of the affected nerve
- Coarse and pale appearance of the nerve fascicle

Microscopic Features (Fig. 71.14a–c)
- Neoplastic perineurial cells
  - Proliferate throughout the endoneurium
  - Form multiple concentric layers around nerve fibers
  - Enlarges fascicles
  - Pseudo-onion bulbs
- Myelin might be scant or absent.
- Hyalinization is possible.

Immunophenotype
- A list of antibodies with positive or negative immunostaining results is given in Table 71.2.

Proliferation Markers
- Mitotic activity: rare
- MIB-1 LI range between 5 and 15%

Ultrastructural Features
- Myelinated nerve fibers surrounded by normal-appearing perineurial cells
- Perineurial cells
  - Long, thin cytoplasmic processes with numerous pinocytic vesicles
  - Lined by patchy surface basement membrane
- Abundant stromal collagen

71.4.4 Molecular Neuropathology

- Monosomy of chromosome 22
- Loss of chromosome 10
- Small chromosome 22q deletion involving *NF2*

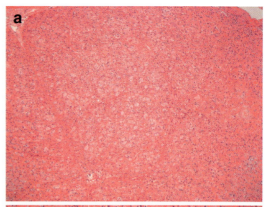
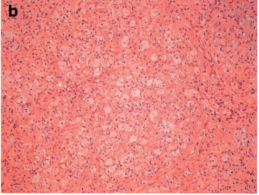
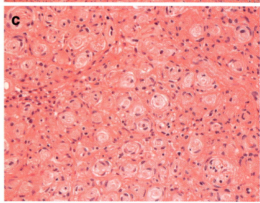

Fig. 71.14 Perineurioma: neoplastic perineurial cells proliferate throughout the endoneurium and form multiple concentric layers around nerve fibers (**a–c**)

Pathogenesis
- Unknown

71.4.5 Treatment and Prognosis

Treatment
- Surgical excision

Table 71.2 Immunophenotype of perineurioma

Positivity	Negativity
• Vimentin • EMA (membranous staining) • Collagen IV • Laminin • S-100 (residual Schwann cells) • Neurofilament (axons at the center of pseudo-onion bulbs) • P53 • Claudin-1 • Glut-1	• CD34 • S-100

Biologic Behavior–Prognosis–Prognostic Factors
- Benign tumor
- No tendency for recurrence or metastasis

71.5 Hybrid Nerve Sheath Tumors

WHO Definition
2016—Benign peripheral nerve sheath tumors (PNSTs) with combined features of more than one conventional type (i.e., neurofibroma, schwannoma, and perineurioma) (Antonescu et al. 2016c). Two of the more common types of hybrid nerve sheath tumors are schwannoma/perineurioma, which typically occurs sporadically, and neurofibroma/schwannoma, which is typically associated with schwannomatosis, neurofibromatosis type 1 (NF1) or neurofibromatosis type 2 (NF2). Rare cases of neurofibroma/perineurioma have also been described, usually associated with NF1.

71.5.1 Neuropathology Findings

Macroscopic Findings
- Indistinguishable from schwannoma or neurofibroma

Microscopic Findings (Fig. 71.15a–n)
- Hybrid schwannoma/perineurioma
  - Predominantly Schwannian cytomorphology
  - Perineurioma-like architecture
  - Spindle cells with
    ○ Plump, tapering nuclei
    ○ Pale eosinophilic cytoplasm
  - Storiform, whorled, and/or lamella architecture
  - Myxoid stromal changes
- Hybrid schwannoma/neurofibroma
  - Schwannoma-like component
    ○ Nodular Schwann cell proliferation
    ○ Mainly Antoni A areas
    ○ Verocay bodies
  - Neurofibroma-like component
    ○ Mixed cellular population
    ○ Myxoid change
    ○ Collagen
- Hybrid neurofibroma/perineurioma
  - Plexiform neurofibroma
  - Areas with perineuriomatous differentiation

Immunophenotype
- A list of antibodies with positive or negative immunostaining results is given in Table 71.3.

71.6 Malignant Peripheral Nerve Sheath Tumor (MPNST)

WHO Definition
2016—A malignant tumor with evidence of Schwann cell or perineurial cell differentiation, commonly arising in a peripheral nerve or in extraneural soft tissue (Reuss et al. 2016a).

2007—A malignant tumor arising from a peripheral nerve, or in extraneural soft tissue if it shows nerve sheath differentiation, excluding tumors originating from epineurial tissue or from peripheral nerve vasculature; somewhat over 50% of malignant peripheral nerve sheath tumors are associated with neurofibromatosis type 1 (Scheithauer et al. 2007a).

2000—Any malignant tumor arising from a peripheral nerve or showing nerve sheath differentiation, with the exception of tumors originating from epineurium or the peripheral nerve vasculature. Approximately 50% of cases are

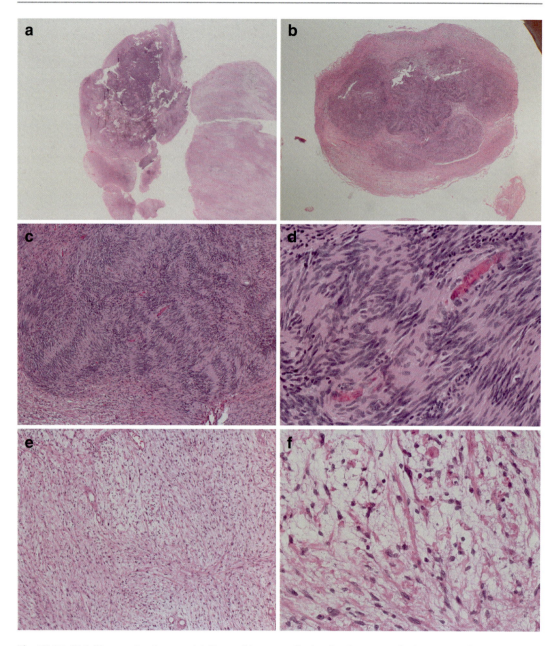

Fig. 71.15 Hybrid nerve sheath tumor (**a**). Parts of the tumor display the phenotype of schwannoma (**b–d**) and neurofibroma (**e–j**). Immunophenotype: tumor cells are positive for S-100 (**k–n**)

71.6 Malignant Peripheral Nerve Sheath Tumor (MPNST)

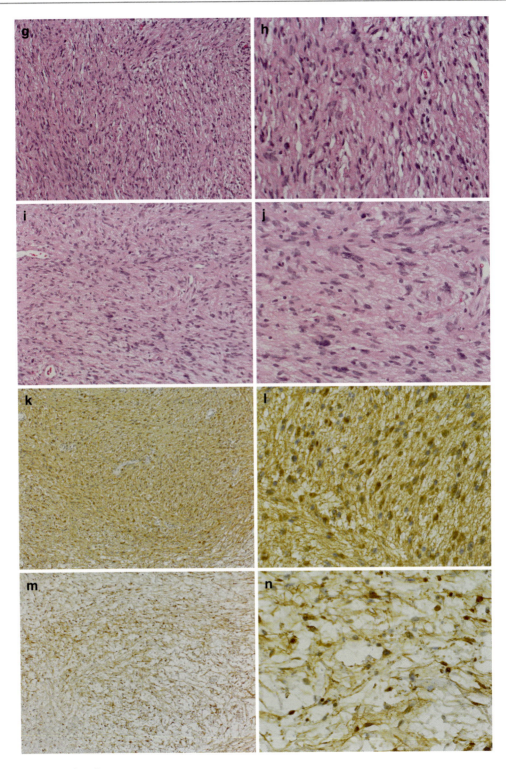

Fig. 71.15 (continued)

Table 71.3 Immunophenotype of hybrid nerve sheath tumors

Schwannoma/ perineurioma	Neurofibroma/ schwannoma	Neurofibroma/ perineurioma
• S-100 (S) • EMA (P) • Claudin-1 (P) • GLUT1 (P)	• S-100 (S) • SOX10 (S)	• EMA (P) • GLUT1 (P) • Claudi-1 (P)

(S) Schwannoma, *(P)* perineuriomas, *(N)* neurofibroma

associated with neurofibromatosis 1 (NF1) (Woodruff et al. 2000a).

1993—Generally, the malignant counterpart of neurofibroma since malignant forms of schwannomas are extremely rare (Kleihues et al. 1993).

1979—Anaplastic [malignant] Neurilemmoma [Schwannoma, Neurinoma]: A rare malignant counterpart of the neurilemmoma characterized by loss of the usual architecture and by excessive numbers of mitotic figures. This tumor corresponds histologically to grade III (Zülch 1979).

Anaplastic [malignant] Neurofibroma (Neurofibrosarcoma, Neurogenic Sarcoma): The malignant counterpart of the neurofibroma. The transformation of a neurofibroma into a sarcoma is a recognized complication of von Recklinghausen's disease. These tumors correspond to grades III and IV (Zülch 1979).

WHO Grade
- WHO grades II or III

71.6.1 Epidemiology

Incidence
- Rare
- 50–70% arise from neurofibroma

Age Incidence
- 3rd–6th decade

Sex Incidence
- Male:Female ratio: 1.1:1

Localization
- Large and medium-size nerves
- Nerves of the buttock, thigh, brachial plexus, upper arm, paraspinal region
- Sciatic nerve
- Rarely cranial nerves

71.6.2 Neuroimaging Findings

General Imaging Findings
- Malignant peripheral nerve sheath tumors are difficult to distinguish from neurofibromas, MPNST tend to be in a larger dimension, peripheral enhancement pattern, perilesional edema, and intratumoral cystic lesion.

CT non-contrast-enhanced
- Hypo- to isodense

CT contrast-enhanced
- Heterogeneous enhancement

MRI-T2
- Heterogeneous, cysts possible
- Hypointense due to high collagen content
- Perilesional edema-like zone described

MRI-FLAIR
- Heterogeneous
- Perilesional edema-like zone described

MRI-T1
- Isointense to muscle
- Heterogeneity helps to differentiate from neurofibroma in cases with NF1

MRI-T1 Contrast-Enhanced
- Peripheral enhancement

MRI-T2∗/SWI
- Hemorrhages possible

MR-Diffusion Imaging
- No restricted diffusion

71.6.3 Neuropathology Findings

Macroscopic Features
- Wide variation of fusiform, expansible masses lacking encapsulation
- Infiltrating surrounding structures
- Large tumors 5–10 cm
- Firm to hard consistency
- Colored or gray cut surface
- Foci of necroses and hemorrhage common

Microscopic Features (Fig. 71.16a–h)
- The following histological types are distinguished:
- MPNST with divergent differentiation (malignant triton tumor, glandular MPNST)
- Epithelioid MPNST
- MPNST with perineurial differentiation (malignant perineurioma)

The common histological features are:

- Herringbone or interwoven-fasciculated pattern of cell growth
- Tightly packed spindle cells with variable quantities of cytoplasm
- Elongate, waved nuclei
- Alternating loose and densely cellular areas or diffuse growth pattern
- Grow within nerve fascicles
- Invade through perineurium and epineurium into adjacent soft tissue
- Geographic necrosis in 75% of cases
- Mitotic activity with >4 mitotic figures per high field
- WHO low-grade tumor:
  - Increased cellularity as compared to neurofibroma
  - Increased nuclear size >3 times that of neurofibroma
  - Hyperchromasia
  - Increased mitotic activity
- WHO high-grade tumor:
  - Presence of necroses
  - High pleomorphism

MPNST with Divergent Differentiation (Malignant Triton Tumor, Glandular MPNST)
- Contains a variety of mesenchymal tissues:
  - Cartilage, bone, skeletal muscle
  - Angiosarcoma-like areas
- Glandular MPNST:
  - Contains glandular epithelium which resembles that of intestines and is histologically benign.
- Myoid elements, chondro, and/or osteosarcoma.
- Neoplastic epithelium.
- Neuroendocrine differentiation frequently seen.
- 75% of cases have neurofibromatosis type 1.
- Rhabdomyosarcomatous differentiation: malignant triton tumor.
- 60% of triton tumor have neurofibromatosis type 1.

Epithelioid MPNST
- Multiple nodules of polygonal epithelioid cells separated by fibrovascular septa.
- Tumor cells form trabeculae or cords separated by myxoid stroma.
- Tumor cells have
  - Large nuclei
  - Prominent nucleoli
  - Moderate amount of eosinophilic or amphophilic cytoplasm
- No association with neurofibromatosis type 1.
- Superficial and deep seated.

MPNST with Perineurial Differentiation (Malignant Perineurioma)
- Histological features of perineurial differentiation
- Hypercellularity
- Nuclear atypia
- Increased mitotic activity

Immunophenotype (Fig. 71.17a–d)
- S-100
  - positive in 50–70%
  - grade-related: patchy or in individual cells in high-grade tumors

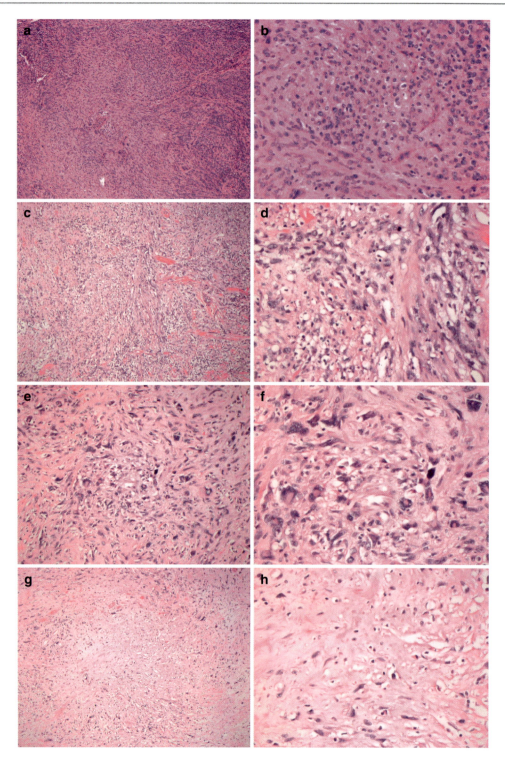

Fig. 71.16 Malignant peripheral nerve sheath tumor displays a herringbone or interwoven-fasciculated pattern of cell growth with tightly packed spindle cells with variable quantities of cytoplasm and elongated, waved nuclei (**a–h**). Note the cellular pleomorphism (**d–f**). Some areas are paucicellular

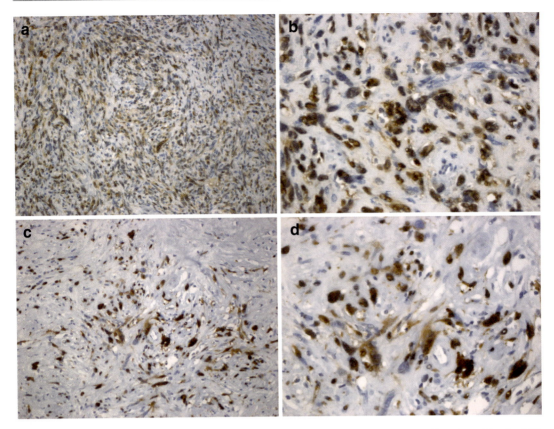

Fig. 71.17 Malignant peripheral nerve sheath tumor (MPNST). Immunophenotype: tumor cells stain-positive for S100 (**a–d**). Note their bizarre forms (**c, d**)

- p53
  - present in a majority of cases
- p27 and p16 uncommon
- CEA positivity in MPNST with divergent differentiation (i.e., glandular MPNST)

Proliferation Markers
- Ki-67: 5–65%

Ultrastructural Features
- Poor differentiation of tumor cells
- Gland formation is seen in glandular MPNST with terminal bars and luminal microvilli
- Dense core granules

Differential Diagnosis
- Malignant fibrosarcoma

71.6.4 Molecular Neuropathology

- 50% of MPNSTs manifest in patients with NF1
- Complex numerical and structural karyotypic abnormalities
  - Near-triploid or hypodiploid chromosome numbers
  - Chromosomal losses
  - Recombinations involving almost all chromosomes
- Chromosome 17 with abnormalities in NF1 and *TP53* loci
- Losses of chromosomes 13, 17, 18, 22
- Gains of chromosomes 2, 14
- Inactivation of both *NF1* alleles in MPNSTs of NF1 patients
- *TP53* with mutations and altered protein expression

- *CDKN2A* on chromosome 9p21:
  - homozygous deletions in the gene encoding p16^{INK4a} and p12^{ARF}
  - in 50% of the cases
  - inactivates the neighboring gene *CDKN2B* (encodes the p15 inhibitory molecule)
- Inactivation of the p53 and pRb regulatory pathways in 75% of cases

71.6.5 Treatment and Prognosis

Treatment
- Surgical excision
- LINAC radiation
- Gamma knife

Biologic Behavior–Prognosis–Prognostic Factors
- Highly aggressive tumor
- Poor prognosis
- 60% of patients die of the disease
- 5- and 10-year survival rate: 34% and 23%
- Triton tumor:
  - Poor prognosis
  - 2- and 5-year survival rates: 33 and 12%

71.7 Neurofibromatosis Type 1 (NF1)

WHO Definition
2016—An autosomal dominant disorder characterized by neurofibromas, multiple café-au-lait spots, axillary and inguinal freckling, optic gliomas, osseous lesions, and iris hamartomas (Lisch nodules). Patients with neurofibromatosis type 1 (NF1) have an increased risk for malignant peripheral nerve sheath tumor (MPNST), gastrointestinal stromal tumor, rhabdomyosarcoma, juvenile chronic myeloid leukemia, duodenal carcinoids, C-cell hyperplasia/medullary thyroid carcinomas, other carcinomas, and pheochromocytoma. The disorder is caused by mutations of the NF1 gene on chromosome 17q11.2 (Reuss et al. 2016b).

2007—An autosomal dominant disorder characterized by neurofibromas, multiple café-au-lait spots, axillary and inguinal freckling, optic gliomas, osseous lesions, and iris hamartomas (Lisch nodules); caused by mutations of the NF1 gene on chromosome 17q11.2 (von Deimling and Perry 2007).

2000—Neurofibromatosis type 1 (NF1) is an autosomal dominant disorder characterized by multiple neurofibromas, malignant peripheral nerve sheath tumors, optic nerve gliomas and other astrocytomas, multiple café-au-lait spots, axillary and inguinal freckling, iris hamartomas (Lisch nodules), and various osseous lesions (von Deimling et al. 2000).

71.7.1 Incidence and Diagnostic Criteria

Incidence
- 1:3000

Diagnostic Criteria
- The presence of two or more of the following signs identifies the NF1 patient (Gutmann et al. 1997):
- Six or more café-au-lait macules (1.5 cm or larger in postpubertal individuals, 0.5 cm or larger in prepubertal individuals)
- Two or more neurofibromas of any type or
- One or more plexiform neurofibromas
- Freckling of armpits or groin
- Pilocytic astrocytoma of optic pathway ("optic glioma")
- Two or more Lisch nodules (iris hamartomas)
- Dysplasia/absence of the sphenoid bone or dysplasia/thinning of long bone cortex
- First-degree relative with NF1

Tumors Associated with NF1
- Tumor associated with neurofibromatosis 1 are listed in Table 71.4.

Other Lesions Encountered in NF1
- Other lesions encountered in neurofibromatosis 1 are listed in Table 71.5.

71.8 Neurofibromatosis Type 2 (NF2)

Table 71.4 Tumor associated with neurofibromatosis 1

Tumor group	Tumor type
Neurofibromas	• Dermal • Nodular • Plexiform
Gliomas	• Optic glioma • Astrocytoma • Glioblastoma
Sarcomas	• Malignant peripheral nerve sheath tumor • Rhabdomyosarcoma • Triton tumor • Gastrointestinal stromal tumor (GIST)
Neuroendocrine/neuroectodermal tumors	• Pheochromocytoma • Carcinoid tumor • Medullary thyroid carcinoma • C-cell hyperplasia
Hematopoietic tumors	• Juvenile chronic myeloid leukemia • Juvenile xanthogranuloma

Table 71.5 Other lesions encountered in neurofibromatosis 1

Osseous lesions	• Scoliosis • Height reduction • Macrocephaly • Pseudoarthrosis • Sphenoid wing dysplasia
Nervous system	• Intellectual handicap • Epilepsy • Neuropathy • Hydrocephalus due to aqueductal stenosis
Vascular lesions	• Fibromuscular dysplasia/hyperplasia of renal artery and other arteries
Skin	• café-au-lait spots

71.7.2 Neuroimaging Findings

General Imaging Findings
- Plexiform neurofibromas (PNF) and optic nerve gliomas (ONG), see neurofibromas.
- Focal areas of signal intensity (FASI) in white matter and deep gray matter present until 10 years and then disappear.

CT non-contrast-enhanced (Bone)
- Enlargement of orbital fissure or foramen ovale due to ONG or PNF
- Hypoplastic sphenoid wing, enlarged middle cerebral fossa

MRI-T2 (Fig. 71.18a, e, h)
- Hyperintense FASI
- Proliferate in 10%, then tumefactive

MRI-FLAIR (Fig. 71.18b)
- Hyperintense FASI best seen

MRI-T1 (Fig. 71.18c, f)
- Variable signal of FASI, increasing signal with age

MRI-T1 Contrast-Enhanced (Fig. 71.19d, g)
- Rare enhancement of FASI, predictor of proliferation

MR-Diffusion Imaging
- FASI: ADC elevated

71.7.3 Neuropathology Findings

Macroscopic Findings (Figs. 71.19 and 71.20)
- Subcutaneous bulging lesion
- Neurofibromas on the skin

71.7.4 Molecular Neuropathology

- Mutations at chromosome 17q11.2
  - Encoded protein: Neurofibromin
    - Tumor suppressor gene
    - Plays a role in cell proliferation and differentiation

71.8 Neurofibromatosis Type 2 (NF2)

WHO Definition
2016—An autosomal dominant disorder characterized by neoplastic and dysplastic lesions that primarily affect the nervous system, with bilateral vestibular schwannomas as a diagnostic hallmark. Other manifestations include schwannomas of other cranial nerves, spinal and peripheral nerves, and the skin; intracranial and spinal meningiomas; gliomas, in particular spinal epen-

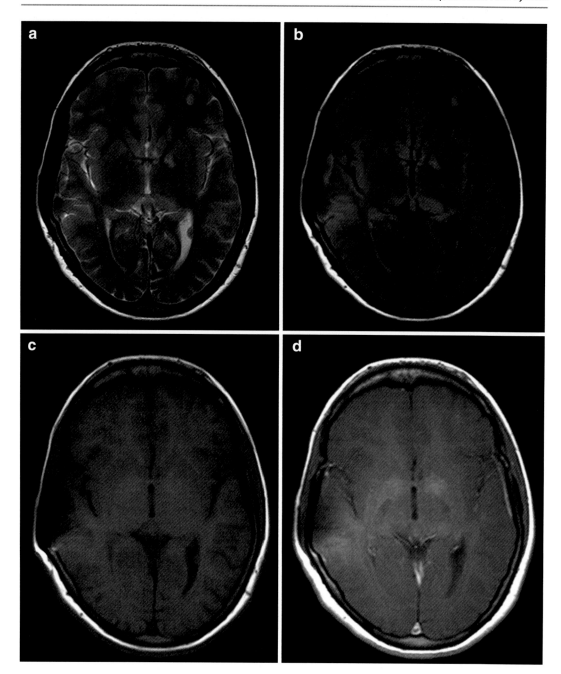

Fig. 71.18 NF1 with FASI left hemispheric T2 (**a**), FLAIR (**b**), T1 (**c**), and slight enhancement left frontal T1 contrast (**d**). Optic nerve glioma right T2 cor (**e**), T1 cor (**f**), T1 contrast (**g**). Additional tectal glioma in T2 sag (**h**)

71.8 Neurofibromatosis Type 2 (NF2)

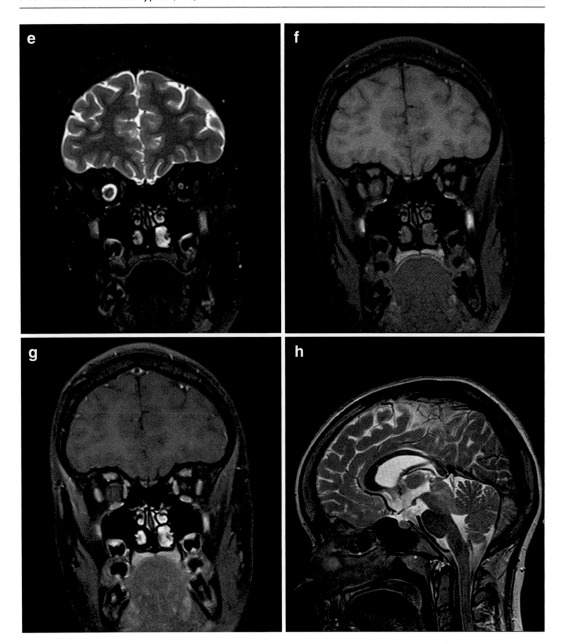

Fig. 71.18 (continued)

dymomas; and a variety of non-tumoral and dysplastic/development lesions, including meningiomatosis, glial hamartomas, ocular abnormalities (e.g., posterior subcapsular cataracts, retinal hamartomas, and epiretinal membranes), and neuropathies. NF2 is caused by mutations of the NF2 gene on chromosome 22q12 (Stemmer-Rachamimov et al. 2016b).

2007—An autosomal dominant disorder characterized by neoplastic and dysplastic lesions that primarily affect the nervous system; bilateral vestibular schwannomas are the hallmark, with other manifestations, including schwannomas of other cranial nerves, spinal and cutaneous schwannomas, intracranial and spinal meningiomas, gliomas, meningioangiomatosis,

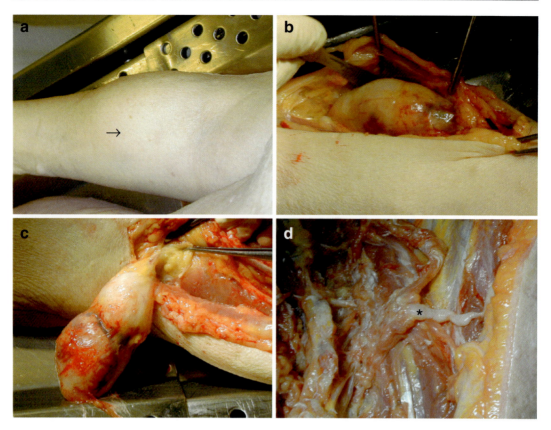

Fig. 71.19 Neurofibroma affecting the right upper arm with a bulging lesion (→) (**a**). Massive enlargement of the nerve is seen (**b**, **c**). Visceral organs are also involved (∗)

glial hamartomas, ocular abnormalities, and neuropathies, caused by mutations of the *NF2* gene on chromosome 22q12 (Stemmer-Rachamimov et al. 2007).

2000—Neurofibromatosis type 2 (NF2) is an autosomal dominant disorder characterized by neoplastic and dysplastic lesions of Schwann cells (schwannomas and schwannosis), meningeal cells (meningiomas und meningioangiomatosis) and glial cells (gliomas and glial microhamartomas). Bilateral vestibular, schwannomas are diagnostic. Additional lesions include posterior lens opacities and cerebral calcifications (Louis et al. 2000).

71.8.1 Incidence and Diagnostic Criteria

Incidence
- 1:25,000–1:40,000

Diagnostic Criteria for Neurofibromatosis Type 2
- The diagnostic criteria for neurofibromatosis type 2 are given as follows (Gutmann et al. 1997):
- Definite NF2
    - Bilateral schwannomas or
    - First-degree relative with NF2 and either
        - Unilateral vestibular schwannoma at <30 years or

71.8 Neurofibromatosis Type 2 (NF2)

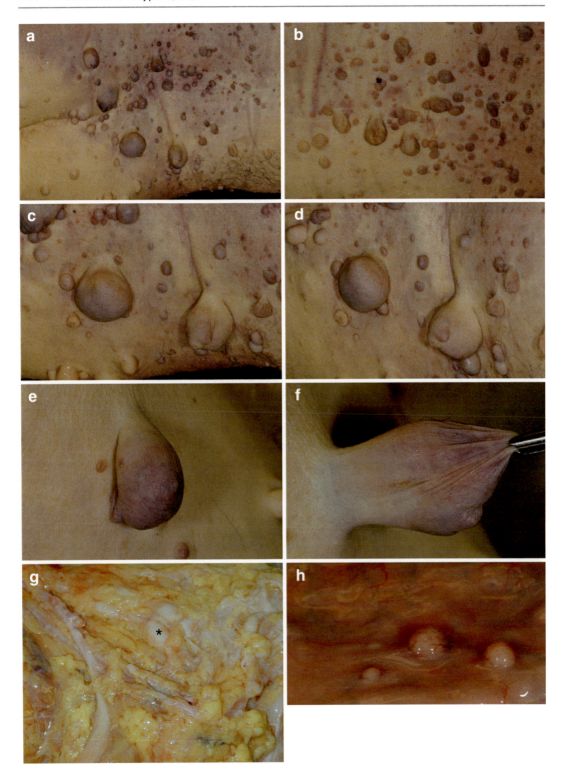

Fig. 71.20 The whole body is covered with multiple neurofibromas of various sizes (**a–f**). The nerves of the abdomen show thickening (∗) (**g**). Three neurofibromas are evident in the lumen of the stomach (**h**)

- Any two of the following:
  - Meningioma
  - Schwannoma
  - Glioma
  - Posterior subcapsular lens opacity
- Probable NF2
  - Unilateral vestibular schwannoma at <30 years and at least one of the following:
    - Meningioma
    - Schwannoma
    - Glioma
    - Posterior lens opacity or
  - Two or more meningiomas and either
    - Unilateral vestibular schwannoma at <30 years or
    - One of the following:
      - Schwannoma
      - Glioma
      - Posterior lens opacity

71.8.2 Neuroimaging Findings

General Imaging Findings
- See intracranial schwannomas, meningiomas, and ependymomas

71.9 Schwannomatosis

WHO Definition
2016—A usually sporadic and sometimes autosomal dominant disorder characterized by multiple schwannomas (spinal, cutaneous, and cranial) and multiple meningiomas (cranial and spinal), associated with inactivation of the NF2 gene in tumors but not in the germline, and caused by mutations in SMARCB1 on 22q or LZTR1 on 22q (Stemmer-Rachamimov et al. 2016a).

2007—A usually sporadic and sometimes autosomal dominant disorder characterized by multiple spinal, cutaneous, and cranial nerve schwannomas, without vestibular schwannomas or other manifestations of NF1 or NF1; associated with inactivation of the NF2 gene in tumors but not in the germline (Stemmer-Rachamimov et al. 2007).

71.9.1 Incidence and Diagnostic Criteria

Incidence
- 1: 40,000–1.80,000

Diagnostic Criteria for Schwannomatosis
- Diagnostic criteria for schwannomatosis have been described as follows (MacCollin et al. 2005):
- Definite schwannomatosis
  - Two or more (pathologically proven) schwannomas and lack of vestibular schwannomas on MRI study at >30 years and no known constitutional NF2 mutation or
  - One (pathologically proven) schwannoma and first-degree relative with schwannomatosis
- Probable schwannomatosis
  - Two or more schwannomas and age < 30 years and no evidence of vestibular schwannomas on MRI scan and no known constitutional NF2 mutation or
  - Two or more schwannomas and age < 45 years and no symptoms of cranial nerve VII dysfunction and no known constitutional NF2 mutation or
  - Radiographic evidence of one schwannoma and first-degree relative with schwannomatosis

Clinical overlap and differences between NF2 and schwannomatosis are given in Table 71.6.

71.10 Molecular Neuropathology

The neurofibromatoses comprise a group of hereditary tumor syndromes including the three genetically distinct diseases neurofibromatosis type 1 (NF1), neurofibromatosis type 2 (NF2), and schwannomatosis. Since specific tumor suppressor genes could be identified that are correlated with each of these syndromes, their molecular pathology is now well established:

71.10 Molecular Neuropathology

Table 71.6 Clinical overlap and differences between NF2 and schwannomatosis: Frequency of clinical feature in %, modified after Kehrer-Sawatzki et al. (2017), data reproduced with kind permission by Springer Nature

Clinical features	NF2	Schwannomatosis
Bilateral vestibular schwannoma	90–95	Absent
Unilateral vestibular schwannoma	18	Rare
Intracranial nonvestibular schwannoma	24–51	9–10
Intracranial meningioma	45–58	5
Spinal tumor	63–90	74
Ependymoma	18–58	Absent
Peripheral nerve schwannoma	68	89
Subcutaneous tumor	43–48	23
Skin plaques	41–48	Absent
Intradermal tumor	27	Absent
Retinal hamartoma	6–22	Absent
Epiretinal membrane	12–40	Absent
Subcapsular cataract	60–81	Absent

- The *NF1* (neurofibromin 1) gene, located at chromosome 17q11.2, is affected in NF1 patients; *NF1* encodes the tumor suppressor neurofibromin which acts as a negative regulator of the Ras (Rat sarcoma) protein.
- The *NF2* (neurofibromin 2) gene, encoding the tumor suppressor "Merlin" (moesin-ezrin-radixin-like protein), also termed schwannomin, is involved in NF2 and schwannomatosis; *NF2* is located at chromosome 22q12.2.
- The *SMARCB1* (SWI/SNF-related, matrix-associated, actin-dependent regulator of chromatin, subfamily b, member 1) gene is associated with schwannomatosis; *SMARCB1* is located at chromosome 22q11.23.

71.10.1 Neurofibromatosis Type 1 (NF1)

Genetics

The molecular genetic events observed in NF1 occur according to the "two-hit" model:

1. germline mutations inactivating the *NF1* gene on one allele (*NF1+/−*), resulting in decreased cellular levels of functional neurofibromin; in a subsequent step ("second-hit")
2. somatic *NF1* gene alterations in the other allele occur (loss of heterozygosity; LOH), leading to the complete absence of active neurofibromin protein (*NF1−/−* cells)

Reduced or abolished activity of neurofibromin triggers deregulation and ultimately constitutive activation of the Ras signaling pathway, thereby also affecting members of downstream signaling cascades driving cell proliferation, such as:

- MAPK (mitogen-activated protein kinase)
- PI3K (phosphatidylinositol 3-kinase)
- PKB (protein kinase B; also known as Akt)
- mTOR (mammalian target of rapamycin)

71.10.2 Neurofibromatosis Type 2 (NF2)

The genetic background underlying neurofibromatosis type 2 (NF2) is linked to changes in the *NF2* (neurofibromin 2) gene, which is located on chromosome 22q12.2 and encodes the tumor suppressor protein merlin (schwannomin). The aberrations observed in *NF2* include missense mutations, frameshifts resulting in truncated gene products, small base insertions/deletions, and large deletions. The genetic mechanism driving the development of NF2 involves an initial monoallelic inactivating germline mutation in the *NF2* gene, followed by an inactivating somatic *NF2* mutation in the second allele ("two-hit" model). Together, both events lead to a complete loss of functional merlin protein.

Merlin is involved in the regulation of several cellular processes, depending on its subcellular location (Uhlmann and Plotkin 2012; Carroll 2012; Zhou and Hanemann 2012; Plotkin et al. 2013):

- *Nucleus*: Merlin is able to translocate to the nucleus where it inhibits the pro-proliferative E3 ubiquitin ligase CRL4/DCAF1
- At the *cell membrane*, active merlin inhibits the activities of RTKs (receptor tyrosine

kinases) and integrins, thereby participating in the regulation of downstream intracellular signal cascades; loss of merlin results in enhanced signaling of the oncogenic
- PI3K/Akt (phosphoinositide 3 kinase/Akt, or protein kinase B) pathway
- Raf/ERK/MAPK (rat fibrosarcoma/extracellular signal-regulated kinase/mitogen-activated protein kinase) pathway
- Rac/PAK (rac GTPase/p21-activated kinase) pathway
• Merlin is a key regulator of the Hippo pathway which governs organ size and cell number by controlling the proliferation/apoptosis ratio; mutations inactivating merlin function result in increased cellular proliferation and survival.

Genetics and Molecular Biologic Findings
• Mutations at chromosome 22q12; NF2 gen
  - Encoded protein: Merlin (schwannomin)
• Mosaic genetic alterations in 30% of de novo NF2 patients

Merlin: Functions
• Is an ERM (Ezrin/Radixin/Moesin) protein.
• Tumor suppressor gene.
• Multi-suppressor from cell membrane to nucleus.
• Linker between extracellular cues and intracellular signaling pathways that regulate cell motility, proliferation, and survival.
• Regulator of receptor distribution and signaling at the cell cortex.
• Coordinator of receptor signaling and intercellular contact.
• Regulation of angiogenesis in schwannomas through a Rac1/semaphorin 3F-dependent mechanism.
• Functions upstream of the nuclear E3 ubiquitin ligase CRL4DCAF1 to suppress oncogenic gene expression.
• Regulates the Hippo signaling pathway, which plays important roles in organ size control and cancer development.
• Promotes Schwann cell elongation and influences myelin segment length.
• Degraded through multistep phosphorylation by oncogenic kinases.

• Inhibits cell proliferation by modulating the growth activities of its binding partners, including the cell surface glycoprotein CD44, membrane-cytoskeleton linker protein ezrin and PIKE (PI 3-kinase enhancer) GTPase, etc.
• Merlin exerts its growth suppressive activity through a folded conformation that is tightly controlled through phosphorylation by numerous protein kinases including PAK, PKA, and Akt. Merlin inhibits PI 3-kinase activity through binding to PIKE-L.
• Proliferation repressive activity of merlin is also partially regulated by S518 phosphorylation.

71.10.3 Schwannomatosis

Although NF2 and schwannomatosis are recognized as two clinically distinct syndromes, it appears that aberrations in the *NF2* gene are involved in both diseases. However, inactivating germline *NF2* mutations, typically found in NF2, are lacking in schwannomatosis where only somatic mutations in tumor tissues have been observed. Mutations in the *NF2* gene are frequently detected in schwannomatosis-associated schwannoma tissue, but are absent in the germline.

As the major predisposing factor in schwannomatosis, however, the tumor suppressor gene *SMARCB1* (SWI/SNF-related, matrix-associated, actin-dependent regulator of chromatin, subfamily b, member 1) has been identified. Germline mutations of the *SMARCB1* gene were reported in 45% of familial cases and 7% of sporadic cases.

The gene is located on chromosome 22q11.2, which is in proximity to the *NF2* gene (22q12.2). In fact, germline *SMARCB1* mutations associated with somatic *NF2* mutations were frequently described in patients developing schwannomas. This observation led to the proposition of a "four-hit" mechanism which is thought to trigger tumorigenesis:

1. presence of a germline *SMARCB1* mutation on one of the two alleles
2. deletion of the chromosome 22 region spanning the second (wild-type)
3. *SMARCB1* allele and one of the *NF2* alleles
4. mutation of the second (wild-type) *NF2* allele

71.10 Molecular Neuropathology

Table 71.7 microRNAs involved in the pathogenesis of malignant tumors of the peripheral nervous system (MPNST) (Sedani et al. 2012), data reproduced with kind permission by Springer Nature

	Activity	miR expression: • Upregulated (↑) • Downregulated (↓)	Associated expression: • Upregulated (↑) • Downregulated (↓)
miR-10b	Oncogenic	↑	• Neurofibromin ↓ • twist basic helix-loop-helix transcription factor 1 (TWIST1) ↑
miR-21	Oncogenic	↑	• Programmed cell death 4 (neoplastic transformation inhibitor) (PDCD4) ↓
miR-29c	Tumor suppressor	↓	• Collagen, type I, alpha 1 (COL1A1) ↓ • Collagen, type XXI, alpha 1 (COL21A1) ↓ • Collagen, type V, alpha 2 (COL5A2) ↓ • Thymine-DNA glycosylase (TDG) ↓
miR-34a	Tumor suppressor	↓	• Tp53 ↓
miR-204	Tumor suppressor	↓	• High-mobility group AT-hook 2 (HMGA2) ↑
miR-214	Oncogenic	↑	• twist basic helix-loop-helix transcription factor 1 (TWIST1)
miR-214	Oncogenic	↓	• Phosphatase and tensin homolog (PTEN)

The physiological function of the *SMARCB1* gene product is its involvement in the regulation of gene expression by participating in chromatin remodeling. To date, however, it is unclear by which mechanism(s) the mutated and/or missing proteins promote tumorigenesis.

Genetic and Molecular Biology Findings
- *NF2* mutations in schwannomatosis-associated schwannomas, absent in non-tumor tissue.
- Germline mutations of the *SMARCB1* (*INI1*) gene
  - Exon 1 mutation c.41C>A.
  - 3′ untranslated region mutation c.*82C>T.
  - Mutant SMARCB1 proteins retain the ability to suppress cyclin D1 activity.
- Further causative genes might be found.

71.10.4 Malignant Peripheral Nerve Sheath Tumor (MPNST)

Clinical manifestations of NF1 range from benign *neurofibromas*, representing the most common Schwann cell neoplasms, to different malignant transformations, including *malignant peripheral nerve sheath tumors* (MPNST) which develop in up to 8–13% of NF1 patients.

It has been observed that MPNSTs predominantly arise from plexiform neurofibromas and are associated with the *NF1*−/− genotype. Listed below are some of the major molecular biology findings in MPNSTs:

- 50% of MPNSTs manifest in patients with NF1
- Complex numerical and structural karyotypic abnormalities
  - Near-triploid or hypodiploid chromosome numbers, chromosomal losses, recombinations involving almost all chromosomes
- Chromosome 17 with abnormalities in *NF1*- and *TP53* (tumor protein 53) loci
- Losses of chromosomes 13, 17, 18, 22
- Gains of chromosomes 2, 14
- *TP53* with mutations and altered protein expression
- *CDKN2A* (cyclin-dependent kinase inhibitor 2A) on chromosome 9p21:
  - homozygous deletions in the gene encoding the tumor suppressors p16INK4A and p14ARF
    - in 50% of the cases
    - inactivates the neighboring gene *CDKN2B* (cyclin-dependent kinase inhibitor 2B; encoding the tumor suppressor p15INK4B)
- inactivation of the p53- and Rb (retinoblastoma) regulatory pathways in 75% of cases

71.10.5 Epigenetics

MicroRNAs (miRs) regulating expression of oncogenes or tumor suppressor genes have been shown to participate in the malignant transformation of benign neurofibromas to MPNSTs, a process which is reflected in altered miR expression levels in the MPNST cells. Table 71.7 shows a selection of several miRs including some associated protein-coding genes (compiled from Sedani et al. (2012)).

Selected References

Abramowicz A, Gos M (2014) Neurofibromin in neurofibromatosis type 1—mutations in NF1gene as a cause of disease. Dev Period Med 18(3):297–306

Ahlawat S, Fayad LM, Khan MS, Bredella MA, Harris GJ, Evans DG, Farschtschi S, Jacobs MA, Chhabra A, Salamon JM, Wenzel R, Mautner VF, Dombi E, Cai W, Plotkin SR, Blakeley JO (2016) Current whole-body MRI applications in the neurofibromatoses: NF1, NF2, and schwannomatosis. Neurology 87(7 Suppl 1):S31–S39. https://doi.org/10.1212/wnl.0000000000002929

Anderson JL, Gutmann DH (2015) Neurofibromatosis type 1. Handb Clin Neurol 132:75–86. https://doi.org/10.1016/b978-0-444-62702-5.00004-4

Antonescu CR, Louis DN, Hunter S, Perry A, Reuss DE, Stemmer-Rachamimov AO (2016a) Schwannoma. In: Louis DN, Ohgaki H, Wiestler OD, Cavenee WK (eds) WHO classification of tumours of the central nervous system, Revised 4th edn. IARC, Lyon, pp 214–218

Antonescu CR, Perry A, Reuss DE (2016b) Perineurioma. In: Louis DN, Ohgaki H, Wiestler OD, Cavenee WK (eds) WHO classification of tumours of the central nervous system, Revised 4th edn. IARC, Lyon, pp 222–224

Antonescu CR, Stemmer-Rachamimov AO, Perry A (2016c) Hybrid nerve sheath tumours. In: Louis DN, Ohgaki H, Wiestler OD, Cavenee WK (eds) WHO classification of tumours of the central nervous system, Revised 4th edn. IARC, Lyon, pp 224–225

Bakker AC, La Rosa S, Sherman LS, Knight P, Lee H, Pancza P, Nievo M (2017) Neurofibromatosis as a gateway to better treatment for a variety of malignancies. Prog Neurobiol 152:149–165. https://doi.org/10.1016/j.pneurobio.2016.01.004

Beltrami S, Kim R, Gordon J (2013) Neurofibromatosis type 2 protein, NF2: an unconventional cell cycle regulator. Anticancer Res 33(1):1–11

Carroll SL (2012) Molecular mechanisms promoting the pathogenesis of Schwann cell neoplasms. Acta Neuropathol 123(3):321–348

Evans DG (2015) Neurofibromatosis type 2. Handb Clin Neurol 132:87–96. https://doi.org/10.1016/b978-0-444-62702-5.00005-6

Evans DG, Huson SM, Donnai D, Neary W, Blair V, Newton V, Harris R (1992) A clinical study of type 2 neurofibromatosis. Q J Med 84(304):603–618

Ferner RE, Gutmann DH (2013) Neurofibromatosis type 1 (NF1): diagnosis and management. Handb Clin Neurol 115:939–955. https://doi.org/10.1016/b978-0-444-52902-2.00053-9

Gutmann DH, Aylsworth A, Carey JC, Korf B, Marks J, Pyeritz RE, Rubenstein A, Viskochil D (1997) The diagnostic evaluation and multidisciplinary management of neurofibromatosis 1 and neurofibromatosis 2. JAMA 278(1):51–57

Helfferich J, Nijmeijer R, Brouwer OF, Boon M, Fock A, Hoving EW, Meijer L, den Dunnen WF, de Bont ES (2016) Neurofibromatosis type 1 associated low grade gliomas: a comparison with sporadic low grade gliomas. Crit Rev Oncol Hematol 104:30–41. https://doi.org/10.1016/j.critrevonc.2016.05.008

Jouhilahti EM, Peltonen S, Heape AM, Peltonen J (2011) The pathoetiology of neurofibromatosis 1. Am J Pathol 178(5):1932–1939. https://doi.org/10.1016/j.ajpath.2010.12.056

Karajannis MA, Ferner RE (2015) Neurofibromatosis-related tumors: emerging biology and therapies. Curr Opin Pediatr 27(1):26–33. https://doi.org/10.1097/mop.0000000000000169

Kehrer-Sawatzki H, Farschtschi S, Mautner VF, Cooper DN (2017) The molecular pathogenesis of schwannomatosis, a paradigm for the co-involvement of multiple tumour suppressor genes in tumorigenesis. Hum Genet 136(2):129–148. https://doi.org/10.1007/s00439-016-1753-8

Kleihues P, Burger PC, Scheithauer BW (1993) Histological typing of tumours of the central nervous system, 2nd edn. Springer-Verlag, Berlin

Koontz NA, Wiens AL, Agarwal A, Hingtgen CM, Emerson RE, Mosier KM (2013) Schwannomatosis: the overlooked neurofibromatosis? AJR Am J Roentgenol 200(6):W646–W653. https://doi.org/10.2214/ajr.12.8577

Kresak JL, Walsh M (2016) Neurofibromatosis: a review of NF1, NF2, and Schwannomatosis. J Pediatr Genet 5(2):98–104. https://doi.org/10.1055/s-0036-1579766

Lloyd SK, Evans DG (2013) Neurofibromatosis type 2 (NF2): diagnosis and management. Handb Clin Neurol 115:957–967. https://doi.org/10.1016/b978-0-444-52902-2.00054-0

Louis DN, Stemmer-Rachamimov AO, Wiestler OD (2000) Neurofibromatosis type 2. In: Kleihues P, Cavenee WK (eds) Pathology and genetics of tumours of the nervous system, 3rd edn. IARC Press, Lyon, pp 219–222

Lu-Emerson C, Plotkin SR (2009) The neurofibromatoses. Part 2: NF2 and schwannomatosis. Rev Neurol Dis 6(3):E81–E86

Selected References

MacCollin M, Chiocca EA, Evans DG, Friedman JM, Horvitz R, Jaramillo D, Lev M, Mautner VF, Niimura M, Plotkin SR, Sang CN, Stemmer-Rachamimov A, Roach ES (2005) Diagnostic criteria for schwannomatosis. Neurology 64(11):1838–1845. https://doi.org/10.1212/01.wnl.0000163982.78900.ad

MacCollin M, Woodfin W, Kronn D, Short MP (1996) Schwannomatosis: a clinical and pathologic study. Neurology 46(4):1072–1079

Pasmant E, Vidaud M, Vidaud D, Wolkenstein P (2012) Neurofibromatosis type 1: from genotype to phenotype. J Med Genet 49(8):483–489. https://doi.org/10.1136/jmedgenet-2012-100978

Patil S, Chamberlain RS (2012) Neoplasms associated with germline and somatic NF1 gene mutations. Oncologist 17(1):101–116. https://doi.org/10.1634/theoncologist.2010-0181

Perry A, von Deimling A, Louis DN, Hunter S, Reuss DE, Antonescu CR (2016) Neurofibroma. In: Louis DN, Ohgaki H, Wiestler OD, Cavenee WK (eds) WHO classification of tumours of the central nervous system, Revised 4th edn. IARC, Lyon, pp 219–221

Plotkin SR, Blakeley JO, Evans DG, Hanemann CO, Hulsebos TJ, Hunter-Schaedle K, Kalpana GV, Korf B, Messiaen L, Papi L, Ratner N, Sherman LS, Smith MJ, Stemmer-Rachamimov AO, Vitte J, Giovannini M (2013) Update from the 2011 International Schwannomatosis Workshop: from genetics to diagnostic criteria. Am J Med Genet A 161A(3):405–416. https://doi.org/10.1002/ajmg.a.35760

Rad E, Tee AR (2016) Neurofibromatosis type 1: fundamental insights into cell signalling and cancer. Semin Cell Dev Biol 52:39–46. https://doi.org/10.1016/j.semcdb.2016.02.007

Reuss DE, Louis DN, Hunter S, Perry A, Hirose T, Antonescu CR (2016a) Malignant peripheral nerve sheath tumour. In: Louis DN, Ohgaki H, Wiestler OD, Cavenee WK (eds) WHO classification of the central nervous system, Revised 4th edn. IARC, Lyon, pp 226–229

Reuss DE, von Deimling A, Perry A (2016b) Neurofibromatosis type 1. In: Louis DN, Ohgaki H, Wiestler OD, Cavenee WK (eds) WHO classification of tumours of the central nervous system, Revised 4th edn. IARC, Lyon, pp 294–296

Rodriguez FJ, Stratakis CA, Evans DG (2012) Genetic predisposition to peripheral nerve neoplasia: diagnostic criteria and pathogenesis of neurofibromatoses, Carney complex, and related syndromes. Acta Neuropathol 123(3):349–367. https://doi.org/10.1007/s00401-00011-00935-00407

Salamon J, Mautner VF, Adam G, Derlin T (2015) Multimodal imaging in neurofibromatosis type 1-associated nerve sheath tumors. Rofo 187(12):1084–1092. https://doi.org/10.1055/s-0035-1553505

Scheithauer BW, Giannini C, Woodruff JM (2000) Perineurioma. In: Kleihues P, Cavenee WK (eds) Pathology and genetics of tumours of the nervous system, 3rd edn. IARC Press, Lyon, pp 169–171

Scheithauer BW, Louis DN, Hunter S, Woodruff JM, Antonescu CR (2007a) Malignant peripheral nerve sheath tumour (MPNST). In: Louis DN, Ohgaki H, Wiestler OD, Cavenee WK (eds) WHO classification of tumours of the central nervous system, 4th edn. International Agency for Research on Cancer, Lyon, pp 160–162

Scheithauer BW, Louis DN, Hunter S, Woodruff JM, Antonescu CR (2007b) Neurofibroma. In: Louis DN, Ohgaki H, Wiestler OD, Cavenee WK (eds) WHO classification of tumours of the central nervous system, 4th edn. International Agency for Research on Cancer, Lyon, pp 156–157

Scheithauer BW, Louis DN, Hunter S, Woodruff JM, Antonescu CR (2007c) Schwannoma. In: Louis DN, Ohgaki H, Wiestler OD, Cavenee WK (eds) WHO classification of tumours of the central nervous system, 4th edn. International Agency for Research on Cancer, Lyon, pp 152–155

Scheithauer BW, Woodruff JM, Antonescu CR (2007d) Perineurioma. In: Louis DN, Ohgaki H, Wiestler OD, Cavenee WK (eds) WHO classification of tumours of the central nervous system, 4th edn. International Agency for Research on Cancer, Lyon, pp 158–159

Sedani A, Cooper DN, Upadhyaya M (2012) An emerging role for microRNAs in NF1 tumorigenesis. Hum Genomics 6:23. https://doi.org/10.1186/1479-7364-1186-1123

Shofty B, Constantini S, Ben-Shachar S (2015) Advances in molecular diagnosis of Neurofibromatosis type 1. Semin Pediatr Neurol 22(4):234–239. https://doi.org/10.1016/j.spen.2015.10.007

Slattery WH (2015) Neurofibromatosis type 2. Otolaryngol Clin N Am 48(3):443–460. https://doi.org/10.1016/j.otc.2015.02.005

Stemmer-Rachamimov AO, Hulsebos TJM, Wesseling P (2016a) Schwannomatosis. In: Louis DN, Ohgaki H, Wiestler OD, Cavenee WK (eds) WHO classification of tumours of the central nervous system, Revised 4th edn. IARC, Lyon, pp 301–303

Stemmer-Rachamimov AO, Wiestler OD, Louis DN (2007) Neurofibromatosis type 2. In: Louis DN, Ohgaki H, Wiestler OD, Cavenee WK (eds) WHO classification of tumours of the central nervous system, 4th edn. International Agency for Research on Cancer, Lyon, pp 210–214

Stemmer-Rachamimov AO, Wiestler OD, Louis DN (2016b) Neurofibromatosis type 2. In: Louis DN, Ohgaki H, Wiestler OD, Cavenee WK (eds) WHO classification of tumours of the central nervous system, Revised 4th edn. IARC, Lyon, pp 297–300

Uhlmann EJ, Plotkin SR (2012) Neurofibromatoses. Adv Exp Med Biol 724:266–277

von Deimling A, Foster R, Krone W (2000) Neurofibromatosis type 1. In: Kleihues P, Cavenee WK (eds) Pathology and genetics of tumours of the nervous system, 3rd edn. IARC Press, Lyon, pp 216–218

von Deimling A, Perry A (2007) Neurofibromatosis type 1. In: Louis DN, Ohgaki H, Wiestler OD, Cavenee WK (eds) WHO classification of tumours of the central nervous system, 4th edn. International Agency for Research on Cancer, Lyon, pp 206–209

Wasa J, Nishida Y, Tsukushi S, Shido Y, Sugiura H, Nakashima H, Ishiguro N (2010) MRI features in the differentiation of malignant peripheral nerve sheath tumors and neurofibromas. AJR Am J Roentgenol 194(6):1568–1574. https://doi.org/10.2214/ajr.09.2724

Woodruff JM, Kourea HP, Louis DN, Scheithauer BW (2000a) Malignant peripheral nerve sheath tumour (MPNST). In: Kleihues P, Cavenee WK (eds) Pathology and genetics of tumours of the nervous system, 3rd edn. IARC Press, Lyon, pp 172–174

Woodruff JM, Kourea HP, Louis DN, Scheithauer BW (2000b) Neurofibroma. In: Kleihues P, Cavenee WK (eds) Pathology and genetics of tumours of the nervous system, 3rd edn. IARC Press, Lyon, pp 167–168

Woodruff JM, Kourea HP, Louis DN, Scheithauer BW (2000c) Schwannoma. In: Kleihues P, Cavenee WK (eds) Pathology and genetics of tumours of the nervous system, 3rd edn. IARC Press, Lyon, pp 164–166

Zhou L, Hanemann CO (2012) Merlin, a multi-suppressor from cell membrane to the nucleus. FEBS Lett 586(10):1403–1408

Zülch KJ (1979) Histological typing of tumours of the central nervous system. World Health Organization, Geneva

Tumors of Meningothelial Cells: Meningiomas

72.1 Introduction

Meningiomas are usually benign tumors arising from meningeal or arachnoithelial cells. They occur frequently and make up 40–45% of tumors seen in the daily clinical practice.

According to biologic behavior, the following three groups of meningiomas are distinguished:

• Meningioma (with various histologic subtypes)	WHO grade I
• Atypical meningioma	WHO grade II
• Anaplastic meningioma	WHO grade III

72.2 General Aspects

72.2.1 Clinical Signs and Symptoms

- Headache
- Seizures
- Visual disturbances
- Based on tumor location
  - Cerebellar signs
- Symptoms due to compression of specific anatomic structures

72.2.2 Epidemiology

Incidence
- 25–30% of primary intracranial tumors
- Annual incidence rate: 13 per 100,000
- Frequencies by WHO grade (Table 72.1):
  - WHO grade I 85%
  - WHO grade II 12%
  - WHO grade III 3%

Table 72.1 Frequencies of histological meningioma subtype

Meningioma type	WHO grade	Frequency in %
Meningothelial	I	43
Transitional	I	38
Fibroblastic	I	9
Angiomatous	I	4
Metaplastic	I	2
Psammomatous	I	1
Secretory	I	1
Microcystic	I	1
Lymphoplasmacyte-rich	I	<1
Atypical	II	12
Clear cell	II	<1
Chordoid	II	<1
Anaplastic	III	3
Rhabdoid	III	<1
Papillary	III	<1

Age Incidence
- Middle-aged and elderly patients
- sixth to seventh decade
- Childhood rare: more aggressive tumors

Sex Incidence

• Male:Female ratio	1:2
• Male:Female aged 40–49 years	1:3.5
• Spinal meningiomas	female predominance
• Atypical and anaplastic meningiomas	male predominance

Localization
- Intracranial
  - Over the cerebral convexities
  - Parasagittal in connection with the falx and venous sinus
  - Sphenoid ridges
  - Petrous ridges
  - Para/suprasellar region
  - Olfactory grooves
- Intraspinal
  - Predominantly thoracic level
- Orbita
  - Optic nerve
- Rare locations:
  - Intraventricular
  - Epidural
  - Other organs (e.g., lung, pleura, liver, bone)

72.2.3 Neuroimaging Features

General Imaging Findings
- Extra-axial, well-defined mass, attached to the dura.
- Round, lobulated, or en plaque configuration.
- Tumor grading on the basis of imaging findings is in the majority of the cases impossible. In anaplastic meningioma (WHO grade III), infiltration of the bone with extracranial mass and extinguished border to the brain is more frequent.

CT non-contrast-enhanced (Figs. 72.1a, b, 72.2a, c, 72.3a, 72.4c, 72.5a)

- Well-defined, hyperdense tumor.
- Variable surrounding edema.
- Variable Calcifications are seen in 20% of the cases.
- Bone changes include hyperostosis, lysis, or destruction.

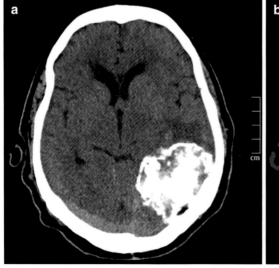 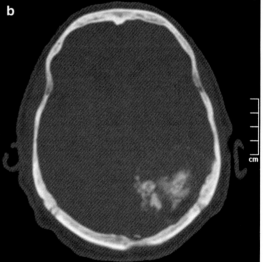

Fig. 72.1 Non-enhanced CT scan demonstrates a strongly calcified dural based mass (**a**) with bone CT (**b**)

72.2 General Aspects

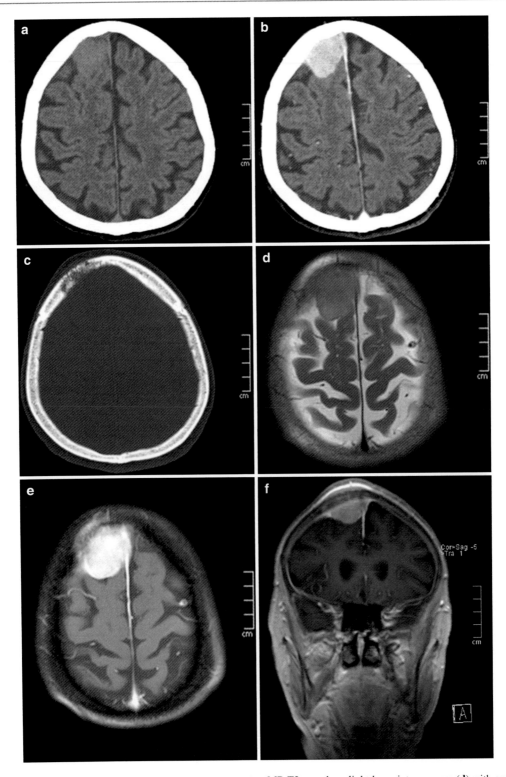

Fig. 72.2 Classic CT appearance of a right frontal meningioma WHO grade I, which is slightly hyperdense (**a**) with intense enhancement (**b**) and bone infiltration (**c**). MR T2 reveals a slight hyperintense mass (**d**) with corresponding strong enhancement (**e, f**)

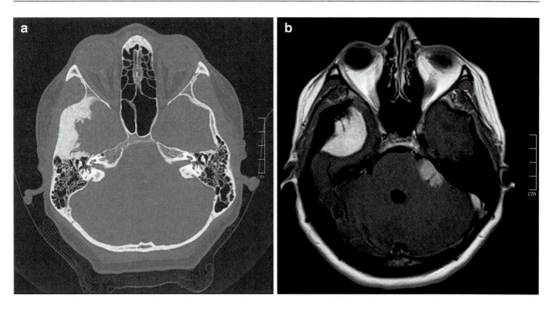

Fig. 72.3 On CT scan hyperostosis of the temporal bone is seen due to the right-sided meningioma (**a**), MR with T1 postcontrast demonstrates a second meningioma at the left cerebellopontine angle (**b**)

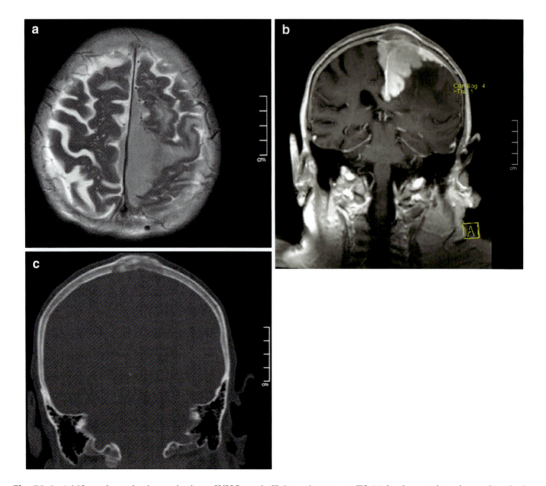

Fig. 72.4 A bifrontal anaplastic meningioma WHO grade II, hyperintense on T2 (**a**) leads to an invasion and occlusion of the superior sagittal sinus on T1 contrast (**b**), also invading the calvaria with extracranial mass on bone CT (**c**)

72.2 General Aspects

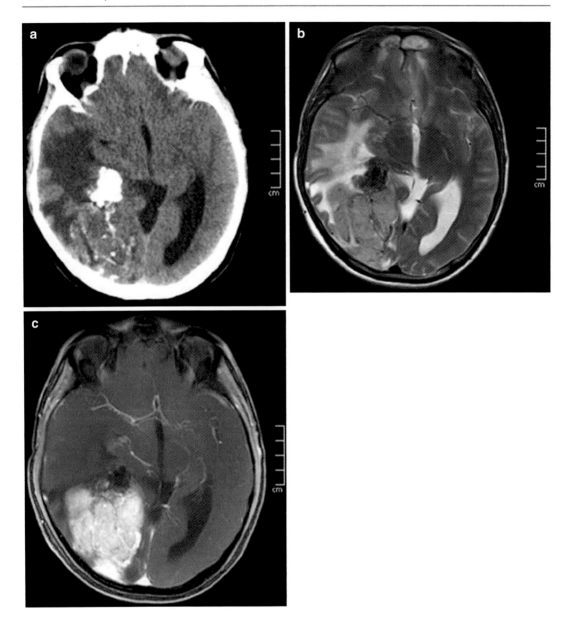

Fig. 72.5 CT shows a calcified anaplastic meningioma WHO grade III (**a**) leading to mass effect with surrounding edema on T2 image (**b**) and has partly irregular borders to the brain on T1 contrast (**c**)

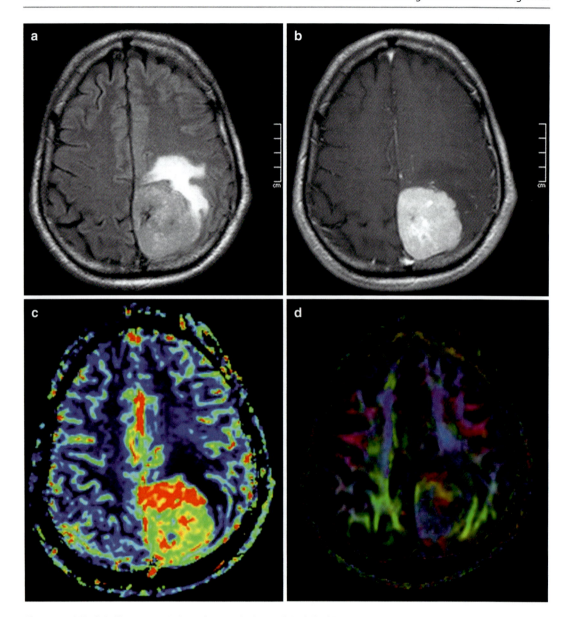

Fig. 72.6 MR-flair illustrates (**a**) the peritumoral edema of the left-sided homogenously enhancing meningioma on T1 contrast (**b**) with elevated rCBV (**c**) and displaced fibers according to the extra-axial mass with cortical buckling (**d**)

72.2 General Aspects

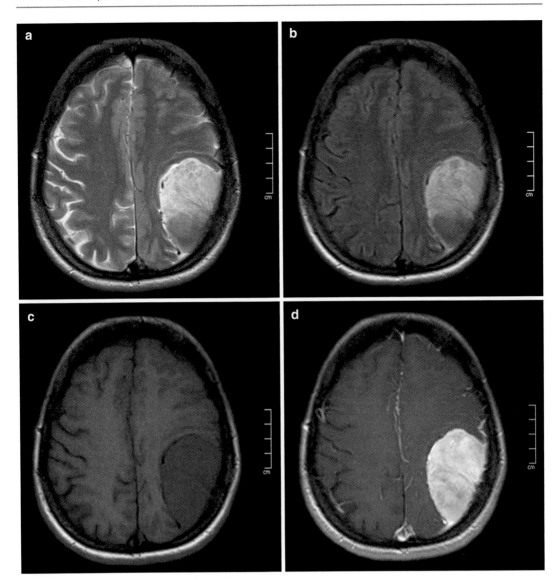

Fig. 72.7 Atypical meningioma WHO grade II with typical radial appearance of the vessels in T2 and Flair (**a**, **b**). On T1 the tumor is commonly isointense to the cortex (**c**). The dural tail is well demonstrated on the posterior base of the meningioma on T1 contrast (**d**). Digital angiography of selective external artery injection shows spoke-wheel pattern of meningeal vessels (**e**), which were embolized with onyx (**f**) initiating necrosis of the tumor with reduced contrast on T1 (**g**)

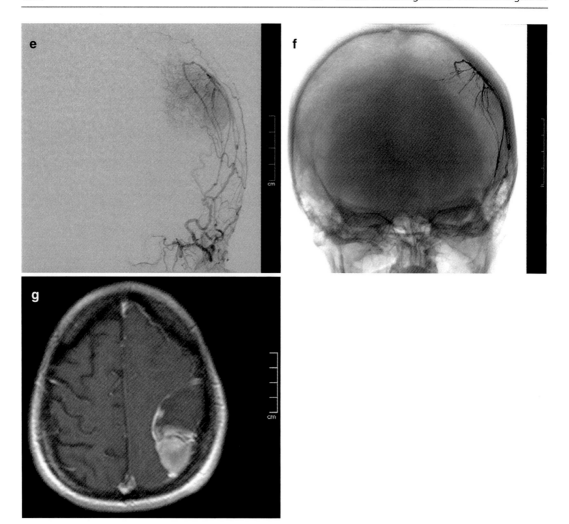

Fig. 72.7 (continued)

CT contrast-enhanced (Fig. 72.2b)

- Strong, homogeneous enhancement

MRI-T2/FLAIR (Figs. 72.2d, e, 72.6a, 72.7a, b, 72.4a, 72.5b, 72.8)

- Iso- to hyperintense

MRI-T1 (Fig. 72.7c)

- Iso- to hypointense

MRI-T1 Contrast-Enhanced (Figs. 72.3b, 72.4b, 72.5c, e, f, 72.6b, and 72.7d, g)

- Homogeneous, strong enhancement.
- Adjacent dural thickening—dural tail—is common, but not pathognomonic, it is reactive and has not to be resected.

MRI-T2∗/SWI

- Identifies calcifications.
- Hemorrhage is rare.

MR-Diffusion Imaging

- Variable diffusion restriction
- ADC lower in malignant meningiomas

72.2 General Aspects

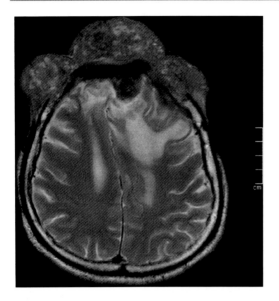

Fig. 72.8 Expansive extracranial growth of a recurrent bifrontal meningothelial meningioma (WHO grade I) on T2

MRI-Perfusion (Fig. 72.6c)

- Increasing rCBV in peritumoral edma may indicate malignant meningioma.

MR-Diffusion Tensor Imaging (Fig. 72.6d)

- Increased mean FA within the perifocal edema

MR-Spectroscopy

- Elevated Alanin peak

Angiography (Fig. 72.7e, f)

- CTA/MRA
  - Demonstrates invasion or occlusion of dural sinuses
- DSA
  - Primary supply from meningeal arteries (external carotid artery) showing a radial pattern.
  - Pial vessels from the internal carotid artery are more frequent at the skull base.
  - Early dense tumor blush that persists into the venous phase is typical.
  - Preoperative embolization reduces blood loss and makes neurosurgical resection less difficult.

Nuclear Medicine Imaging Findings (Figs. 72.9, 72.10, 72.11, 72.12, 72.13, 72.14, 72.15, 72.16, 72.17, and 72.18)

- Meningiomas express somatostatin receptors and thereby can be visualized with radioactively labeled somatostatin analogs. Normal brain tissue expresses no SSR (except the pituitary gland—this has to be taken into account) resulting in a very good tracer to background ratio.
- These radiotracers are available for SPECT (111In-octreotide and 99Tc-tectrotyde) and for PET (68Ga-DOTA-NOC/TOC/TATE, etc.).
- The somatostatin expression can be used for nuclear medicine therapy too (labeled with yttrium-90 or lutetium-177).
- Differences in resolution, half-life, and tracer-kinetics between the different SPECT and PET tracers have to be taken into account (e.g., the indium-labeled SPECT tracers causes a higher radiation burden than the technetium-labeled one, gallium-68 has a half-life of 68 min).
- There are small differences in the binding to the different SSR between the different radiotracers which play only a minor role in nuclear medicine practice.
- As meningiomas dedifferentiate they lose more and more of the somatostatin receptors and increase their metabolism, thus, FDG shows an increased uptake in these lesions although there is no possibility of grading with FDG.
- FET, thallium, MIBI, or CBF-tracers can show an increased uptake (especially depending on the dedifferentiation) but are not the radiotracers of choice to evaluate a possible meningioma.
- The possibility of a meningioma has to be taken into account if there is an uptake of these tracers and a SSR-PET or SPECT should be performed if there is the clinical suspicion for meningioma.

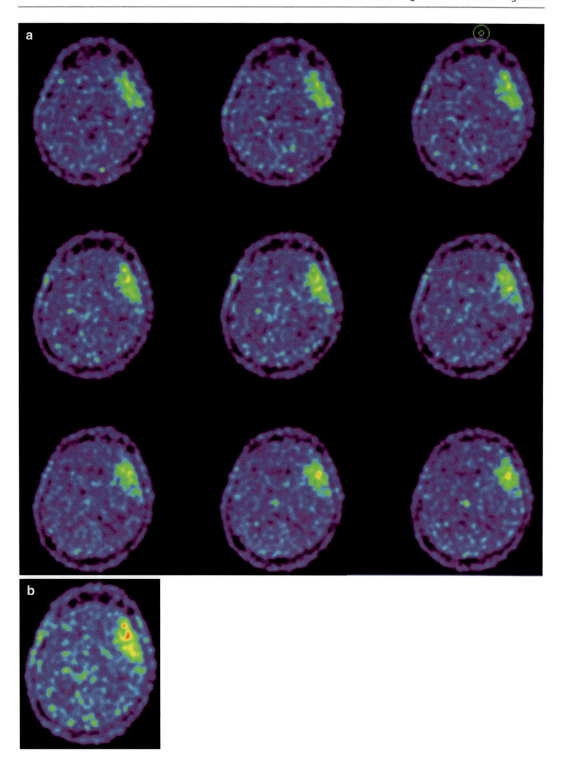

Fig. 72.9 FET uptake in a meningioma WHO grade I left sphenoid wing (**a**, **b**)

72.3 Meningioma

WHO Definition

2016—A group of mostly benign, slow-growing neoplasms that are most likely derived from the meningothelial cells of the arachnoid layer (Perry et al. 2016b).

2007—Meningothelial (arachnoidal) cell neoplasms, typically attached to the inner surface of the dura mater (Perry et al. 2007).

2000—Meningiomas are generally slowly growing, benign tumors attached to the dura mater and composed of neoplastic meningothelial (arachnoidal) cells. They typically manifest in adults and show a predominance for women (Louis et al. 2000).

1993—A benign tumor composed of neoplastic meningothelial (arachnoidal) cells (Kleihues et al. 1993).

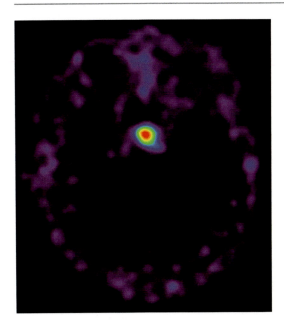

Fig. 72.10 Physiological uptake in the pituitary gland; somatostatin receptor PET

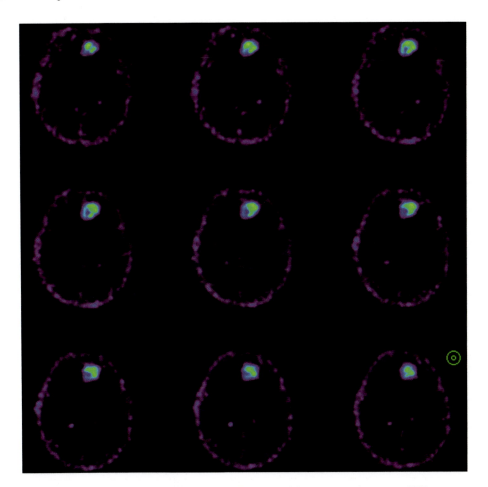

Fig. 72.11 Slices of a meningioma WHO grade I left located at the falx; somatostatin receptor PET

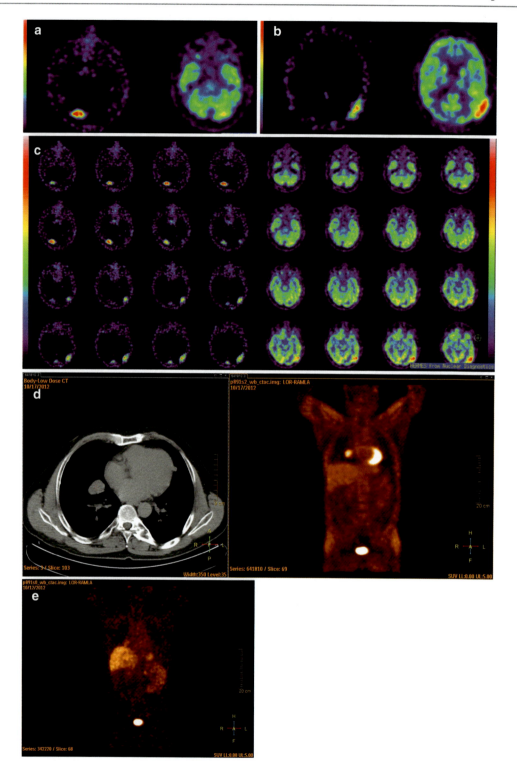

Fig. 72.12 Anaplastic meningioma WHO grade III with different biological behaving meningiomas. Somatostatin receptor-positive and FDG-negative meningioma (**a**), somatostatin receptor and FDG-positive meningioma (**b**), slices of the patients head (**c**), clear FDG-positive metastasis of the right lung (**d**), only faint SSR expression in the metastasis of the right lung (**e**)

72.3 Meningioma

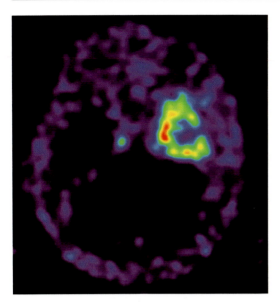

Fig. 72.13 Patient with a left sphenoid meningioma WHO grade II after surgery (2 times) and radiation therapy; somatostatin receptor PET

1979—A tumor originating from cellular elements of the meninges (Zülch 1979).

WHO Grade
- WHO grade I

72.3.1 Neuropathology Findings

Macroscopic Features (Figs. 72.19, 72.20, and 72.21)
- Rubber or firm
- Well demarcated
- Nodular or lobulated appearance
- Gritty surface (calcifications in form of psammomatous bodies)
- Plaque-like appearance, i.e., flat, carpet-like growth
- Invasion of dura, venous sinuses, skull (hyperostosis)
- Can reach appreciable sizes. Kerschner 1928 described a meningioma in a 34-year-old man weighing 1300 g and measuring 18 × 14 × 9 cm. Since 2 years prior to death, a trepanation was performed, a considerable part of the tumor did prolabate through the trepanation opening.

Microscopic Features

From a histological point of view, the subdivision of meningiomas into the following categories can be done:

- Meningothelial meningioma
- Fibrous (fibroblastic) meningioma
- Transitional meningioma
- Psammomatous meningioma
- Angiomatous meningioma
- Microcystic meningioma
- Secretory meningioma
- Clear cell meningioma
- Chordoid meningioma
- Lymphoplasmacyte-rich meningioma
- Metaplastic meningioma

One should always keep in mind that the histological subtyping has no clinical relevance regarding outcome, survival, and recurrences.

Meningothelial Meningioma (Fig. 72.22a–h)
A classic and common variant of meningioma, with medium-sized epithelioid tumor cells forming lobules, some of which are partly demarcated by thin collagenous septa (Perry et al. 2016a).

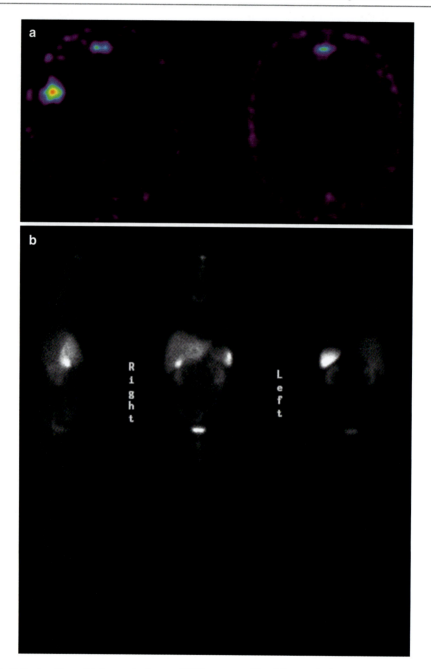

Fig. 72.14 Patient with multiple meningiomas WHO grade I. (**a**) Before and after resection of one meningioma, (**b**) technetium-labeled somatostatin receptor whole body scan with a faint uptake in the meningiomas, (**c**) slices of the suprasellar meningioma

72.3 Meningioma

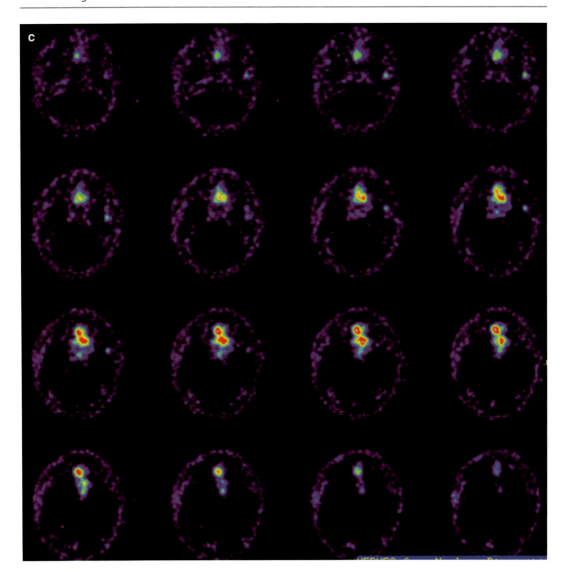

Fig. 72.14 (continued)

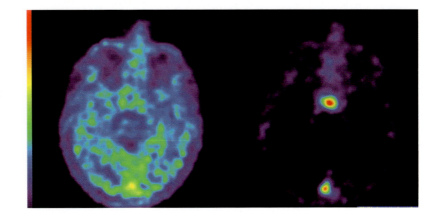

Fig. 72.15 Faint FET uptake and clear somatostatin receptor-positive PET of an atypical meningioma WHO grade II left occipital (physiological uptake in the pituitary gland)

Fig. 72.16 MIBI and thallium-positive fibroblastic meningioma WHO grade I (physiological uptake in the pituitary gland)

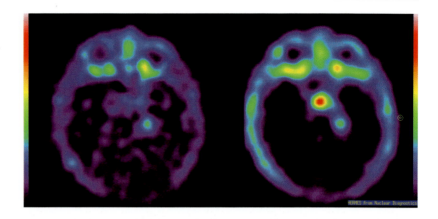

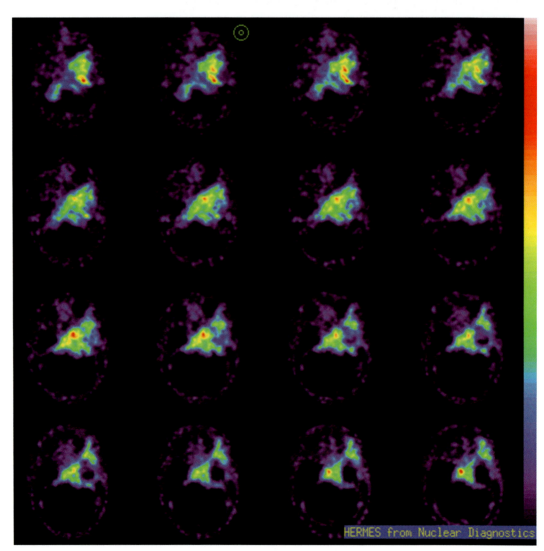

Fig. 72.17 SSR-PET of a large infiltrative atypical meningioma WHO grade II

72.3 Meningioma

Fig. 72.18 Atypical meningioma WHO grade II left parietal. SSR-scintigraphy before and SSR-PET after resection (**a**), whole body SSR-scintigraphy showing the uptake in the meningioma (**b**)

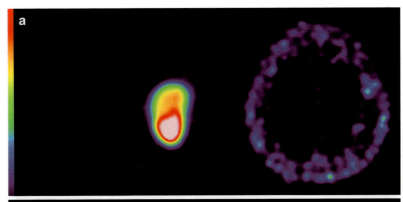

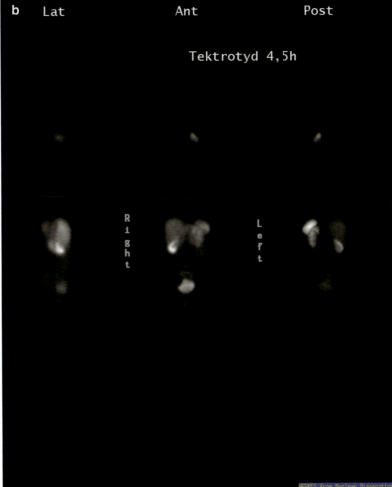

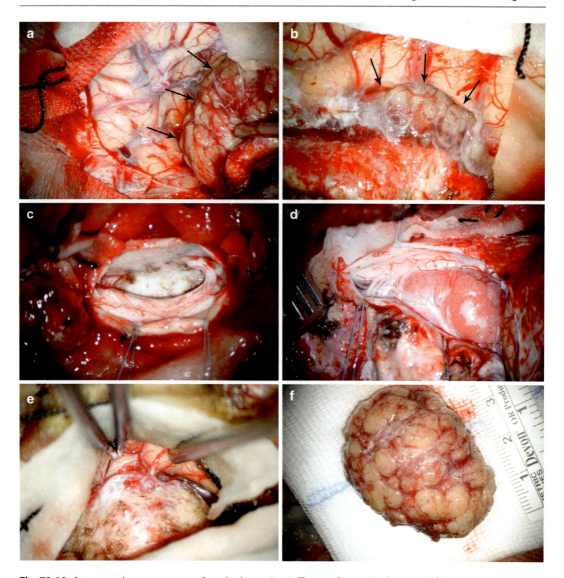

Fig. 72.19 Intraoperative appearances of meningiomas (**a**–**e**). Tumor after surgical removal (**f**)

72.3 Meningioma

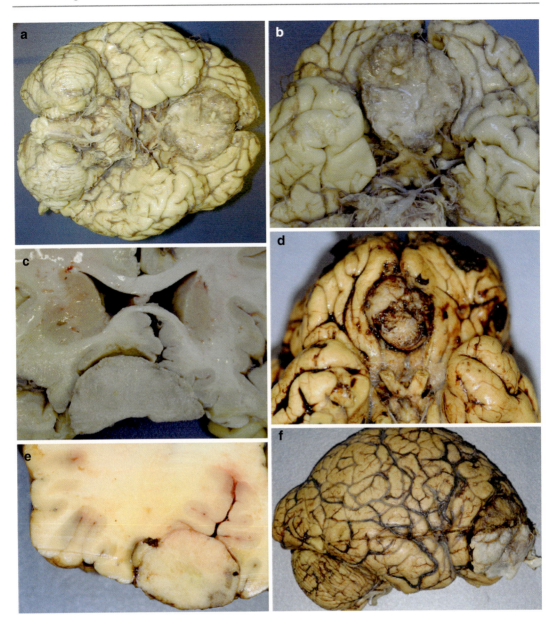

Fig. 72.20 Macroscopic appearances of meningiomas on autopsy brains. Typical olfactory meningiomas (**a–e**) frontobasal meningioma (**f, g**) with compression of the brain (**h, i**), falcine meningiomas (**j–m**) sphenoid wing meningioma (**n–p**), multiple meningiomas (**q–r**), meningioma en plaque with brain infiltration (**s–t**)

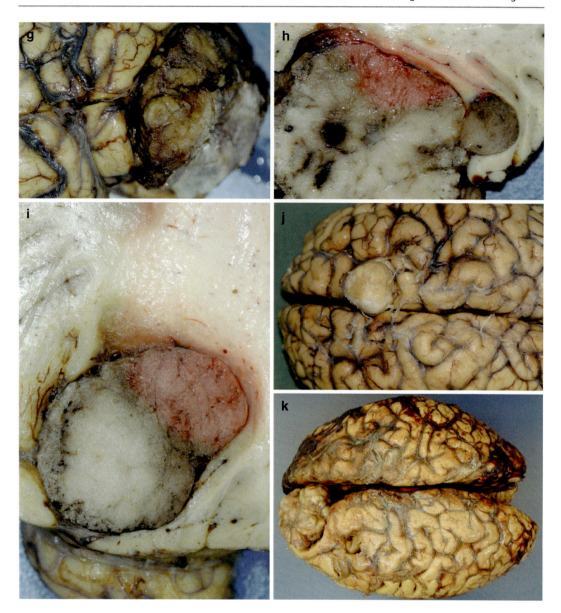

Fig. 72.20 (continued)

72.3 Meningioma

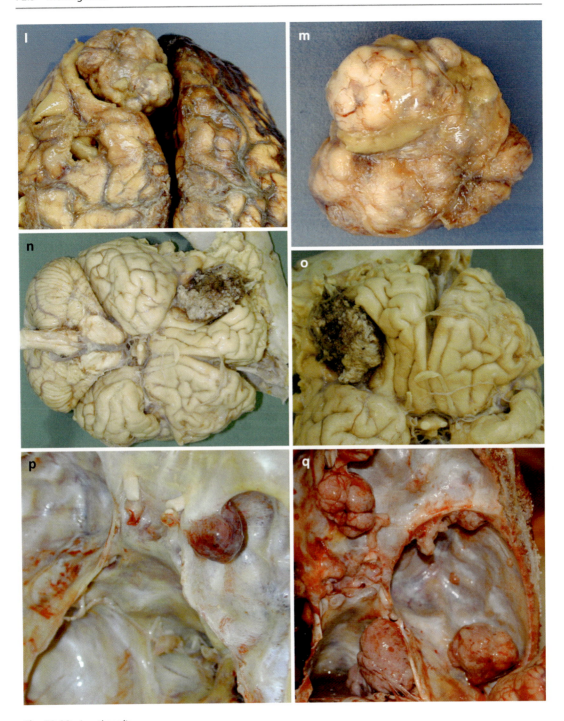

Fig. 72.20 (continued)

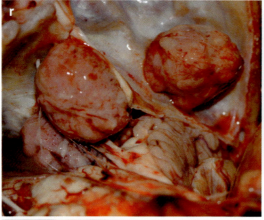
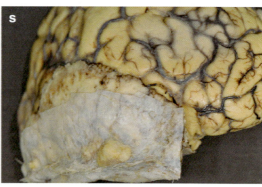
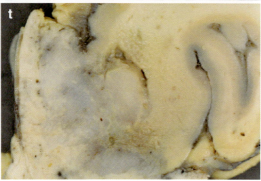

Fig. 72.20 (continued)

- Tumor cells with
  - uniform size
  - oval nuclei
  - delicate chromatin
  - resemblance of arachnoid cap cells
- Tumor cells form
  - Syncytium
  - Undiscernible cell processes
- Tumor cells form
  - lobules, separated by thin collagenous septae
- Whorl formation infrequent
- Psammoma body formation rare

Fibrous (Fibroblastic) Meningioma (Fig. 72.23a–h)
A variant of meningioma that consist of spindled cells forming parallel, storiform, and interlacing bundles in a collagen-rich matrix (Perry et al. 2016a).

- Spindle cells forming
  - parallel, storiform, and interlacing bundles in a collagen-rich matrix
- Tumor cells form
  - wide fascicles with varying amounts of intercellular collagen

72.3 Meningioma

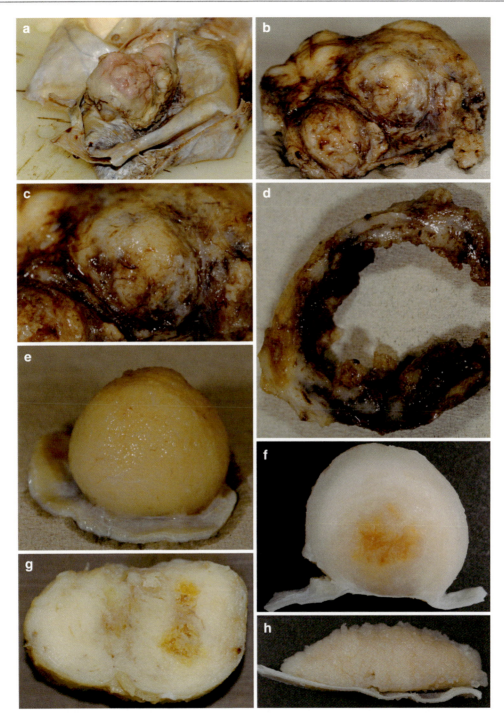

Fig. 72.21 Meningioma attached to the dura mater (**a**), lobulation is possible (**b**, **c**), cystic formation in the inner part of the meningioma (**d**), meningioma attached to the dura after en bloc removal (**e**), the cut surface might be of different color and consistency (**f**, **g**), en plaque growth pattern (**h**), soft consistency (**i**, **j**), thickening of the skull bone due to tumor infiltration (**k**, **l**), infiltration of the superior sagittal sinus (**m**, **n**)

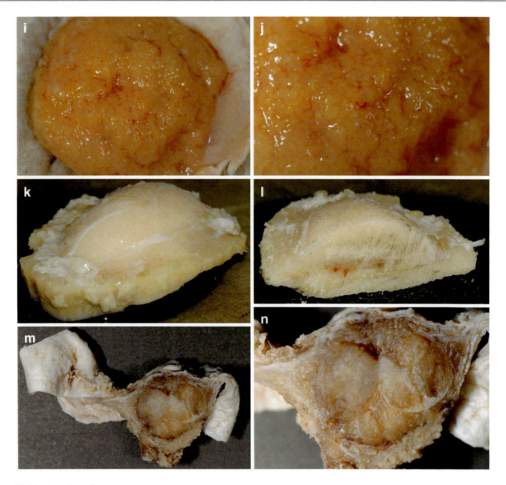

Fig. 72.21 (continued)

Transitional Meningioma (Fig. 72.24 a, b)

A common variant of meningioma that contains meningothelial and fibrous patterns as well as transitional features (Perry et al. 2016a).

- Coexistence of meningothelial and fibrous patterns
- Lobular or fascicular arrangements
- Whorl and psammoma body formation possible

Psammomatous Meningioma (Fig. 72.25a–e)

A designation applied to meningiomas (usually of the transitional type) containing a predominance of psammoma bodies over tumor cells (Perry et al. 2016a).

- Tumors containing more psammoma bodies than tumor cell mass
- Psammoma bodies:
  - Irregular calcified masses
  - May become confluent
- Some tumors consist exclusively of psammoma bodies.

Angiomatous Meningioma (Fig. 72.26a–h)

A variant of meningioma that features numerous blood vessels, which often constitute a greater proportion of the tumor mass than do the intermixed meningioma cells (Perry et al. 2016a).

- Predominance of blood vessels
- Vascular channels may be

72.3 Meningioma

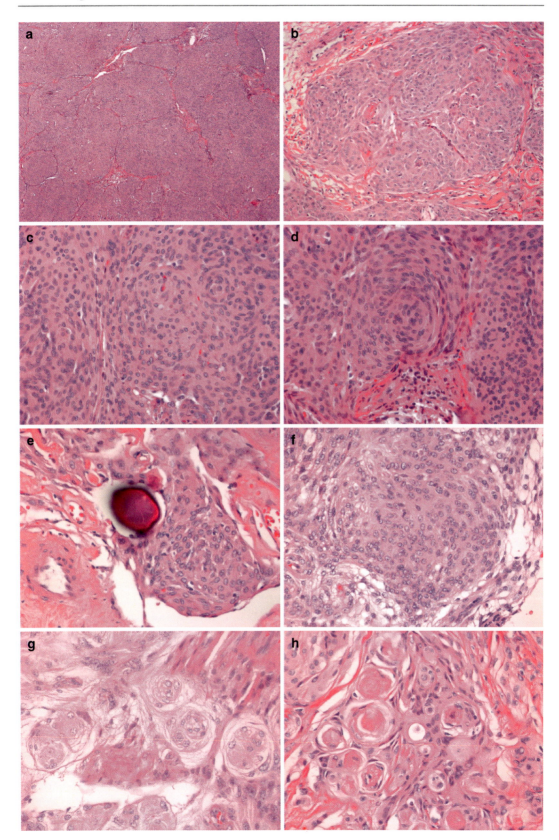

Fig. 72.22 Meningothelial meningioma WHO grade I (**a**–**h**)

- Small- or medium sized
- Thin-walled or thick
- Hyalinized walls
- Marked degenerative nuclear atypia

Microcystic Meningioma (Fig. 72.27a–f)

A variant of meningioma characterized by cells with thin, elongated processes encompassing microcysts and creating a cobweb-like background (Perry et al. 2016a).

- Tumor cells with thin elongate processes containing
- Microcysts with pale, eosinophilic mucinous fluid
- Presence of pleomorphic cells

Secretory Meningioma (Fig. 72.28a–j)

A variant of meningioma characterized by the presence of focal epithelial differentiation in the form of intracellular lumina containing periodic acid-Schiff-positive eosinophilic secretions called pseudopsammoma bodies (Perry et al. 2016a).

- Presence of intracellular lumina containing PAS-positive eosinophilic secretion (sign of focal epithelial differentiation)
  - Called "pseudopsammoma bodies"
  - Immunoreactive for carcinoembryonic antigen (CEA)

Metaplastic Meningioma

A variant of meningioma with striking focal or widespread mesenchymal components including osseous, cartilaginous, lipomatous, myxoid, and xanthomatous tissue, either singly or in combinations (Perry et al. 2016a).

- Focal presence of either singly or combined mesenchymal components like
  - Osseous
  - Cartilaginous
  - Lipomatous
  - Myxoid
  - Xanthomatous

Lymphoplasmacyte-Rich Meningioma (Fig. 72.29a–d)

A rare variant of meningioma that features extensive chronic inflammatory infiltrates, often overshadowing the inconspicuous meningothelial component (Perry et al. 2016a).

- Extensive chronic inflammatory infiltrates
- Immunoreactivities for
  - CD45
  - CD3
  - CD4

72.3 Meningioma

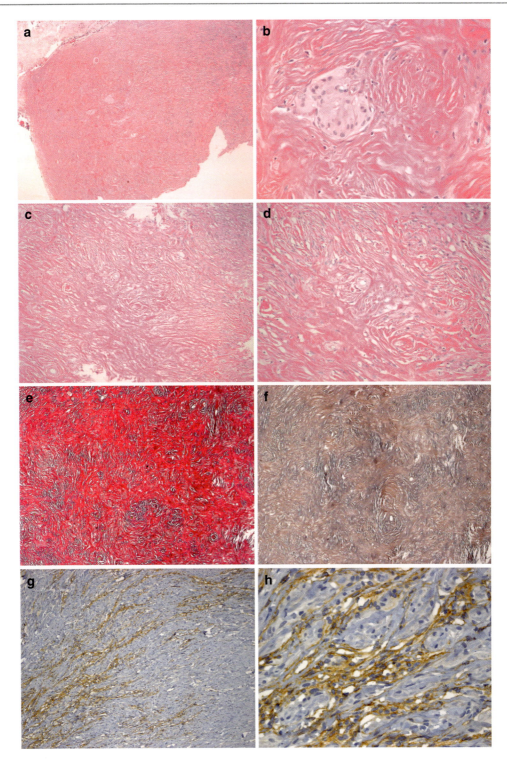

Fig. 72.23 Fibrous meningioma WHO grade I. Presence of tumor cells located between fibrous tissue (**a–d**). Spindle cells stain red with the Elastica van Gieson stain (**e**) and black with the reticulin stain (**f**). Tumor cells are immunopositive for EMA (**g**, **h**)

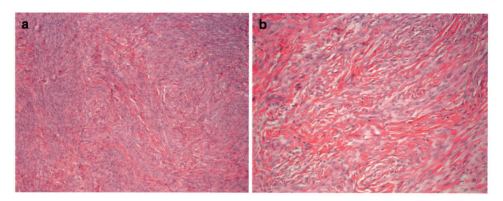

Fig. 72.24 Transitional meningioma WHO grade I with features of meningothelial (asterisk) and fibrous (+) meningiomas (**a**, **b**)

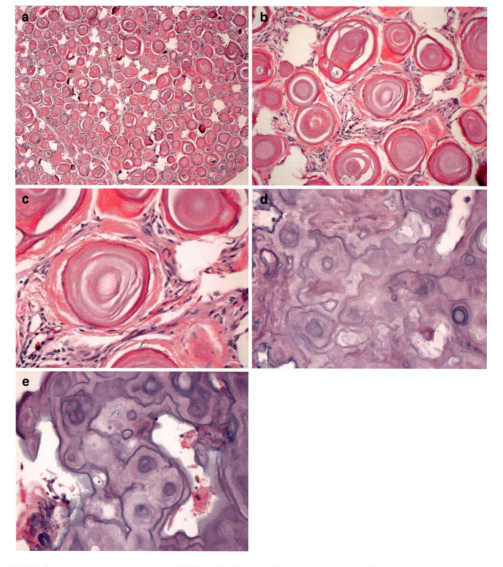

Fig. 72.25 Psammomatous meningioma WHO grade I (**a–c**) with large areas of calcifications (**d**, **e**)

72.3 Meningioma

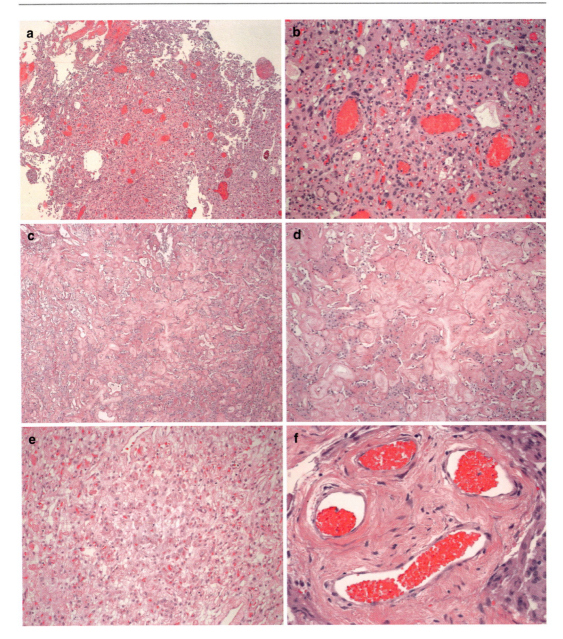

Fig. 72.26 Angiomatous meningioma WHO grade I. Vessels are present in high number (**a**, **b**). Hyalinization of vessel wall might be encountered (**c**, **d**). Might be mistaken for clear cell type (**e**). Rarely "smilies" might be identified (**f**). The vessels stain immunohistochemically for CD34 (**g**, **h**)

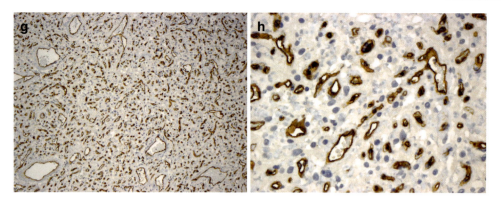

Fig. 72.26 (continued)

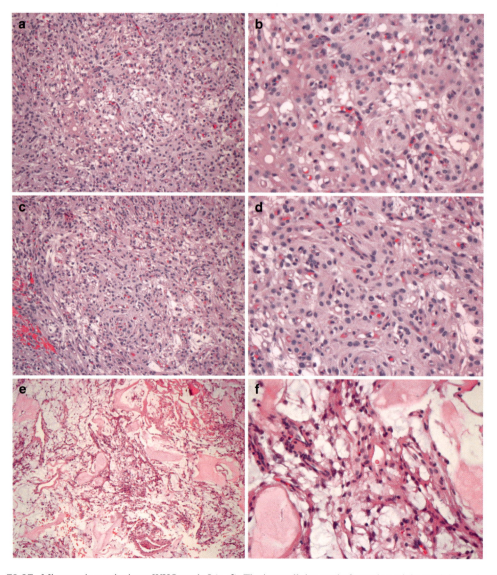

Fig. 72.27 Microcystic meningioma WHO grade I (**a–d**). The intracellular cystic formation might reach large size (**e**, **f**)

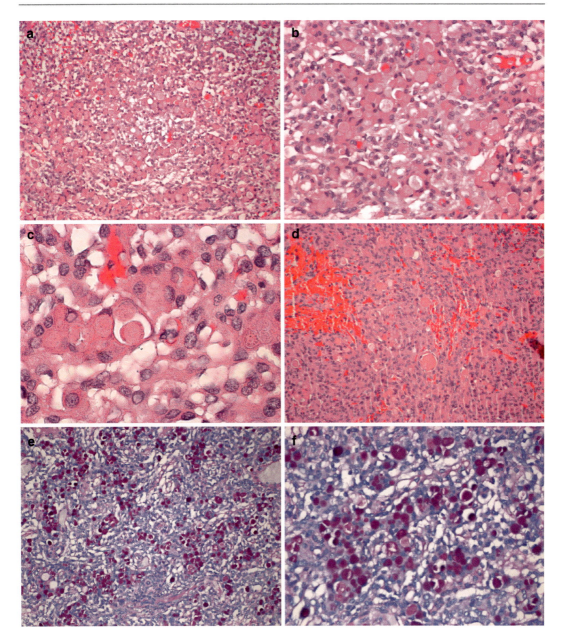

Fig. 72.28 Secretory meningioma WHO grade I. The round, ball-like eosinophilic secretions (**a–d**) are PAS-positive (**e**, **f**) and immunohistochemically positive for carcinoembryonic antigen (CEA) (**g**, **h**), and pancytokeratin AE1/AE3 (**i**, **j**)

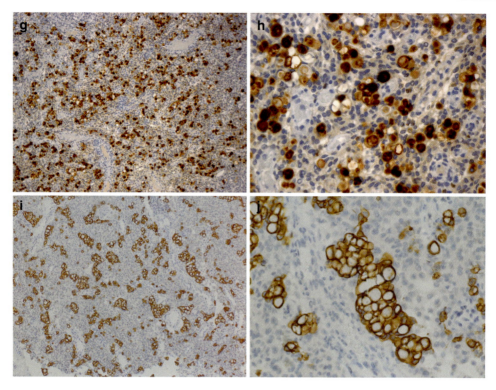

Fig. 72.28 (continued)

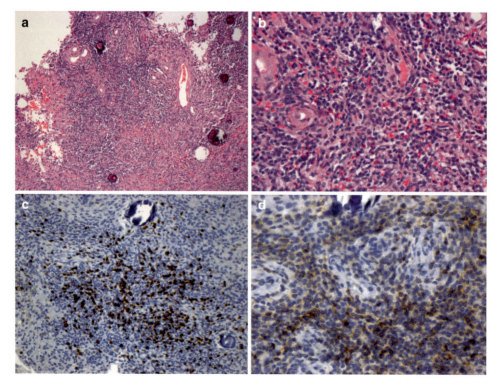

Fig. 72.29 Lymphocyte-rich meningioma WHO grade I (**a**, **b**). The lymphocytes are immunohistochemically identified as CD3-positive T-lymphocytes (**c**, **d**)

72.4 Atypical Meningioma

WHO Definition

2016—A meningioma of intermediate grade between benign and malignant forms, with increased mitotic activity, brain invasion on histology, or at least three of the following features: increased cellularity, small cells with a high nuclear-to-cytoplasmic ratio, prominent nucleoli, sheeting (i.e., uninterrupted patternless or sheet-like growth), and foci of spontaneous (i.e., not iatrogenically induced) necrosis (Perry et al. 2016a).

2007—A meningioma with increased mitotic activity or three or more of the following histologic features: increased cellularity, small cells with a high nuclear: cytoplasmic ratio, prominent nucleoli, uninterrupted patternless or sheet-like growth, and foci of "spontaneous" or "geographic" necrosis (Perry et al. 2007).

2000—A meningioma with increased mitotic activity or three or more of the following features: increased cellularity, small cells with high nucleus: cytoplasmic ratio, prominent nucleoli, uninterrupted patternless or sheet-like growth, and foci of "spontaneous" or "geographic necrosis" (Louis et al. 2000).

1993—Meningiomas in which several of the following features are evident: frequent mitoses, increased cellularity, small cells with high nuclear-cytoplasmic ratios and/or prominent nucleoli, uninterrupted patternless or sheet-like growth and foci of "spontaneous" or geographic necrosis (Kleihues et al. 1993).

WHO Grade
- WHO grade II

72.4.1 Neuropathology Findings

Microscopic Features (Fig. 72.30a–d)
Atypical meningiomas are characterized by:

- increased mitotic activity
  - 4 or more mitoses per 10 high-power (40×) fields
- three or more of the following histologic features:
  - increased cellularity
  - small cells with a high nuclear: cytoplasmic ratio
  - prominent nucleoli
  - uninterrupted patternless or sheet-like growth
  - foci of "spontaneous" or "geographic" necrosis

In addition to atypical meningioma WHO grade II per se and based on their biologic behavior, the following two meningiomas are included in the group of atypical meningioma and correspond to WHO grade II:

- Chordoid meningioma
- Clear cell meningioma

Chordoid Meningioma (WHO Grade II)
A rare variant of meningioma that histologically resembles chordoma, featuring cords or trabeculae of eosinophilic, often vacuolated cells set in an abundant mucoid matrix (Perry et al. 2016a).

- Tumor composed of cords or trabeculae of eosinophilic often vacuolated cells in an abundant mucoid background
- Resembling chordoma
- Chronic inflammatory infiltrates

Clear Cell Meningioma (WHO Grade II)
(Fig. 72.31a, b)
A rare variant of meningioma with a patternless (commonly) or sheeting architecture and round to polygonal cells with clear, glycogen-rich cytoplasm and prominent blocky perivascular and interstitial collagen (Perry et al. 2016a).

- patternless tumor composed of
- polygonal cells with clear, glycogen-rich cytoplasm
- prominent blocky perivascular and interstitial collagen

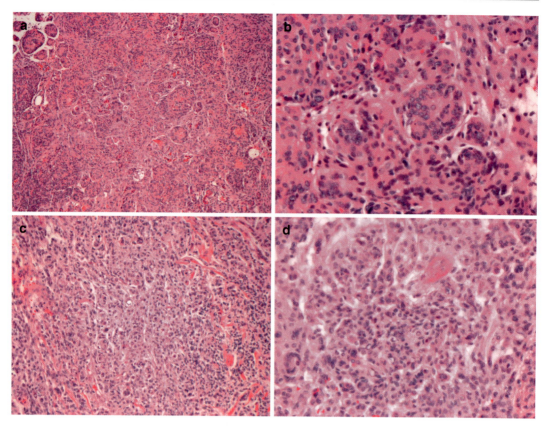

Fig. 72.30 Atypical meningioma WHO grade II (**a–d**)

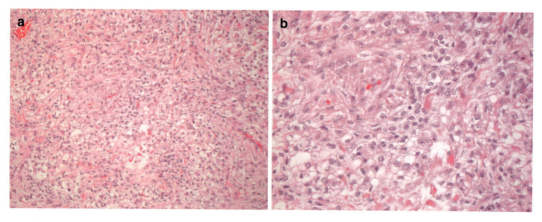

Fig. 72.31 Clear cell meningioma WHO grade II (**a, b**)

- PAS-positive, diastase-sensitive cytoplasmic clearing
- Rare classic features of meningioma
- Whorl and psammoma body formation rare

72.5 Anaplastic (Malignant) Meningioma

WHO Definition
2016—A meningioma that exhibits overtly malignant cytology (resembling that of carcinoma, melanoma, or high-grade sarcoma) and/or markedly elevated mitotic activity (Perry et al. 2016a).
2007—A meningioma exhibiting histological features of frank malignancy far in excess of the abnormalities present in atypical meningioma (Perry et al. 2007).
2000—A meningioma exhibiting histological features of frank malignancy far in excess of the abnormalities present in atypical meningioma (Louis et al. 2000).
1993—A meningioma exhibiting histological features of frank malignancy far in excess of the abnormalities noted in atypical meningioma. These include obviously malignant cytology, a high mitotic index, and conspicuous necrosis (Kleihues et al. 1993).
1979—Any meningioma that displays anaplastic features yet has not developed into a frank sarcoma. Some of the features of a meningioma are retained. It corresponds histologically to grades II and III (Zülch 1979).

WHO Grade
- WHO grade III

72.5.1 Microscopic Features

Anaplastic meningiomas are characterized by (Fig. 72.32a–j)

- histological features of frank malignancy with
  - malignant cytology resembling carcinoma, melanoma, or high-grade sarcoma
  - marked elevated mitotic index (20 or more mitoses per 10 high-power fields)

In addition to anaplastic meningioma WHO grade III per se and based on their biologic behavior, the following two meningiomas are included in the group of anaplastic meningioma and correspond to WHO grade III:

- Papillary meningioma
- Rhabdoid meningioma

Papillary Meningioma (WHO Grade III)
- Highly cellular meningioma composed of
- Perivascular pseudopapillary pattern

Rhabdoid Meningioma (WHO Grade III) (Fig. 72.33a–d)
- Contains sheets of rhabdoid cells
  - i.e., plump cells with eccentric nuclei
  - open chromatin
  - prominent nucleolus
  - prominent inclusion-like eosinophilic cytoplasm
- Histological features of malignancy

72.6 Common Neuropathology Aspects

Immunophenotype (Fig. 72.34a–h)
- Epithelial membrane antigen (EMA) vast majority
- Vimentin in all meningiomas
- S-100 varying positivity
- Carcinoembryonic antigen (CEA)—secretory meningioma
- Claudin-1
- CD45—lymphoplasmacyte-rich meningioma

Proliferation Markers (Fig. 72.35a–d)
- Mitotic index:
  - Grade I 0.03–1.3
  - Grade II 3.5–5.5
  - Grade III 15–23
- MIB-1 or Ki-67 labeling index
  - Grade I 0.03–1.3
  - Grade II 3.5–5.5
  - Grade III 15–23
- Moderate high MIB-1 labeling index in atypical meningioma

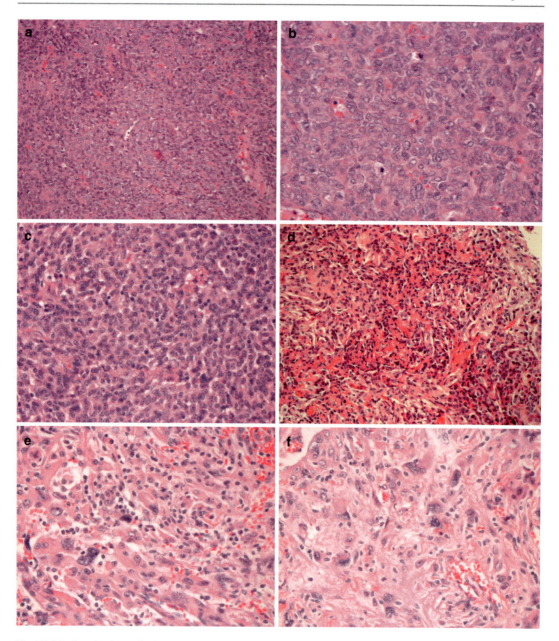

Fig. 72.32 Anaplastic meningioma WHO grade III characterized by high cell density (**a–d**) nuclear atypia and pleomorphism (**e–f**). Necroses might be encountered (**h**). Infiltration into brain tissue (**i**). High Ki-67 proliferation index (**j**)

72.6 Common Neuropathology Aspects

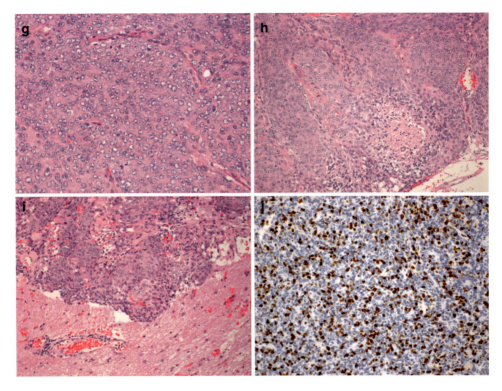

Fig. 72.32 (continued)

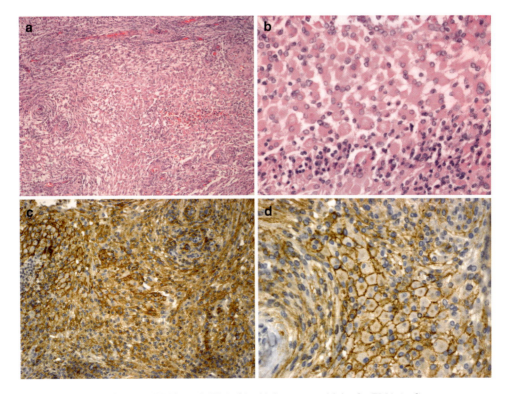

Fig. 72.33 Rhabdoid meningioma WHO grade III (**a**, **b**) with immunopositivity for EMA (**c**, **d**)

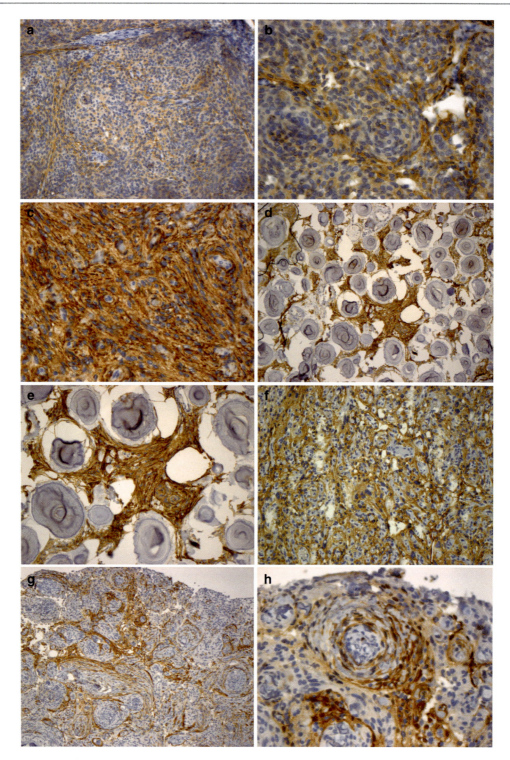

Fig. 72.34 Immunopositivity of meningiomas for epithelial membrane antigen (EMA) (**a–f**) and for S-100 (**g–h**). Weak staining (**a–b**) and strong immunoreactivity (**c**) in meningothelial meningioma, in psammomatous meningioma (**d–e**), in angiomatous meningioma (**f**). Some cases of meningioma show additional staining for S-100 (**g–h**)

72.7 Molecular Neuropathology

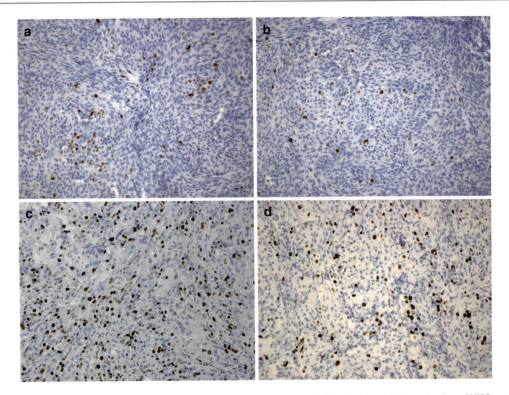

Fig. 72.35 Proliferating cells in meningothelial meningioma WHO grade I (**a**, **b**), in atypical meningioma WHO grade II (**c**), and in anaplastic meningioma WHO grade III (**d**)

Ultrastructural Features
- abundance of intermediate filaments (vimentin)
- complex interdigitating cellular processes
- desmosomal intercellular junctions

Differential Diagnosis
- Schwannoma
- S100 positive
- mostly EMA-negative
- Vascular malformations, capillary hemangioblastoma
  - Angiomatous meningioma

72.7 Molecular Neuropathology

72.7.1 Pathogenesis

- Radiation (low, moderate, and high dose) → atypical or aggressive multifocal highly proliferative meningiomas
- Sex hormones (overrepresentation of women)
- Hormonal medications

72.7.2 Genetics

In contrast to glioblastoma, where comprehensive information on the underlying molecular pathology is available, studies on genetic mechanisms involved in meningioma development and progression have been intensified only more recently. Below, some current major findings in this field are summarized (Table 72.2).

72.7.3 Signaling Pathways

Several signaling pathways were shown to malfunction in meningioma; among those, the hedgehog (Hh) and the Wnt ("wingless") pathways appear to be most frequently affected.

72.7.4 Hh (Hedgehog) Pathway

The primary physiological role of the Hh signaling cascade is its regulatory function in embryonic development and differentiation. Defects in this pathway are often associated with tumorigenesis. In meningioma, several affected Hh pathway-related genes were identified, including:

72.7.5 Wnt (Wingless) Pathway

Aberrant functions of the Wnt pathway in meningioma are listed in Table 72.3.

Additional signaling cascades that were found to be affected in meningioma include (Choy et al. 2011):

- the RB (retinoblastoma)/TP53 (tumor protein 53) pathways (see Chap. 51)
- the PI3K (phosphatidylinositol 3-kinase)/Akt pathway (see Chap. 51)

- the MAPK (mitogen-activated protein kinase) pathway
- the Notch signaling pathway

72.7.6 Chromosomal Aberrations and Mutations (Table 72.4)

- The best studied chromosomal abnormality in meningioma is loss of heterozygosity (LOH) of chromosome region 22q12.2 where the tumor suppressor gene *NF2* (neurofibromin 2), encoding the merlin (schwannomin) protein, is located. Additional somatic mutations in the second *NF2* allele lead to complete loss of functional merlin, thus triggering tumorigenesis. *NF2* somatic mutations in meningiomas were reported at frequencies of 30–60% in WHO grade I, and 70–80% in WHO grades II/III.
- Loss of chromosome 1p is found more often in higher grade than in benign meningiomas, suggesting an association with tumor progres-

Table 72.2 Genes involved in the genesis of meningiomas

Gene	Gene characteristics
SMO (smoothened)	• oncogenic properties • chromosome 7q32.3
GLI1, *GLI2* (GLI family zinc finger proteins)	• oncogenic properties • chromosome regions 12q13.2-q13.3 and 2q14, respectively
GLIS2 (GLI-similar zinc finger 2)	• oncogenic properties • chromosome 16p13.3
FOXM1 (forkhead box protein M1)	• oncogenic properties • chromosome 12p13
IGF2 (insulin-like growth factor 2)	• oncogenic properties • chromosome 11p15.5
SPP1 (secreted phosphoprotein 1)	• encoding osteopontin • oncogenic properties • chromosome 4q22.1
PTCH1 (patched)	• tumor suppressor • chromosome 9q22.3

Table 72.3 Aberrant functions of the Wnt pathway in meningioma are related to the downregulation of the following genes

Gene	Gene characteristics
APC (adenomatous polyposis coli)	• tumor suppressor • chromosome region 5q21-q22 • LOH in benign meningioma
BCR (breakpoint cluster region)	• putative tumor suppressor • chromosome 22q11.23
CDH1 (cadherin 1)	• encoding E-cadherin • tumor suppressor • chromosome 16q22.1
SFRP1 (secreted frizzled-related protein 1)	• tumor suppressor • chromosome 8p11.21

Table 72.4 Short overview of the described chromosomal aberrations in meningioma

Chromosomal abnormality	Genes affected	
	Oncogenes	Tumor suppressor genes
LOH in chromosome regions 1p32/1p36		*CDKN2C/ALPL*
LOH in chromosome region 9p		*CDKN2A, CDKN2B*
LOH in chromosome regions 14q11/14q32		*NDRG2/MEG3*
Amplification of chromosome 17q23	*RPS6K*	
LOH in chromosome region 18p11.32		*DAL-1*
LOH in chromosome regions 22q12.2/22q12.3		*NF2/TIMP-3*

72.7 Molecular Neuropathology

sion and recurrence. Possible tumor suppressor candidate genes are, e.g., *CDKN2C* (cyclin-dependent kinase inhibitor 2C) at 1p32-encoding protein p18INK4C, or *ALPL* (alkaline phosphatase, liver/bone/kidney) at 1p36.12.

- Losses of chromosome 9p regions are found predominantly in the more aggressive tumors, with the highest incidence in WHO grade III meningiomas. At region 9p21, two tumor suppressor genes are lost: *CDKN2A* (cyclin-dependent kinase inhibitor 2A) encoding proteins p16INK4A and p14ARF, and *CDKN2B* (cyclin-dependent kinase inhibitor 2B) encoding p16INK4B.
- Loss of chromosome 14q regions is associated more frequently with increasing tumor grade. Genes that are affected include the tumor suppressors *MEG3* (maternally expressed gene 3) at 14q32, or *NDRG2* (N-Myc downstream-regulated gene 2) at 14q11.2.
- Amplification of chromosome 17q23 encompassing the oncogene *RPS6K* (ribosomal protein S6 kinase) was identified in some malignant meningiomas.
- Another genetic aberration is LOH at chromosome 18p11.32 which was reported at frequencies between 20 and 70%. This locus contains the *DAL-1* (differentially expressed in adenocarcinoma of the lung-1) gene, encoding tumor suppressor protein 4.1B, which in turn interacts with the tumor suppressor in lung cancer-1 protein (TSLC1; cf. Chap. 51 "Gene Expression").
- A germline missense mutation was reported in the tumor suppressor gene *SMARCB1* (SWI/SNF-related matrix-associated actin-dependent regulator of chromatin subfamily B member 1) in members of a single family suffering from schwannomas and multiple meningiomas. Additional losses of the *SMARCB1* wild-type allele was demonstrated in these patients, frequently accompanied by somatic *NF2* mutations and loss of the *NF2* wild-type allele (van den Munckhof et al. 2012).

72.7.7 Epigenetics

72.7.7.1 DNA Methylation

Promoter hypermethylation as a means of inhibiting gene expression in meningioma has been reported for several tumor suppressor genes, e.g.,

- *TIMP-3* (tissue inhibitor of metalloproteinase-3)
  – Located on chromosome 22q12.3.
  – *TIMP-3* hypermethylation is almost exclusively accompanied by LOH at 22q12.3.
- *MEG3* (maternally expressed gene 3)
  – Chromosome 14q32.
  – Methylation is associated more frequently with LOH at 14q32 in higher grade meningiomas.
- *NDRG2* (N-Myc downstream-regulated gene 2)
  – Chromosome 14q11.2.
  – Downregulated expression is consistently observed in meningiomas WHO grade III.
- *HOX* (homeobox) genes of the *HOXA* cluster:
  – *HOXA7*, *9*, and *10* hypermethylation appears to be associated with higher grades of meningioma and recurrence (Kishida et al. 2012; Di Vinci et al. 2012).

72.7.7.2 MicroRNAs

Several studies focused on dysregulated microRNA (miRNA) expression in meningiomas:

- Downregulated *miR-200a* was reported in a limited number of benign meningiomas and was identified as a tumor suppressor molecule (Saydam et al. 2009).
- miR-335 overexpression was demonstrated in meningiomas of all grades, with the highest levels found in WHO grade III tumors. The miR-335 molecule exhibits oncogenic properties by decreasing expression of the tumor suppressor protein Rb-1 (retinoblastoma 1) (Shi et al. 2012).
- In a more recent study (Zhi et al. 2013), a signature of 14 differentially expressed miRNAs was proposed to discriminate meningeal from

normal tissue. Some of those, *miR-96-5p*, *miR-190a* (both upregulated), *miR-29c-3p*, and *miR-219-5p* (both downregulated) were associated with tumor progression and higher recurrence rates.

72.7.8 Gene Expression

Genes involved in the Hh and Wnt pathways are closely associated with meningioma development and/or -progression which is illustrated by distinct expression patterns (Pham et al. 2011; Laurendeau et al. 2010).

- For the hedgehog pathway, elevated mRNA levels were determined for pathway-activating genes such as *SMO*, *FOXM1*, *SPP1*, *IGF2*, and the *GLI* family genes, whereas *DHH* (desert hedgehog), *PTH1R* (parathyroid hormone 1 receptor), and the tumor suppressor *PTCH1* appear to be downregulated, the latter, however, only in low-grade meningiomas.
- Wnt pathway-related genes frequently underexpressed include, e.g., *CDH1* in atypical and malignant meningioma, and *BCR* in all grades of meningioma; *SFRP1* was found to be downregulated in recurrent vs. primary meningiomas and thus is considered a putative marker for recurrent meningiomas.
- Downregulation of the *DLC1* gene (deleted in liver cancer 1) was observed in benign meningiomas and interpreted as a potential tumor suppressor.
- Loss of expression was reported for TSLC1, a tumor suppressor interacting with protein 4.1B; this phenomenon was more pronounced in higher grade meningiomas where it correlated with increased proliferation rates and poorer prognosis.
- A comprehensive microarray-based study identified differentially expressed genes (DEGs) in original and recurrent meningiomas. Most DEGs were located on chromosomes 1p, 6q, and 14q, and the majority were found to be underexpressed in recurrent meningiomas. On the other hand, genes of the histone cluster 1, located on chromosome 6p, were overexpressed in recurrent meningiomas (Perez-Magan et al. 2010).
- In microcystic meningiomas, a tissue inhibitor of metalloproteinases, TIMP-1 (TIMP metallopeptidase inhibitor 1) interacting with matrix metalloproteinase 9 (MMP-9), was shown to be underexpressed, as compared to a control group. In contrast, high levels of MMP-9 were detected in the tumor tissues; therefore, it was speculated that increased MMP-9/TIMP-1 ratios might be involved in the pathogenesis of microcystic meningioma (Paek et al. 2006).
- Expression of *STAT3* (signal transducer and activator of transcription 3), an oncogene, was found to be upregulated in meningiomas WHO grade II, with concomitant induction of VEGF (vascular endothelial growth factor) expression.
- Several oncogenes, upregulated in some meningiomas, include *c-sis* (encodes the platelet-derived growth factor beta polypeptide; PDGFB), the transcription factors *c-myc* and *c-fos*, *bcl-2* (bcl-2 protein, a regulator of apoptosis) or *TP73* (tumor protein p73).
- *hTERT* mRNA, encoding the telomerase catalytic subunit of human telomerase reverse transcriptase, is more frequently detected in grade II and III than in benign meningiomas which correlates well with the high levels of telomerase activity found in the aggressive tumors.

72.8 Treatment and Prognosis

Treatment
- Surgery
- Radiation

Biologic Behavior–Prognosis–Prognostic Factors
- Brain invasion:
- Irregular, tongue-like protrusion of tumor cells infiltrating brain parenchyma without intervening layer of leptomeninges
- Occurs in benign, atypical, or anaplastic meningiomas
- Signifies greater likelihood of recurrence
- Meningiomas with brain invasion should be considered WHO grade II tumors

72.8 Treatment and Prognosis

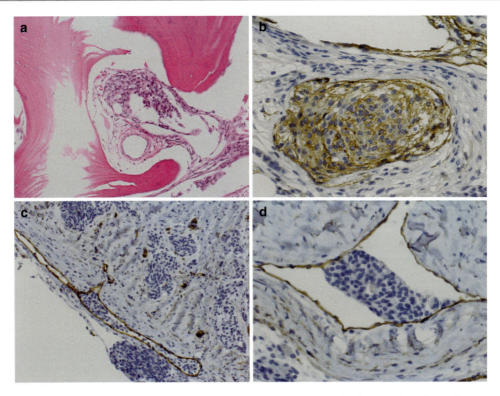

Fig. 72.36 Meningioma cells infiltrate the bone (**a**) immunopositive for EMA (**b**). Invasion of vascular structures (CD34 stain) (**c, d**)

- Metastases (Fig. 72.36a–d):
  - Very rare, 1 in 1000 meningiomas
  - Often in anaplastic meningiomas
- **Simpson grading** defining extend of tumor resection (Simpson 1957)
  - *Grade I*: Gross total resection of tumor, dural attachments, and abnormal bone
  - *Grade II*: Gross total resection of tumor, coagulation of dural attachments
  - *Grade III*: Gross total resection of tumor without resection or coagulation of dural attachments or extradural extensions (e.g., invaded or hyperostotic bone)
  - *Grade IV*: Partial resection of tumor
  - *Grade V*: Simple decompression (biopsy)
- **Modified Shinshu grade** (revised Simpson grading system based on a microsurgical perspective) (Kobayashi et al. 1992)
  - *Grade I*: Complete microscopic removal of tumor and dural attachment with any abnormal bone
  - *Grade II*: Complete microscopic removal of tumor with diathermy coagulation of its dural attachment
  - *Grade IIIA*: Complete microscopic removal of intradural and extradural tumor without resection or coagulation of its dural attachments
  - *Grade IIIB*: Complete microscopic removal of intradural tumor without resection or coagulation of its dural attachments or of any extradural extensions
  - *Grade IVA*: Intentional subtotal removal to preserve cranial nerves or blood vessels with complete microscopic removal of dural attachment
  - *Grade IVB*: Partial removal, leaving tumor of <10% in volume
  - *Grade V*: Partial removal, leaving tumor >10% in volume, or decompression with or without biopsy

- Increased risk of recurrence: index >4%
- Fatal outcome: index >20%
- Poor outcome:
  - Progesterone receptor score 0
  - Mitotic index >6
  - WHO grade III
- Anaplastic meningioma: median survival: less than 2 years
- Papillary meningiomas:
  - local invasion and brain invasion
  - recurrence in 55%
  - metastases in 20%
- Rhabdoid meningioma:
  - Aggressive clinical course

Selected References

Agrawal V, Ludwig N, Agrawal A, Bulsara KR (2007) Intraosseous intracranial meningioma. AJNR Am J Neuroradiol 28(2):314–315

Al-Faham Z, Kassir MA, Wood D, Balon HR (2016) Appearance of meningioma on 99mTc-HMPAO SPECT: correlation with MRI. J Nucl Med Technol 44(2):90–91. https://doi.org/10.2967/jnmt.115.163287

Bi WL, Mei Y, Agarwalla PK, Beroukhim R, Dunn IF (2016a) Genomic and epigenomic landscape in meningioma. Neurosurg Clin N Am 27(2):167–179. https://doi.org/10.1016/j.nec.2015.11.009

Bi WL, Zhang M, Wu WW, Mei Y, Dunn IF (2016b) Meningioma genomics: diagnostic, prognostic, and therapeutic applications. Front Surg 3:40. https://doi.org/10.3389/fsurg.2016.00040

Choy W, Kim W, Nagasawa D, Stramotas S, Yew A, Gopen Q, Parsa AT, Yang I (2011) The molecular genetics and tumor pathogenesis of meningiomas and the future directions of meningioma treatments. Neurosurg Focus 30(5):E6. https://doi.org/10.3171/2011.3172.FOCUS1116

Cimino PJ (2015) Malignant progression to anaplastic meningioma: neuropathology, molecular pathology, and experimental models. Exp Mol Pathol 99(2):354–359. https://doi.org/10.1016/j.yexmp.2015.08.007

Cornelius JF, Langen KJ, Stoffels G, Hanggi D, Sabel M, Jakob Steiger H (2012) Positron emission tomography imaging of meningioma in clinical practice: review of literature and future directions. Neurosurgery 70(4):1033–1041. https://doi.org/10.1227/NEU.0b013e31823bcd87; discussion 1042

Di Vinci A, Brigati C, Casciano I, Banelli B, Borzi L, Forlani A, Ravetti GL, Allemanni G, Melloni I, Zona G, Spaziante R, Merlo DF, Romani M (2012) HOXA7, 9, and 10 are methylation targets associated with aggressive behavior in meningiomas. Transl Res 160(5):355–362. https://doi.org/10.1016/j.trsl.2012.1005.1007. Epub 2012 Jun 1023

Ellis JA, D'Amico R, Sisti MB, Bruce JN, McKhann GM, Lavine SD, Meyers PM, Strozyk D (2011) Preoperative intracranial meningioma embolization. Expert Rev Neurother 11(4):545–556. https://doi.org/10.1586/ern.11.29

Hallinan JT, Hegde AN, Lim WE (2013) Dilemmas and diagnostic difficulties in meningioma. Clin Radiol 68(8):837–844. https://doi.org/10.1016/j.crad.2013.03.007

Kishida Y, Natsume A, Kondo Y, Takeuchi I, An B, Okamoto Y, Shinjo K, Saito K, Ando H, Ohka F, Sekido Y, Wakabayashi T (2012) Epigenetic subclassification of meningiomas based on genome-wide DNA methylation analyses. Carcinogenesis 33(2):436–441. https://doi.org/10.1093/carcin/bgr1260 Epub 2011 Nov 1018

Kleihues P, Burger PC, Scheithauer BW (1993) Histological typing of tumours of the central nervous system, 2nd edn. Springer, Berlin

Kobayashi K, Okudera H, Tanaka Y (1992) Surgical considerations in skull base meningioma, 1st edn. International Skull Base Congress

Laurendeau I, Ferrer M, Garrido D, D'Haene N, Ciavarelli P, Basso A, Vidaud M, Bieche I, Salmon I, Szijan I (2010) Gene expression profiling of the hedgehog signaling pathway in human meningiomas. Mol Med 16(7–8):262–270. https://doi.org/10.2119/molmed.2010.00005. Epub 02010 Mar 00026

Louis DN, Scheithauer BW, Budka H, von Deimling A, Kepes JJ (2000) Meningiomas. In: Kleihues P, Cavenee WK (eds) Pathology and genetics of tumours of the nervous system, 3rd edn. IARC Press, Lyon, pp 176–184

Maclean J, Fersht N, Short S (2014) Controversies in radiotherapy for meningioma. Clin Oncol (R Coll Radiol) 26(1):51–64. https://doi.org/10.1016/j.clon.2013.10.001

Paek SH, Kim DG, Park CK, Phi JH, Kim YY, Im SY, Kim JE, Park SH, Jung HW (2006) The role of matrix metalloproteinases and tissue inhibitors of matrix metalloproteinase in microcystic meningiomas. Oncol Rep 16(1):49–56

Paldor I, Awad M, Sufaro YZ, Kaye AH, Shoshan Y (2016) Review of controversies in management of non-benign meningioma. J Clin Neurosci 31:37–46. https://doi.org/10.1016/j.jocn.2016.03.014

Perez-Magan E, Rodriguez de Lope A, Ribalta T, Ruano Y, Campos-Martin Y, Perez-Bautista G, Garcia JF, Garcia-Claver A, Fiano C, Hernandez-Moneo JL, Mollejo M, Melendez B (2010) Differential expression profiling analyses identifies downregulation of 1p, 6q, and 14q genes and overexpression of 6p histone cluster 1 genes as markers of recurrence in meningiomas. Neuro-Oncology 12(12):1278–1290. https://doi.org/10.1093/neuonc/noq1081. Epub 2010 Aug 1274

Perry A, Louis DN, Scheithauer BW, Budka H, von Deimling A (2007) Meningiomas. In: Louis DN, Ohgaki H, Wiestler OD, Cavenee WK (eds) WHO classification of tumours of the central nervous system, 4th edn. International Agency for Research on Cancer, Lyon, pp 164–172

Perry A, Louis DN, Budka H, von Deimling A, Sahm F, Mawrin C, Rushing EJ (2016a) Meningioma variants. In: Louis DN, Ohgaki H, Wiestler OD, Cavenee WK (eds) WHO classification of tumours of the central nervous system, revised 4th edn. IARC, Lyon, pp 237–245

Perry A, Louis DN, Budka H, von Deimling A, Sahm F, Rushing EJ, Mawrin C, Claus EB, Loeffler J, Sadetzki S (2016b) Meningioma. In: Louis DN, Ohgaki H, Wiestler OD, Cavenee WK (eds) WHO classification of tumours of the central nervous system, revised 4th edn. IARC, Lyon, pp 232–237

Pham MH, Zada G, Mosich GM, Chen TC, Giannotta SL, Wang K, Mack WJ (2011) Molecular genetics of meningiomas: a systematic review of the current literature and potential basis for future treatment paradigms. Neurosurg Focus 30(5):E7. https://doi.org/10.3171/2011.3172.FOCUS1117

Saloner D, Uzelac A, Hetts S, Martin A, Dillon W (2010) Modern meningioma imaging techniques. J Neuro-Oncol 99(3):333–340. https://doi.org/10.1007/s11060-010-0367-6

Saydam O, Shen Y, Wurdinger T, Senol O, Boke E, James MF, Tannous BA, Stemmer-Rachamimov AO, Yi M, Stephens RM, Fraefel C, Gusella JF, Krichevsky AM, Breakefield XO (2009) Downregulated microRNA-200a in meningiomas promotes tumor growth by reducing E-cadherin and activating the Wnt/beta-catenin signaling pathway. Mol Cell Biol 29(21):5923–5940. https://doi.org/10.1128/MCB.00332-00309. Epub 02009 Aug 00324

Shi L, Jiang D, Sun G, Wan Y, Zhang S, Zeng Y, Pan T, Wang Z (2012) miR-335 promotes cell proliferation by directly targeting Rb1 in meningiomas. J Neuro-Oncol 110(2):155–162. https://doi.org/10.1007/s11060-11012-10951-z. Epub 12012 Aug 11014

Shibuya M (2015) Pathology and molecular genetics of meningioma: recent advances. Neurol Med Chir 55(1):14–27. https://doi.org/10.2176/nmc.ra.2014-0233

Shiroishi MS, Boxerman JL, Pope WB (2016a) Physiologic MRI for assessment of response to therapy and prognosis in glioblastoma. Neuro-Oncology 18(4):467–478. https://doi.org/10.1093/neuonc/nov179

Shiroishi MS, Cen SY, Tamrazi B, D'Amore F, Lerner A, King KS, Kim PE, Law M, Hwang DH, Boyko OB, Liu CS (2016b) Predicting meningioma consistency on preoperative neuroimaging studies. Neurosurg Clin N Am 27(2):145–154. https://doi.org/10.1016/j.nec.2015.11.007

Simpson D (1957) The recurrence of intracranial meningiomas after surgical treatment. J Neurol Neurosurg Psychiatry 20(1):22–39

Toh CH, Castillo M, Wong AM, Wei KC, Wong HF, Ng SH, Wan YL (2008) Differentiation between classic and atypical meningiomas with use of diffusion tensor imaging. AJNR Am J Neuroradiol 29(9):1630–1635. https://doi.org/10.3174/ajnr.A1170

van den Munckhof P, Christiaans I, Kenter SB, Baas F, Hulsebos TJ (2012) Germline SMARCB1 mutation predisposes to multiple meningiomas and schwannomas with preferential location of cranial meningiomas at the falx cerebri. Neurogenetics 13(1):1–7. https://doi.org/10.1007/s10048-10011-10300-y. Epub 12011 Oct 10026

Vranic A, Peyre M, Kalamarides M (2012) New insights into meningioma: from genetics to trials. Curr Opin Oncol 24(6):660–665. https://doi.org/10.1097/CCO.0b013e3283571a06

Yao A, Pain M, Balchandani P, Shrivastava RK (2018) Can MRI predict meningioma consistency?: a correlation with tumor pathology and systematic review. Neurosurg Rev 41(3):745–753. https://doi.org/10.1007/s10143-016-0801-0

Yuzawa S, Nishihara H, Tanaka S (2016) Genetic landscape of meningioma. Brain Tumor Pathol 33(4):237–247. https://doi.org/10.1007/s10014-016-0271-7

Zhang H, Rodiger LA, Shen T, Miao J, Oudkerk M (2008) Perfusion MR imaging for differentiation of benign and malignant meningiomas. Neuroradiology 50(6):525–530. https://doi.org/10.1007/s00234-008-0373-y

Zhi F, Zhou G, Wang S, Shi Y, Peng Y, Shao N, Guan W, Qu H, Zhang Y, Wang Q, Yang C, Wang R, Wu S, Xia X, Yang Y (2013) A microRNA expression signature predicts meningioma recurrence. Int J Cancer 132(1):128–136. https://doi.org/10.1002/ijc.27658. Epub 22012 Jun 27626

Zülch KJ (1979) Histological typing of tumours of the central nervous system. World Health Organization, Geneva

Tumors of the Sellar Region

73.1 Classification of Tumors of the Sellar Region

Tumors affecting the sellar region are listed in Table 73.1.

Tumors of the pituitary gland are discussed in Chap. 74, while cystic lesions are discussed in Chap. 75.

Table 73.1 Tumors of the sellar region encompass a multitude of tumor entities

Type of tumor	Tumor entity
Pituitary tumors	• Pituitary adenoma • Pituitary carcinoma • Pituitary hyperplasia • Pituitary apoplexia
Craniopharyngioma	
Other tumors	• Gangliocytoma • Paraganglioma • Spindle cell oncocytoma of the adenohypophysis • Pituicytoma • Granular cell tumor of the neurohypophysis • Meningioma • Glioma • Lipoma • Postirradiation neoplasia • Metastatic neoplasms
Cystic lesions	• Rathke's cleft cyst

73.2 Craniopharyngioma

WHO Definition
2016—A histologically benign, partly cystic epithelial tumor of the sellar region presumably derived from embryonic remnants of the Rathke's pouch epithelium, with two clinicopathological variants (adamantinomatous and papillary) that have distinct phenotypes and characteristic mutations (Buslei et al. 2016).

2007—A benign, partly cystic epithelial tumor of the sellar region presumably derived from Rathke's pouch epithelium (Rushing et al. 2007).

2000—A benign, partly cystic epithelial tumor of the sellar region presumably derived from Rathke's pouch epithelium. Two clinicopathological forms are distinguished, the adamantinomatous and the papillary craniopharyngioma. Xanthogranuloma of the sellar region is a related but distinct clinicopathological entity (Janzer et al. 2000).

1993—A benign, partly cystic epithelial tumor of the sellar region presumably derived from Rathke's pouch epithelium. Two clinicopathological forms are distinguished, the adamantinomatous and the papillary craniopharyngioma. Xanthogranuloma of the sellar region is a related but distinct clinicopathological entity (Kleihues et al. 1993).

1979—A tumor considered by some to originate from vestigial remnants of the craniopharyngeal duct (Rathke's pouch) (Zülch 1979).

WHO grade
- WHO grade I

73.2.1 Clinical Signs and Symptoms

- Visual disturbances (60–84% of patients)
- Endocrine deficiencies 50–87% of patients
  - Growth hormone (75% of cases)
  - LH/FSH (40% of cases)
  - ACTH (25% of cases)
  - TSH (25% of cases)
- Diabetes insipidus (30% of adults, 15% of children)
- Cognitive impairment
- Personality change
- Signs of increased intracranial pressure

73.2.2 Epidemiology

Incidence
- 1–4.5% of all intracranial tumors
- 0.5–2.5 new cases per million population
- 5–10% of intracranial tumors in children

Age Incidence
- Children: 5–15 years of age
- Adults: 45–75 years of age

Sex Incidence
- Male:Female ratio: 1:1

Localization
- Suprasellar (majority of cases)
- Intrasellar component (minority of cases)

73.2.3 Neuroimaging Findings

General Imaging Findings
- Adamantinomatous type: solid and cystic components, calcifications
- Papillary type: homogeneous, calcifications rare

CT non-contrast-enhanced (Fig. 73.1a)
- Adamantinomatous:
  - solid portion isodense, cysts hypodense, calcifications
- Papillary:
  - isodense

CT contrast-enhanced
- Homogeneous enhancement of solid components and cyst wall

MRI-T2/FLAIR (Figs. 73.1b, c, 73.2a, b, and 73.3a, b)
- Solid component heterogeneous iso- to hyperintense
- Cyst hyperintense
- Calcifications hypointense
- Hyperintensities of adjacent brain parenchyma may indicate
  - Gliosis
  - Edema
  - CSF diapedesis
  - Tumor infiltration

MRI-T1 (Figs. 73.1d and 73.2c, e)
- Solid component isointense or heterogeneous
- Cyst hyperintense, depends on protein content

MRI-T1 contrast-enhanced (Figs. 73.1e–g, 73.2d, f, and 73.3c, d)
- Heterogeneous enhancement of solid portions
- Strong enhancement of cyst wall

MRI-T2∗/SWI
- Reveals calcifications in adamantinomatous types

MR-Diffusion Imaging
- Depends on cyst fluid
- ADC value lower than in Rathke's cleft cyst

MR-Spectroscopy
- Lipid peaks in cysts

Nuclear Medicine Imaging Findings (Fig. 73.4a, b)
- Craniopharyngiomas are reported to be MIBI and Tl201 negative.
- FDG shows often no significant elevated uptake in contrast to background, but case reports describe a high uptake in some patients.
- MET is reported to be more useful, indicating that FET which has similar uptake mechanism will be helpful as well.
- C11-Cholin PET is reported to be positive.

73.2.4 Neuropathology Findings

Macroscopic Features (Figs. 73.5a–d and 73.6a–f)
- Lobulated solid mass
- Dark brownish-green appearance on sections
- Penetrate neighboring brain
- Adhere to adjacent blood vessels and nerves

Microscopic Features (Fig. 73.7a–n)
- The following two forms of craniopharyngiomas are distinguished:
- Adamantinomatous (adaCP)
- Papillary (papCP)

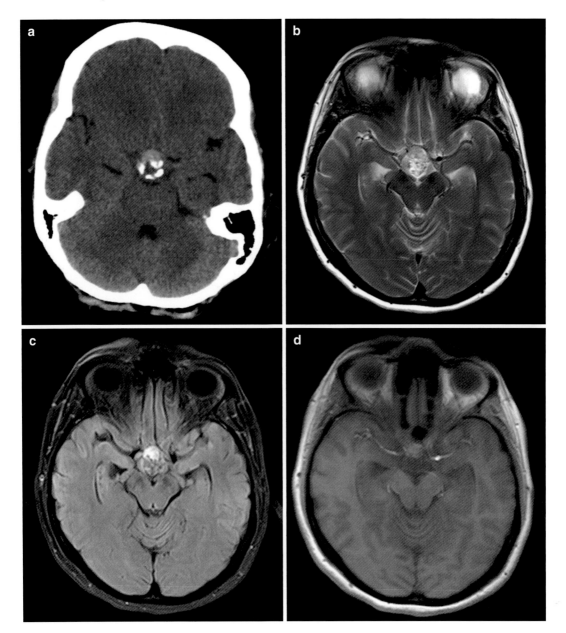

Fig. 73.1 Adamantinomatous craniopharyngioma: CT (**a**), T2 (**b**), FLAIR (**c**), T1 (**d**), T1 contrast ax/sag/cor (**e–g**)

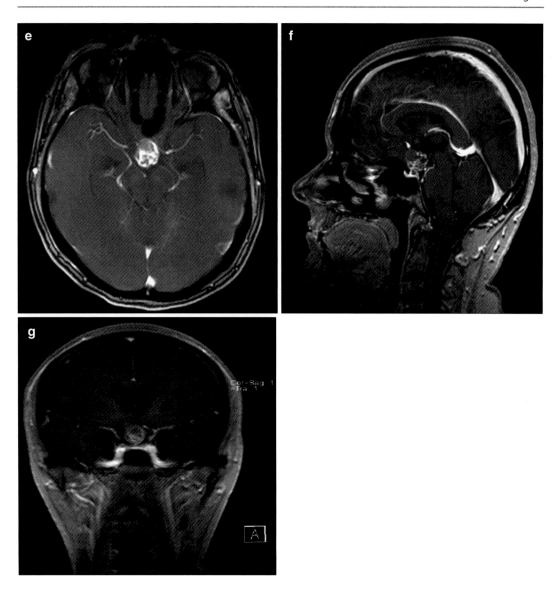

Fig. 73.1 (continued)

Adamantinomatous craniopharyngioma
- Squamous epithelium disposed in cords, lobules
- Distinctive epithelium that form stellate reticulum
- Irregular trabeculae bordered by palisaded columnar epithelium
- Nodules of wet keratin, i.e., remnants of pale nuclei embedded within an eosinophilic keratinous mass wet keratin
- Basal palisades
- Cystic cavities with squamous debris lined by flattened epithelium
- Granulomatous inflammation
- Cholesterol clefts
- Giant cells
- Calcifications
- Piloid gliosis and Rosenthal fibers at the infiltrative interface between tumor and brain

73.2 Craniopharyngioma

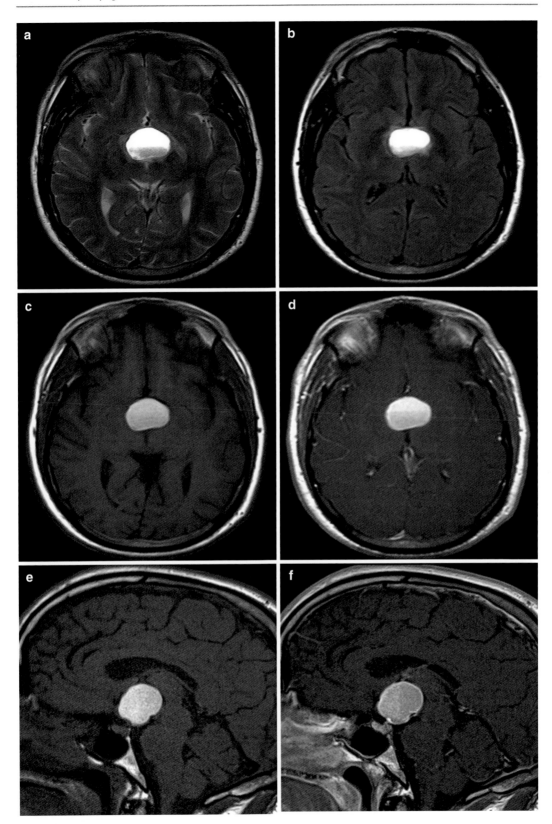

Fig. 73.2 Adamantinomatous craniopharyngioma rich in protein: T2 (**a**), FLAIR (**b**), T1 (**c**), T1 contrast (**d**), T1 sag (**e**), T1 contrast sag (**f**)

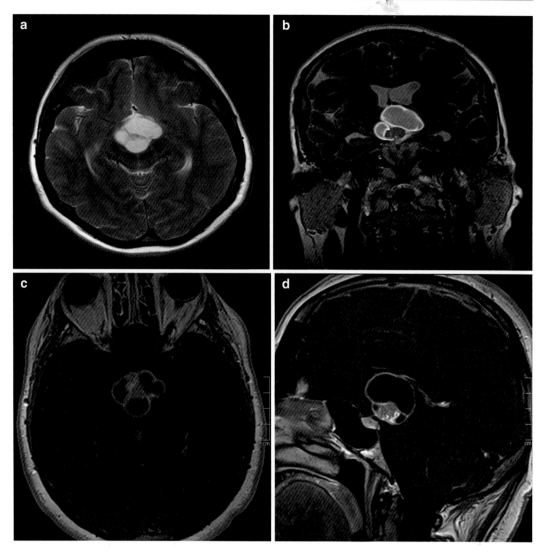

Fig. 73.3 Predominantly cystic craniopharyngioma: T2 (**a**), T2 cor (**b**), T1 contrast (**c**), T1 contrast sag (**d**)

Papillary craniopharyngioma
- Monomorphous mass of well-differentiated squamous epithelium lacking surface maturation
- Picket-fence like palisades
- Fibrovascular cores lined by non-keratinizing squamous epithelium
- Wet keratin, i.e., remnants of pale nuclei embedded within an eosinophilic keratinous mass
- Absence of calcification

Immunophenotype (Fig. 73.8a–j)
- High- and low-molecular weight keratins
- P-glycoprotein
- Somatostatin receptor
- Estrogen receptor
- Adamantinomatous craniopharyngiomas
  – aberrant nuclear expression of beta-catenin
- Papillary craniopharyngiomas
  – BRAF V600E mutations

73.2 Craniopharyngioma

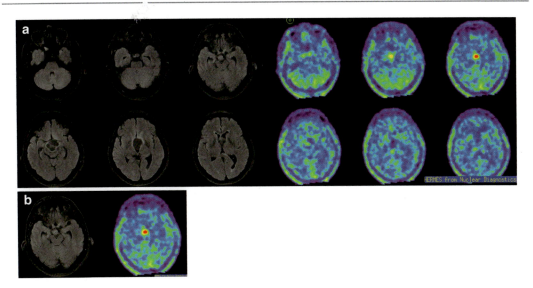

Fig. 73.4 FET-PET and corresponding MRI (FLAIR) of an adamantinomatous craniopharyngioma with clear uptake in the solid part of the tumor (**a**, **b**)

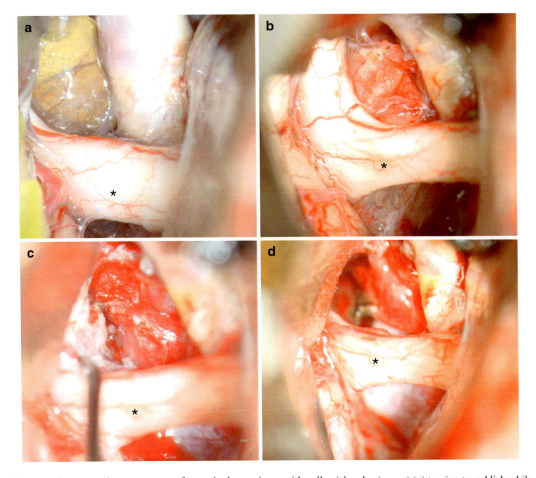

Fig. 73.5 Intraoperative appearance of a craniopharyngioma with yellowish color (arrow) (**a**) turning to reddish while being removed (**b**, **c**). After surgical removal (**d**). Note the close proximity to the optic nerve (asterisk)

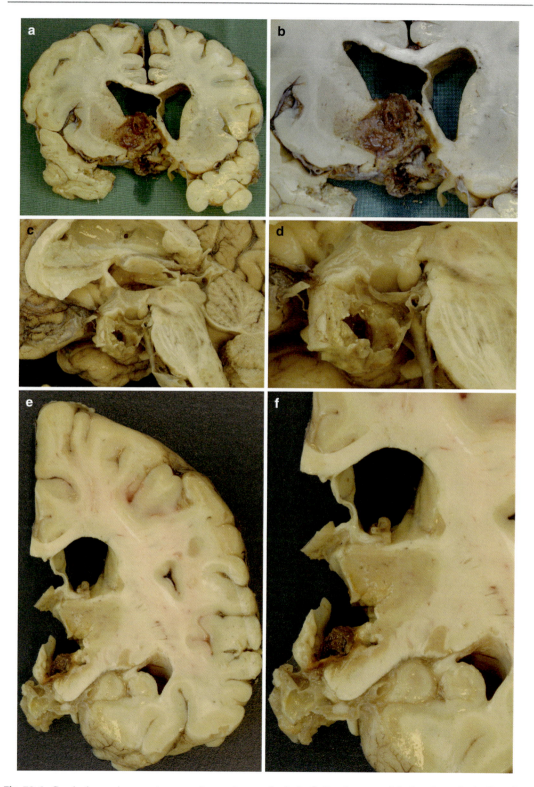

Fig. 73.6 Craniopharyngioma: autopsy specimens showing remnants of the tumor in form of a lobulated dark brownish-green solid mass penetrating the neighboring brain (**a–f**). Involvement of the basal ganglia (**a, b**), sellar region (**c, d**), and thalamus (**e, f**)

73.2 Craniopharyngioma

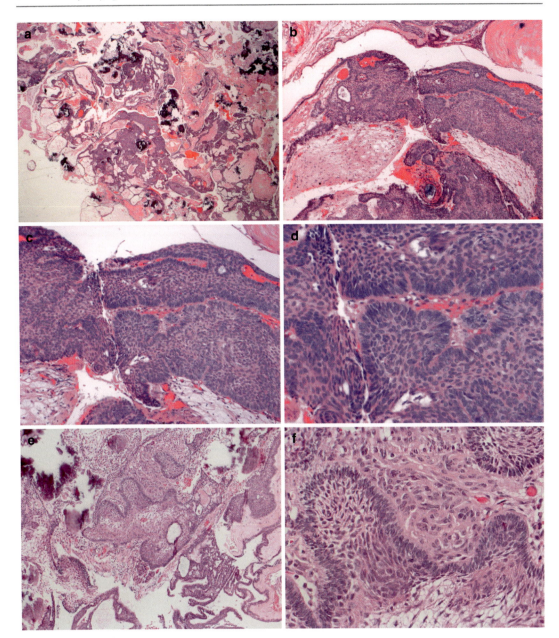

Fig. 73.7 Craniopharyngioma: tumor of moderate cellularity composed of distinctive epithelium that form stellate reticulum, irregular trabeculae bordered by palisaded columnar epithelium and squamous epithelium disposed in cords, lobules (**a–f**). Cystic cavities with squamous debris lined by flattened epithelium (**g, h**). Peculiar gland formations with palisading (**i, j**). Nodules of wet keratin, i.e., remnants of pale nuclei embedded within an eosinophilic keratinous mass wet keratin (**k–n, m, n**; PAS: **m, n**)

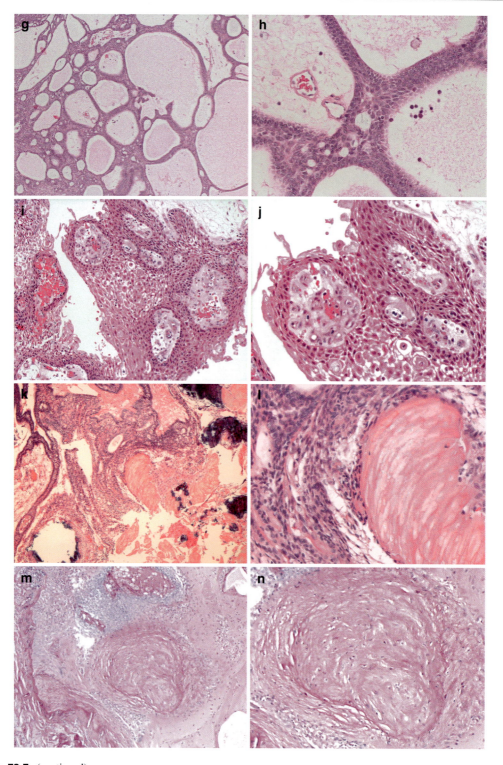

Fig. 73.7 (continued)

73.2 Craniopharyngioma

Proliferation Markers
- Ki-67 reactivity in peripherally palisaded cells
- High interindividual variability
- No correlation between Ki-67 LI and recurrence

Ultrastructural Features
- Epithelial cells contain:
  - Usual organelles
  - Glycogen
  - Tonofilaments

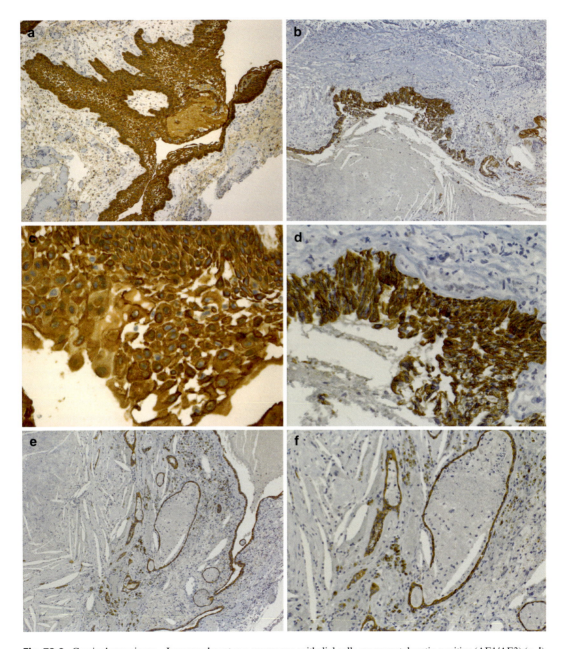

Fig. 73.8 Craniopharyngioma—Immunophenotype: squamous epithelial cells are pancytokeratin-positive (AE1/AE3) (**a–j**)

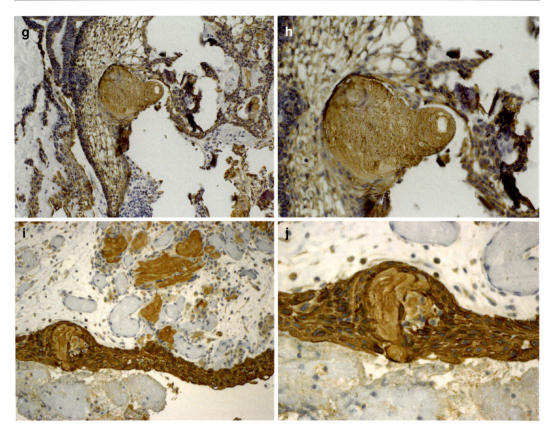

Fig. 73.8 (continued)

- Joined by desmosomes
- Connective tissue stroma characterized by:
  - Fenestrated capillary endothelium
  - Amorphous ground matrix
  - Collagen fibrils
- Mineral precipitates in membrane-bound vesicles

Differential Diagnosis
- Xantogranuloma of the sellar region
- Cholesterol clefts
- Macrophages
- Chronic inflammatory cellular reaction
- Necrotic debris
- Hemosiderin deposits
- Lack of β-catenin immunoreactivity
- Rathke's cleft cyst/epidermoid cyst
  - Presence of a uniloculated cyst lined by squamous epithelium and filled with flaky, dry keratin
  - Single layer of flattened either ciliated or mucin-producing epithelium

73.2.5 Molecular Neuropathology

- Neoplastic transformation of ectodermal-derived epithelial cell remnants of Rathke's pouch and the craniopharyngeal duct
- Metaplasia of
  - tooth primordial cells give rise to the adamantinomatous variant
  - buccal mucosa primordial cells give rise to the papillary variant
- Contain neuroendocrine lineage demonstrated by:
  - Expression of one or more pituitary hormones
  - Chromogranin A
  - Human chorionic gonadotropin
- Mutation of the *β-catenin* (*CTNNB1*) gene in adamantinomatous craniopharyngioma
  - Exon 3 encoding the degradation targeting box of β-catenin leading to an accumulation of β-catenin
  - Abnormalities on chromosome 2 and 12

- *BRAF*V600E mutations were solely found in the papCP subgroup
- *BRAF*V600E mutations were not detectable in adaCP samples
- *CTNNB1* mutations were exclusively detected in adaCP (Holsken et al. 2016)
- The methylome fingerprints distinguished correctly between papCP and adaCP
- No significant difference in methylation signature by age.
- Differential gene expression and methylation reveal a distinct upregulation of Wnt- and SHH signaling pathway genes in adaCP.

73.2.6 Treatment and Prognosis

Treatment
- Surgery

Biologic Behavior–Prognosis–Prognostic Factors
- Indolent tumor
- 60–95% of patients with 10-year recurrence-free survival
- 65–96% of patients with 10-year survival
- Extent of surgical resection
  - Incomplete resection leads to higher recurrence rates because of infiltrative tumor behavior.
- Brain invasion not correlated with higher recurrence

73.3 Pituicytoma

WHO Definition
2016—A circumscribed and generally solid low-grade glial neoplasm that originates in the neurohypophysis or infundibulum and is composed of bipolar spindled cells arranged in a fascicular or storiform pattern (Brat et al. 2016).

2007—A rare, circumscribed, and generally solid, low-grade, spindle cell, glial neoplasm of adults that originates in the neurohypophysis or infundibulum (Wesseling et al. 2007).

2000—Considered to be a synonym of granular cell tumor of the neurohypophysis (Warzok et al. 2000).

1993—An intra- or suprasellar neoplasm composed of finely granular cells similar to those occurring incidentally as clusters and "tumorlets" in the normal pituitary stalk and posterior pituitary. This lysosome-rich, astrocyte-derived tumor is not related to the granular tumor of soft tissue (Kleihues et al. 1993).

WHO grade
- WHO grade I

73.3.1 Epidemiology

Incidence
- Extremely rare

Age Incidence
- Adulthood

Sex Incidence
- Male:Female ratio: 1.6:1

Localization
- Neurohypophysis including pituitary stalk and posterior pituitary
- Intra- and/or suprasellar

73.3.2 Neuroimaging Findings

General Imaging Findings
- Intra- or suprasellar enhancing mass

CT non-contrast-enhanced
- Hyperdense

CT contrast-enhanced
- Homogeneous enhancement

MRI-T2/FLAIR (Fig. 73.9a, b)
- Hyperintense

MRI-T1 (Fig. 73.9c, e)
- Isointense

MRI-T1 contrast-enhanced (Fig. 73.9d, f)
- Homogeneous enhancement

MRI-T2∗/SWI
- Calcification rare

73.3.3 Neuropathology Findings

Macroscopic Features
- Solid mass
- Well-demarcated
- Rarely cyst formation
- Adheres to the adjacent suprasellar structures

Microscopic Features (Fig. 73.10a–d)
- Bipolar, short to elongate spindle-shaped cells
- With oval to elongate nuclei
- Rare or no mitoses

Immunophenotype (Fig. 73.10e–j)
- A list of antibodies with positive or negative immunostaining results is given in Table 73.2.

Spindle cell oncocytomas, granular cell tumors of the sellar region, and pituicytomas show nuclear expression of TTF1, suggesting that these three tumors may constitute a spectrum of a single nosological entity.

Proliferation Markers
- Ki-67 LI: 1–2%

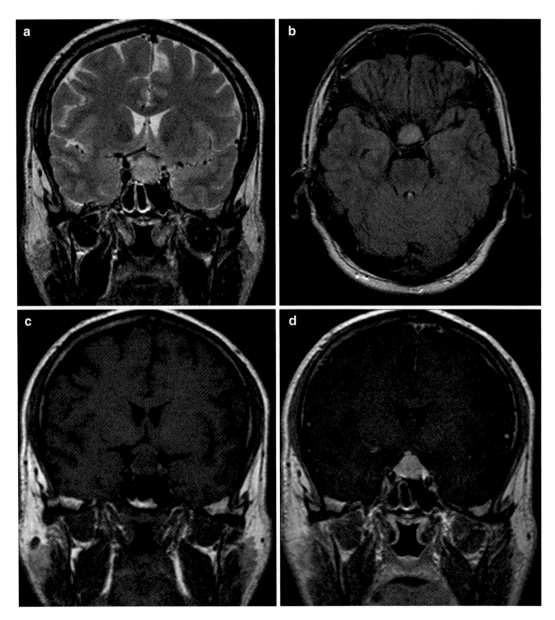

Fig. 73.9 MR pituicytoma: T2 cor (**a**), FLAIR (**b**), cor T1/T1 contrast (**c/d**), and sag T1/T1 contrast (**e/f**)

73.3 Pituicytoma

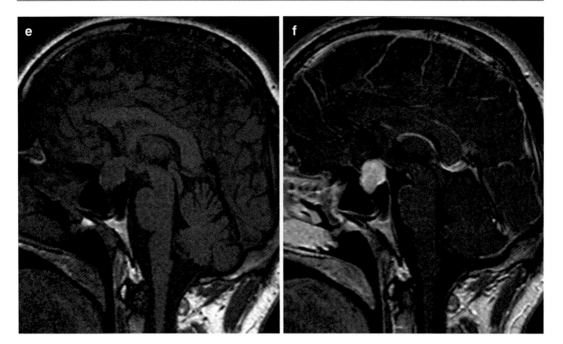

Fig. 73.9 (continued)

Ultrastructural Features
- Elongated spindle cells containing in the Golgi area abundant aggregates of intermediate filaments in a concentric pathway
- Absence of neurosecretory granules
- Absence of pericellular deposition of basal lamina-like material like that seen in schwannomas
- Scattered intercellular junctions

Differential Diagnosis
- Spindle cell oncocytoma
- Granular cell tumor of the infundibulum
- Fibrous meningioma
- Pilocytic astrocytoma
- Schwannomas
- Pituitary adenoma

73.3.4 Molecular Neuropathology

- Originate from:
  - pituicytes of the neurohypophysis
  - alternatively from folliculostellate stromal cells of the adenohypophysis
- Due to nuclear expression of TTF1, pituicytomas, granular cell tumors of the sellar region, and spindle cell oncocytomas may form a spectrum of a single nosological entity.

73.3.5 Treatment and Prognosis

Treatment
- Surgical removal

Biologic Behavior–Prognosis–Prognostic Factors
- No malignant transformation

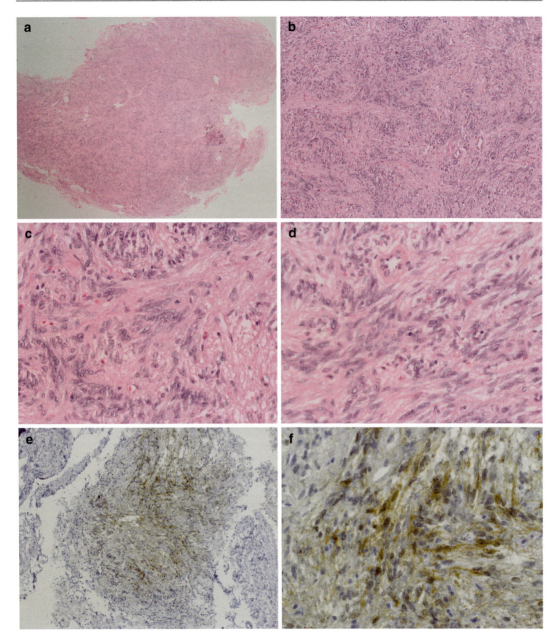

Fig. 73.10 Pituicytoma: Moderately cellular tumor composed of bipolar, short to elongate spindle-shaped cells with oval to elongate nuclei (**a–d**). The tumor cells are immunopositive for S-100 (**e, f**), vimentin (**g, h**), and thyroid transcription factor 1 (TTF1) (**i, j**)

73.4 Granular Cell Tumor of the Sellar Region

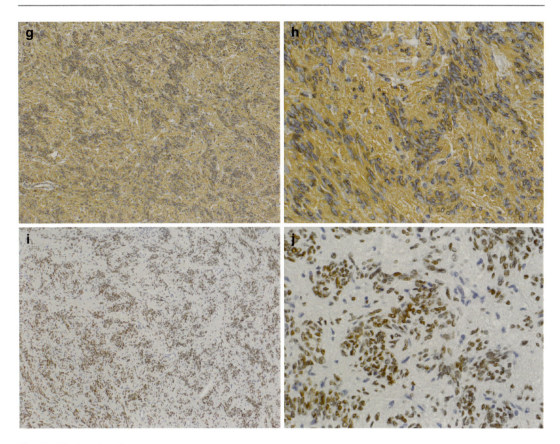

Fig. 73.10 (continued)

Table 73.2 Immunophenotype of pituicytoma

IHC-positivities	IHC-negativities

• Vimentin
• S100
• TTF1 (nuclear)
• Bcl-2
• Variable positivities
  – GFAP
  – Galectin 3
	• EMA
	• Annexin-A1
	• Synaptophysin
	• Chromogranin
	• Pituitary hormones

73.4 Granular Cell Tumor of the Sellar Region

WHO Definition

2016—A circumscribed tumor that is composed of large epitheloid to spindled cells with distinctively granular, eosinophilic cytoplasm (due to an abundance of intracytoplasmic lysosomes) and that arises from the neurohypophysis or infundibulum (Fuller et al. 2016).

2007—An intrasellar and/or suprasellar mass arising from the neurohypophysis or infundibulum, composed of nests of large cells with granular, eosinophilic cytoplasm due to abundant intracytoplasmic lysosomes (Fuller and Wesseling 2007).

2000—An intrasellar and/or suprasellar mass arising from the neurohypophysis or infundibulum, composed of nests of large cells with granular, eosinophilic cytoplasm due to abundant intracytoplasmic lysosomes (Warzok et al. 2000).

1993—An intra- or suprasellar neoplasm composed of finely granular cells similar to those occurring incidentally as clusters and "tumorlets" in the normal pituitary stalk and posterior pituitary. This lysosome-rich, astrocyte-derived tumor is not related to the granular tumor of soft tissue (Kleihues et al. 1993).

WHO grade
- WHO grade I

73.4.1 Epidemiology

Incidence
- Rare

Age Incidence
- Adulthood

Sex Incidence
- Male:Female ratio: 1:2

Localization
- Neurohypophysis including
- Posterior pituitary
- Pituitary stalk/infundibulum

73.4.2 Neuroimaging Findings

General Imaging Findings
- Typically suprasellar enhancing mass

CT non-contrast-enhanced
- Hyperdense

CT contrast-enhanced
- Homogeneous enhancement

MRI-T2/FLAIR (Fig. 73.11a, b)
- Isointense

MRI-T1 (Fig. 73.11c)
- Isointense

MRI-T1 contrast-enhanced (Fig. 73.11d–f)
- Strong enhancement

73.4.3 Neuropathology Findings

Macroscopic Features
- Lobulated
- Well circumscribed
- Soft but rubbery consistency
- Gray to yellow color

Microscopic Features (Fig. 73.12a–j)
- Densely packed polygonal cells.
- Abundant granular eosinophilic cytoplasm.
- Arrangement of cells in nodules, sheets, fascicles.
- Foamy cells may be present.
- Cytoplasmic granules are positive for PAS, and diastase-resistant PAS.
- Perivascular lymphocytic infiltrates.

Atypical granular cell tumor characterized by:

- Nuclear polymorphism
- Prominent nucleoli
- Multinucleated cell
- Increased mitotic activity (five mitoses per ten high power field)
- Ki-67 labeling index of 7%
- Uncertain clinical behavior

Immunophenotype (Fig. 73.12k–p)
- A list of antibodies with positive or negative immunostaining results is given in Table 73.3.

Spindle cell oncocytomas, granular cell tumors of the sellar region, and pituicytomas show nuclear expression of TTF1, suggesting that these three tumors may constitute a spectrum of a single nosological entity.

Proliferation Markers
- Mitotic activity inconspicuous
- Low LI for Ki-67

Ultrastructural Features
- Tumor cells contain phagolysosomes
  - Which contain unevenly distributed electron-dense material and membranous debris
- Absence of neurosecretory granules

73.4 Granular Cell Tumor of the Sellar Region

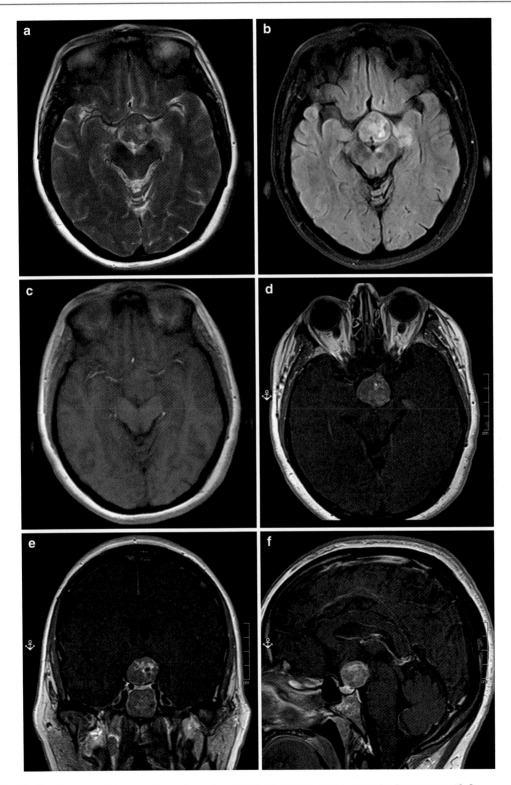

Fig. 73.11 Granular cell tumor of the sellar region: T2 (**a**), FLAIR (**b**), T1 (**c**), T1 ax/cor/sag contrast (**d–f**)

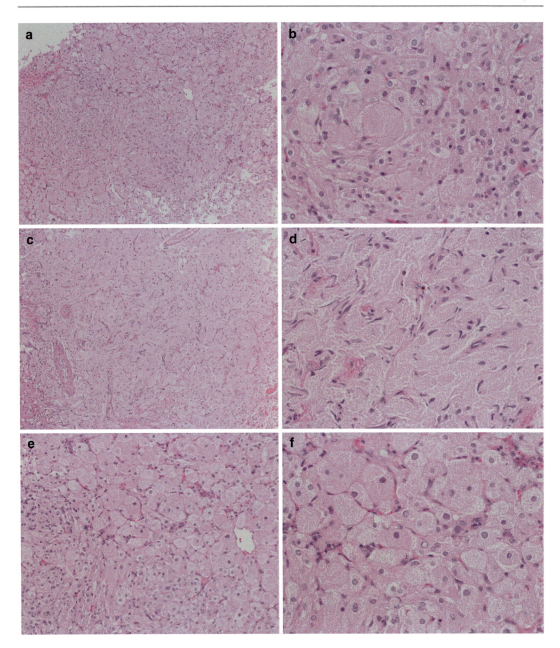

Fig. 73.12 Granular cell tumor: Tumor of low cellularity composed of densely packed polygonal cells with abundant granular eosinophilic cytoplasm arrangement of cells in nodules, sheets, fascicles (**a–d**), foamy cells are present (**e, f**). Cytoplasmic granules are positive for PAS, and diastase-resistant PAS (**g, h**). Reticulin stain highlights the nodular architecture (**i, j**). Immunophenotype: tumor cells are positive for S-100 (**k, l**), CD68 (**m, n**). A few GFAP-astroglial cells might be seen (**o, p**)

73.4 Granular Cell Tumor of the Sellar Region

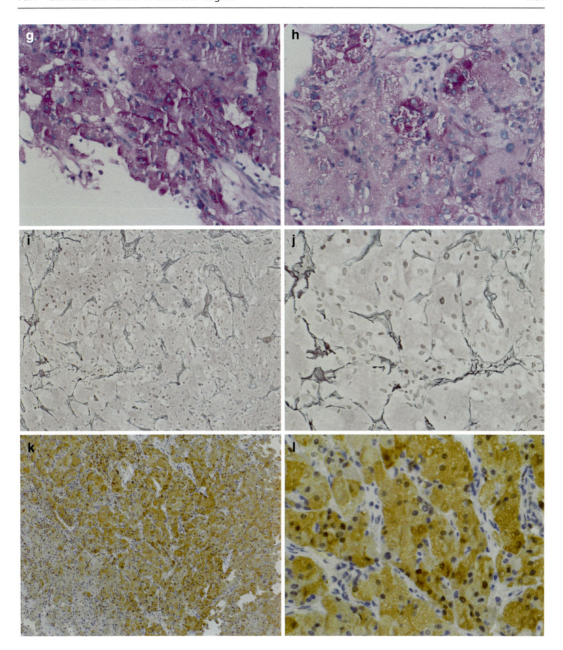

Fig. 73.12 (continued)

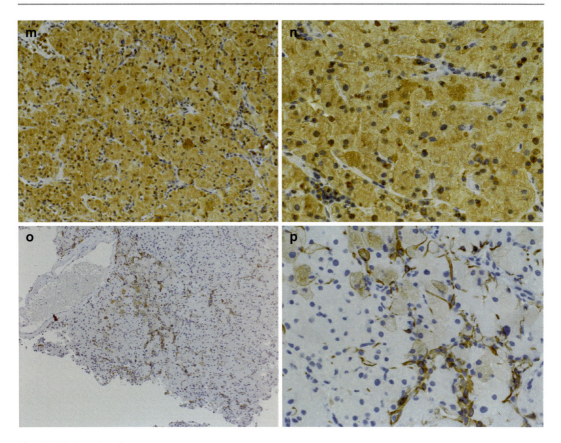

Fig. 73.12 (continued)

Table 73.3 Immunophenotype of granular cell tumor of the sellar region

IHC-positivity	IHC-negativity
• CD68 • S-100 • α-1-antitrypsin • α-1-antichimotrypsin • Cathepsin B • TTF1 (nuclear)	• Neurofilament • Cytokeratins • Chromogranin A • Synaptophysin • Desmin • Smooth muscle actin • Pituitary hormones • GFAP

Differential Diagnosis
- Pituicytoma
- Spindle cell oncocytoma
- Granular cell astrocytoma

73.4.4 Molecular Neuropathology

- Arise from pituicytes (i.e., glial element in the posterior lobe and stalk of the pituitary gland).

- Due to nuclear expression of TTF1, pituicytomas, granular cell tumors of the sellar region, and spindle cell oncocytomas may form a spectrum of a single nosological entity.

73.4.5 Treatment and Prognosis

Treatment
- Total resection if possible

Biologic Behavior–Prognosis–Prognostic Factors
- Benign
- Slow progression
- Lack of invasive growth
- *Atypical granular cell tumor* characterized by:
  – Uncertain clinical behavior

73.5 Spindle Cell Oncocytoma

WHO Definition
2016—A spindled to epithelioid, oncocytic, non-neuroendocrine neoplasm of the pituitary gland (Lopes et al. 2016).

2007—A spindled to epitheloid, oncocytic, non-endocrine neoplasm of the adenohypophysis that manifests in adults and follows a benign clinical course (Fuller et al. 2007).

WHO grade
- WHO grade I

73.5.1 Epidemiology

Incidence
- Rare
- <1% of pituitary tumors

Age Incidence
- Third to seventh decade

Sex Incidence
- Male:Female ratio: 1:1

Localization
- Pituitary
  - Suprasellar extension possible
  - Invasion of the cavernous sinus possible

73.5.2 Neuroimaging Findings

General Imaging Findings
- Intra-suprasellar, infiltrating, enhancing mass, cannot be separated from pituitary gland.

CT non-contrast-enhanced
- Hyperdense

CT contrast-enhanced
- Heterogeneous enhancement

MRI-T2/FLAIR
- Hypointense

MRI-T1
- Isointense

MRI-T1 contrast-enhanced
- Heterogeneous enhancement

73.5.3 Neuropathology Findings

Macroscopic Features
- Soft tissue
- No clear delineation from pituitary parenchyma
- Invasion of the sellar floor possible

Microscopic Features
- Spindle cells
  - With eosinophilic, granular cytoplasm
  - Arranged in fascicles
  - Mild nuclear pleomorphism
  - Dense chromatin
- Admixed with epithelioid cells
- No mitoses
- Positivity of tumor cells for PTAH (cytoplasmic, granular staining)
- Negative staining for PAS and Alcian blue
- Patchy lymphocytic infiltration

Immunophenotype
- A list of antibodies with positive or negative immunostaining results is given in Table 73.4.

Spindle cell oncocytomas, granular cell tumors of the sellar region, and pituicytomas show nuclear expression of TTF1, suggesting that these three tumors may constitute a spectrum of a single nosological entity.

Table 73.4 Immunophenotype of spindle cell oncocytoma

Positivity	Negativity
• EMA	• GFAP
• S100	• Cytokeratin
• Vimentin	• CD34
• Galectin-3	• Bcl-2
• Annexin A1	• Smooth muscle actin
• Anti-mitochondrial antibodies	• Desmin
• TTF1 (nuclear)	• Pituitary hormones
	• Synaptophysin
	• Chromogranin

Proliferation Markers
- Ki-67 LI: mean 3%, range 1–10%

Ultrastructural Features
- Spindled or polygonal tumor cells:
  - Contain a large number of mitochondria
  - Well-formed desmosomes without tonofilaments and intermediate junctions
  - No secretory granules

Differential Diagnosis
- Pituicytoma
- Granular cell tumor of the adenohypophysis
- Pituitary adenoma
- Meningioma

73.5.4 Molecular Neuropathology

- Uncertain origin.
- Derivation from folliculostellate cells of the anterior hypophysis.
- Due to nuclear expression of TTF1, pituicytomas, granular cell tumors of the sellar region, and spindle cell oncocytomas may form a spectrum of a single nosological entity.

73.5.5 Treatment and Prognosis

Treatment
- Surgical resection
- Radiosurgery possible

Biologic Behavior–Prognosis–Prognostic Factors
- Benign clinical course
- Rare recurrences
- Local aggressive behavior

Selected References

Alexandrescu S, Brown RE, Tandon N, Bhattacharjee MB (2012) Neuron precursor features of spindle cell oncocytoma of adenohypophysis. Ann Clin Lab Sci 42(2):123–129

Brat DJ, Wesseling P, Fuller GN, Roncaroli F (2016) Pituicytoma. In: Louis DN, Ohgaki H, Wiestler OD, Cavenee WK (eds) WHO classification of tumours of the central nervous system, Revised 4th edn. IARC, Lyon, pp 332–333

Buslei R, Rushing EJ, Giangaspero F, Paulus W, Burger PC, Santagata S (2016) Craniopharyngioma. In: Louis DN, Ohgaki H, Wiestler OD, Cavenee WK (eds) WHO classification of tumours of the central nervous system, Revised 4th edn. IARC, Lyon, pp 324–328

Covington MF, Chin SS, Osborn AG (2011) Pituicytoma, spindle cell oncocytoma, and granular cell tumor: clarification and meta-analysis of the world literature since 1893. AJNR Am J Neuroradiol 32(11):2067–2072. https://doi.org/10.3174/ajnr.A2717

El Hussein S, Vincentelli C (2017) Pituicytoma: review of commonalities and distinguishing features among TTF-1 positive tumors of the central nervous system. Ann Diagn Pathol 29:57–61. https://doi.org/10.1016/j.anndiagpath.2017.05.004

Farooq MU, Bhatt A, Chang HT (2008) Teaching neuroimage: spindle cell oncocytoma of the pituitary gland. Neurology 71(2):e3. https://doi.org/10.1212/01.wnl.0000316805.30694.4f

Fuller GN, Brat DJ, Wesseling P, Roncaroli F (2016) Granular cell tumour of the sellar region. In: Louis DN, Ohgaki H, Wiestler OD, Cavenee WK (eds) WHO classification of tumours of the central nervous system, Revised 4th edn. IARC, Lyon, pp 329–331

Fuller GN, Scheithauer BW, Roncaroli F, Wesseling P (2007) Spindle cell oncocytoma of the adenohypophysis. In: Louis DN, Ohgaki H, Wiestler OD, Cavenee WK (eds) WHO classification of tumours of the central nervous system, 4th edn. International Agency for Research on Cancer, Lyon, pp 245–246

Fuller GN, Wesseling P (2007) Granular cell tumour of the sellar region. In: Louis DN, Ohgaki H, Wiestler OD, Cavenee WK (eds) WHO classification of tumours of the central nervous system, 4th edn. International Agency for Research on Cancer, Lyon, pp 241–242

Furtado SV, Ghosal N, Venkatesh PK, Gupta K, Hegde AS (2010) Diagnostic and clinical implications of pituicytoma. J Clin Neurosci 17(7):938–943. https://doi.org/10.1016/j.jocn.2009.09.047

Gibbs WN, Monuki ES, Linskey ME, Hasso AN (2006) Pituicytoma: diagnostic features on selective carotid angiography and MR imaging. AJNR Am J Neuroradiol 27(8):1639–1642

Hasiloglu ZI, Ure E, Comunoglu N, Tanriover N, Oz B, Gazioglu N, Mihmanli I (2016) New radiological clues in the diagnosis of spindle cell oncocytoma of the adenohypophysis. Clin Radiol 71(9):937.e935–937.e911. https://doi.org/10.1016/j.crad.2016.04.022

Holsken A, Sill M, Merkle J, Schweizer L, Buchfelder M, Flitsch J, Fahlbusch R, Metzler M, Kool M, Pfister SM, von Deimling A, Capper D, Jones DT, Buslei R (2016) Adamantinomatous and papillary craniopharyngiomas are characterized by distinct epigenomic as well as mutational and transcriptomic profiles. Acta Neuropathol Commun 4:20. https://doi.org/10.1186/s40478-016-0287-6

Janzer RC, Burger PC, Giangaspero F, Paulus W (2000) Craniopharyngioma. In: Kleihues P, Cavenee WK (eds) Pathology and genetics of tumours of the nervous system, 3rd edn. IARC Press, Lyon, pp 244–246

Selected References

Karamchandani J, Syro LV, Uribe H, Horvath E, Kovacs K (2012) Pituicytoma of the neurohypophysis: analysis of cell proliferation biomarkers. Can J Neurol Sci 39(6):835–837

Kleihues P, Burger PC, Scheithauer BW (1993) Histological typing of tumours of the central nervous system, 2nd edn. Springer, Berlin

Kosuge Y, Hiramoto J, Morishima H, Tanaka Y, Hashimoto T (2012) Neuroimaging characteristics and growth pattern on magnetic resonance imaging in a 52-year-old man presenting with pituicytoma: a case report. J Med Case Rep 6:306. https://doi.org/10.1186/1752-1947-6-306

Kowalski RJ, Prayson RA, Mayberg MR (2004) Pituicytoma. Ann Diagn Pathol 8(5):290–294

Kwon MJ, Suh YL (2011) Pituicytoma with unusual histological features. Pathol Int 61(10):598–602. https://doi.org/10.1111/j.1440-1827.2011.02708.x

Lopes MBS, Fuller GN, Roncaroli F, Wesseling P (2016) Spindle cell oncocytoma. In: Louis DN, Ohgaki H, Wiestler OD, Cavenee WK (eds) WHO classification of tumours of the central nervous system, Revised 4th edn. IARC, Lyon, pp 334–336

Machado I, Cruz J, Lavernia J, Llombart-Bosch A (2016) Solitary, multiple, benign, atypical, or malignant: the "granular cell tumor" puzzle. Virchows Arch 468(5):527–538. https://doi.org/10.1007/s00428-015-1877-6

Manoranjan B, Koziarz A, Kameda-Smith MM, Provias JP (2017) Multiple recurrences require long-term follow-up in patients diagnosed with spindle cell oncocytoma of the Sella turcica. J Clin Neurosci 43:134–146. https://doi.org/10.1016/j.jocn.2017.05.017

Mende KC, Matschke J, Burkhardt T, Saeger W, Buslei R, Buchfelder M, Fahlbusch R, Westphal M, Flitsch J (2017) Pituicytoma-an outlook on possible targeted therapies. CNS Neurosci Ther 23(7):620–626. https://doi.org/10.1111/cns.12709

Neidert MC, Leske H, Burkhardt JK, Kollias SS, Capper D, Schrimpf D, Regli L, Rushing EJ (2016) Synchronous pituitary adenoma and pituicytoma. Hum Pathol 47(1):138–143. https://doi.org/10.1016/j.humpath.2015.08.017

Ogiwara H, Dubner S, Shafizadeh S, Raizer J, Chandler JP (2011) Spindle cell oncocytoma of the pituitary and pituicytoma: two tumors mimicking pituitary adenoma. Surg Neurol Int 2:116. https://doi.org/10.4103/2152-7806.83932

Ordonez NG (1999) Granular cell tumor: a review and update. Adv Anat Pathol 6(4):186–203

Ordonez NG, Mackay B (1999) Granular cell tumor: a review of the pathology and histogenesis. Ultrastruct Pathol 23(4):207–222

Piccirilli M, Maiola V, Salvati M, D'Elia A, Di Paolo A, Campagna D, Santoro A, Delfini R (2014) Granular cell tumor of the neurohypophysis: a single-institution experience. Tumori 100(4):160e–164e. https://doi.org/10.1700/1636.17940

Romero-Rojas AE, Melo-Uribe MA, Barajas-Solano PA, Chinchilla-Olaya SI, Escobar LI, Hernandez-Walteros DM (2011) Spindle cell oncocytoma of the adenohypophysis. Brain Tumor Pathol 28(4):359–364. https://doi.org/10.1007/s10014-011-0051-3

Roncaroli F, Scheithauer BW (2007) Papillary tumor of the pineal region and spindle cell oncocytoma of the pituitary: new tumor entities in the 2007 WHO classification. Brain Pathol 17(3):314–318. https://doi.org/10.1111/j.1750-3639.2007.00081.x

Rushing EJ, Giangaspero F, Paulus W, Burger PC (2007) Craniopharyngioma. In: Louis DN, Ohgaki H, Wiestler OD, Cavenee WK (eds) WHO classification of tumours of the central nervous system, 4th edn. International Agency for Research on Cancer, Lyon, pp 238–240

Sali A, Epari S (2017) Spindle cell oncocytoma of adenohypophysis: review of literature and report of another recurrent case. Neuropathology 37(6):535–543. https://doi.org/10.1111/neup.12393

Tampi C, Goel A, Mathkour M, Garces J, Scullen T, Valle-Giler E, Halat S, Arrington T, Ware M (2017) Spindle cell oncocytoma of the pituitary gland. Neuropathology 61(5):554–557. https://doi.org/10.1111/neup.12393

Teti C, Castelletti L, Allegretti L, Talco M, Zona G, Minuto F, Boschetti M, Ferone D (2015) Pituitary image: pituicytoma. Pituitary 18(5):592–597. https://doi.org/10.1007/s11102-014-0612-7

Vuong HG, Kondo T, Tran TM, Oishi N, Nakazawa T, Mochizuki K, Inoue T, Kasai K, Tahara I, Jieying W, Katoh R (2016) Spindle cell oncocytoma of adenohypophysis: report of a case and immunohistochemical review of literature. Pathol Res Pract 212(3):222–225. https://doi.org/10.1016/j.prp.2015.07.014

Wang J, Liu Z, Du J, Cui Y, Fang J, Xu L, Li G (2016) The clinicopathological features of pituicytoma and the differential diagnosis of sellar glioma. Neuropathology 36(5):432–440. https://doi.org/10.1111/neup.12291

Warzok RW, Vogelsang S, Feiden W, Shuangshoti S (2000) Granular cell tumour of the neurohyophysis. In: Kleihues P, Cavenee WK (eds) Pathology and genetics of tumours of the nervous system, 3rd edn. IARC Press, Lyon, pp 247–248

Wesseling P, Brat DJ, Fuller GN (2007) Pituicytoma. In: Louis DN, Ohgaki H, Wiestler OD, Cavenee WK (eds) WHO classification of tumours of the central nervous system, 4th edn. International Agency for Research on Cancer, Lyon, pp 243–244

Yoshimoto T, Takahashi-Fujigasaki J, Inoshita N, Fukuhara N, Nishioka H, Yamada S (2015) TTF-1-positive oncocytic sellar tumor with follicle formation/ependymal differentiation: non-adenomatous tumor capable of two different interpretations as a pituicytoma or a spindle cell oncocytoma. Brain Tumor Pathol 32(3):221–227. https://doi.org/10.1007/s10014-015-0219-3

Zhi L, Yang L, Quan H, Bai-ning L (2009) Pituicytoma presenting with atypical histological features. Pathology 41(5):505–509

Zülch KJ (1979) Histological typing of tumours of the central nervous system. World Health Organization, Geneva

Zunarelli E, Casaretta GL, Rusev B, Lupi M (2011) Pituicytoma with atypical histological features: are they predictive of unfavourable clinical course? Pathology 43(4):389–394. https://doi.org/10.1097/PAT.0b013e32834687b3

Tumors of the Pituitary Gland

WHO Definition
2017—Pituitary adenoma is a neoplastic proliferation of anterior pituitary hormone-producing cells. The tumors are typically benign, but can be aggressive and invasive into adjacent structures (OSAMURA et al. 2017a).

2004—Pituitary tumors are defined as neoplasms located in the sella turcica. The vast majority are pituitary adenomas derived from adenohypophysial cells with only a very small percentage of these tumors representing pituitary carcinomas. Other lesions located in the sella include mesenchymal, neural, or epithelial tumors and metastases (Lloyd et al. 2004).

74.1 Epidemiology

Incidence
- 10–15% of intracranial neoplasms

Age Incidence
- Depending on adenoma type
Age range: 20–80 years

Sex Incidence
- Depending on adenoma type
Male:Female ratio: Range: 1:1 up to 1:8

74.2 Classification of Pituitary Tumors

An accurate classification of tumors of the pituitary gland is based on its hormonal activity both at the clinical level and in histological specimens (Table 74.1):

- Pituitary adenoma
  - Somatotroph adenoma
    - Densely granulated somatotroph adenoma
    - Sparsely granulated somatotroph adenoma
    - Mammosomatotroph adenoma
    - Mixed somatotroph and lactotroph adenoma
    - Plurihormonal adenomas
  - Lactotroph adenoma
    - Densely granulated lactotroph adenoma
    - Sparsely granulated lactotroph adenoma
    - Acidophil stem cell adenoma (ASCA)
  - Thyrotroph adenoma
  - Corticotroph adenoma
    - Densely granulated corticotroph adenoma
    - Sparsely granulated corticotroph adenoma
    - Crooke cell adenoma
    - Silent corticotroph adenoma
  - Gonadotroph adenoma
  - Null cell adenoma
  - Plurihormonal and double adenoma

Table 74.1 2017 WHO classification of pituitary adenomas (Lopes 2017)

Adenoma type	Morphological variants	Pituitary hormones and other immunomarkers	Transcription factors and other co-factors
Somatotroph adenomas	Densely granulated adenoma	GH ± PRL ± α-subunit	PIT-1
	Sparsely granulated adenoma	GH ± PRL, [CK]	PIT-1
	Mammosomatotroph adenoma	GH + PRL (in same cells) ± α-subunit	PIT-1, ERα
	Mixed somatotroph–lactotroph adenoma	GH + PRL (in different cells) ± α-subunit	PIT-1, ERα
Lactotroph adenomas	Sparsely granulated adenoma	PRL	PIT-1, ERα
	Densely granulated adenoma	PRL	PIT-1, ERα
	Acidophilic stem cell adenoma	PRL, GH (focal and variable)	PIT-1, ERα
Thyrotroph adenoma		β-TSH, α-subunit	PIT-1
Corticotroph adenomas	Densely granulated adenoma	ACTH, [CK]	T-PIT
	Sparsely granulated adenoma	ACTH, [CK]	T-PIT
	Crooke cell adenoma	ACTH, [CK]	T-PIT
Gonadotroph adenoma		β-FSH, β-LH, α-subunit (various combinations)	SF-1, GATA2, ERα
Null cell adenoma		None	None
Plurihormonal adenomas	Plurihormonal PIT-1-positive adenoma (previously called silent subtype 3 adenoma)	GH, PRL, β-TSH ± α-subunit	PIT-1
	Adenomas with unusual immunohistochemical combinations	Various combinations: ACTH/GH, ACTH/PRL	N/A

- Atypical pituitary adenoma
- Pituitary carcinoma
- Pituitary blastoma
- Pituitary hyperplasia

The distribution of various adenoma types from an unselected series is shown in Table 74.2 while that derived from surgical series is given in Table 74.3.

74.2.1 Clinical Classification of Pituitary Tumors

The clinical classification of pituitary tumors is based on the hormonal activity of the tumor:

- GH-producing adenomas (acromegaly and/or gigantism)
- Hyperprolactinemia-producing adenomas
- ACTH-producing adenomas (Cushing syndrome or Nelson syndrome)
- TSH-producing tumors
- Gonadotroph adenomas (rare)
- Non-functioning adenomas

74.2.2 Radiologic Classification of Pituitary Tumors

MRI is the most appropriate method to visualize pituitary tumors.

- 3 mm thick T1-weighted images pre- and post-administration of IV gadolinium

In general, the classification is based on:

- Tumor size
- Degree of local invasion

Based on tumor size, two types of tumor are distinguished:

- Microadenoma <1 cm in diameter
- Macroadenoma 1–4 cm in diameter
- Giant adenoma >4 cm in diameter

Table 74.2 Distribution of various adenoma types based on an unselected series of 2091 biopsies modified after (Lloyd et al. 2004) from (Horvath et al. 2002)

Adenoma type	Frequency	Male:Female	Immunoprofile
Sparsely granulated PRL cell adenoma	27.0	1:2.5	PRL
Densely granulated PRL cell adenoma	0.4		PRL
Sparsely granulated GH cell adenoma	7.6	1:1.2	GH, α-SU, PRL
Densely granulated GH cell adenoma	7.1	1:0.7	GH, α-SU, PRL, TSH
Mixed (GH cell—PRL cell) adenoma	3.5	1:1.1	GH, PRL, α-SU, TSH
Mammosomatotroph cell adenoma	1.2	1:1.1	GH, PRL, α-SU, TSH
Acidophil stem cell adenoma	1.6	1:1.5	PRL, GH
Corticotroph cell adenoma	9.6	1:5.4	ACTH, (LH, α-SU)
Thyrotroph cell adenoma	1.1	1:1.3	TSH, α-SU, (GH, PRL)
Gonadotroph cell adenoma	9.8	1:0.8	FSH, LH, α-SU, (ACTH)
Silent corticotroph adenoma, subtype 1	2.0	1:0.2	ACTH
Silent corticotroph adenoma, subtype 2	1.5	1:1.7	β-endorphin, ACTH
Silent corticotroph adenoma, subtype 3	1.4	1:1.1	None
Null cell adenoma	12.4	1:0.7	FSH, LH, α-SU, TSH
Oncocytoma	13.4	1:0.5	FSH, LH, α-SU, TSH
Unclassified	1.8		

Table 74.3 Frequencies pituitary adenoma types based on surgical material only, modified after Fahlbusch and Buchfelder (2011) data reproduced with kind permission by Elsevier

Pituitary adenoma type	Number of tumors	Percent
Non-functioning adenomas	1537	41.40
GH-omas	877	23.62
Prolactinomas	730	19.66
ACTH-producing adenomas	537	14.46
TSH-omas	32	0.86
Total	3713	

The following grading of pituitary tumors was proposed:

- Grade I—microadenoma
  - <1 cm in diameter
  - no bony changes
- Grade II—macroadenoma
  - 1 cm diameter
  - no bony destruction
  - intrasellar localization
  - extrasellar expansion without invasion
- Grade III
  - small or large
  - locally invasive
  - diffuse sellar enlargement
  - suprasellar extension
  - bony erosion of the sella turcica
- Grade IV
  - large tumor
  - invade extrasellar structures (bone, hypothalamus, cavernous sinus)
- Giant adenoma
  - 4 cm diameter

74.3 Radiological Features of Pituitary Tumors

74.3.1 Microadenoma

General Imaging Findings
- Round, well demarcated, less than 10 mm in size, enhancement delayed compared to surrounding normal gland.

CT non-contrast-enhanced
- Invisible, isodense

CT contrast-enhanced
- May be hypodense

MRI-T2/FLAIR (Fig. 74.1a)
- Isointense, without pathological findings

MRI-T1 (Fig. 74.1b)
- Isointense
Hyperintense if hemorrhage

MRI-T1 Contrast-Enhanced (Fig. 74.1c, d)
- Enhancement less rapid than normal pituitary

MRI-T2∗/SWI
- Hypointense if hemorrhage

74.3.2 Macroadenoma

General Imaging Findings
- >10 mm in diameter by definition, pituitary gland not circumscribable, cysts and necrosis possible, internal carotid arteries in cavernous sinus are typically encased but rarely compressed

CT non-contrast-enhanced (Fig. 74.2a)
- Isodense to cortex
- Inhomogeneous if cysts or necrosis

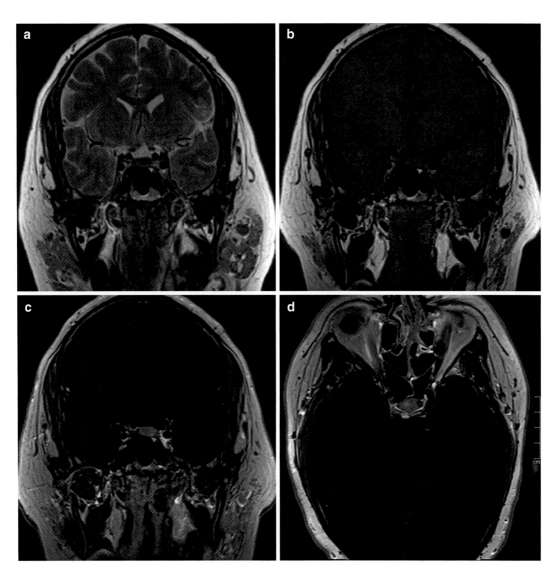

Fig. 74.1 MR of a left endosellar microadenoma T2 coronal (**a**), T1 coronal (**b**), with lack of enhancement in T1 coronal contrast (**c**), and T1 axial contrast (**d**)

74.3 Radiological Features of Pituitary Tumors

- Thinning of sellar floor
- Less calcifications than in craniopharyngiomas

CT contrast-enhanced
- Moderate, inhomogeneous enhancement

MRI-T2 (Fig. 74.2b)
- Isointense, hyperintense cyst, hypointense if hemorrhage

MRI-FLAIR (Fig. 74.2c)
- Hyperintense to cortex

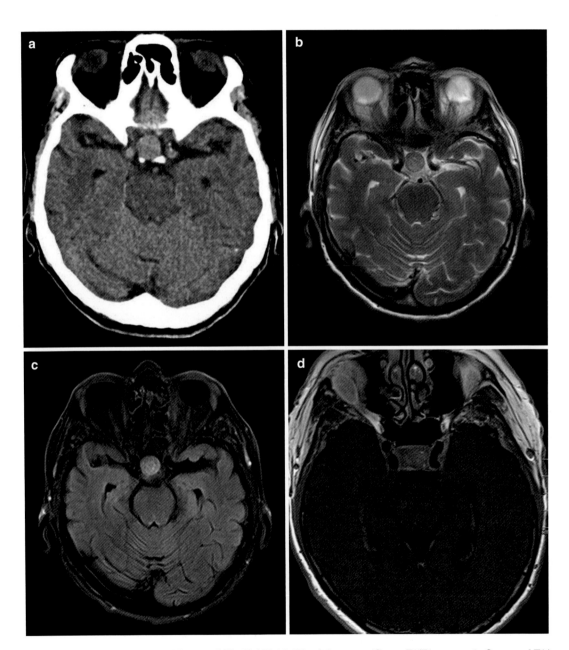

Fig. 74.2 Macroadema: CT (**a**), T2 coronal (**b**), FLAIR (**c**), T1 axial contrast (**d**), sag T1/T1 contrast (**e, f**), coronal T1/T1 contrast (**g, h**)

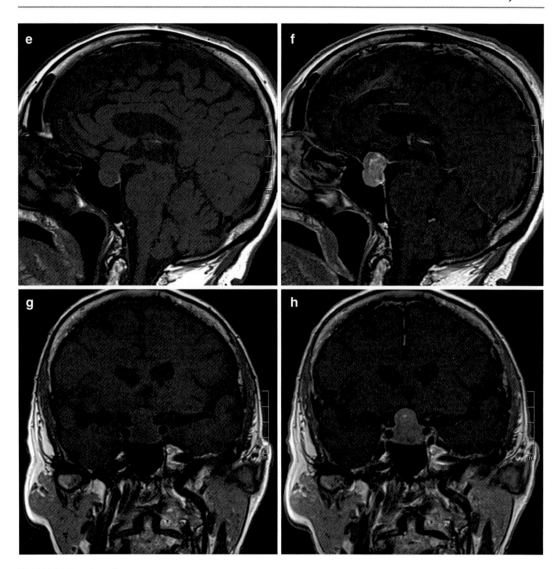

Fig. 74.2 (continued)

MRI-T1 (Fig. 74.2e, g)
- Isointense
- Hyperintense if hemorrhage

MRI-T1 Contrast-Enhanced (Fig. 74.2d, f, h)
- Strong, heterogeneous enhancement
- "Dural tail" possible

MRI-T2∗/SWI
- Hypointense if hemorrhage

Nuclear Medicine Imaging Findings (Fig. 74.3)
- D2-receptor PET can be used to assess the D2-receptor status of pituitary adenomas due to possible therapeutic options.
- Somatostatin receptor PET can be used to assess the SSR-status of adenomas.
- FET-PET can be used to assess the activity and extent of pituitary carcinomas.

74.3 Radiological Features of Pituitary Tumors

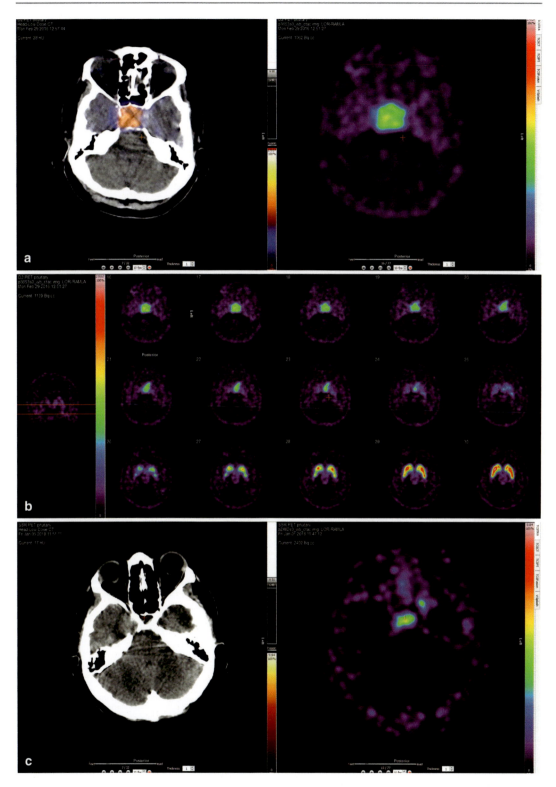

Fig. 74.3 Pituitary macroadenoma with positive D2 receptor imaging (**a**), D2 pituitary slices of the same patient and imaging of the striatum (positive control for D2 receptors) (**b**), pituitary microadenoma with somatostatin receptor (SSR) imaging (**c**)

74.4 Neuropathology Classification of Pituitary Tumors

74.4.1 Historical Histological Classification of Pituitary Tumors

Before the application of immunohistochemical methods, the classification of pituitary tumors was based on tinctorial properties of tumor cells as follows:

- Acidophilic adenoma
  - Associated with acromegaly or gigantism
- Basophilic
  - Associated with Cushing disease
- Chromophobic
  - Associated with non-functioning adenomas

CAVE:

- Chromophobic adenomas were associated with hormone excess.
- Some acidophilic and basophilic adenomas were hormonally inactive.

74.4.2 Immunohistochemical Classification of Pituitary Tumors

Panels of antibodies used in the diagnosis of pituitary lesions are given in Tables 74.4 and 74.5.

74.5 Molecular Neuropathology

Pathogenetic mechanisms include:

- Oncogenes (Lloyd et al. 2004)
- *GSP*
- *CREB*
- *Ras*
- *PTTG*
- *Cyclin D1*
- *ptd-FGFR4*

Table 74.4 Panels of antibodies used in the diagnosis of pituitary lesions

Classification	
Classification	• ACTH • GH • PRL • TSH • FSH • LH • alpha subunit
Proliferation	• p53 • KI-67
Transcription factors	• Pit-1 • ER-alpha • TPIT • SF1 • GATA2 • NeuroD1
Predictive markers	• SSTR2 • SSTR5 • MGMT • MSH6

Table 74.5 Adenohypophyseal cell lineage basis for the 2017 classification of pituitary adenomas (Lopes 2017)

Lineage	Main transcription factors and other co-factors	Adenohypophyseal cell
Acidophilic lineage	PIT-1	Somatotrophs
	PIT-1, ERα	Lactotrophs
	PIT-1, GATA-2	Thyrotrophs
Corticotroph lineage	T-PIT	Corticotrophs
Gonadotroph lineage	SF-1; GATA-2, ERα	Gonadotrophs

PIT-1 pituitary-specific POU-class homeodomain transcription factor 1, *ERα* estrogen receptor α, *GATA-2* member of the GATA family of zinc finger transcriptional regulatory proteins, *T-PIT* T-box family member TBX19, *SF-1* steroidogenic factor 1

- Tumor suppressor genes (Table 74.6)
  - *MEN1*
  - *RB1*
  - *TP53*
  - *ZAC*
  - *GADD45*
  - *p16/CDKN2A*
  - *p27/KIP1*
- Activating and inactivating factors (Table 74.7)
- Genetic predisposition (Table 74.8)
- Biological systems/pathways (Table 74.9)

Table 74.6 Tumor suppressor genes involved in the pathogenesis of pituitary tumors, modified from Zhou et al. (2014) data reproduced with kind permission by Elsevier

Gene	Description	Function	Changed in percent of cases
AIP	Aryl hydrocarbon receptor-interacting protein	• Predisposition gene for FIPA • Inactivated by genetic mutations	3.8
BMP-4	Bone morphogenetic protein 4	• Cytokine of the TGFb superfamily • Downregulated	45
CDKN2A	Cyclin-dependent kinase inhibitor 2A p16Ink4a	• Inhibits CDK4/6 • Activates RB • Silenced by promoter methylation	56
CDKN2A	Alternative open reading frame of CDKN2A transcripts, p14Arf	• Inhibits MDM2 • Activates p53 • Silenced by promoter	12
CDKN2B	Cyclin-dependent kinase inhibitor 2B, p15Ink4b	• Inhibits CDK4/6 • Activates RB • Silenced by promoter methylation	38
CDKN2C	Cyclin-dependent kinase inhibitor 2C, p18Ink4c	• Inhibits CDK4/6 • Activates RB • Silenced by promoter methylation	20
CDKN1A	Cyclin-dependent kinase inhibitor 1A, p21Cip1	• A p53 target gene • Inhibits CDK2, CDK4 • Activates RB • Component of the RB pathway • Downregulated	
CDKN1B	Cyclin-dependent kinase inhibitor 1B, p27Kip1	• A predisposition gene for MEN4 • Inhibits CDK2, CDK4 • Activates RB • Downregulated	45
CDH1	E-cadherin	• Classical epithelial cadherin • Cell adhesion protein • Inhibitor of epithelial–mesenchymal transition • Silenced by promoter methylation	36
CDH13	H-cadherin	• A nonclassical cadherin • Silenced by promoter methylation	30
GADD45B	Growth arrest and DNA-damage-inducible protein GADD45b	• Inhibits CDK1/cyclin B1 • Interacts with PCNA • Downregulated	
GADD45G	Growth arrest and DNA-damage-inducible protein GADD45c	• Inhibits CDK1/cyclin B1 • Interacts with p21Cip1 and PCNA • Silenced by promoter methylation	58
MEG3	Maternally expressed gene 3	• A long non-coding RNA • A p53 activator • Silenced in 96% of NFAs • Downregulated in 30% of functioning adenomas	96
MEN1	menin	• Predisposition gene for multiple endocrine neoplasia type I syndrome • Encodes menin • Inactivated in 3% of sporadic pituitary tumors by genetic mutations	3
MGMT	O-6-methylguanine–DNA methyltransferase	• Involved in DNA repair • Silenced by promoter methylation	18

(continued)

Table 74.6 (continued)

Gene	Description	Function	Changed in percent of cases
PLAGL1	Pleomorphic adenoma gene-like 1	• Also known as ZAC (zinc finger protein) • Regulates apoptosis and cell cycle arrest • Downregulated	64
RASSF1	Ras association (RalGDS/AF-6) domain family member 1	• A p53 activator • Silenced by promoter methylation	38
RASSF3	Ras association (RalGDS/AF-6) domain family member 3, also known as RASSF5	• A p53 activator • Silenced by promoter methylation in all pituitary tumors	100
RB1	Retinoblastoma 1	• The core member of the RB pathway • A negative cell cycle regulator • Silenced by promoter methylation	27
SOCS1	Suppressor of cytokine signaling 1	• Inhibitor of JAK/STAT pathways • A p53 activator • Silenced by promoter methylation	51

Table 74.7 Activating and inactivating factors in the pathogenesis of pituitary adenomas, modified from Donangelo and Melmed (2012) data reproduced with kind permission by Elsevier

	Tumor type	Mechanism
Activating		
Gsp (mutation in guanine nucleotide-activating α-subunit (*GNAS*))	GH adenoma	Activating mutation
CREB (cAMP response element (CRE) binding protein)	GH adenoma	Increased Ser-phosphorylated CREB promoted by gsp overexpression
Cyclin B2 (CCNB2)	All tumor types	Overexpression
Cyclin D1 (CCND1)	Non-functioning adenoma	Overexpression
EGF/EGFR	Non-functioning adenoma	Overexpression
PTTG (pituitary tumor-transforming gene)	All tumor types	Overexpression
HMGA2 (high motility group agene)	Non-functioning ACTH adenoma Prolactinoma	Overexpression
FGF-4 (fibroblast growth factor)	Prolactinoma	Overexpression
Inactivating		
AIP (aryl hydrocarbon receptor-interacting protein gene)	20% of FIPA 2% sporadic adenomas	Inactivation mutation
BMP-4 bone morphogenetic protein 4	Downregulated in 45% of pituitary tumors	Cytokine of the TGFb superfamily
CDKN2A Cyclin-dependent kinase inhibitor 2A	In 56% of pituitary tumors	p16Ink4a, inhibits CDK4/6 and activates RB, silenced by promoter methylation
CDKN2A alternative open reading frame of CDKN2A transcripts, p14Arf	In 12% of pituitary tumors	Inhibits MDM2 and activates p53, silenced by promoter methylation
CDKN2B Cyclin-dependent kinase inhibitor 2B, p15Ink4b	In 38% of pituitary tumors	Inhibits CDK4/6 and activates RB, silenced by promoter methylation
CDKN2C Cyclin-dependent kinase inhibitor 2C, p18Ink4c	In 20% of pituitary tumors	Inhibits CDK4/6 and activates RB, silenced by promoter methylation

74.5 Molecular Neuropathology

Table 74.7 (continued)

	Tumor type	Mechanism
CDKN1A Cyclin-dependent kinase inhibitor 1A, p21Cip1	Downregulated in 47% of pituitary tumors	A p53 target gene, inhibits CDK2, CDK4, and activates RB, component of the RB pathway
CDKN1B Cyclin-dependent kinase inhibitor 1B, p27Kip1	Downregulated in 45% of sporadic pituitary adenomas	A predisposition gene for MEN4, inhibits CDK2, CDK4, and activates RB
CDH1 E-cadherin, classical epithelial cadherin	In 36% of pituitary tumors	Cell adhesion protein, inhibitor of epithelial–mesenchymal transition, silenced by promoter methylation
CDH13 H-cadherin, a non-classical cadherin	In 30% of tumors	Silenced by promoter methylation
GADD45B growth arrest and DNA-damage-inducible protein GADD45b	Downregulated in pituitary tumors	Inhibits CDK1/cyclin B1 and interacts with PCNA
GADD45G growth arrest and DNA-damage-inducible protein GADD45c	In 58% of tumors	Inhibits CDK1/cyclin B1, interacts with p21Cip1 and PCNA, silenced by promoter methylation
Gadd45-γ (growth arrest and DNA-damage-inducible gene 45-γ	Non-functioning GH adenomas Prolactinomas	Promoter methylation
MEG3a (maternally expressed 3 gene)	Silenced in 96% non-functioning GH adenomas	a long non-coding RNA, a p53 activator promoter methylation
MEG3 maternally expressed gene 3	Downregulated in 30% of functioning adenomas	
MEN1 (multiple endocrine neoplasia 1)	Inactivated in 3% of sporadic pituitary tumors by genetic mutations Prolactinoma in familial MEN1	Inactivation mutation encodes menin
MGMT O-6-methylguanine–DNA methyltransferase	In 18% of tumors	Involved in DNA repair, silenced by promoter methylation
PLAGL1 Pleomorphic adenoma gene-like 1, also known as ZAC	Downregulated in 64% of pituitary tumors	Zinc finger protein which regulates apoptosis and cell cycle arrest
RASSF1 Ras association (RalGDS/AF-6) domain family member 1	In 38% of pituitary tumors	A p53 activator, silenced by promoter methylation
RASSF3 Ras association (RalGDS/AF-6) domain family member 3, also known as RASSF5	In all pituitary tumors	A p53 activator, silenced by promoter methylation
RB1 (retinoblastoma susceptibility gene)	Negative pRB in 25% GH adenomas	A negative cell cycle regulator, silenced by promoter methylation
P16NK4a (CDKN2A)	All tumor types	Promoter methylation
P27KIP1 (CDKN1B)	All tumor types	Reduced expression
SOCS1 suppressor of cytokine signaling 1	In 51% of pituitary tumors	Inhibitor of JAK/STAT pathways, a p53 activator, silenced by promoter methylation
13q14	Aggressive tumors	13q14 loss of heterozygosity

Table 74.8 Genetic predisposition to pituitary adenomas

Disease	Associated genes
Multiple endocrine neoplasia type 1	*MEN1*
Multiple endocrine neoplasia type 4	*CDKN1B*
SDH-related familial paraganglioma and pheochromocytoma Syndromes	*SDHA* *SDHB* *SDHC* *SDHD* *SDHAF2*
Carney complex	*PRKAR1A* *PRKACA*
McCure-Albright syndrome	Mosaic *GNAS*
Neurofibromatosis	*NF1*
DICER1 syndrome	*DICER1*
Familial isolated pituitary adenoma (somatotroph)	*AIP*
X-linked acrogigantism	*GRP101*

Table 74.9 Biological systems that operate in pituitary adenomas, modified after Zhan et al. (2016) data reproduced with kind permission by Frontiers journals, open access

Systems	Differentially expressed proteins	Differentially expressed genes
Hormones		
GH	Somatotropin	GHRH receptor
TSH		TSH β
PRL	Prolactin	PRL
LH		LH β
FSH		FSH β
Signal transduction		
G-proteins	G0 subunits 1, 2a	• G-protein • G-binding protein • Regulator of G-protein signaling 16 • Regulator of G-protein bind signaling 2, 5 • Rho-GTPase-activating protein 5
Cytokine receptors		
IGF	IGF binding	• IGF • IGF binding • IGF binding 5 • IGF binding 3 • Protease Ser 11 IGF binding
IL	Splice isoform IL-15	
EGF		• EGF-containing fibulin • ECM protein 1
TGF		• TGFα receptor III
IFN		• Interferon-induced protein 56

74.5 Molecular Neuropathology

Table 74.9 (continued)

Systems	Differentially expressed proteins	Differentially expressed genes
Signal-system enzymes		
		• MAPK 4 • Phospholipase A2-IB • Protein kinase cAMP-dependent β
Retinoic acid		• Cellular retinoic acid-binding protein 2
Phosphorylation	Ser/Thr protein phosphatase 2A	
Others	Rab GDP dissociation inhibitor α	• SH3-domain GRB2-like 2 • XIST nuclear receptor 1, 3
Reactive oxygen species		
Cytochrome P450		Cytochrome P450, III A
HSP	HSP27	HSP 105 kDa
GST	GSTμ-2	
Peroxidase	Phospholipidhydroperoxide glutathione peroxidase	
DNA/mRNA methylation		
	6 N-adenosine methyltransferase	• RNA-binding protein 2 • Eukaryotic translation initiation factor 3–5 • U4/U6-associated RNA splicing factor
Tumor genes		
Proto-oncogenes	• Proto-oncogene Tyr protein kinase FYN • L-myc-1 proto-oncogene protein	
Oncogenes		Neuroblastoma overexpressed gene
Tumor suppressor genes	Tumor rejection antigen (endoplasmin)	
Excitatory (tachykinins)		
	Secretagogin	• Reticulocalbin 1, EF-hand calcium-binding domain • Peptidylglycine α-amidating monooxygenase
Energy		
	• ATP synthase, mitochondrial • ATP-binding protein	• ATPase
Immune system		
	Ig κ, λ	• IgG • Pre-B cell leukemia transcription factor 3 • CD58 • MHC class 1
Intermediate filaments		
	Vimentin	• Vimentin
Transcription factors		
		Pit 1 Basic transcription factor 3
Cell cycle (G1-S-G2-M)		
		• Death-associated protein • Folate receptor C1

Table 74.10 Genes that altered consistently in the levels of protein and mRNA with comparison of proteomics data and transcriptomic data, modified after Zhan et al. (2016) data reproduced with kind permission by Frontiers journals, open access

Protein name	NF	PRL	Gene name	NF	PRL
Secretagogin (SCGN)	−	− (weak)	*SCGN*: secretagogin	−	
Guanine nucleotide-binding protein G(I)/G(S)/G(T) β-subunit 3	+		Guanine nucleotide-binding protein (G-protein), β polypeptide	+	
Tissue transglutaminase (TGM2)	−	−	*TGM2*: transglutaminase 2	−	−
Isocitrate dehydrogenase (NADP) cytoplasmic (IDH1)	+	+ (weak)	*IDH1*: isocitrate dehydrogenase (NADP+), soluble	+	
Calreticulin precursor	+		*KDEL*: endoplasmic reticulum (ER) protein	+	
Somatotropin (GH1)	−	−	*GH1*: growth hormone 1	−	−
			GH2: growth hormone 2	−	−
			GHRHR: growth hormone-releasing hormone receptor	−	−
Prolactin (PRL)	−	±	Prolactin	−	±
Cellular retinoic acid-binding protein II	+		Cellular retinoic acid-binding protein 2	+	
Hemoglobin β chain (HBB)	−	−	*HBB*: hemoglobin β	−	−
			HBD: hemoglobin δ	−	

- Genes with altered levels of protein and mRNA (Table 74.10)

microRNAs
- In GH and prolactin cell adenomas and in ACTH cell adenomas
  - Underexpression of six miRNAs (*miR-542–3p, miR-629, miR-450b-5p, miR-424, miR-503,* and *miR-214*).
  - *miR-629* and *miR-214* target the antiapoptotic protein bcl2, and therefore may stimulate growth.
- miRNAs targeting HMGA proteins are downregulated.
  - inhibited proliferation of pituitary cell line GH3
  - direct targeting of HMGA A1 by miR-16
  - downregulation regardless of histologic subtype
- Sporadic NFPS
  - 162 miRNAs underexpressed or overexpressed.
  - Overexpressed miRNAs specific for the Wee1 transcript.
    ○ Wee1 kinase is an inhibitor of CDK1 and therefore a regulator of the checkpoint at G2/M.
  - Downregulation of miR-134, miR-323, miR-370, miR-410 and miR-432.

Others
- Dysregulation of the feedback loops in GH and adrenocorticotrophic hormone (ACTH) cell adenomas.
  - promote cell proliferation, hypothalamic hormone stimulation, or loss of autofeedback mechanisms
- Genetic alterations in pituitary stem cells may result in adenoma development,

74.6 Treatment

- Surgery
  - Transsphenoidal approach
  - Indications for surgery
    ○ Tumors with mass effect on neighboring structures, i.e., visual loss due to compression of the optic nerve
    ○ Hyperfunctioning tumors in Cushing disease, acromegaly, or hyperthyroidism
    ○ Failure of prior medical treatment

- Massive acute hemorrhagic necrosis of an adenoma (pituitary apoplexy)
- Medication
  - Prolactinomas:
    - Dopamine agonists reduce tumor size and hyperprolactinemia.
  - GH adenomas:
    - long acting somatostatin decrease pituitary GH secretion and inhibit GH-induced IGF-1 generation
    - GH receptor antagonists
  - TSH adenomas:
    - somatostatin analogs
- Radiotherapy
  - In case of incomplete tumor resection or tumor recurrence
  - CAVE: side effects include hypopituitarism, radiation-induced glioma or sarcoma
- Stereotactic radiosurgery (Gamma knife, LINAC)

74.7 Prognostic Clinicopathological Classification of Pituitary Tumors

A recently proposed new prognostic clinicopathological classification of pituitary adenomas is shown in Table 74.11 (Trouillas et al. 2013).

Table 74.11 A new prognostic clinicopathological classification of pituitary adenomas was recently proposed (Trouillas et al. 2013), data reproduced with kind permission by Springer Nature

Tumor diameter	• Micro (<10 mm) • Macro (≥10 mm) • Giant (>40 mm)
Tumor type	• GH • PRL • ACTH • FSH/LH • TSH
Tumor grade	• Grade 1a: noninvasive tumor • Grade 1b: noninvasive and proliferative tumor • Grade 2a: invasive tumor • Grade 2b: invasive and proliferative tumor • Grade 3: metastatic tumor

The two parameters used for grading, i.e., tumor invasion and proliferation are defined as follows:

- Invasion
  - Signs of cavernous or sphenoid sinus invasion (histology or radiology)
- Proliferation
  - Presence of at least two of three criteria
    - Ki-67 LI >1% (Bouin-Hollande fixation) or ≥3% (formalin fixation)
    - Mitoses: >2 per 10 high-power fields
    - P53: >10 strongly positive nuclei per 10 HPF

74.8 Pituitary Adenomas

74.8.1 Somatotroph Adenoma

WHO Definition

2017—Somatotroph adenoma is a pituitary adenoma that expresses mainly growth hormone (GH) and arises from PIT1-lineage cells. These tumors often result in GH excess, leading to gigantism and/or acromegaly. Pure somatotroph adenomas are divided into two clinically relevant histological subtypes: densely granulated somatotroph adenoma (DGSA) and sparsely granulated somatotroph adenoma (SGSA). Other adenomas leading to acromegaly and/or gigantism cosecrete GH and prolactin (PRL); these include mammosomatotroph adenomas, mixed somatotroph and lactotroph adenomas, and plurihormonal adenomas (Mete et al. 2017b).

2004—Pituitary adenomas secreting growth hormone (GH) in excess are clinically associated with either gigantism or acromegaly, depending on patient age at onset of disease. Well-documented non-functioning cases are very rare (Kontogeorgos et al. 2004). Pure GH-producing tumors, solely consisting of somatotrophs are separated into well-defined types: densely granulated and sparsely granulated somatotroph adenomas (Kontogeorgos et al. 2004). Mixed GH-PRL cell adenoma and mammosomatotroph adenomas produce excess GH and prolactin

(PRL); acidophil stem cell adenomas are typically associated with hyperprolactinemia in the absence of stigmata of acromegaly (Kontogeorgos et al. 2004).

74.8.1.1 Clinical Signs and Symptoms
- Prepubertal onset:
  - Gigantism: unrestrained somatic growth
- Postpubertal onset:
  - Acromegaly: enlargement of acral parts of the body

74.8.1.2 Epidemiology
Incidence
- 25–30% of surgically removed pituitary tumors

Age Incidence
- Younger patients (gigantism)
- Patients aged 25–35 years (acromegaly)

Sex Incidence
- Mostly males

Localization
- Within the sella turcica
- Lateral wings

74.8.1.3 Neuropathology Findings
Macroscopic Features (Fig. 74.4a–d)
- White to gray-red.
- Soft.
- Invasion of meninges, cavernous sinus, sella turcica, and sphenoid sinus is possible.
- Seldom: protrusion as polyp in the nasal cavity.

Microscopic Features (Fig. 74.5a–h)
- Densely granulated somatotroph adenomas
  - Medium sized, round, or polyhedral acidophilic cell
  - Granular cytoplasm

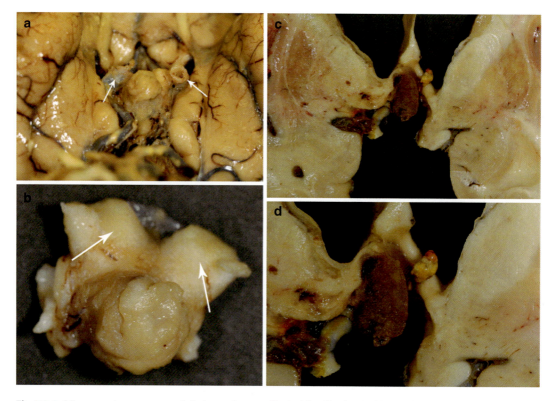

Fig. 74.4 Macroscopic appearance of pituitary adenoma. Typical localization (**a**, **b**) (asterisk), note the close proximity to the internal carotid artery (arrow) (**a**) and the optic chiasm (arrow) (**b**). Hemorrhagic pituitary adenoma (**c**, **d**)

74.8 Pituitary Adenomas

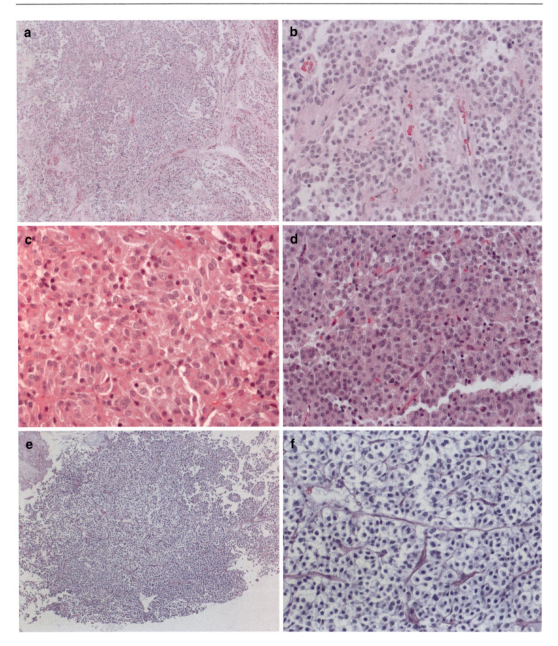

Fig. 74.5 Somatotroph adenoma composed of medium sized, round, or polyhedral acidophilic cell with granular cytoplasm, round nuclei with finely dispersed chromatin. Diffuse pattern of growth (**a–h**) (**a–d, g**: HE; **e, f, h**: PAS). Immunohistochemical detection of growth hormone-producing tumor cells (**i, j**). Moderate proliferation (**k, l**: Ki-67)

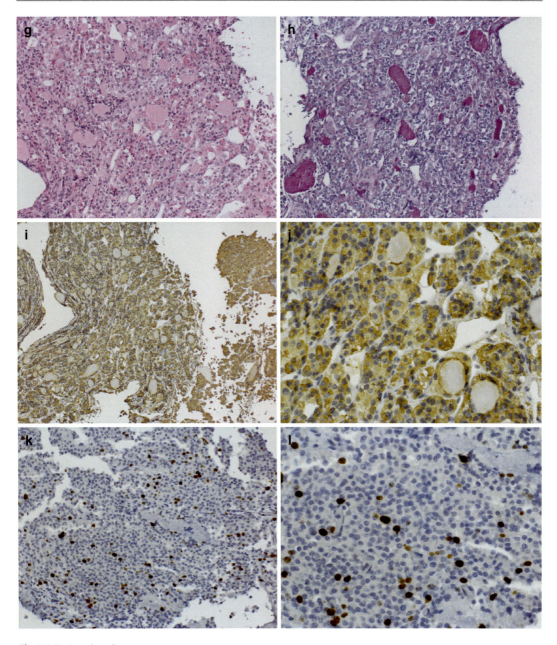

Fig. 74.5 (continued)

- Diffuse pattern of growth
- Round nuclei with finely dispersed chromatin
- Sparsely granulated somatotroph adenomas
  - Cellular, chromophobic tumor
  - Small, round, partly irregular cells
  - Fibrous body: pale, acidophilic, spherical inclusion in the paranuclear cytoplasmic region
- Mixed-somatotroph-lactotroph adenomas
  - Two populations of acidophilic and chromophobic cell populations
- Mammosomatotroph adenomas
  - Polyhedral, strongly acidophilic cells
  - Diffuse growth pattern
- Acidophil stem cell adenomas
  - Chromophobic cells with some degree of acidophilia

- Diffuse growth pattern
- Nuclear pleomorphism
- Plurihormonal GH-producing adenomas
- Effects of somatostatin treatment
  - Increase number and size of secretory granules
  - Increase number and size of lysosomes
  - Increased tumor cell apoptosis
  - Mild to moderate stromal fibrosis and hyalinosis

Immunophenotype (Fig. 74.5i, j)
- Densely granulated somatotroph adenomas
  - Positive for GH
  - α-subunit of glycoprotein hormones (50%)
- Sparsely granulated somatotroph adenomas
  - Fibrous body: positive for low molecular weight cytokeratin (CK8)
- Mixed-somatotroph-lactotroph adenomas
  - Positive for GH and prolactin
- Mammosomatotroph adenomas
  - Positivity for GH and prolactin within one single cell
- Acidophil stem cell adenomas
  - Positivity for PRL
  - Faint staining for GH
- Plurihormonal GH-producing adenomas
  - Positivity for GH
  - Additional positivity for PRL, α-subunit, β-TSH
  - Rare positivity for β-FSH and β-LH

Proliferation Markers (Fig. 74.5k, l)
- low
- KI-67 LI <3%

Ultrastructural Features
- Densely granulated somatotroph adenomas
  - Similar to normal somatotrophs
  - Well-developed Golgi apparatus and RER
  - abundant, round, and regular granules of 300–450 nm size
- Sparsely granulated somatotroph adenomas
  - Cell type not present in normal pituitary
  - Variably developed RER
  - Secretory granules: 100–250 nm in size
  - Fibrous body:
    - Concentric aggregates of intermediate filaments
- Mammosomatotroph adenomas
  - Resemble densely granulated somatotroph cells
  - Secretory granules: abundant and large (1500 nm)
- Acidophil stem cell adenomas
  - Giant mitochondria (hallmark)
  - Accumulation of intermediate filaments (fibrous bodies)
  - Secretory granules: 150–200 nm

74.8.2 Lactotroph Adenoma

WHO Definition
2017—Lactotroph adenoma is a pituitary adenoma that expresses mainly prolactin (PRL) and arises from PIT1-lineage adenohypophyseal cells. These tumors are classified into three distinct histological subtypes: sparsely granulated lactotroph adenoma (SGLA), densely granulated lactotroph adenoma (DGLA), and acidophil stem cells adenoma (ASCA) (Nosé et al. 2017).

2004—A benign pituitary tumor-producing prolactin (PRL), originating from the prolactin adenohypophysial cell (Saeger et al. 2004).

74.8.2.1 Clinical Signs and Symptoms
Hyperprolactinemia

74.8.2.2 Epidemiology
Incidence
- 10–25% of pituitary adenomas

Age Incidence
- Females: 21–40 years

Sex Incidence
- Male:Female ratio: 1:2.6

Localization
- Lateral and posterior part of the pituitary

74.8.2.3 Neuropathology Findings
Macroscopic Features
- Red-tan color
- Soft consistency

Microscopic Features (Fig. 74.6a–d)
- Sparsely granulated lactotroph adenomas
  - Diffuse or papillary growth pattern
  - Relatively large, elongated cells
  - Chromophobic to slightly acidophilic cytoplasm
- Densely granulated lactotroph adenomas
  - Similar to sparsely granulated lactotroph adenomas
  - Stronger cytoplasmic acidophilia

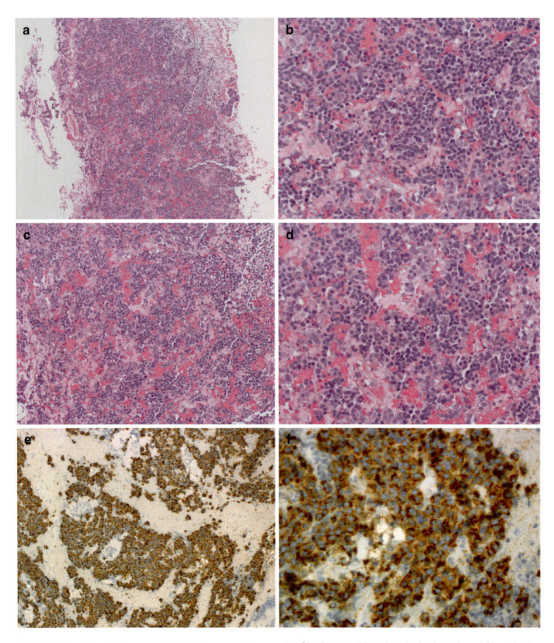

Fig. 74.6 Lactotroph adenoma with a diffuse or papillary growth pattern is made up of relatively large, elongated cells with chromophobic to slightly acidophilic cytoplasm (**a–d**). Immunohistochemical detection of prolactin-producing tumor cells (**e, f**)

74.8 Pituitary Adenomas

- Acidophil stem cell adenomas
  - Chromophobic cells with some degree of acidophilia
  - Diffuse growth pattern
  - Nuclear pleomorphism
  - Considered to be a variant of PRL-producing adenomas or a subtype of GH-producing adenomas
- Effects of dopamine agonists
  - Smaller cells with increased nuclear:cyoplasmic ratio
  - Hyperchromatic nuclei
  - Extensive perivascular and interstitial fibrosis

Immunophenotype (Fig. 74.6e, f)
- Sparsely granulated lactotroph adenomas
  - Paranuclear PRL positivity
- Densely granulated lactotroph adenomas
  - Strong cytoplasmic PRL reactivity

Proliferation Markers
- Low
- Ki-67 LI <3%

Ultrastructural Features
- Sparsely granulated lactotroph adenomas
  - Large euchromatic nuclei, prominent nucleoli
  - Extremely developed RER forming concentric whorls
  - Large Golgi areas
  - Many immature granules
  - Sparse mature granules: 150–300 nm
- Densely granulated lactotroph adenomas
  - Many irregular large secretory granules
  - Well-developed Golgi complexes
- Acidophil stem cell adenomas

74.8.2.4 Prognosis
Biologic Behavior–Prognosis–Prognostic Factors
- Good prognosis
- Recurrence demonstrated by hyperprolactinemia

74.8.3 Thyrotroph Adenoma

WHO Definition
2017—Thyrotroph adenoma expresses mainly TSH and arises from PIT1-lineage adenohypophyseal cells (Osamura et al. 2017b).

2004—A benign pituitary tumor-producing thyrotropin (TSH), originating from the adenohypophysial cells (Osamura et al. 2004).

74.8.3.1 Clinical Signs and Symptoms
- Goiter
- Hyperthyroidism (hypermetabolic state, tachycardia, tremor, proximal myopathy, neuropsychiatric abnormalities)

74.8.3.2 Epidemiology
Incidence
- Rare
- 1% of pituitary adenomas

Age Incidence
- 23–62 years

Sex Incidence
- Male:Female ratio: 1:3

Localization
- In the mucoid wedge

74.8.3.3 Neuropathology Findings
Macroscopic Features
- Firm tumor
- Invasive growth
- fibrotic

Microscopic Features (Fig. 74.7a–f)
- chromophobic cells
- varying degree of nuclear pleomorphism
- solid or sinusoidal growth pattern
- stromal fibrosis
- psammoma bodies
- strong PAS-positive cytoplasmic globules (lysosomes)

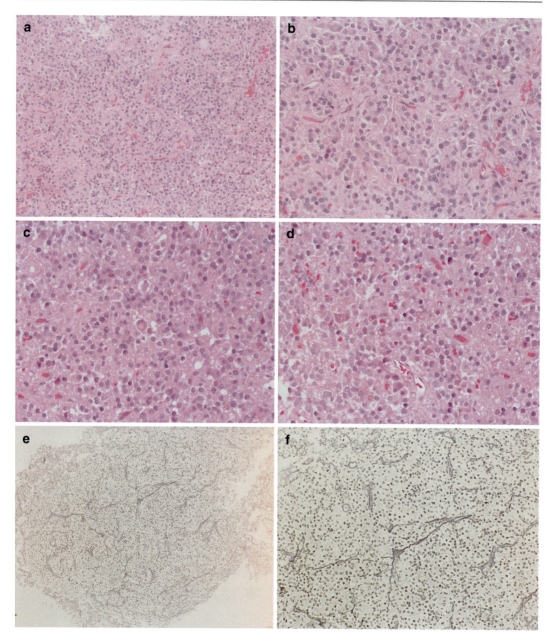

Fig. 74.7 Thyrotroph adenoma with a solid to sinusoidal growth pattern of chromophobic cells with varying degree of nuclear pleomorphism (**a–d**: HE). Reticulin fiber distribution pattern normal (**e**, **f**: Reticulin). Immunohistochemical detection of thyrotroph-producing tumor cells (**g, h**). Moderate proliferation (**i, j**: Ki-67)

74.8 Pituitary Adenomas

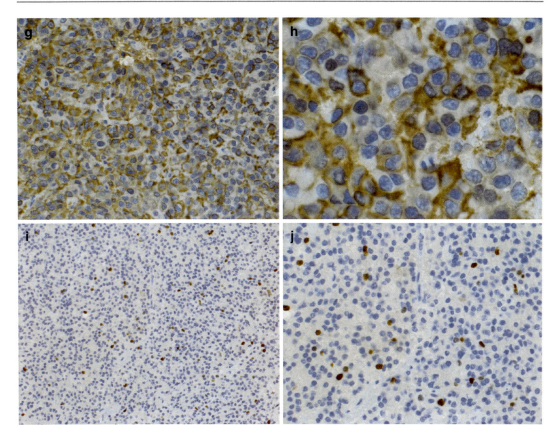

Fig. 74.7 (continued)

Immunophenotype (Fig. 74.7g, h)
- Variable reactivities for TSH and α-subunit

Proliferation Markers (Fig. 74.7i, j)
- Can be high → aggressive behavior

Ultrastructural Features
- resembles normal thyrotrophs
- secretory granules: 150–200 nm

74.8.4 Corticotroph Adenoma

WHO Definition
2017—Corticotroph adenoma is a pituitary adenoma that expresses ACTH and other proopiomelanocortin-derived peptides and arises from TPIT-lineage adenohypophyseal cells. These neoplasms are histologically classified into these subtypes: densely granulated corticotroph adenoma, sparsely granulated corticotroph adenoma, and Crooke cell adenoma (Mete et al. 2017a).

2004—The ACTH-producing adenoma is a benign tumor, derived from corticotrophs of the anterior pituitary, that synthesize proopiomelanocortin (POMC) from which several peptides including ACTH, β-LPH, and β-endorphin are cleaved (Trouillas et al. 2004).

74.8.4.1 Clinical Signs and Symptoms
- Cushing disease
  - Weight gain
  - High blood pressure
  - Poor short-term memory
  - Irritability
  - Excess hair growth (women)
  - Impaired immunological function
  - Red, ruddy face
  - Extra fat around neck

- Moon face
- Fatigue
- Red stretch marks
- Poor concentration
- Irregular menstruation

74.8.4.2 Epidemiology
Incidence
- 10–15% of pituitary adenomas
- 3–10 cases per one million population

Age Incidence
- 30–40 years

Sex Incidence
- Male:Female ratio: 1:8

Localization
- intrasellar

74.8.4.3 Neuropathology Findings
Macroscopic Features
- red color
- soft consistency

Microscopic Features (Fig. 74.8a–d)
- monomorphic round cells
- sinusoidal pattern around capillaries
- basophilic tumor
- strongly PAS-positive
- round central nuclei

Crooke Cell Adenoma
- ACTH-producing tumor cells with prominent cytoplasmic cytokeratin filaments

Immunophenotype (Fig. 74.8e, f)
- Positive for
  - ACTH, β LPH, and/or β-endorphin

Proliferation Markers
- Ki67 LI: <3%

Ultrastructural Features
Two variants are distinguished:
- Cells resemble normal corticotrophs
  - Moderately developed Golgi complex and RER
  - Perinuclear bundles of 7 nm intermediate filaments of cytokeratins
  - Secretory granules: numerous, 200–500 nm in size
- Silent subtype 2
  - Smaller than average size polyhedral cells
  - Secretory granules: sparse, 150–300 nm

74.8.5 Gonadotroph Adenoma

WHO Definition
2017—Gonadotroph adenoma produces FSH-beta, LH-beta, and/or alpha subunit and arises from SF1-lineage adenohypophyseal cells. The most relevant criteria for the diagnosis of gonadotroph adenoma are immunohistochemical findings (Yamada et al. 2017).

2004—Gonadotropin-producing adenoma is a benign pituitary neoplasm composed of adenohypophysial gonadotrophs, cells that produce the gonadotropic hormones follicle-stimulating hormone (FSH) and/or luteinizing hormone (LH), or that show evidence of differentiation along the pathway of gonadotroph differentiation (Asa et al. 2004).

74.8.5.1 Clinical Signs and Symptoms
- Hormonally inactive
- Visual disturbances
- Hypopituitarism
- Headaches

74.8.5.2 Epidemiology
Incidence
- unknown

Age Incidence
- adults

74.8 Pituitary Adenomas

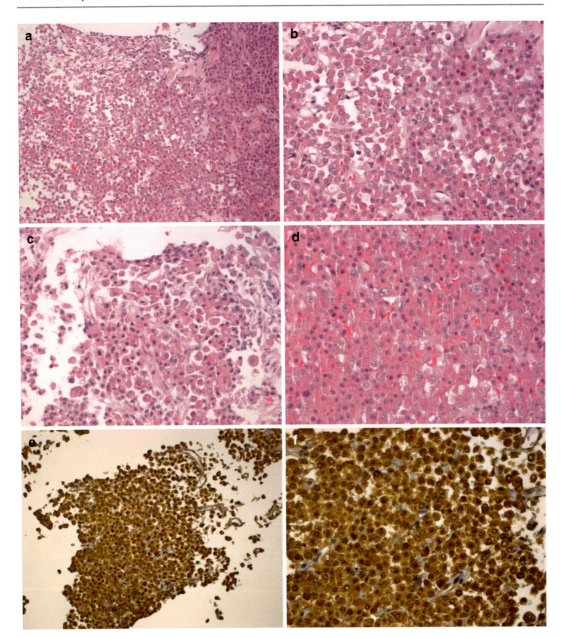

Fig. 74.8 Corticotroph adenoma composed of monomorphic round cells with round central nuclei arranged in a sinusoidal pattern around capillaries (**a–d**). Immunohistochemical detection of ACTH-producing tumor cells (**e, f**)

Sex Incidence
- Male predominance
- Rare in females

Localization
- Macroadenoma
- Suprasellar extension
- Parasellar invasion
- Cavernous sinus invasion

74.8.5.3 Neuropathology Findings
Macroscopic Features
- Macroadenoma
- Tan to brown color
- Soft
- Hemorrhage or necroses
- Multilobulated

Microscopic Features (Fig. 74.9a–d)
- Histologic pattern
  - Uniform, tall, polar cells forming sinusoidal pattern with pseudorosettes around vessels
  - Papillary growth pattern
  - Diffuse growth pattern
- Chromophobe tumor
- Middle sized to large non-polar cells with uniform spherical nuclei and low density cytoplasm
- No PAS-reactivity

Immunophenotype (Fig. 74.9e, f)
- Immunopositivity for FSH and LH
- FSH immunoreactivity stronger and more widely distributed than LH

Proliferation Markers
- Ki-67 LI: <3%

Ultrastructural Features
- No similarity to normal gonadotroph cells
- Uniform, markedly polar cell with
  - Long, attenuated interwoven processes
  - Uniform and largely euchromatic nuclei
  - Cytoplasm with well-developed RER
  - Secretory granules: 50–150 nm
- Vacuolar transformation of the Golgi apparatus in women

74.8.5.4 Prognosis
Biologic Behavior–Prognosis–Prognostic Factors
- Dependent on the success of surgical removal

74.8.6 Null Cell Adenoma

WHO Definition
2017—Null cell adenoma is an adenoma composed of adenohypophyseal cells that show no evidence of cell-type-specific differentiation by immunohistochemistry for pituitary hormones and transcription factors (Nishioka et al. 2017).

2004—Null cell adenoma have no hormone immunoreactivity, and no other immunohistochemical or ultrastructural markers of specific adenohypophysial cell differentiation. There is controversy about the classification of tumors with only few scattered hormone immunoreactive cells (Sano et al. 2004).

74.8.6.1 Clinical Signs and Symptoms
- No clinical features of a syndrome of anterior pituitary hormone hypersecretion.
- Mild hyperprolactinemia due to stalk section effect.
- Mass effects are possible.

74.8.6.2 Epidemiology
Incidence
- 33% of pituitary adenomas
- 60–80% of all operated pituitary macroadenomas

Age Incidence
- Elderly patients
- Mean age sixth decade
- Very rare in patients under 40 years of age

Sex Incidence
- Slight male preponderance

Localization
- adenohypophysis

74.8 Pituitary Adenomas

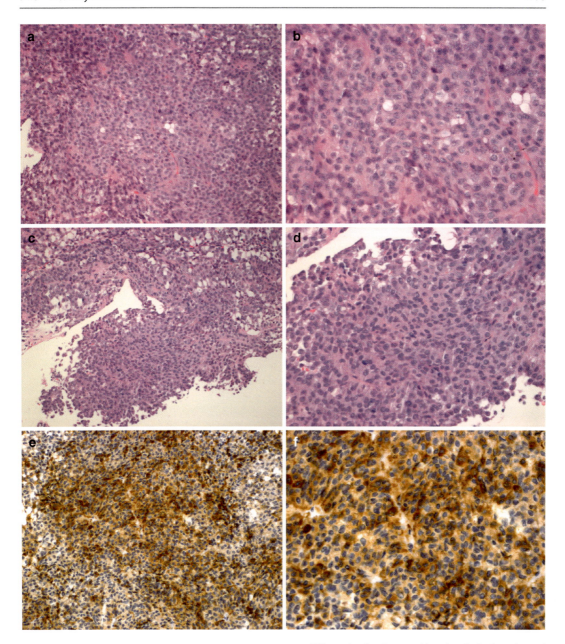

Fig. 74.9 Gonadotroph adenoma made up of uniform, tall, polar cells which form sinusoidal pattern with pseudorosettes around vessels. The growth pattern is papillary to diffuse (**a–d**). Immunohistochemical detection of luteinizing hormone-producing tumor cells (**e, f**)

74.8.6.3 Neuropathology Findings
Macroscopic Features
- yellow-tan
- soft

Microscopic Features (Fig. 74.10a–j)
- chromophobic tumor
- varying degrees of acidophilia
- round to polyhedral cells
- diffuse or papillary growth pattern
- pseudorosette formation
- no PAS-reactivity

Immunophenotype
- negative for pituitary hormones
- a few scattered cells positive for β-FSH and α-subunit of glycoprotein hormones

Proliferation Markers
- Ki-67 LI: <2%

Ultrastructural Features
- small, polyhedral cells
- cytoplasm with inconspicuous scattered rough endoplasmatic reticulum
- numerous microtubules
- secretory granules: 100–250 nm

Differential Diagnosis
- Gonadotroph adenoma
Oncocytoma

74.8.6.4 Prognosis
Biologic Behavior–Prognosis–Prognostic Factors
- Slowly growing tumor

74.8.7 Plurihormonal and Double Adenoma

WHO Definition
2017—Plurihormonal adenomas are adenohypophyseal tumors that produce more than one hormone. They can be monomorphous, consisting of a single cell type producing two (or rarely more) hormones, or plurimorphous, consisting of two or more different cell lineages. Plurihormonal adenomas include plurihormonal PIT1-positive adenoma (previously called silent subtype 3 adenoma), clinically functioning adenomas such as growth hormone (GH)/prolactin (PRL)/TSH-producing adenomas with acromegaly and thyroid dysfunction, and adenomas with unusual immunohistochemical combinations that cannot be explained by cytodifferentiation. Adenomas that produce combinations of GH and PRL, or FSH and LH, are not considered plurihormonal in this sense. Double adenomas are composed of two separate tumors with two different cell types in the same gland. More than two tumors can also coexist (multiple adenomas) (Kontogeorgos et al. 2017).

2004—Plurihormonal adenomas are usual tumors that have immunoreactivities for more than one pituitary hormone which are not explained by normal cytophysiology or developmental mechanisms. They do not include the combinations of GH, PRL, and TSH, or of FSH and LH (Horvath et al. 2004).

74.8.7.1 Clinical Signs and Symptoms
Depends on hormones produced by adenoma

74.8.7.2 Epidemiology
Incidence
- rare
- 0.9% of all adenomas

Age Incidence
- middle ages
- female patients: 20–35 years

Sex Incidence
- Male:Female ratio: 1:1

Localization
- pituitary

74.8 Pituitary Adenomas

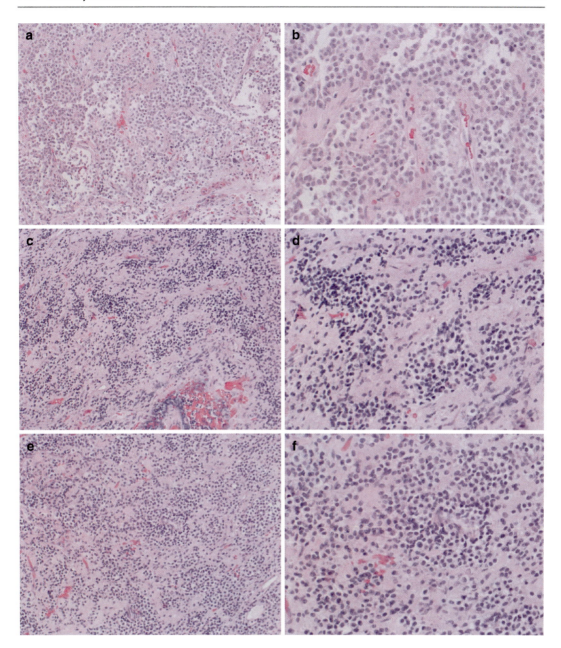

Fig. 74.10 Null cell adenoma composed of chromophobic round to polyhedral tumor cells with varying degrees of acidophilia. Diffuse or papillary growth pattern (**a–f**). Chromophobic cytoplasm is more obvious on PAS-stained section (**g**, **h**). Lobular structure as revealed by reticulin stain (**i**, **j**)

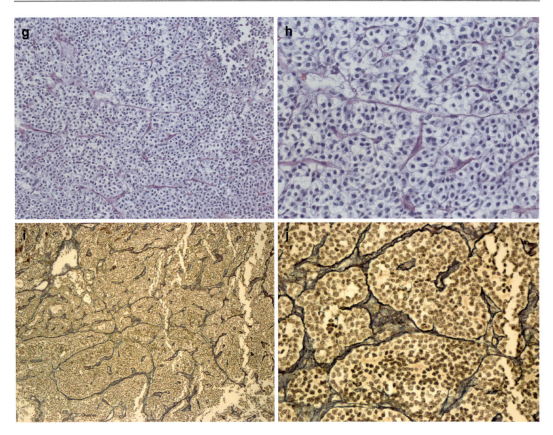

Fig. 74.10 (continued)

74.8.7.3 Neuropathology Findings
Macroscopic Features
- macroadenoma
- yellow-tan
- soft to firm

Microscopic Features
- chromophobic tumor
- slightly acidophilic
- no PAS-positivity
- spindle-shaped cells
- fibrous stroma

Immunophenotype
- Immunoreactivities of unrelated hormones.
- CAVE: few scattered positive cells are insufficient evidence for true plurihormonality.
- Common patterns:
  - TSH + FSH + GH
  - PRL + TSH

Ultrastructural Features
- ultrastructure of well differentiated glycoprotein hormone-producing adenomas
- large polar cells with
  - euchromatic nucleus
  - prominent nucleolus
  - fragments of nuclear inclusions (spheridia)
- sparse secretory granules: 100–200 nm

74.8.7.4 Prognosis
Biologic Behavior–Prognosis–Prognostic Factors
- Aggressive behavior of lesion

74.9 Atypical Pituitary Adenoma

Atypical adenomas are characterized by (Asa 2011) (Fig. 74.11a–f):

74.9 Atypical Pituitary Adenoma

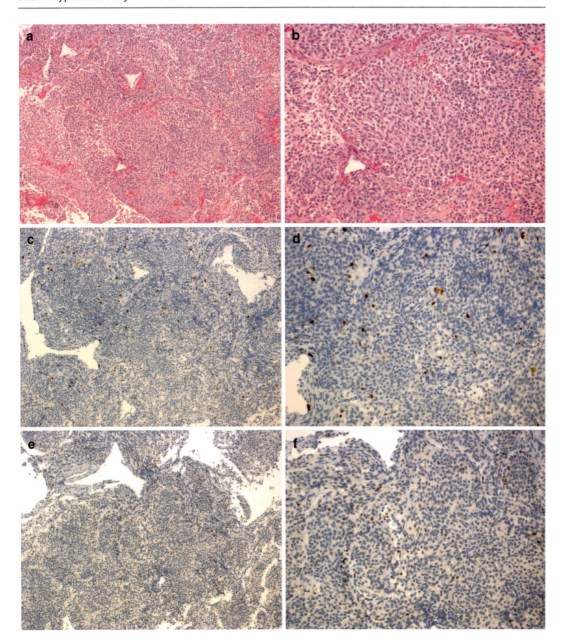

Fig. 74.11 Atypical adenoma with invasive growth (**a**, **b**), high mitotic index, MIB-1 labeling >3% (**c**, **d**), and extensive nuclear reactivity for p53 (**e**, **f**)

- invasive growth
- high mitotic index
- MIB-1 labeling >3%
- extensive nuclear reactivity for p53

Introduced for the first time in the WHO Classification in 2004:

- Its distinction from pituitary adenoma is still not entirely clear.
- Is associated with higher potential for recurrence.
- is associated with possible transformation into pituitary carcinoma.
- Close monitoring of the patient is advisable.

Not anymore recommended in the 2017 WHO Classification

74.10 Pituitary Carcinoma

WHO Definition
2017: Pituitary carcinoma is strictly defined as a tumor of adenohypophyseal cells that metastasizes craniospinally or is associated with systemic metastasis. The definition is independent of the histological appearance (Roncaroli et al. 2017).

2004: The term pituitary carcinoma is restricted to a tumor of adenohypophysial cells that exhibit cerebrospinal and/or systemic metastasis (Scheithauer et al. 2004).

74.10.1 Clinical Signs and Symptoms

- Might be hormone active and endocrinologically functional (75%)
- Most commonly produce: ACTH and PRL
- Silent ACTH-producing, gonadotropin-producing carcinomas

74.10.2 Epidemiology

Incidence
- Very rare
- 0.2 % of all operated pituitary tumors

Age Incidence
- Adults at any age

Sex Incidence
- Male:Female ratio: 1:1

Localization
- Anterior lobe

74.10.3 Neuroimaging Findings

General Neuroimaging Findings (Fig. 74.12)
- Rare, not to distinguish from invasive macroadenoma.
- Intraspinal metastasis are described.

74.10.4 Neuropathology Findings

Macroscopic Features
- Discontinuous spread with single or multiple nodular subarachnoidal deposits
- Invasive of underlying brain or overlying dura mater
- Indistinguishable from metastases of carcinomas from other organs

Microscopic Features
- Cell pleomorphism
- Nuclear abnormalities
- Mitotic activity
- Necroses
- Invasion

Immunophenotype
- Positive for hormones
  - PRL, ACTH
- Positive for neuroendocrine markers
  - Synaptophysin, chromogranin

Proliferation Markers
- KI-67 LI: 66.7% in carcinomas

Ultrastructural Features
- Ultrastructural findings consistent with immunophenotype

Differential Diagnosis
- Invasive adenomas
- Metastases from carcinomas from other organs

74.10 Pituitary Carcinoma

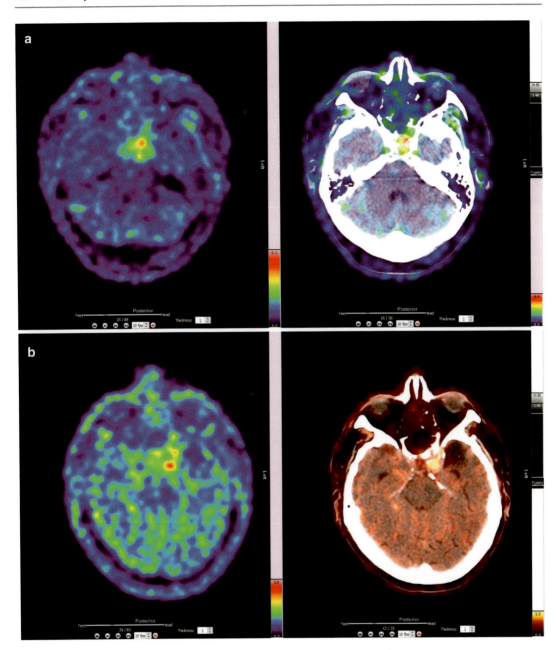

Fig. 74.12 FET accumulation in a pituitary carcinoma (**a**), FET-PET of the pituitary performed in the same patient 2 years later shows a central necrosis and infiltrative tumor growth (**b**), D2 PET showing in the same patient a D2 receptor-positive metastasis in close proximity to the cerebellum (right panel shows an MIP image including the striatum) (**c**), and D2 PET of the same patient with D2-positive receptors of the pituitary carcinoma

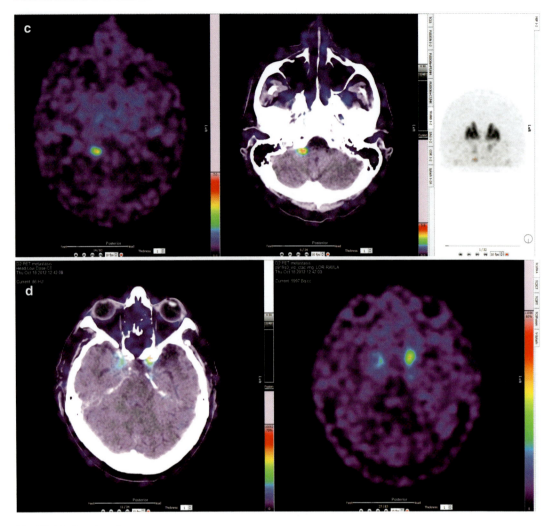

Fig. 74.12 (continued)

74.10.5 Molecular Neuropathology

Originate from
- previously normal adenohypophysial cells
- adenomas

74.10.6 Prognosis

Biologic Behavior–Prognosis–Prognostic Factors
- Poor prognosis

74.11 Pituitary Blastoma

WHO Definition

2017—Pituitary blastoma (PitB) is a rare developmental early childhood neoplasm, arising within the fetal anterior pituitary. It consists of cells resembling primordial Rathke epithelium, small folliculostellate cells, and a limited range of partially differentiated secretory adenohypophyseal cells. Pituitary blastoma is usually associated with Cushing disease (Rotondo et al. 2017).

74.11 Pituitary Blastoma

74.11.1 Clinical Signs and Symptoms

- Features of Cushing disease
  - elevated blood ACTH levels
  - hypercortisolism
- Ophthalmoplegia

74.11.2 Epidemiology

Incidence
- Very rare

Age Incidence
- neonatal period
- early childhood

Sex Incidence
- Male:Female ratio: 1:1

Localization
- sellar region
- parasellar region
- suprasellar region

74.11.3 Neuropathology Findings

Macroscopic Features
- lobulated
- partly cystic

Microscopic Features
- Composed of three cell types:
  - small, chromophobic, and undifferentiated blastemal-like cells
  - larger, patternless secretory cells with
    - round to oval nuclei
    - inconspicuous nucleoli
    - abundant cytoplasm
  - cuboidal or columnar cells making up glandular-like structures
- Large, polygonal amphophilic cells are PAS-positive.

Table 74.13 Immunophenotype of pituitary blastoma

Positivities	Negativities
• ACTH • GH	• TSH • FSH • LH • alpha subunit

Immunophenotype
- A list of antibodies with positive or negative immunostaining results is given in Table 74.13.

Proliferation Markers
- KI-67 LI:
  - higher in follicular cells than in the hormone-producing cells
  - marked variation

Ultrastructural Features
- resemble fetal pituitary of 10–12 weeks gestational age
- fully differentiated corticotrophs and somatotrophs
- scant cytoplasm of glycoprotein hormone-producing type
- small secretory granules
- glandular epithelial cells consistent with undifferentiated Rathke-type epithelium

Differential Diagnosis
- Retinoblastoma
- Neuroblastoma

74.11.4 Molecular Neuropathology

- at least one *DICER1* mutation (usually germline)
- somatic mutation affecting the RNase IIIb domain of *DICER1*

74.11.5 Prognosis

Biologic Behavior–Prognosis–Prognostic Factors
- Poor prognosis

74.12 Apoplexia of the Pituitary

Following the AFIP definition, pituitary apoplexy is an acute hemorrhagic necrosis of pituitary adenoma which leads to rapid tumor expansion and cause severe headache, lethargy, coma, or other signs of increased intracranial pressure.

74.12.1 Clinical Signs and Symptoms

- Acute headache
- Nausea
- Vomiting
- Altered consciousness
- Visual disturbances, mainly ocular motor deficits
- Partial pituitary insufficiency

74.12.2 Epidemiology

Incidence
- 0.6–1% of all pituitary adenomas

Age Incidence
- Mea age: 46.7 years

Sex Incidence
- Slight male preponderance

Localization
- Pituitary gland

74.12.3 Neuroimaging Findings

General Imaging Findings
- Endo−/suprasellar mass +/−hemorrhage

CT non-contrast-enhanced (Fig. 74.13a)
- Insensitive
- Homogeneous to inhomogeneous hyperdense
- Hemorrhage may be seen, even subarachnoidal

MRI-T2/FLAIR (Fig. 74.13b, c)
- Acute: hypointense (bleeding)
- Subacute: hyperintense

MRI-T1 (Figs. 74.13d, f, h and 74.14a, c, e)
- Hyperintense if hemorrhagic

MRI-T1 Contrast-Enhanced (Figs. 74.13e, g, i and 74.14b, d, f)
- Peripheral enhancement

MRI-T2∗/SWI
- Hypointense if hemorrhagic

MR-DWI
- Restricted diffusion in solid components possible

Nuclear Medicine Imaging Findings
- lack of normal uptake

74.12.4 Neuropathology Findings

Macroscopic Features
- Brownish to reddish color
- Soft consistency

Microscopic Features (Fig. 74.15a–h)
- Large areas of necrotic tissue.
- Hemorrhagic infarction.
- Residues of a pituitary adenoma might be seen.

Proliferation Markers
- No proliferation

Differential Diagnosis
- Intratumoral hemorrhage

74.12.5 Molecular Neuropathology

- No identifiable predisposing factor

74.12 Apoplexia of the Pituitary

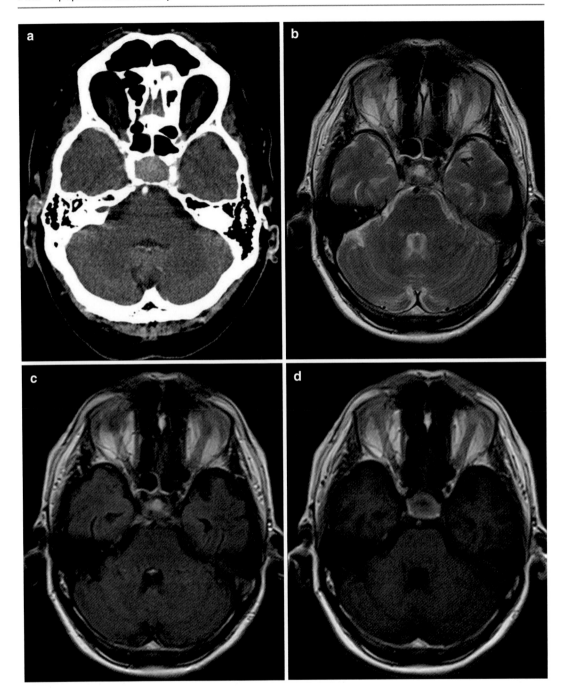

Fig. 74.13 Pituitary apoplexy/adenoma CT (**a**), T2 (**b**), FLAIR (**c**), T1 (**d**), T1 contrast (**e**), sag T1/T1 gd (**f, g**), and cor T1/T1gd (**h, i**)

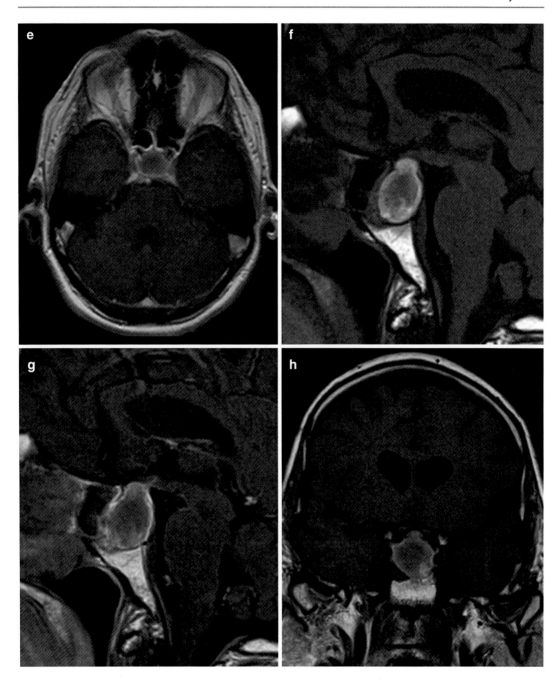

Fig. 74.13 (continued)

74.12 Apoplexia of the Pituitary

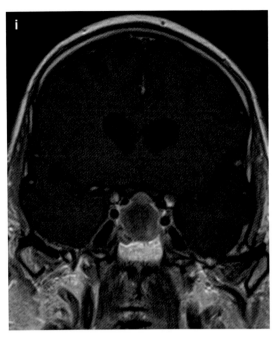

Fig. 74.13 (continued)

74.12.6 Treatment and Prognosis

Treatment
- Surgery mandatory in case of visual loss or neurologic deficit
- Achieve homeostasis for electrolytes and anterior pituitary functions

Biologic Behavior–Prognosis–Prognostic Factors
- Good recovery

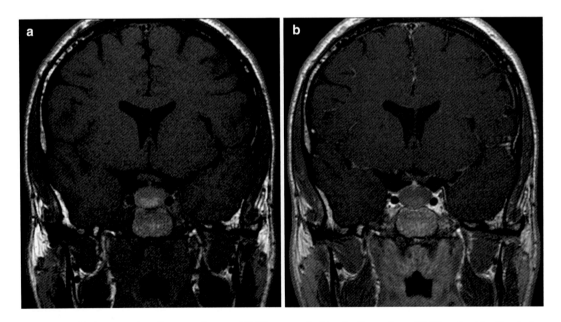

Fig. 74.14 Pituitary apoplexy in acute phase cor T1/T1contrast (**a**, **b**), after 3 month cor T1/T1contrast (**c**, **d**) and after 3 years cor T1/T1contrast (**e**, **f**)

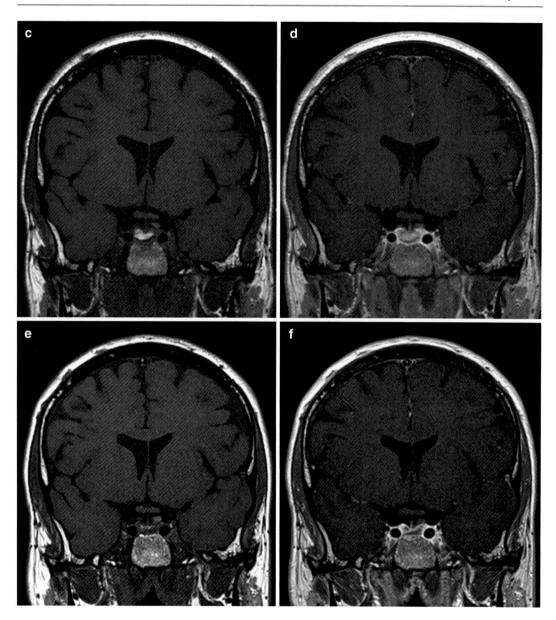

Fig. 74.14 (continued)

74.12 Apoplexia of the Pituitary

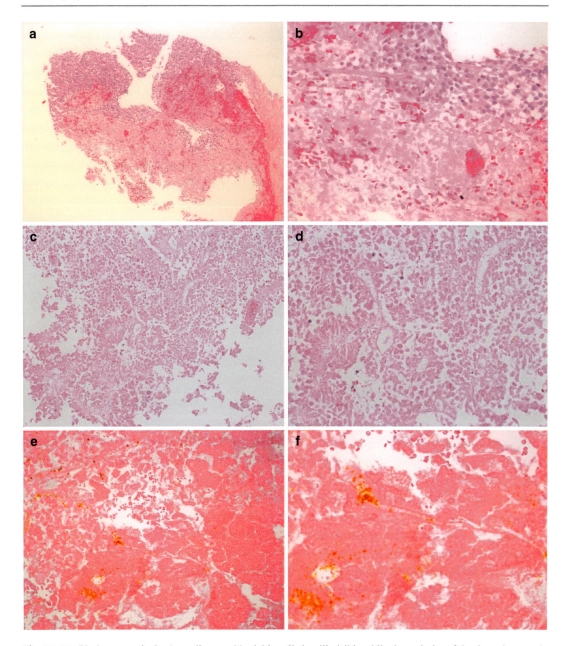

Fig. 74.15 Pituitary apoplexia. A small area with viable cells is still visible while the majority of the tissue is necrotic (**a**, **b**). "Shadows" of cells are still discernible (**c**, **d**). Signs of past hemorrhages might be seen (**e**–**h**)

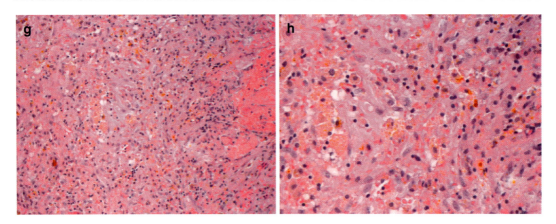

Fig. 74.15 (continued)

Selected References

Asa SL (2011) Tumors of the pituitary gland. In: APFIP atlas of tumor pathology, vol 15. ARP Press, Washington, DC

Asa SL, Ezzat S, Watson RE, Lindell EP, Horvath E (2004) Gonadotropin producing adenoma. In: DeLellis RA, Lloyd RV, Heitz PU, Eng C (eds) Pathology and genetics of tumours of endocrine organs. IARCC Press, Lyon, pp 30–32

Castinetti F, Dufour H, Gaillard S, Jouanneau E, Vasiljevic A, Villa C, Trouillas J (2015) Non-functioning pituitary adenoma: when and how to operate? What pathologic criteria for typing? Ann Endocrinol 76(3):220–227. https://doi.org/10.1016/j.ando.2015.04.007

Chanson P, Raverot G, Castinetti F, Cortet-Rudelli C, Galland F, Salenave S (2015) Management of clinically non-functioning pituitary adenoma. Ann Endocrinol 76(3):239–247. https://doi.org/10.1016/j.ando.2015.04.002

Chesnokova V, Zonis S, Ben-Shlomo A, Wawrowsky K, Melmed S (2010) Molecular mechanisms of pituitary adenoma senescence. Front Horm Res 38:7–14. https://doi.org/10.1159/000318489

de Kock L, Sabbaghian N, Plourde F, Srivastava A, Weber E, Bouron-Dal Soglio D, Hamel N, Choi JH, Park SH, Deal CL, Kelsey MM, Dishop MK, Esbenshade A, Kuttesch JF, Jacques TS, Perry A, Leichter H, Maeder P, Brundler MA, Warner J, Neal J, Zacharin M, Korbonits M, Cole T, Traunecker H, McLean TW, Rotondo F, Lepage P, Albrecht S, Horvath E, Kovacs K, Priest JR, Foulkes WD (2014) Pituitary blastoma: a pathognomonic feature of germ-line DICER1 mutations. Acta Neuropathol 128(1):111–122. https://doi.org/10.1007/s00401-014-1285-z

Donangelo I, Melmed S (2012) Pituitary adenomas. In: Fink G, Pfaff DW, Levine JE (eds) Handbook of neuroendocrinology. Elsevier, New York, pp 739–760

Fahlbusch R, Buchfelder M (2011) Pituitary surgery. In: Melmed S (ed) The pituitary, 3rd edn. Elsevier Academic Press, New York, pp 703–719

Gadelha MR, Kasuki L, Denes J, Trivellin G, Korbonits M (2013) MicroRNAs: suggested role in pituitary adenoma pathogenesis. J Endocrinol Investig 36(10):889–895. https://doi.org/10.1007/bf03346759

Grizzi F, Borroni EM, Vacchini A, Qehajaj D, Liguori M, Stifter S, Chiriva-Internati M, Di Ieva A (2015) Pituitary adenoma and the chemokine network: a systemic view. Front Endocrinol 6:141. https://doi.org/10.3389/fendo.2015.00141

Horvath E, Lloyd RV, Kovacs K, Sano T, Kontogeorgos G, Trouillas J, Asa SL (2004) Plurihormonal adenoma. In: DeLellis RA, Lloyd RV, Heitz PU, Eng C (eds) Pathology and genetics of tumours of endocrine organs. IARCC Press, Lyon, p 35

Horvath E, Scheithauer B, Kovacs K, Lloyd RV (2002) Hypothalamus and pituitary. In: Graham DI, Lantos P (eds) Greenfield's neuropathology, 7th edn. Edward Arnold, London, pp 983–1062

Jaffe CA (2006) Clinically non-functioning pituitary adenoma. Pituitary 9(4):317–321. https://doi.org/10.1007/s11102-006-0412-9

Kaltsas GA, Grossman AB (1998) Malignant pituitary tumours. Pituitary 1(1):69–81

Kontogeorgos G, Kovacs K, Lloyd RV, Righi A (2017) Plurihormonal and double adenomas. In: Lloyd RV, Osamura RY, Klöppel G, Rosai J (eds) WHO classification of tumours of endocrine organs, 4th edn. IARC, Lyon, pp 39–40

Kontogeorgos G, Watson RE, Lindell EP, Barkan AL, Farrell WE, Lloyd RV (2004) Growth hormone producing adenoma. In: DeLellis RA, Lloyd RV, Heitz PU, Eng C (eds) Pathology and genetics of tumours of endocrine organs. IARCC, Lyon, pp 14–19

Lloyd RV, Kovacs K, Young WF, Farrell WE, Asa SL, Truillas J, Kontogeorgos G, Sano T, Scheithauer BW, Horvath E (2004) Pituitary tumours: introduction. In: DeLellis RA, Lloyd RV, Heitz PU, Eng C (eds) Pathology and genetics of tumours of endocrine organs. IARCC Press, Lyon, pp 10–13

Lopes MBS (2017) The 2017 World Health Organization classification of tumors of the pituitary gland: a summary. Acta Neuropathol 134(4):521–535. https://doi.org/10.1007/s00401-017-1769-8

Mete O, Grossman A, Trouillas J, Yamada S (2017a) Corticotroph adenoma. In: Lloyd RV, Osamura RY, Klöppel G, Rosai J (eds) WHO classification of tumours of endocrine organs, 4th edn. IARCC Press, Lyon, pp 30–33

Mete O, Korbonits M, Osamura RY, Trouillas J, Yamada S (2017b) Somatotroph adenoma. In: Lloyd RV, Osamura RY, Klöppel G, Rosai J (eds) WHO classification of tumours of endocrine organs, 4th edn. IARC, Lyon, pp 19–23

Nishioka H, Kontogeorgos G, Lloyd RV, Lopes MBS, Mete O, Nosé V (2017) Null cell adenoma. In: Lloyd RV, Osamura RY, Klöppel G, Rosai J (eds) WHO classification of tumours of endocrine organs, 4th edn. IARC, Lyon, pp 37–38

Nosé V, Grossman A, Mete O (2017) Lactotroph adenoma. In: Lloyd RV, Osamura RY, Klöppel G, Rosai J (eds) WHO classification of tumours of endocrine organs, 4th edn. IARC, Lyon, pp 24–27

Oki Y (2014) Medical management of functioning pituitary adenoma: an update. Neurol Med Chir 54(12):958–965

Osamura RY, Grossman A, Korbonits M, Kovacs K, Lopes MBS, Matsuno A, Trouillas J (2017a) Pituitary adenoma. In: Lloyd RV, Osamura RY, Klöppel G, Rosai J (eds) WHO classification of tumours of endocrine organs, 4th edn. IARC, Lyon, pp 14–18

Osamura RY, Grossman A, Nishioka H, Trouillas J (2017b) Thyrotroph adenoma. In: Lloyd RV, Osamura RY, Klöppel G, Rosai J (eds) WHO classification of tumours of endocrine organs, 4th edn. IARC, Lyon, pp 28–29

Osamura RY, Sano T, Ezzat S, Asa SL, Barkan AL, Watson RE, Lindell EP (2004) TSH producing adenoma. In: DeLellis RA, Lloyd RV, Heitz PU, Eng C (eds) Pathology and genetics of tumours of endocrine organs. IARCC Press, Lyon, pp 24–25

Platta CS, Mackay C, Welsh JS (2010) Pituitary adenoma: a radiotherapeutic perspective. Am J Clin Oncol 33(4):408–419. https://doi.org/10.1097/COC.0b013e31819d878d

Ragel BT, Couldwell WT (2004) Pituitary carcinoma: a review of the literature. Neurosurg Focus 16(4):E7

Raverot G, Assie G, Cotton F, Cogne M, Boulin A, Dherbomez M, Bonneville JF, Massart C (2015) Biological and radiological exploration and management of non-functioning pituitary adenoma. Ann Endocrinol 76(3):201–209. https://doi.org/10.1016/j.ando.2015.04.005

Roncaroli F, Kovacs K, Lloyd RV, Matsuno A, Righi A (2017) Pituitary carcinoma. In: Lloyd RV, Osamura RY, Klöppel G, Rosai J (eds) WHO classification of tumours of endocrine organs, 4th edn. IARC, Lyon, pp 41–44

Rostad S (2012) Pituitary adenoma pathogenesis: an update. Curr Opin Endocrinol Diabetes Obes 19(4):322–327. https://doi.org/10.1097/MED.0b013e328354b2e2

Rotondo F, Syro LV, Lloyd RV, Foulkes WD, Kovacs K (2017) Pituitary blastoma. In: Lloyd RV, Osamura RY, Klöppel G, Rosai J (eds) WHO classification of tumours of endocrine organs, 4th edn. IARC, Lyon, p 45

Saeger W, Horvath E, Kovacs K, Nose V, Farrell WE, Lloyd RV, Watson RE, Lindell EP (2004) Prolactin producing adenoma. In: DeLellis RA, Lloyd RV, Heitz PU, Eng C (eds) Pathology and genetics of tumours of endocrine organs. IARCC Press, Lyon, pp 20–23

Sano T, Yamada S, Watson RE, Lindell EP, Ezzat S, Asa SL (2004) Null cell adenoma. In: DeLellis RA, Lloyd RV, Heitz PU, Eng C (eds) Pathology and genetics of tumours of endocrine organs. IARCC Press, Lyon, pp 33–34

Scheithauer B, Kovacs K, Horvath E, Roncaroli F, Ezzat S, Asa SL, Lloyd RV, Nose V, Watson RE, Lindell EP (2004) Pituitarcy carcinoma. In: DeLellis RA, Lloyd RV, Heitz PU, Eng C (eds) Pathology and genetics of tumours of endocrine organs. IARCC Press, Lyon, pp 36–39

Scheithauer BW, Horvath E, Abel TW, Robital Y, Park SH, Osamura RY, Deal C, Lloyd RV, Kovacs K (2012) Pituitary blastoma: a unique embryonal tumor. Pituitary 15(3):365–373. https://doi.org/10.1007/s11102-011-0328-x

Scheithauer BW, Kovacs K, Horvath E, Kim DS, Osamura RY, Ketterling RP, Lloyd RV, Kim OL (2008) Pituitary blastoma. Acta Neuropathol 116(6):657–666. https://doi.org/10.1007/s00401-008-0388-9

Shi X, Tao B, He H, Sun Q, Fan C, Bian L, Zhao W, Lu YC (2012) MicroRNAs-based network: a novel therapeutic agent in pituitary adenoma. Med Hypotheses 78(3):380–384. https://doi.org/10.1016/j.mehy.2011.12.001

Shin M (2002) Gamma knife radiosurgery for pituitary adenoma. Biomed Pharmacother 56(suppl 1):178s–181s

Suhardja A, Kovacs K, Rutka J (2001) Genetic basis of pituitary adenoma invasiveness: a review. J Neurooncol 52(3):195–204

Trouillas J, Barkan AL, Watson RE, Lindell EP, Farrell WE, Lloyd RV (2004) ACTH producing adenoma. In: DeLellis RA, Lloyd RV, Heitz PU, Eng C (eds) Pathology and genetics of tumours of endocrine organs. IARCC Press, Lyon, pp 26–29

Trouillas J, Roy P, Sturm N, Dantony E, Cortet-Rudelli C, Viennet G, Bonneville JF, Assaker R, Auger C, Brue T, Cornelius A, Dufour H, Jouanneau E, Francois P, Galland F, Mougel F, Chapuis F, Villeneuve L, Maurage CA, Figarella-Branger D, Raverot G, Barlier A, Bernier M, Bonnet F, Borson-Chazot F, Brassier G, Caulet-Maugendre S, Chabre O, Chanson

P, Cottier JF, Delemer B, Delgrange E, Di Tommaso L, Eimer S, Gaillard S, Jan M, Girard JJ, Lapras V, Loiseau H, Passagia JG, Patey M, Penfornis A, Poirier JY, Perrin G, Tabarin A (2013) A new prognostic clinicopathological classification of pituitary adenomas: a multicentric case-control study of 410 patients with 8 years post-operative follow-up. Acta Neuropathol 126(1):123–135. https://doi.org/10.1007/s00401-013-1084-y

Vance ML (2008) Pituitary adenoma: a clinician's perspective. Endocr Pract 14(6):757–763. https://doi.org/10.4158/ep.14.6.757

Wang YQ, Fan T, Zhao XG, Liang C, Qi XL, Li JY (2015) Pituitary carcinoma with intraspinal metastasis: report of two cases and review of the literature. Int J Clin Exp Pathol 8(8):9712–9717

Yamada S, Osamura RY, Righi A, Trouillas J (2017) Gonadotroph adenoma. In: Lloyd RV, Osamura RY, Klöppel G, Rosai J (eds) WHO classification of tumours of endocrine organs, 4th edn. IARC, Lyon, pp 34–36

Zhan X, Wang X, Cheng T (2016) Human pituitary adenoma proteomics: new progresses and perspectives. Front Endocrinol 7:54. https://doi.org/10.3389/fendo.2016.00054

Zhou Y, Zhang X, Klibanski A (2014) Genetic and epigenetic mutations of tumor suppressive genes in sporadic pituitary adenoma. Mol Cell Endocrinol 386(1–2):16–33. https://doi.org/10.1016/j.mce.2013.09.006

Cystic Lesions

75.1 Introduction

The following primary non-neoplastic cystic lesions of the nervous system with space-occupying character can be distinguished:

- Epidermoid cyst
- Dermoid cyst
- Colloid cyst of the third ventricle
- Rathke's cleft cyst
- Enterogeneous cyst
- Neuroglial cyst
- Congenital arachnoid cyst
- Pineal cyst
- Choroid plexus cyst
- Perineurial cyst

75.2 General Aspects

Clinical Signs and Symptoms
- Long history and gradual onset of symptoms
- Headache
- Seizures
- Suprasellar lesions
  - Visual deficits
  - Pituitary or hypothalamic dysfunction
- Cerebellopontine lesions
  - Ataxia
  - Nystagmus
  - Palsies of cranial nerves V and VIII

Nuclear Medicine Imaging Findings
- In general, cystic lesions appear as a defect in nuclear medicine studies (mainly in FDG-PET or perfusion SPECT) due to the lack of perfusion and metabolism.
- In small cystic lesions, the resolution limit of the system has to be taken into account.

75.3 Epidermoid Cyst

WHO Definition
1993—Thin-walled and "pearly," these cysts are lined by a delicate layer of keratin-producing squamous epithelial cells containing keratohyalin granules. The underlying stroma is scant (Kleihues et al. 1993).

1979—A cyst lined by keratin-producing squamous epithelium. The contents are brittle, white, and pearly (Zülch 1979).

75.3.1 Epidemiology

Incidence
- 1–2% of all intracranial tumors

Age Incidence
- Birth to old age
- 20–50 years

Sex Incidence
- Slight male predominance

Localization
- Sellar region
- Cerebellopontine angle
- Cerebral hemispheres
- Lateral ventricles
- Spine (rare):
  – Thoracolumbar (epidermoid cyst)
  – Lumbosacral (dermoid cyst)
  – Posterior
  – Intradural
  – Intra/extramedullary
- Involvement of bone of the middle ear and cranial vault possible

75.3.2 Neuroimaging Findings

General Imaging Findings
- Cisternal, CSF-like mass with restricted diffusion

CT non-contrast-enhanced (Figs. 75.1a and 75.2a)
- Hypodense
- In rare cases hyperdense
- Calcifications are rare
- Erosions of the bone, if located at diploic space

CT contrast-enhanced
- No enhancement

MRI-T2 (Figs. 75.1b and 75.2b)
- Usually isointense to CSF

MRI-FLAIR (Figs. 75.1c and 75.2c)
- Slightly hyperintense to CSF

MRI-T1 (Figs. 75.1d and 75.2d)
- Isointense to CSF
- Rarely hypo- or hyperintense (depends on cholesterol or triglyceride content)

MRI-T1 Contrast-Enhanced (Figs. 75.1e, f and 75.2e)
- Usually no enhancement
- Peripheral enhancement described

MRI-T2*/SWI
- Depends on calcifications

MR-Diffusion Imaging (Figs. 75.1g, h and 75.2f, g)
- Restricted diffusion causes high signal intensity and is pathognomonic

MRI-Perfusion (Fig. 75.1i)
- No elevation of rCBV

75.3.3 Neuropathology Findings

Macroscopic Features (Figs. 75.3a, b and 75.4a–j)
- Rounded, slightly fluctuant mass
- Smooth whitish capsule
  – "Mother of pearl": shining, silky appearance
- Cyst if filled with
  – Lamellated flakes of pearly white keratin with friable, wax texture
  – Arranged in strikingly concentric layers
  – Greasy brownish fluid

Microscopic Features (Fig. 75.5a–h)
- Cyst lining consists of:
  – Keratinizing stratified squamous epithelium
    ○ Forms germinal, granular, and corneal layers (similar to skin)
    ○ Rests on an outer thin layer of collagen
    ○ Devoid of glands and dermal appendages
- Patchy chronic inflammatory infiltrates
- Focal degeneration of the epithelial lining
- Granulomatous reaction with foreign-body multinucleated giant cells
- Surrounding gliotic brain tissue

75.3 Epidermoid Cyst

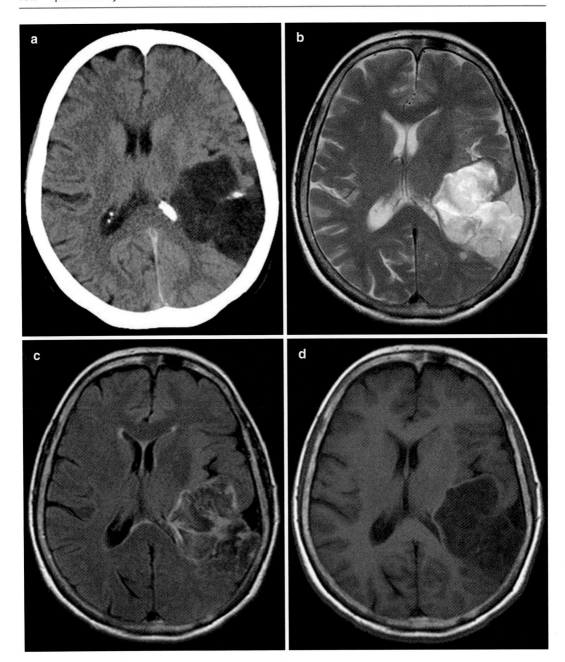

Fig. 75.1 Epidermoid cyst, left hemisphere on CT (**a**), T2 (**b**), FLAIR (**c**), T1 (**d**), T1 contrast ax/cor (**e, f**), DWI (**g**), ADC (**h**), rCBV (**i**)

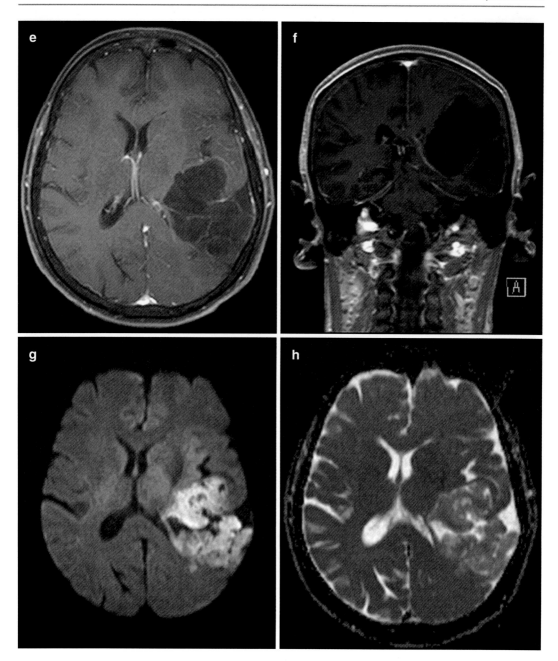

Fig. 75.1 (continued)

75.3 Epidermoid Cyst

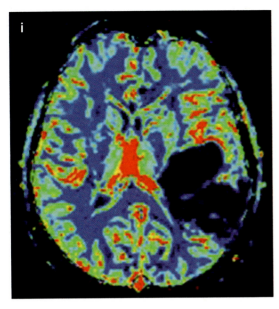

- Cholesteatoma: epidermoid cyst in the petrous bone
  - Reactive inward growth of epithelial elements following chronic mastoid or middle ear infection
- Epidermoid cyst of the suprasellar region considered to be a variant of craniopharyngioma

Immunophenotype

- Cyst epithelium positive for:
  - Cytokeratin (AE1/AE3)
  - Epithelial membrane antigen (EMA)

Proliferation Markers

- Very low

Fig. 75.1 (continued)

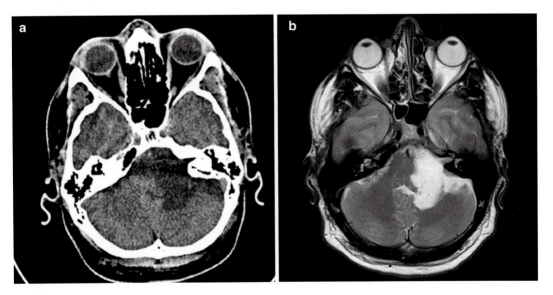

Fig. 75.2 Epidermoid cyst in typical location of cerebellopontine angle left CT (**a**), T2 (**b**), FLAIR (**c**), T1 (**d**), T1 contrast (**e**), DWI (**f**), ADC (**g**), CISS (**h**)

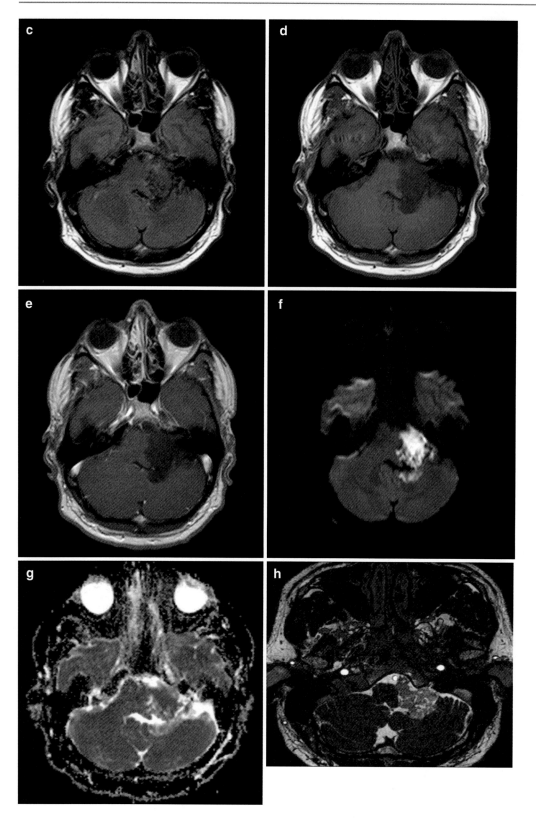

Fig. 75.2 (continued)

75.3.4 Molecular Neuropathology

- Arise from inclusions of embryonal ectodermal elements during closure of the primitive neural groove or the secondary cerebral vesicles.
- Occurs at a late point of embryogenesis.
- Cholesteatoma: epidermoid cyst in the petrous bone.
  - Reactive inward growth of epithelial elements following chronic mastoid or middle ear infection
- Spinal lesions result possibly from penetrating trauma or multiple lumbar punctures through mechanical implantation of skin fragments into the spinal canal.
- Association with other disorders as spina bifida, other congenital abnormalities (diastematomyelia).

75.3.5 Treatment and Prognosis

Treatment
- Surgical excision
  - CAVE: strong adherence of the capsule to the brain
  - Partial stripping of the capsule
  - Removal of keratinous material

Biologic Behavior–Prognosis–Prognostic Factors
- Good prognosis
- Rare symptomatic recurrences
- Malignant transformation rare

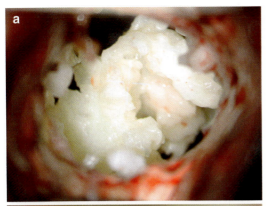
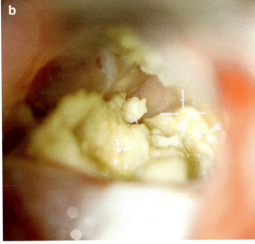

Fig. 75.3 Intraoperative appearance of the whitish-yellow content of an epidermoid cyst after incisure (**a**, **b**)

Ultrastructural Features
- Intracellular osmiophilic, crystalline inclusions
- Gliosis with Rosenthal fibers in brain parenchyma adjacent to the tumor capsule
- Dermal structures
- Skin appendages

Differential Diagnosis
- Craniopharyngioma
- Teratoma
- Dermoid cyst
- Metastatic carcinoma
- Enterogeneous cyst
- Colloid cyst
- Neuroglial cyst

75.4 Dermoid Cyst

WHO Definition
1993—A cyst lined by squamous epithelium with underlying dermal appendages, including hair follicles and adnexae (Kleihues et al. 1993).

1979—A cyst lined by keratin-producing squamous epithelium and containing skin appendages. It frequently occurs in a median location.

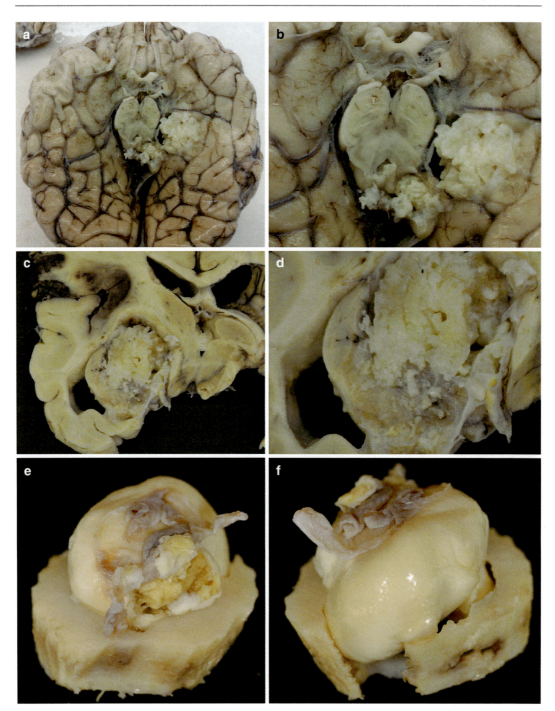

Fig. 75.4 Macroscopic appearance of an epidermal cyst destroying parts of the temporal lobe (**a**, **b**) and hippocampal formation (**c**, **d**). Epidermal cyst of the bone (**e–g**). Smooth whitish capsule "Mother of pearl" with shining, silky appearance (**e**, **f**). Rounded, slightly fluctuant mass (**h**) with lamellated flakes of pearly white keratin with friable, wax texture (**i**, **j**), and arranged in strikingly concentric layers

75.4 Dermoid Cyst

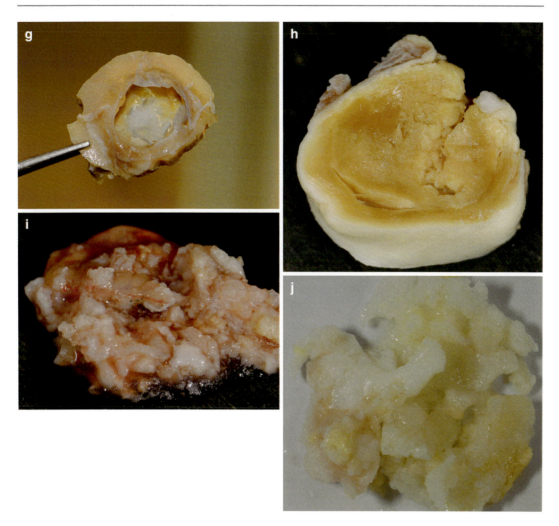

Fig. 75.4 (continued)

The contents are smeary or cheesy and hair and rarely teeth may be included (Zülch 1979).

75.4.1 Epidemiology

Incidence
- 0.3–0.5% of all intracranial tumors

Age Incidence
- Birth to old age
- Childhood adolescence

Sex Incidence
- No sex predominance

Localization
- Midline sites
- Posterior fossa
- Cerebellopontine angle
- Cerebral hemispheres
- Lateral ventricles
- Spine:
  - Thoracolumbar (epidermoid cyst)
  - Lumbosacral (dermoid cyst)
  - Posterior
  - Intradural
  - Intra/extramedullary
- Involvement of bone of the middle ear and cranial vault possible

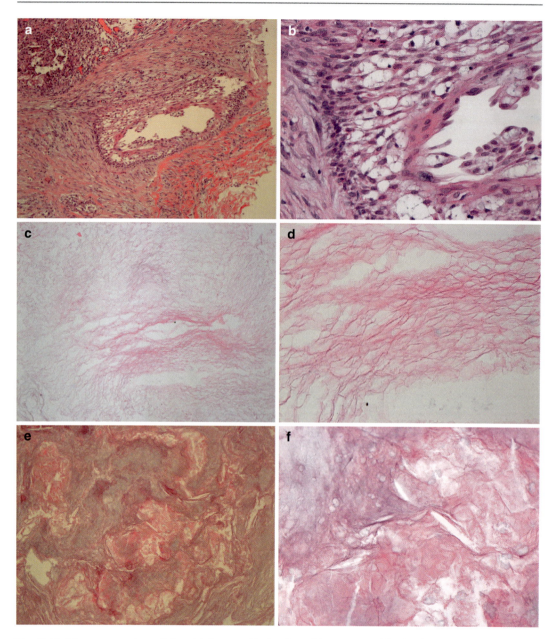

Fig. 75.5 The cyst consists of keratinizing stratified squamous epithelium (**a**, **b**) keratin layers (**c–f**). Patchy chronic inflammatory infiltrates and granulomatous reaction with presence of foreign-body multinucleated giant cells (**g**, **h**)

75.4 Dermoid Cyst

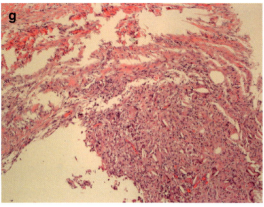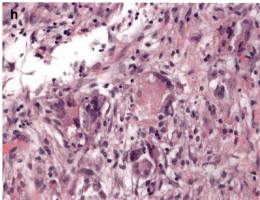

Fig. 75.5 (continued)

75.4.2 Neuroimaging Findings

General Imaging Findings
- Well-defined, "fatty" mass, in cases of rupture subarachnoidal/intraventricular spreading

CT non-contrast-enhanced (Fig. 75.6a)
- Isodense to fat
- Peripheral calcifications possible
- Rupture: fat-isodense drops subarachnoidal or intraventricular with fat-fluid levels

CT contrast-enhanced
- No enhancement

MRI-T2 (Fig. 75.6b)
- Heterogeneous

MRI-FLAIR (Fig. 75.6c)
- Heterogeneous

MRI-T1 (Fig. 75.6d)
- Hyperintense
- Rupture: hyperintense drops subarachnoidal/intraventricular

MRI-T1 Contrast-Enhanced (Fig. 75.6e)
- No enhancement
- Rupture: reactive meningeal enhancement

MRI-T2∗/SWI
- Peripheral calcifications hypointense

MR-Diffusion Imaging (Fig. 75.6f, g)
- No restricted diffusion (helps to distinguish from epidermoid)

MRI-Perfusion (Fig. 75.6h)
- No elevation of rCBV

MR-Spectroscopy (Fig. 75.6i)
- Lipid peak

75.4.3 Neuropathology Findings

Macroscopic Features (Figs. 75.7a–c and 75.8a–d)
- Well-defined rounded mass
- Firm outer capsule
- Adherent to surrounding brain structures
- Cyst filled with
  - Thick, greasy, yellow sebaceous material
  - Matted, tangled hair
  - Rarely teeth
- Calcifications

Microscopic Features (Fig. 75.9a–l)
- Cyst lined by:
  - Stratified squamous epithelium
- Collagenous tissue of varying size
  - Resembling dermis
  - Containing skin appendages (hair follicles, sebaceous glands, sweat glands)

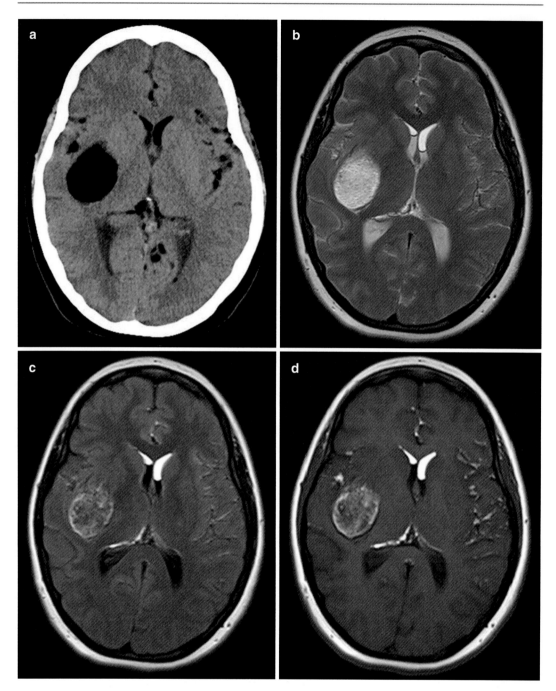

Fig. 75.6 Ruptured dermoid cyst right temporal with subarachnoidal and intraventricular spreading on CT (**a**), T2 (**b**), FLAIR (**c**), T1 (**d**), T1 contrast (**e**), DWI (**f**), ADC (**g**), rCBV (**h**), spectroscopy (270 ms) with lactate peak (**i**). FDG-PET with lack of accumulation in the cyst and faint reactive uptake of the surrounding structures (**j**)

75.4 Dermoid Cyst

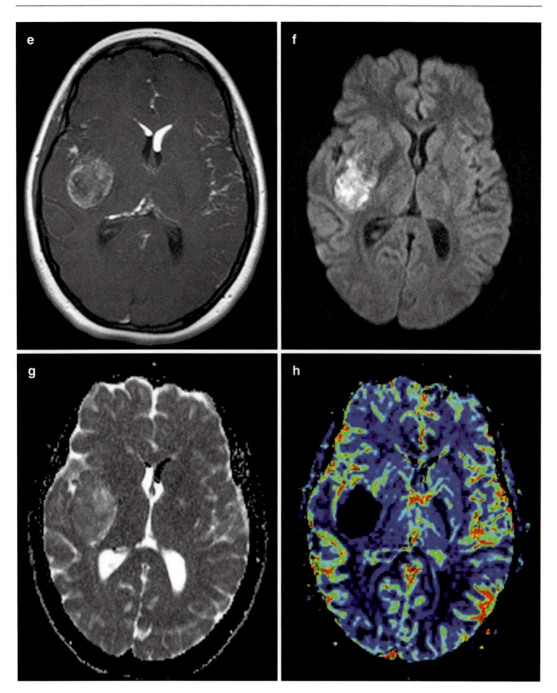

Fig. 75.6 (continued)

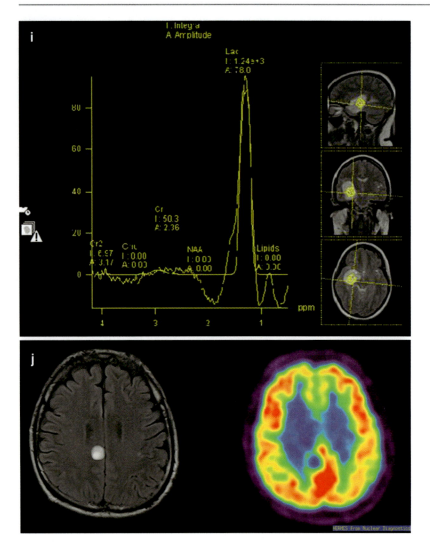

Fig. 75.6 (continued)

- Rarely bone or cartilage
- Granulomatous inflammatory reaction

Immunophenotype (Fig. 75.9m, n)
- Cyst epithelium positive for:
  - Cytokeratin (AE1/AE3)
  - Epithelial membrane antigen (EMA)

Proliferation Markers
- Low

Ultrastructural Features
- Intracellular osmiophilic, crystalline inclusions
- Gliosis with Rosenthal fibers in brain parenchyma adjacent to the tumor capsule

- Dermal structures
- Skin appendages

Differential Diagnosis
- Craniopharyngioma
- Teratoma
- Epidermoid cyst
- Metastatic carcinoma
- Enterogeneous cyst
- Colloid cyst
- Neuroglial cyst

A variety of differences between dermoid and epidermoid tumors is shown in Table 75.1.

75.5 Rathke's Cleft Cyst

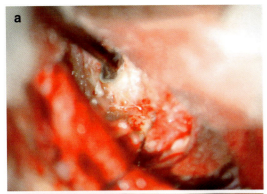
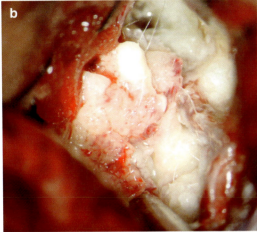
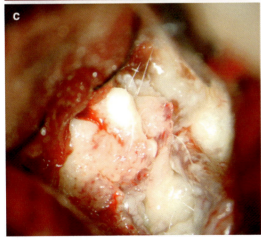

Fig. 75.7 Intraoperative appearance of a dermoid cyst. Note the presence of whitish-glistening hair (**a**–**c**)

75.4.4 Molecular Neuropathology

- Arise from inclusions of embryonal ectodermal elements during closure of the primitive neural groove or the secondary cerebral vesicles.

- Entrapment of ectodermal cells occurs at an early point of embryogenesis.
- Spinal lesions occurred after surgical closure of myelomeningoencephaloceles (iatrogenic implantation of inadequately excised dermal elements).
- Association with other disorders as spina bifida occulta or myelomeningoencephaloceles.

75.4.5 Treatment and Prognosis

Treatment
- Surgical excision
  - CAVE: strong adherence of the capsule to the brain
  - Partial stripping of the capsule
  - Removal of keratinous material

Biologic Behavior–Prognosis–Prognostic Factors
- Good prognosis.
- Rare symptomatic recurrences.
- Malignant transformation very rare.

75.5 Rathke's Cleft Cyst

WHO Definition
1993—An intra- or suprasellar cyst lined by ciliated, cuboidal to columnar epithelium, goblet cells, and occasional pituitary endocrine cells (Kleihues et al. 1993).

1979—An intrasellar cyst lined by cuboidal or ciliated epithelium identical with that lining the small cyst frequently found between the pars anterior and the infundibular process (Zülch 1979).

75.5.1 Epidemiology

Incidence
- Rare

Age Incidence
- Second to eighth decade
- Mean: fourth decade

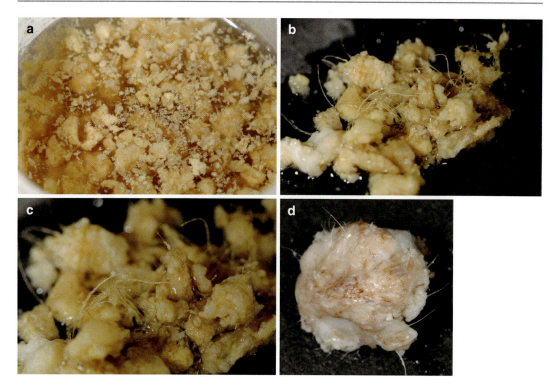

Fig. 75.8 Macroscopic appearance of dermoid cyst. Thick, greasy, yellow sebaceous material contains matted, tangled hair (**a–c**). Firm outer capsule (**d**)

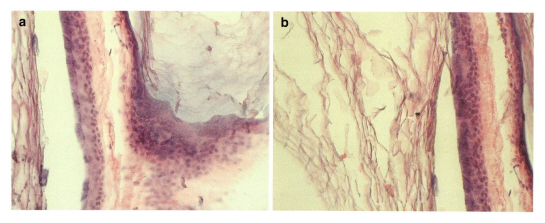

Fig. 75.9 Dermoid cyst: The cyst is lined by stratified squamous epithelium (**a–d**). Collagenous tissue of varying size resembles dermis (**c, d**) and contains skin appendages [hair follicles (**e, f, i, j**) sebaceous glands (**i, j**), sweat glands (**g**)] (**e–j**). Granulomatous inflammatory reaction with presence of numerous multinucleated giant cells (**k, l**). The epithelial elements are immunopositive for pancytokeratin AE1/AE3 (**m, n**)

75.5 Rathke's Cleft Cyst

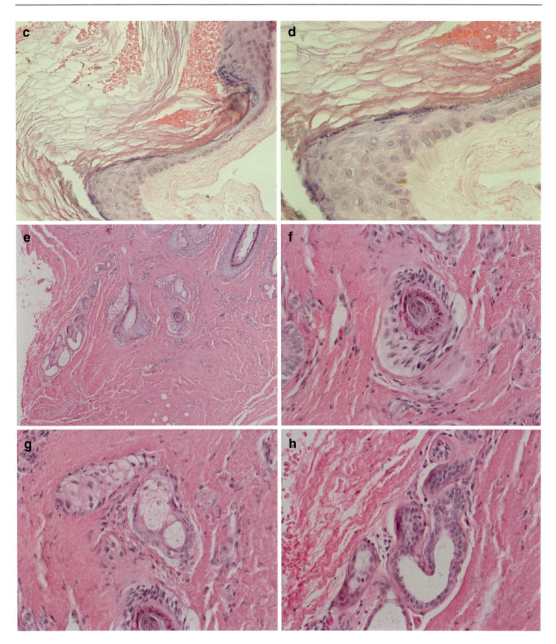

Fig. 75.9 (continued)

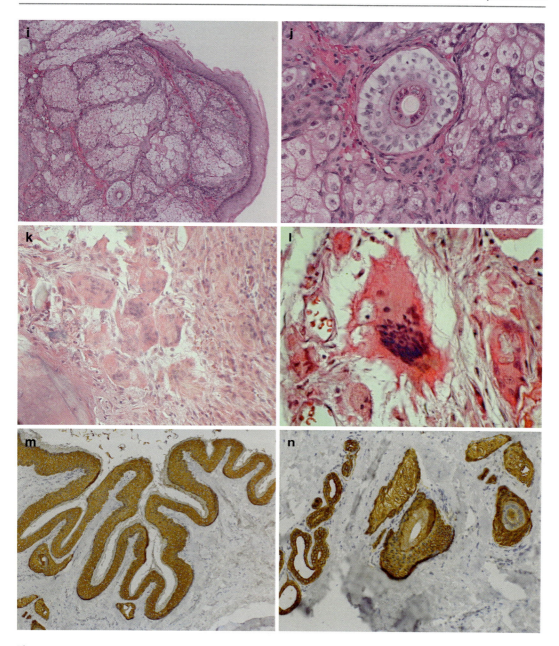

Fig. 75.9 (continued)

75.5 Rathke's Cleft Cyst

Table 75.1 Differences between dermoid and epidermoid tumors, modified after Kavar and Kaye (2011)

Feature	Dermoid	Epidermoid
Incidence	0.3% of brain tumors	0.5–1.8% of brain tumors
Sex	M = F	M > F
Age	Childhood	20–50 years
Origin	Ectoderm	Ectoderm
Location	More common midline	More common laterally
Associated anomalies	Associated with other congenital anomalies in up to 50% of cases	Tend to be isolated lesions
CT	Very low density	Low density
MRI	Very high T1, Iso–/high T2	Higher on T1 and T2 than CSF
Enhancement	Mild, thicker, and nodular	Very thin enhancing capsule
MR pattern	Generally heterogeneous	Generally homogeneous
Wall	Also includes dermal appendages (hair follicles, sebaceous sweat glands)	Stratified squamous epithelium
Contents	As epidermoid plus hair and sebum	Keratin, cellular debris, and cholesterol
Meningitis	May have repeated bouts of bacterial meningitis	May have brief recurrent episodes of aseptic meningitis
Malignancy	Rare than epidermoid	Documented
Growth	Desquamation and gland secretion	Desquamation

Sex Incidence
- F > M

Localization
- Intrasellar
- Significant suprasellar extension

75.5.2 Neuroimaging Findings

General Imaging Findings
- Intrasellar cyst usually between anterior and intermediate lobe of hypophysis

CT non-contrast-enhanced
- Round mass of variable density

CT contrast-enhanced
- No enhancement
- Calcifications in cyst wall rare

MRI-T2 (Fig. 75.10a)
- Depends on cyst content
- ¾ hyperintense
- ¼ iso-hypointense

MRI-FLAIR (Fig. 75.10b)
- Hyperintense

MRI-T1 (Fig. 75.10c)
- 50% hyperintense due to proteins
- 50% hypo-isointense

MRI-T1 Contrast-Enhanced (Fig. 75.10d–f)
- Usually no enhancement
- Non enhancing intracystic nodule pathognomonic

MRI-T2∗/SWI
- Peripheral calcifications rare

MRI-Perfusion
- No elevation

75.5.3 Neuropathology Findings

Macroscopic Features
- Small in size (<5 mm)
- Smooth glistening membrane
- Thin and translucent wall
- Contain opalescent mucous, clear colorless fluid, altered blood, creamy purulent material

Microscopic Features (Fig. 75.11a–j)
- Lined by columnar or cuboidal sometimes stratified epithelium

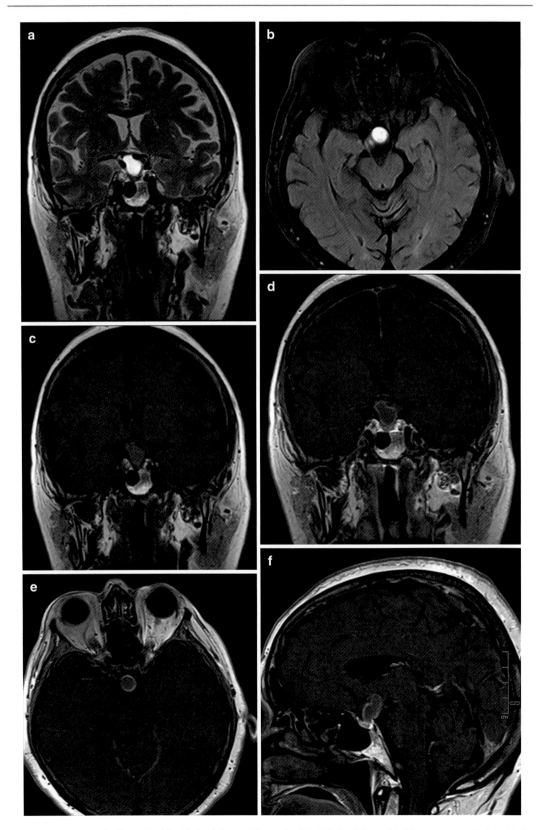

Fig. 75.10 Histologically verified Rathke's cleft cyst T2 cor (**a**), FLAIR (**b**), T1 cor (**c**), T1 contrast cor/ax/sag (**d–f**)

75.5 Rathke's Cleft Cyst

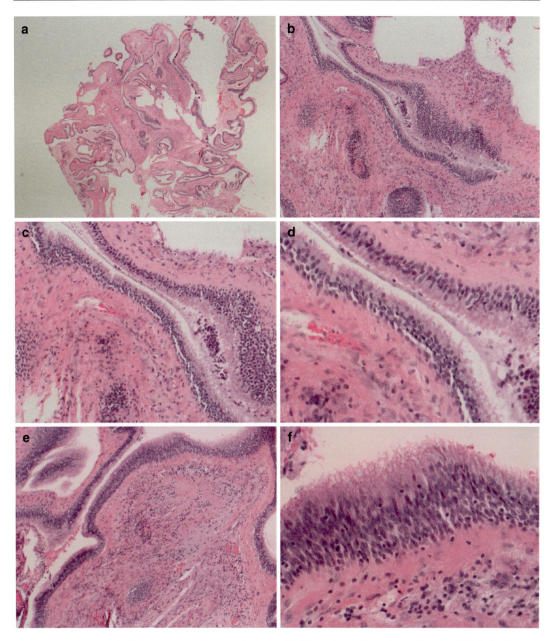

Fig. 75.11 The cyst is lined by columnar or cuboidal sometimes stratified epithelium (**a–h**). The epithelial cells bear apical cilia (**d**, **f**) and have goblet cell appearance (**g**, **h**). The goblet cells stain-positive for PAS (**i**, **j**). The epithelium is immunopositive for the pancytokeratin AE1/AE3 (**k–n**)

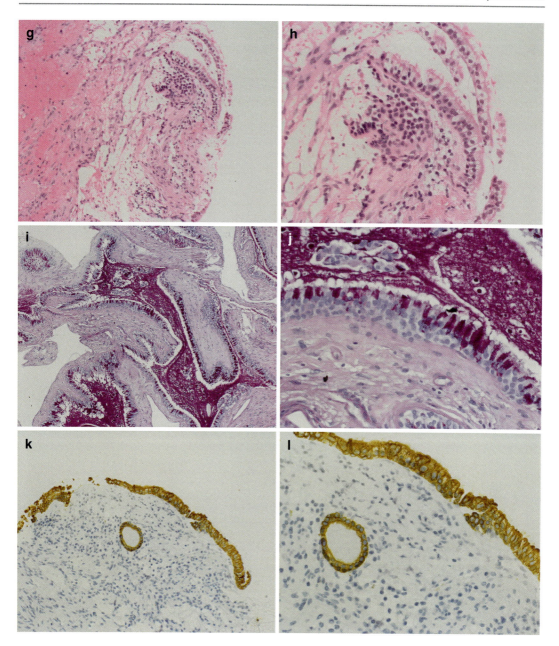

Fig. 75.11 (continued)

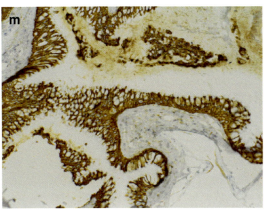 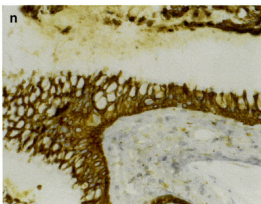

Fig. 75.11 (continued)

- Bear apical cilia
- Have goblet cell appearance
• Rest on a sparse connective tissue layer containing simple gland-like structures

Immunophenotype (Fig. 75.11k–n)
• Positive for:
  - Cytokeratins
  - Epithelial membrane antigen
• Occasional expression of:
  - GFAP
  - S-100
  - Carcinoembryonic antigen

Proliferation Markers
• Very low

Ultrastructural Features
• Columnar (secretory) epithelial cells with
  - Abundant apical cilia
  - Luminal-surface microvilli
  - Membrane-bound secretory granules in the apical cytoplasm
  - Cytoplasmic tonofilaments, desmosomes, and intercellular bridges

Differential Diagnosis
• Craniopharyngioma
• Pituitary cyst
• Teratoma
• Dermoid cyst
• Arachnoid cyst
• Mucocele

75.5.4 Molecular Neuropathology

• Fragments of a blind-ended evagination of the ectodermally lined stomatodeum
• Neuroepithelial origin

75.5.5 Treatment and Prognosis

Treatment
• Surgical removal

Biologic Behavior–Prognosis–Prognostic Factors
• Good outcome

75.6 Colloid Cyst of the Third Ventricle

WHO Definition
1993—A cyst occurring in the anterior third ventricle near the foramen of Monro. The lesion is lined by cuboidal to columnar, ciliated and/or goblet cells which may become flattened and atrophic under pressure (Kleihues et al. 1993).

1979—A cyst occurring in the region of the foramen of Monro, near the choroid plexus, and lined by ciliated columnar or cuboidal epithelium which may become flattened under pressure. Paraphyseal cyst and neuroepithelial cyst are synonyms (Zülch 1979).

75.6.1 Epidemiology

Incidence
- 0.5–1% of all intracranial tumors
- 18% of tumors affecting the third ventricle

Age Incidence
- Young
- Middle age
- 4–5 decade

Sex Incidence
- Male > female

Localization
- Third ventricle
- Foramen of Monro

75.6.2 Neuroimaging Findings

General Imaging Findings
- Well-defined, round mass, located at the foramen of Monro, hydrocephalus rare

CT non-contrast-enhanced (Fig. 75.12a)
- Hyperdense rarely iso- to hypodense
- Calcifications and hemorrhage possible

CT contrast-enhanced
- No enhancement
- Rarely rim enhancement

MRI-T2 (Fig. 75.12b, c)
- Variable, isointense to CSF

MRI-FLAIR (Fig. 75.12d)
- Hyperintense to CSF

MRI-T1 (Fig. 75.12e)
- Depends on cyst content
- Hyperintense to CSF
- Rarely isointense

MRI-T1 Contrast-Enhanced (Fig. 75.12f, g)
- Usually no enhancement
- Rim enhancement rare

MRI-T2∗/SWI
- Calcifications and hemorrhage described

MR-Diffusion Imaging (Fig. 75.12h)
- No diffusion restriction

MRI-Perfusion
- No elevation of rCBV

75.6.3 Neuropatholog Findings

Macroscopic Features (Fig. 75.13a–c)
- 1–3 cm in diameter
- Unilocular
- Grape-like structure
- Smooth, thin, membranous capsule
- Colloid contents

Microscopic Features (Fig. 75.14a–j)
- Lined by flattened cuboidal or low columnar cells
- Only one cell layer thick
- Stratification possible
- Ciliated cells present
- Goblet cells
- Rest on a collagenous layer of varying thickness
- Colloid, gelatinous contents
- Calcospherites
- Focal chronic inflammation

Immunophenotype (Fig. 75.14k, l)
- A list of antibodies with positive or negative immunostaining results is given in Table 75.2.

Proliferation Markers
- Very low

75.6 Colloid Cyst of the Third Ventricle

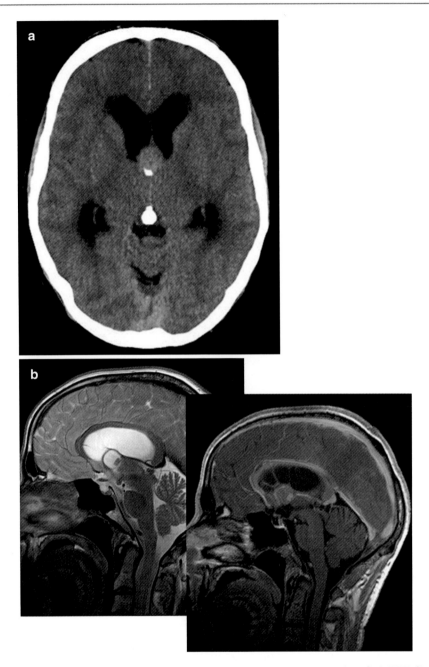

Fig. 75.12 Colloid cyst on CT (**a**), T2 sag (**b**), T2 (**c**), FLAIR (**d**), T1 (**e**), T1 contrast ax/sag (**f, g**), DWI (**h**), 3D Ciss (**i**)

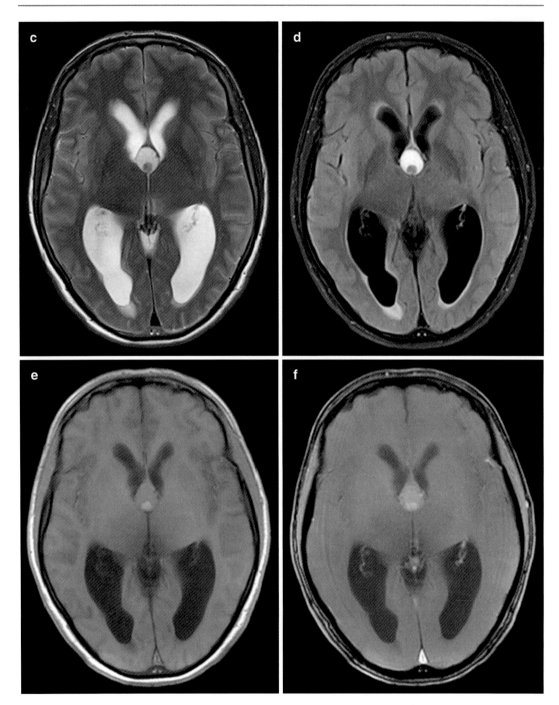

Fig. 75.12 (continued)

75.6 Colloid Cyst of the Third Ventricle

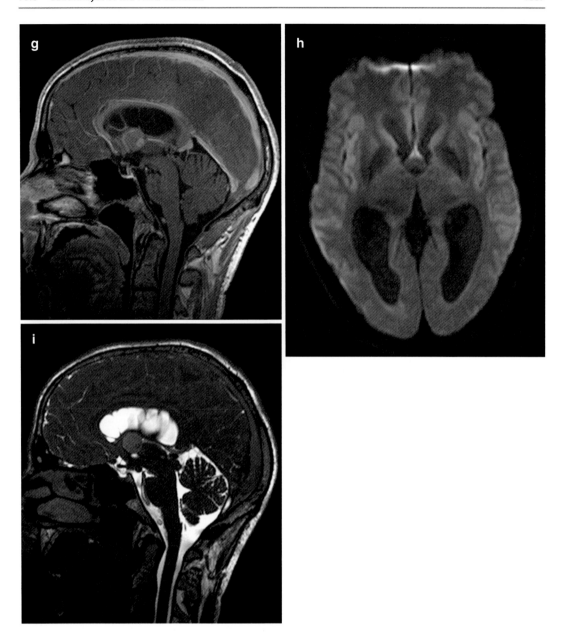

Fig. 75.12 (continued)

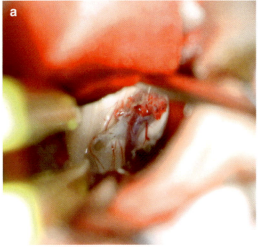
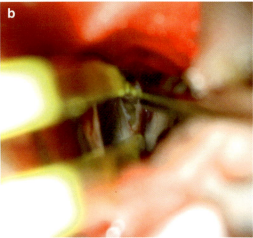
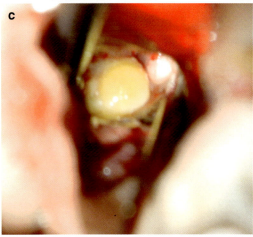

Fig. 75.13 Colloid cyst: Intraoperative appearance of the cyst wall (whitish) (**a**), the opened cyst wall (**b**), and the yellowish cyst content (**c**)

Ultrastructural Features
- Various distinct cell types are recognized:
  - ciliated cells with occasional abnormal cilia
  - non-ciliated cells with microvilli coated with granulofibrillary material
  - goblet cells showing discharge of secretory granules
  - basal cells with prominent tonofilaments and desmosomes
  - basal-located cells with elongated electron-lucent cytoplasm and scattered membrane-bound dense core granules (150–350 nm)
  - small undifferentiated cells with scanty organelles
- Junctional complexes were present in the first four cell types and absent in the other two cell types.
- The types of epithelial cells and their topographic distribution within the epithelium are both very similar to those of normal respiratory epithelium.

Differential Diagnosis
- Epidermoid cyst
- Dermoid cyst
- Craniopharyngioma
- Rathke's cleft cyst

75.6.4 Molecular Neuropathology

- Originate from persisting embryological remnants
- Unclear if of endodermal or neuroglial origin

75.6.5 Treatment and Prognosis

Treatment
- Surgery

Biologic Behavior–Prognosis–Prognostic Factors
- Good outcome
- Seldom recurrences

75.6 Colloid Cyst of the Third Ventricle

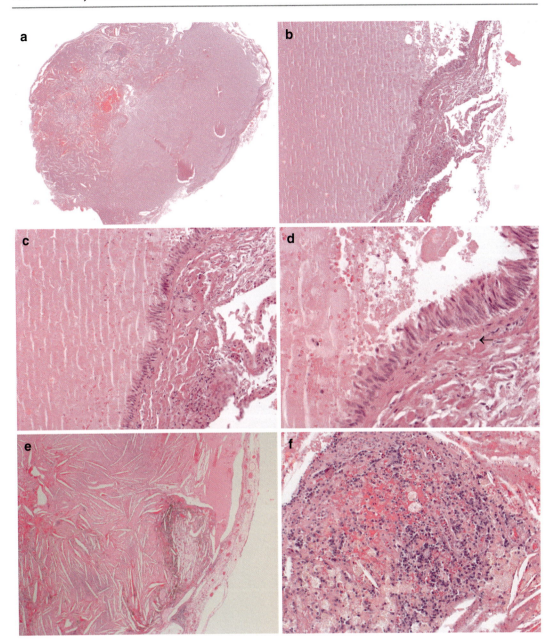

Fig. 75.14 The colloid, gelatinous contents are lined by flattened cuboidal or low columnar cells (arrow) (**a–d**). Cellular debris is surrounded by mononuclear cells (**e, f**) and macrophages (**g, h**) representing focal chronic inflammation. The cuboidal cells rest on a collagenous layer of varying thickness (arrow) (**d**). The cellular debris is partly PAS-positive (**i, j**). The cuboidal cells are immunopositive for pancytokeratin AE1/AE3 (**k, l**)

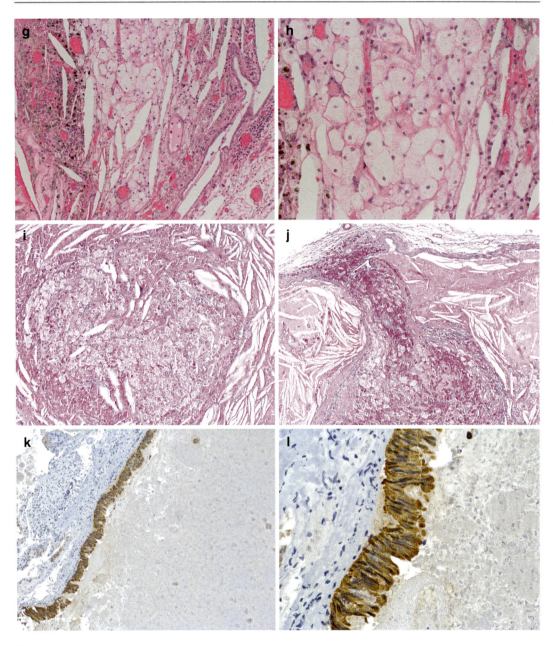

Fig. 75.14 (continued)

Table 75.2 Immunophenotype of a colloid cyst of the third ventricle

IHC-positivity	IHC-negativity
• EMA • Cytokeratins	• GFAP

75.7 Enterogeneous cyst

WHO Definition
1993—A cyst lined by mucin-secreting and/or ciliated, cuboidal to columnar epithelium resembling that of the respiratory and intestinal tract (Kleihues et al. 1993).

1979—A cyst lined by mucin-secreting epithelium, resembling that of the gastrointestinal tract. These cysts are usually intraspinal (Zülch 1979).

75.7.1 Epidemiology

Incidence
- Rare

Age Incidence
- Birth to fifth decade

Sex Incidence
- M > F

Localization
- Spinal canal
- Intradural extramedullary

75.7.2 Neuroimaging Findings

General Imaging Findings
- Well-demarcated extra-axial cyst, bright in T2 and Flair, more often in spine

CT non-contrast-enhanced
- Iso- to hyperdense compared to CSF

CT contrast-enhanced
- No enhancement

MRI-T2/FLAIR (Fig. 75.15a–c)
- Hyperintense compared to CSF

MRI-T1 (Fig. 75.15d)
- CSF-isointense, slightly hyperintense

MRI-T1 Contrast-Enhanced (Fig. 75.15e)
- No enhancement

MRI-T2∗/SWI
- No calcification or hemorrhage

MR-Diffusion Imaging (Fig. 75.15f)
- No diffusion restriction

MRI-Perfusion
- No elevation of rCBV

75.7.3 Neuropathology Findings

Macroscopic Features
- Transparent, thin-walled, smooth rounded structure
- Can compress the spinal cord
- Focal thickening possible
- Contain clear colorless fluid

Microscopic Features (Fig. 75.16a–f)
- Simple, low, or high columnar epithelium
- Frequently ciliated
- Cytoplasm positive for mucin stains (PAS diastase, Alcian blue, mucicarmine)
- Interspersed goblet cells
- Stratification or pseudostratification possible resembling adult respiratory tract epithelium
- Focal non-keratinizing squamous metaplasia
- Rests on a thin outer layer of sparsely cellular collagen

Immunophenotype (Fig. 75.16g, h)
- Positive for:
  – Cytokeratins
  – EMA

Proliferation Markers
- Nil to very low

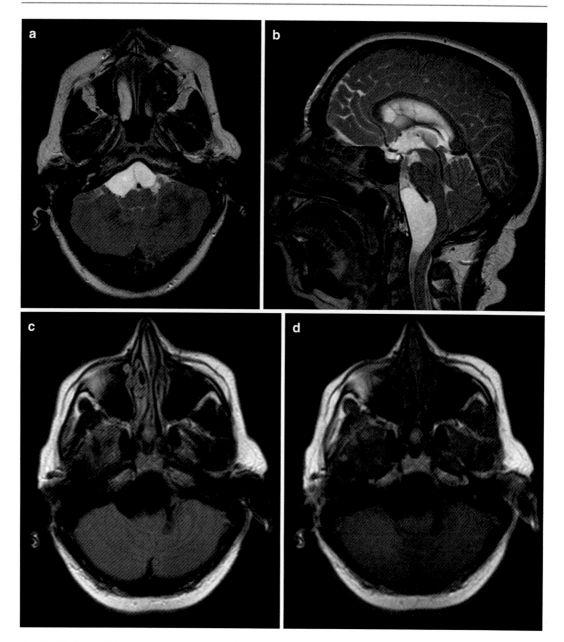

Fig. 75.15 Premedullary enterogeneous cyst: T2 (**a**), T2 sag (**b**), FLAIR (**c**), T1 (**d**), T1 contrast (**e**), DWI (**f**)

75.7 Enterogeneous cyst

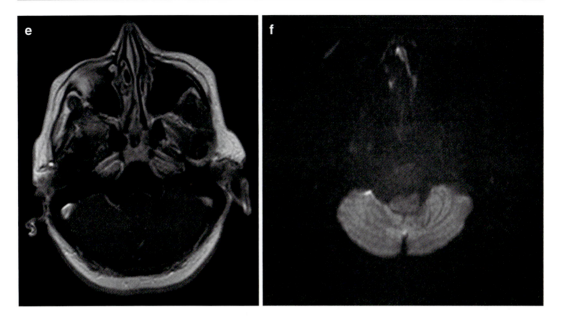

Fig. 75.15 (continued)

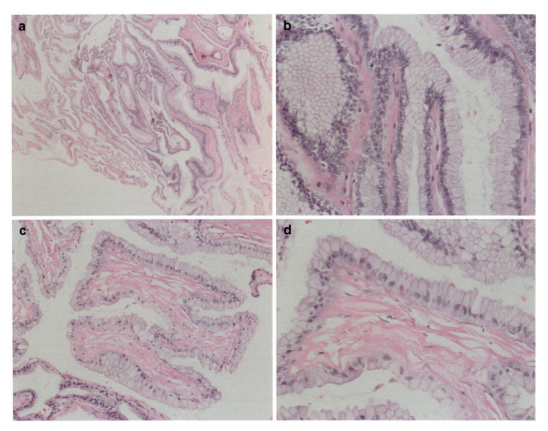

Fig. 75.16 Enterogeneous cyst: The cyst forms palisades made up of simple, low, or high columnar epithelium (**a–d**). The cytoplasm is positive for PAS (**e, f**). The basal parts of the epithelial cells are immunopositive for pancytokeratin AE1/AE3 (**g, h**)

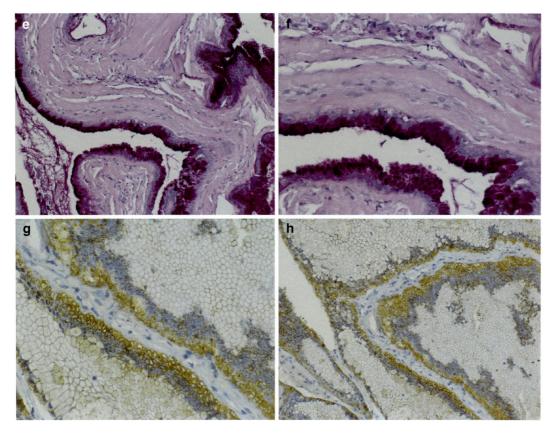

Fig. 75.16 (continued)

Ultrastructural Features
- Epithelial cells with abundant cilia protruding from their apical surface
- Microvilli coated by a layer of electron-dense material
- Membrane-bound secretory granules
- Cytoplasmic interdigitations
- Basement membrane separates epithelial layer from underlying collagen

Differential Diagnosis
- Teratoma
- Dermoid and epidermoid cysts
- Neuroglial cysts
- Arachnoid cyst

75.7.4 Molecular Neuropathology

- Anomalous embryological connection between the primitive foregut and the developing neural tube
- Associated with vertebral malformations

75.7.5 Treatment and Prognosis

Treatment
- Surgical excision

Biologic Behavior–Prognosis–Prognostic Factors
- Benign
- Potentially curable

75.8 Arachnoidal Cyst

75.8.1 Epidemiology

Incidence
- Rare

Age Incidence
- Young age

Sex Incidence
- M > F

Localization
- Supratentorial (2/3 of cases)
- Sylvian fissure
- Parasagittal convexity of a cerebral hemisphere
- Posterior fossa
- Spine
- Intra- or extradural

75.8.2 Neuroimaging Findings

General Imaging Findings
- Extra-axial, CSF-isointense cyst

CT non-contrast-enhanced (Fig. 75.17a)
- CSF isodense
- Hemorrhages rare
- Thinning of adjacent bone

CT contrast-enhanced
- No enhancement

MRI-T2 (Fig. 75.17b–d)
- CSF-isointense

MRI-FLAIR (Fig. 75.17e)
- CSF-isointense

MRI-T1 (Fig. 75.17f)
- CSF-isointense

MRI-T2∗/SWI
- Hemorrhages rare

MRI-T1 Contrast-Enhanced (Fig. 75.17g)
- No enhancement

MR-Diffusion Imaging (Fig. 75.17h)
- No diffusion restriction

MRI-Perfusion
- No elevation of rCBV

Nuclear Medicine Imaging Findings (Fig. 75.18)
- Hypometabolism in FDG-PET

75.8.3 Neuropathology Findings

Macroscopic Features (Fig. 75.19a–f)
- Rounded sac-like structure filled with clear fluid resembling CSF
- Thin and transparent wall with smooth surface
- Can reach 10 cm in diameter

Microscopic Features (Fig. 75.20a–d)
- Flattened arachnoidal cells
- Rest on a thin, vascularized collagenous membrane
- Indistinguishable from normal leptomeningeal membrane
- Arachnoidal cell whorls
- Psammoma bodies
- No evidence of old hemorrhage
- No evidence of inflammatory infiltrates

Immunophenotype (Fig. 75.20e–h)
- Positive for EMA

Proliferation Markers
- Low

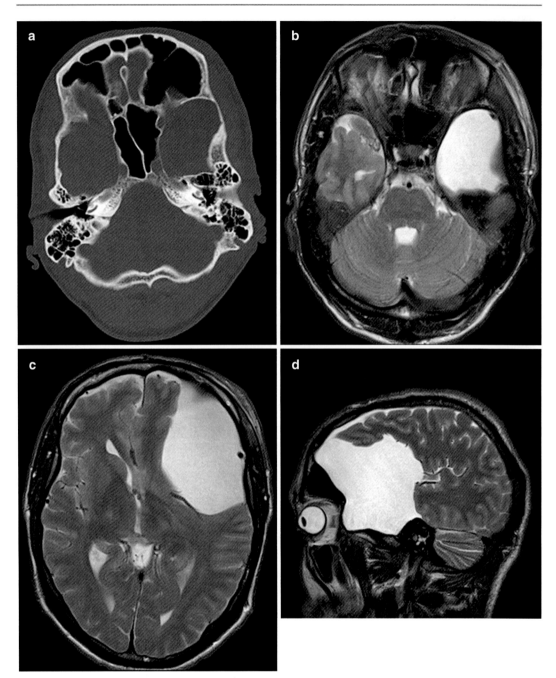

Fig. 75.17 Arachnoidal cyst left temporal: CT demonstrates thinning of temporal bone (**a**), T2 (**b**, **c**), T2 sag (**d**), FLAIR (**e**), T1 (**f**), T1 contrast (**g**), DWI (**h**)

75.8 Arachnoidal Cyst cyst

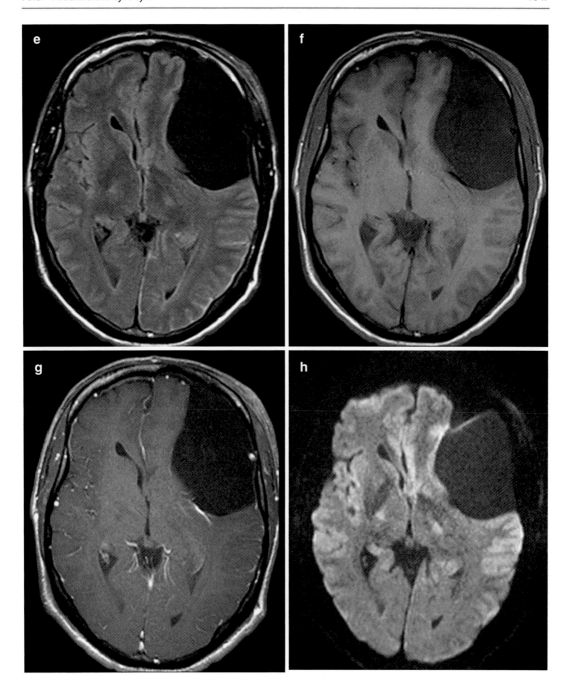

Fig. 75.17 (continued)

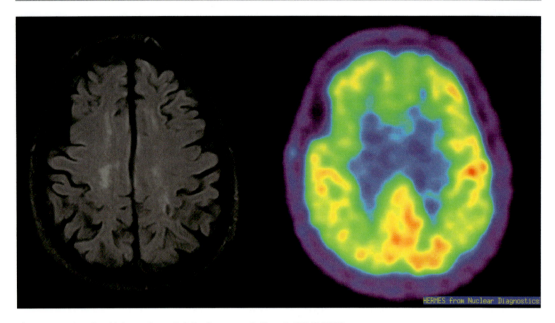

Fig. 75.18 Arachnoidal cyst frontal right (hypometabolism in FDG-PET)

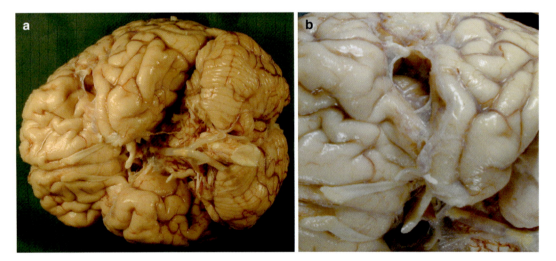

Fig. 75.19 Arachnoidal cysts: macroscopical appearances, (**a**, **b**) small cyst fronto-orbital left, (**c**, **d**) large cyst covering the whole left frontal lobe, (**e**, **f**) large cyst covering the left frontal lobe and central region extending into the lateral sulcus

75.8 Arachnoidal Cyst cyst

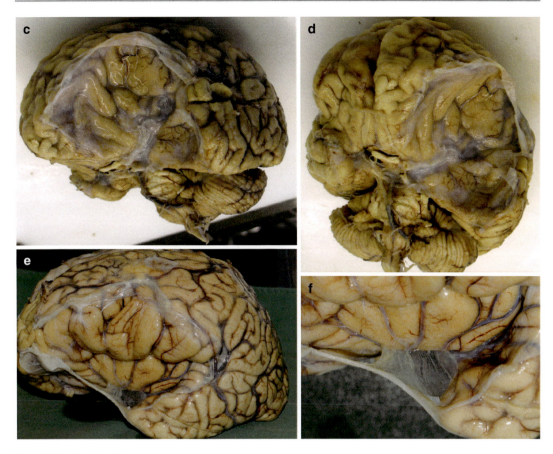

Fig. 75.19 (continued)

Ultrastructural Features
- Arachnoidal cell type
- Abundant intermediate type cytoplasmic filaments
- Desmosomes

Differential Diagnosis
- Porencephalic defect
- Subdural hygroma
- Dandy-Walker syndrome cyst
- Neuroglial cyst
- Rathke's cyst
- Enterogeneous cyst

75.8.4 Molecular Neuropathology

- Results from the focal splitting of the arachnoid membrane

75.8.5 Treatment and Prognosis

Treatment
- Surgical excision

Biologic Behavior–Prognosis–Prognostic Factors
- Contents may reaccumulate after simple aspiration.

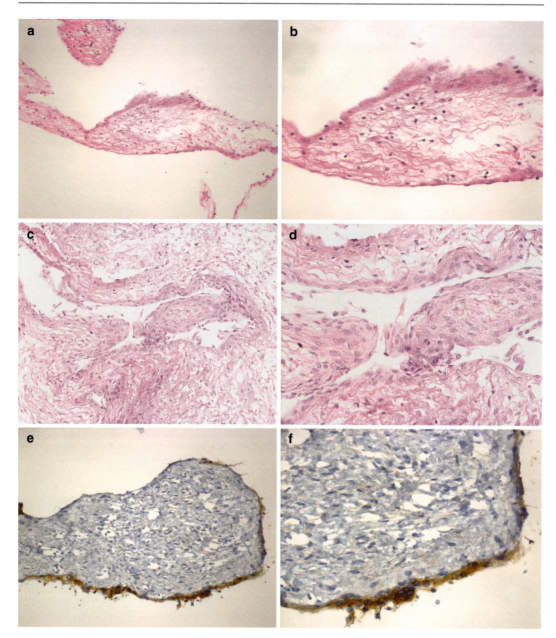

Fig. 75.20 Arachnoidal cyst: Flattened arachnoidal cells rest on a thin (**a**, **b**) to large (**c**, **d**) vascularized collagenous membrane/tissue. The arachnoidal cells stain-positive for EMA (**e–h**)

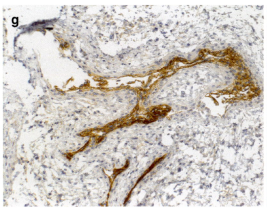
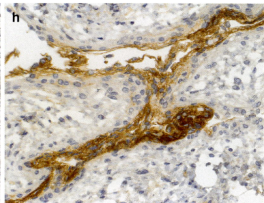

Fig. 75.20 (continued)

Selected References

Armao D, Castillo M, Chen H, Kwock L (2000) Colloid cyst of the third ventricle: imaging-pathologic correlation. AJNR Am J Neuroradiol 21(8):1470–1477

Awaji M, Okamoto K, Nishiyama K (2007) Magnetic resonance cisternography for preoperative evaluation of arachnoid cysts. Neuroradiology 49(9):721–726. https://doi.org/10.1007/s00234-007-0248-7

Bhatia R, Anderson S, Bradley V, Akinwunmi JA (2008) Neuropsychological profiling of ischemic deficit secondary to ruptured dermoid cyst: a case report. Appl Neuropsychol 15(4):293–297. https://doi.org/10.1080/09084280802312478

Bhatoe HS, Mukherji JD, Dutta V (2006) Epidermoid tumour of the lateral ventricle. Acta Neurochir 148(3):339–342;. , discussion 342. https://doi.org/10.1007/s00701-005-0678-0

Byun WM, Kim OL, Kim D (2000) MR imaging findings of Rathke's cleft cysts: significance of intracystic nodules. AJNR Am J Neuroradiol 21(3):485–488

Christov C, Chretien F, Brugieres P, Djindjian M (2004) Giant supratentorial enterogenous cyst: report of a case, literature review, and discussion of pathogenesis. Neurosurgery 54(3):759–763. discussion 763

Chung LK, Beckett JS, Ong V, Lagman C, Nagasawa DT, Yang I, Kim W (2017) Predictors of outcomes in fourth ventricular epidermoid cysts: a case report and a review of literature. World Neurosurg 105:689–696. https://doi.org/10.1016/j.wneu.2017.06.037

Cobbs CS, Pitts LH, Wilson CB (1997) Epidermoid and dermoid cysts of the posterior fossa. Clin Neurosurg 44:511–528

El-Bahy K, Kotb A, Galal A, El-Hakim A (2006) Ruptured intracranial dermoid cysts. Acta Neurochir 148(4):457–462. https://doi.org/10.1007/s00701-005-0722-0

Eyselbergs M, Cheecharoen P, Bali A, Venstermans C, De Belder F, Ozsarlak O, Van Goethem J, Menovsky T, Lammens M, Vanhoenacker F, Parizel PM (2015) Arachnoidal cyst arising from the oculomotor cistern. JBR-BTR: organe de la Societe royale belge de radiologie (SRBR) = orgaan van de Koninklijke Belgische Vereniging voor Radiologie (KBVR) 98(1):54

Gabelic T, Klepac N, Mubrin Z, Ozretic D, Habek M (2009) Giant arachnoidal cyst. Acta Neurol Belg 109(3):244

Hu XY, Hu CH, Fang XM, Cui L, Zhang QH (2008) Intraparenchymal epidermoid cysts in the brain: diagnostic value of MR diffusion-weighted imaging. Clin Radiol 63(7):813–818. https://doi.org/10.1016/j.crad.2008.01.008

Kaido T, Okazaki A, Kurokawa S, Tsukamoto M (2003) Pathogenesis of intraparenchymal epidermoid cyst in the brain: a case report and review of the literature. Surg Neurol 59(3):211–216

Kavar B, Kaye AH (2011) Dermoid, epidermoid, and neurenteric cysts. In: Kaye AH, Laws ER (eds) Brain tumors, 3rd edn. Elsevier, New York, pp 831–848

Khandelwal N, Malik N, Khosla VK, Radotra B (1993) Intramedullary enterogenous cyst. Australas Radiol 37(3):272–273

Kleihues P, Burger PC, Scheithauer BW (1993) Histological typing of tumours of the central nervous system, 2nd edn. Springer, Berlin

Krishnamurthy G, Roopesh Kumar VR, Rajeswaran R, Rao S (2010) Supratentorial enterogenous cyst: a report of two cases and review of literature. Neurol India 58(5):774–777. https://doi.org/10.4103/0028-3886.72200

Lavrador JP, Brogna C, Vergani F, Hasegawa H, Aizpurua M, Bhangoo R (2017) Third-ventricle enterogenous cyst presentation mimicking a colloid cyst: uncommon presentation of a rare disease and literature review. Acta Neurochir 159(3):465–468. https://doi.org/10.1007/s00701-016-3052-5

Li ZJ, Miao YX, Sun P, Li YJ, Dou YH, Xu J, Chen X, Jiang YX (2011) Unusual CT hyperattenuating dermoid cyst of cerebellum: a new case report and literature review. Cerebellum (London, England) 10(3):536–539. https://doi.org/10.1007/s12311-011-0268-z

Liu JK, Gottfried ON, Salzman KL, Schmidt RH, Couldwell WT (2008) Ruptured intracranial dermoid cysts: clinical, radiographic, and surgical features. Neurosurgery 62(2):377–384.; , discussion 384. https://doi.org/10.1227/01.neu.0000316004.88517.29

Marshman LA, Chawda SJ, David KM (2004) Change in CT radiodensity of a colloid cyst of the third ventricle: case report and literature review. Neuroradiology 46(12):984–987. https://doi.org/10.1007/s00234-004-1303-2

Mortini P, Bailo M, Spina A, Acerno S, Boari N, Gagliardi F (2016) Cyst-cisternal shunting for cystic multirecurrent brainstem epidermoid: case report and literature review. Acta Neurochir 158(6):1197–1201. https://doi.org/10.1007/s00701-016-2813-5

Nagasawa D, Yew A, Safaee M, Fong B, Gopen Q, Parsa AT, Yang I (2011) Clinical characteristics and diagnostic imaging of epidermoid tumors. J Clin Neurosci 18(9):1158–1162. https://doi.org/10.1016/j.jocn.2011.02.008

Nguyen JB, Ahktar N, Delgado PN, Lowe LH (2004) Magnetic resonance imaging and proton magnetic resonance spectroscopy of intracranial epidermoid tumors. Crit Rev Comput Tomogr 45(5–6):389–427

Orakcioglu B, Halatsch ME, Fortunati M, Unterberg A, Yonekawa Y (2008) Intracranial dermoid cysts: variations of radiological and clinical features. Acta Neurochir 150(12):1227–1234;. discussion 1234. https://doi.org/10.1007/s00701-008-0152-x

Osborn AG, Preece MT (2006) Intracranial cysts: radiologic-pathologic correlation and imaging approach. Radiology 239(3):650–664. https://doi.org/10.1148/radiol.2393050823

Ozutemiz C, Ada E, Ersen A, Ozer E (2017) Imaging findings of an epidermoid cyst with malignant transformation to squamous cell carcinoma. Turk Neurosurg 27(2):312–315. https://doi.org/10.5137/1019-5149.jtn.12722-14.0

Park JK, Lee EJ, Kim SH (2012) Optimal surgical approaches for Rathke cleft cyst with consideration of endocrine function. Neurosurgery 70(2 suppl Operative):250–256.; , discussion 256–257. https://doi.org/10.1227/NEU.0b013e3182418034

Patibandla MR, Yerramneni VK, Mudumba VS, Manisha N, Addagada GC (2016) Brainstem epidermoid cyst: an update. Asian J Neurosurg 11(3):194–200. https://doi.org/10.4103/1793-5482.145163

Peeters SM, Daou B, Jabbour P, Ladoux A, Abi Lahoud G (2016) Spontaneous regression of a third ventricle colloid cyst. World Neurosurg 90:704.e719–704.e722. https://doi.org/10.1016/j.wneu.2016.02.116

Pikis S, Margolin E (2016) Malignant transformation of a residual cerebellopontine angle epidermoid cyst. J Clin Neurosci 33:59–62. https://doi.org/10.1016/j.jocn.2016.04.008

Preece MT, Osborn AG, Chin SS, Smirniotopoulos JG (2006) Intracranial neurenteric cysts: imaging and pathology spectrum. AJNR Am J Neuroradiol 27(6):1211–1216

Rao VJ, James RA, Mitra D (2008) Imaging characteristics of common suprasellar lesions with emphasis on MRI findings. Clin Radiol 63(8):939–947. https://doi.org/10.1016/j.crad.2007.10.003

Ren X, Lin S, Wang Z, Luo L, Jiang Z, Sui D, Bi Z, Cui Y, Jia W, Zhang Y, Yu L, Chen S (2012) Clinical, radiological, and pathological features of 24 atypical intracranial epidermoid cysts. J Neurosurg 116(3):611–621. https://doi.org/10.3171/2011.10.jns111462

Sanchez-Mejia RO, Limbo M, Tihan T, Galvez MG, Woodward MV, Gupta N (2006) Intracranial dermoid cyst mimicking hemorrhage. Case report and review of the literature. J Neurosurg 105(4 Suppl):311–314. https://doi.org/10.3171/ped.2006.105.4.311

Schneider UC, Koch A, Stenzel W, Thomale UW (2012) Intracranial, supratentorial dermoid cysts in paediatric patients—two cases and a review of the literature. Childs Nerv Syst 28(2):185–190. https://doi.org/10.1007/s00381-011-1646-z

Shetty DS, Lakhkar BN (2000) Cervico-dorsal spinal enterogenous cyst. Indian J Pediatr 67(4):304–306

Spears RC (2004) Colloid cyst headache. Curr Pain Headache Rep 8(4):297–300

Stendel R, Pietila TA, Lehmann K, Kurth R, Suess O, Brock M (2002) Ruptured intracranial dermoid cysts. Surg Neurol 57(6):391–398, discussion 398

Turgut M (2009) Klippel-Feil syndrome in association with posterior fossa dermoid tumour. Acta Neurochir 151(3):269–276. https://doi.org/10.1007/s00701-009-0203-y

Two A, Christian E, Mathew A, Giannotta S, Zada G (2016) Giant, calcified colloid cyst of the lateral ventricle. J Clin Neurosci 24:6–9. https://doi.org/10.1016/j.jocn.2015.05.044

Urso JA, Ross GJ, Parker RK, Patrizi JD, Stewart B (1998) Colloid cyst of the third ventricle: radiologic-pathologic correlation. J Comput Assist Tomogr 22(4):524–527

van Burken MM, Sarioglu AC, O'Donnell HD (1992) Supratentorial arachnoidal cyst with intracystic and subdural haematoma. Neurochirurgia 35(6):199–203. https://doi.org/10.1055/s-2008-1052278

Vellutini EA, de Oliveira MF, Ribeiro AP, Rotta JM (2014) Malignant transformation of intracranial epidermoid cyst. Br J Neurosurg 28(4):507–509. https://doi.org/10.3109/02688697.2013.869552

Wang L, Zhang J, Wu Z, Jia G, Zhang L, Hao S, Geng S (2011) Diagnosis and management of adult intracranial neurenteric cysts. Neurosurgery 68(1):44–52;. discussion 52. https://doi.org/10.1227/NEU.0b013e3181fc5ee0

Werder EA, Haertel M, Bekier A, Weber JR, Siegfried J (1984) Suprasellar arachnoidal cyst as a cause of early puberty. Helv Paediatr Acta 39(3):261–264

Yadav YR, Yadav N, Parihar V, Kher Y, Ratre S (2015) Management of colloid cyst of third ventricle. Turk Neurosurg 25(3):362–371. https://doi.org/10.5137/1019-5149.jtn.11086-14.1

Zada G (2011) Rathke cleft cysts: a review of clinical and surgical management. Neurosurg Focus 31(1):E1. https://doi.org/10.3171/2011.5.focus1183

Zara G, Ponza I, Citton V, Manara R (2010) Temporosylvian arachnoidal cyst and an extreme pneumatization of the cranial sinuses: a case report. Clin Neurol Neurosurg 112(9):821–823. https://doi.org/10.1016/j.clineuro.2010.06.015

Zülch KJ (1979) Histological typing of tumours of the central nervous system. World Health Organization, Geneva

Germ Cell Tumors

WHO Definition

2016—In the CNS, the morphological, immunophenotypic, and (in some respects) genetic homologs of gonadal and other extraneuraxial germ cell neoplasms (Rosenblum et al. 2016).

2007—Morphological and immunophenotypic homologs of gonadal and other extraneuraxial germ cell tumors (Rosenblum et al. 2007).

2000—Morphological homologs of germinal neoplasms arising in the gonads and in other extragonadal sites (Rosenblum et al. 2000).

1993—The classification and features of these tumors are the same as are described in the WHO Histological Typing of Testis Tumours (Zülch 1979).

76.1 General Aspects

Classification of germ cell tumors into the following types:

- Germinoma
- Yolk sac tumor
- Embryonal carcinoma
- Choriocarcinoma
- Teratoma
  - Mature teratoma
  - Immature teratoma
  - Teratoma with malignant transformation
- Mixed germ cell tumors
  - Harbor multiple types

76.1.1 Epidemiology

Incidence
- 2–3% of all primary intracranial tumors
- 8–15% of pediatric intracranial tumors
- Most prevalent in far-east Asia
  - Japan: 0.17 cases per 100,000 person-years
  - USA: 0.09 per 100,000 person-years

Age Incidence
- Patients under 25 years of age
- Mean age: 10–14 years

Sex Incidence
- M > F 3:1
- M:F ratio varies with tumor localization and histology

Localization
- Affect midline structures
  - Third ventricle
  - Pineal gland
  - Suprasellar compartment
- Other regions possible

76.1.2 Nuclear Medicine Imaging Findings

- Only case reports are available at the moment on germ cell tumors. They are mainly found in studies dealing with brain tumors whereby histology revealed germ cell tumor.
- Case reports state that
  - Germinomas are FDG, FET, and FLT-positive
  - Teratoma: altered brain perfusion SPECT (mainly due to the disrupted blood–brain barrier), and defect in brain perfusion SPECT.
  - Malignant teratoma: Tl201-positive.

76.1.3 Immunophenotype (Tables 76.1 and 76.2)

Antibodies used:
- PLAP—Placenta-like alkaline phosphatase
  - A membrane-bound enzyme of 120 kDa
  - Synthesized by placental syncytiotrophoblast
  - Produced by many neoplasms
- AFP—α-fetoprotein
  - Normally produced by fetal yolk sac, liver, and gastrointestinal epithelium
- β-HCG—Human chorionic gonadotrophin
  - A 37 kDa glycoprotein
  - Synthetized by benign and malignant syncytiotrophoblasts
  - Important diagnostic, staging, therapeutic monitoring, and follow-up serum marker
- HPL—Human placental lactogen
  - A 22-kDA protein with partial homology to growth hormone
  - Secreted by syncytiotrophoblasts
- c-kit
  - Transmembrane glycoprotein receptor tyrosine kinase
  - Role in survival of germ cells, and other cells
- Oct-4
  - Stem cell transcription regulator
  - Maintains pluripotency in embryonic stem cells and germ cells
- NANOG
  - Stemness factor

Table 76.1 The immunohistochemical profile of germinal cell tumors

	PLAP	AFP	β-HCG	HPL	AE1/AE3	c-kit	EMA	CD30
Germinoma	+++ M/C	–	–	–	± C	++++ M	–	–
Embryonal carcinoma	++ M/C	±	–	–	++ C	± C	± M	++++ M/C
Yolk sac tumor	±	++++ C	–	–	+++ C	± C	–	–
Choriocarcinoma	±	–	+++ C	+++ C	+++ C	–	+++	–
Mature teratoma	±	±	–	–	+++ C	–	+++ M	–
Immature teratoma	–	–	±	–	–	±	–	–

M membranous, *C* cytoplasmic

Table 76.2 The immunohistochemical profile of transcription factors and podoplanin in germinal cell tumors

	Transcription factors				Podoplanin	
	OCT4	NANOG	AP-2γ	SOX2	D2–40	YM-1
Germinoma	+++ N	+++ N	+++ N	–	++++ M	++++ M
Embryonal carcinoma	+++ N	+++ N	+++ N	++++ N	± C	–
Yolk sac tumor	–	–	–	–	–	–
Choriocarcinoma	–	–	–	–	–	–
Mature teratoma	–	–	–	± N	–	–
Immature teratoma	–	–	–	++++ N	–	+ M

M membranous, *C* cytoplasmic, *N* nuclear

76.1 General Aspects

- Determines cell fate in both embryonic and cancer stem cells
- Activated Nanog results in cancer stem cells rather than normal pluripotent stem cells or differentiated somatic cells
- Regulates tumor cell proliferation, self-renewal, motility, epithelial–mesenchymal transition, immune evasion, and drug resistance
- Activator protein-2γ (Ap-2γ)
  - Nuclear transcription factor
  - Involved in embryonic morphogenesis
  - Functionally related to c-kit and PLAP
- Podoplanin
  - Onco-fetal transmembrane mucoprotein
  - Expressed by fetal germ cells and testicular GCTs

- Displaced embryonic tissues misincorporated in the developing neural tube
  - Germinoma is derived from misrouted primordial germ cells.
  - Choriocarcinoma arises from misplaced trophoblast.
  - Yolk sac tumor arises from malpositioned elements of the secondary yolk sac proper.
  - Embryonal carcinoma is derived from primitive constituents of the trophoblastic embryo.
  - Teratoma is derived from differentiating tissues of the later embryonic period.
- Toti- or pluripotent stem cells with selective genetic programming along germ cell differentiation and subsequent neoplastic transformation

76.1.4 Differential Diagnosis

- Germinoma
- Embryonal carcinoma
- Yolk sac tumor
- Choriocarcinoma
- Teratoma
- Gliomas
- Lymphoma
- Sarcoidosis
- Infection
- Metastatic carcinoma

76.1.5 Molecular Neuropathology

- Elevated circulating gonadotropin levels (tumors localized to diencephalic centers regulating gonadal activity)
- Chromosome X overdosage (increased incidence of tumors in Klinefelter syndrome)
- Neoplastic offspring of primordial germ cells that migrate in aberrant fashion or home to the embryonic CNS rather than the developing genital ridges

76.1.6 Treatment and Prognosis

Treatment
- Surgical resection
- Adjuvant chemotherapy
- Radiotherapy
  - germinoma

Biologic Behavior–Prognosis–Prognostic Factors
- Germinoma
  - less malignant than choriocarcinoma
  - prone to recurrence
  - remarkably radiosensitive
  - 10-year survival rate 85%
- Immature teratomas
  - might undergo spontaneous differentiation into fully mature, somatic-type tissues over time
- Mature teratoma
  - potentially curable
- Poor prognosis
  - Yolk sac tumor, embryonal carcinoma, choriocarcinoma
- Disease progression characterized by:
  - Local recurrence
  - CSF-borne dissemination

76.2 Germinoma

WHO Definition

2016—A malignant germ cell tumor histologically characterized by the presence of large primordial germ cells with prominent nucleoli and variable cytoplasmic clearing (Rosenblum et al. 2016).

2007—The pure germinoma, the most common CNS germ cell tumor, is populated by large cells that appear undifferentiated and that resemble primordial germinal elements (of which, in theory, they present the neoplastic counterparts) (Rosenblum et al. 2007).

2000—The tumor is composed of uniform cells resembling primitive germ cells, with large, vesicular nuclei, prominent nucleoli and a clear, glycogen-rich cytoplasm (Rosenblum et al. 2000).

1993—Histopathologically identical to the testicular seminoma, the germinoma is composed of uniform cells resembling primitive germ cells (Kleihues et al. 1993).

1979—A tumor composed of large primitive, spheroidal cells indistinguishable from the testicular seminoma and ovarian dysgerminoma. Lymphoid cells are a prominent feature in its stroma. Fibrous and granulomatous reactions, including multinucleated giant cells, may be found (Zülch 1979).

76.2.1 Neuroimaging Findings

General Imaging Findings
- Well-defined, enhancing mass, most common site is the pineal region, hydrocephalus und CSF spreading possible

CT non-contrast-enhanced (Fig. 76.1a)
- Hyperdense mass

CT contrast-enhanced
- Strong enhancement
- Calcifications of pineal gland surrounded by tumor

MRI-T2 (Fig. 76.1b–d)
- Iso- to hyperintense
- Cysts or necrosis hyperintense

MRI-FLAIR (Fig. 76.1e)
- Hyperintense

MRI-T1 (Fig. 76.1f)
- Iso- to hyperintense

MRI-T1 Contrast-Enhanced (Fig. 76.1g, h)
- Homogeneous enhancement

MRI-T2∗/SWI
- Hemorrhages rare

MR-Diffusion Imaging (Fig. 76.1i)
- Restricted diffusion

MR-Spectroscopy
- Cho elevated
- NAA low
- Lactate peaks

76.2.2 Neuropathology Findings

Macroscopic Features
- Solid tumor
- Tan-white tissue

Microscopic Features (Fig. 76.2a–f)
- Biphasic population of
  - Larger germinoma cells
  - Mature lymphocytes
- Germinoma cells:
  - Large undifferentiated cells resembling primordial germinal elements
  - Disposed in monomorphous sheets, lobules, regimented cords, or trabeculae
  - With round vesicular and centrally positioned nuclei, prominent nucleoli
  - Discrete cell membranes
  - Relatively abundant cytoplasm, sometimes clear due to glucogen accumulation
- T-lymphocytes:
  - helper/inducer T-lymphocytes
  - cytotoxic/suppressor T-lymphocytes

76.2 Germinoma 1859

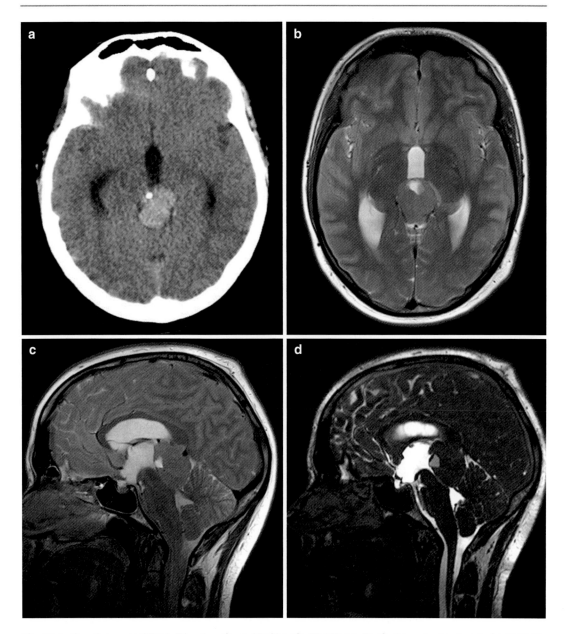

Fig. 76.1 Germinoma on CT (**a**), T2 ax/sag (**b**, **c**), 3D Ciss (**d**), FLAIR (**e**), T1 (**f**), T1 contrast ax/sag (**g**, **h**), DWI (**i**)

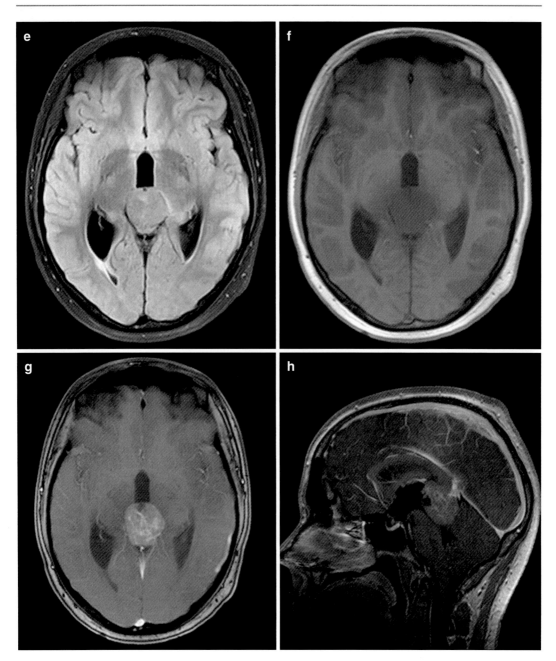

Fig. 76.1 (continued)

76.3 Yolk Sac tumor

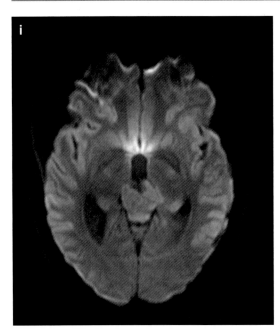

Fig. 76.1 (continued)

- Mitoses present
- Fibrovascular septae
- Granulomatous reaction (DD: sarcoidosis, tuberculosis)
- Syncytiotrophoblastic giant cells

Immunophenotype (Fig. 76.2g–j)
- Positive for:
  - C-kit (CD117)
  - OCT4 (nuclear)
  - PLAP (cytoplasmic)
  - β-HCG (syncytiotrophoblastic giant cells)
  - HPL
  - T-cell markers

Proliferation Markers
- Moderate to high

Ultrastructural Features
- Similar to testicular seminoma
- Large tumor cells 15 μm diameter
- abundant, well-defined perikaryal cytoplasm

- nuclei: large, irregularly shaped, pale chromatin
- prominent nucleoli
- scant rough endoplasmic reticulum
- abundant polyribosomes
- large mitochondria
- well-developed Golgi bodies
- lipid vacuoles
- glycogen granules

76.3 Yolk Sac tumor

WHO Definition
2016—An aggressive non-germinomatous malignant germ cell tumor composed of primitive germ cells arranged in various patterns, which can recapitulate the yolk sac, allantois, and extra-embryonic mesenchyme and produce alpha fetoprotein (Rosenblum et al. 2016).

2007—This neoplasm is composed of primitive-appearing epithelial cells—putatively representing yolk sac endoderm—set in a loose, variably cellular, and often conspicuous myxoid matrix resembling extra-embryonic mesoblast (Rosenblum et al. 2007).

2000—This neoplasm is composed of primitive-appearing epithelial cells—putatively representing yolk sac endoderm—set in a loose, variably cellular, and often conspicuously myxoid matrix resembling extra-embryonic mesoblast. Eosinophilic hyaline globules immunoreactive for AFP are a diagnostic feature (Rosenblum et al. 2000).

1993—A tumor composed of cells of primitive-appearing cells, typically growing in a loosely knit or reticular network. Tubular, papillary, and solid patterns may also be present. Eosinophilic intracytoplasmic or stromal globules containing α-fetoprotein are a diagnostic feature (Kleihues et al. 1993).

1979—No specific definition provided. Considered to be an embryonal carcinoma (Zülch 1979).

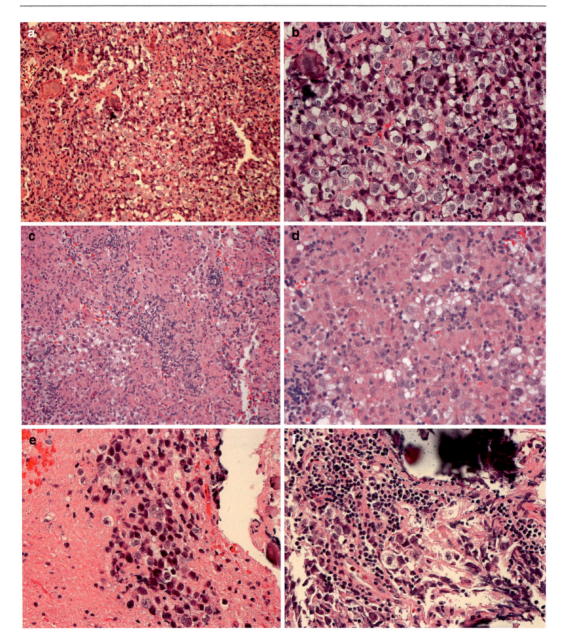

Fig. 76.2 Germinoma is made up of a biphasic population of larger germinoma cells and mature lymphocytes (**a–f**). The germinoma cells are large undifferentiated cells resembling primordial germinal elements disposed in monomorphous sheets, lobules, regimented cords, or trabeculae with round vesicular and centrally positioned nuclei, prominent nucleoli discrete cell membranes relatively abundant cytoplasm, sometimes clear due to glucogen accumulation (**a–d**). The T-lymphocytes are helper/inducer T-lymphocytes and cytotoxic/suppressor T-lymphocytes (**g–h**). Immunoprofile: positive for PLAP (**i, j**)

76.3 Yolk Sac tumor

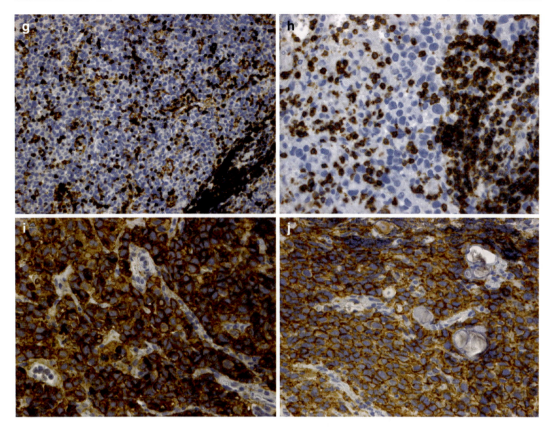

Fig. 76.2 (continued)

76.3.1 Neuropathology Findings

Macroscopic Features
- Solid tumor
- Tan-white tissue

Microscopic Features (Fig. 76.3a–f)
- primitive-appearing epithelial cells—putatively representing yolk sac endoderm
- cell arrangement in:
  - meshwork of irregular tissue spaces, i.e., reticular pattern
  - line anastomosing sinusoidal channels
  - cover delicate fibrovascular projections forming distinctive papillae, i.e., Schiller-Duval bodies
  - solid sheets
- loose, variably cellular, and often conspicuous myxoid matrix resembling extra-embryonic mesoblast
- may contain:
  - eccentrically constricted cysts delimited by flattened epithelial elements, i.e., polyvesicular vitelline pattern
  - enteric-type glands lined by goblet cells
  - hepatocellular differentiation, i.e., hepatoid variant
- bright, eosinophilic, PAS-positive, diastase-resistant hyaline globules within the cytoplasm or free in the stroma
- variable mitotic activity

Immunophenotype (Fig. 76.3g, h)
- A list of antibodies with positive or negative immunostaining results is given in Table 76.3.

Proliferation Markers
- Moderate to high

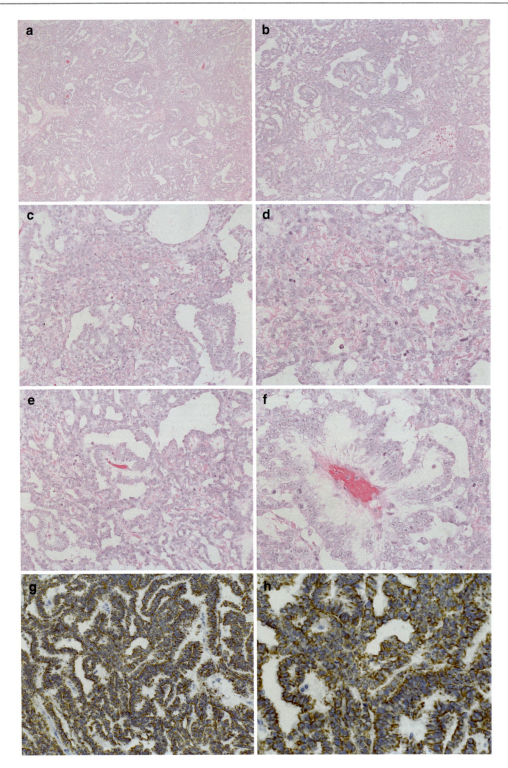

Fig. 76.3 Yolk sac tumor is composed of primitive-appearing epithelial cells, putatively representing yolk sac endoderm. The cells are arranged in a meshwork of irregular tissue spaces, i.e., reticular pattern and line anastomosing sinusoidal channels (**a–f**). They cover delicate fibrovascular projections forming distinctive papillae, i.e., Schiller-Duval bodies (**e–f**). Immunoprofile: positive for pancytokeratin AE1/AE3 (**g, h**)

Table 76.3 Immunophenotype of yolk sac tumor

Positivities	Negativities
• AFP	• C-kit
	• OCT4

Ultrastructural Features
– Glandular epithelial cells with nuclear and cytoplasmic features difficult to distinguish from the cells of Müllerian endometrioid and endometrial adenocarcinoma.
– A minor component of mucinous adenocarcinoma was confirmed as intestinal by the epithelial cells having characteristic microvilli with filamentous cores and rootlets.
– Neuroendocrine cells present in the glands and in nests with dense core granules.

76.4 Embryonal Carcinoma

WHO Definition
2016—An aggressive non-germinomatous malignant germ cell tumor characterized by large epithelioid cells resembling those of the embryonic germ disc (Rosenblum et al. 2016).
2007—The embryonal carcinoma is composed of large cells that proliferate in cohesive nests and sheets, form abortive papillae, or line irregular, gland-like spaces (Rosenblum et al. 2007).
2000—The embryonal carcinoma is composed of large cells that proliferate in cohesive nests and sheets, form abortive papillae, or line irregular, gland-like spaces (Rosenblum et al. 2000).
1993—A tumor composed of cells of primitive epithelial appearance, sometimes with clear cytoplasm, growing in a variety of patterns, including solid sheets or poorly formed glands. The tumor is highly mitotic active and often shows foci of necrosis (Kleihues et al. 1993).
1979—A tumor composed of cells of primitive epithelial appearance, often with clear cytoplasm, growing in a variety of patterns—acinar, tubular, papillary, and solid (Zülch 1979).

76.4.1 Neuroimaging Findings

General Imaging Findings
• Difficult to distinguish form other germ cell tumors

CT non-contrast-enhanced
• Iso- to hyperdense

CT contrast-enhanced
• Enhancement of solid components

MRI-T2 (Fig. 76.4a, b)
• Iso- to hyperintense solid portion

MRI-FLAIR (Fig. 76.4c)
• Hyperintense solid portion

MRI-T1 (Fig. 76.4d)
• Iso- to hypointense

MRI-T2∗/SWI
• Hemorrhages possible

MRI-T1 Contrast-Enhanced (Fig. 76.4e–g)
• Heterogeneous enhancement

MR-Diffusion Imaging
• Restriction

MR-Spectroscopy
• Cho high, NAA decreased, lactate, and lipid peaks

76.4.2 Neuropathology Findings

Macroscopic Features
• Solid tumor
• Tan-white tissue

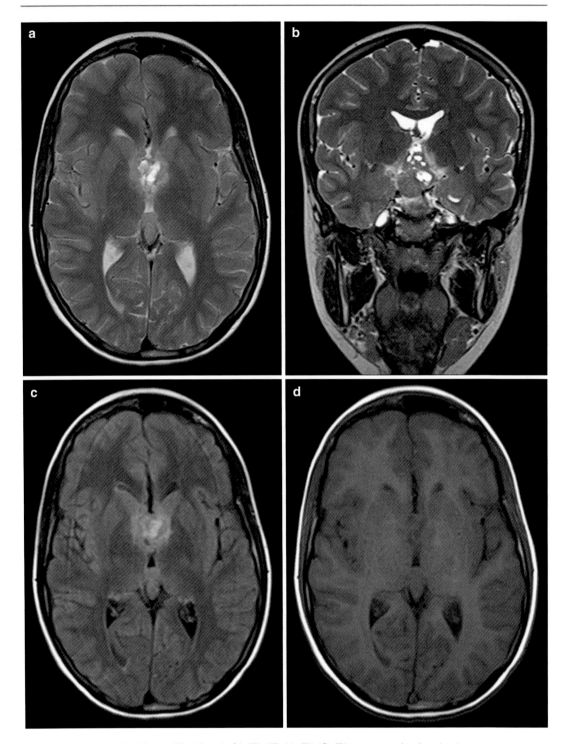

Fig. 76.4 Embryonal carcinoma T2 ax/sag (**a**, **b**), FLAIR (**c**), T1 (**d**), T1 contrast ax/cor/sag (**e–g**)

76.4 Embryonal Carcinoma

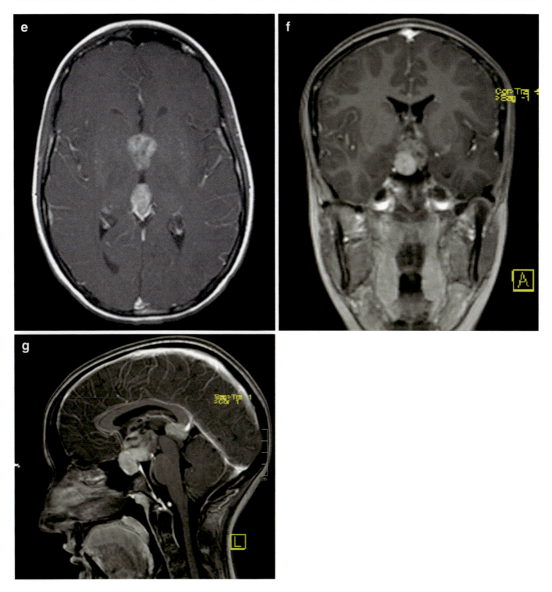

Fig. 76.4 (continued)

Microscopic Features (Fig. 76.5a–f)
- Composed of large cells with
  - enlarged nucleoli
  - abundant clear to violet cytoplasm
- Tissue pattern:
  - proliferate in cohesive nests and sheets
  - form abortive papillae
  - line irregular, gland-like spaces
- May replicate the structure of the early embryo
  - form embryoid bodies, i.e., germ discs and miniature amniotic cavities
- Pseudoglandular or pseudopapillary structures
- Mitotic rate high
- Areas of coagulative necrosis

Immunophenotype (Fig. 76.5g–l)
- A list of antibodies with positive or negative immunostaining results is given in Table 76.4.

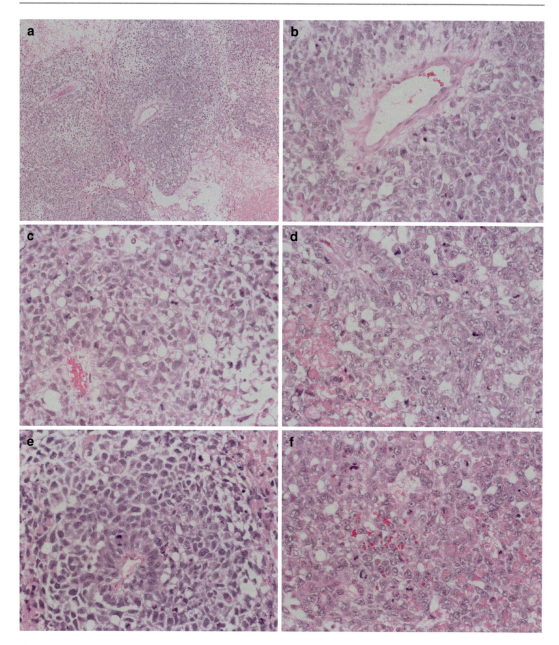

Fig. 76.5 Embryonal carcinoma is composed of large cells with enlarged nucleoli and abundant clear to violet cytoplasm (**a–f**). The tumor cells proliferate in cohesive nests and sheets, form abortive papillae, and line irregular, gland-like spaces (**a–f**). Mitotic rate is high (**d, f**). Immunoprofile: positive for PLAP (**g, h**), and pancytokeratin AE1/AE3 (**i, j**)

76.5 Choriocarcinoma

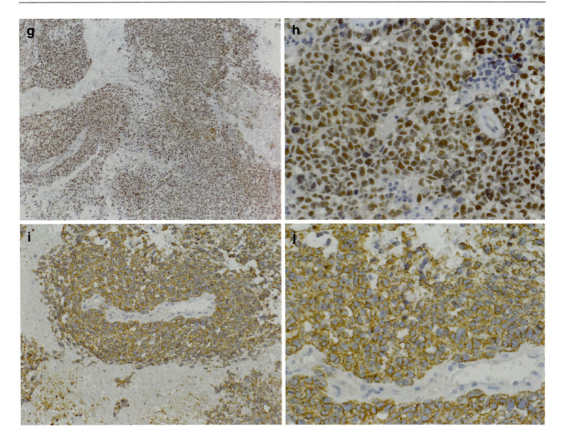

Fig. 76.5 (continued)

Table 76.4 Immunophenotype of embryonal carcinoma

Positivities	Negativities
• Cytokeratins • PLAP • OCT4	• C-kit

Ultrastructural Features
- Differentiated type:
  - The differentiated cells contain well-developed mitochondria, Golgi apparatus, rough endoplasmic reticulum, and some contained secretory granules.
- Intermediate type:
  - The intermediate cells possess dilated and irregularly shaped mitochondria but still retained large numbers of free polysomes.
- Undifferentiated type:
  - The undifferentiated show scanty cytoplasmic organelles and numerous free polysomes.

76.5 Choriocarcinoma

WHO Definition

2016—An aggressive non-germinomatous malignant germ cell tumor composed of syncytiotrophoblasts, cytotrophoblasts, and occasionally intermediate trophoblasts (Rosenblum et al. 2016).

2007—The choriocarcinoma is characterized by extra-embryonic differentiation along trophoblastic lines (Rosenblum et al. 2007).

2000—The choriocarcinoma is characterized by extra-embryonic differentiation along trophoblastic lines (Rosenblum et al. 2000).

1993—A highly malignant tumor composed of both syncytiotrophoblast and cytotrophoblast, arranged in a characteristic bilayered pattern. Immunoreactivity for HCG is strong (Kleihues et al. 1993).

1979—A highly malignant tumor composed of elements identical with syncytiotrophoblast and cytotrophoblast. It corresponds histologically to grade IV (Zülch 1979).

76.5.1 Neuroimaging Findings

General Imaging Findings
- Unspecific, similar to other germ cell tumors

76.5.2 Neuropathology Findings

Macroscopic Features
- Solid tumor
- Tan-white tissue
- Hemorrhagic necrosis

Microscopic Features (Fig. 76.6a–d)
- Cells with extra-embryonic differentiation along trophoblastic lines, i.e.,
  - Cytotrophoblastic elements
  - Syncytiotrophoblastic giant cells
- Cytotrophoblastic cells
  - Large mononucleated cells
  - With vesicular nuclear features and
  - Clear or acidophilic cytoplasm
- Syncytiotrophoblastic giant cells
  - Reach large to enormous size
  - Contain multiple, densely hyperchromatic nuclei
  - Large basophilic cytoplasm
- Ectatic stromal vascular channels
- Blood lakes
- Extensive hemorrhagic necroses

Immunophenotype (Fig. 76.6e, f)
- Positive for:
  - β-HCG
  - HPL

Ultrastructural Features
- Classical choriocarcinoma shows
  - well-defined cytotrophoblasts
  - syncytiotrophoblasts
- Cytotrophoblasts are
  - primitive epithelial cells
- Syncytiotrophoblasts are
  - Complex cells with multiple nuclei and dense cytoplasm containing dilated endoplasmic reticulum, lysosomes, vesicles, and tonofilaments.
  - The syncytiotrophoblast cell membranes often contained numerous microvilli.
- Scattered intermediate trophoblasts showed features transitional between the cytotrophoblasts and the syncytiotrophoblasts, with moderately complex cytoplasm containing some of the organelles found in the syncytiotrophoblasts.

76.6 Teratoma

The following types of teratoma are distinguished:

- Immature teratoma
- Mature teratoma
- Teratoma with malignant transformation

WHO Definition
2016—A germ cell tumor composed of somatic tissues is derived from two or three of the germ layers (i.e., the ectoderm, endoderm, and mesoderm) (Rosenblum et al. 2016).
- Mature teratoma:
  - Mature teratomas consist entirely of fully differentiated, adult-type tissue elements that exhibit little or no mitotic activity (Rosenblum et al. 2016).
- Immature teratoma:
  - Immature teratomas consist of incompletely differentiated elements resembling fetal tissues (Rosenblum et al. 2016).
- Teratoma with malignant transformation:
  - Teratoma containing intracranial germ cell tumors can include a variety of somatic-type cancers; the most commonly encountered are rhabdomyosarcomas and undifferentiated sarcomas followed by enteric-type adenocarcinomas, squamous carcinomas, and primitive neuroectodermal tumors (Rosenblum et al. 2016).

76.6 Teratoma

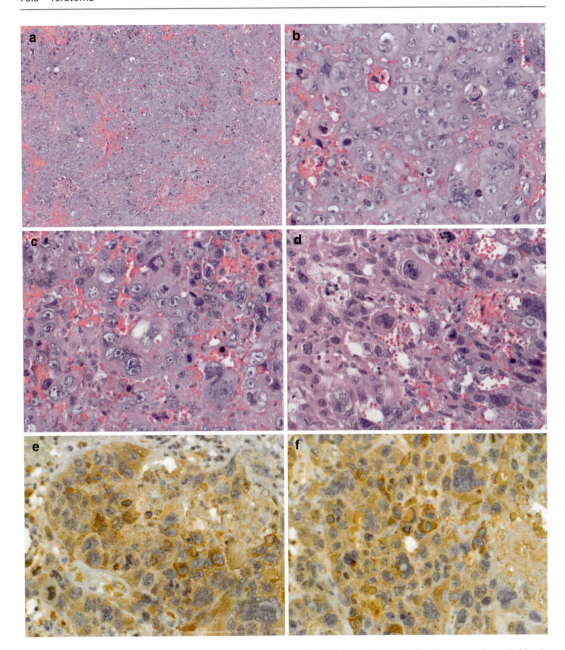

Fig. 76.6 Choriocarcinoma is made up of cells with extra-embryonic differentiation along trophoblastic lines, i.e., cytotrophoblastic elements and syncytiotrophoblastic giant cells. The cytotrophoblastic cells are large mononucleated cells with vesicular nuclear features and clear or acidophilic cytoplasm (**a–d**). The syncytiotrophoblastic giant cells reach large to enormous size, contain multiple, densely hyperchromatic nuclei and large basophilic cytoplasm (**a–d**). Immunoprofile: positive for HCG (**e–f**)

2007—Teratomas differentiate long ectodermal, endodermal, and mesodermal lines (e.g., they recapitulate somatic development from the three embryonic layers). Mature and immature variants require distinction (Rosenblum et al. 2007).

- Mature teratoma:
  - Mature teratomas are composed exclusively of fully differentiated, "adult – type" tissue elements (Rosenblum et al. 2007).
- Immature teratoma:
  - This teratoma variant contains incompletely differentiated components resembling fetal tissue (Rosenblum et al. 2007).
- Teratoma with malignant transformation:
  - These are generic designations for the occasional teratomatous neoplasm that contains as an additional malignant component a cancer of conventional somatic type (Rosenblum et al. 2007).

2000—Teratomas differentiate along ectodermal, endodermal, and mesodermal lines (e.g., they recapitulate somatic development from the three embryonic germ layers) (Rosenblum et al. 2000).

- Mature teratoma:
  - Mature teratomas are composed exclusively of fully differentiated, "adult-type" tissue elements that are sometimes arranged in a pattern resembling normal tissue relationships. Mitotic activity is low or absent (Rosenblum et al. 2000).
- Immature teratoma:
  - This teratoma variant is composed of incompletely differentiated components resembling fetal tissues (Rosenblum et al. 2000).
- Teratoma with malignant transformation:
  - This is the generic designation for the occasional teratomatous neoplasm that contains as an additional malignant component a cancer of conventional somatic type (Rosenblum et al. 2000).

1993—A tumor composed of an admixture of different tissue types representative of ectoderm, endoderm, and mesoderm. Accordingly, the immunoreactivity of teratomas is that of the various component tissues (Kleihues et al. 1993).

- Immature teratoma
  - A teratoma composed of incompletely differentiated tissues resembling those of the fetus. Mitoses are typically present.
- Mature teratoma
  - A teratoma composed exclusively of fully differentiated tissues, sometimes arranged in such a manner as to resemble normal tissue relationships. Mitoses are absent or rare.
- Teratoma with malignant transformation
  - A rare form of teratoma containing malignant components of the type typically encountered in other organs and tissues. Sarcomas of various types, or epithelial malignancies such as squamous cell or adenocarcinomas are most common.

1979—A tumor that is typically composed of several types of tissue representing more than one germinal layer. Histologically, it corresponds to grade I (Zülch 1979).

76.6.1 Neuroimaging Findings

General Imaging Findings
- Small to huge holocephalic mass with "mixed picture," round or lobulated

CT non-contrast-enhanced
- Mixture of fat (hypodense), soft tissue (hyperdense), and calcifications

CT contrast-enhanced
- Enhancement of solid components

MRI-T2/FLAIR (Fig. 76.7a, b)
- Solid: Iso- to hyperintense
- Cysts: hyperintense

76.6 Teratoma

MRI-T1 (Fig. 76.7c)
- Inhomogeneous, fat hyperintense, cysts hypointense, calcifications

MRI-T2∗/SWI
- Calcifications—low signal
- Hemorrhages

MRI-T1 Contrast-Enhanced (Fig. 76.7d–f)
- Solid portions enhance

MR-Spectroscopy
- Lipid peaks

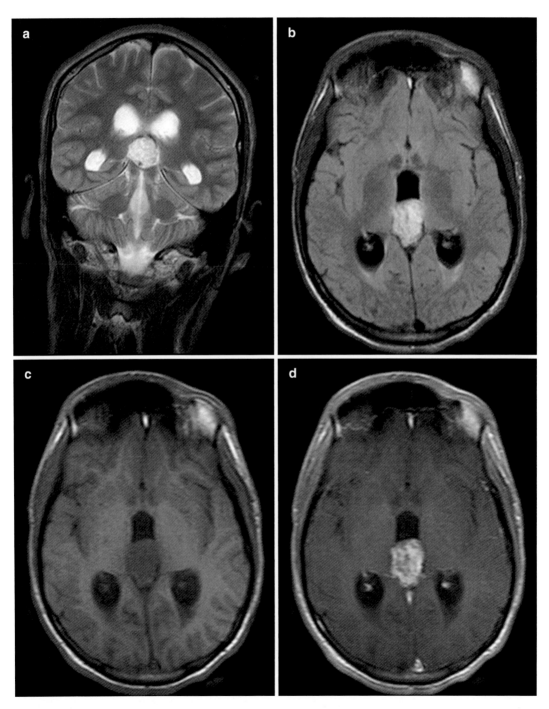

Fig. 76.7 Teratoma: T2 cor (**a**), FLAIR (**b**), T1 (**c**), T1 contrast ax/cor/sag (**d–f**), DWI (**g**)

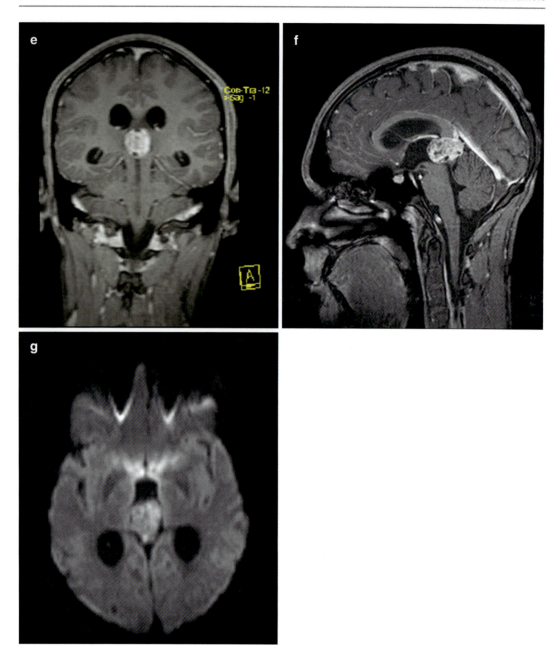

Fig. 76.7 (continued)

76.6.2 Neuropathology Findings

Macroscopic Features (Fig. 76.8a–d)
- Mucous-laden cysts
- Contain
  - Fat
  - Chondroid nodule
  - Bony spicules

Microscopic Features (Fig. 76.9a–n)
- Mature teratoma
  - Composed exclusively of fully differentiated, "adult-type" tissue elements.
  - Ectodermal components include skin, brain, and choroid plexus.
  - Mesodermal component include cartilage, bone, fat, and muscle.

76.6 Teratoma

- Endodermal component include cysts lined by respiratory or enteric epithelium.
- Immature teratoma
  - Contains incompletely differentiated components resembling fetal tissue
  - Might constitute only a minor part of an otherwise differentiated tumor.
  - Hypercellular and mitotically active stroma reminiscent of embryonic mesenchyme.
  - Primitive neuroectodermal elements might form neuroepithelial rosettes and canalicular arrays mimicking the developing neural tube.
  - Clefts lined by melanotic neuroepithelium represent abortive retinal differentiation.
- Teratoma with malignant transformation
  - Teratomatous neoplasm contains an additional malignant cancer of conventional somatic type like:
    - Rhabdomyosarcoma
    - Undifferentiated sarcoma
    - Squamous cell carcinoma
    - Enteric-type adenocarcinoma

Immunophenotype (Fig. 76.9o–r)
- Constituent elements express their appropriate native somatic counterparts.

Proliferation Markers
- Moderate to high

Ultrastructural Features
- Ultrastructural similarities to their normal counterparts in the nervous system, i.e.,
  - "meningeal" and "ependymal" surfaces, between astrocytes, ependymal cells, neurones with synapses and microglia
- Oligodendrocytes with parallel bundles of cytoplasmic intermediate filaments.
- Squamous epithelium with abnormal maturation and keratinization of surface cells with keratinous flakes occasionally in polypoid configurations.
- Respiratory epithelium shows an abundance of microvillous and ciliated cells and areas with disorganized surface structures.
- Piling up of squamous cells in heaps, piles, cauliflower- or onion-like arrangements.

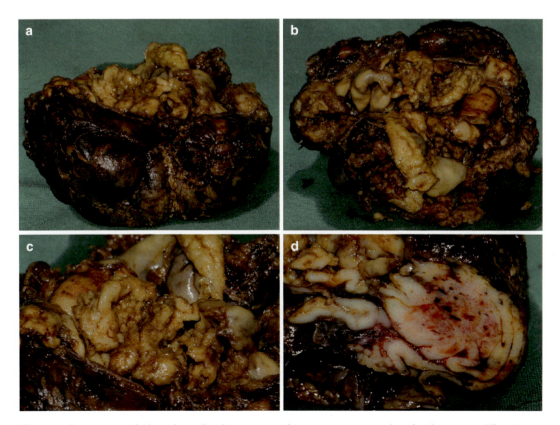

Fig. 76.8 Teratoma: surgical specimen showing macroscopic appearances suggestive of various organ differentiation (ovary) (**a**), intestines (**b**, **c**), cerebrum (**d**)

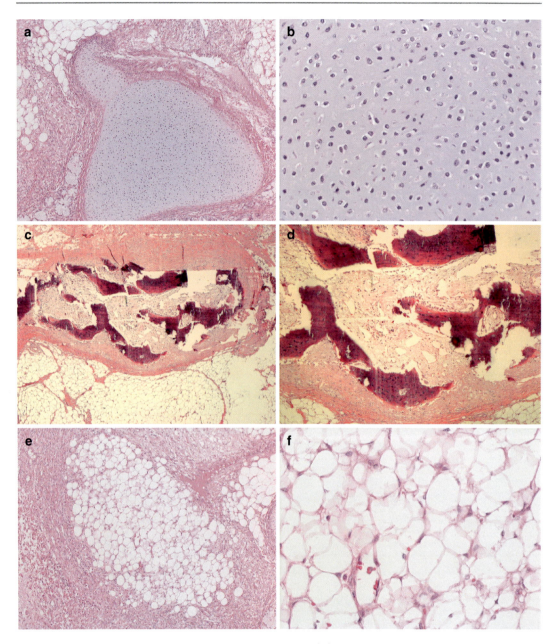

Fig. 76.9 Teratoma: This mature teratoma consists of foci with various tissue differentiation: cartilage (**a**, **b**), bone (**c**, **d**), adipose tissue (**e**, **f**), intestinal (**g**, **h**), squamous (**i**, **j**), glandular (**k**, **l**), neuronal (**m**, **n**). The tissue with neuronal differentiation shows immunopositivity for synaptophysin (**o**, **p**) and GFAP (**q**, **r**)

76.6 Teratoma 1877

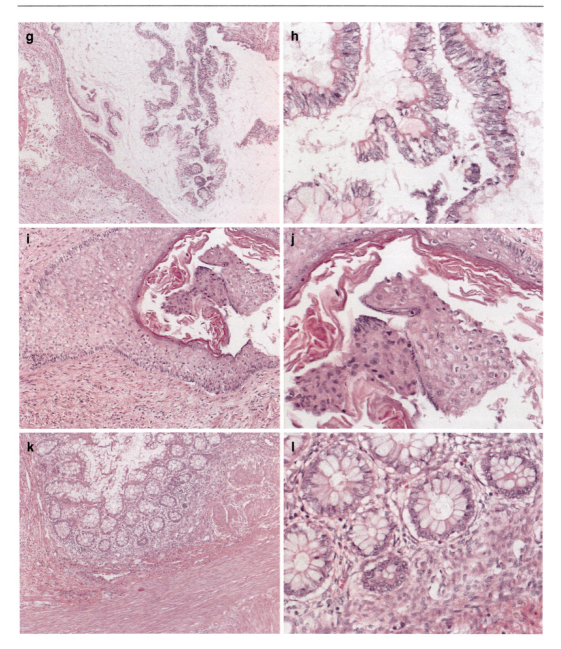

Fig. 76.9 (continued)

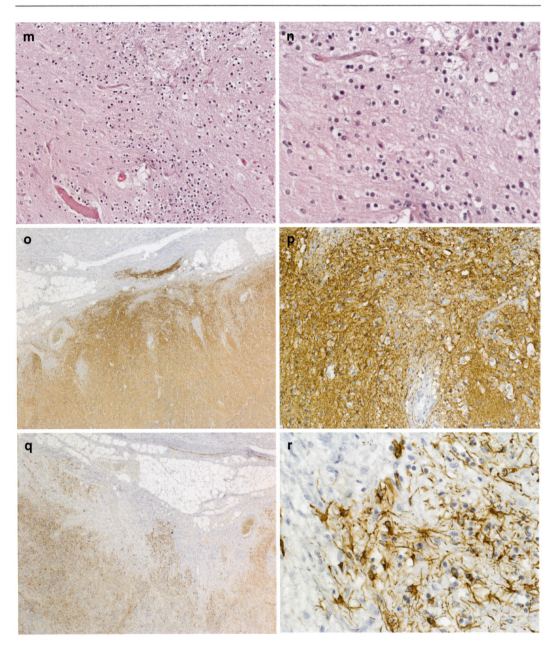

Fig. 76.9 (continued)

Selected References

Aleckovic M, Simon C (2008) Is teratoma formation in stem cell research a characterization tool or a window to developmental biology? Reprod Biomed Online 17(2):270–280

Bain G, Ray WJ, Yao M, Gottlieb DI (1994) From embryonal carcinoma cells to neurons: the P19 pathway. Bioessays 16(5):343–348. https://doi.org/10.1111/j.1365-2184.2006.00385.x

Bulic-Jakus F, Katusic Bojanac A, Juric-Lekic G, Vlahovic M, Sincic N (2016) Teratoma: from spontaneous tumors to the pluripotency/malignancy assay. Wiley Interdiscip Rev Dev Biol 5(2):186–209. https://doi.org/10.1002/wdev.219

Cassart M, Bosson N, Garel C, Eurin D, Avni F (2008) Fetal intracranial tumors: a review of 27 cases. Eur Radiol 18(10):2060–2066. https://doi.org/10.1007/s00330-008-0999-5

Chiloiro S, Giampietro A, Bianchi A, De Marinis L (2016) Clinical management of teratoma, a rare hypothalamic-pituitary neoplasia. Endocrine 53(3):636–642. https://doi.org/10.1007/s12020-015-0814-4

De Giorgi U, Pupi A, Fiorentini G, Rosti G, Marangolo M (2005) FDG-PET in the management of germ cell tumor. Ann Oncol 16(Suppl 4):iv90–iv94. https://doi.org/10.1093/annonc/mdi915

Dormeyer W, van Hoof J, Mummery CL, Krijgsveld J, Heck AJ (2008) A practical guide for the identification of membrane and plasma membrane proteins in human embryonic stem cells and human embryonal carcinoma cells. Proteomics 8(19):4036–4053. https://doi.org/10.1002/pmic.200800143

Forquer JA, Harkenrider M, Fakiris AJ, Timmerman RD, Cavaliere R, Henderson MA, Lo SS (2007) Brain metastasis from non-seminomatous germ cell tumor of the testis. Expert Rev Anticancer Ther 7(11):1567–1580. https://doi.org/10.1586/14737140.7.11.1567

Fu H, Guo X, Li R, Xing B (2017) Radiotherapy and chemotherapy plus radiation in the treatment of patients with pure intracranial germinoma: a meta-analysis. J Clin Neurosci 43:32–38. https://doi.org/10.1016/j.jocn.2017.05.024

Gordeeva OF (2011) Pluripotent cells in embryogenesis and in teratoma formation. J Stem Cells 6(1):51–63

Jessberger R (2008) New insights into germ cell tumor formation. Horm Metab Res 40(5):342–346. https://doi.org/10.1055/s-2008-1073168

Kelly GM, Gatie MI (2017) Mechanisms regulating stemness and differentiation in embryonal carcinoma cells. Stem Cells Int 2017:3684178. https://doi.org/10.1155/2017/3684178

Kleihues P, Burger PC, Scheithauer BW (1993) Histological typing of tumours of the central nervous system, 2nd edn. Springer, New York

Kortmann RD (2014) Current concepts and future strategies in the management of intracranial germinoma. Expert Rev Anticancer Ther 14(1):105–119. https://doi.org/10.1586/14737140.2014.856268

Lu NH, Chen CY, Chou JM, Kuo TH, Yeh CH (2009) MR imaging of primary spinal germinoma: a case report and review of the literature. J Neuroimaging 19(1):92–96. https://doi.org/10.1111/j.1552-6569.2007.00214.x

Manivel JC, Pambuccian S (2003) Germ cell tumor-like neoplasms occurring outside the anatomic midline. Semin Diagn Pathol 20(4):260–271

Osorio DS, Allen JC (2015) Management of CNS germinoma. CNS Oncol 4(4):273–279. https://doi.org/10.2217/cns.15.13

Oya S, Saito A, Okano A, Arai E, Yanai K, Matsui T (2014) The pathogenesis of intracranial growing teratoma syndrome: proliferation of tumor cells or formation of multiple expanding cysts? Two case reports and review of the literature. Childs Nerv Syst 30(8):1455–1461. https://doi.org/10.1007/s00381-014-2396-5

Rogers SJ, Mosleh-Shirazi MA, Saran FH (2005) Radiotherapy of localised intracranial germinoma: time to sever historical ties? Lancet Oncol 6(7):509–519. https://doi.org/10.1016/s1470-2045(05)70245-x

Rosenblum MK, Matsutani M, Van Meir EG (2000) CNS germ cell tumours. In: Kleihues P, Cavenee WK (eds) Pathology and genetics of tumours of the nervous system, 3rd edn. IARC Press, Lyon, pp 208–214

Rosenblum MK, Nakazato Y, Matsutani M (2007) CNS germ cell tumours. In: Louis DN, Ohgaki H, Wiestler OD, Cavenee WK (eds) WHO classification of tumours of the central nervous system, 4th edn. International Agency for Research on Cancer, Lyon, pp 198–204

Rosenblum MK, Nakazato Y, Matsutani M, Ichimura K, Leuschner I, Huse JT (2016) Germ cell tumours. In: Louis DN, Ohgaki H, Wiestler OD, Cavenee WK (eds) WHO classification of tumours of the central nervous system, Revised 4th edn. IARC, Lyon, pp 286–291

Secil M, Altay C, Basara I (2016) State of the art in germ cell tumor imaging. Urol Oncol 34(3):156–164. https://doi.org/10.1016/j.urolonc.2015.06.017

Shibamoto Y (2009) Management of central nervous system germinoma: proposal for a modern strategy. Prog Neurol Surg 23:119–129. https://doi.org/10.1159/000210058

Silvan U, Diez-Torre A, Arluzea J, Andrade R, Silio M, Arechaga J (2009) Hypoxia and pluripotency in embryonic and embryonal carcinoma stem cell biology. Differentiation 78(2–3):159–168. https://doi.org/10.1016/j.diff.2009.06.002

Smirniotopoulos JG, Chiechi MV (1995) Teratomas, dermoids, and epidermoids of the head and neck. Radiographics 15(6):1437–1455. https://doi.org/10.1148/radiographics.15.6.8577967

Ulrich H, Majumder P (2006) Neurotransmitter receptor expression and activity during neuronal differentiation of embryonal carcinoma and stem cells: from basic research towards clinical applications. Cell Prolif 39(4):281–300. https://doi.org/10.1002/pmic.200800143

Waber DP (2011) CNS germinoma: one more piece of the puzzle. Pediatr Blood Cancer 57(4):537–538. https://doi.org/10.1002/pbc.23207

Yu L, Krishnamurthy S, Chang H, Wasenko JJ (2010) Congenital maturing immature intraventricular teratoma. Clin Imaging 34(3):222–225. https://doi.org/10.1016/j.clinimag.2008.06.037

Zhang WY, de Almeida PE, Wu JC (2008) Teratoma formation: a tool for monitoring pluripotency in stem cell research. In: Zhang WY, de Almeida PE, Wu JC (eds) StemBook. Harvard Stem Cell Institute, Cambridge. https://doi.org/10.3824/stembook.1.53.1

Zhu R, Bhattacharya C, Matin A (2007) The role of dead-end in germ-cell tumor development. Ann N Y Acad Sci 1120:181–186. https://doi.org/10.1196/annals.1411.006

Zülch KJ (1979) Histological typing of tumours of the central nervous system. World Health Organization, Geneva

Lymphomas

77.1 Introduction

The most frequently encountered hematopoietic neoplasms of the brain encompass:
- Primary CNS lymphoma
- Intravascular lymphoma
- Post-transplant T-cell lymphoproliferation
- Intraocular lymphoma
- Neurolymphomatosis
- Plasmacytoma

Simplified Classification of CNS lymphomas:
- B-cell lymphoma
  - Diffuse large B-cell lymphoma
  - Low-grade B-cell lymphoma
  - Marginal zone B-cell lymphoma
  - MALT lymphoma
  - Intravascular B-cell lymphoma
  - Other types of B-cell lymphoma
- T-cell lymphoma
  - Anaplastic large cell lymphoma
  - NK-/T-cell lymphoma
- Hodgkin disease

The 2017 WHO classification lists the following entities (Table 77.1) (Swerdlow et al. 2017a):
- Diffuse large B-cell lymphoma of the CNS
- Immunodeficiency-associated CNS lymphomas
  - AIDS-related diffuse large B-cell lymphoma
  - EBV+ diffuse large B-cell lymphoma, NOS
  - Lymphomatoid granulomatosis
- Intravascular large B-cell lymphoma
- Miscellaneous rare lymphomas in the CNS
  - Low-grade B-cell lymphoma of the CNS
  - T-cell and NK-/T-cell lymphoma of the CNS
  - Anaplastic large cell lymphoma
    - Primary CNS anaplastic large cell lymphoma, ALK-positive
    - Primary CNS anaplastic large cell lymphoma, ALK-negative
- Extranodal marginal zone lymphoma of mucosa-associated lymphoid tissue (MALT lymphoma) of the dura

Plasma Cell Neoplasms
WHO classification (Swerdlow et al. 2017a)

- Non-IgM monoclonal gammopathy of undetermined significance
- Plasma cell myeloma
- Plasma cell myeloma variants
  - Smoldering (asymptomatic) plasma cell myeloma
  - Non-secretory myeloma
  - Plasma cell leukemia
- Plasmacytoma
  - Solitary plasmacytoma of bone
  - Extraosseous plasmacytoma

Table 77.1 The 2017 WHO classification of mature lymphoid, histiocytic, and dendritic neoplasms (Swerdlow et al. 2016, 2017a)

Mature B-cell neoplasms	• Chronic lymphocytic leukemia/small lymphocytic lymphoma
	  – Monoclonal B-cell lymphocytosis
	• B-cell prolymphocytic leukemia
	• Splenic marginal zone lymphoma
	• Hairy cell leukemia
	• Splenic B-cell lymphoma/leukemia, unclassifiable
	  – Splenic diffuse red pulp small B-cell lymphoma
	  – Hairy cell leukemia-variant
	• Lymphoplasmacytic lymphoma
	  – Waldenström macroglobulinemia
	• IgM monoclonal gammopathy of undetermined significance
	• Heavy-chain disease
	  – μ heavy-chain disease
	  – γ heavy-chain disease
	  – α heavy-chain disease
	• Plasma cell neoplasms (see below)
	• Extranodal marginal zone lymphoma of mucosa-associated lymphoid tissue (MALT lymphoma)
	• Nodal marginal zone lymphoma
	  – Pediatric nodal marginal zone lymphoma
	• Follicular lymphoma
	  – Testicular follicular lymphoma
	  – In situ follicular neoplasia
	  – Duodenal-type follicular lymphoma
	• Pediatric-type follicular lymphoma
	• Large B-cell lymphoma with IRF4 rearrangement
	• Primary cutaneous follicle center lymphoma
	• Mantle cell lymphoma
	  – Leukemic non-nodal mantle cell lymphoma
	  – In situ mantle cell neoplasia
	• Diffuse large B-cell lymphoma (DLBCL), NOS
	• T-cell/histiocyte-rich large B-cell lymphoma
	• Primary DLBCL of the central nervous system (CNS)
	• Primary cutaneous DLBCL, leg type
	• EBV+ DLBCL, NOS
	• *EBV+* mucocutaneous ulcer
	• DLBCL associated with chronic inflammation
	  – Fibrin-associated diffuse large B-cell lymphoma
	• Lymphomatoid granulomatosis
	• Primary mediastinal (thymic) large B-cell lymphoma
	• Intravascular large B-cell lymphoma
	• ALK1 large B-cell lymphoma
	• Plasmablastic lymphoma
	• Primary effusion lymphoma
	• HHV8-associated lymphoproliferative disorders
	  – Multicentric Castleman disease
	  – HHV8-positive diffuse large B-cell lymphoma, NOS
	  – HHV8-positive germinotropic lymphoproliferative disorder
	• Burkitt lymphoma
	• Burkitt-like lymphoma with 11q aberration
	• High-grade B-cell lymphoma
	  – High-grade B-cell lymphoma with MYC and BCL2 and/or BCL6 rearrangements
	  – High-grade B-cell lymphoma, NOS
	• B-cell lymphoma, unclassifiable, with features intermediate between DLBCL and classical Hodgkin lymphoma

Table 77.1 (continued)

Mature T and NK neoplasms	• T-cell prolymphocytic leukemia
	• T-cell large granular lymphocytic leukemia
	• Chronic lymphoproliferative disorder of NK-cells
	• Aggressive NK-cell leukemia
	• EBV-positive T-cell lymphoma and NK-cell lymphoproliferative diseases of childhood
	   – Systemic EBV+ T-cell lymphoma of childhood
	   – Chronic active EBV infection of T- and NK-cell type, systemic form
	   – Hydroa vacciniforme-like lymphoproliferative disorder
	   – Severe mosquito bite allergy
	• Adult T-cell leukemia/lymphoma
	• Extranodal NK-/T-cell lymphoma, nasal type
	• Intestinal T-cell lymphoma
	   – Enteropathy-associated T-cell lymphoma
	   – Monomorphic epitheliotropic intestinal T-cell lymphoma
	   – Intestinal T-cell lymphoma
	   – Indolent T-cell lymphoproliferative disorder of the GI tract
	• Hepatosplenic T-cell lymphoma
	• Subcutaneous panniculitis-like T-cell lymphoma
	• Mycosis fungoides
	• Sézary syndrome
	• Primary cutaneous CD301 T-cell lymphoproliferative disorders
	   – Lymphomatoid papulosis
	   – Primary cutaneous anaplastic large cell lymphoma
	• Primary cutaneous peripheral T-cell lymphomas, rare subtypes
	   – Primary cutaneous γδ T-cell lymphoma
	   – Primary cutaneous CD8+ aggressive epidermotropic cytotoxic T-cell lymphoma
	   – Primary cutaneous acral CD8+ T-cell lymphoma
	   – Primary cutaneous CD4+ small-/medium T-cell lymphoproliferative disorder
	• Peripheral T-cell lymphoma, NOS
	• Angioimmunoblastic T-cell lymphoma and other nodal lymphomas of T follicular helper (TFH) cell origin
	   – Angioimmunoblastic T-cell lymphoma
	   – Follicular T-cell lymphoma∗
	   – Nodal peripheral T-cell lymphoma with TFH phenotype
	• Anaplastic large cell lymphoma, ALK-positive
	• Anaplastic large cell lymphoma, ALK-negative
	• Breast implant-associated anaplastic large cell lymphoma

Hodgkin lymphoma	• Nodular lymphocyte-predominant Hodgkin lymphoma
	• Classical Hodgkin lymphoma
	   – Nodular sclerosis classical Hodgkin lymphoma
	   – Lymphocyte-rich classical Hodgkin lymphoma
	   – Mixed cellularity classical Hodgkin lymphoma
	   – Lymphocyte-depleted classical Hodgkin lymphoma

Post-transplant lymphoproliferative disorders (PTLD)	• Plasmacytic hyperplasia PTLD • Infectious mononucleosis PTLD • Florid follicular hyperplasia PTLD • Polymorphic PTLD • Monomorphic PTLD (B- and T-/NK-cell types) • Classical Hodgkin lymphoma PTLD
Histiocytic and dendritic cell neoplasms	• Histiocytic sarcoma • Langerhans cell histiocytosis • Langerhans cell sarcoma • Indeterminate dendritic cell tumor • Interdigitating dendritic cell sarcoma • Follicular dendritic cell sarcoma • Fibroblastic reticular cell tumor • Disseminated juvenile xanthogranuloma • Erdheim-Chester disease

- Monoclonal immunoglobulin deposition diseases
  - Primary amyloidosis
  - Light chain and heavy-chain deposition diseases
- Plasma cell neoplasms with associated paraneoplastic syndrome
  - POEMS syndrome
  - TEMPI syndrome

77.2 Primary CNS Lymphoma:

WHO Definition
2016—Diffuse large B-cell lymphoma of the CNS: A diffuse large B-cell lymphoma (DLBCL) confined to the CNS at presentation (Deckert et al. 2016).
2007—Extranodal malignant lymphomas arising in the CNS in the absence of lymphoma outside the nervous system at the time of diagnosis; these tumors need to be differentiated from secondary involvement of the nervous system in systemic lymphomas (Deckert and Paulus 2007).
2000—Primary CNS lymphomas are extranodal malignant lymphomas arising in the CNS in the absence of obvious lymphoma outside the nervous system at the time of diagnosis. They are to be differentiated from secondary involvement of the nervous system in systemic lymphomas (Paulus et al. 2000).
1993—Malignant lymphoma: Histologically, CNS lymphomas resemble systemic lymphomas; they are almost exclusively non-Hodgkin lymphomas with a diffuse rather than a follicular/nodular growth pattern (Kleihues et al. 1993).

77.2.1 Clinical Symptoms and Signs

- Neurocognitive, motor, or constitutional symptoms (in the majority)
- Seizures (in 20% of the cases)
- Symptoms associated with increased intracranial pressure (in 1/3 of the cases)
- Leptomeningeal involvement (in 15–20% of cases)
- Visual symptoms: nonspecific and binocular-blurred vision, decreased acuity, floaters, pain, photophobia (in 30% of cases)
- Personality changes (24% of cases)
- Cerebellar signs (21% of cases)
- Rapid response to glucocorticoids: both in clinical symptoms and in radiographic features

77.2.2 Epidemiology

Incidence
- 0.8–6.6% of primary intracranial neoplasms

Age Incidence
- All age groups affected
- Immunocompetent: sixth to seventh decade
- Inherited immunodeficiency: 10 years
- Transplant recipients: 37 years
- AIDS patients: 39 years

Sex Incidence
- Male:Female ratio 3:2

Localization
- Supratentorial space (60%)
  - Frontal (15%)
  - Temporal (8%)
  - Parietal (7%)
  - Occipital (3%)
  - Basal ganglia/periventricular regions (10%)
- Posterior fossa (13%)
- Spinal cord (1%)

77.2.3 Neuroimaging Findings

General Imaging Findings
- Lesions depend on immune status.
- Single or multiple lesions, well defined or infiltrative
- Mild perifocal edema
- Usually supratentorial
- Hemorrhages or necrosis in immunocompromised patients

CT non-contrast-enhanced (Fig. 77.1a)
- Typically hyperdense, in rare cases isodense

CT contrast-enhanced (Fig. 77.1b)
- Homogeneous enhancement
- Peripheral enhancement—immunocompromised

MRI-T2/FLAIR (Fig. 77.1c, d)
- Iso/hypointense to cortex
- Inhomogeneous in immunocompromised due to hemorrhages and necrosis
- Slight edema

MRI-T1 (Fig. 77.1e)
- Iso/hypointense to cortex
- Inhomogeneous in immunocompromised (hemorrhages, necrosis)

MRI-T2∗/SWI
- Hypointense hemorrhages particularly in immunocompromised
- Immunocompetent: less hypointensities compared to glioblastoma

MRI-T1 contrast-enhanced (Fig. 77.1f)
- Homogeneous enhancement
- Immunocompromised: ring enhancement

MR-Diffusion Imaging (Fig. 77.1g)
- Diffusion restricted with ADC lowering

MRI-Perfusion (Fig. 77.1h)
- rCBV elevated, less than in glioblastoma

MR-Diffusion Tensor Imaging
- FA and ADC values of lymphoma lower compared to glioblastoma

MR-Spectroscopy
- Choline elevated
- NAA reduced—unspecific
- Lactate peak

Nuclear Medicine Imaging Findings (Fig. 77.2)
- Primary CNS lymphoma is usually FDG avid (in contrast to toxoplasmosis).
- FDG-PET can be used to assess the damage to healthy brain tissue.
- FDG-PET can be used to screen the body for other lymphoma manifestations.
- Steroids can reduce FDG uptake in these patients. It has been discussed, to use FDG-PET for risk stratification of patients with primary CNS lymphoma.
- Historically, I123-IMP, Tc99m-MIBI, and Tl201 were used to assess primary CNS lymphoma.
- Radiotracers like FET (a marker of amino acid uptake (L-system)) or FLT (a marker of DNA biosynthesis) have the advantage of nearly no uptake in the healthy brain tissues resulting in a much better tumor-to-background ratio. Studies demonstrated the ability to differentiate high-grade gliomas and primary CNS lymphomas from low-grade gliomas and non-neoplastic lesions.

77.2.4 Neuropathology Findings

Macroscopic Features (Figs. 77.3 and 77.4a–j)
- Single or multiple masses
- Deep seated
- Firm, friable, granular, central necrosis
- Gray-tan, yellow

Microscopic Features (Figs. 77.5a–j, 77.6, 77.7, and 77.8)
- Angiocentric infiltration
  - Tumor cells form collars within concentric perivascular reticulin deposits
- Invasion of the cerebral parenchyma by tumor cells
- Diffuse growth pattern
- Large areas of necrosis
- Prominent astrocytic and microglial response
- Presence of:
  - Large CD68-positive macrophages
  - Reactive CD4- and CD8-positive T-cells

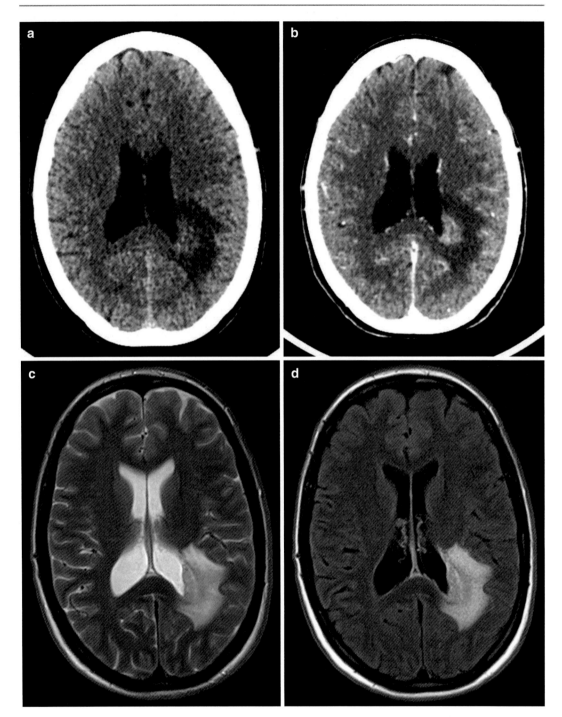

Fig. 77.1 Left periventricular primary CNS lymphoma. CT (**a**), CT contrast (**b**), T2 (**c**), FLAIR (**d**), T1 (**e**), T1 contrast (**f**), DWI (**g**), rCBV (**h**)

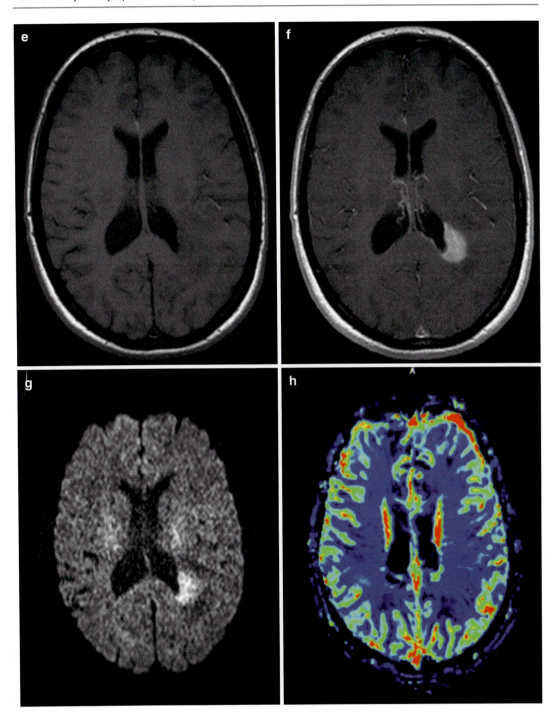

Fig. 77.1 (continued)

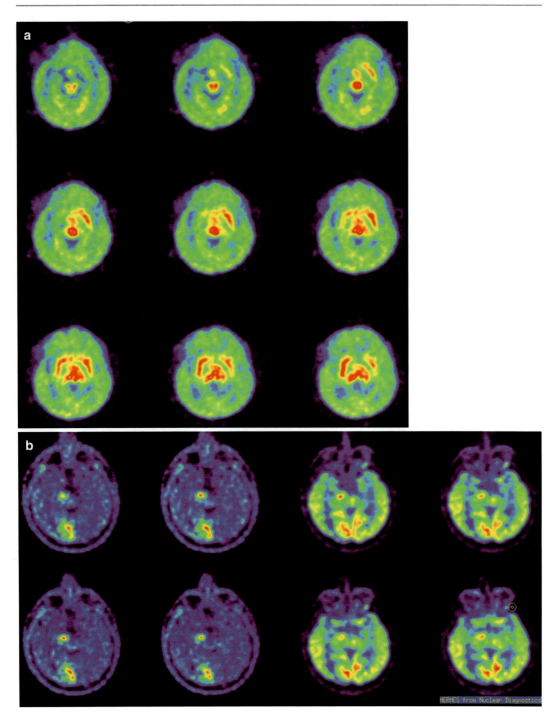

Fig. 77.2 PCNS-DLCBL: FDG-PET showing hypermetabolism in the brainstem and basal ganglia (**a**). FDG and FET show hypermetabolism in the right thalamus and right occipital lobe. A surrounding hypometabolism is observed due to edema (**b**)

Immunophenotype (Figs. 77.5k–p, 77.6c, d, 77.7c, d, and 77.8c, d)

Antibodies used to differentiate the various lymphoma types are listed in Table 77.2.

Frequently used immunostaining markers in lymphoid and histiocytic neoplasms (Table 77.3), markers for mature B-lymphocytic lymphoma (Table 77.4), and markers for mature T-lymphocytic and natural killer (NK)-cell lymphoma (Tables 77.5 and 77.6) are given below.

Proliferation Markers (Fig. 77.5o, p)
- Mitotic activity high
- Ki-67 LI: 50–70%

Ultrastructural Features
- Nuclear pleomorphism
- Nuclear convolution
- Multilobulation and fragmentation of the nucleus
- Slight to marked nuclear irregularity with convoluted-shape predominance
- Cleaved or indented nucleus with an even heterochromatin distribution
- An absent or inconspicuous nucleolus
- Specked chromatin pattern of the large cells
- Prominent lysosomes
- Glycogen accumulation
- Low nuclear/cytoplasmic ratio

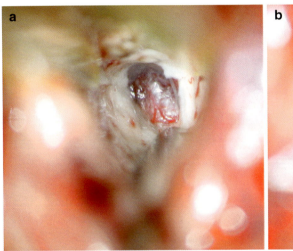
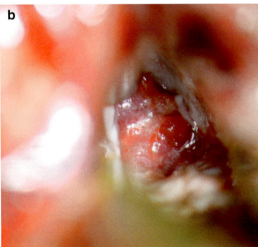

Fig. 77.3 PCNS-DLCBL: Intraoperative appearance of a reddish to grayish mass (**a**, **b**)

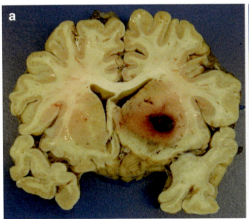
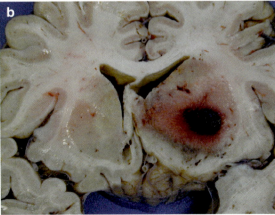

Fig. 77.4 PCNS-DLCBL: Macroscopic features of lymphoma with hemorrhagic component (**a–j**) affecting the basal ganglia (**a**, **b**), parietal lobe (**c**, **d**), splenium of the corpus callosum (**e**, **f**), occipital lobe (**g**, **h**), and multifocally in the cerebellum (**i**, **j**), and cerebral aqueduct (**i**)

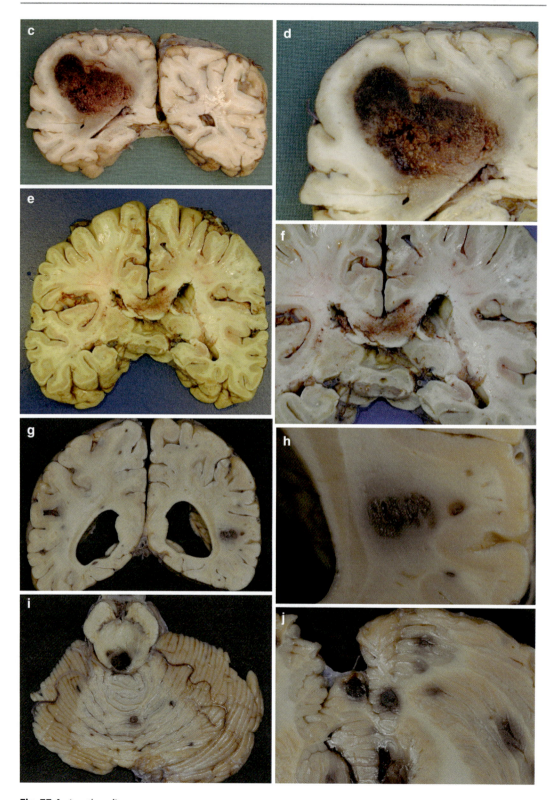

Fig. 77.4 (continued)

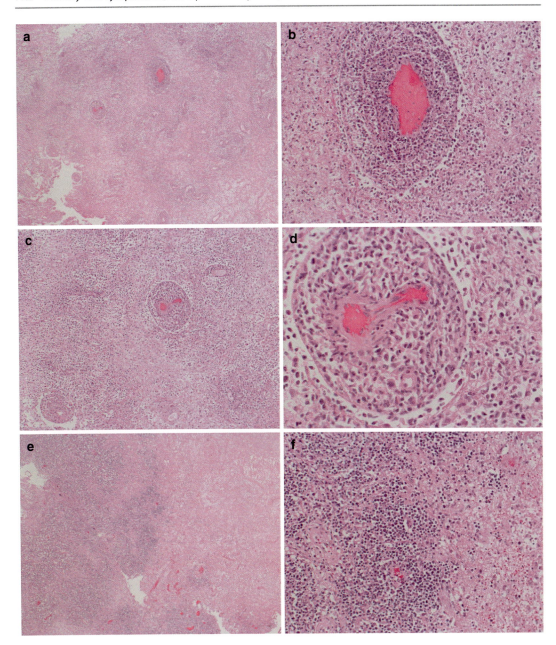

Fig. 77.5 PCNS-DLCBL: Histology shows a moderate to high cellular tumor with angiocentric infiltration by tumor cells (**b–d**). The tumor cells form collars within concentric perivascular reticulin deposits (**i, j**). The cerebral parenchyma is diffusely infiltrated by tumor cells (**a–h**). Large areas of necrosis are present (∗) (**e**). The tumor cells are immunopositive for CD20 (**k, l**), and MUM1 (**m, n**). High Ki67 proliferation index (**o, p**)

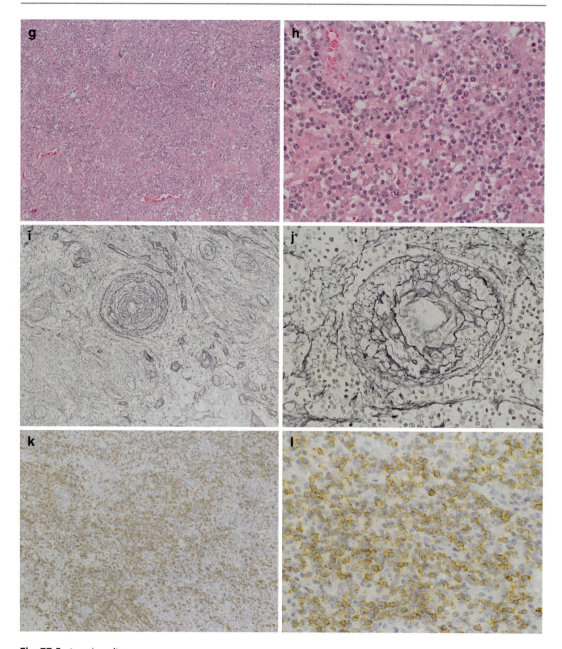

Fig. 77.5 (continued)

77.2 Primary CNS Lymphoma: [Hemopoetic Neoplasms]

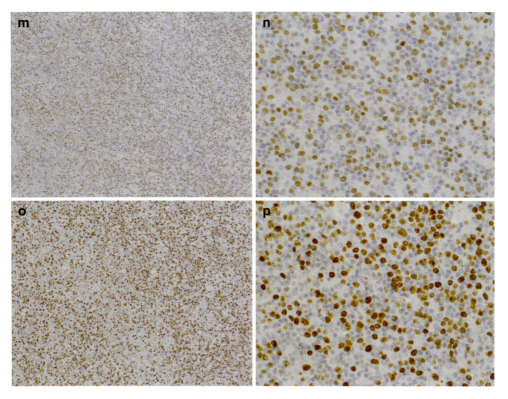

Fig. 77.5 (continued)

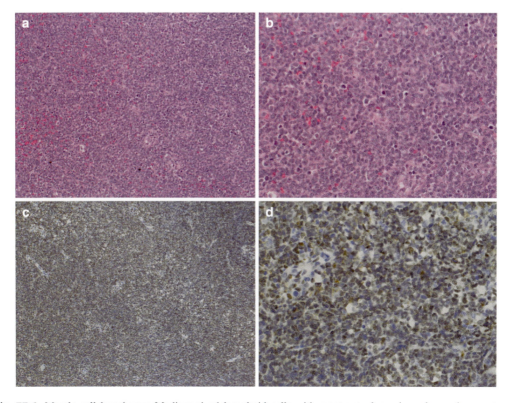

Fig. 77.6 Mantle cell lymphoma: Medium-sized lymphoid cells with scant cytoplasm, irregular nuclear contours, condensed chromatin, and inconspicuous nucleoli. The tumor cells are immunopositive for CyclinD1 (**c, d**)

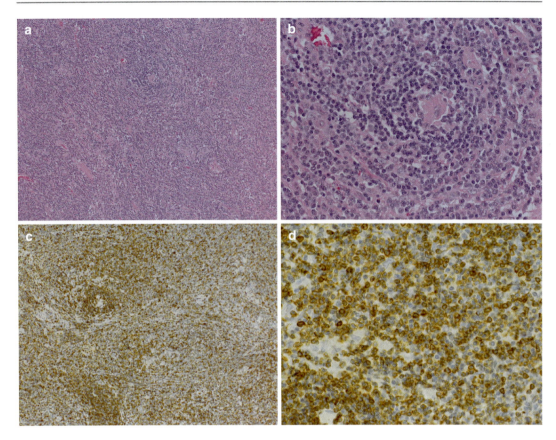

Fig. 77.7 Marginal zone lymphoma: Polymorphous infiltrate of centrocyte-like cells, monocytoid cells, small lymphocytes, and lymphoid cells with plasmacytic differentiation. The tumor cells are immunopositive for Bcl-2 (**c, d**)

- Abundant mitochondria
- Well-developed Golgi zone
- Profiles of endoplasmic reticulum and centrioles

Differential Diagnosis
- Metastatic carcinoma
- Glioblastoma
- Anaplastic oligodendroglioma
- Primitive neuroectodermal tumor (PNET)
- Encephalitis
- Abscess
- Demyelinating disease

77.2.5 Molecular Neuropathology

- Inherited or acquired immunodeficiency
- Epstein-Barr virus (EBV) in immunocompromised patients
  - Lymphoma cells are latently infected with EBV
    - 95% of tumor cells in immunodeficient patients
    - 0–20% of tumor cells in immunocompetent patients
  - Infected cells express:
    - EBNA-1-6
    - LMP1
    - EBER1, EBER2

77.2 Primary CNS Lymphoma: [Hemopoetic Neoplasms]

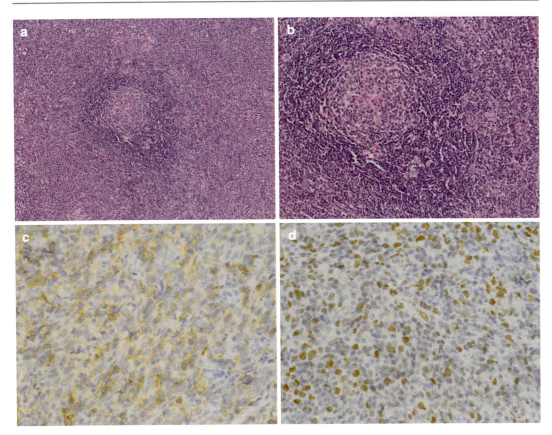

Fig. 77.8 Follicular lymphoma: follicular pattern of closely packed neoplastic fascicles mimicking germinal centers of secondary follicles composed of either small cleaved centrocytes or large centroblasts interspersed with T-cells. The tumor cells are immunopositive for Bcl-6 (**c**, **d**)

Table 77.2 Antibodies used to differentiate the various lymphoma types

Tumor type	IHC-positivity	IHC-negativity
B-cell Non-Hodgkin Lymphoma	• CD20 • CD79a • CD19 • Bcl-2	
Diffuse large B-cell lymphoma	• CD19 • CD20 • CD22 • CD79a • CD45 • PAX-% • CD10 (20–40%) • CD5 (10%) • CD30 (10%) • Bcl-2 (50%) • Bcl-6 (60%) • IRF4/MUM1 • FOXP1 • P53 • MIB-1 ≥80%	• CD5 • Bcl-1

(continued)

Table 77.2 (continued)

Tumor type	IHC-positivity	IHC-negativity
B-CLL (chronic lymphocytic leukemia)	• CD5 • CD20 • CD23 • CD22 • CD11c • CD45 • CD79a • CD19 • CD43 • PAX-5 • Bcl-2 • LEF1 • CD160 • CD200 • CD11c	• CD10 • CD79b • FMC-7 • CD138 • BCL-1 • Cyclin D1 • CD38 (+/−) • Zap70 (+/−)
Mantle cell lymphoma	• Cyclin D1(hallmark) • CD20 • CD79a • CD19 • CD23 • CD5 • CD43 • Bcl-2 • Sox11 • IgM • IgD • Bcl-2	• CD23 • CD10 • CD11c • Bcl-6
B-cell lymphoblastic lymphoma	• TdT • CD34 • CD10 • CD19 • Bcl-6 • CD99	• CD20
Marginal zone lymphoma	• CD20 • CD79a • CD43 • CD21 • CD35 • IgD • MNDA • Bcl-2 • CD19 • CD45 • p27 • IgM	• CD3 • CD5 • CD10 • CD23 • CD43 • Cyclin D1 • Bcl-1 • Bcl-6 • AnnexinA1 • IgD

Table 77.2 (continued)

Tumor type	IHC-positivity	IHC-negativity
Follicular lymphoma	• CD19 • CD20 • CD22 • CD79a • CD10 • CD21 • Cd23 • Pax-5 • Bcl-2 • Bcl-6 • HGAL • GCET-1 (centrin) • LMO2 • Ig • STMN1	• CD5 • CD43 • CD11c • CyclinD1 • Bcl-1 • Bcl-2 (follicular center B-cells) • IRF4/MUM1
Mucosa-associated lymphoid tissue (MALT) lymphoma	• IgM • CD20 • CD79a • CD21 • CD35 • CD43 • CD11c • IRTA1 • MNDA	• CD5 • CD10 • CD23 • Bcl-1
Burkitt lymphoma	• CD19 • CD20 • CD22 • CD79a • CD10 • CD38 • CD43 • CD77 • Bcl-6 • C-MYC • MIB-1 ≥90% • EBV ± (15–30%)	• CD5 • CC23 • Cyclin D1 • TdT • Bcl-2 • MUM1
Hairy cell leukemia	• CD19 • CD20 • CD22 • CD25 • CD11c • CD103 • CD123 • CD160 • CD200 • SOX1BRAF V600E • DBA.44 • TRAP • Annexin A1 (ANXA1) • FMC-7 • T-bet (weak) • Bcl-1 (weak)	• CD5 • CD10 • CD23
Immunocytoma	• CD20 • CD23	• CD5
T-cell non-Hodgkin lymphoma	• CD3	

Table 77.2 (continued)

Tumor type	IHC-positivity	IHC-negativity
Anaplastic large cell lymphoma (ALCL), ALK-positive	• CD30 • ALK • EMA • CD2 (70% of cases) • CD4 (70% of cases) • CD5 (70% of cases) • CD43 • CD25 • CD15 • TIA1 • Granzyme B • Perforin	• CD3 • CD8 • CD68 • Bcl-2 • EBV
Anaplastic large cell lymphoma (ALCL), ALK-negative	• CD30 • EMA • CD3 • CD2 • CD43 • CD4 • TIA1 • Granzyme B • Perforin • Clusterin	• ALK • CD5 • CD8 • EMA • EBV
Hodgkin lymphoma classical	• CD30 (>90%) • CD15 (75–85%) • IMP3 • TNFAIP2 • CD200 • Pax5 • IRF4/MUM-1 • Fascin • Vimentin • CD25 • CD40 • LMP-1 (20–50%)	• CD45RO • CD43 • CD75 • CD68 • CD138 • EMA • Cytokeratin • ALK1 • J-chain • Bcl-6 • BOB-1 • CD20 • CD79a • TIA-1 • Oct.2 • PU.1
Hodgkin lymphoma non-classical	• CD20 • CD79a • EMA • CD45RO • J-chain • Bcl-6	• CD30 • CD15 • LMP

77.2 Primary CNS Lymphoma: [Hemopoetic Neoplasms]

Table 77.3 Frequently used immunostaining markers in lymphoid and histiocytic neoplasms, modified after Zhang and Aguilera (2015) data reproduced with kind permission by Springer Nature

Markers	B-cell acute lymphoblastic leukemia/lymphoma (B lymphoblastic leukemia/lymphoma) B-ALL	T-cell acute lymphoblastic leukemia/lymphoma (T lymphoblastic leukemia/lymphoma) T-ALL	Mature B-cell neoplasms BCN	Mature T-/NK-cell neoplasms	Classical Hodgkin lymphoma CHL	Histocytic and dendritic cell neoplasms HDCN
CD3	−	+	−	+	−	−
CD20	+ or −	−	+	−	−	−
CD79a	+ or −	− or +	+	−	−	−
PAX-5	+ or −	−	+	−	+ weak	−
CD5	−	+ or −	+	+	−	−
CD23	−	−	+	−	−	−
CD10	+	+ or −	+	−	−	ND
CD2	−	+ or −	−	+	−	−
CD4	−	+ or −	−	+	−	+
CD8	−	+	−	+	−	−
CD7	−	+	−	+	−	−
CD34	+	+	−	−	−	−
TdT	+	+	−	−	−	−
CD99	ND	+	−	−	ND	−
CD15	+	ND	−	−	+	−
CD30	ND	ND	+	+	+	−
CD68	ND	ND	−	−	−	+
S-100	ND	ND	−	−	ND	+
CD1a	−	+	−	−	ND	+
CD123	ND	ND	−	−	ND	+
CD163	ND	ND	−	−	ND	+
MIB(Ki67)	+	+	+ or −	+ or −	ND	ND

- Pathogenetic factors in PNCSL (Paydas 2017)
  - Angiocentricity and angiotropism
  - Alterations and translocations in copy number of 9p.24/PD-L1/PD-L2
  - Neurotropic factors: CXCL12 (SDF-1), CXCL-13, IL-10
  - JAK/STAT signaling pathway
  - Dysregulation in B-cell receptor signaling pathway: IL-4, CD79B (mutated in 20% of the cases)
  - Dysregulation in NF-κB pathway
  - Dysregulation in Toll-like receptor signaling pathway: MYD88 (mutated in 35–80% of cases)
  - Recurrent mutations in *PIM1* (in 69%), *TBL1XR1* (in 24%), *TRDM1* (in 24%), *BTG2* (in 29%), *PRDM1* (in 24%)
  - Protein-changing mutations with next-generation sequencing analyses: *CTNN1, PIK3CA, PTEN, ATM, KRAS, PTPN11, TP53, SMO* (in more than 80% of the cases)
- Chromosomal translocations involving the following oncogenes
  - *BcL-2* (anti-apoptosis) in follicular NHL
  - *CCND1* (cyclin D1) (cell cycle regulator) in mantle cell NHL

Table 77.4 Markers for mature B-lymphocytic lymphoma, modified after Zhang and Aguilera (2015) data reproduced with kind permission by Springer Nature

	Chronic lymphocytic leukemia/small lymphocytic lymphoma CLL/SLL	Mantle cell lymphoma MCL	Follicular lymphoma FL	Marginal zone lymphoma MZL	Lymphoplasmacytic lymphoma/ Waldenström macroglobulinemia LPL/WM	Hairy cell leukemia HCL	Prolymphocytic leukemia PLL
CD3	−	−	−	−	−	−	−
CD5	+	+	−	−	−	−	−
CD10	−	−	+	−	− or +	− or +	−
CD20	+	+	+	+	+	+	+
CD23	+	−	+ or −	− or +	− or +	− or +	−
BCL-1	−	+	−	−	−	+	−
BCL-2	+	+	+	+	+	+	+
BCL-6	−	−	+	−	−	−	−
MIB	+	+	+	+	+	+	+
κ/λ	Monotypic	Monotypic	Monotypic	Monotypic	Monotypic	Monotypic	Monotypic

Table 77.5 Additional markers for mature B-lymphocytic lymphoma (Zhang and Aguilera 2015) data reproduced with kind permission by Springer Nature

	Chronic lymphocytic leukemia/ small lymphocytic lymphoma CLL/SLL	Mantle cell lymphoma MCL	Follicular lymphoma FL	Marginal zone lymphoma MZL	Lymphoplasmacytic lymphoma/ Waldenström macroglobulinemia LPL/WM	Hairy cell leukemia HCL
LEF-1 lymphoid enhancer binding factor-1	+	−	−	−	−	ND
CD160	+	−	−	−	−	+
CD200	+	−	−	−	+	+
SOX11	−	+	−	−	−	+
BRAF V600E	−	−	−	−	ND	+
HGAL human germinal center-associated lymphoma	−	−	+	−	−	ND
LMO2 LIM-only transcription factor 2	−	−	+	−	−	ND
Stathmin	−	+	+	−	−	ND
GCET1 germinal center B-cell expressed transcript-1	−	−	+	−	−	ND
IRTA1 immunoglobulin superfamily receptor translocation-associated 1	−	−	−	+	−	ND
MNDA myeloid cell nuclear differentiation antigen	+	+	−	+	+	ND
MYD88 myeloid differentiation primary response gene 88	−	−	−	−	+	ND

Table 77.6 Markers for mature T-lymphocytic and natural killer (NK)-cell lymphoma, modified after Zhang and Aguilera (2015) data reproduced with kind permission by Springer Nature

	T-cell prolymphocytic leukemia (TPLL)	T-cell large granular lymphocytic leukemia (TLGL)	Adult T-cell leukemia/ lymphoma (ATLL)	Enteropathy-associated T-cell lymphoma (EATL)	Hepatosplenic T-cell lymphoma (HSTL)	Subcutaneous panniculitis-like T-cell lymphoma (SPTCL)	Mycosis fungoides/ Sézary syndrome (MF/SS)	Angioimmunoblastic T-cell lymphoma (AITL)	Anaplastic large cell lymphoma (ALCL)	Peripheral T-cell lymphoma (PTCL)	Extranodal NK-/T-cell lymphoma, nasal type ENK/T, nasal
CD2	+	+	+	+	+	+	+	+	+ or −	+	+
CD3	+	+	+	+	+	+	+	+	+ or −	+	−
CD4	+	−	+	−	−	−	+	+	+ or −	+ or −	−
CD8	+ or −	+	−	− or +	+ or −	+	− or +	−	− or +	− or +	− or +
CD5	+	− or +	+	−	−	+	+ or −	+	+ or −	− or +	−
CD7	+	− or +	−	+	+	+	− or +	+	− or +	− or +	+
TIA	−	+	−	+	+	+	−	−	+	−	+
GrB	−	+	−	+	−	+	−	−	+	−	+
CD25	−	+	+	− or +	−	ND	−	−	+	−	−
CD30	−	−	− or +	− or +	−	−	−	−	+	− or +	−
CD56	−	−	−	− or +	+	−	−	−	+ or −	− or +	+
CD57	−	+	−	−	−	−	−	−	−	−	−
EBV	−	−	−	−	−	−	−	+	−	−	+
CD20	−	−	−	−	−	−	−	−	−	−	−

- *BcL-2* (anti-apoptosis) in diffuse large B-cell NHL
- *Bcl-6* (transcription deregulation) in diffuse large B-cell NHL
- *C-myc* (transcription deregulation) in Burkitt lymphoma
- *NPM/ALK* (tyrosine kinase) in anaplastic large T-cell NHL
- *API2/MLT* (anti-apoptosis) in MALT

77.2.6 Treatment and Prognosis

Treatment
- Immunocompetent PCNSL
  - Glucocorticoids
  - Radiation therapy
  - Chemotherapy (CHOP: cyclophosphamide, doxorubicin, vincristine, prednisone)
  - Combined-modality therapy
  - Intrathecal methotrexate
  - High-dose methotrexate
  - Autologous stem cell therapy
- AIDS-related PCNSL
  - High-dose intravenous methotrexate
- Essential points in the management of PCNSL
  - Treatment consists of induction with CT and consolidation with WBRT or HDCT with ASCT support.
  - CHOP or derivatives are not recommended in PCNSL.
  - CT should include HD-MTX at doses of at least 3 g/m^2, optimal dose of MTX has not been identified.
  - There is no consensus on the optimal dose of HD-MTX on the role of radiation.
  - MTX should be given by IV infusion for 2–3 h for a minimum of 4–6 injections and intervals should not exceed 2–3 weeks. It is not known the optimal number of HD-MTX cycles in PCNSL, but it is proposed that it must be more than 4 before consolidation.
  - Responses improve with the use of combination of HD-MTX with other CT agents which are known to be active to cross the BBB.
  - HD-MTX is feasible in elderly patients with good PS and adequate renal function.
  - Intra-arterial MTX is an alternative experimental approach for selected cases but must be done only with experienced teams.
  - Prevention and management of HD-MTX toxicity are critical.
  - Rituximab combined with CT is recommended only as an experimental regimen within clinical trials.
  - Intrathecal chemotherapy (IT-CT) is not recommended as a prophylaxis, but may be considered in cases with leptomeningeal involvement.

Biologic Behavior–Prognosis–Prognostic Factors
- Secondary meningeal spread in 30–40%
- 5-year survival: 29.3%
- 10-year survival: 21.6%
- If CNS prophylaxis is to be given,
  - it should be preferably administered during primary chemotherapy.
  - there is no strong evidence that supports any single approach for CNS prophylaxis.
- Predictive markers for DLBCL
  - Adverse prognosis
    o Bcl-2 and c-myc
    o X-linked inhibitor of apoptosis (XIAP)
    o IRF4/MUM1
    o Cyclin D2
    o Cyclin D3
    o P53
    o CD5
    o FOXP1
    o PKC-ß
    o ICAM1
    o HLA-DR
    o C-Flip
    o EBV
    o DcR3 and sutvivin
    o KI67 high index
  - Favorable outcome
    o Bcl-6
    o CD10
    o LMO2

77.3 Intravascular Lymphoma

WHO Definition
2016—A distinctive lymphoma characterized by exclusively intravascular growth (Deckert et al. 2016).

Synonyms used:
- intravascular lymphomatosis
- angiotropic lymphoma
- malignant angioendotheliomatosis

77.3.1 Clinical Signs and Symptoms

- Highly variable clinical presentation as:
  - Dementia
  - Creutzfeldt–Jacob disease
  - Aphasia
  - Dystonia
  - Multiple cerebral infarctions
  - Status epilepticus as the initial presentation
  - Acute hemorrhagic leukoencephalopathy
  - Pituitary apoplexy
  - Cerebral stroke
  - Acute hemispheric dysfunction
  - Longitudinally extensive myelitis
  - Cerebral infarction and a high serum MPO-ANCA level
  - Recurrent cerebral hemorrhages
  - Progressive paraparesis

77.3.2 Epidemiology

Incidence
- unusually rare disorder

Age Incidence
- middle-aged to elderly patients

Localization
- predilection site: CNS and skin

77.3.3 Neuroimaging Findings

General
- Scattered multifocal hyperintensities with enhancement

CT non-contrast-enhanced (Fig. 77.9a)
- Usually normal
- Focal hypodensities possible

CT contrast-enhanced (Fig. 77.9b)
- No enhancement

MRI-T2/FLAIR (Fig. 77.9c, d)
- Focal, multiple hyperintensities

MRI-T1 (Fig. 77.9e)
- Multifocal hypointensities

MRI-T1 Contrast-Enhanced (Fig. 77.9f)
- Linear enhancement along perivascular spaces
- Meningeal enhancement

MRI-T2∗/SWI
- Microhemorrhages possible

MR-Diffusion Imaging (Fig. 77.9g)
- Restricted diffusion in lesions described

Nuclear Medicine Imaging Findings
- FDG-PET can be positive.
- FDG-PET can be used to screen the whole body for other lymphoma manifestations.

77.3.4 Neuropathology Findings

Macroscopic Features
- Normal appearing
- Areas of
  - brain softening
  - infarction
  - hemorrhages
  - necroses

77.3 Intravascular Lymphoma

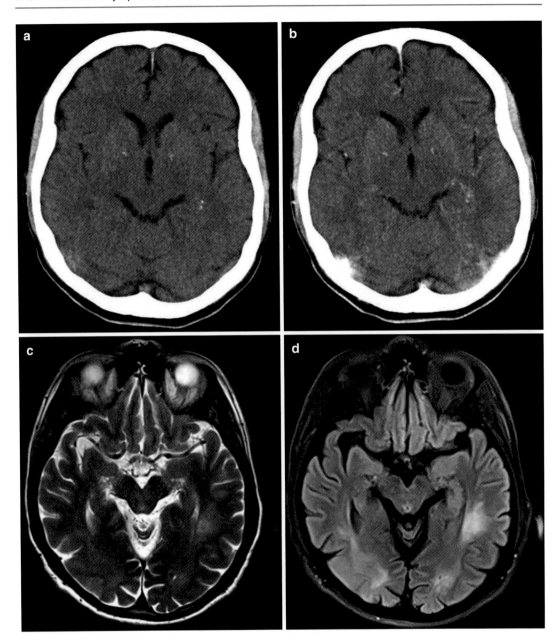

Fig. 77.9 Intravascular lymphoma in CT (**a**), CT contrast (**b**), T2 (**c**), FLAIR (**d**), T1 (**e**), T1 contrast (**f**), DWI (**g**), rCBV (**h**)

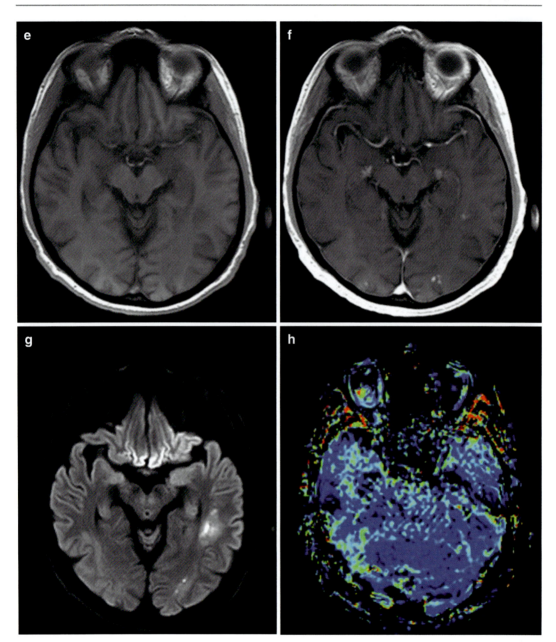

Fig. 77.9 (continued)

Microscopic Features (Fig. 77.10a–d)
- Intravascular growth of
  - large lymphoma cells
    - with vesicular nuclei
    - prominent nucleoli
- B-cell lymphoma
- Necroses after vessel occlusion

Immunophenotype (Fig. 77.10e–j)
A list of antibodies with positive or negative immunostaining results is given in Table 77.7.

Proliferation Markers
- High labeling index for Ki67

77.3 Intravascular Lymphoma

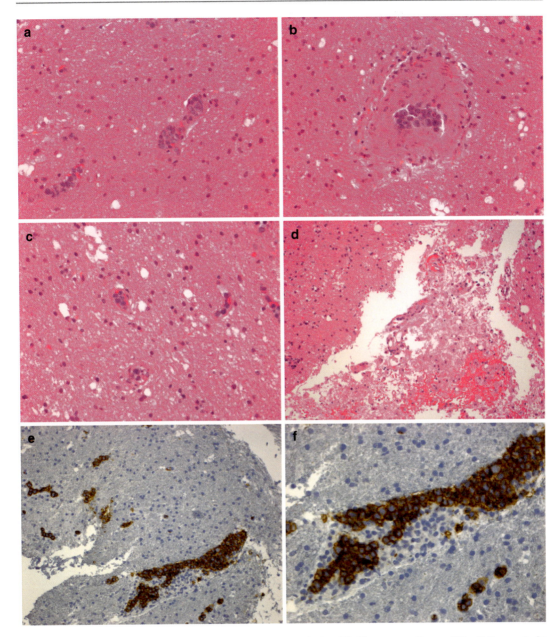

Fig. 77.10 Intravascular lymphoma. Intravascular growth of large lymphoma cells with vesicular nuclei and prominent nucleoli (**a–c**). Necroses occur after vessel occlusion (**d**). The tumor cells are of B-cell lineage (**e–h**) (IHC for CD20). Few T-cell lymphocytes are located in perivascular spaces (**i, j**) (IHC for CD3)

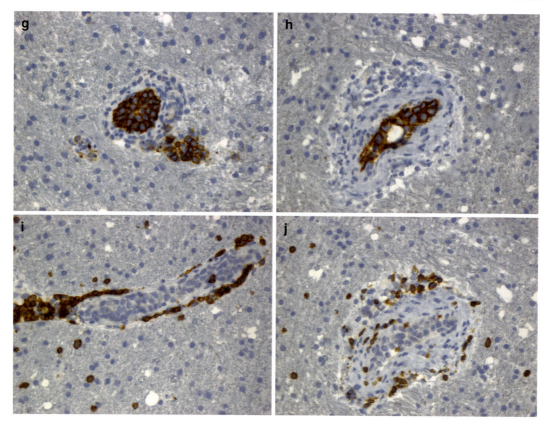

Fig. 77.10 (continued)

Table 77.7 Immunophenotype of intravascular lymphoma

Positivities	Negativities
B-cell markers • CD19 • CD20 • CD22 • CD79a • MUM1 87% cases • CD5 (38% cases positive) • CD10 (13% cases positive)	• CD29 • ICAM1 (CD54) • CD10

Differential Diagnosis
- Primary CNS lymphoma
- Progressive multifocal leukoencephalopathy
- Encephalomyelitis
- Chronic inflammation
- Creutzfeldt–Jacob disease
- Infarction

77.3.5 Molecular Neuropathology

- Immunoglobulin gene rearrangement
- Altered expression of adhesion molecules, i.e., CD44, ß-1 integrin

77.3.6 Treatment and Prognosis

Treatment
- Combination of chemotherapy (combination of MTX-based intrathecal chemotherapy and R-CHOP)
- Intrathecal therapy with cytarabine
- Prednisolone
- Intravascular use of unfractionated heparin
- Bone marrow transplantation

Biologic Behavior–Prognosis–Prognostic Factors
- Aggressive behavior
- Short survival (14 months–2 years)

77.4 Post-Transplant Lymphoproliferative Disorder (PTLD)

WHO Definition

2017—Post-transplant lymphoproliferative disorders (PTLDs) are lymphoid or plasmacytic proliferations that develop as a consequence of immunosuppression in a recipient of a solid organ or stem cell allograft. They constitute a spectrum ranging from usually EBV-driven polyclonal proliferations to EBV-positive or EBV-negative proliferations indistinguishable from a subset of B-cell or (less often) T-/NK-cell lymphomas that occur in immunocompetent individuals (Swerdlow et al. 2017b).

2008—Post-transplant lymphoproliferative disorders (PTLDs) are lymphoid or plasmacytic proliferations that develop as a consequence of immunosuppression in a recipient of a solid organ, bone marrow, or stem cell allograft. PTLD comprise a spectrum ranging from usually Epstein-Barr virus (EBV)-driven infectious mononucleosis-type polyclonal proliferations to EBV-positive or EBV-negative proliferations indistinguishable from a subset of B-cell or less often T-cell lymphomas that occur in immunocompetent individuals (Swerdlow et al. 2008)

2001—Post-transplant lymphoproliferative disorder (PTLD) is a lymphoid proliferation or lymphoma that develops as a consequence of immunosuppression in a recipient of a solid organ or bone marrow allograft. PTLDs comprise a spectrum ranging from early, Epstein-Barr virus (EBV)-driven polyclonal proliferations resembling infectious mononucleosis to EBV-positive or EBV-negative lymphomas of predominantly B-cell or less often T-cell type.

77.4.1 Epidemiology

Incidence
- Rare
- Kind of allograft:
  - <1% in patients with renal allografts
  - 5% in patients with heart/lung or intestinal allografts

Age Incidence
- middle age

Sex Incidence
- no gender predominance

Localization
- Any part of the brain

77.4.2 Neuroimaging Findings

General
Similar to AIDS-related lymphoma.

CT non-contrast-enhanced
- Hypodense lesions

CT contrast-enhanced
- Peripheral enhancement

MRI-T1
- Hypointense lesions

MRI-T2/FLAIR
- Heterogeneous masses

MRI-T1 contrast-enhanced
- Peripheral enhancement

MR-Diffusion Imaging
- Restricted diffusion

MRI-T2*/SWI
- Hemorrhages and necrosis common

MRI-Perfusion
- rCBV elevated

77.4.3 Neuropathology Findings

Macroscopic Features
- Single or multiple masses
- Deep seated
- Firm, friable, granular, central necrosis
- Gray-tan, yellow

Microscopic Features (Fig. 77.11a–h)
- Early lesions:
- Plasmacytic hyperplasia
- Infectious mononucleosis-like changes
- Polymorphic PLTD
  - Heterogeneous cell populations
    - Immunoblasts
    - Plasma cells
    - Small- to medium-sized lymphocytes
- Monomorphic PLTD
  - B-cell neoplasms
    - Diffuse large B-cell lymphoma
    - Burkitt lymphoma
    - Plasma cell neoplasm
    - Plasmacytoma-like lesion
  - B-cell neoplasms
    - Transformed monoclonal B-lymphocytes or plasma cells
    - Qualify as diffuse large B-cell lymphoma
    - IgG gene rearrangements
    - EBV-positivity
  - T-cell neoplasms
    - Peripheral T-cell lymphoma, NOS
    - Hepatosplenic T-cell lymphoma
  - Classical Hodgkin lymphoma-type PLTD
    - Resembles classical Hodgkin lymphoma
    - EBV-positive

Immunophenotype (Fig. 77.11i–t)
- Positive for
  - EBV
  - B-cell markers
  - T-cell markers

Proliferation Markers (Fig. 77.11u, v)
- Medium to high

Differential Diagnosis
- Primary CNS lymphoma

77.4.4 Molecular Neuropathology

- Immunosuppressive treatment after solid organ transplant, bone marrow, or stem cell allograft
- Infection with Epstein-Barr virus (EBV)
  - Infected host lymphocytes in organ recipients
  - Infected donor lymphocytes in bone marrow or stem cell allograft recipients

77.4.5 Treatment and Prognosis

Treatment
- Surgical resection
- Reduction in immunosuppression
- Steroids
- Radiotherapy
- High-dose methotraxate
- Immunotherapy
- Rituximab
- Anti-Cd21 and anti-CD24 monoclonal antibodies
- Cellular therapy
- Antiviral therapy
- Cytokine therapy
- Intrathecal treatments

Biologic Behavior–Prognosis–Prognostic Factors
- Poor prognosis
- CNS PTLDs more aggressive than PTLDs of other organs
- Median survival: 13 weeks
- Mortality rate: 60–90%

77.4 Post-Transplant Lymphoproliferative Disorder (PTLD)

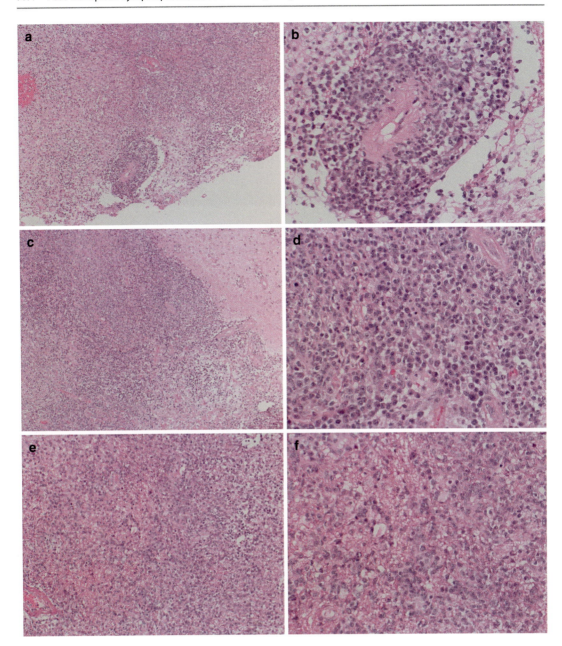

Fig. 77.11 Post-transplant lymphoproliferative disorder—polymorphic subtype: tumor of moderate cellularity with partly diffuse growth pattern, partly perivascular cuffing (**a–h**). The tumor cells are partly CD-20-positive B-lymphocytes (**i, j**), partly CD-3-positive T-lymphocytes (**k, l**). Tumor cells are positive for Epstein-Barr virus (EBV) (**m, n**). Presence of cells of plasmacytic origin (CD138) (**o, p**). Reactive astrogliosis in the surrounding tissue (GFAP: **q, r**; S-100: **s, t**). High Ki67 proliferation rate (**u, v**)

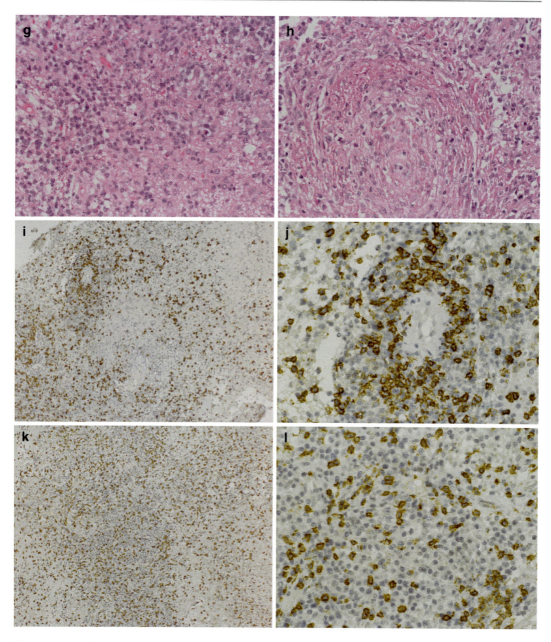

Fig. 77.11 (continued)

77.4 Post-Transplant Lymphoproliferative Disorder (PTLD)

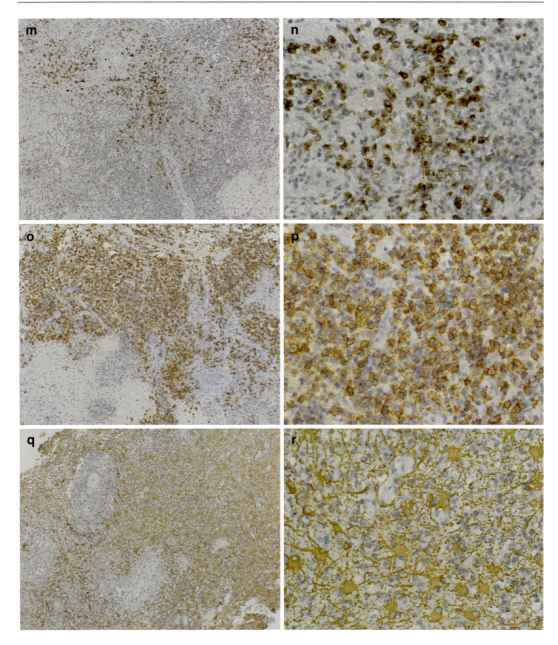

Fig. 77.11 (continued)

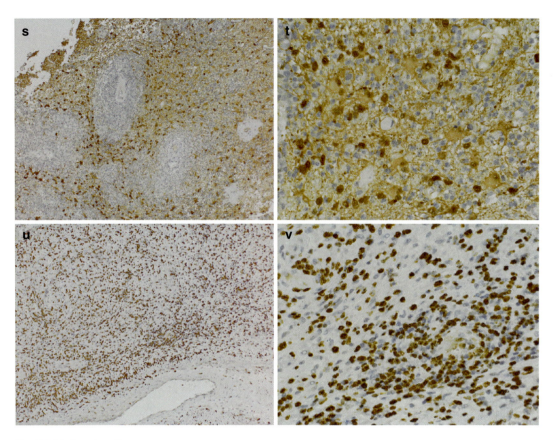

Fig. 77.11 (continued)

77.5 Plasmacytoma

WHO Definition
2016—not mentioned anymore.

2007—In its purely extraosseous for, intracranial plasmacytoma most often appears as a nodular or plaque-like dural mass, with variable infiltration of the underlying brain (Deckert and Paulus 2007)

2001—In its purely extraosseous for, intracranial plasmacytoma most often appears as a nodular or plaque-like dural mass, with variable infiltration of the underlying brain (Paulus et al. 2000).

1993—A tumor composed of mature-appearing neoplastic plasma cells (Kleihues et al. 1993).

77.5.1 Epidemiology

Incidence
- 10% of hematologic malignancies

Age Incidence
- Older than 50 years of age

Sex Incidence
- Male:Female ratio: 2:1

Localization
- Osseous
- Extraosseous

77.5.2 Neuroimaging Findings

General
- Intracranial involvement is rare.
- Destructive osseous lesions in calvarium, skull, nose, or paranasal sinuses with dural or leptomeningeal involvement.

CT non-contrast-enhanced (Fig. 77.12a)
- Iso- to hyperdense lesion

CT contrast-enhanced
- Enhancement

MRI-T2/FLAIR (Fig. 77.12b, c)
- Hypointense lesion

MRI-T1 (Fig. 77.12d)
- Iso- to hyperintense lesion

MRI-T2∗/SWI
- Usually no hemorrhages

MRI-T1 Contrast-Enhanced (Fig. 77.12e, f)
- Lesion enhances

MR-Diffusion Imaging (Fig. 77.12g)
- Restricted diffusion in lesions described

MRI-Perfusion
- rCBV increased

Nuclear Medicine Imaging Findings
- Plasmacytomas are described to be FDG-positive (despite of their indolent characteristics).
- Studies showed the value of FDG-PET in differentiating MGUS patients from plasmacytoma.
- Tc99m-MIBI is an alternative in evaluating plasmacytoma patients if FDG-PET is not available, but the poorer tumor to background ratio and the lower spatial resolution have to be taken into account. In one case an intense uptake of Tc99m-HMPAO in a plasmacytoma was reported.
- In bone scan, plasmacytoma shows reduced uptake (with a possible increased uptake in the margin due to reparation processes) but the resolution limit of the system has to be taken into account.

77.5.3 Neuropathology Findings

Macroscopic Features
- Destructive bone lesion
- Nodular or plaque-like dural mass
- Single or multiple masses
- Deep seated
- Firm, friable, granular, central necrosis
- Gray-tan, yellow
- Infiltration of the underlying brain tissue

Microscopic Features (Fig. 77.13a–f)
- Plasma cell differentiation
  - Resembling normal plasma cell with abundant cytoplasm
  - Immature features
  - Pleomorphic features
- Bone lesions
  - Filling of medullary cavity
  - Erosion of cancellous bone
  - Destruction of bone cortex
- Diffuse infiltration of brain or surrounding soft tissues

Immunophenotype (Fig. 77.13g–j)
A list of antibodies with positive or negative immunostaining results is given in Table 77.8.

Proliferation Markers (Fig. 77.13k, l)
- Moderate to high

Ultrastructural Features
- prominent rER
- prominent enlarged nucleolus

Differential Diagnosis
- Lymphoma
- Metastatic carcinoma

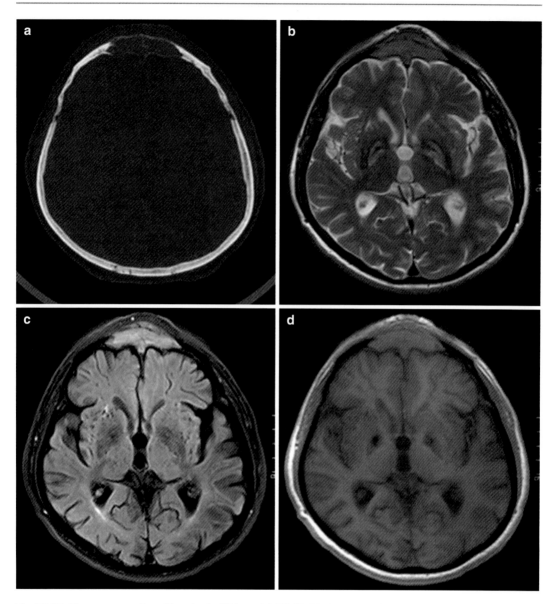

Fig. 77.12 Plasmocytoma: frontal location in CT bone (**a**), T2 (**b**), FLAIR (**c**), T1 (**d**), T1 contrast ax/sag (**e, f**), DWI (**g**)

77.5 Plasmacytoma

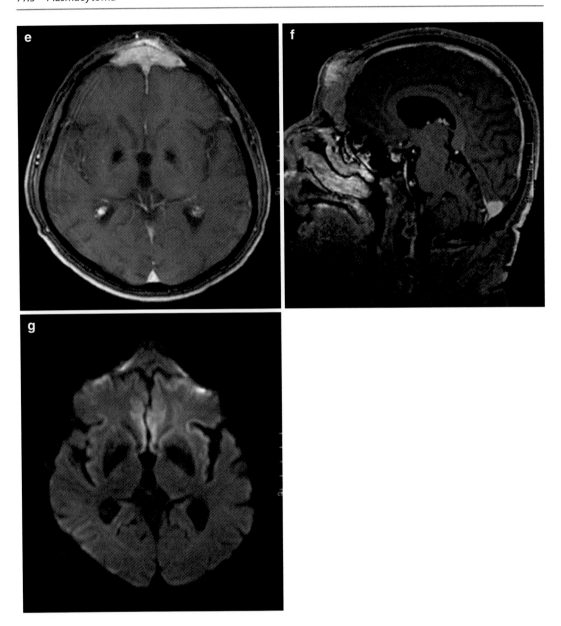

Fig. 77.12 (continued)

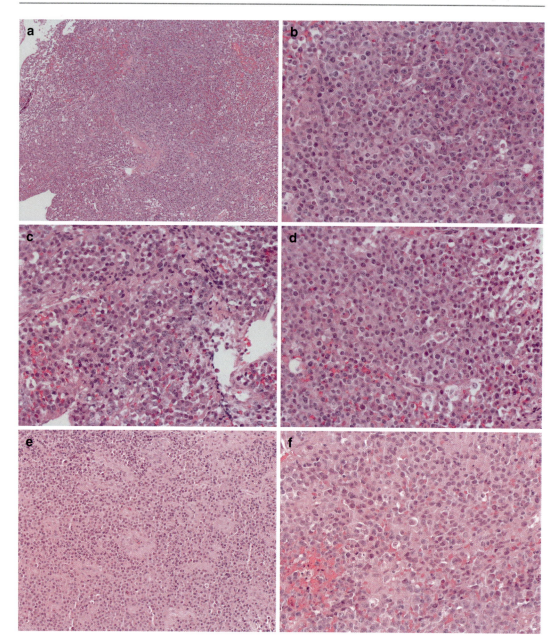

Fig. 77.13 Plasmocytoma: Tumor of high cellularity composed of cells with plasma cell, differentiation with abundant cytoplasm, immature features, and pleomorphic features (**a–f**). The tumor cells are immunopositive for CD138 (**g**, **h**). Restriction of kappa light chain demonstrated by immunohistochemistry (**i**) or of lambda light chain as demonstrated by color in situ hybridization (CISH) (**j**). High Ki67 proliferation rate (**k**, **l**)

77.5 Plasmacytoma

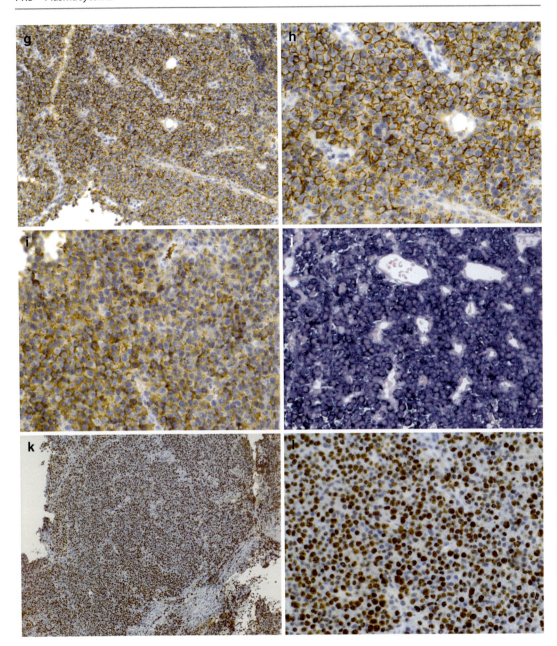

Fig. 77.13 (continued)

Table 77.8 Immunophenotype of plasmacytoma

Positivities	Negativities

• Plasma cell marker
  – CD138, CD38
• B-cell marker
  – CD79a
• Either kappa or lambda light chain restriction
• Bcl-1
• Possible:
  – CD56, CD117, CD52, CD10, CD45
	• CD19
	• CD20

77.5.4 Molecular Neuropathology

- Postgerminal center origin of the neoplastic cells
- Clonal rearrangement of the IgL- and IgH-chain genes

77.5.5 Treatment and Prognosis

Treatment
- Surgical resection
- Radiation therapy
- In case of progression in multiple myeloma:
  - High-dose chemotherapy with bone marrow rescue by autologous hematopoietic-cell transplantation in patients diagnosed before age 65
  - Combination of chemotherapy with thalidomide
  - Treatment of complications (anemia, infections, hypercalcemia)

Biologic Behavior–Prognosis–Prognostic Factors
- 66% progress within 3 years to generalized myeloma
- Poor prognostic features include:
  - Low level of serum albumin
  - Anemia
  - C-reactive protein
  - Serum calcium
  - Large tumor burden

Selected References

Adachi K, Yamaguchi F, Node Y, Kobayashi S, Takagi R, Teramoto A (2013) Neuroimaging of primary central nervous system lymphoma in immunocompetent patients: comparison of recent and previous findings. J Nippon Med Sch 80(3):174–183

Agarwal A (2014) Neuroimaging of plasmacytoma. A pictorial review. Neuroradiol J 27(4):431–437. https://doi.org/10.15274/nrj-2014-10078

Anastasi J (2009) Another great medical mimic: intravascular lymphoma. Leuk Lymphoma 50(11):1742–1743. https://doi.org/10.3109/10428190903350439

Baehring JM, Henchcliffe C, Ledezma CJ, Fulbright R, Hochberg FH (2005) Intravascular lymphoma: magnetic resonance imaging correlates of disease dynamics within the central nervous system. J Neurol Neurosurg Psychiatry 76(4):540–544. https://doi.org/10.1136/jnnp.2003.033662

Batchelor TT (2016) Primary central nervous system lymphoma. Hematology Am Soc Hematol Educ Program 2016(1):379–385. https://doi.org/10.1182/asheducation-2016.1.379

Bierman PJ (2014) Surgery for primary central nervous system lymphoma: is it time for reevaluation? Oncology 28(7):632–637

Brandao LA, Castillo M (2016a) Lymphomas-Part 1. Neuroimaging Clin N Am 26(4):511–536. https://doi.org/10.1016/j.nic.2016.06.004

Brandao LA, Castillo M (2016b) Lymphomas-part 2. Neuroimaging Clin N Am 26(4):537–565. https://doi.org/10.1016/j.nic.2016.06.005

Brennan KC, Lowe LH, Yeaney GA (2005) Pediatric central nervous system posttransplant lymphoproliferative disorder. Am J Neuroradiol 26(7):1695–1697

Carnevale J, Rubenstein JL (2016) The challenge of primary central nervous system lymphoma. Hematol Oncol Clin North Am 30(6):1293–1316. https://doi.org/10.1016/j.hoc.2016.07.013

Cerase A, Tarantino A, Gozzetti A, Muccio CF, Gennari P, Monti L, Di Blasi A, Venturi C (2008) Intracranial involvement in plasmacytomas and multiple myeloma: a pictorial essay. Neuroradiology 50(8):665–674. https://doi.org/10.1007/s00234-008-0390-x

Citterio G, Reni M, Ferreri AJ (2015) Present and future treatment options for primary CNS lymphoma. Expert Opin Pharmacother 16(17):2569–2579. https://doi.org/10.1517/14656566.2015.1088828

Citterio G, Reni M, Gatta G, Ferreri AJM (2017) Primary central nervous system lymphoma. Crit Rev Oncol Hematol 113:97–110. https://doi.org/10.1016/j.critrevonc.2017.03.019

Clarke JL, Deangelis LM (2012) Primary central nervous system lymphoma. Handb Clin Neurol 105:517–527. https://doi.org/10.1016/b978-0-444-53502-3.00006-9

Selected References

Daras M, DeAngelis LM (2013) Management of elderly patients with primary central nervous system lymphoma. Curr Neurol Neurosci Rep 13(5):344. https://doi.org/10.1007/s11910-013-0344-5

DeAngelis LM (2014) Whither whole brain radiotherapy for primary CNS lymphoma? Neuro Oncol 16(8):1032–1034. https://doi.org/10.1093/neuonc/nou122

Deckert M, Paulus W (2007) Malignant lymphomas. In: Louis DN, Ohgaki H, Wiestler OD, Cavenee WK (eds) WHO Classification of Tumours of the Central Nervous System, 4th edn. International Agency for Research on Cancer, Lyon, pp 188–192

Deckert M, Brunn A, Montesinos-Rongen M, Terreni MR, Ponzoni M (2014) Primary lymphoma of the central nervous system—a diagnostic challenge. Hematol Oncol 32(2):57–67. https://doi.org/10.1002/hon.2087

Deckert M, Paulus W, Kluin PM, Ferry JA (2016) Lymphomas. In: Louis DN, Ohgaki H, Wiestler OD, Cavenee WK (eds) WHO classification of tumours of the central nervous system, Revised 4th edn. IARC, Lyon, pp 272–277

Di Micco P, Di Micco B (2005) Up-date on solitary plasmacytoma and its main differences with multiple myeloma. Exp Oncol 27(1):7–12

Fonkem E, Dayawansa S, Stroberg E, Lok E, Bricker PC, Kirmani B, Wong ET, Huang JH (2016) Neurological presentations of intravascular lymphoma (IVL): meta-analysis of 654 patients. BMC Neurol 16:9. https://doi.org/10.1186/s12883-015-0509-8

Fraser E, Gruenberg K, Rubenstein JL (2015) New approaches in primary central nervous system lymphoma. Chin Clin Oncol 4(1):11. https://doi.org/10.3978/j.issn.2304-3865.2015.02.01

Gan LP, Ooi WS, Lee HY, Ng WH (2013) A case of large B-cell intravascular lymphoma in the brain. Surg Neurol Int 4:99. https://doi.org/10.4103/2152-7806.115709

Giannini C, Dogan A, Salomao DR (2014) CNS lymphoma: a practical diagnostic approach. J Neuropathol Exp Neurol 73(6):478–494. https://doi.org/10.1097/nen.0000000000000076

Haldorsen IS, Espeland A, Larsson EM (2011) Central nervous system lymphoma: characteristic findings on traditional and advanced imaging. Am J Neuroradiol 32(6):984–992. https://doi.org/10.3174/ajnr.A2171

Hottinger AF, Alentorn A, Hoang-Xuan K (2015) Recent developments and controversies in primary central nervous system lymphoma. Curr Opin Oncol 27(6):496–501. https://doi.org/10.1097/cco.0000000000000233

Illerhaus G (2015) III. Current concepts in primary central nervous lymphoma. Hematol Oncol 33(Suppl 1):25–28. https://doi.org/10.1002/hon.2211

Kageyama T, Yamanaka H, Nakamura F, Suenaga T (2017) Persistent lesion hyperintensity on brain diffusion-weighted MRI is an early sign of intravascular lymphoma. BMJ Case Rep 2017. https://doi.org/10.1136/bcr-2017-220099

Kerbauy MN, Moraes FY, Lok BH, Ma J, Kerbauy LN, Spratt DE, Santos FP, Perini GF, Berlin A, Chung C, Hamerschlak N, Yahalom J (2017) Challenges and opportunities in primary CNS lymphoma: a systematic review. Radiother Oncol 122(3):352–361. https://doi.org/10.1016/j.radonc.2016.12.033

Kleihues P, Burger PC, Scheithauer BW (1993) Histological typing of tumours of the central nervous system, 2nd edn. Springer-Verlag, Berlin

Kloc G, Budziak M, Wieckiewicz A, Plesniak M, Bartosik-Psujek H (2016) Intravascular lymphoma mimicking multiple sclerosis. Neurol Neurochir Pol 50(4):313–317. https://doi.org/10.1016/j.pjnns.2016.04.007

Ko CC, Tai MH, Li CF, Chen TY, Chen JH, Shu G, Kuo YT, Lee YC (2016) Differentiation between glioblastoma multiforme and primary cerebral lymphoma: additional benefits of quantitative diffusion-weighted MR imaging. PLoS One 11(9):e0162565. https://doi.org/10.1371/journal.pone.0162565

Korfel A, Schlegel U (2013) Diagnosis and treatment of primary CNS lymphoma. Nat Rev Neurol 9(6):317–327. https://doi.org/10.1038/nrneurol.2013.83

Nabavizadeh SA, Vossough A, Hajmomenian M, Assadsangabi R, Mohan S (2016) Neuroimaging in central nervous system lymphoma. Hematol Oncol Clin North Am 30(4):799–821. https://doi.org/10.1016/j.hoc.2016.03.005

Nayak L, Pentsova E, Batchelor TT (2015) Primary CNS lymphoma and neurologic complications of hematologic malignancies. Continuum 21(2 Neuro-oncology):355–372. https://doi.org/10.1212/01.CON.0000464175.96311.0a

Nizamutdinov D, Patel NP, Huang JH, Fonkem E (2017) Intravascular lymphoma in the CNS: options for treatment. Curr Treat Options Neurol 19(10):35. https://doi.org/10.1007/s11940-017-0471-4

Panda AK, Malik S (2014) CNS intravascular lymphoma: an underappreciated cause of rapidly progressive dementia. BMJ Case Rep 2014. https://doi.org/10.1136/bcr-2014-203772

Patrick LB, Mohile NA (2015) Advances in primary central nervous system lymphoma. Curr Oncol Rep 17(12):60. https://doi.org/10.1007/s11912-015-0483-8

Paulus W, Jellinger K, Morgello S, Deckert-Schlüter M (2000) Malignant lymphomas. In: Kleihues P, Cavenee WK (eds) Pathology and genetics of tumours of the nervous system, 3rd edn. IARC, Lyon, pp 198–203

Paydas S (2017) Primary central nervous system lymphoma: essential points in diagnosis and management. Med Oncol 34(4):61. https://doi.org/10.1007/s12032-017-0920-7

Phillips EH, Fox CP, Cwynarski K (2014) Primary CNS lymphoma. Curr Hematol Malig Rep 9(3):243–253. https://doi.org/10.1007/s11899-014-0217-2

Prayson RA (2016) Intravascular lymphoma mimicking vasculitis. J Clin Neurosci 34:224–225. https://doi.org/10.1016/j.jocn.2016.06.010

Roohi F (2013) Diagnosis of intravascular lymphoma. JAMA Neurol 70(7):941. https://doi.org/10.1001/jamaneurol.2013.307

Roth P, Korfel A, Martus P, Weller M (2012) Pathogenesis and management of primary CNS lymphoma. Expert Rev Anticancer Ther 12(5):623–633. https://doi.org/10.1586/era.12.36

Schaafsma JD, Hui F, Wisco D, Staugaitis SM, Uchino K, Kouzmitcheva E, Jaigobin C, Hazrati LN, Mikulis DJ, Mandell DM (2017) High-resolution vessel wall MRI: appearance of intravascular lymphoma mimics central nervous system vasculitis. Clin Neuroradiol 27(1):105–108. https://doi.org/10.1007/s00062-016-0529-9

Schafer N, Glas M, Herrlinger U (2012) Primary CNS lymphoma: a clinician's guide. Expert Rev Neurother 12(10):1197–1206. https://doi.org/10.1586/ern.12.120

Slone HW, Blake JJ, Shah R, Guttikonda S, Bourekas EC (2005) CT and MRI findings of intracranial lymphoma. Am J Roentgenol 184(5):1679–1685. https://doi.org/10.2214/ajr.184.5.01841679

Sugiyama A, Kobayashi M, Daizo A, Suzuki M, Kawashima H, Kagami SI, Tanaka H, Suzuki Y, Matsunaga T, Kuwabara S (2017) Diffuse cerebral vasoconstriction in a intravascular lymphoma patient with a high serum MPO-ANCA level. Intern Med 56(13):1715–1718. https://doi.org/10.2169/internalmedicine.56.8051

Sureka B, Bansal K, Arora A (2015) Intravascular lymphoma. Am J Roentgenol 205(3):W387. https://doi.org/10.2214/ajr.15.14741

Swerdlow SH, Webber SA, Chadburn A, Ferry JA (2008) Post-transplant lymphoproliferative disorders. In: Swerdlow SH, Campo E, Harris NL et al (eds) WHO classification of tumours of haematopoietic and lymphoid tissues. IARC, Lyon, pp 343–349

Swerdlow SH, Campo E, Pileri SA, Harris NL, Stein H, Siebert R, Advani R, Ghielmini M, Salles GA (2016) The 2016 revision of the World Health Organization classification of lymphoid neoplasms. Blood 127(20):2375–2390. https://doi.org/10.1182/blood-2016-01-643569

Swerdlow SE, Campo E, Harris NL, Jaffe ES, Pileri SA, Stein H, Thiele J, Arber DA, Hasserjian RP, Le Beau MM, Orazi A, Siebert R (2017a) WHO classification of tumours of haematopoietic and lymphoid tissues. IARC, Lyon

Swerdlow SH, Webber SA, Chadburn A, Ferry JA (2017b) Post-translplant lymphoproliferative disorders. In: Swerdlow SE, Campo E, Harris NL et al (eds) WHO classification of tumours of haematopoietic and lymphoid tissues. IARC, Lyon, pp 453–462

Szczepanek D, Wasik-Szczepanek E, Stoma F, Sokolowska B, Trojanowski T (2017) Primary central nervous system lymphoma as a neurosurgical problem. Neurol Neurochir Pol 51(4):319–323. https://doi.org/10.1016/j.pjnns.2017.04.004

Tahsili-Fahadan P, Rashidi A, Cimino PJ, Bucelli RC, Keyrouz SG (2016) Neurologic manifestations of intravascular large B-cell lymphoma. Neurol Clin Pract 6(1):55–60. https://doi.org/10.1212/cpj.0000000000000185

Toh CH, Castillo M, Wong AM, Wei KC, Wong HF, Ng SH, Wan YL (2008) Primary cerebral lymphoma and glioblastoma multiforme: differences in diffusion characteristics evaluated with diffusion tensor imaging. Am J Neuroradiol 29(3):471–475. https://doi.org/10.3174/ajnr.A0872

Usuda D, Arahata M, Temaru R, Iinuma Y, Kanda T, Hayashi S (2016) Autopsy-proven intravascular lymphoma presenting as rapidly recurrent strokes. Case Rep Oncol 9(1):148–153. https://doi.org/10.1159/000444632

Wavre A, Baur AS, Betz M, Muhlematter D, Jotterand M, Zaman K, Ketterer N (2007) Case study of intracerebral plasmacytoma as an initial presentation of multiple myeloma. Neuro Oncol 9(3):370–372. https://doi.org/10.1215/15228517-2007-008

Williams RL, Meltzer CC, Smirniotopoulos JG, Fukui MB, Inman M (1998) Cerebral MR imaging in intravascular lymphomatosis. Am J Neuroradiol 19(3):427–431

Yang XL, Liu YB (2017) Advances in pathobiology of primary central nervous system lymphoma. Chin Med J (Engl) 130(16):1973–1979. https://doi.org/10.4103/0366-6999.211879

Yang M, Sun J, Bai HX, Tao Y, Tang X, States LJ, Zhang Z, Zhou J, Farwell MD, Zhang P, Xiao B, Yang L (2017) Diagnostic accuracy of SPECT, PET, and MRS for primary central nervous system lymphoma in HIV patients: a systematic review and meta-analysis. Medicine 96(19):e6676. https://doi.org/10.1097/md.0000000000006676

Yap KK, Sutherland T, Liew E, Tartaglia CJ, Pang M, Trost N (2012) Magnetic resonance features of primary central nervous system lymphoma in the immunocompetent patient: a pictorial essay. J Med Imaging Radiat Oncol 56(2):179–186. https://doi.org/10.1111/j.1754-9485.2012.02345.x

Zacharia TT, Law M, Naidich TP, Leeds NE (2008) Central nervous system lymphoma characterization by diffusion-weighted imaging and MR spectroscopy. J Neuroimaging 18(4):411–417. https://doi.org/10.1111/j.1552-6569.2007.00231.x

Zahid MF, Khan N, Hashmi SK, Kizilbash SH, Barta SK (2016) Central nervous system prophylaxis in diffuse large B-cell lymphoma. Eur J Haematol 97(2):108–120. https://doi.org/10.1111/ejh.12763

Zhang XM, Aguilera NS (2015) Lymph node. In: Lin F, Prichard J (eds) Handbook of practical immunohistochemistry. frequently asked questions, 2nd edn. Springer, Berlin, pp 591–628

Histiocytic Tumors

78.1 General Considerations

78.1.1 Definitions

Histiocytic tumors affecting the nervous system include:
- Langerhans cell histiocytosis
- Non-Langerhans cell histiocytosis
  - Rosai–Dorfman disease
  - Erdheim–Chester disease
  - Juvenile xanthogranuloma and xanthoma disseminatum
  - Histiocytic sarcoma

Histiocytes/Macrophages
- Derived from monocytes
- Involved in host defence and tissue repair including
  - Phagocytosis
  - Cytotoxic activities
  - Regulation of inflammatory and immune responses
  - Wound healing

Dendritic Cells
- Most potent cells for antigen processing and antigen presentation to B- and T-lymphocytes
- Capable of initiating the adaptive immune response
- Three major subclasses
  - Langerhans cells (LC)
  - Interdigitating dendritic cells (IDC)
  - Follicular dendritic cells (FDC)

Langerhans Cells
- Mobile, dendritic, antigen-presenting cells
- Present in all stratified epithelium and predominantly in the mid to upper parts of squamous layers
- Positive for CD1a and S-100

78.1.2 Epidemiology

Incidence
- Langerhans cell histiocytosis
  - 0.5 per 100.000 children
- Non-Langerhans cell histiocytosis
  - 1:1,000,000 per year

Age Incidence
- Langerhans cell histiocytosis
  - Children
  - Mean age: 12 years
- Non-Langerhans cell histiocytosis
  - Adolescence, mean age: 39.4 years

Sex Incidence
- Male:Female ratio
  - Langerhans cell histiocytosis
  - Non-Langerhans cell histiocytosis: 1.5:1

Localization
- Leptomeninges
- Dura mater
- Intracerebral
- Intraventricular

78.1.3 Nuclear Medicine Imaging Findings

- Langerhans cell histiocytosis
  - SSR-scintigraphy has been shown to be useful in detecting pulmonary disease, but insensitive for central nervous lesions. Bone involvement can be assessed by bone scintigraphy, but with less sensitivity than with radiographic skeletal surveys. Thyroid involvement can lead to increased uptake in thyroid scintigraphy with Tc99m.
  - FDG is also positive in these patients, but with some false negative findings (hypometabolism was reported too).
  - Patients with neurodegenerative Langerhans cell histiocytosis presented with hypometabolism in the cerebellum, basal ganglia, frontal cortex and increased uptake in the amygdalae.
- Lesions of patients with Erdheim–Chester disease are described to be positive in FDG-PET.

78.2 Langerhans Cell Histiocytosis (LCH)

WHO Definition
2016—A clonal proliferation of Langerhans-type cells that express CD1a, langerin (CD207), and S100 protein (Paulus et al. 2016).

2007—A heterogeneous group of tumors and tumor-like masses composed of histiocytes that are commonly associated with histologically identical extracranial lesions. Langerhans cell histiocytosis shows features of dendritic Langerhans cells (Paulus and Perry 2007).

2000—Histiocytic tumors
A heterogeneous group of tumors and tumor-like masses composed of histiocytes that are commonly associated with histologically indentical extracranial lesions. Langerhans cell histiocytosis (LCH) shows features of dendritic Langerhans cells, whereas the various types of non-LCH show macrophage differentiation (Paulus et al. 2000).

78.2.1 Clinical Signs and Symptoms

- Neurological problems
  - Deficits in cognition
  - Behavioral disturbances
  - Neuromotor dysfunction
- Diabetes insipidus
- Radiological neurodegeneration—clinical neurodegeneration
  - Mild abnormalities of the reflexes
  - Discrete gait disturbances
  - Dysarthria
  - Dysphagia
  - Motor spasticity
  - Ataxia
  - Behavioral disturbances
  - Learning difficulties
  - Severe psychiatric disease

Three types of CNS involvement are evident
- Hypothalamic-pituitary
- Space occupying
  - Intracerebral
  - Meninges
  - Choroid plexus
- Neurodegenerative

78.2.2 Epidemiology

Incidence
- Langerhans cell histiocytosis
  - 0.5 per 100.000 children

Age Incidence
- Langerhans cell histiocytosis
  - Children
  - Mean age: 12 years

Sex Incidence
- Male:Female ratio
  - Langerhans cell histiocytosis: 1:1

Localization
- Leptomeninges
- Dura mater
- Intracerebral
- Intraventricular

78.2.3 Neuroimaging Findings

General
- Lysis of craniofacial bones and skull base with or without soft tissue extension
- Changes in hypothalamic-pituitary region, meninges, circumventricular organs
- Variable white matter and gray matter changes
- Cerebral atrophy

CT non-contrast-enhanced (Fig. 78.1a)
- Lytic skull lesions without sclerosis
- Associated soft tissue extension

MRI-T2 (Fig. 78.2a)
- Dilated Virchow–Robin spaces (60%)—hyperintense
- Cysts in pineal gland (28%)
- Patchy, confluent white matter hyperintensities
- Pontine and dentate nucleus hyperintensities
- Bilateral choroid-plexus lesions—hypointense
- Epi-subdural, dura-based masses—iso- to hypointense

MRI-FLAIR (Fig. 78.2b)
- Patchy, confluent white matter hyperintensities
- Pontine and dentate nucleus hyperintensities

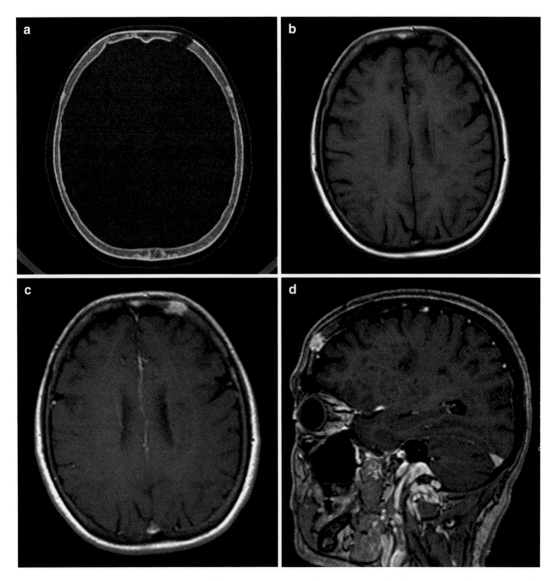

Fig. 78.1 Langerhans cell histiocytosis left frontal intraosseous. CT bone (**a**), T1 (**b**), T1 contrast axial and sag (**c, d**)

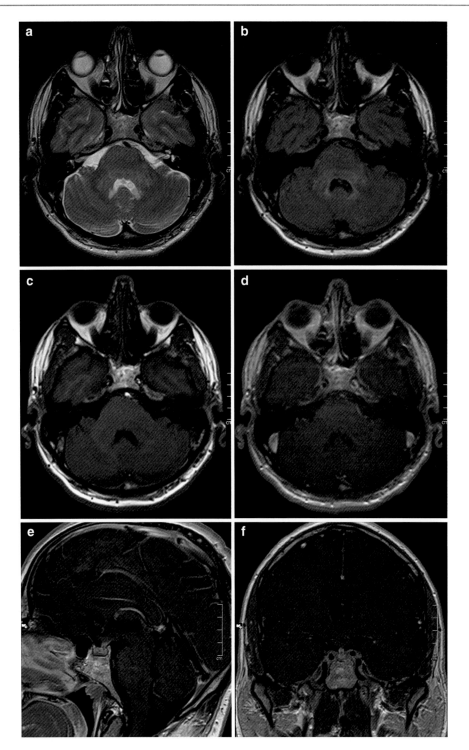

Fig. 78.2 Langerhans cell histiocytosis with thickening of pituitary stalk and periventricular white matter lesions. T2 (**a**), Flair (**b**), T1 (**c**), T1 contrast ax, sag and cor (**d**, **e**, **f**)

78.2 Langerhans Cell Histiocytosis (LCH)

MRI-T1 (Figs. 78.1b and 78.2c)
- Epi-subdural, dura-based masses—isointense
- Bilateral choroid-plexus lesions—hypointense
- Thickening of pituitary stalk
- Lacking of hyperintense neurohypophysis
- Poorly defined, hypointense lesions in white matter
- Dentate nucleus hyperintensities

MRI-T1 contrast-enhanced (Figs. 78.1c, d and 78.2d–f)
- White matter lesions without enhancement
- Dura-based masses with inconstant enhancement
- Thickened infundibular stalk enhance

Nuclear Medicine Imaging Findings (Fig. 78.3)
- SSR-scintigraphy has been shown to be useful in detecting pulmonary disease, but insensitive for central nervous lesions. Bone involvement can be assessed by bone scintigraphy, but with less sensitivity than with radiographic skeletal surveys. Thyroid involvement can lead to increased uptake in thyroid scintigraphy with Tc99m.
- FDG is also positive in these patients, but with some false negative findings (hypometabolism was reported too).
- Patients with neurodegenerative Langerhans cell histiocytosis presented with hypometabolism in the cerebellum, basal ganglia, frontal cortex and increased uptake in the amygdalae.

78.2.4 Neuropathology Findings

Macroscopic Features
- Yellow to white color
- Discrete dural-based nodules
- Granular parenchymal infiltrates
- Either well-delineated or ill-defined

Microscopic Features (Fig. 78.4a–h)
- Langerhans cells
  - Eccentric, ovoid, reniform, or convoluted nuclei
  - Inconspicuous nucleoli
  - Large, pale to eosinophilic cytoplasm
- Macrophages
- Lymphocytes
- Collagen deposits
- Touton giant cells
- No Birbeck granules

Immunophenotype (Fig. 78.4i–l)
A list of antibodies with positive or negative immunostaining results is given in Table 78.1.

Proliferation Markers
- KI-67 LI: 4–16%

Ultrastructural Features
- Birbeck granules in Langerhans cells
  - 34 nm wide rod-shaped intracytoplasmic pentalaminar structures with cross-striation and a zipper-like central core

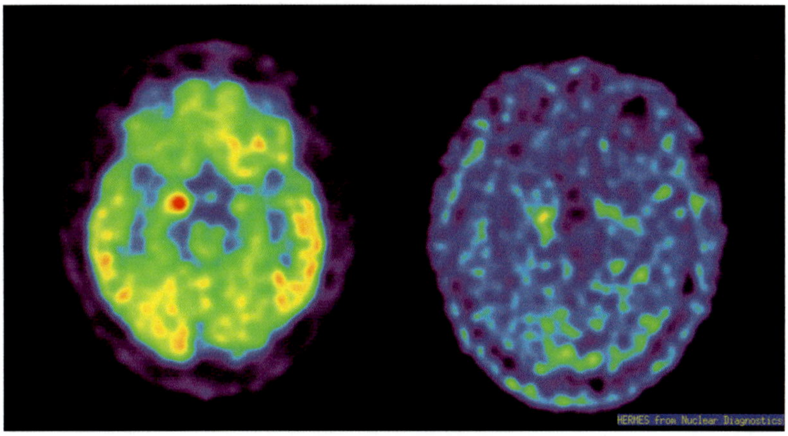

Fig. 78.3 FDG positive (left) histiocytic lesion affecting the right hippocampus with only faint FET uptake (right)

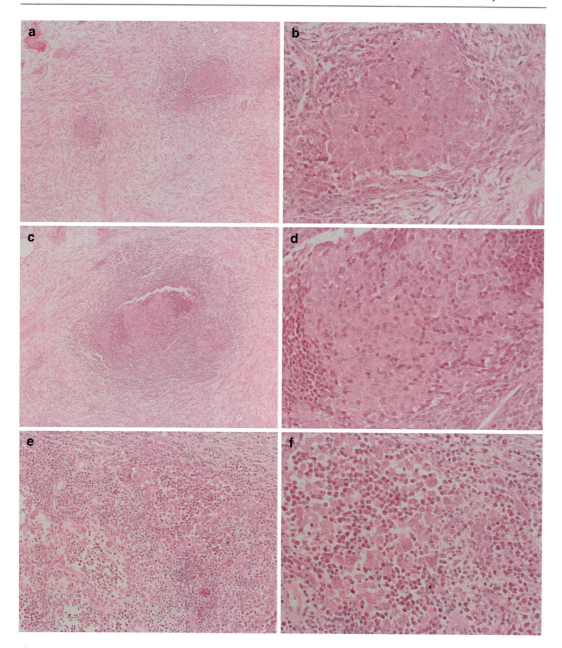

Fig. 78.4 Langerhans disease: Diffuse infiltration of large mononuclear cells with abundant eosinophilic cytoplasm, eccentric, ovoid, reniform or convoluted nuclei, inconspicuous nucleoli, and large, pale to eosinophilic cytoplasm (**a–h**), partly arranged in nodules (eosinophilic granulomas) (**a–d**). The Langerhans cells stain immunopositive for CD1a (**i, j**), and S-100 (**k, l**)

78.2 Langerhans Cell Histiocytosis (LCH)

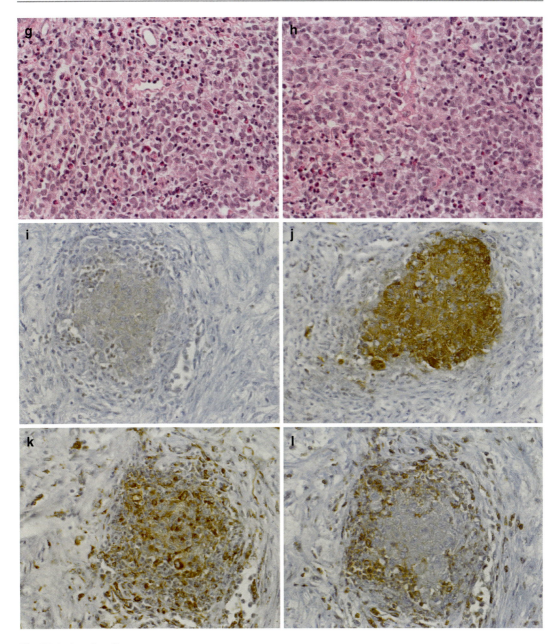

Fig. 78.4 (continued)

Table 78.1 Immunophenotype of Langerhans cell histiocytosis

Positive	Negative
• S-100	• CD1a
• Vimentin	• CD45
• Langerin (CD207)	• CD15
• HLA-DR	• Lysozyme
• ß2-microglobulin	

Differential Diagnosis
- Lymphoma
- Inflammation
- Infection

78.2.5 Molecular Neuropathology

- Immature, partially activated dendritic Langerhans cells
- Clonal proliferation
- Immune dysfunction
- Aberrant expression of chemokine receptors (CCR6, CCR7)

78.2.6 Treatment and Prognosis

Treatment
- Surgical removal
- Radiotherapy
- Chemotherapy
- Combinations of all three

Biologic Behavior–Prognosis–Prognostic Factors
- Survival rates:
  - 5 years: 88%
  - 15 years: 88%
  - 20 years: 77%
- Event-free survival at 15 years: 30%

78.3 Non-Langerhans Cell Histiocytoses

The following non-Langerhans histiocytoses are distinguished:
- Rosai–Dorfman disease
- Erdheim–Chester disease
- Juvenile xanthogranuloma and xanthoma disseminatum
- Histiocytic sarcoma
- Hemophagocytic lymphohistiocytosis

WHO Definition
2016—Erdheim–Chester disease: Erdheim–Chester disease manifesting in the brain or the meninges (Paulus et al. 2016).

Rosai–Dorfman disease: Rosai–Dorfman disease manifesting in the brain or the meninges (Paulus et al. 2016).

Juvenile xanthogranuloma: Juvenile xanthogranuloma arising in the brain or the meninges, either with or without cutaneous lesions (Paulus et al. 2016).

Histiocytic sarcoma: A rare, aggressive, malignant neoplasm with the histological and immunophenotypic characteristics of mature histiocytes (Paulus et al. 2016).

2007—A heterogeneous group of tumors and tumor-like masses composed of histiocytes that are commonly associated with histologically identical extracranial lesions. This group of diseases differs from LCH by the absence of features of dendritic Langerhans cells. Most but not all exhibit macrophage differentiation (Paulus and Perry 2007).

2000—Histiocytic tumors
A heterogeneous group of tumors and tumor-like masses composed of histiocytes that are commonly associated with histologically indentical extracranial lesions. Langerhans cell histiocytosis (LCH) shows features of dendritic Langerhans cells, whereas the various types of non-LCH show macrophage differentiation (Paulus et al. 2000).

78.3.1 Epidemiology

Incidence
- Non-Langerhans cell histiocytosis
  - 1:1,000,000 per year

Age Incidence
- Non-Langerhans cell histiocytosis
  - Adolescence, mean age: 39.4 years
- *Rosai–Dorfman disease*
  - Children and young adults
- *Erdheim–Chester disease*
  - Adults (mean age: 55 years)
- *Hemophagocytic lymphohistiocytosis*
  - Autosomal recessive systemic disease
- *Juvenile xanthogranuloma*
  - Young children
- *Xanthoma disseminatum*
  - Young adults
- *Histiocytic sarcoma*

78.3 Non-Langerhans Cell Histiocytoses

Sex Incidence
- Male:Female ratio
  - Non-Langerhans cell histiocytosis: 1.5:1

Localization
- Leptomeninges
- Dura mater
- Intracerebral
- Intraventricular

78.3.2 Neuroimaging Findings

78.3.2.1 Rosai–Dorfman Disease
General Imaging Findings
- Occurs in 5% as intracranial, dura-based masses, thickening of pituitary stalk less common

CT non-contrast-enhanced
- Hyperdense dura-based masses

CT contrast-enhanced
- Dura-based masses enhance

MRI-T2 (Fig. 78.5a)
- Iso- to hypointense dural masses

MRI-FLAIR (Fig. 78.5b)
- Iso- to hypointense dural masses

MRI-T1 (Fig. 78.5c)
- Dura-based masses isointense

MRI-T1 contrast-enhanced (Fig. 78.5d)
- Dura-based masses enhance homogeneously

MRI-Perfusion
- rCBV decreased

78.3.2.2 Erdheim–Chester Disease: General Imaging Findings
In 10% intracranial spectrum of following:
Osteosclerosis of skull and spine
Dura-based masses
Multifocal hyperintense parenchymal lesions
Thickening of infundibulum

CT non-contrast-enhanced
- Sclerosis of craniofacial bones or spine with thickening

CT contrast-enhanced
- Enhancement of dura-based masses

MRI-T2
- Pontine and dentate nucleus hyperintensities
- Dura-based masses—iso- to hypointense
- Hypointense perivascular thickening along carotid arteries into cavernous sinus
- Multifocal hyperintense lesions

MRI-FLAIR
- Pontine and dentate nucleus hyperintensities

MRI-T1
- Nodular thickening of pituitary stalk
- Lacking of hyperintense neurohypophysis
- Dura-based masses—isointense

MRI-T1 contrast-enhanced (Fig. 78.6a, b)
- Thickened pituitary stalk enhances
- Enhancement of perivascular thickening along carotid arteries
- Dura-based masses enhance
- Ependymal enhancement
- Hyperintense lesions can enhance

Nuclear Medicine Imaging Findings
- Lesions of patients with Erdheim–Chester disease are described to be positive in FDG-PET.

78.3.3 Neuropathology Findings

Macroscopic Features
- Yellow to white color
- Discrete dural-based nodules
- Granular parenchymal infiltrates
- Either well-delineated or ill-defined

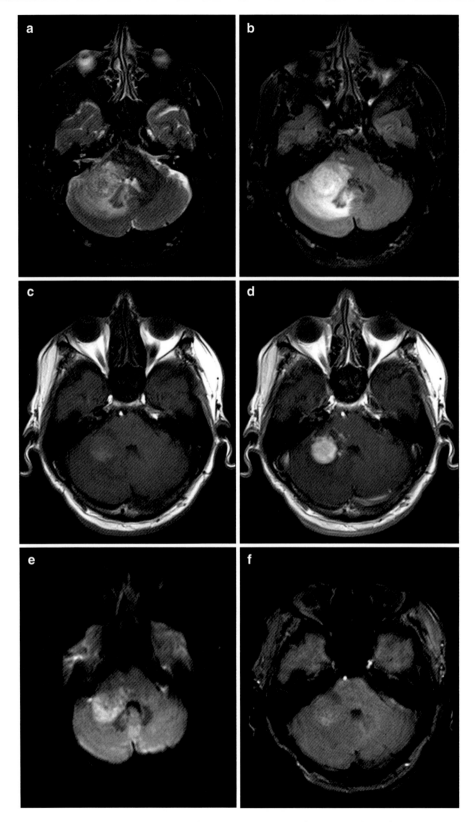

Fig. 78.5 Rosai–Dorfman disease: T2 (**a**), Flair (**b**), T1 (**c**), T1 contrast (**d**), DWI (**e**), SWI (**f**)

78.3 Non-Langerhans Cell Histiocytoses

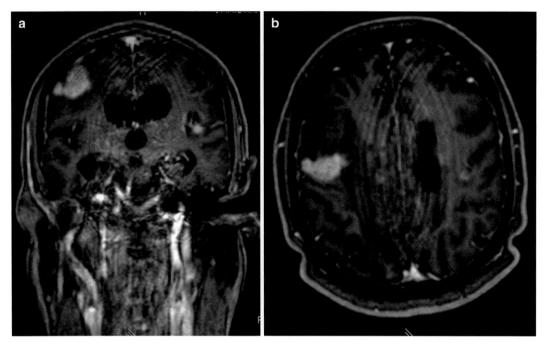

Fig. 78.6 Erdheim–Chester with T1 contrast-enhanced cor and ax (**a, b**) (kindly provided by R McCoy, Division of Neuroradiology, Christian Doppler University Hospital, Salzburg, Austria)

- *Rosai–Dorfman disease*
  - Dural-based solitary or multiple masses
  - Intracerebral and intrasellar lesions
- *Erdheim–Chester disease* (Fig. 78.7a–d)
  - Brain, spinal cord, meninges, orbit
- *Hemophagocytic lymphohistiocytosis*
  - Leptomeninges and multifocal brain lesions
- *Juvenile xanthogranuloma*
  - Brain or meninges
- *Xanthoma disseminatum*
  - Hypothalamus, pituitary gland, or dura mater
- *Histiocytic sarcoma*

Microscopic Features
- *Rosai–Dorfman disease* (Fig. 78.8a–f)
  - corresponds histologically and immunohistochemically to its counterparts occurring elsewhere
  - Sheets or nodules of histiocytes with vacuolated or eosinophilic cytoplasm
  - Emperipolesis:
    - Well-preserved lymphocytes and plasma cells within the cytoplasm of histiocytes
  - Foci of lymphocytes
  - Plasma cells
  - Fibrosis

- *Erdheim–Chester disease* (Fig. 78.9a–j)
  - corresponds histologically and immunohistochemically to its counterparts occurring elsewhere.
  - Systemic lesions may be present or absent.
  - Lipid-laden histiocytes with small nuclei.
  - Touton-like multinucleated giant cells.
  - Lymphocytic infiltrates.
  - Eosinophilic granulocytes.
  - Fibrosis.
- *Juvenile xanthogranuloma*
  - corresponds histologically and immunohistochemically to its cutaneous counterpart
  - Composed of histiocytes
  - Scattered Touton giant cells
  - Lymphocytes
  - Eosinophils
- *Xanthoma disseminatum*
  - Composed of histiocytes
  - Scattered Touton giant cells
  - Lymphocytes
  - Eosinophils

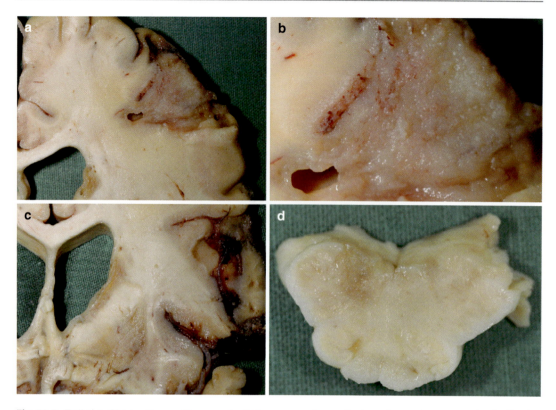

Fig. 78.7 Erdheim–Chester disease: Macroscopically large areas of necrotic tissue destruction are seen (**a–d**) affecting the precentral gyrus (**a, b**), caudate nucleus (**c**), and medulla oblongata (**d**)

- *Histiocytic sarcoma*
  - Intrafollicular dendritic cell sarcoma
- *Hemophagocytic lymphohistiocytosis*
  - Diffuse infiltration of lymphocytes and macrophages with hemophagocytosis

Immunophenotype (Figs. 78.8g–l and 78.10a–n)
A list of antibodies with positive or negative immunostaining results is given in Table 78.2.

Proliferation Markers
- Low to moderate

Differential Diagnosis
- Langerhans cell histiocytosis

78.3.4 Molecular Neuropathology

- Arise from bone marrow derived mononuclear macrophages at various stages of development and activation

78.3.5 Treatment and Prognosis

Treatment
- Surgery
- Corticosteroids
- Antimetabolites
- Interferon alpha

Biologic Behavior–Prognosis–Prognostic Factors
- Rosai–Dorfman
  - Clinical course may be chronic or fluctuating.
  - Usually self-limiting.
  - 70–80% of individuals have spontaneous resolution.
  - Mortality rate is low.
  - Death may result from CNS or renal involvement, immune dysfunction, and opportunistic infections.
- Erdheim–Chester disease
  - Prognosis depends on the extent and distribution of the extraskeletal manifestations.
  - Death due to respiratory distress, extensive pulmonary fibrosis, and cardiac failure.

78.3 Non-Langerhans Cell Histiocytoses

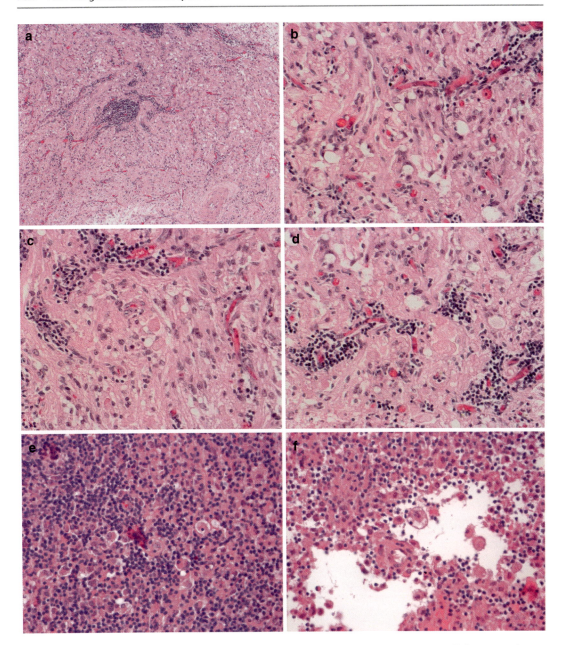

Fig. 78.8 Rosai–Dorfman disease: Sheets or nodules of histiocytes with vacuolated or eosinophilic cytoplasm (**a–e**). Emperipolesis: Well-preserved lymphocytes and plasma cells within the cytoplasm of histiocytes (**f**). Foci of lymphocytes are evident (**a–e**). Histiocytes are immunopositive for S-100 (**g–j**). Low to moderate Ki67 proliferation rate (**k, l**)

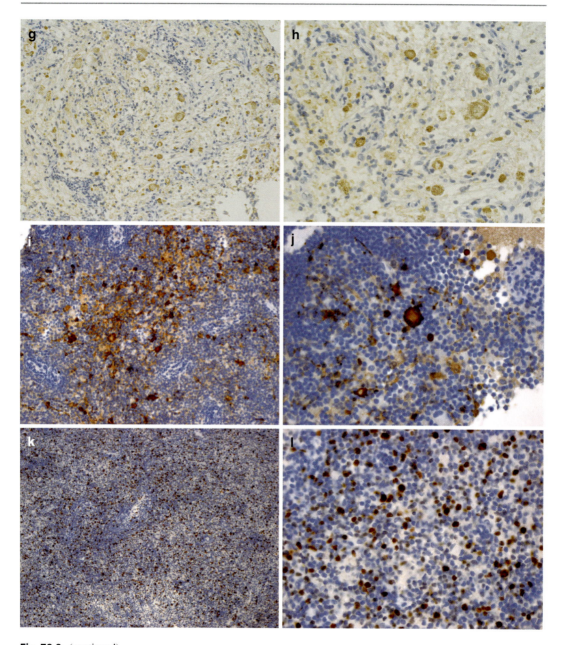

Fig. 78.8 (continued)

78.3 Non-Langerhans Cell Histiocytoses

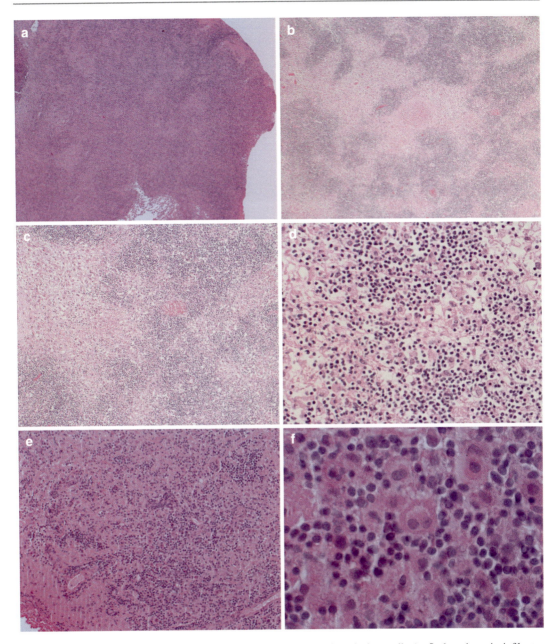

Fig. 78.9 Erdheim–Chester disease: Microscopically, the lesion is of moderate cellularity made up of lipid-laden histiocytes with small nuclei (**a**–**c**), Touton-like multinucleated giant cells (**e**, **f**), lymphocytic infiltrates (**b**–**d**), eosinophilic granulocytes (**d**), perivascular lymphocytic cuffing (**g**, **h**), and reactive astrogliosis (**i**, **j**)

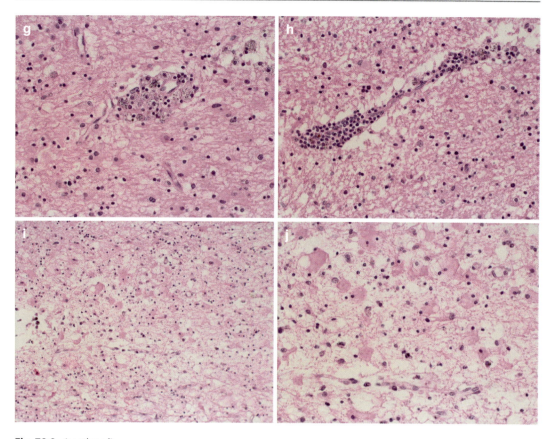

Fig. 78.9 (continued)

Table 78.2 Antibodies used in the differential diagnosis of Non-Langerhans histiocytoses

Entity	Positive	Negative
Rosai–Dorfman disease	• CD11c • CD68 • MAC387 • S-100	• CD1a
Erdheim–Chester disease	• CD68	• CD1a • S-100
Hemophagocytic lymphohistiocytosis	• CD11c • CD68 Variable results for: • CD1a • S-100	
Juvenile xanthogranuloma and xanthoma disseminatum	• CD11c • CD68 • Factor VIIIa Variable result • MAC387	• CD1a • Lysozyme • S-100
Malignant histiocytic disorders	• CD68 • CD163 • CD11c • CD14 • Lysozyme	• Myeloid markers • Dendritic markers • CD30 • ALK1

78.3 Non-Langerhans Cell Histiocytoses

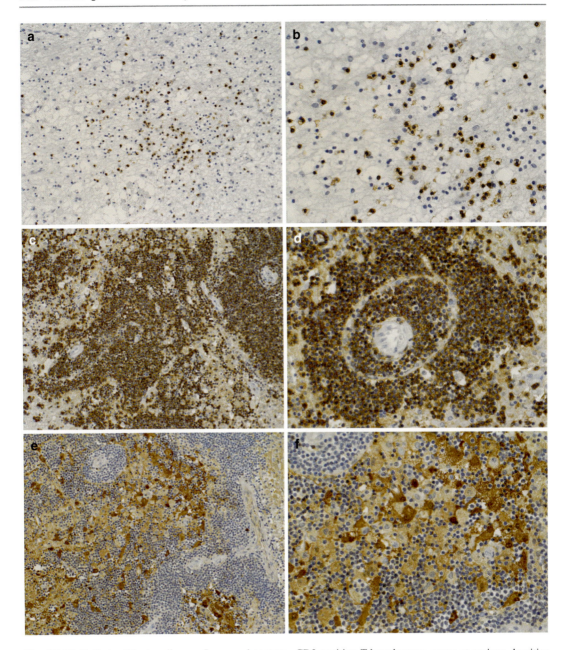

Fig. 78.10 Erdheim–Chester disease: Immunophenotype. CD3-positive T-lymphocytes occur at various densities (**a–d**). S-100 large histiocytes (**e–h**). CD68-positive macrophages (**i–l**). Moderate Ki67 proliferation rate (**m, n**)

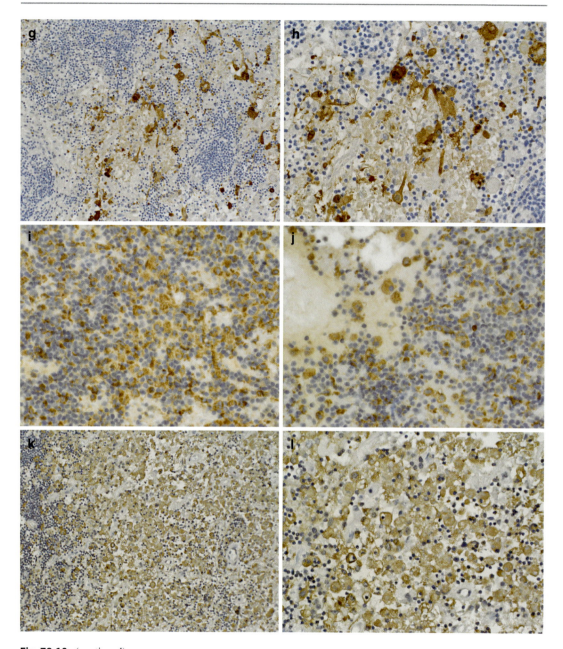

Fig. 78.10 (continued)

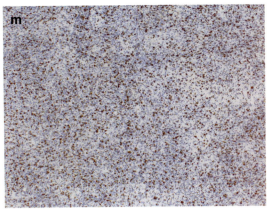 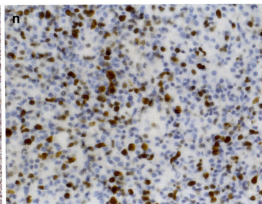

Fig. 78.10 (continued)

Selected References

Abdelfattah AM, Arnaout K, Tabbara IA (2014) Erdheim-Chester disease: a comprehensive review. Anticancer Res 34(7):3257–3261

Adeleye AO, Amir G, Fraifeld S, Shoshan Y, Umansky F, Spektor S (2010) Diagnosis and management of Rosai-Dorfman disease involving the central nervous system. Neurol Res 32(6):572–578. https://doi.org/10.1179/016164109x12608733393836

Agarwal KK, Seth R, Behra A, Jana M, Kumar R (2016) 18F-Fluorodeoxyglucose PET/CT in Langerhans cell histiocytosis: spectrum of manifestations. Jpn J Radiol 34(4):267–276. https://doi.org/10.1007/s11604-016-0517-7

Alfieri A, Gazzeri R, Galarza M, Neroni M (2010) Surgical treatment of intracranial Erdheim-Chester disease. J Clin Neurosci 17(12):1489–1492. https://doi.org/10.1016/j.jocn.2010.03.062

Badalian-Very G, Vergilio JA, Fleming M, Rollins BJ (2013) Pathogenesis of Langerhans cell histiocytosis. Annu Rev Pathol 8:1–20. https://doi.org/10.1146/annurev-pathol-020712-163959

Campochiaro C, Tomelleri A, Cavalli G, Berti A, Dagna L (2015) Erdheim-Chester disease. Eur J Intern Med 26(4):223–229. https://doi.org/10.1016/j.ejim.2015.03.004

Cavalli G, Biavasco R, Borgiani B, Dagna L (2014) Oncogene-induced senescence as a new mechanism of disease: the paradigm of erdheim-chester disease. Front Immunol 5:281. https://doi.org/10.3389/fimmu.2014.00281

Chaudhary V, Bano S, Aggarwal R, Narula MK, Anand R, Solanki RS, Singh P (2013) Neuroimaging of Langerhans cell histiocytosis: a radiological review. Jpn J Radiol 31(12):786–796. https://doi.org/10.1007/s11604-013-0254-0

Cives M, Simone V, Rizzo FM, Dicuonzo F, Cristallo Lacalamita M, Ingravallo G, Silvestris F, Dammacco F (2015) Erdheim-Chester disease: a systematic review. Crit Rev Oncol Hematol 95(1):1–11. https://doi.org/10.1016/j.critrevonc.2015.02.004

Collin M, Bigley V, McClain KL, Allen CE (2015) Cell(s) of origin of Langerhans cell histiocytosis. Hematol Oncol Clin North Am 29(5):825–838. https://doi.org/10.1016/j.hoc.2015.06.003

Cooper SL, Jenrette JM (2012) Rosai-Dorfman disease: management of CNS and systemic involvement. Clin Adv Hematol Oncol 10(3):199–202

Dalia S, Sagatys E, Sokol L, Kubal T (2014) Rosai-Dorfman disease: tumor biology, clinical features, pathology, and treatment. Cancer Control 21(4):322–327

Drutz JE (2011) Histiocytosis. Pediatr Rev 32(5):218–219. https://doi.org/10.1542/pir.32-5-218

Eksi MS, Demirci Otluoglu G, Uyar Bozkurt S, Sav A, Bayri Y, Dagcinar A (2013) Cerebral Erdheim-Chester disease mimicking high-grade glial tumor: a case report. Pediatr Neurosurg 49(3):179–182. https://doi.org/10.1159/000360424

El Demellawy D, Young JL, de Nanassy J, Chernetsova E, Nasr A (2015) Langerhans cell histiocytosis: a comprehensive review. Pathology 47(4):294–301. https://doi.org/10.1097/pat.0000000000000256

Gabbay LB, Leite Cda C, Andriola RS, Pinho Pda C, Lucato LT (2014) Histiocytosis: a review focusing on neuroimaging findings. Arq Neuropsiquiatr 72(7):548–558

Grana N (2014) Langerhans cell histiocytosis. Cancer Control 21(4):328–334

Grois N, Fahrner B, Arceci RJ, Henter JI, McClain K, Lassmann H, Nanduri V, Prosch H, Prayer D (2010) Central nervous system disease in Langerhans cell histiocytosis. J Pediatr 156(6):873–881.e1. https://doi.org/10.1016/j.jpeds.2010.03.001

Harmon CM, Brown N (2015) Langerhans cell histiocytosis: a clinicopathologic review and molecular pathogenetic update. Arch Pathol Lab Med 139(10):1211–1214. https://doi.org/10.5858/arpa.2015-0199-RA

Haroche J, Arnaud L, Cohen-Aubart F, Hervier B, Charlotte F, Emile JF, Amoura Z (2013) Erdheim-Chester disease. Rheum Dis Clin North Am 39(2):299–311. https://doi.org/10.1016/j.rdc.2013.02.011

Haroche J, Arnaud L, Cohen-Aubart F, Hervier B, Charlotte F, Emile JF, Amoura Z (2014) Erdheim-Chester disease. Curr Rheumatol Rep 16(4):412. https://doi.org/10.1007/s11926-014-0412-0

Haroche J, Cohen-Aubart F, Charlotte F, Maksud P, Grenier PA, Cluzel P, Mathian A, Emile JF, Amoura Z (2015) The histiocytosis Erdheim-Chester disease is an inflammatory myeloid neoplasm. Expert Rev Clin Immunol 11(9):1033–1042. https://doi.org/10.1586/1744666x.2015.1060857

Haroun F, Millado K, Tabbara I (2017) Erdheim-Chester disease: comprehensive review of molecular profiling and therapeutic advances. Anticancer Res 37(6):2777–2783. https://doi.org/10.21873/anticanres.11629

Hutter C, Minkov M (2016) Insights into the pathogenesis of Langerhans cell histiocytosis: the development of targeted therapies. ImmunoTargets Ther 5:81–91. https://doi.org/10.2147/itt.s91058

Imashuku S, Arceci RJ (2015) Strategies for the prevention of central nervous system complications in patients with Langerhans cell histiocytosis: the problem of neurodegenerative syndrome. Hematol Oncol Clin North Am 29(5):875–893. https://doi.org/10.1016/j.hoc.2015.06.006

Kroft SH (2016) Rosai-Dorfman disease: familiar yet enigmatic. Semin Diagn Pathol 33(5):244–253. https://doi.org/10.1053/j.semdp.2016.05.008

La Barge DV III, Salzman KL, Harnsberger HR, Ginsberg LE, Hamilton BE, Wiggins RH III, Hudgins PA (2008) Sinus histiocytosis with massive lymphadenopathy (Rosai-Dorfman disease): imaging manifestations in the head and neck. Am J Roentgenol 191(6):W299–W306. https://doi.org/10.2214/ajr.08.1114

Luo Z, Zhang Y, Zhao P, Lu H, Yang K, Zhang Y, Zeng Y (2017) Characteristics of Rosai-Dorfman disease primarily involved in the central nervous system: 3 case reports and review of literature. World Neurosurg 97:58–63. https://doi.org/10.1016/j.wneu.2016.09.084

Mar WA, Yu JH, Knuttinen MG, Horowitz JM, David O, Wilbur A, Menias CO (2017) Rosai-Dorfman disease: manifestations outside of the head and neck. Am J Roentgenol 208(4):721–732. https://doi.org/10.2214/ajr.15.15504

Mazor RD, Manevich-Mazor M, Shoenfeld Y (2013) Erdheim-Chester disease: a comprehensive review of the literature. Orphanet J Rare Dis 8:137. https://doi.org/10.1186/1750-1172-8-137

Mimouni-Bloch A, Schneider C, Politi KE, Konen O, Gothelf D, Stark B, Yaniv I, Shuper A (2010) Neuropsychiatric manifestations in Langerhans' cell histiocytosis disease: a case report and review of the literature. J Child Neurol 25(7):884–887. https://doi.org/10.1177/0883073809351317

Moulis G, Sailler L, Bonneville F, Wagner T (2014) Imaging in Erdheim-Chester disease: classic features and new insights. Clin Exp Rheumatol 32(3):410–414

Murray D, Marshall M, England E, Mander J, Chakera TM (2001) Erdheim-chester disease. Clin Radiol 56(6):481–484. https://doi.org/10.1053/crad.2001.0681

Nakamine H, Yamakawa M, Yoshino T, Fukumoto T, Enomoto Y, Matsumura I (2016) Langerhans cell histiocytosis and langerhans cell sarcoma: current understanding and differential diagnosis. J Clin Exp Hematop 56(2):109–118. https://doi.org/10.3960/jslrt.56.109

Paulus W, Perry A (2007) Histiocytic tumours. In: Louis DN, Ohgaki H, Wiestler OD, Cavenee WK (eds) WHO classification of tumours of the central nervous system, 4th edn. International Agency for Research on Cancer, Lyon, pp 193–196

Paulus W, Kepes JJ, Jellinger K (2000) Histiocytic tumours. In: Kleihues P, Cavenee WK (eds) Pathology and genetics of tumours of the nervous system, 3rd edn. IARC, Lyon, pp 204–206

Paulus W, Perry A, Sahm F (2016) Histiocytic tumours. In: Louis DN, Ohgaki H, Wiestler OD, Cavenee WK (eds) WHO classification of tumours of the central nervous system, Revised 4th edn. IARC, Lyon, pp 280–283

Perry VH (2011) Central nervous system involvement in Langerhans cell histiocytosis: the importance of long term follow-up. Pediatr Blood Cancer 56(2):175–176. https://doi.org/10.1002/pbc.22869

Picarsic J, Jaffe R (2015) Nosology and pathology of Langerhans cell histiocytosis. Hematol Oncol Clin North Am 29(5):799–823. https://doi.org/10.1016/j.hoc.2015.06.001

Prayer D, Grois N, Prosch H, Gadner H, Barkovich AJ (2004) MR imaging presentation of intracranial disease associated with Langerhans cell histiocytosis. Am J Neuroradiol 25(5):880–891

Prayson RA, Rowe JJ (2014) Dural-based Rosai-Dorfman disease: differential diagnostic considerations. J Clin Neurosci 21(11):1872–1873. https://doi.org/10.1016/j.jocn.2014.07.011

Rollins BJ (2015) Genomic alterations in Langerhans cell histiocytosis. Hematol Oncol Clin North Am 29(5):839–851. https://doi.org/10.1016/j.hoc.2015.06.004

Russo N, Giangaspero F, Beccaglia MR, Santoro A (2009) Intracranial dural histiocytosis. Br J Neurosurg 23(4):449–454. https://doi.org/10.1080/02688690902756173

Sedrak P, Ketonen L, Hou P, Guha-Thakurta N, Williams MD, Kurzrock R, Debnam JM (2011) Erdheim-Chester disease of the central nervous system: new manifestations of a rare disease. Am J Neuroradiol 32(11):2126–2131. https://doi.org/10.3174/ajnr.A2707

Zaveri J, La Q, Yarmish G, Neuman J (2014) More than just Langerhans cell histiocytosis: a radiologic review of histiocytic disorders. Radiographics 34(7):2008–2024. https://doi.org/10.1148/rg.347130132

Zinn DJ, Chakraborty R, Allen CE (2016) Langerhans cell histiocytosis: emerging insights and clinical implications. Oncology 30(2):122–132. 139

Soft Tissue Tumors: Mesenchymal, Non-meningothelial Tumors

79.1 General Aspects

In the WHO Classification of Tumours of the Central Nervous System (Louis et al. 2016), soft tissue tumors are listed under the heading of "mesenchymal, non-meningothelial tumors."

Following Goldblum et al. (2014), soft tissues can be defined as non-epithelial extra-skeletal tissue of the body exclusive of the reticuloendothelial system, glia, and supporting tissue of various parenchymal organs.

Soft tissue is represented by:
- Voluntary muscle
- Fat
- Fibrous tissue
- Vessels serving these tissues
- Peripheral nervous system (see Chap. 71)

Soft tissue tumors are:
- Heterogeneous group of tumors
- Classified along the line of differentiation according to the adult tissue they resemble
- Benign tumors
  - Closely resemble normal tissue
  - Have limited capacity for autonomous growth
  - Low tendency for invasion
  - Low rate of recurrence
- Malignant tumors or sarcomas
  - Local aggressive behavior
  - Invasive and destructive growth
  - Radical surgery required

79.1.1 Classification of Soft tissue tumors

The recent WHO classification of tumors of tissue and bone is shown in Appendix B (Fletcher et al. 2013). Soft tissue tumors occur with a very low incidence affecting the brain. The most common tumors will be presented in this chapter. Although the histogenesis of hemangioblastoma is still unclear, this tumor entity is included in this chapter. Table 79.1 lists the most commonly encountered entities in surgical neuropathology.

79.1.2 Grading of Soft Tissue Tumors

Histologic grade is a means of quantitating the degree of differentiation by applying a set of histologic criteria (Coindre et al. 1986) (Table 79.2).
- Grading: assessment of the degree of malignancy of a sarcoma based on evaluation of several histologic parameters.
- Staging: information regarding the extent of disease at a designated time (time of diagnosis).
- Histologic grade is defined as follows:
- Grade 1
  - Total score: 2–3
- Grade 2
  - Total score: 4–5
- Grade 3
  - Total score: 6–8

Table 79.1 Selection of soft tissue tumors based on the origin of the tumor cell

Origin of tumor cells	Tumor entities
Adipose tissue tumors	• Lipoma • Angiolipoma • Complex lipomatous lesions • Epidural lipomatosis • Intracranial liposarcoma
Fibrous tumors	• Fibromatosis • Solitary fibrous tumor • Inflammatory myofibroblastic tumor • Fibrosarcoma
Fibrohistiocytic tumors	• Benign fibrous histiocytoma • Malignant fibrous histiocytoma (MFH)
Myogenic tumors	• Leiomyoma • Leiomyosarcoma • Rhabdomyoma • Rhabdomyosarcoma
Vascular tumors	• Hemangioma • Epithelioid hemangioendothelioma • Angiosarcoma • Kaposi sarcoma

Table 79.2 Grading of soft tissue sarcomas most often follows the guidelines of French Federation of Cancer Centers sarcoma Group (FNCLCC)

Parameter	Score	Criterion
Tumor differentiation	1	Sarcoma closely resembling normal adult mesenchymal tissue
	2	Sarcomas for which histologic typing is certain
	3	Embryonal and undifferentiated sarcomas, sarcoma of uncertain type
Mitosis count	1	0–9/10 HPF
	2	10–19/10 HPF
	3	≥20/10 HPF
Tumor necrosis (microscopic)	0	No necrosis
	1	≤50% tumor necrosis
	2	>50% tumor necrosis

79.1.3 Incidence

More benign soft tissue tumors than malignant forms

Malignant soft tissue tumors
- Rare.
- Annual incidence: 6 per 100,000 persons.
- 1.5% of all cancers.
- 5% of soft tissue tumors affect the head and neck region.

79.1.4 Pathogenesis

- Unknown
- Physical and chemical agents
- Environmental factors
- Oncogenic viruses
- Immunologic factors
- Genetic factors

79.2 Solitary Fibrous Tumor/Hemangiopericytoma

The term *Hemangiopericytoma* was coined in 1942 by Stout & Murray for a tumor thought to originate from pericytes. The term *Solitary Fibrous Tumor* was used in 1931 by Klemperer & Rabin to describe a pleura based lesion.

The WHO classification for soft tissue tumors considers hemangiopericytoma as cellular phase of SFT; it also discourages the further use of hemangiopericytoma.

The WHO classification for Tumors of the CNS list:
- Solitary fibrous tumor/hemangiopericytoma—Grade 1
- Solitary fibrous tumor/hemangiopericytoma—Grade 2
- Solitary fibrous tumor/hemangiopericytoma—Grade 3

WHO Definition
Solitary Fibrous Tumor/Hemangiopericytoma
2016—A mesenchymal tumor of fibroblastic type, often showing a rich branching vascular pattern, encompassing a histological spectrum of tumors previously classified separately as meningeal solitary fibrous tumor and hemangiopericytoma (Giannini et al. 2016).
Hemangiopericytoma

79.2 Solitary Fibrous Tumor/Hemangiopericytoma

2007—A highly cellular and vascularized mesenchymal tumor exhibiting a characteristic monotonous low-power appearance and a well-developed, variable thick-walled, branching "staghorn" vasculature; almost always attached to the dura and having a high tendency to recur and to metastasize outside the CNS (Giannini et al. 2007).

2000—Hemangiopericytoma (HPC) of the central nervous system is a highly cellular and richly vascularized tumor, almost always attached to the dura, and indistinguishable histologically from hemangiopericytomas occurring in somatic soft tissues, with a tendency to recur and to metastasize outside the CNS (Jääskeläinen et al. 2000).

1993—A monotonous cellular tumor composed of plump or polygonal cells with oval nuclei and scant, ill-defined cytoplasm accompanied by an often dense intercellular pattern of reticulin staining, typically surrounding vascular spaces lined by normal endothelium (Kleihues et al. 1993).

79.2.1 Epidemiology

Incidence
- Rare
- 1% of all primary CNS tumors

Age Incidence
- Adults
- Fourth to sixth decade of life
- Mean age: 43 years

Sex Incidence
- Male:Female ratio: 1:1

Localization
- Solitary
- Supratentorial
- Cranial or spinal (10%) dura
- Rare:
  - Intraparenchymal
  - Intraventricular

79.2.2 Neuroimaging Findings

General Imaging Findings
Extra-axial mass arising from the dura with strong enhancement, well defined with lobulating contour, similar to meningiomas

CT non-contrast-enhanced
- Heterogeneous, hyperattenuated mass
- Iso- to hyperdense
- Bone invasions described
- Erosion of calvarium
- No calcifications or hyperostosis (DD: meningioma)

CT contrast-enhanced (Fig. 79.1a)
- Strong enhancement
- Heterogeneous in case of cysts or necrosis

MRI-T2 (Figs. 79.1b and 79.2a, b)
- Variable, heterogeneous isointense
- "black-and-white mixed" pattern
- Prominent flow voids common
- Cysts possible

MRI-FLAIR (Figs. 79.1c and 79.2c)
- Surrounding edema possible

MRI-T1 (Figs. 79.1d and 79.2d)
- Heterogeneous hypo-, isointense

MRI-T1 contrast-enhanced (Figs. 79.1e, f and 79.2e)
- Strong homo- to heterogeneous enhancement
- In cases of cysts—rim enhancement
- Thickening of the meninges
- Non-enhancing necrosis
- Dural tail possible

MRI-T2∗/SWI (Fig. 79.2f)
- No calcifications

MR-Diffusion Imaging
- No restricted diffusion

MRI-Perfusion
- Elevated rCBV (Fig. 79.1g)

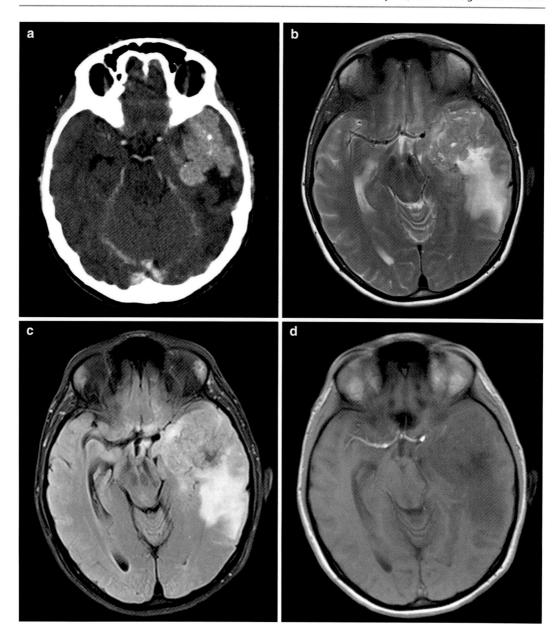

Fig. 79.1 Anaplastic hemangiopericytoma left temporal in CT contrast (**a**), T2 (**b**), FLAIR (**c**), T1 (**d**), T1 contrast (**e**), T1 contrast cor (**f**), rCBV (**g**), MR-spectroscopy (**h**), DSA of external carotid artery with feeders form the middle meningeal arteries sag/cor (**i, j**)

79.2 Solitary Fibrous Tumor/Hemangiopericytoma

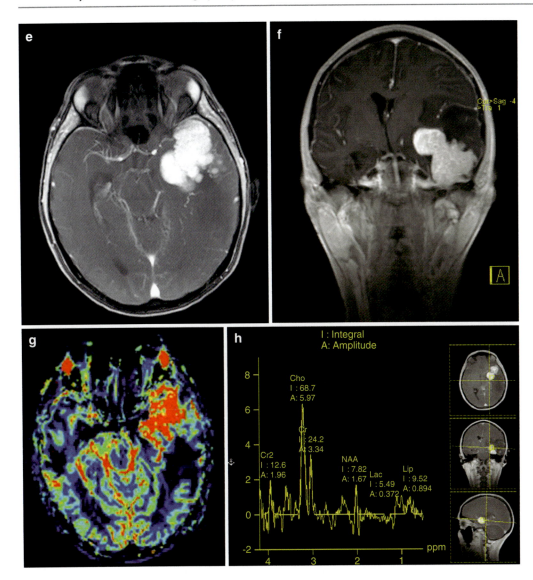

Fig. 79.1 (continued)

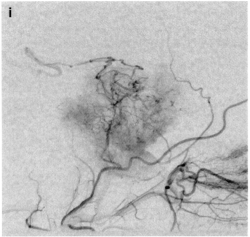
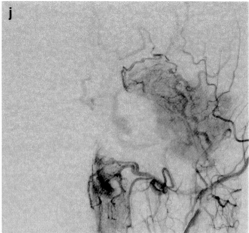

Fig. 79.1 (continued)

MR-Spectroscopy (Fig. 79.1h)
- Myoinositol peaks

DSA
- Delayed tumor blushing
- In half of the cases dysplastic dilation of tumor vessels

Nuclear Medicine Imaging Findings
- There are no systematic studies dealing with solitary fibrous tumor affecting the nervous system.
- In one study, a malignant solitary fibrous tumor as found as pleural thickening was described to be negative in FDG-PET.
- Hemangiopericytoma is expressing SSR and thereby positive in SSR-scintigraphy and SSR-PET, but less stronger than meningiomas.
- FDG is reported to show hypometabolism or as reported in one case hypermetabolism.
- Amino acid PET with MET is reported to be positive.

79.2.3 Neuropathology Findings

Macroscopic Features
- Brownish, grayish, whitish
- Solid and firm tumor
- Well-demarcated
- Globoid, slightly lobulated
- Grayish to red-brown
- Hemorrhages possible

Microscopic Features
- SFT phenotype (Fig. 79.3a–d)
  - patternless architecture
  - short fascicular pattern composed of spindle cells
  - Arranged in fascicles
  - Prominent, alternating hypocellular and hypercellular eosinophilic thick bands of collagen
- Hemangiopericytoma phenotype (Fig. 79.4a–d)
  - Monomorphous tumor
  - High cellularity

79.2 Solitary Fibrous Tumor/Hemangiopericytoma

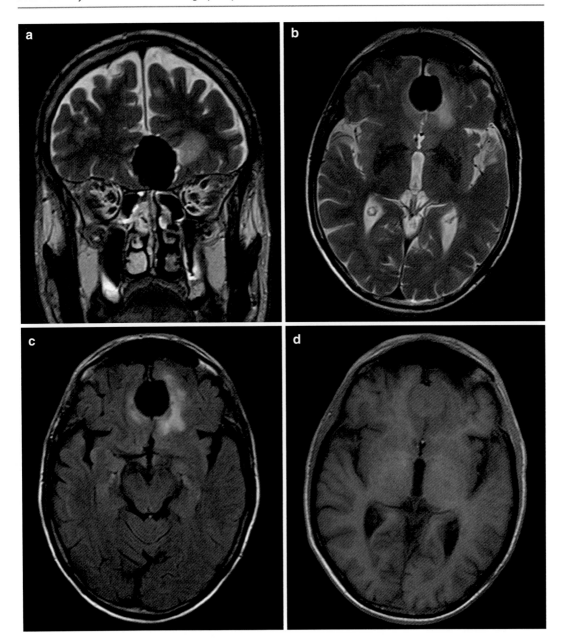

Fig. 79.2 Solid fibrous tumor mid-frontal similar to meningioma in T2 cor (**a**), T2 (**b**), FLAIR (**c**), T1 (**d**), T1 contrast (**e**), T2∗ (**f**)

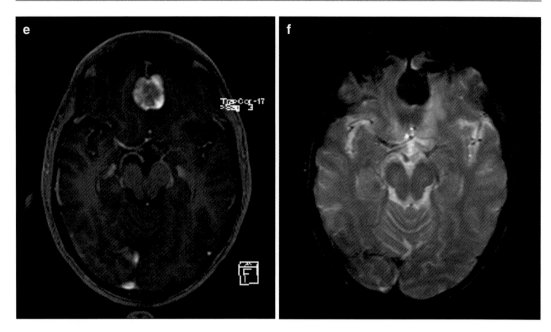

Fig. 79.2 (continued)

- Closely packed, randomly oriented tumor cells with
  - Scant cytoplasm
  - Distinct cell borders
  - Round to oval nuclei
  - Moderately dense chromatin
- Nuclear atypia low
- Mitoses low
- Fibrosis mild
- Anaplastic hemangiopericytoma (WHO grade III)
  - Increased mitotic activity, at least 5 mitoses per 10 HPF
  - And/or necrosis
  - At least two of the following:
    - Hemorrhage
    - Moderate to high nuclear atypia and cellularity
- Rich network of reticulin fibers investing tumor cells
- Highly vascularized tumor with
  - Slit-like vascular channels
  - Lined by flattened endothelial cells
  - Gaping, thin-walled and branching vascular spaces, so-called "staghorn sinusoids"
- Calcifications absent
- Infiltration of adjacent brain tissue and invasion with bone destruction possible

Grades
- Grade I
  - Benign
  - SFT phenotype
  - Hypocellular, collagenized tumor
- Grade II malignant (Fig. 79.5a–h)
  - Hemangiopericytoma phenotype
  - Densely cellular tumor
  - Mitoses <5 per 10 high-power fields
- Grade III malignant (Fig. 79.5a–h)
  - Hemangiopericytoma phenotype
  - Densely cellular tumor
  - Mitoses ≥ 5 per 10 high-power fields

Immunophenotype (Figs. 79.3e–j and 79.4e–j)
A list of antibodies with positive or negative immunostaining results is given in Table 79.3.

79.2 Solitary Fibrous Tumor/Hemangiopericytoma

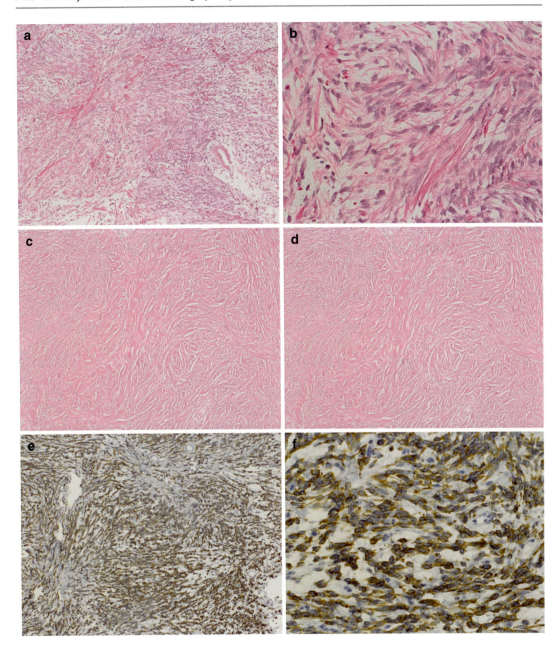

Fig. 79.3 Solitary fibrous tumor (SFT) with cellular areas (**a**, **b**: H&E) and acellular areas (**c**, **d**: H&E). Immunophenotype shows reactivities of tumor cells for bcl2 (**e**, **f**), CD34 (**g**, **h**), and CD99 (**i**, **j**)

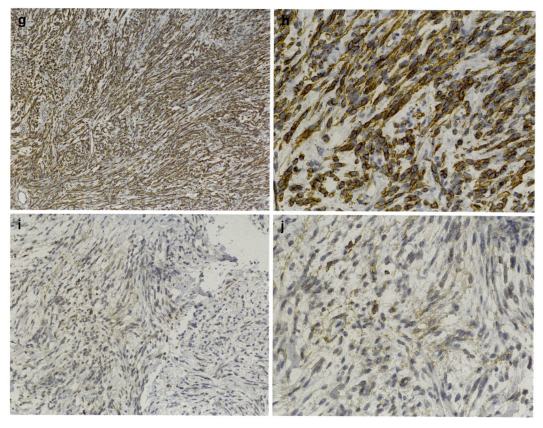

Fig. 79.3 (continued)

Proliferation Markers
- Low to high
- Ki-67 LI: 0.6–39%

Ultrastructural Features
- Elongated cells with
  - Short processes
  - Small bundles of intracytoplasmic intermediate filaments
  - Absence of true desmosomes and gap junctions
- Extracellular basement membrane-like material

Differential Diagnosis
- Meningioma
- Fibroma
- Fibrosarcoma
- Histiocytoma

79.2.4 Molecular Pathology

- Uncertain
- No evidence of pericytic differentiation (contrary to what the name might suggest)
- Fibroblastic differentiation
- Morphological continuum with solitary fibrous tumor
- Genomic inversion at the 12q13 locus
  - Fusing the *NAB2* und *STAT6* genes
  - Leading to STAT6 nuclear expression detectable by immunohistochemistry

79.2.5 Treatment and Prognosis

- Grade I:
  - Surgical excision

79.2 Solitary Fibrous Tumor/Hemangiopericytoma

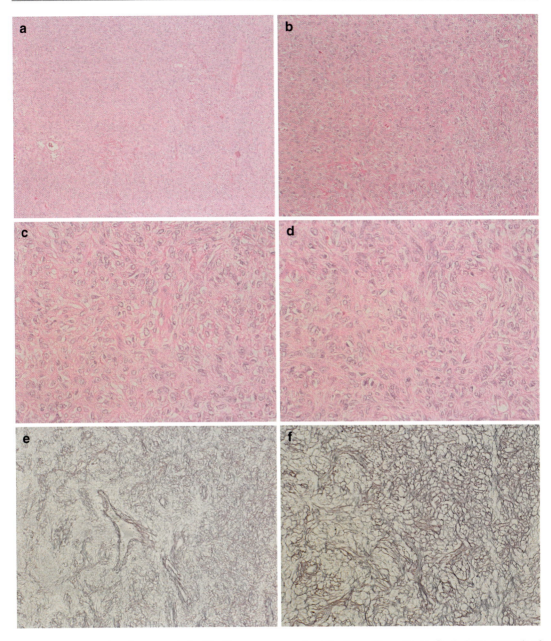

Fig. 79.4 Hemangiopericytoma grade II: The tumor shows increased cellularity and is composed of monomorphous cells which are closely packed and randomly oriented with scant cytoplasm, round to oval nuclei and moderately dense chromatin (**a–d**). A dense network of reticulin fibers is note (stain: Reticulin) (**e, f**). Immunophenotype shows reactivities of tumor cells for bcl2 (**g, h**), and CD99 (**i, j**)

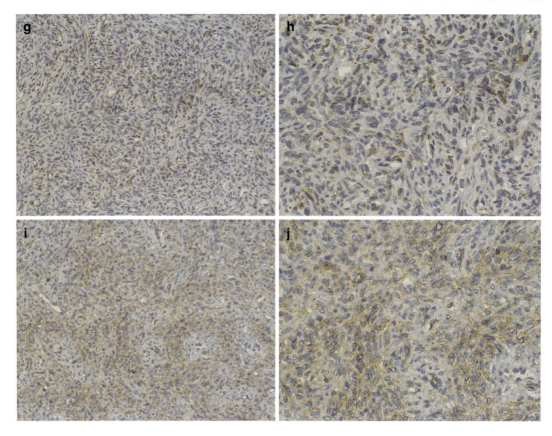

Fig. 79.4 (continued)

Table 79.3 Immunophenotype of solitary fibrous tumor/hemangiopericytoma

Positivities	Negativities
• STAT6 • CD34 (33–100%) • CD99 • Bcl2 • Vimentin (85%) • ß-catenin • Factor XIIIa (80–100%) • Leu-7 (70%)	• EMA • S-100 • Desmin • CD117 • Pancytokeratin • CD31 • Progesterone receptor

- Grade II and III:
  - Surgery
  - Radiotherapy
  - Chemotherapy

Biologic Behavior–Prognosis–Prognostic Factors
- SFT phenotype
  - Time to recurrence: 40–40 months
  - Benign, provided gross total resection can be achieved
  - Gross total removal possible

- Hemangiopericytoma phenotype
  - Local recurrences in 85–91% of the cases after 15 years
  - High rate of recurrence (>75% at 10 years)
  - Median recurrence:
    58 months after irradiation
    29 months without irradiation
  - Aggressive behavior in 15% of the cases
  - Extracranial metastases (in ~20% of cases) possible to
    Bone
    Lung
    Liver
  - Mean survival after metastases: 2 years

79.2 Solitary Fibrous Tumor/Hemangiopericytoma

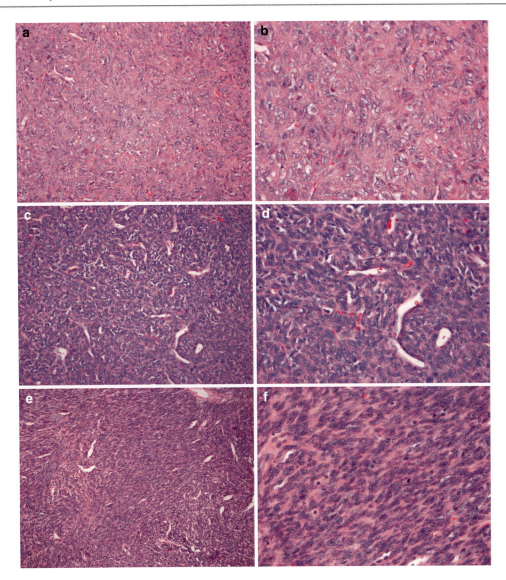

Fig. 79.5 Hemangiopericytoma grade III: Highly cellular tumor; the tumor cells with high nuclear atypia and presence of mitoses (**f**). Proliferation is high (Ki67: **g**, **h**)

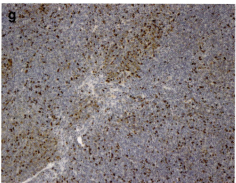
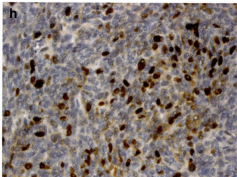

Fig. 79.5 (continued)

79.3 Hemangioblastoma

WHO Definition

2016—A tumor histologically characterized by neoplastic stromal cells and abundant small vessels (Plate et al. 2016).

2007—A slowly growing, highly vascular tumor of adults, occurring in the cerebellum, brain stem, or spinal cord; histologically comprised of stromal cells and small blood vessels; occurring in sporadic forms and in association with von Hippel–Lindau (VHL) syndrome (Aldape et al. 2007).

2000—A WHO grade I tumor of uncertain histogenesis, composed of stromal cells and abundant capillaries. Approximately 25% of hemangioblastomas are associated with von Hippel–Lindau disease (Böhling et al. 2000).

1993—A well-demarcated, highly vascular and occasionally multifocal tumor that often has an associated cyst and typically connects with the leptomeninges (Kleihues et al. 1993).

1979—A tumor composed of blood vessels that are separated by stromal cells with clear cytoplasm. The stromal cells often contain sudanophilic material (Zülch 1979).

79.3.1 Epidemiology

Incidence
- Rare tumor
- Familial forms associated with von Hippel–Lindau disease

Age Incidence
- Adults

Sex Incidence
- Male:Female ratio: 1:1

Localization
- Any part of the nervous system
- Predominantly cerebellar hemispheres
- Brain stem, spinal cord, and nerve roots

79.3.2 Neuroimaging Findings

General Imaging Findings
- Intra-axial cyst with enhancing mural nodule
- Typically in posterior fossa

CT non-contrast-enhanced (Fig. 79.6a)
- Hypodense cyst, hyperdense nodule

CT contrast-enhanced (Fig. 79.6b)
- Enhancing nodule
- Typically no enhancement of cyst wall

MRI-T2/FLAIR (Fig. 79.6c, d, g)
- Hyperintense cyst and nodule
- Flow voids possible

MRI-T1 (Fig. 79.6e)
- Cyst slightly hyperintense
- Isointense nodule

MRI-T1 Contrast-Enhanced (Fig. 79.6f, h)
- Strong enhancement of nodule
- Typically no enhancement of cyst wall

79.3 Hemangioblastoma

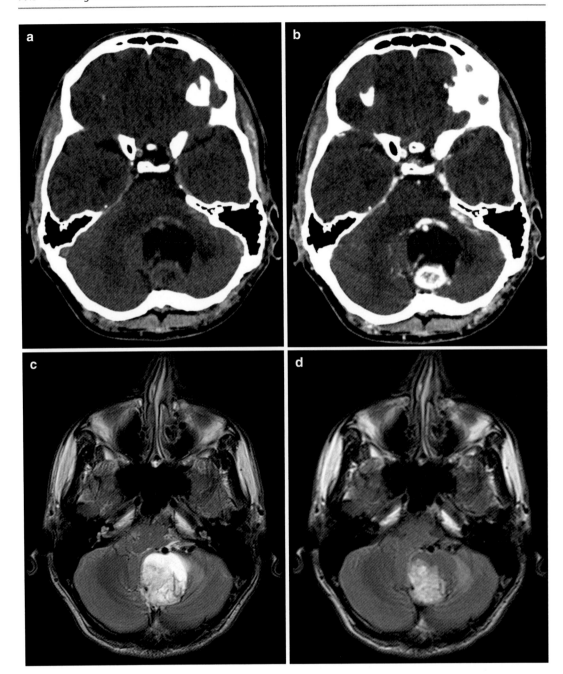

Fig. 79.6 Hemangioblastoma in CT native (**a**), CT contrast (**b**), T2 (**c**), FLAIR (**d**), T1 (**e**), T1 contrast (**f**), T2 sag (**g**), T1 contrast sag (**h**), Digital subtractive angiography (DSA) of left vertebral artery with cor/sag (**i, j**)

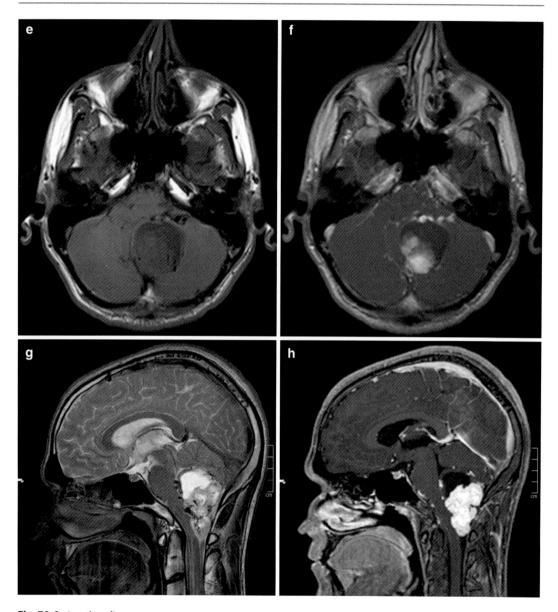

Fig. 79.6 (continued)

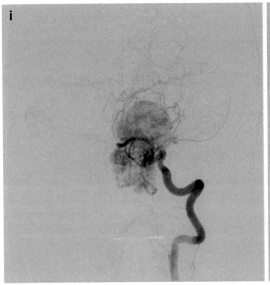
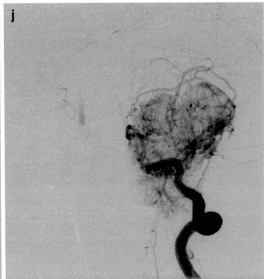

Fig. 79.6 (continued)

MRI-T2∗/SWI
- Hypointense hemorrhages possible

MR-Diffusion Imaging
- No restricted diffusion

MRI-Perfusion
- Elevated rCBV, higher than in pilocytic astrocytoma

Nuclear Medicine Imaging Findings (Fig. 79.7)
- Hemangioblastoma was historically addressed by scintiangiography with Tc99m-DTPA.
- Today studies dealing with the assessment of hypoxia with F18-FMISO are performed.
- FET-PET is positive in these patients.

79.3.3 Neuropathology Findings

Macroscopic Features (Figs. 79.8a–f and 79.9a, b)
- Well-delineated, nodular tumor
- Highly vascularized
- Cyst formation in the tumor wall
- Reddish to yellowish

Microscopic Features (Fig. 79.9c–n)
- Two main components:
  - Stromal cells
  - Vascular cells
- Stromal cells
  - Large, vacuolated cells.
  - Considerable cytologic variation.
  - Variable nuclear size.
  - Atypical, hyperchromatic nuclei might be seen.
  - Lipid-containing vacuoles (clear cell appearance).
- Vascular cells
  - Abundant
- Variants based on the abundance of stromal cells:
  - Cellular variant
  - Reticular variant
- Abundant thin-walled vessels
- Rosenthal fibers frequent
- Extensive sclerosis possible

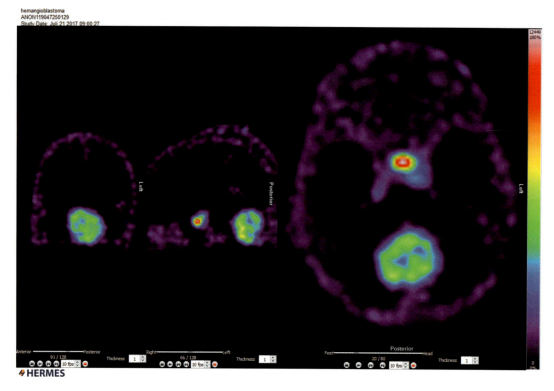

Fig. 79.7 SSR-PET of a hemangioblastoma of the posterior fossa. No background accumulation leads to good discrimination of the tumor (coronal, sagittal, transversal). Physiological uptake of the pituitary gland

Immunophenotype (Fig. 79.10)
- A list of antibodies with positive or negative immunostaining results is given in Table 79.4.

Proliferation Markers
- Low
- Ki-67 LI: 0–2%

Ultrastructural Features
- Stromal cells:
  - Abundant electron-lucent cytoplasm containing lipid droplets

Differential Diagnosis
- Clear cell renal carcinoma
- Meningioma

79.3.4 Molecular Pathology

- Uncertain.
- Stromal cell is the neoplastic cell.
  - Origin: controversial, includes glial, endothelial arachnoidal, embryonic choroid plexus, neuroendocrine, fibrohistiocytic, neuroectodermal, embryonal hemangioblast progenitor cells
- Occur in sporadic forms (~70% of cases) and in association with the inherited von Hippel–Lindau disease (VHL) (~30% of cases).
- The VHL tumor suppressor gene is inactivated both in VHL-associated cases and in most sporadic cases.

79.3.5 Treatment and Prognosis

Treatment
- Surgery

Biologic Behavior–Prognosis–Prognostic Factors
- Benign slow-growing tumor
- Excellent prognosis if total surgical excision can be achieved
- Improved outcome in sporadic cases as compared to von Hippel–Lindau syndrome
- Multiple lesion in von Hippel–Lindau syndrome

79.4 Lipoma

79.4.1 Definition

A benign lesion that microscopically resembles normal adipose tissue.

Intracranial lipomas are believed to be congenital malformations rather than true neoplasms, resulting from abnormal differentiation of the meninx primitive (the undifferentiated mesenchyme).

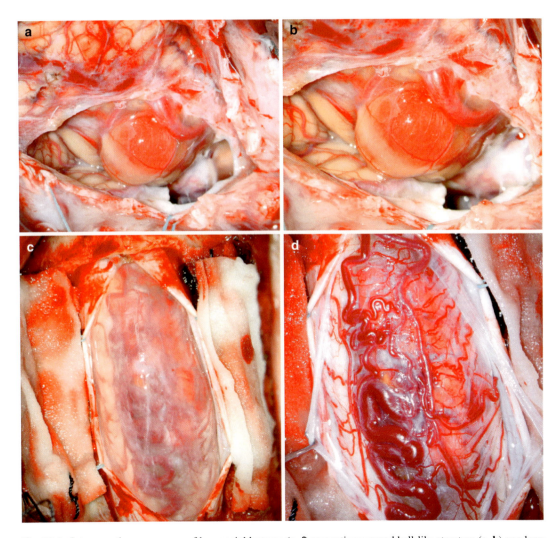

Fig. 79.8 Intraoperative appearance of hemangioblastoma (**a–f**) presenting a round ball-like structure (**a, b**) or a long mass (**c**) covered by leptomeninges, (**d**) covered by numerous tortuous vessels (**e** and **f**) exposed for surgical removal

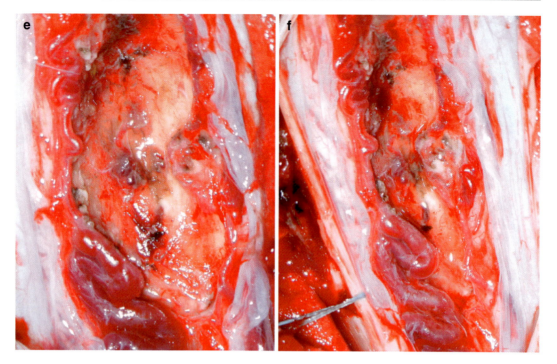

Fig. 79.8 (continued)

79.4.2 Neuroimaging Findings

General Imaging Features
Mass with imaging features similar to fat on CT and MRI

CT non-contrast-enhanced (Fig. 79.11a–d)
- Hypodense mass with negative HU, calcifications possible

CT contrast-enhanced
- No enhancement

MRI: T2 (Fig. 79.11e)
- Hyperintense

MRI: FLAIR (Fig. 79.11f)
- Hyperintense

MRI: T1 (Fig. 79.11g)
- Hyperintense

MRI: T1 contrast-enhanced (Fig. 79.11h, i)
- No enhancement

79.4.3 Neuropathology Findings

Macroscopic Features (Fig. 79.12a, b)
- Well-circumscribed lesion
- Yellow, greasy, cut surface

Microscopic Features (Fig. 79.12c–h)
- Lobules of mature adipocytes
- Immunopositive for S100
- May contain areas of
    - Bone formation (osteolipoma)
    - Cartilage (chondrolipoma)
    - Fibrous tissue (fibrolipoma)

79.4 Lipoma

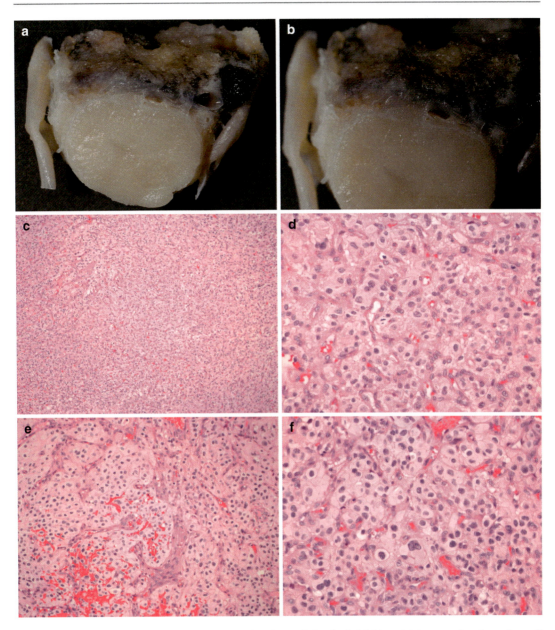

Fig. 79.9 Hemangioblastoma: Brownish-black colored lesion surrounding the spinal cord (autopsy finding) (**a**, **b**). Tumor of moderate cellularity is composed of large, vacuolated cells stromal cells with considerable cytologic variation (**c–j**). Lipid-containing vacuoles give a clear cell appearance (**g–j**). Reticular variant is demonstrated by reticulin stain (**k–n**)

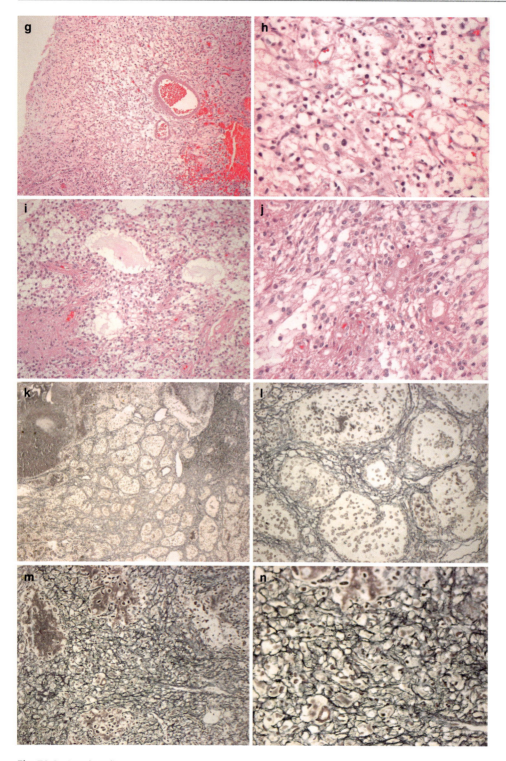

Fig. 79.9 (continued)

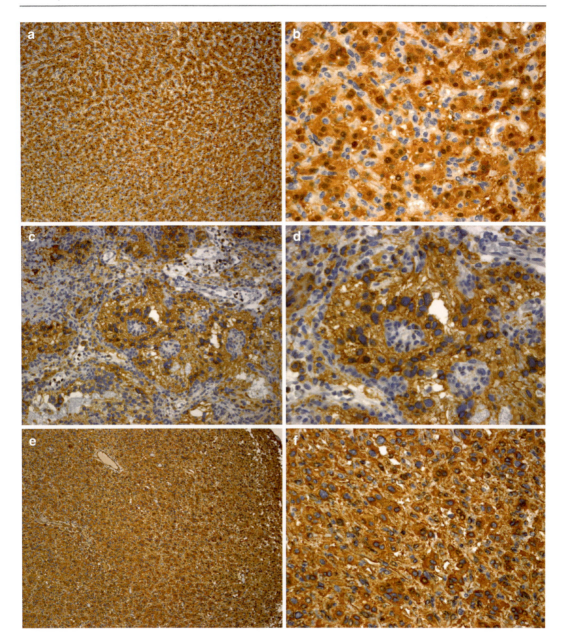

Fig. 79.10 Hemangioblastoma: Immunoprofile showing reactivities of tumor cells with S-100 (**a**, **b**), ezrin (**c**, **d**), vimentin (**e**, **f**), CD56 (**g**, **h**), and CD34 (**i**, **j**). GFAP-positive astrocytes and their ramifications are intermingled between tumor cells. Proliferation might be moderate (**m**, **n**) Ki67)

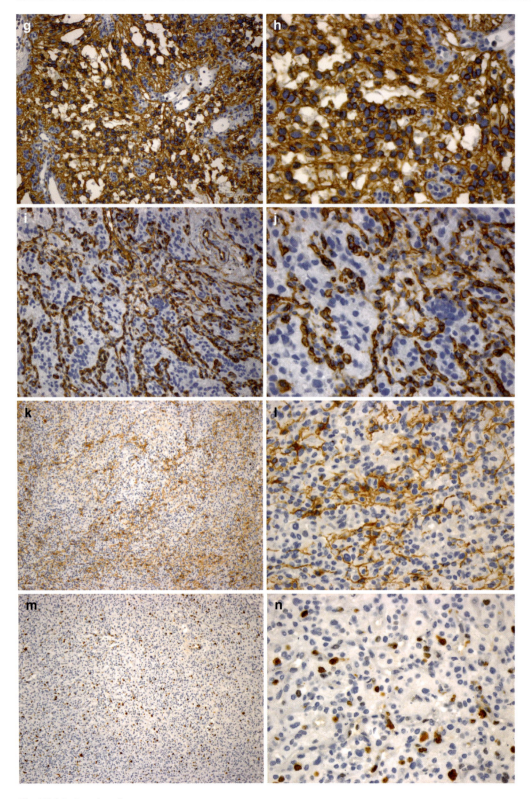

Fig. 79.10 (continued)

Table 79.4 Immunophenotype of hemangioblastoma

Stromal cells positive for	Stromal cell negative for	Vascular cell positive for
• Neuron-specific enolase • Neural cell adhesion molecule • S-100 • CD56 • Ezrin • Vimentin • CXCR4 • Aquaporin-1 • Brachyury • Inhibin alpha • EGFR • VEGF • VEGFR-1 and VEGFR-2 • Tie-1 • Carbonic anhydrase isoenzymes	• Von Willebrand factor • CD34 • CD31	• VEGFR-1 and VEGFR-2 • Tie-1 • Platelet-derived growth factor

79.5 Undifferentiated High-Grade Pleomorphic Sarcoma: Malignant Fibrous Histiocytoma (MFH)

79.5.1 Neuropathology Findings

Macroscopic Features
- Tan to grayish-white color
- Soft to firm consistency

Microscopic Features
- Spindle-shaped cells with abundant cytoplasm
  - Pleomorphic nuclei
  - Numerous atypical mitoses
- Spindle cell storiform pattern
- Multinucleated giant cells
- Inflammatory infiltrate of lymphocytes and histiocytes
- Differential diagnoses include:
  - Pleomorphic fibrosarcoma
  - Osteosarcoma
  - Leiomyosarcoma
  - Metastatic carcinoma
  - Melanoma

79.6 Other Mesenchymal Tumors

79.6.1 Hemangioma

- A benign vascular neoplasm of variable size.
- Are primary lesions of bone that impinge on the CNS secondarily.
- Dural and parenchymal hemangiomas are rare.
- Histologically, hemangiomas have predominantly capillary-type growth and occur mostly in the pediatrics age group.
- Infantile hemangiomas are consistently positive for GLUT1.

79.6.2 Epithelioid Hemangioendothelioma

- A low-grade malignant vascular neoplasm.
- Presence of epithelioid endothelial cells, arranged in cords and single cells embedded in a distinctive chondromyxoid or hyalinized stroma.
- Rarely located in the skull base, dura, or brain parenchyma.
- Its cells contain relatively abundant eosinophilic cytoplasm, which may be vacuolated.
- In general, the nuclei are round or occasionally indented or vesicular, and show only minor atypia.
- Mitoses and limited necrosis may be seen.
- Small intracytoplasmic lumina (blister cells) are seen, but well-formed vascular channels are typically absent.
- Immunohistochemical studies (e.g., for CD31 and ERG) confirm the endothelial nature of this tumors.
- Approximately 90% of epithelioid hemangioendotheliomas harbor the recurrent t(1;3)(p36;q25) translocation, which results in a WWTR1-CAMTA1 fusion.
- A smaller subset of epithelioid hemangioendotheliomas have a t(x;11)(p11;q22) translocation, which results in a YAP1-TFE3 fusion.

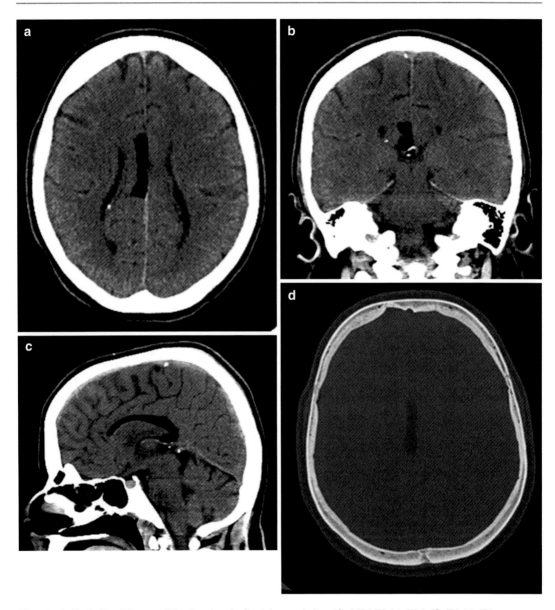

Fig. 79.11 Pericallosal lipoma; CT ax/ cor/sag (**a**, **b**, **c**), bone window (**d**), MRI T2 (**e**), Flair (**f**), T1 (**g**), T1 contrast ax and cor (**h**, **i**), DWI (**j**)

79.6 Other Mesenchymal Tumors

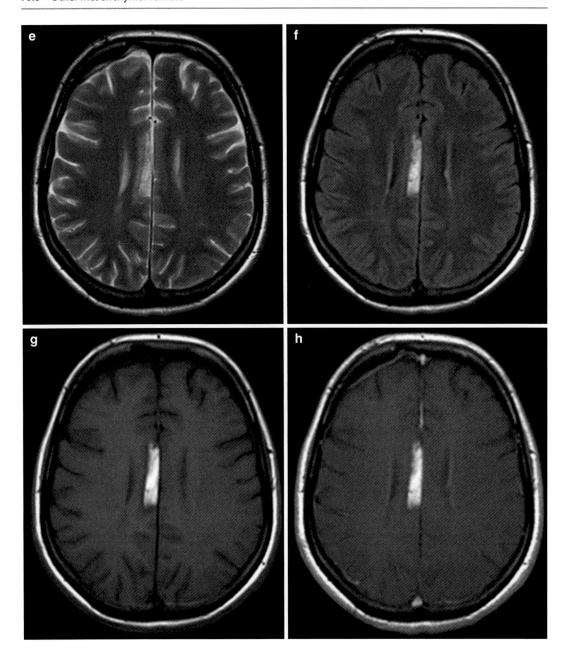

Fig. 79.11 (continued)

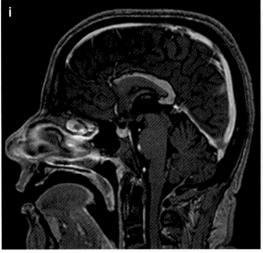
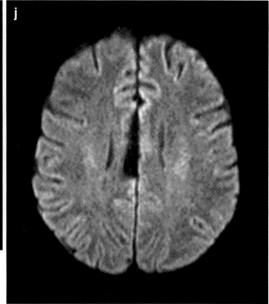

Fig. 79.11 (continued)

79.6.3 Angiosarcoma

- A high-grade malignant neoplasm with evidence of endothelial differentiation.
- The rare examples of angiosarcoma that originate in brain or meninges vary in differentiation from patently vascular tumors with anastomosing vascular channels lined by mitotically active, cytologically atypical endothelial cells to poorly differentiated, often epithelioid solid lesions, in which immunoreactivity for vascular markers (e.g., CD31, CD4, ERG, and FLI1) is required for definitive diagnosis.
- No genetic abnormalities have been described for CNS angiosarcomas.

79.6.4 Kaposi Sarcoma

- A malignant neoplasm
- Spindle-shaped cells forming slit-like blood vessels, which is only rarely encountered as a parenchymal or meningeal tumor,
- Typically in the setting of HIV type 1 infection or AIDS.
- The tumor is almost always immunopositive for HHV8.

79.6.5 Ewing Sarcoma/Peripheral Primitive Neuroectodermal Tumor

- A small round blue cell tumor of neuroectodermal origin.
- involves the CNS either as a primary dural neoplasm or by direct extension from contiguous bone or soft tissue (e.g., skull, vertebra, or paraspinal soft tissue).
- Radiologically, the tumor can mimic meningioma.
- Wide patient age range; peak incidence in the second decade of life.
- The histology, immunophenotype, and biology are essentially identical to those of tumors encountered in bone or soft tissue.
- The tumor is composed of sheets of small, round, primitive-appearing cells with scant clear cytoplasm and uniform nuclei with fine chromatin and smooth nuclear contours.
- Homer Wright rosettes are occasionally seen.

79.6 Other Mesenchymal Tumors

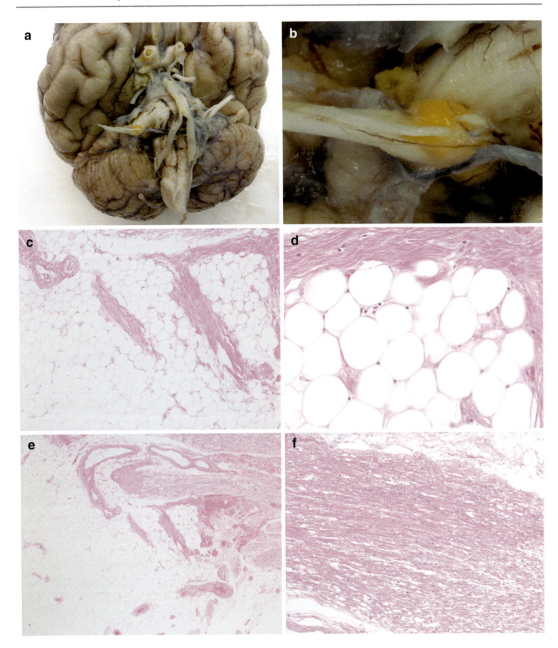

Fig. 79.12 Lipoma: A yellowish mass located near the vestibulocochlear nerve (**a**, **b**). Mass consists of lobules of mature adipocytes partly separated by bundles of collagen fibers (→) (**c**, **d**), containing a longitudinal section of a small nerve fiber bundle (→) (**e**, **f**) and supplied by vessels (**g**, **h**)

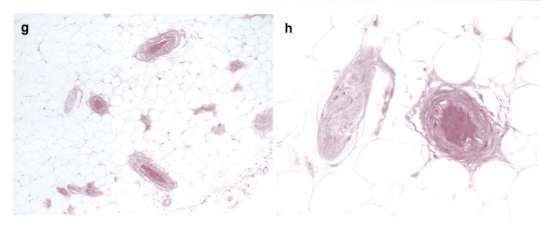

Fig. 79.12 (continued)

- Stains at least focally with synaptophysin and neuron-specific enolase.
- Cytokeratin is only focally seen (20% of cases).
- CD99 shows strong and diffuse membranous immunoreactivity in most cases.
- Tumor must be confirmed at the molecular level by:
  - RT-PCR for the presence of an *EWSR1-FLI1* or *EWSR1-ERG* fusion transcript
  - FISH for *EWSR1* gene rearrangement
- Alternative gene fusion includes:
  - *CIC-DUX4* inversion
  - *BCOR-CCNB3* intrachromosomal inversion

79.6.6 Angiolipoma

- A lipoma variant with prominent vascularity
- Vessels are:
  - by definition of capillary type
  - most prominent in the periphery
  - often contain dispersed fibrin thrombi
- The proportions of adipose cells and vasculature in angiolipoma vary
- Interstitial fibrosis may ensue

79.6.7 Hibernoma

- A very rare lipoma variant within the CNS
- Composed of uniform granular or multivacuolated cells with small, centrally located nuclei, resembling brown fat

79.6.8 Liposarcoma

- A malignant tumor composed entirely or partly of neoplastic adipocytes.
- Intracranial liposarcoma is extremely rare.

79.6.9 Desmoid-Type Fibromatosis

- A locally infiltrative lesion
- Cytologically benign lesion
- Composed of
  - uniform myofibroblastic-type cells
  - in an abundant collagenous stroma
  - arranged in intersecting fascicles

79.6.10 Myofibroblastoma

- A benign mesenchymal neoplasm
- Composed of
  - spindle-shaped cells with features of myofibroblasts
  - embedded in a stroma that contains coarse band of hyalinized collagen and conspicuous mast cells
  - admixed with a variable amount of adipose tissue

- Immunohistochemistry:
  - CD34-positive lesion
  - Positive for desmin
- Molecular findings:
  - 13q14 losses
  - Loss of RB

79.6.11 Inflammatory Myofibroblastic Tumor

- A distinctive neoplastic proliferation
- Composed of
  - bland myofibroblastic-type cells
  - intimately associated with a variable lymphoplasmacytic infiltrate
  - arranged in loose fascicles within an oedematous stroma
- Rare tumor
- Occur in patients of any age
- Radiological characteristics similar to those of meningiomas
- Three patterns occur:
  - myxoid-nodular fasciitis-like
  - fibromatosis-like
  - scar-like
- Molecular findings:
  - ALK gene rearrangement and overexpress ALK (50% of cases)
  - Gene fusions in ROS1, PDGFRB, and RET
- Favorable outcomes after gross total resection

79.6.12 Benign Fibrous Histiocytoma

- A lesion composed of
  - mixture of spindled (fibroblast-like) and plump (histiocyte-like) cells
  - arranged in a storiform pattern
- Involves the dura or cranial bone
- Scattered giant cells and/or inflammatory cells are common

79.6.13 Fibrosarcoma

- A rare sarcoma type showing
  - monomorphic spindle cells
  - arranged in intersecting fascicles (a so-called herringbone pattern)
  - marked cellularity
  - brisk mitotic activity
  - necrosis

79.6.14 Undifferentiated Pleomorphic Sarcoma/ Malignant Fibrous Histiocytoma

- A malignant neoplasm composed of
  - spindled, plump, and pleomorphic giant cells
  - arranged in a storiform or fascicular pattern
  - numerous mitoses
  - presence of necroses
- Malignant behavior

79.6.15 Leiomyoma

- A benign smooth muscle tumor
  - intersecting fascicles
  - composed of eosinophilic spindle cells with blunt-ended nuclei
  - lack mitotic activity
  - lack cytological atypia

79.6.16 Leiomyosarcoma

- A malignant neoplasm with
  - predominantly smooth muscle differentiation
  - intersecting fascicles at 90° angles
  - eosinophilic cytoplasm
  - marked nuclear pleomorphism
  - increased mitotic activity
  - presence of necroses
- The morphological variants
  - epithelioid leiomyosarcoma
  - myxoid leiomyosarcoma
  - granular cell leiomyosarcoma
  - inflammatory leiomyosarcoma

- Arise in or adjacent to the dura (e.g., in the paraspinal region or epidural space)
- Association with EBV and immunosuppression
- Most leiomyosarcomas diffusely express desmin and SMA

79.6.17 Rhabdomyoma

- A benign lesion consisting of mature striated muscle
- DD: skeletal muscle heterotopia, occur within prepontine leptomeninges

79.6.18 Rhabdomyosarcoma

- A malignant neoplasm with predominantly skeletal muscle differentiation.
- Nearly all primary CNS rhabdomyosarcomas are of the embryonal type.
- Consist primarily of undifferentiated small cells, whereas strap cells with cross striations are only occasionally observed.
- Immunostaining for desmin and myogenin.
- Differential diagnosis: medullomyoblastomas, gliosarcomas, MPNSTs, germ cell tumors.

Selected References

Aldape KD, Plate KH, Vortmeyer AO, Zagzag D, HPH N (2007) Haemangioblastoma. In: Louis DN, Ohgaki H, Wiestler OD, Cavenee WK (eds) WHO classification of tumours of the central nervous system, 4th edn. International Agency for Research on Cancer, Lyon, pp 184–186

Bamps S, Calenbergh FV, Vleeschouwer SD, Loon JV, Sciot R, Legius E, Goffin J (2013) What the neurosurgeon should know about hemangioblastoma, both sporadic and in Von Hippel-Lindau disease: a literature review. Surg Neurol Int 4:145. https://doi.org/10.4103/2152-7806.121110

Barresi V, Vitarelli E, Branca G, Antonelli M, Giangaspero F, Barresi G (2012) Expression of brachyury in hemangioblastoma: potential use in differential diagnosis. Am J Surg Pathol 36(7):1052–1057. https://doi.org/10.1097/PAS.0b013e31824f4ce3

Bing F, Kremer S, Lamalle L, Chabardes S, Ashraf A, Pasquier B, Le Bas JF, Krainik A, Grand S (2009) Value of perfusion MRI in the study of pilocytic astrocytoma and hemangioblastoma: preliminary findings. J Neuroradiol 36(2):82–87. https://doi.org/10.1016/j.neurad.2008.09.002

Bisceglia M, Galliani C, Giannatempo G, Lauriola W, Bianco M, D'Angelo V, Pizzolitto S, Vita G, Pasquinelli G, Magro G, Dor DB (2011) Solitary fibrous tumor of the central nervous system: a 15-year literature survey of 220 cases (August 1996-July 2011). Adv Anat Pathol 18(5):356–392. https://doi.org/10.1097/PAP.0b013e318229c004

Böhling T, Plate KH, Haltia MJ, Alitalo K, Neumann HPH (2000) Von Hippel-Lindau disease and capillary haemangioblastoma. In: Kleihues P, Cavenee WK (eds) Pathology and genetics of tumours of the nervous system, 3rd edn. IARC, Lyon, pp 215–217

Clarencon F, Bonneville F, Rousseau A, Galanaud D, Kujas M, Naggara O, Cornu P, Chiras J (2011) Intracranial solitary fibrous tumor: imaging findings. Eur J Radiol 80(2):387–394. https://doi.org/10.1016/j.ejrad.2010.02.016

Coindre JM, Trojani M, Contesso G, David M, Rouesse J, Bui NB, Bodaert A, De Mascarel I, De Mascarel A, Goussot JF (1986) Reproducibility of a histopathologic grading system for adult soft tissue sarcoma. Cancer 58(2):306–309

Fargen KM, Opalach KJ, Wakefield D, Jacob RP, Yachnis AT, Lister JR (2011) The central nervous system solitary fibrous tumor: a review of clinical, imaging and pathologic findings among all reported cases from 1996 to 2010. Clin Neurol Neurosurg 113(9):703–710. https://doi.org/10.1016/j.clineuro.2011.07.024

Fletcher CDM, Bridge JA, Hogendoorn PCW, Mertens F (2013) WHO classification of tumors of soft tissue and bone, 4th edn. IARC, Lyon

Ghose A, Guha G, Kundu R, Tew J, Chaudhary R (2017) CNS hemangiopericytoma: a systematic review of 523 patients. Am J Clin Oncol 40(3):223–227. https://doi.org/10.1097/coc.0000000000000146

Giannini C, Rushing EJ, Hainfellner JA (2007) Heamangiopericytoma. In: Louis DN, Ohgaki H, Wiestler OD, Cavenee WK (eds) WHO classification of tumours of the central nervous system, 4th edn. International Agency for Research on Cancer, Lyon, pp 178–180

Giannini C, Rushing EJ, Hainfellner JA, Bouvier C, Figarella-Branger D, von Deimling A, Wesseling P, Antonescu CR (2016) Solitary fibrous tumour/heamangiopericytoma. In: Louis DN, Ohgaki H, Wiestler OD, Cavenee WK (eds) WHO classification of tumours of the central nervous system, Revised 4th edn. IARC, Lyon, pp 249–254

Ginat DT, Bokhari A, Bhatt S, Dogra V (2011) Imaging features of solitary fibrous tumors. Am J Roentgenol 196(3):487–495. https://doi.org/10.2214/ajr.10.4948

Glasker S, Smith J, Raffeld M, Li J, Oldfield EH, Vortmeyer AO (2014) VHL-deficient vasculogenesis in hemangioblastoma. Exp Mol Pathol 96(2):162–167. https://doi.org/10.1016/j.yexmp.2013.12.011

Goldblum JR, Weis SW, Folpe AL (2014) Enzinger and Weis's soft tissue tumors, 6th edn. Elsevier, Oxford

Ho VB, Smirniotopoulos JG, Murphy FM, Rushing EJ (1992) Radiologic-pathologic correlation: hemangioblastoma. Am J Neuroradiol 13(5):1343–1352

Isobe T, Yamamoto T, Akutsu H, Anno I, Shiigai M, Zaboronok A, Masumoto T, Takano S, Matsumura A (2010) Proton magnetic resonance spectroscopy findings of hemangioblastoma. Jpn J Radiol 28(4):318–321. https://doi.org/10.1007/s11604-010-0421-5

Jääskeläinen J, Louis DN, Paulus W, Haltia MJ (2000) Haemangiopericytoma. In: Kleihues P, Cavenee WK (eds) Pathology and genetics of tumours of the nervous system, 3rd edn. IARC, Lyon, pp 190–192

Jimenez-Heffernan JA, Barcena C, Pascual-Gallego M, Canizal JM (2015) Hemangioblastoma stromal cells. Diagn Cytopathol 43(12):987–989. https://doi.org/10.1002/dc.23313

Keraliya AR, Tirumani SH, Shinagare AB, Zaheer A, Ramaiya NH (2016) Solitary fibrous tumors: 2016 imaging update. Radiol Clin North Am 54(3):565–579. https://doi.org/10.1016/j.rcl.2015.12.006

Kleihues P, Burger PC, Scheithauer BW (1993) Histological typing of tumours of the central nervous system, 2nd edn. Springer-Verlag, Berlin

Louis DN, Ohgaki H, Wiestler OD, Cavenee WK, Ellison DW, Figarella-Branger D, Perry A, Reifenberger G, Von Deimling A (2016) WHO classification of tumours of the central nervous system, Revised 4th edn. IARC, Lyon

Mukherjee A, Karunanithi S, Bal C, Kumar R (2014) 68Ga DOTANOC PET/CT aiding in the diagnosis of von Hippel-Lindau syndrome by detecting cerebellar hemangioblastoma and adrenal pheochromocytoma. Clin Nucl Med 39(10):920–921. https://doi.org/10.1097/rlu.0000000000000486

Muscarella LA, la Torre A, Faienza A, Catapano D, Bisceglia M, D'Angelo V, Parrella P, Coco M, Fini G, Tancredi A, Zelante L, Fazio VM, D'Agruma L (2014) Molecular dissection of the VHL gene in solitary capillary hemangioblastoma of the central nervous system. J Neuropathol Exp Neurol 73(1):50–58. https://doi.org/10.1097/nen.0000000000000024

Park MS, Araujo DM (2009) New insights into the hemangiopericytoma/solitary fibrous tumor spectrum of tumors. Curr Opin Oncol 21(4):327–331. https://doi.org/10.1097/CCO.0b013e32832c9532

Plate KH, Aldape KD, Vortmeyer AO, Zagzag D, Neumann HPH (2016) Haemangioblastoma. In: Louis DN, Ohgaki H, Wiestler OD, Cavenee WK (eds) WHO classification of tumours of the central nervous system, Revised 4th edn. IARC, Lyon, pp 254–257

Rapalino O, Smirniotopoulos JG (2016) Extra-axial brain tumors. Handb Clin Neurol 135:275–291. https://doi.org/10.1016/b978-0-444-53485-9.00015-5

Raz E, Zagzag D, Saba L, Mannelli L, Di Paolo PL, D'Ambrosio F, Knopp E (2012) Cyst with a mural nodule tumor of the brain. Cancer Imaging 12:237–244. https://doi.org/10.1102/1470-7330.2012.0028

Rutkowski MJ, Sughrue ME, Kane AJ, Aranda D, Mills SA, Barani IJ, Parsa AT (2010) Predictors of mortality following treatment of intracranial hemangiopericytoma. J Neurosurg 113(2):333–339. https://doi.org/10.3171/2010.3.jns091882

Sibtain NA, Butt S, Connor SE (2007) Imaging features of central nervous system haemangiopericytomas. Eur Radiol 17(7):1685–1693. https://doi.org/10.1007/s00330-006-0471-3

Surendrababu NR, Chacko G, Daniel RT, Chacko AG (2006) Solitary fibrous tumor of the lateral ventricle: CT appearances and pathologic correlation with follow-up. Am J Neuroradiol 27(10):2135–2136

Thway K, Ng W, Noujaim J, Jones RL, Fisher C (2016) The current status of solitary fibrous tumor: diagnostic features, variants, and genetics. Int J Surg Pathol 24(4):281–292. https://doi.org/10.1177/1066896915627485

Truwit CL, Barkovich AJ (1990) Pathogenesis of intracranial lipoma: an MR study in 42 patients. Am J Roentgenol 155(4):855–864.; discussion 865. https://doi.org/10.2214/ajr.155.4.2119122

Weon YC, Kim EY, Kim HJ, Byun HS, Park K, Kim JH (2007) Intracranial solitary fibrous tumors: imaging findings in 6 consecutive patients. Am J Neuroradiol 28(8):1466–1469. https://doi.org/10.3174/ajnr.A0609

Yalcin CE, Tihan T (2016) Solitary fibrous tumor/hemangiopericytoma dichotomy revisited: a restless family of neoplasms in the CNS. Adv Anat Pathol 23(2):104–111. https://doi.org/10.1097/pap.0000000000000103

Zhou J, Wang J, Li N, Zhang X, Zhou H, Zhang R, Ma H, Zhou X (2010) Molecularly genetic analysis of von Hippel-Lindau associated central nervous system hemangioblastoma. Pathol Int 60(6):452–458. https://doi.org/10.1111/j.1440-1827.2010.02540.x

Zülch KJ (1979) Histological typing of tumours of the central nervous system. World Health Organization, Geneva

Bone Tumors

80.1 General Aspects of Bone Tumors

Bone tumors are in general rare diseases; more rarely are they encountered as lesions affecting the skull and vertebral column.

80.1.1 Classification of Bone tumors

Classifications of tumors affecting the bone are given in Tables 80.1 and 80.2.

80.1.2 Incidence

Age Incidence
- Adults

The most commonly encountered bone tumors affecting the skull and vertebral column are given in Table 80.3 while the frequencies (in %) of various bone tumors affecting the skull or vertebral column are listed in Table 80.4.

80.1.3 Nuclear Medicine Imaging Findings

- Bone tumors can be visualized by bone scan with Tc99m-labelled tracers like MDP or DPD.
- The mineralization phase images in these studies are taken 2–4 h (but not longer than 6 h) after administration of the tracer.
- Several tumors are positive in these scans and include: osteosarcoma, osteoid osteoma, osteoblastoma, chondrosarcoma, enchondroma, chrondroblastoma, Ewing sarcoma, or osteoblastic bone metastasis.
- Cystic bone lesions can be seen as a central defect with an osteoplastic rim.
- Some other causes of increased tracer uptake have to be taken into account: dental focus, fracture, postoperative changes, osteomyelitis, sinusitis, Paget disease.
- FDG can be positive (see Fig. 80.1).

80.1.4 Molecular Pathogenesis

Osteosarcoma
- Mutations in tumor suppressor genes:
  - Germline mutation in Retinoblastoma gene (*RB1*) (66%)
  - Germline mutation in *TP53* gene
- Wnt/catenin pathway.
- GSK-3ß/NF-κB.
- Cyclin-dependent kinases (CDKs).
- Regulation downstream of the p53 gene.
- Downregulation of the PI3K/AT pathway.

Table 80.1 Bone tumors as distinguished based on the WHO classification of tumors of soft tissue and bone (Fletcher et al. 2013)

Tumor origin	Behavior	Tumor type
Chondrogenic	Benign	• Osteochondroma • Chondroma • Osteochondromyxoma • Subungual exostosis
	Intermediate	• Chondroblastoma
	Malignant	• Chondrosarcoma (grade II, III) • Dedifferentiated chondrosarcoma • Mesenchymal chondrosarcoma • Clear cell chondrosarcoma
Osteogenic	Benign	• Osteoma • Osteoid osteoma
	Intermediate	• Osteoblastoma
	Malignant	• Low-grade central osteosarcoma • Conventional osteosarcoma • Osteosarcoma subtypes (see WHO)
Fibrogenic	Intermediate	• Desmoplastic fibroma of bone
	Malignant	• Fibrosarcoma of bone
Fibrohistiocytic		• Benign fibrous histiocytoma/non-ossifying fibroma
Hematopoietic	Malignant	• Plasma cell myeloma • Solitary plasmacytoma of bone • Primary non-Hodgkin lymphoma of bone
Osteoclastic giant cell rich	Benign	• Giant cell lesion of the small bones
	Intermediate	• Giant cell tumor of bone
	Malignant	• Malignancy in giant cell tumor of bone
Notochordal	Benign	• Benign notochordal tumor
	Malignant	• Chordoma
Vascular	Benign	• Hemangioma
	Intermediate	• Epithelioid hemangioma
	Malignant	• Epithelioid hemangioendothelioma • Angiosarcoma
Myogenic	Benign	• Leiomyoma of bone
	Malignant	• Leiomyosarcoma of bone
Lipogenic	Benign	• Lipoma of bone
	Malignant	• Liposarcoma of bone
Undefined neoplastic nature	Benign	• Simple bone cyst • Fibrous dysplasia • Osteofibrous dysplasia • Chondromesenchymal hamartoma • Rosai–Dorfman disease
	Intermediate	• Aneurysmal bone cyst • Langerhans cell histiocytosis • Erdheim–Chester disease
Miscellaneous		• Ewing sarcoma (PNET) • Adamantinoma • Undifferentiated high-grade pleomorphic sarcoma of bone

80.1 General Aspects of Bone Tumors

Table 80.2 A similar approach for the classification of bone tumors is given by Nielsen et al. (2017)

Benign bone-forming tumors	• Bone island/osteopoikilosis • Osteoma • Osteoid osteoma • Osteoblastoma
Malignant bone-forming tumors	• Osteosarcoma
Benign cartilage-forming tumors	• Osteochondroma • Enchondroma • Chondroma • Chondroblastoma • Chondromyxoid fibroma
Malignant cartilage-forming tumors	• Conventional chondrosarcoma • Dedifferentiated chondrosarcoma • Clear cell chondrosarcoma • Mesenchymal chondrosarcoma
Fibrous and fibrohistiocytic tumors	• Non-ossifying fibroma • Desmoplastic fibroma • Myofibroma • Fibrosarcoma • Benign fibrous histiocytoma • Solitary fibrous tumor/hemangiopericytoma
Fibro-osseous tumors	• Fibrous dysplasia • Liposclerosing myxofibrous tumor
Malignant small round cell tumors	• Ewing sarcoma • Melanotic neuroectodermal tumor
Notochordal tumors	• Ecchordosis • Benign notochordal cell tumor • Chordoma
Giant cell-rich tumors	• Giant cell tumor • Brown tumor • Giant cell reparative granuloma
Cystic lesions of bone	• Intra-osseous ganglion • Unicameral bone cyst • Aneurysmal bone cyst • Epidermoid inclusion cyst
Vascular tumors	• Conventional hemangioma • Lymphangioma/lymphangiomatosis • Epithelioid hemangioma • Epithelioid hemangioendothelioma • Angiosarcoma
Hematopoietic tumors	• Langerhans cell histiocytosis • Primary lymphoma • Plasma cell myeloma • Mast cell disease • Erdheim–Chester disease • Rosai–Dorman disease
Miscellaneous mesenchymal tumors	• Osteofibrous dysplasia • Adamantinoma • Adipocytic tumors • Leiomyosarcoma • Myoepithelioma • Schwannoma • Myxopapillary ependymoma • Phosphaturic mesenchymal tumor
Bone tumor mimics	• Bizarre parosteal osteochondromatous proliferation • Melorheostosis • Amyloidoma • Gaucher disease
Metastatic tumors	• Metastatic tumors

Table 80.3 The most commonly encountered bone tumors affecting the skull and vertebral column; patterned after Nielsen et al. (2017)

Benign bone-forming tumors	• Osteoma • Osteoid osteoma • Osteoblastoma
Malignant bone-forming tumors	• Osteosarcoma
Benign cartilage-forming tumors	• Osteochondroma • Enchondroma • Chondroma • Chondroblastoma
Malignant cartilage-forming tumors	• Chondrosarcoma
Fibrous and fibrohistiocytic tumors	• Benign fibrous histiocytoma • Solitary fibrous tumor/hemangiopericytoma
Fibro-osseous tumors	• Fibrous dysplasia
Malignant small round cell tumors	• Ewing sarcoma/Primitive neuroectodermal tumor (PNET)
Notochordal tumors	• Chordoma
Giant cell-rich tumors	• Giant cell tumors
Cystic lesions of bone	• Aneurysmal bone cyst • Epidermoid inclusion cyst
Vascular tumors	• Conventional hemangioma
Hematopoietic tumors	• Langerhans cell histiocytosis • Plasmacytoma/myeloma • Erdheim–Chester disease • Rosai–Dorman disease
Miscellaneous mesenchymal tumors	• Osteofibrous dysplasia • Adipocytic tumors
Bone tumor mimics	• Amyloidoma
Metastatic tumors	• Metastatic tumors

Table 80.4 Frequencies (in %) of various bone tumors affecting the skull or vertebral column (based on Vigorita (2016))

Tumor entity	Skull	Vertebral column
Osteoma		
Osteoid osteoma	<1	7
Osteoblastoma	3	21
Osteosarcoma	2	<1
Osteochondroma	<<1	<1
Enchondroma	<<1	<1
Chondroma		
Chondroblastoma	1	<1
Chondromyxoid fibroma	<1	1
Chondrosarcoma	2	4
Benign fibrous histiocytoma	<1	<1
Fibrous dysplasia	8–10	<1
Ewing sarcoma/Primitive neuroectodermal tumor (PNET)	<1	2
Chordoma		
Giant cell tumors	<1	2
Aneurysmal bone cyst	<1	5
Myeloma	20	20

80.1 General Aspects of Bone Tumors

- GLI2 transcription factor accelerates the progression of OSA through Hedgehog pathway.
- Role of SPHK1/ASK1/JNK/CHK1,2 in the differentiation, proliferation, and apoptosis.
- PEDF.

Chondroma

Fibrous dysplasia
- Mutations in the GNAS1 gene encoding

Chondrosarcoma (Table 80.5)
- Isocitrate dehydrogenase (IDH)
- Tyrosine kinase
- Phosphoinositide 3-Kinase/AKT/
- Mammalian target of rapamycin (mTOR)
- Tumor suppressor pathways: retinoblastoma and p53
- Hedgehog

Chordoma (Table 80.6)
- Originate from remnants of embryonic notochord along the spine, more frequently at the skull base and sacrum.

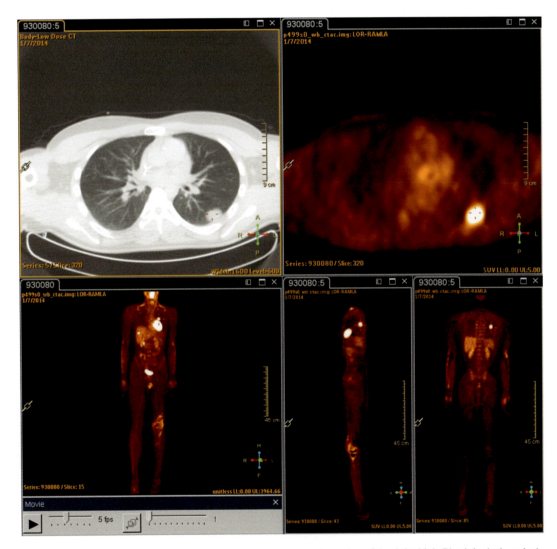

Fig. 80.1 Patient with pulmonal metastasized osteosarcoma of the right tibia with clear FDG uptake in the metastasis and inhomogeneous uptake after surgery around the right knee with additional FDG uptake in a soft tissue formation of the right thigh. Physiological uptake in brown fat as it is often seen in young patients. Unspecific artifactual FDG uptake outside the body in front of the liver due to the injection site

Table 80.5 Summary of genetic profiles of chordoma and chondrosarcoma (Kitamura et al. 2017)

Chordoma	Chondrosarcoma
Key tumorigenesis-related genes	
T (Brachyury)	*IDH1/2*
Other key genes	
SMARCB1/INI1	*COL2A1, TP53, CDKN2A/p16*
Major chromosomal copy number alterations	
Gains on 1p, 3, 4, 9, 10, 13, 14, 18	Gains on 2p, 5p, 7, 8q, 14q, 19, 20, 21q
Losses on 1q, 7	Losses on 4q, 6q, 9p, 13q, 17
Major dysregulated RTKs and ligands	
EGFR	EGFR
PDGFRα	PDGFRα
PDGFRβ	PDGFRβ
FGFRs	IGF-1
MET	VEGF
IGF-1R, IGF-1	
KIT	
p75 receptor, TrkA, NGF	
VEGF	
Major dysregulated downstream effectors	
PDK1	Akt, s6
Akt	mTOR
TSC2, mTOR, s6	Src
PTEN	HIF1α
PIK3CA	RB
ERK1/2	CDKN2A/p16
FRS2a	CDK4
STAT3	CDK6
Src	Cyclin D1
CDKN2A/p16	PTCH1, HHIP, GLI1, SUFO
	RUNX2
NRAS	
TP53	
Bcl-2	
Genes with dysregulated methylation statuses	
TNFRSF8	*Maspin, 14-3-3σ*
CDKN2A/p16, PTEN	*CDKN2A/p16*
C3, XIST, TACSTD2, FMR1, HIC1, RARB, DLEC1, KL, RASSF1	*3-OST*
FAM181B, NPR3, PON3, RAB32, RAI1, SLC16A5, ZNF397OS	*RUNX3*
Dysregulated miRNAs (predicted target)	
miR-1, miR-206 (MET)	*miR-10b (BDNF)*
miR-31 (MET), miR-140-3p (ERK2, GOLT1B, CBL, SCAMP1), miR-148a (BCL2L11, USP33), miR-222-3p (KIT, CDKN1B)	*miR-30a, miR-335 (RUNX2, SOX4)*
miR-149-3p, miR-663a, miR-1908, miR-2861, miR-3185 (MAPK signaling pathway)	
miR-1237-3p (MMP2)	*miR-100 (mTOR)*
miR-155 (SOCS1, TP53INP1)	*miR-145, miR-494 (SOX9)*
miR-181a (VEGF)	
miR-519d (p38)	

80.1 General Aspects of Bone Tumors

Table 80.6 Differential diagnosis of chordoma by molecular markers (Gulluoglu et al. 2016), data reproduced with kind permission by Springer Nature

Marker	Chromosomal region	Role in cancer
EMA	1q21	Promoting chemoresistance and cancer growth, invasion, inhibition of apoptosis
Galectin-3	14q22.3	Malignant transformation, cancer growth, angiogenesis, invasion and metastasis
E-cadherin	16q22.1	Tumor cell adhesion
Vimentin	10p13	Metastasis, tumor growth
CD24	6q21	Tumor growth, tumor cell invasion and metastasis
CD44	11p13	Tumor growth, tumor cell adhesion, migration, invasion and metastasis
Cytokeratin-19	17q21.2	Prevention of apoptosis, promotion of metastasis
Cytokeratin-8	12q13	Tumor progression, metastasis
Cytokeratin-13	17q12-q21.2	Tumor growth
Cytokeratin-15	17q21.2	Tumor progression
Cytokeratin-18	12q13	Tumor progression
c-met	7q31	Tumor cell invasion and metastasis
Brachyury	6q27	Tumor progression
FOSB	19q13.32	Tumor progression, tumor cell invasion
IL-18	11q22.2-q22.3	Tumor progression, angiogenesis, migration, metastasis, proliferation, and immune escape
FGF 1	5q31	Tumor growth, invasion
Syndecan 4	20q12	Tumor cell migration, invasion
Integrin beta 4	17q25	Tumor progression, tumor cell invasion
Stat3	17q21.31	Tumor progression, angiogenesis, invasion and metastasis, inhibition of apoptosis
SRC	20q12-q13	Tumor progression, metastasis
Bcl-xl	20q11.21	Chemoresistance
MCL1	1q21	Chemoresistance
Survivin 1	7q25	Inhibition of apoptosis
Periplakin 1	6p13.3	Tumor progression
PDGF receptor b	5q33.1	Tumor progression, metastasis
KIT	4q11-q12	Tumor progression
EGFR	7p12	Tumor progression
TGF-alpha	2p13	Tumor progression

- Chordomas highly and generally show a dual epithelial–mesenchymal differentiation.
- These tumors resist chemotherapy and radiotherapy.

Fibrous dysplasia
- Stimulatory alpha subunit of G-protein (Gs) has been found in dysplastic bone lesions.
- Mutations in Gsalpha
- Constitutive elevation in cAMP level induced by the Gsalpha mutations leads to alterations in the expression of several target genes whose promoters contain cAMP-responsive elements, such as c-fos, c-jun, Il-6, and Il-11.

Giant cell tumor (Table 80.7)
- Giant cells are principally responsible for the extensive bone resorption by the tumor.
- The spindle-like stromal cells chiefly direct the pathology of the tumor by:
  - recruiting monocytes and promoting their fusion into giant cells
  - enhancing the resorptive ability of the giant cells

Table 80.7 Functions of key factors expressed in giant cell tumor (GCT)

Function	Cell	Factor	Likely role in GCT
Monocyte recruitment	S	SDF-1	• Chemotactic agent signaling via CXCR4 (M)
	S	MCP-1	• Chemotactic agent signaling via CCR1 (M)
	S	VEGF	• Promote angiogenesis • Promote chemotaxis via Flt-1 (M)
Monocyte proliferation	S	M-CSF	• Stimulates proliferation and RANK expression via CSF1R (M)
	S/G	IL-34	• Stimulates proliferation via CSF1R (M)
Cellular fusion	S	RANKL	• Stimulates RANK (M) to induce giant cell formation
	S	OPG	• Decoy receptor for RANKL that inhibits giant cell formation
	M/G	NFATc1	• Essential transcription factor for osteoclast-specific genes
	M/G	DC-STAMP	• Transmembrane protein essential for cell fusion
	S/G	C/EBPβ	• Transcription factor that promotes RANKL expression • Induces larger osteoclasts to form
	S	CaSR	• Receptor for calcium • Leads to stimulation of RANKL expression
	S	PTHrP	• Stimulates RANKL expression via PTH1R (S)
Bone resorption	G	Cathepsin K	• Degrades organic components of bone
	G	V-ATPase	• Demineralizes the crystals of hydroxyapatite, provides acidic environment for cathepsin K
	G	TRAP	• Dephosphorylates bone matrix proteins, involved in giant cell migration
	G	αvβ3 integrin	• Regulates giant cell cytoskeleton and attachment to bone
	G	MMP-9	• Stimulates bone resorption by giant cells
	S	MMP-13	• Stimulates bone resorption by giant cells
	S	MMP-2	• Involved in vascular invasion
	S	TGF-β1	• Chemotaxis of giant cells via TGFBR2 (G)

Proteins are grouped by general tasks and indicate the cell or cells responsible for their expression: spindle-like stromal cells (S), monocytes (M), or giant cells (G), modified after Cowan and Singh (2013), data reproduced with kind permission from Elsevier

- Receptor activator of nuclear factor-κB ligand (RANKL).
- Proteases, including numerous matrix metalloproteinases.

80.1.5 Treatment and Prognosis

Treatment
- surgery
- chemotherapy
- radiation

Biologic Behavior–Prognosis–Prognostic Factors
- Osteoma
  - slow-growing lesion
  - observation
  - simple excision
  - excellent, no recurrence
- Osteoid osteoma
  - radiofrequency ablation
  - curettage, resection
  - local recurrence rate 0–10%
- Osteosarcoma
  - surgery
  - chemotherapy
  - radiation
  - relapse-free survival rates 70%
  - response to chemotherapy (good vs. poor responders)
- Chondroma
  - excision
  - rare malignant degeneration
  - rarely development of dedifferentiated component
- Chondrosarcoma
  - aggressive curettage to surgical resection
  - radiation

- Grade 1: 5-year survival rate 85%
- Grade 2 and 3: 5-year survival rate 50%
• Fibrous dysplasia
  - observation to surgical removal
  - asymptomatic disease: excellent prognosis
  - symptomatic disease: significant disability, pain, recurrent fractures
  - malignant transformation possible
• Chordoma
  - surgery
  - radiation therapy
  - prognosis affected by tumor location, size, and resectability
  - local progression possible
  - metastatic spread: 5–43%
• Giant cell tumor
  - surgery
  - radiation
  - RANK ligand inhibitors
  - local recurrence rates of about 25%
  - Metastases in 1–2%
• Aneurysmal bone cyst
  - low recurrence rate
  - malignant transformation possible (rare)

80.2 Osteoma

WHO Definition

A benign tumor composed of compact bone arising on the surface of the bone and, when developing in the medullary cavity, known as enostosis (Baumhoer and Bras 2013).

A benign bone-forming tumor composed of cortical-type bone with limited growth potential.

Isolated cases of intracranial osteoma (usually dural-based) have been reported. Outside the CNS, osteomas often develop in the skull and only secondarily displace dura and brain. Histologically, they correspond to similar tumors arising in bone and must be distinguished from asymptomatic dural calcification, ossification related to metabolic disease or trauma, and rare examples of astrocytoma and gliosarcoma with osseous differentiation.

80.2.1 Localization

• Craniofacial skeleton
  - frontal and ethmoid sinuses
  - sphenoid sinus

80.2.2 Neuroimaging Findings

General Imaging Features
• Well-delineated bony mass

CT (Figs. 80.2a–c and 80.3a, b)
• Usually homogeneous bone density

MRI-T1, T2 (Fig. 80.3c)
• All sequences show low signal intensity.

MRI-T1 contrast-enhanced (Fig. 80.3d)
• Usually no pathological enhancement

80.2.3 Pathology Findings

Macroscopic Features (Fig. 80.4a–f)
• Round-oval
• Hard
• Well-circumscribed
• Tan to white

Microscopic Features (Fig. 80.5)
• Lamellar and woven bone with Haversian-like systems
• Cortical-like architecture
• Interconnecting trabeculae
• Inconspicuous small and flat osteoblasts rim the bone
• Osteocytes inconspicuous
• Fibrous component mimicking fibro-osseous tumor

Differential diagnosis
• osteosarcoma
• osteochondroma
• juxtacortical myositis ossificans
• melorheostosis

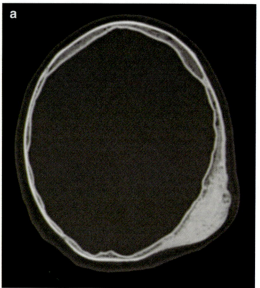
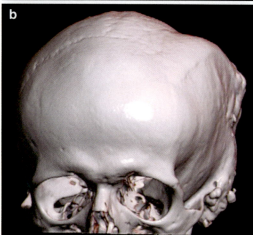
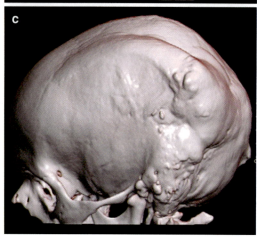

Fig. 80.2 Osteoma of the skull—CT (**a**), 3D reconstruction (**b, c**)

80.3 Osteoid Osteoma

WHO Definition

A benign bone-forming tumor characterized by small size (<2 cm), limited growth potential and disproportionate pain, usually responsive to non-steroidal anti-inflammatory drugs (Horvai and Klein 2013).

Benign bone-forming tumor characterized by its small size, limited growth potential, classic pattern of pain, and composition of woven bone trabeculae rimmed by osteoclasts.

80.3.1 Localization

- vertebral column (10–14% of cases)

80.3.2 Neuroimaging Findings

General Imaging Features
- Lucent nidus (<1.5 cm) with surrounding sclerotic bone (lesions >1.5 cm are called osteoblastoma)

CT non-contrast-enhanced (Fig. 80.6a, b)
- Central hypodense lucency (= nidus) with surrounding hyperdense sclerosis, nidus can be sclerotic

CT contrast-enhanced
- Variable enhancement

MRI-T2/FLAIR
- Variable signal of nidus
- Hyperintense surrounding edema

MRI-T1
- Hypointense nidus

MRI-T1 contrast-enhanced
- Enhancement of nidus.
- Surrounding reactive zone may enhance.

80.3 Osteoid Osteoma

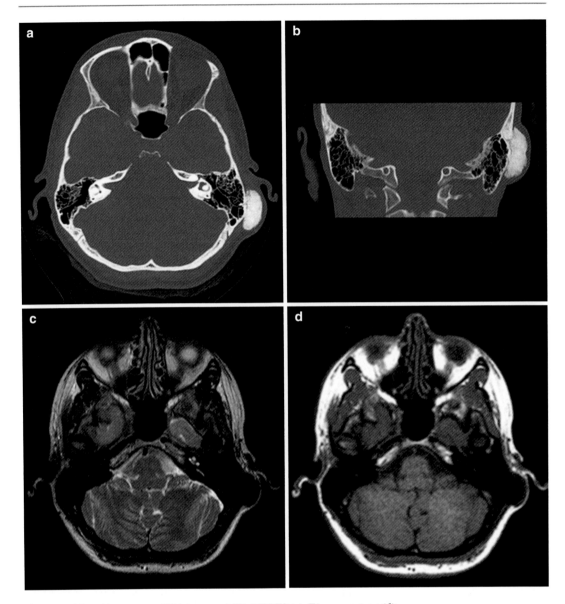

Fig. 80.3 Mastoid osteoma—CT (**a**), coronal (**b**), MRI T2 (**c**), T1 non-contrast (**d**)

80.3.3 Pathology Findings

Macroscopic Features
- Well-circumscribed
- Round
- Gritty
- Dark red to tan
- Central tan-white speckles
- Surrounded by dense sclerotic bone

Microscopic Features (Fig. 80.7)
- Nidus (1–2 cm)
  - Central portion of the lesion
  - Differentiated osteoblastic activity

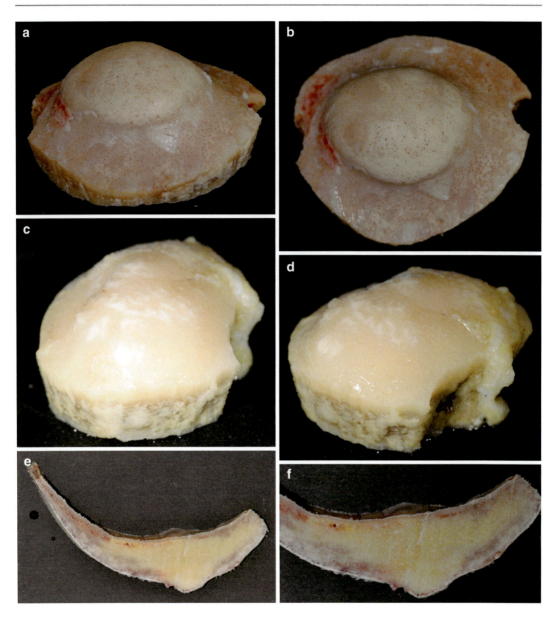

Fig. 80.4 Osteoma: Round-oval, well-circumscribed, hard, tan to white thickened bone (**a–f**)

80.3 Osteoid Osteoma

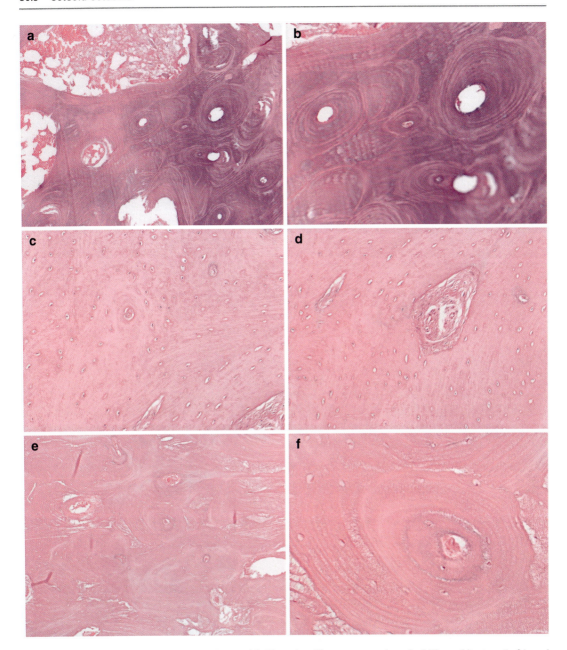

Fig. 80.5 Osteoma: Lamellar and woven bone with Haversian-like systems and cortical-like architecture (**a–h**), and interconnecting trabeculae (**i, j**). Fibrous component mimics fibro-osseous tumor (**g, h**)

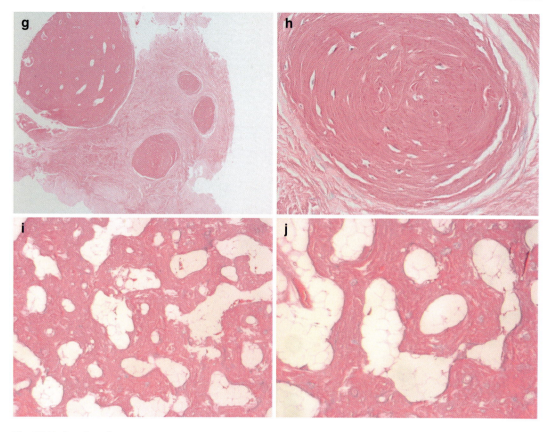

Fig. 80.5 (continued)

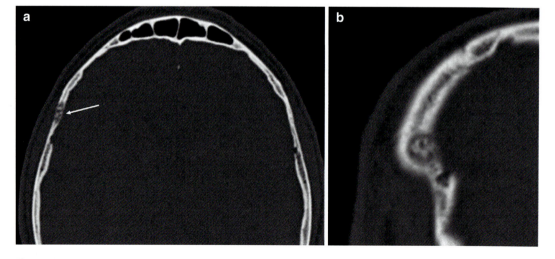

Fig. 80.6 Osteoid osteoma with sclerotic nidus—CT non-contrast (**a**, **b**)

80.3 Osteoid Osteoma

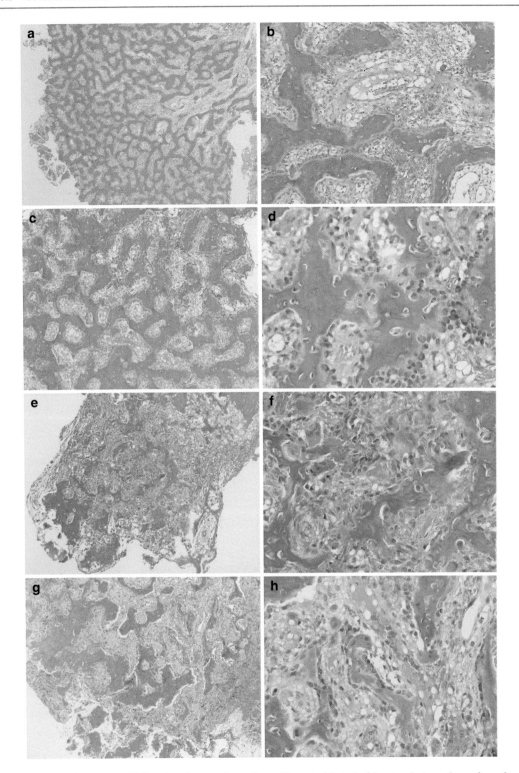

Fig. 80.7 Osteoid osteoma: Trabeculae of woven bone rimmed by osteoblasts (**a–h**); osteoclasts on the surface of trabeculae (**d, h**); intertrabecular spaces filled with loose connective tissue (**e–h**)

- Trabeculae of woven bone rimmed by osteoblasts
- Osteoclasts on the surface of trabeculae
- Intertrabecular spaces filled with loose connective tissue
- Cartilage differentiation possible

Differential diagnosis
- Osteoblastoma
- Intra-osseous abscess
- Stress fracture

80.4 Osteoblastoma

WHO Definition
A benign bone-forming neoplasm, >2 cm, which produces woven bone spicules, which are bordered by prominent osteoblasts (de Andrea et al. 2013).

80.4.1 Localization

- Tubular bones (60%)
- Axial skeleton (30%)
- Craniofacial bones (10%)

80.4.2 Pathology Findings

Macroscopic Features
- solitary
- lesion
- well-circumscribed
- tan-white, dark red
- cystic changes possible

Microscopic Features (Fig. 80.8)
- Trabeculae in haphazard, interconnecting, sheet-like patterns.
- Woven bone rimmed by plump osteoblasts and scattered osteoclasts.
- Vascular connective tissue fills intertrabecular space.

Differential diagnosis
- Osteoid osteoma
- Aneurysmal bone cyst
- Osteoblastoma-like osteosarcoma

80.5 Osteosarcoma

WHO Definition
A high-grade, intra-osseous, malignant neoplasm in which the neoplastic cells produce bone (Rosenberg et al. 2013).

A malignant bone-forming mesenchymal tumor.

Osteosarcoma predominantly affects adolescents and young adults. The preferred sites are the skull and the spine and more rarely the meninges and the brain. Bone matrix or osteoid deposition by the proliferating tumor cells is required for the diagnosis. Osteosarcomatous elements may exceptionally be encountered as components of germ cell tumor and gliosarcoma.

80.5.1 Localization

- affects rarely the skull or vertebral column

80.5.2 Imaging Findings

General Imaging Features
- Aggressive, ill-defined bone tumor with bone destruction and soft tumor mass

CT (Fig. 80.9a–c)
- Blastic or lytic skull mass

MRI-T2 (Fig. 80.9d–f)
- Solid, non-ossified tumor components: hyperintense
- Ossified components: hypointense
- Peritumoral edema hyperintense

80.5 Osteosarcoma

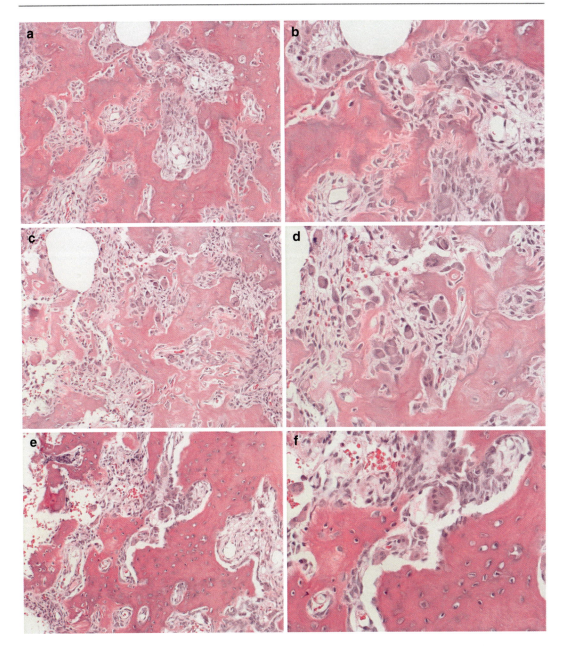

Fig. 80.8 Osteoblastoma: Trabeculae in haphazard, interconnecting, sheet-like patterns (**a–d**); woven bone rimmed by plump osteoblasts and scattered osteoclasts (**e–j**); vascular connective tissue fills intertrabecular space (**g–j**)

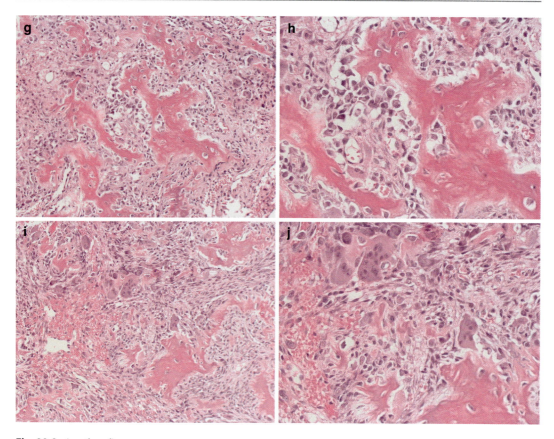

Fig. 80.8 (continued)

MRI-T1
- Solid, non-ossified components: low to intermediate
- Ossified tumor: hypointense

MRI-T1 contrast-enhanced
- Enhancement of solid components

Nuclear Medicine Imaging Finding (Fig. 80.1)
- FDG can be positive.

80.5.3 Pathology Findings

Macroscopic Features
- Intramedullary
- Tan-gray-white color

Microscopic Features (Fig. 80.10)
- Neoplastic bone
  - Woven architecture
  - Primitive disorganized trabeculae
  - Mineralized bone
- Two elements:
  - High-grade sarcoma with epitheloid, plasmacytoid, fusiform, ovoid, small round cells, clear cells, mono- or multinucleated giant cells, or spindle cells
  - Bone matrix produced by tumor
- Various prominent cell types
  - giant cell rich
  - chondroblastic
  - telangiectatic
  - fibroblastic

80.5 Osteosarcoma

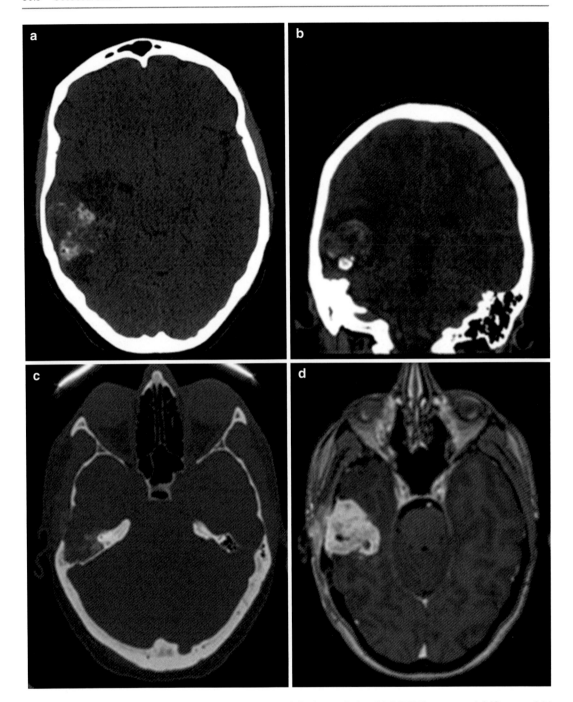

Fig. 80.9 Osteosarcoma—CT non-contrast axial (**a**), coronal (**b**), bone window (**c**), MRI T1-contrast axial (**d**), coronal (**e**)

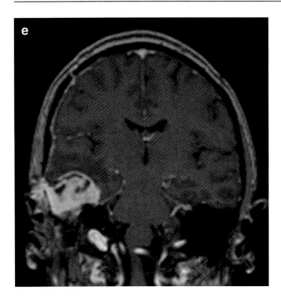

Fig. 80.9 (continued)

Differential diagnosis
- Fibrosarcoma
- Fracture callus
- Osteoblastoma
- Chondrosarcoma
- Dedifferentiated chondrosarcoma
- Myositis ossificans
- Giant cell tumor
- Metastatic carcinoma
- Ewing sarcoma
- Aneurysmal bone cyst

80.6 Chondroma

WHO Definition
A group of benign bone tumours of hyaline cartilage sharing histological features. However, they differ with respect to location and clinical features (Lucas and Bridge 2013).

- Enchondroma is a benign hyaline cartilage neoplasm that arises within the medullary cavity of bone. Most tumours are solitary; however, they occasionally involve more than one bone, or site in a single bone (Lucas and Bridge 2013).
- Periosteal chondroma is a benign hyaline cartilage neoplasm of bone surface that arises beneath the periosteum (Lucas and Bridge 2013).

Chondroma
- A benign, well-circumscribed neoplasm composed of low-cellularity hyaline cartilage.
- Isolated cases of intracranial chondroma (usually dural-based) have been reported.
- Outside the CNS chondromas often develop in the skull and only secondarily displace dura and brain.
- Malignant transformation of a large CNS chondroma to chondrosarcoma has been documented over a long clinical course.

80.6.1 Localization

- Uncommon in spine

80.6.2 Pathology Findings

Macroscopic Features
- Gray-white and opalescent
- Well-marginated
- Firm to hard

Microscopic Features (Fig. 80.11)
- Hypocellular, avascular tumor
- Abundant hyaline cartilage matrix
- Chondrocytes
  - Fine granular eosinophilic cytoplasm
  - Small round nuclei with condensed chromatin
  - Situated within sharp-edged lacunar spaces

Differential diagnosis
- Low-grade chondrosarcoma
- Chondromyxoid fibroma

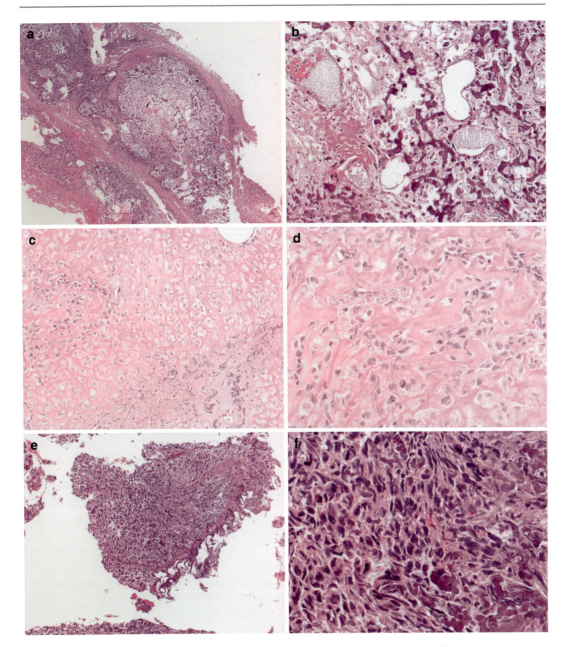

Fig. 80.10 Osteosarcoma: Neoplastic bone shows woven architecture, primitive disorganized trabeculae, and mineralized bone (**a–d**). The second element consists of high-grade sarcoma with epitheloid, plasmacytoid, fusiform, ovoid, small round cells, clear cells, mono- or multinucleated giant cells, or spindle cells (**e–h**). Moderate to high Ki-67 proliferation rate (**i, j**)

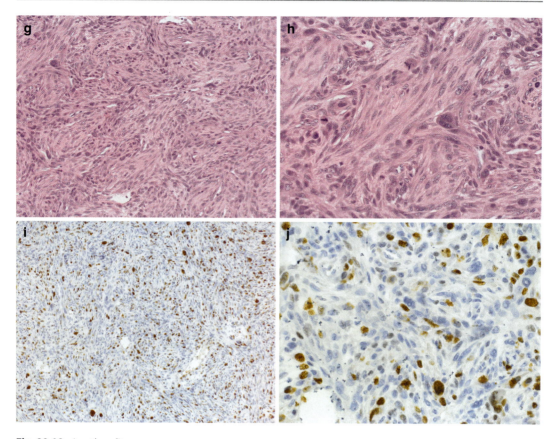

Fig. 80.10 (continued)

80.7 Chondrosarcoma

WHO Definition
A focally aggressive or malignant group of cartilaginous matrix-producing neoplasms with diverse morphological features and clinical behavior (Hogendoorn et al. 2013).

Chondrosarcoma:
- A malignant mesenchymal tumor with cartilaginous differentiation.
- Most chondrosarcomas arise de novo, but some develop in a pre-existing benign cartilaginous lesion.

80.7.1 Localization

- Any bone derived from endochondral ossification

80.7.2 Imaging Findings

General Imaging Features
Lytic tumor with chondroid calcifications

CT non-contrast-enhanced (Fig. 80.12a, b)
- Lytic mass with popcorn-like (chondroid) calcifications

MRI-T2 (Fig. 80.12c)
- Hyperintense

MRI-T1 (Fig. 80.12f)
- Low to intermediate

MRI-T1 contrast-enhanced (Fig. 80.12g, h)
- Heterogeneous enhancement

MRI-T2∗
- Low signal of calcifications

80.7 Chondrosarcoma

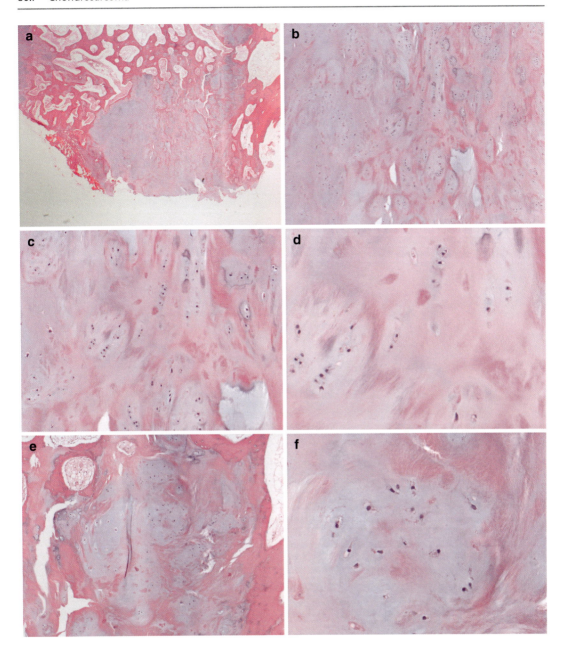

Fig. 80.11 Chondroma: Hypocellular, avascular tumor (**a–j**) consisting of an abundant hyaline cartilage matrix (**a–j**); the chondrocytes have fine granular eosinophilic cytoplasm, small round nuclei with condensed chromatin, and are situated within sharp-edged lacunar spaces (**f, h–j**)

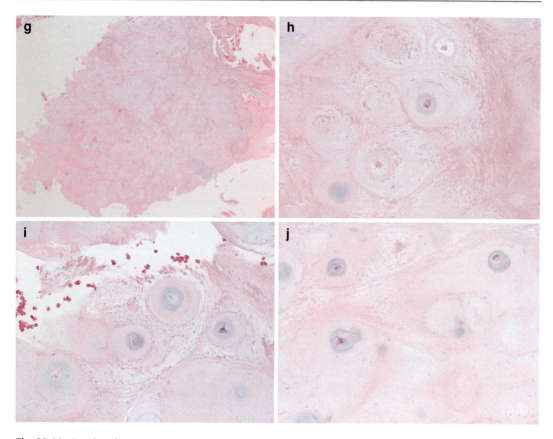

Fig. 80.11 (continued)

80.7.3 Pathology Findings

Macroscopic Features
- gray-tan glistening
- lobulated architecture
- expand bone
- destroy cortex

Microscopic Features (Fig. 80.13)
- Matrix
  - Neoplastic matrix: hyaline or myxoid
  - Hyaline matrix: basophilic
  - Myxoid matrix: frothy or bubbly
- Cells
  - Neoplastic chondrocytes
    ○ variable size
    ○ moderate amounts of eosinophilic cytoplasm
    ○ cytologic atypia
  - Tumor cells in myxoid areas
    ○ bipolar or stellate
    ○ arranged singly or in cords and strands

Grading of chondrosarcoma
- Grade 1
  - Hypocellular.
  - Nuclei are small and dark or slightly enlarged with fine chromatin.
- Grade 2
  - More cellular.
  - Nuclei are larger, irregular, and have coarse chromatin.
  - Mitoses infrequent.
- Grade 3
  - Hypercellular
  - Severe pleomorphism
  - Mitoses

80.7 Chondrosarcoma

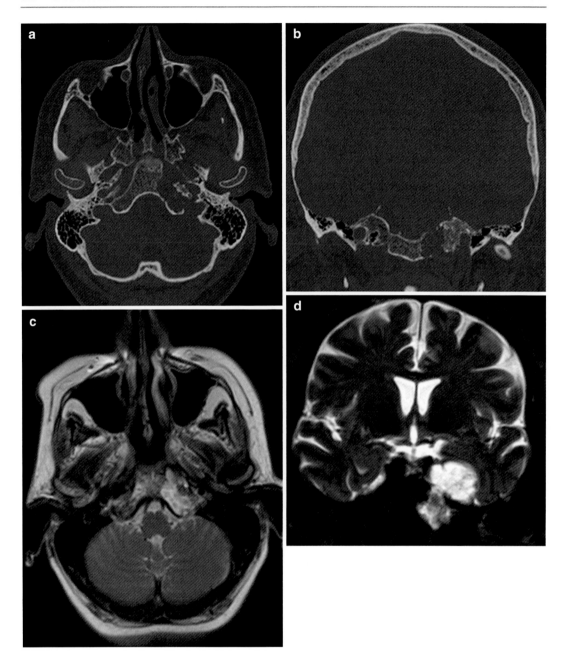

Fig. 80.12 Chondrosarcoma of the skull base—CT axial (**a**), coronal (**b**); MRI T2 axial (**c**), coronal (**d**), FLAIR (**e**), T1 non-contrast (**f**), T1 contrast axial (**g**), coronal (**h**)

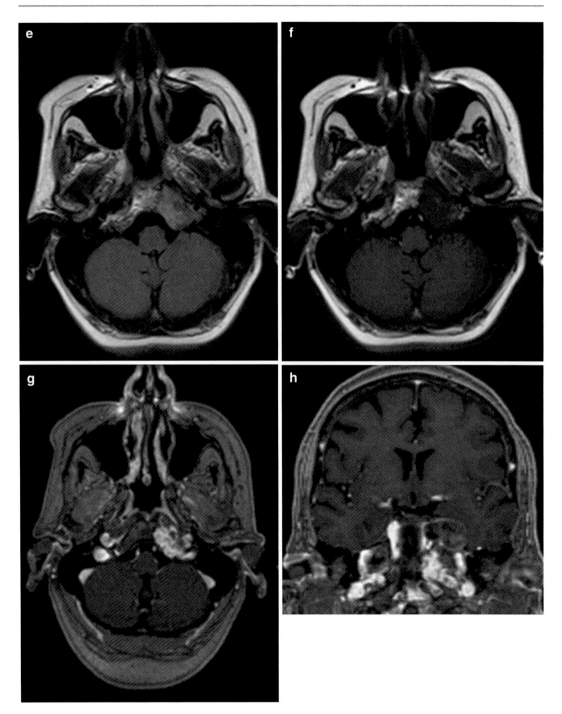

Fig. 80.12 (continued)

80.7 Chondrosarcoma

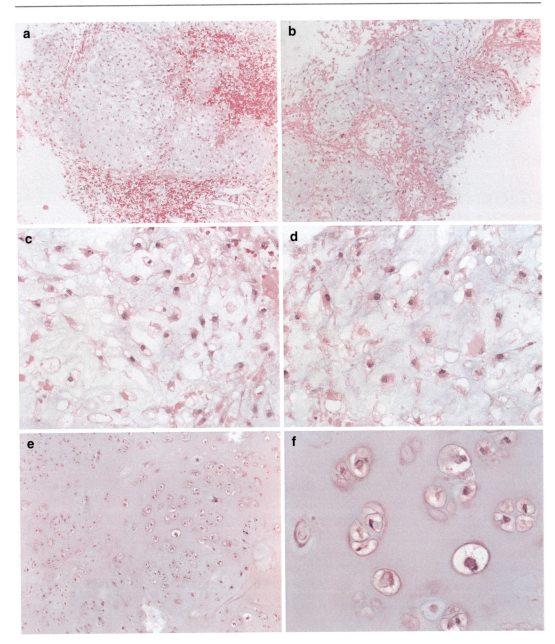

Fig. 80.13 Chondrosarcoma: The tumor matrix consists of a hyaline or myxoid neoplastic matrix and a basophilic hyaline matrix (**a–h**); the neoplastic chondrocytes are of variable size, have moderate amounts of eosinophilic cytoplasm and present cytologic atypia (**i**, **j**). Immunophenotype of chondrosarcoma: tumor cells are positive for vimentin (**k**, **l**) and S-100 (**m**, **n**)

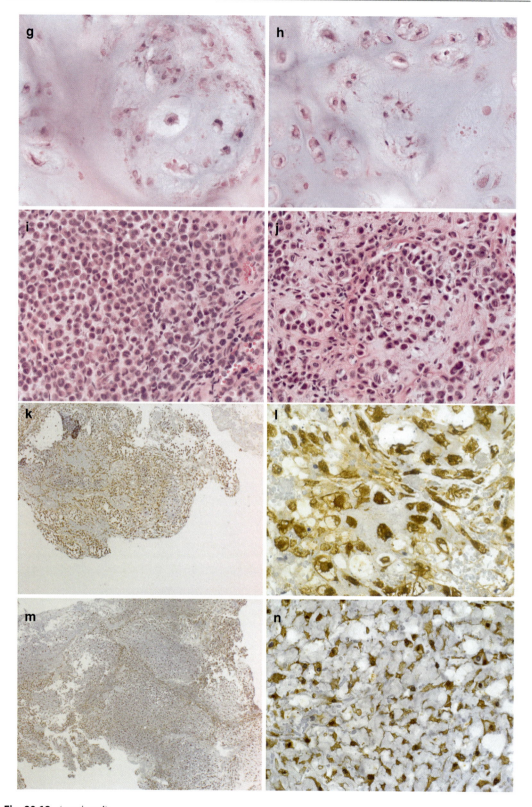

Fig. 80.13 (continued)

Differential diagnosis
- Enchondroma
- Chondromyxoid fibroma
- Clear cell chondrosarcoma
- Chordoma
- Fracture callus

80.8 Fibrous Dysplasia

WHO Definition
A benign, medullary, fibro-osseous lesion, which may involve one or more bones (Siegal et al. 2013).

Fibrous dysplasia
- Common monostotic or polyostotic benign fibro-osseous neoplasm of the bone.

80.8.1 Localization

- Calvarium

80.8.2 Imaging Findings

General Imaging Features
- Tumor-like growth of fibrous tissue replacing normal bone, causing bone deformation

CT non-contrast-enhanced (Fig. 80.14a–c)
- Expansion of bone with ground glass appearance
- Can be cystic or sclerotic

MRI-T2 (Fig. 80.14d)
- Heterogeneous signal, intermediate to high

MRI-T1 (Fig. 80.14e)
- Heterogeneous signal, intermediate to low

MRI-T1 contrast-enhanced (Fig. 80.14f, g)
- Heterogeneous enhancement

80.8.3 Pathology Findings

Macroscopic Features (Fig. 80.15a, b)
- Expanded bone
- Tan-gray color
- Firm to gritty consistency
- Solid or focally cystic
- Erodes and thins the cortex

Microscopic Features (Fig. 80.15c–l)
- Varying proportions of fibrous and osseous tissue
- Fibrous tissue
  – Composed of bland fibroblastic cells
- Osseous component
  – Irregular, curvilinear, trabeculae of woven bone
- Inconspicuous, spindle-shaped osteoblasts
- Nodules of benign hyaline cartilage
- Secondary changes include:
  – Foam cells
  – Multinucleated osteoclastic giant cells
  – Extensive myxoid change

Differential diagnosis
- Well-differentiated osteosarcoma
- Desmoplastic fibroma
- Osteofibrous dysplasia
- Fracture callus
- Paget disease
- Non-ossifying fibroma

80.9 Chordoma

WHO Definition
A malignant tumor showing notochordal differentiation (Flanagan and Yamaguchi 2013).

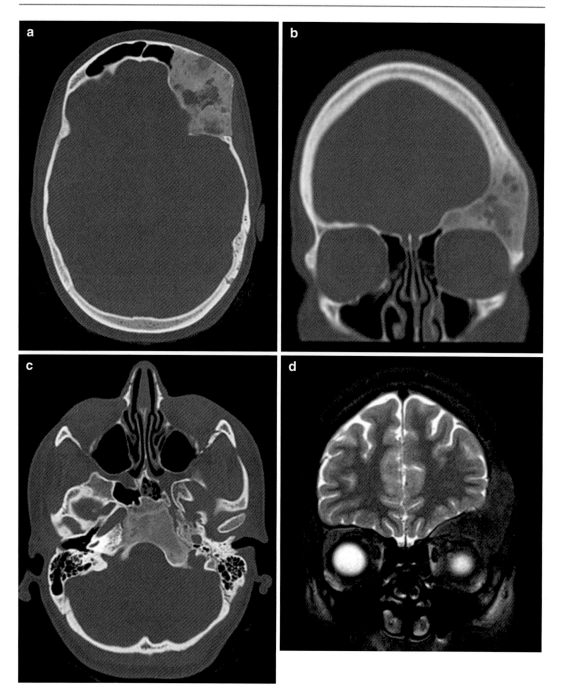

Fig. 80.14 Craniofacial fibrous dysplasia, multiple bones involved—CT non-contrast (**a**, **b**, **c**); MRI T2 (**d**), T1 non-contrast (**e**), T1 contrast coronal (**f**), axial (**g**)

80.9 Chordoma

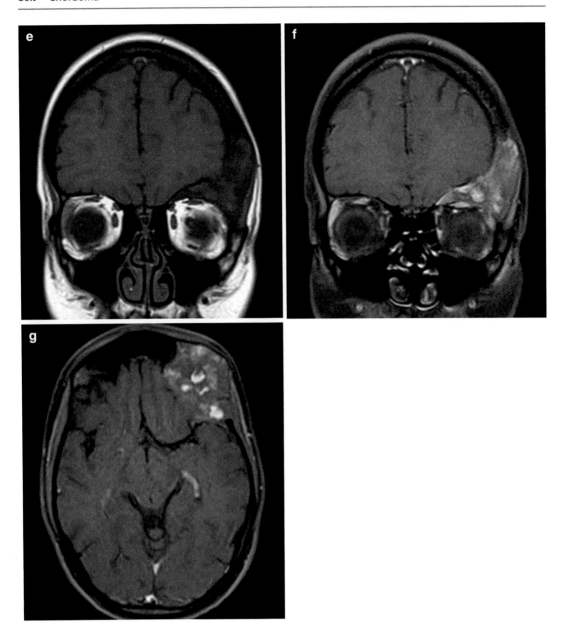

Fig. 80.14 (continued)

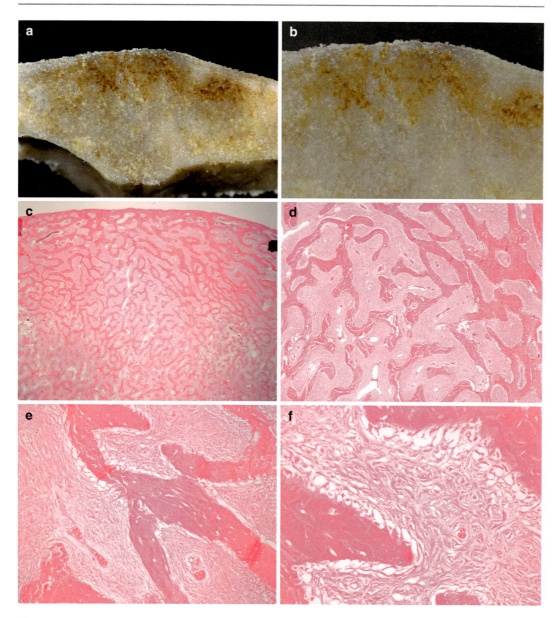

Fig. 80.15 Fibrous dysplasia: Surgical specimen shows expanded bone of tan-gray color, firm to gritty consistency (**a**, **b**). The tumor erodes and thins the cortex (**a**, **b**). The tumor consists of varying proportions of fibrous and osseous tissue. The osseous component is made up of irregular, curvilinear, trabeculae of woven bone (**c–e**, **g**, **h**). The fibrous tissue component is composed of bland fibroblastic cells (**e**, **f**, **i**, **j**). Inconspicuous, spindle-shaped osteoblasts are observed; no osteoblastic rimming (**g**, **h**). The tumor cells are immunopositive for vimentin (**k**, **l**)

80.9 Chordoma

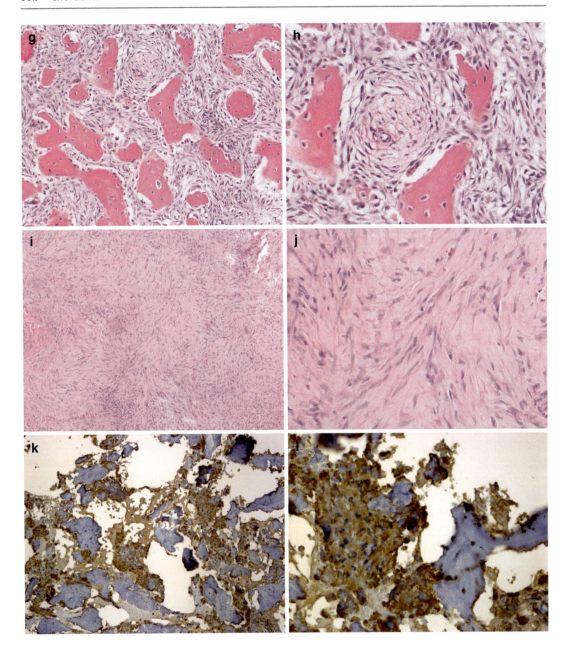

Fig. 80.15 (continued)

Chordoma

- Primary malignant tumor of bone with phenotype that recapitulates notochord and usually arises within bones of axial skeleton

80.9.1 Localization

- Axial skeleton
  - Skull base (35% of cases)
  - Sacral (29% of cases)
  - Spinal (32% of cases)

80.9.2 Imaging Findings

General Imaging Features
Midline tumor in the clival region

CT contrast-enhanced (Fig. 80.16a, b)
- Large soft tissue mass with lytic bone destruction of the clivus

CT contrast-enhanced
- Moderate enhancement

MRI-T2 (Fig. 80.16c, d)
- Hyperintense

MRI-T1 (Fig. 80.16e, f)
- Usually hypointense compared to the high signal of the clivus

MRI-T1 contrast-enhanced (Fig. 80.16g, h)
- Heterogeneous enhancement

MRI-T2*
- Low signal of intratumoral calcifications or hemorrhages

80.9.3 Pathology Findings

Macroscopic Features
- Lobulated structure
- Blue-gray color
- Soft, gelatinous matrix

Microscopic Features (Fig. 80.17)
- Large epithelioid cells with clear eosinophilic cytoplasm.
- Vacuolated cytoplasm, i.e., physaliphorous cells.
- Arrangement of cells in:
  - small ribbons and cords embedded in abundant extracellular matrix
  - densely arranged epithelioid packets
- Lobular architecture with fibrous septae.
- Nuclear atypia defines tumor grade.
- Immunopositive for (Fig. 80.17i, j):
  - EMA
  - CK8
  - CK19
  - S100
  - T-Brachyury

Differential diagnosis
- Metastatic adenocarcinoma
- Chondrosarcoma
- Benign notochordal cell tumor
- Atypical teratoid rhabdoid tumor

80.10 Giant Cell Tumor

WHO Definition
A benign but locally aggressive primary bone neoplasm that is composed of a proliferation of mononuclear cells among which are scattered numerous macrophages and large osteoclast-like giant cells (Athanasou et al. 2013).

Giant cell tumor:
- Neoplasm composed of cytologically benign, oval or polyhedral mononuclear cells that are admixed with numerous, evenly distributed, osteoclast-like cells.

80.10.1 Localization

- Uncommon site: vertebral body

80.10 Giant Cell Tumor

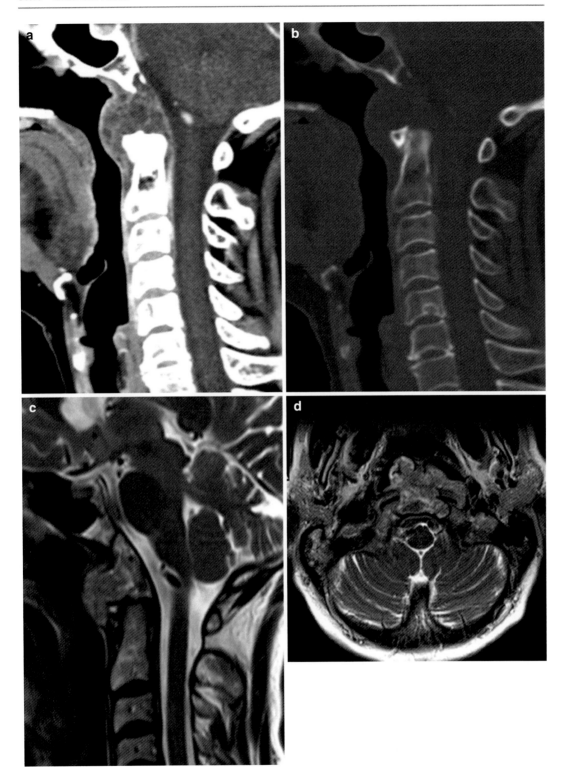

Fig. 80.16 Chordoma—CT sagittal (**a**), bone window (**b**); MRI T2 sagittal (**c**) and axial (**d**), T1 non-contrast sagittal (**e**) and axial (**f**), T1 contrast sagittal (**g**) and axial (**h**)

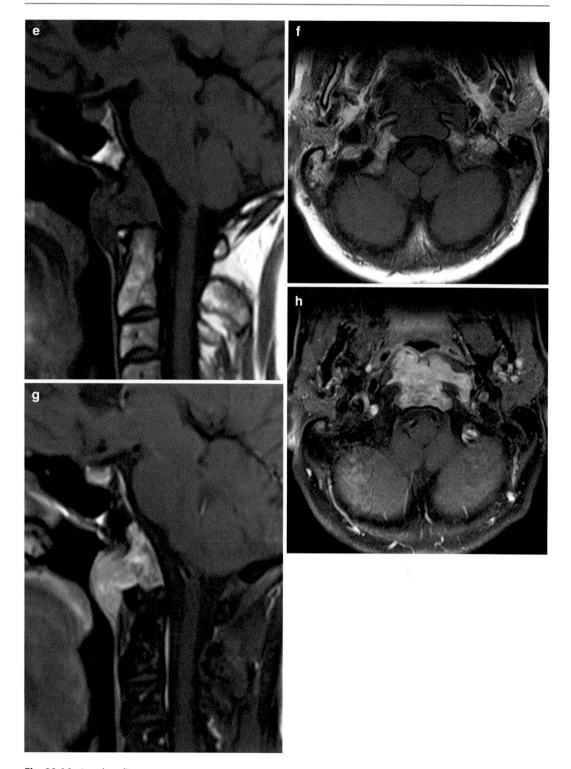

Fig. 80.16 (continued)

80.10 Giant Cell Tumor

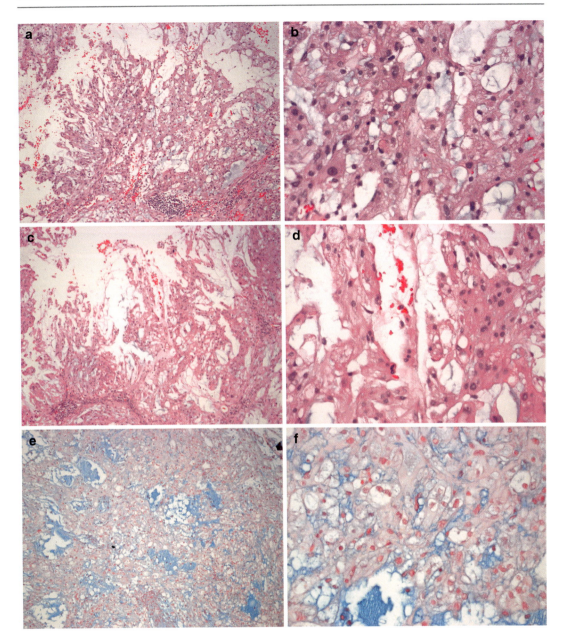

Fig. 80.17 Chordoma: The tumor is composed of large epitheloid cells with clear eosinophilic, vacuolated cytoplasm, i.e., physaliphorous cells (**a–f**). The cells are arranged in small ribbons and cords embedded in abundant extracellular matrix densely arranged epitheloid packets (**a–f**) (**a–d**: HE; **e, f**: Alcian blue). The tumor cells are immunopositive for vimentin (**g, h**) and pancytokeratin AE1/AE3 (**i, j**)

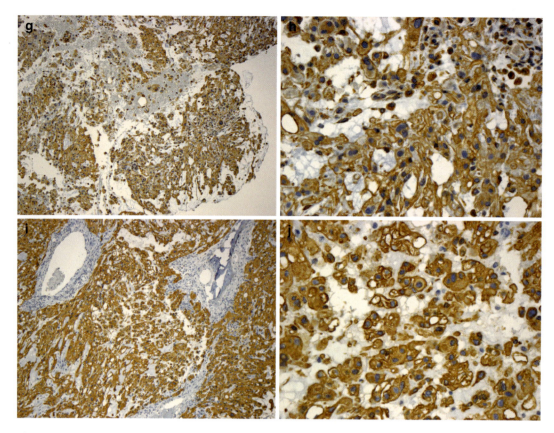

Fig. 80.17 (continued)

80.10.2 Imaging Findings

General Imaging Features
- Well-defined osteolytic lesion usually without sclerotic margin

CT non-contrast-enhanced
- Well-defined osteolytic lesion
- Usually no sclerotic margin
- Cortical thinning, expansion, or destruction
- Pathological fractures possible
- No matrix mineralization

MRI-T2 (Fig. 80.18a, b)
- Areas with hemosiderin and calcifications show low signal.
- Hyperintense signal of cystic components.

MRI-T1 (Fig. 80.18c)
- Hypointense to isointense signal of solid components

MRI-T1 contrast-enhanced (Fig. 80.18d)
- Variable, heterogeneous enhancement
- Enhancement of adjacent bone possible

80.10.3 Pathology Findings

Macroscopic Features
- Well-marginated
- Red-brown color
- Soft
- Hemorrhagic

Microscopic Features (Fig. 80.19)
- Presence of a large number of osteoclast-like giant cells with
  - plump, eosinophilic cytoplasm
  - vesicular nuclei with prominent nucleoli
  - Immunopositive for:
    ○ vitronectin receptor (CD51)

80.10 Giant Cell Tumor

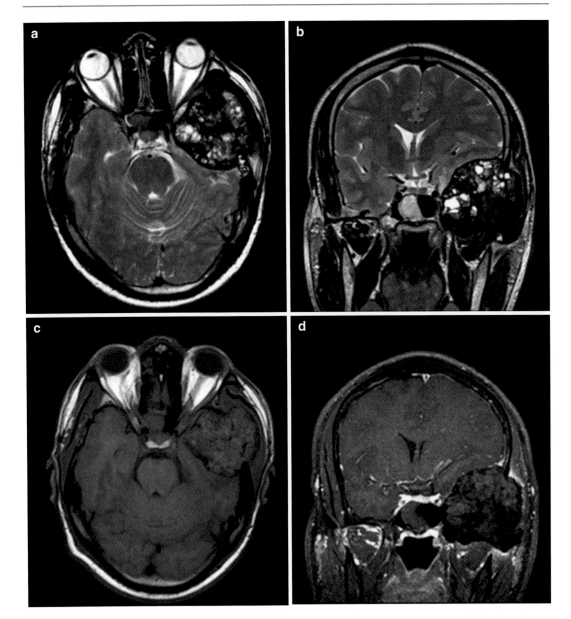

Fig. 80.18 Giant cell tumor—T2 axial (**a**), coronal (**b**), T1 non-contrast axial (**c**), T1 contrast coronal (**d**)

- cathepsin K
- macrophage marker (CD68, CD45, CD33)
– Immunonegative for:
- CD14
- CD163
- HLA-DR
• Numerous round or spindle-shaped mononuclear cells

• Mononuclear stromal cells with poorly-defined cytoplasm and spindle-shaped nucleoli
• Tumor stroma:
– Well vascularized
– Bands of cellular or collagenous fibrous tissue
– Hemorrhage
– Hemosiderin

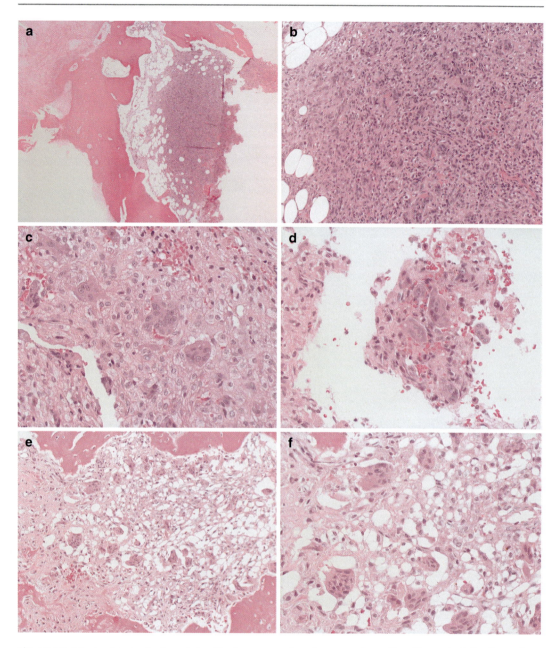

Fig. 80.19 Giant cell tumor is characterized by the presence of a large number of osteoclast-like giant cells with plump, eosinophilic cytoplasm, vesicular nuclei with prominent nucleoli (**a–f**). Numerous round or spindle-shaped mononuclear cells with poorly defined cytoplasm and spindle-shaped nucleoli are evident (**a–f**). Tumor stroma is well vascularized and contains bands of cellular or collagenous fibrous tissue (**a–f**)

Differential diagnosis
- Non-ossifying fibroma
- Chondroblastoma
- Giant cell reparative granuloma
- Aneurysmal bone cyst
- Giant cell-rich osteosarcoma

80.11 Aneurysmal Bone Cyst

WHO Definition
A destructive, expansile, benign neoplasm of bone composed of multiloculated blood-filled cystic spaces (Nielsen et al. 2013).

80.11 Aneurysmal Bone Cyst

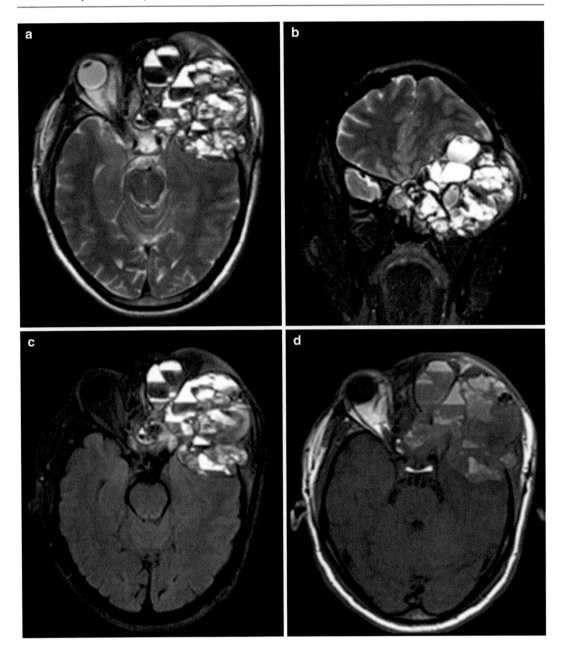

Fig. 80.20 Aneurysmal bone cyst—T2 axial (**a**), coronal (**b**), FLAIR (**c**), T1 non-contrast axial (**d**), coronal (**e**), T1 contrast axial (**f**), coronal (**g**)

Aneurysmal bone cyst:
- Destructive, expansile benign tumor with blood-filled cystic spaces.

80.11.1 Localization

- Craniofacial skeleton

80.11.2 Imaging Findings

General Imaging Features

Lobulated, expansile mass with cystic spaces containing characteristic fluid–fluid levels

CT non-contrast-enhanced
- Well-defined osteolytic, expansile lesion with thin sclerotic margin

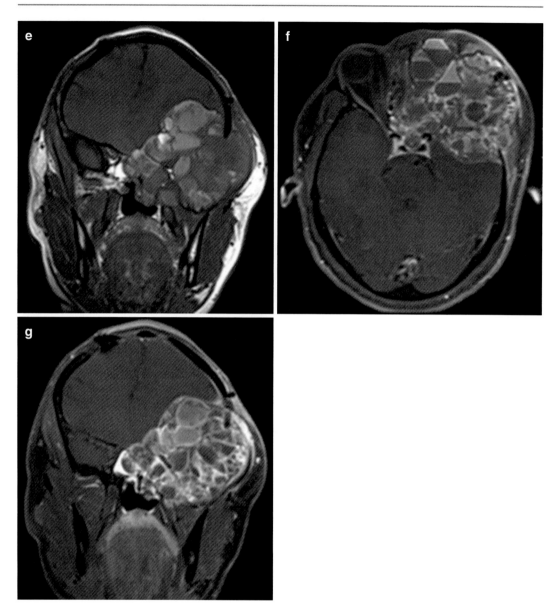

Fig. 80.20 (continued)

- Typical fluid–fluid levels better seen on MRI

MRI-T1/T2 (Fig. 80.20a, b, d, e)
- Cysts with characteristic fluid–fluid levels
- Surrounding hypointense rim

MRI-T1 contrast-enhanced (Fig. 80.20f, g)
- Enhancing septations

80.11.3 Pathology Findings

Macroscopic Features
- well-defined
- blood-filled, cystic spaces
- tan-white, gritty septae

Microscopic Features (Fig. 80.21)
- blood-filled, cystic spaces separated by fibrous septae

80.11 Aneurysmal Bone Cyst

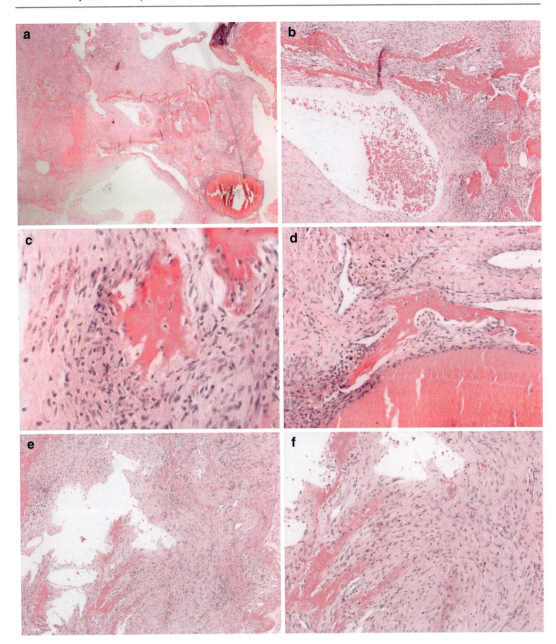

Fig. 80.21 Aneurysmal bone cyst is made up of blood-filled, cystic spaces separated by fibrous septae. The fibrous septae composed of moderately dense, cellular proliferation of bland fibroblasts multinucleated, osteoclast-like giant cells, reactive woven bone rimmed by osteoblasts (**a–h**)

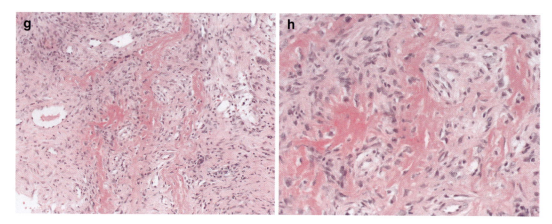

Fig. 80.21 (continued)

- fibrous septae composed of:
  - moderately dense, cellular proliferation of bland fibroblasts
  - multinucleated, osteoclast-like giant cells
  - reactive woven bone rimmed by osteoblasts

Differential diagnosis
- Giant cell reparative granuloma
- Telangiectatic osteosarcoma
- Secondary aneurysmal bone cyst

Selected References

Abarrategi A, Tornin J, Martinez-Cruzado L, Hamilton A, Martinez-Campos E, Rodrigo JP, Gonzalez MV, Baldini N, Garcia-Castro J, Rodriguez R (2016) Osteosarcoma: cells-of-origin, cancer stem cells, and targeted therapies. Stem Cells Int 2016:3631764. https://doi.org/10.1155/2016/3631764

Allen SD, Saifuddin A (2003) Imaging of intra-articular osteoid osteoma. Clin Radiol 58(11):845–852

Amanatullah DF, Clark TR, Lopez MJ, Borys D, Tamurian RM (2014) Giant cell tumor of bone. Orthopedics 37(2):112–120. https://doi.org/10.3928/01477447-20140124-08

Amaral L, Chiurciu M, Almeida JR, Ferreira NF, Mendonca R, Lima SS (2003) MR imaging for evaluation of lesions of the cranial vault: a pictorial essay. Arq Neuropsiquiatr 61(3a):521–532

Anitha N, Sankari SL, Malathi L, Karthick R (2015) Fibrous dysplasia-recent concepts. J Pharm Bioallied Sci 7(Suppl 1):S171–S172. https://doi.org/10.4103/0975-7406.155892

Atesok KI, Alman BA, Schemitsch EH, Peyser A, Mankin H (2011) Osteoid osteoma and osteoblastoma. J Am Acad Orthop Surg 19(11):678–689

Athanasou NA, Bansal M, Forsyth R, Reid RP, Sapi Z (2013) Giant cell tumour of bone. In: Fletcher CDM, Bridge JA, Hogendorn PCW, Mertens F (eds) WHO classification of tumours of soft tissue and bone. IARC, Lyon, pp 321–324

Athwal P, Stock H (2014) Osteoid osteoma: a pictorial review. Conn Med 78(4):233–235

Awad M, Gogos AJ, Kaye AH (2016) Skull base chondrosarcoma. J Clin Neurosci 24:1–5. https://doi.org/10.1016/j.jocn.2015.10.029

Baumhoer D, Bras J (2013) Osteoma. In: Fletcher CDM, Bridge JA, Hogendorn PCW, Mertens F (eds) WHO classification of tumours of soft tissue and bone. IARC, Lyon, p 276

Bielack SS, Hecker-Nolting S, Blattmann C, Kager L (2016) Advances in the management of osteosarcoma. F1000Res 5:2767. https://doi.org/10.12688/f1000research.9465.1

Bloch OG, Jian BJ, Yang I, Han SJ, Aranda D, Ahn BJ, Parsa AT (2009) A systematic review of intracranial chondrosarcoma and survival. J Clin Neurosci 16(12):1547–1551. https://doi.org/10.1016/j.jocn.2009.05.003

Bloch O, Sughrue ME, Mills SA, Parsa AT (2011) Signaling pathways in cranial chondrosarcoma: potential molecular targets for directed chemotherapy. J Clin Neurosci 18(7):881–885. https://doi.org/10.1016/j.jocn.2010.09.025

Boscainos PJ, Cousins GR, Kulshreshtha R, Oliver TB, Papagelopoulos PJ (2013) Osteoid osteoma. Orthopedics 36(10):792–800. https://doi.org/10.3928/01477447-20130920-10

Botter SM, Neri D, Fuchs B (2014) Recent advances in osteosarcoma. Curr Opin Pharmacol 16:15–23. https://doi.org/10.1016/j.coph.2014.02.002

Selected References

Boyce AM, Bhattacharyya N, Collins MT (2013) Fibrous dysplasia and fibroblast growth factor-23 regulation. Curr Osteoporos Rep 11(2):65–71. https://doi.org/10.1007/s11914-013-0144-5

Chakarun CJ, Forrester DM, Gottsegen CJ, Patel DB, White EA, Matcuk GR Jr (2013) Giant cell tumor of bone: review, mimics, and new developments in treatment. Radiographics 33(1):197–211. https://doi.org/10.1148/rg.331125089

Chang L, Shrestha S, LaChaud G, Scott MA, James AW (2015) Review of microRNA in osteosarcoma and chondrosarcoma. Med Oncol 32(6):613. https://doi.org/10.1007/s12032-015-0613-z

Chong VF, Khoo JB, Fan YF (2002) Fibrous dysplasia involving the base of the skull. Am J Roentgenol 178(3):717–720. https://doi.org/10.2214/ajr.178.3.1780717

Collins MT (2006) Spectrum and natural history of fibrous dysplasia of bone. J Bone Miner Res 21(Suppl 2):P99–p104. https://doi.org/10.1359/jbmr.06s219

Cortini M, Avnet S, Baldini N (2017) Mesenchymal stroma: role in osteosarcoma progression. Cancer Lett 405:90–99. https://doi.org/10.1016/j.canlet.2017.07.024

Cottalorda J, Bourelle S (2007) Modern concepts of primary aneurysmal bone cyst. Arch Orthop Trauma Surg 127(2):105–114. https://doi.org/10.1007/s00402-006-0223-5

Cowan RW, Singh G (2013) Giant cell tumor of bone: a basic science perspective. Bone 52(1):238–246. https://doi.org/10.1016/j.bone.2012.10.002

de Andrea CE, Bridge JA, Schiller A (2013) Osteoblastoma. In: Fletcher CDM, Bridge JA, Hogendorn PCW, Mertens F (eds) WHO classification of tumours of soft tissue and bone. IARC, Lyon, pp 279–280

Diaz RJ, Cusimano MD (2011) The biological basis for modern treatment of chordoma. J Neurooncol 104(2):411–422. https://doi.org/10.1007/s11060-011-0559-8

DiCaprio MR, Enneking WF (2005) Fibrous dysplasia. Pathophysiology, evaluation, and treatment. J Bone Joint Surg Am 87(8):1848–1864. https://doi.org/10.2106/jbjs.d.02942

Douis H, Saifuddin A (2013) The imaging of cartilaginous bone tumours. II. Chondrosarcoma. Skeletal Radiol 42(5):611–626. https://doi.org/10.1007/s00256-012-1521-3

Durfee RA, Mohammed M, Luu HH (2016) Review of osteosarcoma and current management. Rheumatol Ther 3(2):221–243. https://doi.org/10.1007/s40744-016-0046-y

Erdem E, Angtuaco EC, Van Hemert R, Park JS, Al-Mefty O (2003) Comprehensive review of intracranial chordoma. Radiographics 23(4):995–1009. https://doi.org/10.1148/rg.234025176

Evola FR, Costarella L, Pavone V, Caff G, Cannavo L, Sessa A, Avondo S, Sessa G (2017) Biomarkers of osteosarcoma, chondrosarcoma, and ewing sarcoma. Front Pharmacol 8:150. https://doi.org/10.3389/fphar.2017.00150

Feller L, Wood NH, Khammissa RA, Lemmer J, Raubenheimer EJ (2009) The nature of fibrous dysplasia. Head Face Med 5:22. https://doi.org/10.1186/1746-160x-5-22

Fernandes GL, Natal MRC, da Cruz CLP, Nascif RL, Tsuno NSG, Tsuno MY (2017) Primary osteosarcoma of the cranial vault. Radiol Bras 50(4):263–265. https://doi.org/10.1590/0100-3984.1914-2014

Fitzpatrick KA, Taljanovic MS, Speer DP, Graham AR, Jacobson JA, Barnes GR, Hunter TB (2004) Imaging findings of fibrous dysplasia with histopathologic and intraoperative correlation. Am J Roentgenol 182(6):1389–1398. https://doi.org/10.2214/ajr.182.6.1821389

Flanagan AM, Yamaguchi T (2013) Chordoma. In: Fletcher CDM, Bridge JA, Hogendorn PCW, Mertens F (eds) WHO classification of tumours of soft tissue and bone. IARC, Lyon, pp 328–329

Fletcher CDM, Bridge JA, Hogendorn PCW, Mertens F (2013) WHO classification of tumours of soft tissue and bone, 4th edn. IARC, Lyon

Florez H, Peris P, Guanabens N (2016) Fibrous dysplasia. Clinical review and therapeutic management. Med Clin 147(12):547–553. https://doi.org/10.1016/j.medcli.2016.07.030

Fountas KN, Stamatiou S, Barbanis S, Kourtopoulos H (2008) Intracranial falx chondroma: literature review and a case report. Clin Neurol Neurosurg 110(1):8–13. https://doi.org/10.1016/j.clineuro.2007.08.020

Georgalas C, Goudakos J, Fokkens WJ (2011) Osteoma of the skull base and sinuses. Otolaryngol Clin North Am 44(4):875–890, vii. https://doi.org/10.1016/j.otc.2011.06.008

Gulluoglu S, Turksoy O, Kuskucu A, Ture U, Bayrak OF (2016) The molecular aspects of chordoma. Neurosurg Rev 39(2):185–196.; discussion 196. https://doi.org/10.1007/s10143-015-0663-x

He JP, Hao Y, Wang XL, Yang XJ, Shao JF, Guo FJ, Feng JX (2014) Review of the molecular pathogenesis of osteosarcoma. Asian Pac J Cancer Prev 15(15):5967–5976

Hogendoorn PCW, Bovée JVMG, Nielsen GP (2013) Chondrosarcoma (grades I-III), including primary and secondary variants and periosteal chondrosarcoma. In: Fletcher CDM, Bridge JA, Hogendorn PCW, Mertens F (eds) WHO classification of tumours of soft tissue and bone. IARC, Lyon, pp 264–268

Hondar Wu HT, Chen W, Lee O, Chang CY (2006) Imaging and pathological correlation of soft-tissue chondroma: a serial five-case study and literature review. Clin Imaging 30(1):32–36. https://doi.org/10.1016/j.clinimag.2005.01.027

Horvai A, Klein M (2013) Osteoid osteoma. In: Fletcher CDM, Bridge JA, Hogendorn PCW, Mertens F (eds) WHO classification of tumours of soft tissue and bone. IARC, Lyon, pp 277–278

Iyer RS, Chapman T, Chew FS (2012) Pediatric bone imaging: diagnostic imaging of osteoid osteoma. Am J Roentgenol 198(5):1039–1052. https://doi.org/10.2214/ajr.10.7313

Jamil N, Howie S, Salter DM (2010) Therapeutic molecular targets in human chondrosarcoma. Int J Exp Pathol 91(5):387–393. https://doi.org/10.1111/j.1365-2613.2010.00749.x

Kan P, Schmidt MH (2008) Osteoid osteoma and osteoblastoma of the spine. Neurosurg Clin N Am 19(1):65–70. https://doi.org/10.1016/j.nec.2007.09.003

Kim Y, Nizami S, Goto H, Lee FY (2012) Modern interpretation of giant cell tumor of bone: predominantly osteoclastogenic stromal tumor. Clin Orthop Surg 4(2):107–116. https://doi.org/10.4055/cios.2012.4.2.107

Kitamura Y, Sasaki H, Yoshida K (2017) Genetic aberrations and molecular biology of skull base chordoma and chondrosarcoma. Brain Tumor Pathol 34(2):78–90. https://doi.org/10.1007/s10014-017-0283-y

Kunimatsu A, Kunimatsu N (2017) Skull base tumors and tumor-like lesions: a pictorial review. Pol J Radiol 82:398–409. https://doi.org/10.12659/pjr.901937

Kushlinskii NE, Fridman MV, Braga EA (2016) Molecular mechanisms and microRNAs in osteosarcoma pathogenesis. Biochem Biokhim 81(4):315–328. https://doi.org/10.1134/s0006297916040027

Leddy LR, Holmes RE (2014) Chondrosarcoma of bone. Cancer Treat Res 162:117–130. https://doi.org/10.1007/978-3-319-07323-1_6

Lee EH, Shafi M, Hui JH (2006) Osteoid osteoma: a current review. J Pediatr Orthop 26(5):695–700. https://doi.org/10.1097/01.bpo.0000233807.80046.7c

Lietman SA, Levine MA (2013) Fibrous dysplasia. Pediatr Endocrinol Rev 10(Suppl 2):389–396

Lin SP, Fang YC, Chu DC, Chang YC, Hsu CI (2007) Characteristics of cranial aneurysmal bone cyst on computed tomography and magnetic resonance imaging. J Formos Med Assoc 106(3):255–259. https://doi.org/10.1016/s0929-6646(09)60249-7

Lin YH, Jewell BE, Gingold J, Lu L, Zhao R, Wang LL, Lee DF (2017) Osteosarcoma: molecular pathogenesis and iPSC modeling. Trends Mol Med 23(8):737–755. https://doi.org/10.1016/j.molmed.2017.06.004

Lindsey BA, Markel JE, Kleinerman ES (2017) Osteosarcoma overview. Rheumatol Ther 4(1):25–43. https://doi.org/10.1007/s40744-016-0050-2

Lisle DA, Monsour PA, Maskiell CD (2008) Imaging of craniofacial fibrous dysplasia. J Med Imaging Radiat Oncol 52(4):325–332. https://doi.org/10.1111/j.1440-1673.2008.01963.x

Liu P, Shen JK, Xu J, Trahan CA, Hornicek FJ, Duan Z (2016) Aberrant DNA methylations in chondrosarcoma. Epigenomics 8(11):1519–1525. https://doi.org/10.2217/epi-2016-0071

Liu X, Zhang Z, Deng C, Tian Y, Ma X (2017) Meta-analysis showing that ERCC1 polymorphism is predictive of osteosarcoma prognosis. Oncotarget 8(37):62769–62779. https://doi.org/10.18632/oncotarget.19370

Logie CI, Walker EA, Forsberg JA, Potter BK, Murphey MD (2013) Chondrosarcoma: a diagnostic imager's guide to decision making and patient management. Semin Musculoskelet Radiol 17(2):101–115. https://doi.org/10.1055/s-0033-1342967

Lu ZH, Cao WH, Qian WX (2013) Aggressive osteoblastoma of the temporal bone: a case report and review of the literature. Clin Imaging 37(2):386–389. https://doi.org/10.1016/j.clinimag.2012.05.017

Lucas DR, Bridge JA (2013) Chondromas: enchondroma, periosteal chondroma. In: Fletcher CDM, Bridge JA, Hogendorn PCW, Mertens F (eds) WHO classification of tumours of soft tissue and bone. IARC, Lyon, pp 252–254

Ma Y, Xu W, Yin H, Huang Q, Liu T, Yang X, Wei H, Xiao J (2015) Therapeutic radiotherapy for giant cell tumor of the spine: a systemic review. Eur Spine J 24(8):1754–1760. https://doi.org/10.1007/s00586-015-3834-0

MacDonald-Jankowski D (2009) Fibrous dysplasia: a systematic review. Dentomaxillofac Radiol 38(4):196–215. https://doi.org/10.1259/dmfr/16645318

Maclean FM, Soo MY, Ng T (2005) Chordoma: radiological-pathological correlation. Australas Radiol 49(4):261–268. https://doi.org/10.1111/j.1440-1673.2005.01433.x

Marie PJ (2001) Cellular and molecular basis of fibrous dysplasia. Histol Histopathol 16(3):981–988

Mascard E, Gomez-Brouchet A, Lambot K (2015) Bone cysts: unicameral and aneurysmal bone cyst. Orthopaed Traumatol Surg Res 101(1 Suppl):S119–S127. https://doi.org/10.1016/j.otsr.2014.06.031

Mavrogenis AF, Igoumenou VG, Megaloikonomos PD, Panagopoulos GN, Papagelopoulos PJ, Soucacos PN (2017) Giant cell tumor of bone revisited. SICOT-J 3:54. https://doi.org/10.1051/sicotj/2017041

McLoughlin GS, Sciubba DM, Wolinsky JP (2008) Chondroma/chondrosarcoma of the spine. Neurosurg Clin N Am 19(1):57–63. https://doi.org/10.1016/j.nec.2007.09.007

Mendenhall WM, Zlotecki RA, Gibbs CP, Reith JD, Scarborough MT, Mendenhall NP (2006a) Aneurysmal bone cyst. Am J Clin Oncol 29(3):311–315. https://doi.org/10.1097/01.coc.0000204403.13451.52

Mendenhall WM, Zlotecki RA, Scarborough MT, Gibbs CP, Mendenhall NP (2006b) Giant cell tumor of bone. Am J Clin Oncol 29(1):96–99. https://doi.org/10.1097/01.coc.0000195089.11620.b7

Morrow JJ, Khanna C (2015) Osteosarcoma genetics and epigenetics: emerging biology and candidate therapies. Crit Rev Oncog 20(3-4):173–197

Murphey MD, Walker EA, Wilson AJ, Kransdorf MJ, Temple HT, Gannon FH (2003) From the archives of the AFIP: imaging of primary chondrosarcoma: radiologic-pathologic correlation. Radiographics 23(5):1245–1278. https://doi.org/10.1148/rg.235035134

Nielsen GP, Fletcher JA, Oliveira AM (2013) Aneurysmal bone cyst. In: Fletcher CDM, Bridge JA, Hogendorn PCW, Mertens F (eds) WHO classification of tumours of soft tissue and bone. IARC, Lyon, pp 348–349

Nielsen GP, Rosenberg AE, Deshpande V, Hornicek FJ, Kattapuram SV, Rosenthal DI (2017) Diagnostic pathology: bone, 2nd edn. Elsevier, Amsterdam

Ozkal E, Erongun U, Cakir B, Acar O, Uygun A, Bitik M (1996) CT and MR imaging of vertebral osteoblastoma. A report of two cases. Clin Imaging 20(1):37–41

Pelargos PE, Nagasawa DT, Ung N, Chung LK, Thill K, Tenn S, Gopen Q, Yang I (2015) Clinical characteristics and diagnostic imaging of cranial osteoblastoma. J Clin Neurosci 22(3):445–449. https://doi.org/10.1016/j.jocn.2014.10.002

Pereira HM, Marchiori E, Severo A (2014) Magnetic resonance imaging aspects of giant-cell tumours of bone. J Med Imaging Radiat Oncol 58(6):674–678. https://doi.org/10.1111/1754-9485.12249

Polychronidou G, Karavasilis V, Pollack SM, Huang PH, Lee A, Jones RL (2017) Novel therapeutic approaches in chondrosarcoma. Future Oncol 13(7):637–648. https://doi.org/10.2217/fon-2016-0226

Pridgeon MG, Grohar PJ, Steensma MR, Williams BO (2017) Wnt signaling in ewing sarcoma, osteosarcoma, and malignant peripheral nerve sheath tumors. Curr Osteoporos Rep 15(4):239–246. https://doi.org/10.1007/s11914-017-0377-9

Pu F, Chen F, Shao Z (2016) MicroRNAs as biomarkers in the diagnosis and treatment of chondrosarcoma. Tumour Biol. https://doi.org/10.1007/s13277-016-5468-1

Rapp TB, Ward JP, Alaia MJ (2012) Aneurysmal bone cyst. J Am Acad Orthop Surg 20(4):233–241. https://doi.org/10.5435/jaaos-20-04-233

Riminucci M, Robey PG, Bianco P (2007) The pathology of fibrous dysplasia and the McCune-Albright syndrome. Pediatr Endocrinol Rev 4(Suppl 4):401–411

Rosenberg AE, Cleton-Jansen A-M, de Pinieux G, Deyrup AT, Hauben E, Squire J (2013) Conventional osteosarcoma. In: Fletcher CDM, Bridge JA, Hogendorn PCW, Mertens F (eds) WHO classification of tumours of soft tissue and bone. IARC, Lyon, pp 282–288

Ruggieri P, McLeod RA, Unni KK, Sim FH (1996) Osteoblastoma. Orthopedics 19(7):621–624

Saccomanni B (2008) Aneurysmal bone cyst of spine: a review of literature. Arch Orthop Trauma Surg 128(10):1145–1147. https://doi.org/10.1007/s00402-007-0477-6

Scotter A (2004) Giant cell tumor. Radiol Technol 75(5):394–396

Serra M, Hattinger CM (2017) The pharmacogenomics of osteosarcoma. Pharmacogenomics J 17(1):11–20. https://doi.org/10.1038/tpj.2016.45

Shah ZK, Peh WC, Koh WL, Shek TW (2005) Magnetic resonance imaging appearances of fibrous dysplasia. Br J Radiol 78(936):1104–1115. https://doi.org/10.1259/bjr/73852511

Siegal GP, Bianco P, Dal Cin P (2013) Fibrous dysplasia. In: Fletcher CDM, Bridge JA, Hogendorn PCW, Mertens F (eds) WHO classification of tumours of soft tissue and bone. IARC, Lyon, pp 352–353

Sobti A, Agrawal P, Agarwala S, Agarwal M (2016) Giant cell tumor of bone—an overview. Arch Bone Joint Surg 4(1):2–9

Soldatos T, McCarthy EF, Attar S, Carrino JA, Fayad LM (2011) Imaging features of chondrosarcoma. J Comput Assist Tomogr 35(4):504–511. https://doi.org/10.1097/RCT.0b013e31822048ff

Speetjens FM, de Jong Y, Gelderblom H, Bovee JV (2016) Molecular oncogenesis of chondrosarcoma: impact for targeted treatment. Curr Opin Oncol 28(4):314–322. https://doi.org/10.1097/cco.0000000000000300

Sprengel SD, Weber MA, Lehner B, Rehnitz C (2015) Osteoidosteoma. From diagnosis to treatment. Radiologe 55(6):479–486. https://doi.org/10.1007/s00117-014-2805-5

Stacy GS, Peabody TD, Dixon LB (2003) Mimics on radiography of giant cell tumor of bone. Am J Roentgenol 181(6):1583–1589. https://doi.org/10.2214/ajr.181.6.1811583

Tamura R, Miwa T, Shimizu K, Mizutani K, Tomita H, Yamane N, Tominaga T, Sasaki S (2016) Giant cell tumor of the skull: review of the literature. J Neurol Surg A Cent Eur Neurosurg 77(3):239–246. https://doi.org/10.1055/s-0035-1554808

Terek RM (2006) Recent advances in the basic science of chondrosarcoma. Orthop Clin North Am 37(1):9–14. https://doi.org/10.1016/j.ocl.2005.09.001

Turcotte RE (2006) Giant cell tumor of bone. Orthop Clin North Am 37(1):35–51. https://doi.org/10.1016/j.ocl.2005.08.005

Van Gompel JJ, Janus JR (2015) Chordoma and chondrosarcoma. Otolaryngol Clin North Am 48(3):501–514. https://doi.org/10.1016/j.otc.2015.02.009

Vigorita VJ (2016) Orthopaedic pathology, 3rd edn. Lippincott Williams & Wilkins, Philadelphia

Walcott BP, Nahed BV, Mohyeldin A, Coumans JV, Kahle KT, Ferreira MJ (2012) Chordoma: current concepts, management, and future directions. Lancet Oncol 13(2):e69–e76. https://doi.org/10.1016/s1470-2045(11)70337-0

Wu PF, Tang JY, Li KH (2015) RANK pathway in giant cell tumor of bone: pathogenesis and therapeutic aspects. Tumour Biol 36(2):495–501. https://doi.org/10.1007/s13277-015-3094-y

Yakkioui Y, van Overbeeke JJ, Santegoeds R, van Engeland M, Temel Y (2014) Chordoma: the entity. Biochim Biophys Acta 1846(2):655–669. https://doi.org/10.1016/j.bbcan.2014.07.012

Yarmish G, Klein MJ, Landa J, Lefkowitz RA, Hwang S (2010) Imaging characteristics of primary osteosarcoma: nonconventional subtypes. Radiographics 30(6):1653–1672. https://doi.org/10.1148/rg.306105524

Yu X, Li Z (2015) Epigenetic deregulations in chordoma. Cell Prolif 48(5):497–502. https://doi.org/10.1111/cpr.12204

Zhang W, Duan N, Song T, Li Z, Zhang C, Chen X (2017) The emerging roles of forkhead box (FOX) proteins in osteosarcoma. J Cancer 8(9):1619–1628. https://doi.org/10.7150/jca.18778

Zou MX, Huang W, Wang XB, Li J, Lv GH, Deng YW (2015) Prognostic factors in spinal chordoma: a systematic review. Clin Neurol Neurosurg 139:110–118. https://doi.org/10.1016/j.clineuro.2015.09.012

Zou MX, Lv GH, Zhang QS, Wang SF, Li J, Wang XB (2018) Prognostic factors in skull base chordoma: a systematic literature review and meta-analysis. World Neurosurg 109:307–327. https://doi.org/10.1016/j.wneu.2017.10.010

Metastatic Tumors

81.1 General Aspects

WHO Definition
2016—Tumors that originate outside the CNS and spread via the hematogenous route to the CNS or (less frequently) directly invade the CNS from adjacent anatomical structures (Wesseling et al. 2016).

2007—Tumors that originate outside the CNS and spread secondarily to the CNS via the hematogenous route (metastasis) or by direct invasion from adjacent tissues (Wesseling et al. 2007).

2000—Tumors involving the CNS that originate from, but are discontinuous with, primary systemic neoplasms (Nelson et al. 2000).

1993—No definition is provided (Kleihues et al. 1993).

81.1.1 Epidemiology

Incidence
- Most common CNS neoplasms
- 11 per 100,000 population per year

Age Incidence
- Adults (30 per 100,000 at age 60 years)
- Children rare (1 per 100,000 at age below 25 years)

Sex Incidence
- In general no sex difference
- Sex-related primary tumors, i.e., breast, prostate

Frequencies by primary site (Table 81.1)
- Respiratory tract
- Breast
- Skin (Melanoma)
- Gastrointestinal tract
- Prostate
- Kidney

Localization (Table 81.2)
- Cerebral hemispheres (80%)
  - in arterial border zones
  - at the junction of cerebral cortex and white matter
- Cerebellum (15%)
- Leptomeninges (4–15%)
- Dura (8–9%)
- Spinal epidural space (5–10%)
- Seeding along the ventricular walls
- Solitary metastasis (i.e., the only metastasis detected in the body)
- Single metastasis (i.e., the only metastasis in the brain)

81.1.2 Neuroimaging Findings

General imaging findings
- Usually round, well-defined enhancing masses with variable edema, 50% multiple

Table 81.1 Approximate frequencies of metastases affecting the brain by primary site

Primary site	Frequency (%)	Range
Skin	48	46–64
Lung	32	23–50
Breast	21	18–22
Thyroid	17	
Soft tissue	15	
Kidney	11	10–17
Leukemia	8	
Prostate	6	
Colon	6	
Liver and pancreas	5	
Lymph nodes	5	
Female genital	2	
Others	19	

Table 81.2 Localization of brain metastasis based on the type of primary tumor

Localization of metastasis	Metastasis from primary tumor
Posterior fossa	• Colorectal • Kidney • Pelvic organs
Dura	• Prostate • Breast • Lung • Hematologic malignancies
Leptomeninges	• Lung • Breast • Melanoma • Hematologic malignancies
Spinal epidural space	• Prostate • Breast • Lung • Kidney • Non-Hodgkin lymphoma • Multiple myeloma
Spine—intramedullary	• Lung (Small cell lung cancer)

CT non-contrast-enhanced (Figs. 81.1a and 81.2a)
- Iso- to hypodense mass
- Variable surrounding edema
- Hemorrhages

CT contrast-enhanced
- Strong, variable enhancement

MRI-T2 (Figs. 81.1b and 81.2b)
- Usually hyperintense
- Variable hyperintense peritumoral edema

MRI-Flair (Figs. 81.1c and 81.2c)
- Usually hyperintense
- Variable hyperintense peritumoral edema

MRI-T1 (Figs. 81.1d and 81.2d)
- Iso- to hypointense mass
- Hemorrhages hyperintense
- Melanomas hyperintense

MRI-T2∗
- Hypointense in case of hemorrhage

MRI-T1 contrast-enhanced (Figs. 81.1e and 81.2e)
- Strong variable enhancement

MR-Diffusion Imaging (Fig. 81.1f)
- No restricted diffusion
- ADC elevation common

MRI-Perfusion (Fig. 81.1h)
- rBCV elevated

MR-Diffusion Tensor Imaging
- Fractional anisotropy values lower than those of glioblastomas were significantly higher than those of brain metastases.

MR-Spectroscopy
- Elevated Cho peak
- Cr peak in 80% of cases missing
- If necrotic: lipid/lactate peaks

Nuclear Medicine Imaging Findings (Fig. 81.3)
- Metastases are normally FDG-avid, often with a hypometabolism surrounding them.
- Radiotracers like FET (a marker of amino acid uptake (L-system)) or FLT (a marker of DNA biosynthesis) demonstrate the increased metabolism as well and have no background activity.

81.1 General Aspects

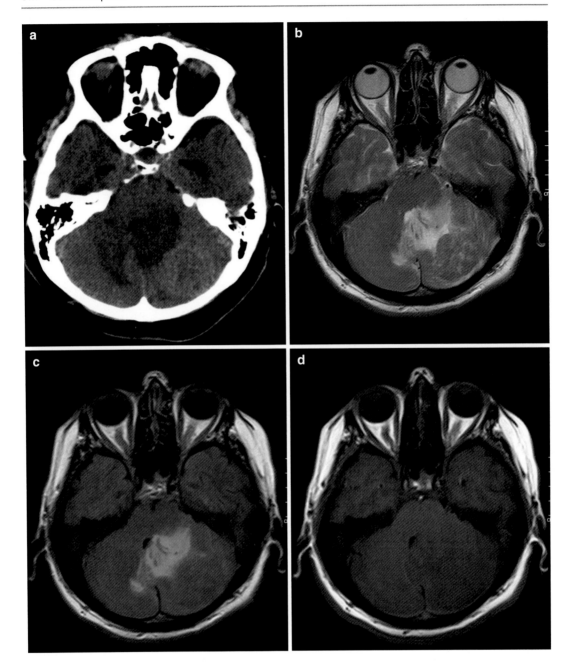

Fig. 81.1 Left cerebellar metastasis in a patient with breast cancer: CT (**a**), T2 (**b**), FLAIR (**c**), T1 (**d**), T1 contrast (**e**), Diffusion (**f**), ADC (**g**), rCBV (**h**)

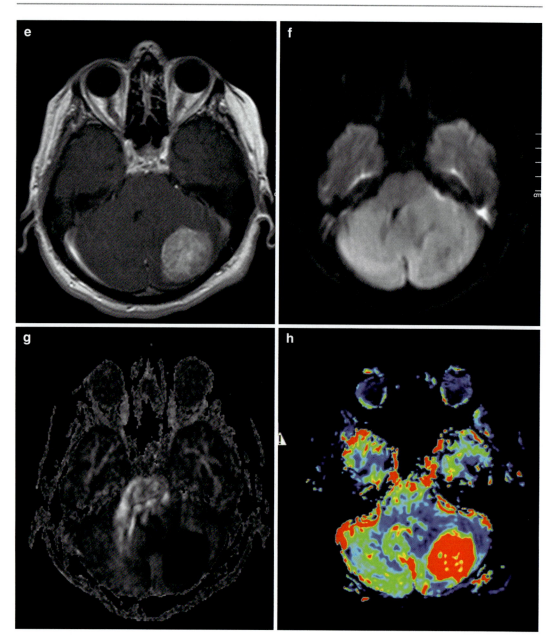

Fig. 81.1 (continued)

81.1 General Aspects

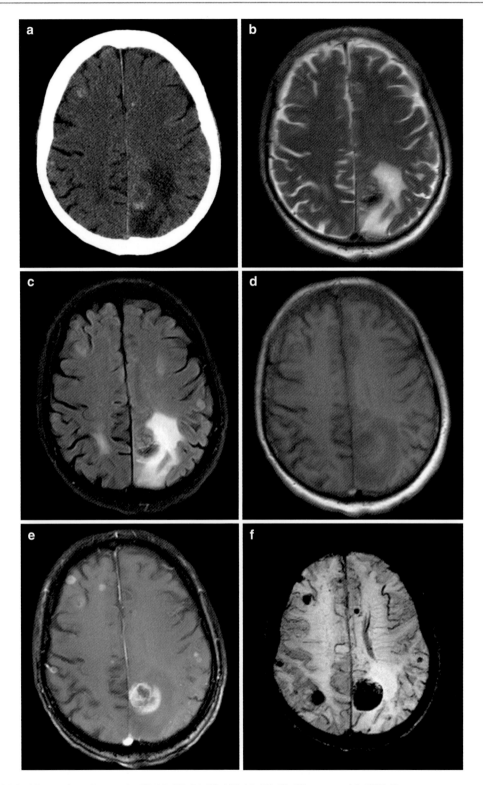

Fig. 81.2 Metastatic melanoma in CT (**a**), T2 (**b**), FLAIR (**c**), T1 (**d**), T1 contrast (**e**), SWI (**f**)

- Images can show homogeneous or heterogeneous uptake representing the tumor biology, often with a homogenous and intense uptake.
- SUV (calculated as ratio of the concentration of the radiotracer corrected by the body weight of the patient) can be used for the assessment of the biologic behavior during therapy.
- Results obtained for MET are similar to FET with the advantage of FET to be taken up in a lesser amount in inflammatory tissue and the longer half-life of 110 min compared to a relatively short half-life of 20 min of C-11 used in MET.

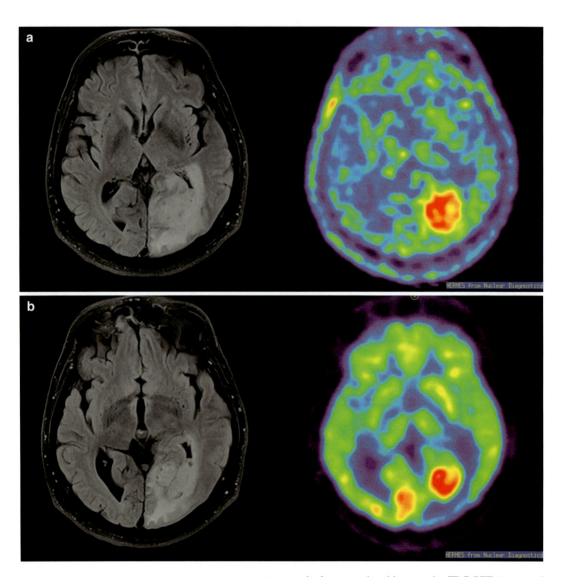

Fig. 81.3 FET-PET of a patient with metastasis left occipital 10 years after operation of a bronchial carcinoma (**a**), FDG-PET of the same metastasis (**b**) (**a, b** same patient); FDG-PET (torso) of a patient with solitary lymphogenic metastasis (**c**), solitary bone metastasis (**d**) and adrenal metastasis (**e**) (**c–e** same patient); FET-PET (brain) (**f**) and FDG-PET (torso) (**g**) of a patient with ovarian cancer with extended metastases including a right cerebral metastasis with necrosis; FDG-PET (torso and brain) (**h, i**) of a patient with cerebellar metastasis and esophageal cancer; bone scan of a patient with prostate cancer and widespread bone metastasis including the vertebral column (**j**); patient with widespread metastasis of a melanoma (bone, lung, lymph node, brain) FET (brain, cerebellum **k**, frontal **l**) (**k, l**) FDG (whole body)-PET (**m**)

81.1 General Aspects

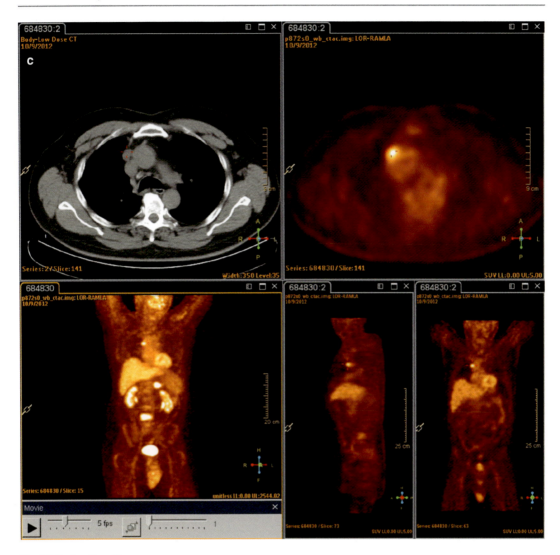

Fig. 81.3 (continued)

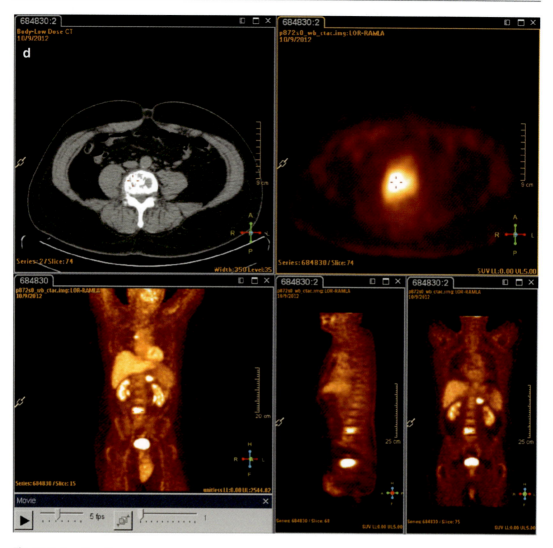

Fig. 81.3 (continued)

81.1 General Aspects

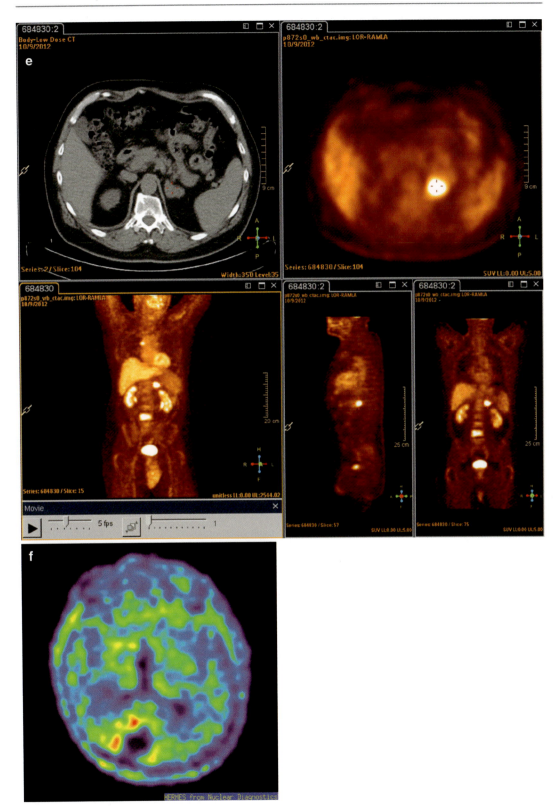

Fig. 81.3 (continued)

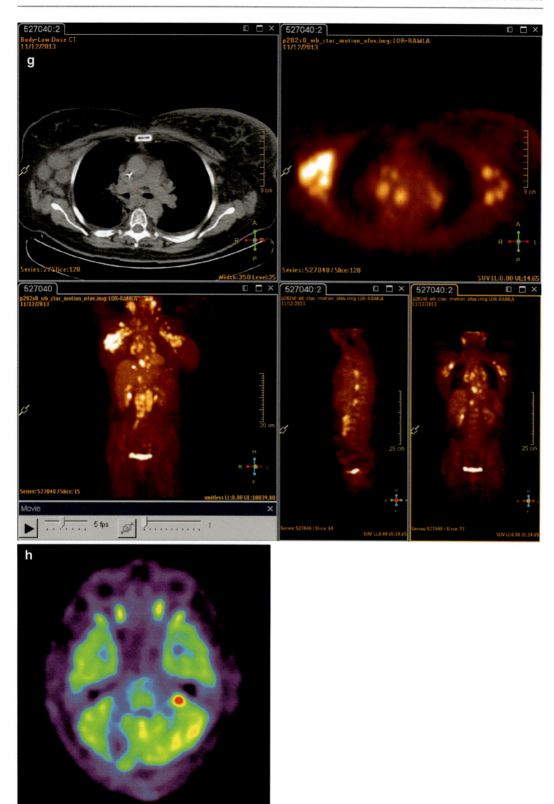

Fig. 81.3 (continued)

81.1 General Aspects

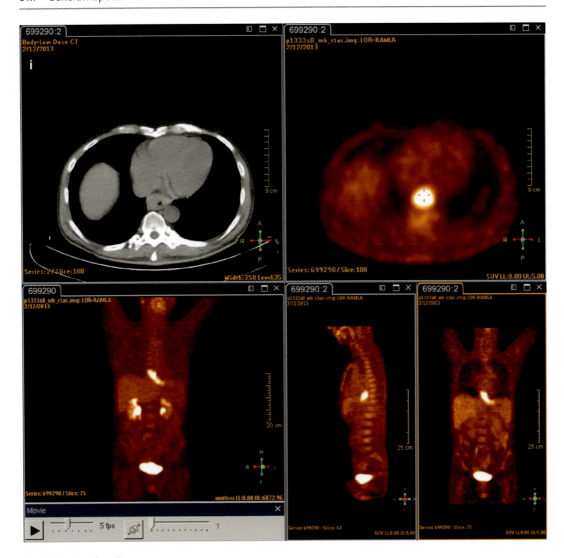

Fig. 81.3 (continued)

Fig. 81.3 (continued)

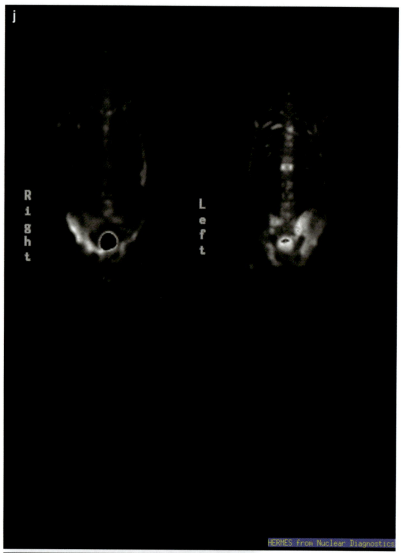

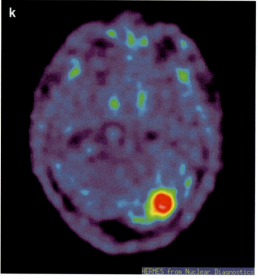

81.1 General Aspects

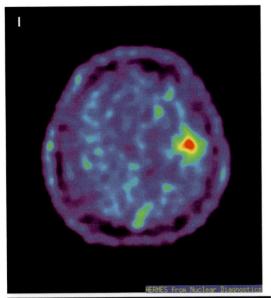

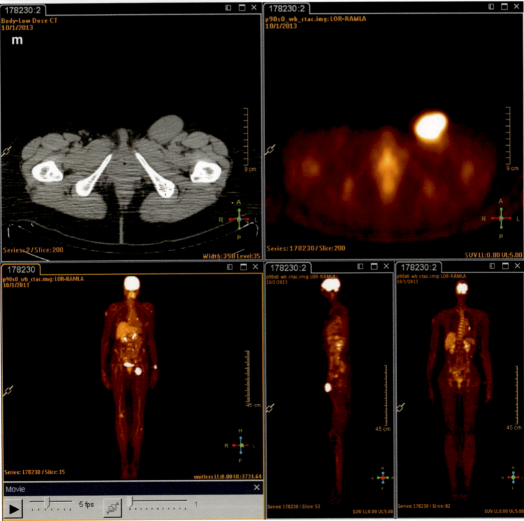

Fig. 81.3 (continued)

- PET (especially FDG) can be chosen for the screening for the primary tumor, if it is not known or the search for other metastasis in the body, thereby allowing the exact staging of the patient and influencing therapy decisions.
  - For renal tumors, it has to be taken into account that FDG is excreted by the kidneys, thereby reducing the sensitivity for the detection of the primary tumor.
  - In prostate cancer, FDG is normally negative (these tumors are investigated by Cholin PET).
  - For breast cancer, FDG is not the modality of choice for screening, but is often positive, especially in metastasis.
  - For the screening of osteoblastic bone metastases, bone scan is a valuable tool for demonstrating a higher uptake in metastases.

81.1.3 Neuropathology Findings

The gross-anatomical features of metastases include: (Figs. 81.4 and 81.5)
- Grossly circumscribed lesions
- Gray white or tan or reddish or brown to black color
- Soft to hard consistency
- Central necrosis
- Peritumoral edema
- Hemorrhages
- Mucoid material (adenocarcinomas)
- Opacification of the leptomeninges
- Plaque-like or nodular or diffuse lesions in the dura
- Bone destruction in case of invasion

81.1.4 Histologic Features

Microscopic Features
- Diverse cellular features
- Relatively well demarcated from surrounding brain tissue
- Invasion of brain tumors by groups of tumor cells (not by single cells) along the Virchow–Robin spaces
- Diffuse infiltration of soft tissues (spine)
- Gliosis
- Inflammation with perivascular lymphocytic cuffing
- Microvascular proliferation
- Necroses

Proliferation Markers
- Variable
- Usually high

Differential Diagnosis
- Glioblastoma
- Other malignant glioma
- Abscess
- Thromboembolic strokes
- Demyelinating diseases

81.1 General Aspects

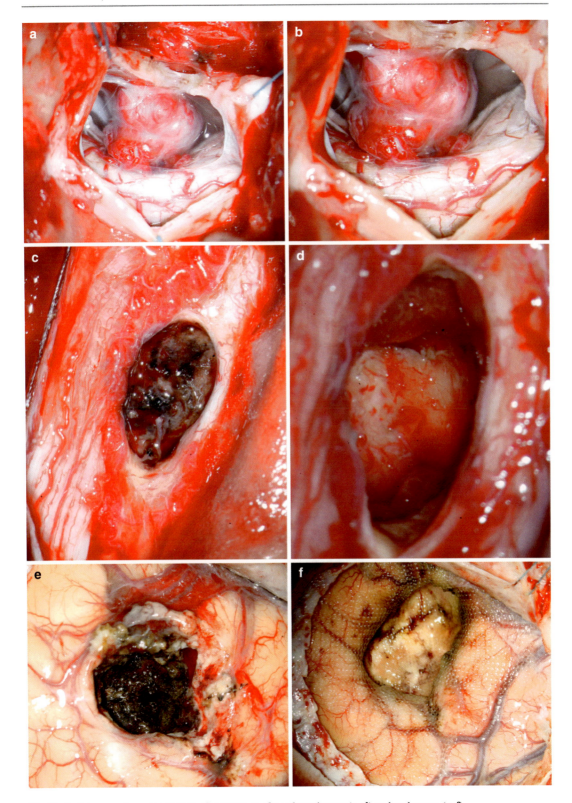

Fig. 81.4 Intraoperative appearances of metastases of renal carcinoma (**a**–**d**) and melanoma (**e**, **f**)

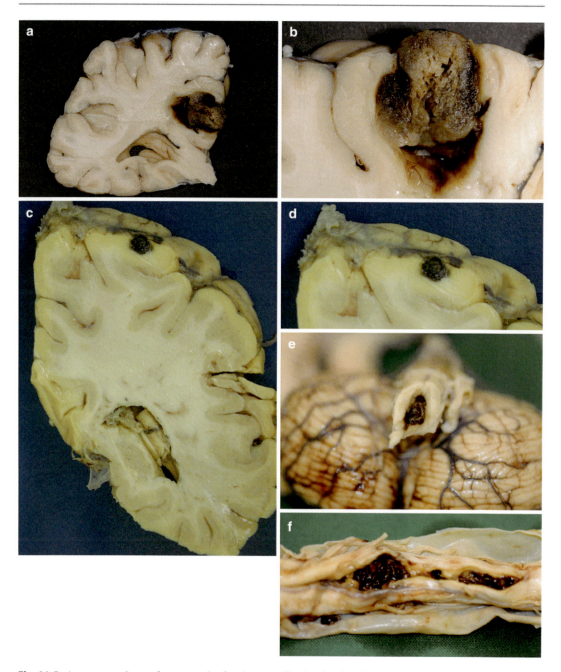

Fig. 81.5 Autopsy specimen of a metastasis of melanoma affecting the cingulate gyrus (**a**, **b**), parietal lobe (**c**, **d**), and spinal cord (**e–h**)

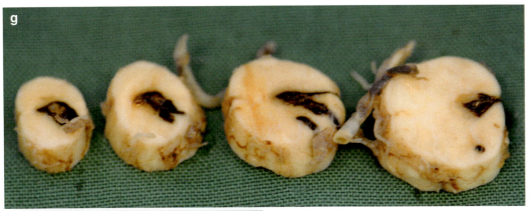
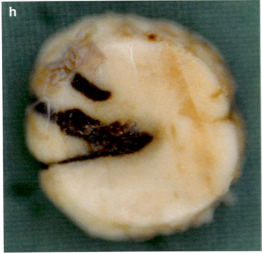

Fig. 81.5 (continued)

81.1.5 Molecular Neuropathology

The following scenario for hematogenous metastases is proposed:
- Seeding from the primary tumor
- Entry into the blood stream
- Survival in the blood stream
- Arrival at the point of destination
- Extravasation into the CNS
- Survival and growth in the CNS microenvironment
- Somatic mutations in various genes (Table 81.3).
- MicroRNAs might help determine the site of primary origin.

Molecular pathways involved in the process of metastasis are shown in Table 81.4.

81.1.6 Treatment and Prognosis

Treatment
- Surgical removal of a single metastasis
- Surgical removal of several metastasis
- Radiotherapy of the whole brain
- Chemotherapy
- Targeted therapy (Table 81.5)

Biologic Behavior–Prognosis–Prognostic Factors
- Karnofsky performance status (KPS)
- Age of patient
- Number of CNS metastases
- Number of sites (CNS and others) for metastases
- Responsiveness of primary tumor to therapy
- Three classes for outcome prediction (Table 81.6)

Table 81.3 Frequencies of the top nine somatic mutations (single nucleotides, or small insertions or deletions (indels)) in common cancers from the Catalogue of Somatic Mutations in Cancer (COSMIC) at the Welcome Trust Sanger Institute (Cambridge, UK), modified after (Schneider et al. 2017) reproduced with kind permission by Springer Nature

Tumor	Gene	Gene name	Frequencies (%)
Breast cancer	PIK3CA	encodes the PI3K catalytic subunit-α	27
	TP53	tumor protein p53	24
	GATA3	GATA-binding 3	11
	CDH1	cadherin 1 (also known as E-cadherin)	10
	KMT2C	lysine methyltransferase 2 family	9
	ESR1	estrogen receptor 1	7
	ARID1A	AT-rich interactive domain 1A	4
	NCOR1	nuclear receptor co-repressor 1	4
	PTEN	phosphatase and tensin homolog	4
Colorectal cancer	APC	adenomatous polyposis coli	48
	TP53	tumor protein p53	45
	KRAS	proto-oncogene, GTPase	34
	FAT4	atypical cadherin	20
	PIK3CA	encodes the PI3K catalytic subunit-a	13
	KMT2C	lysine methyltransferase 2 family	12
	ATM	ataxia telangiectasia mutated	11
	BRAF	B-Raf proto-oncogene, serine/threonine kinase	11
	SMAD4	SMAD family member 4	11
Gastric cancer	TP53	tumor protein p53	34
	FAT4	atypical cadherin	18
	ARID1A	AT-rich interactive domain 1A	14
	CDH1	cadherin 1 (also known as E-cadherin)	13
	KMT2C	lysine methyltransferase 2 family	11
	KMT2D	lysine methyltransferase 2 family	10
	PIK3CA	encodes the PI3K catalytic subunit-a	10
	RNF43	ring finger 43	9
	TRRAP	transformation or transcription domain-associated protein	9
Hepatocellular carcinoma	TP53	tumor protein p53	28
	TERT	telomerase reverse transcriptase	21
	CTNNB1	encoding β-catenin	19
	AXIN1	axin 1	8
	ARID1A	AT-rich interactive domain 1A	7
	CDKN2A	cyclin-dependent kinase inhibitor 2A	6
	KMT2C	lysine methyltransferase 2 family	4
	PIK3CA	encodes the PI3K catalytic subunit-a	3
	TSC2	tuberous sclerosis 2	3
Kidney cancer	VHL	von Hippel–Lindau tumor suppressor	43
	PBRM1	polybromo 1	30
	BAP1	BRCA1-associated protein 1	11
	SETD2	SET domain-containing 2	10
	KDM5C	lysine demethylase 5C	6
	MTOR	mechanistic target of rapamycin	6
	TP53	tumor protein p53	5
	PIK3CA	encodes the PI3K catalytic subunit-a	3
	PTEN	phosphatase and tensin homolog	3

Table 81.3 (continued)

Tumor	Gene	Gene name	Frequencies (%)
Melanoma	BRAF	B-Raf proto-oncogene, serine/threonine kinase	45
	FAT4	atypical cadherin	20
	GRIN2A	glutamate ionotropic receptor NMDA type subunit 2A	20
	CDKN2A	cyclin-dependent kinase inhibitor 2A	19
	TERT	telomerase reverse transcriptase	18
	NRAS	proto-oncogene, GTPase	17
	NF1	neurofibromin 1	16
	TP53	tumor protein p53	14
	ERBB4	erb-b2 receptor tyrosine kinase 4	13
NSCLC (non-small cell lung carcinoma)	EGFR	epidermal growth factor receptor	36
	TP53	tumor protein p53	36
	KRAS	proto-oncogene, GTPase	17
	FAT4	atypical cadherin	11
	KMT2C	lysine methyltransferase 2 family	10
	STK11	serine/threonine kinase 11; T-ALL, T cell acute lymphoblastic leukemia	10
	FAT1	atypical cadherin	9
	CDKN2A	cyclin-dependent kinase inhibitor 2A	8
	SMARCA4	SWI/SNF-related, matrix-associated, actin-dependent regulator of chromatin, subfamily A, member 4	8
Ovarian cancer	TP53	tumor protein p53	48
	KRAS	proto-oncogene, GTPase	11
	PIK3CA	encodes the PI3K catalytic subunit-a	11
	ARID1A	AT-rich interactive domain 1A	9
	CTNNB1	encoding β-catenin	7
	SMARCA4	SWI/SNF-related, matrix-associated, actin-dependent regulator of chromatin, subfamily A, member 4	6
	ATR	ataxia telangiectasia and Rad3-related	5
	BRCA1	DNA repair associated	5
	BRCA2	DNA repair associated	4
Pancreatic duct adenocarcinoma (PDAC)	KRAS	proto-oncogene, GTPase	69
	TP53	tumor protein p53	44
	SMAD4	SMAD family member 4	15
	CDKN2A	cyclin-dependent kinase inhibitor 2A	14
	ARID1A	AT-rich interactive domain 1A	4
	KMT2C	lysine methyltransferase 2 family	4
	ATM	ataxia telangiectasia mutated	3
	GNAS	adenylyl cyclase-stimulating G-protein, alpha subunit	3
	PIK3CA	encodes the PI3K catalytic subunit-a	2
Prostate cancer	TP53	tumor protein p53	11
	PTEN	phosphatase and tensin homolog	8
	SPOP	speckle-type BTB/POZ protein	7
	FOXA1	forkhead box A1	4
	KMT2C	lysine methyltransferase 2 family	4
	KRAS	proto-oncogene, GTPase	4
	CTNNB1	encoding β-catenin	3
	EGFR	epidermal growth factor receptor	3
	PIK3CA	encodes the PI3K catalytic subunit-a	2

Table 81.4 Examples of metastatic events, their molecular processes, and potential targeted chemotherapeutics. (Hardesty and Nakaji 2016) reproduced with kind permission by Frontiers Journals

Cellular event	Pathway(s) implicated	Potential personalized treatments
Migration across BBB	Cathepsin S	Inhibitors in development
	miR-181C	None to date
	miR-105	None to date
Survival in CNS microenvironment	mTOR	Everolimus, temsirolimus
	CDK	Palbociclib, others in development
	VEGF	Bevacizumab
	EGFR	Erlotinib
Establishment of radioresistance	Chk1	Inhibitors in development
	c-met	Cabozantinib

Table 81.5 Overview of actionable mutations in brain metastases of non-small cell lung cancer, breast cancer and melanoma, and potential targeted therapies (Han and Brastianos 2017) reproduced with kind permission by Frontiers Journals

Cancer type	Mutation	Targeted therapy	Objective response rate (%)	Progression-free survival (months)
Non-small cell lung cancer	Activating *EGFR* mutation	First-generation EGFR TKIs: gefitinib, erlotinib	58–83	7–15
		ErbB family inhibitor: afatinib	70–75	8
	EGFR T790M	T790M-specific EGFR TKI: osimertinib	NA	NA Superior blood–brain barrier penetration than gefitinib or afatinib demonstrated in preclinical study
	ALK rearrangement	First-generation ALK TKI: crizotinib	56–85	7–9
		Second-generation ALK TKI: alectinib	75	10–11
	(No specific mutation)	PD-1 inhibitor: pembrolizumab Early analysis showed 33% intracranial response rate	NA	NA
Breast cancer	*HER2* overexpression/*HER2* oncogene amplification	Dual anti-HER2 inhibition: pertuzumab plus trastuzumab	NA	NA
		HER2/EGFR TKI: lapatinib (in combination with capecitabine)	66	5.5
	Mutation in *PI3K/AKT/mTOR* pathway	mTOR inhibitor: everolimus	NA	NA
	Mutation in CDK4/6 pathway	CDK inhibitors	NA	NA

81.1 General Aspects

Table 81.5 (continued)

Cancer type	Mutation	Targeted therapy	Objective response rate (%)	Progression-free survival (months)
Melanoma	Activating *BRAF* mutation	BRAF inhibitors: dabrafenib	39	16
		Vemurafenib	50	4.6
		Dual BRAF/MEK inhibition: dabrafenib + trametinib	NA	NA
		Vemurafenib + cobimetinib	NA	NA
	Mutation in *PI3K/AKT/mTOR* pathway	PI3K inhibitor: BKM120	NA Efficacy demonstrated in preclinical study	NA
	(No specific mutation)	CTLA-4 inhibitor: ipilimumab	24	2.7
		PD-1 inhibitor: pembrolizumab	NA	NA
		Dual CTLA-4/PD-1 inhibition: ipilimumab + nivolumab	NA	NA

EGFR epidermal growth factor receptor; *TKI* tyrosine kinase inhibitor; *ALK* anaplastic lymphoma kinase; *PD-1* programmed death 1; *HER2* human epidermal growth factor receptor 2; *PI3K* phosphoinositide 3-kinase; *mTOR* mammalian target of rapamycin; *CDK4/6* cyclin-dependent kinase 4 and 6; *CTLA-4* cytotoxic T lymphocyte antigen-4; *NA* not available

Table 81.6 The following three classes for outcome prediction were proposed by the Radiation Therapy Oncology Group (RTOG)

Class	Parameters	Median survival (months)
Class 1	• Karnofsky performance status ≥70 • Age ≤65 years • Controlled primary tumor • No extracranial metastases	7.1
Class 3	• Karnofsky performance status <70	2.3
Class 2	• All the other patients	4.2

81.1.7 Immunohistochemical Approach

In the immediate approach of diagnosing a metastasis, the primary should be considered of unknown origin. The primary goal of the next step is to elucidate the derivation of the tumor by using antibodies as shown in Table 81.7. The use of these markers is given in anatomic pathology as well as in the identification of the site of origin of brain metastases in neuropathology.

Cytokeratins
- Intermediate filament proteins
- Present in epithelial cells
- Marker of epithelial differentiation
- 20 distinct types of CKs
- Two categories of CKs based on 2D gel migration properties:
  - Basic (CK1–CK8)
  - Acidic (CK9–CK20)
- Each of the two categories (basic, acidic) contains two groups based on molecular weight:
  - Basic—High Molecular Weight (HMW): (CK1–CK6)
  - Basic—Low Molecular Weight (LMW): (CK7, CK8)
  - Acidic—High Molecular Weight (HMW): (CK9–CK17)
  - Acidic—Low Molecular Weight (LMW): (CK18–CK20)
- Distinction of CKs based on distribution:
  - HMW are squamous keratins (squamous epithelia and basal cells).
  - LMW are simple/non-squamous keratins (in the cytoplasm).
- Distribution patterns of CKs retained in carcinomas

Table 81.7 Markers of differentiation are given as follows

Differentiation	Marker
Mesenchymal	• Vimentin • Desmin
Epithelial	• Cytokeratins (CK) • Epithelial membrane antigen (EMA)
Smooth muscle	• Desmin • Muscle-specific actin • Smooth muscle actin • Calponin • H-caldesmon • Smooth muscle myosin heavy chain (MHC)
Skeletal muscle	• Desmin • Muscle-specific actin • Myogenin • MyoD
Myofibroblastic	• Actins (MSA, SMA) • Calponin
Myoepithelial	• Smooth muscle (SMA, Calponin) • Neural (S100) • Glial (GFAP) • Epithelial (Cytokeratins, CK5/6) • Basal/stem cell factor (p63)
Endothelial	• CD34 • CD31 • Factor VIII • Ulex europaeus I • CD141 • Fli-1 • D2-40 (Lymphatic vessel)
Lipomatous	• S100
Melanocytic	• S100 • HMB45 • Melan-A • MITF • Tyrosinase
Neuroendocrine	• Synaptophysin • Chromogranin A • Neuron-specific enolase • CD56 • CD57
Glial	• GFAP
Neuronal	• Neurofilament • NeuN • Synaptophysin • Chromogranin A
Nerve sheath	• S100
Serous acinar cells	• PAS • Trypsin • Chymotrypsin • Lipase

(continued)

Table 81.7 (continued)

Hematopoietic	• CD45/LCA • CD3 (pan-T-cell) • CD20 • CD79a • PAX5 (pan-B-cell) • CD138 (plasma cells) • CD61 • Myeloperoxidase • Glycophorin A
Histiocytic	• CD68 • CD163 • HAM56 • MAC 387

Examples of frequently used CKs:
1. AE1/AE3
   - Broad-spectrum CK
   - Reacts with HMW-CKs and LMW-CKs
   - Identifies virtually all types of epithelial neoplasms
2. Cam5.2
   - LMW-CK cocktail
   - Reacts with all non-squamous epithelia
3. CK5/6
   - HMW-CK cocktail
   - Reacts with squamous, urothelial, and a few glandular epithelia
4. CK7 and CK20
   - Distinctive patterns of expression in various organs (Tables 81.8 and 81.9)
5. Ber-EP4
   - Reacts with the majority of adenocarcinomas of various sites
6. Epithelial membrane antigen (EMA) (Table 81.10)
   - Present in the majority of non-squamous carcinomas
   - Also present in non-epithelial tissues and neoplasms

Coexpression of cytokeratin and vimentin
- Coexpression common (>50%)
  - Endometrial adenocarcinoma
  - Renal cell carcinoma
  - Salivary gland carcinoma
  - Spindle cell carcinoma
  - Thyroid follicular carcinoma

81.1 General Aspects

Table 81.8 CK7 and CK20 positivity and negativity in various tumor types

CK7-positivity	• Adenocarcinoma of breast, lung, ovary, endometrium, pancreas • Mesothelioma • Urothelial carcinoma • Thymic carcinoma • Cervical squamous cell carcinoma • Fibrolamellar variant of hepatocellular carcinoma
CK7-negativity (rarely positivity)	• Renal carcinoma • Prostate carcinoma • Adrenocortical carcinoma • Squamous carcinoma (except uterine cervix) • Small cell carcinomas • Hepatocellular carcinomas
CK20-positivity	• Colorectal carcinoma • Pancreas carcinoma (60%) • Gastric carcinoma (50%) • Cholangiocarcinoma (40%) • Mucinous ovarian carcinoma • Merkel cell carcinoma • Urothelial carcinomas (30%)
CK20-negativity (rarely positivity)	• Breast carcinoma • Lung carcinoma • Salivary gland carcinoma • Hepatocellular carcinoma • Renal cell carcinoma • Prostate carcinoma • Adrenocortical carcinoma • Squamous carcinoma • Small cell carcinoma

- Coexpression uncommon (<10%)
  - Endocervical adenocarcinoma
  - Colorectal adenocarcinoma
  - Breast ductal-lobular carcinoma
  - Lung non-small cell carcinoma
  - Prostate adenocarcinoma

Staining for carcinoembryonic antigen (CEA) shows positive and negative results in tumors of various organs (Table 81.11). Additional markers are shown in Table 81.12 while a list of markers for sarcomas is given in Table 81.13.

Immunostaining pattern might be (Table 81.14):
- Cytoplasmatic
- Nuclear
- Membranous

Table 81.9 The interplay between CK7 and CK20 positivity or negativity

CK7	CK20	Possible primary
CK7+	CK20+	• Transitional cell carcinoma (bladder) • Pancreas and biliary system • Ovary (mucinous carcinoma) • Stomach (gastric adenocarcinoma)
CK7+	CK20–	• Lung (small and non-small cell carcinoma) • Breast (ductal and lobular carcinoma) • Ovary (non-mucinous carcinoma) • Endometrial adenocarcinoma • Gastric adenocarcinoma • Mesothelioma • Squamous cell carcinoma of cervix • Pancreatic ductal adenocarcinoma • Cholangiocarcinoma • Thyroid • Salivary gland • Kidney (papillary renal cell carcinoma) • Urothelial carcinoma
CK7–	CK20+	• Colorectal carcinoma • Merkel cell carcinoma
CK7–	CK20–	• Lung, squamous cell carcinoma (10% may express focal weak CK7 positivity) • Prostate adenocarcinoma • Kidney (clear cell renal cell carcinoma) • Liver (hepatocellular carcinoma) • Adrenal cortex (adrenocortical carcinoma) • Thymus • Neuroendocrine carcinoma

Table 81.10 The use of CK positivity/negativity in conjunction with EMA positivity/negativity

CK7	EMA	Possible primary
CK+	EMA–	• Hepatocellular carcinoma • Adrenocortical neoplasms • Neuroendocrine neoplasms • Embryonal carcinoma • Yolk sac tumor • Thyroid
CK–	EMA+	• Meningioma • Perineurioma • Plasma cell neoplasms • Anaplastic large cell lymphoma • Hodgkin lymphoma (popcorn or lymphocyte predominant cells) • Renal cell carcinoma

Table 81.11 Carcinoembryonic antigen (CEA): positive and negative staining of tumors in various organs

CEA positive	CEA negative
• Paranasal sinuses	• Prostate
• Lung	• Kidney
• Colon	• Adrenal glands
• Stomach	• Endometrium
• Biliary system	• Ovarian (serous)
• Pancreas	
• Sweat glands	
• Breast	

Table 81.12 Additional immunohistochemical or molecular markers to be used

Primary tumor	Marker
Breast	• ER (estrogen receptor) (60%+) • Progesterone receptor (60%+) • GCDFP-15 (50%+) • MGB (mammaglobin) (50%+) • GATA3 • HER-2 neu (10–25%+) • TFF1 (trefoil factor 1) • CEA
Lung, squamous cell carcinoma	• High molecular weight keratin • CK5/6 • CEA • p40/p63 • Thrombomodulin • Low molecular weight keratin • TTF1 negative • Napsin A negative
Lung, adenocarcinoma	• CAM5.2 • AE1/AE3 • EMA • CEA • CD15 • Ber-Ep4 • CK7 • TTF1 • Napsin A • CK5/6 negative • p63 negative
Lung, small cell carcinoma	• TTF-1 • Synaptophysin • Chromogranin • CD56 • p63 negative

Table 81.12 (continued)

Mesothelioma	• Calretinin • WT1 • CK5/6 • Thrombomodulin • D2-40 • Mesothelin • P63 negative • CEA negative • MOC-31 negative • BerEP4 negative • TTF-1 negative
Melanoma	• Braf (IHC and mutation) • Mart-1 • MiTF • SOX10 • PNL2
Prostate	• PSA (prostate-specific antigen) • PAP • Prostein (P501S) • PSMA • AMACR (P504s) • ERG • NKX3.1 (an androgen-regulated homeodomain) • CEA negative • Uroplakin negative • Thrombomodulin negative • P63 negative • CK5/6 negative
Thyroid—papillary and follicular CA	• TTF-1 • Thyroglobulin • PAX8
Thyroid—medullary CA	• TTF-1 • Calcitonin • Chromogranin A • CEA
Kidney	• RCC • CD10 • PAX2 • PAX8 • CAIX
Adrenocortical carcinoma	• Inhibin • Calretinin • Melan-A • Vimentin • CEA negative
RCC clear cell type	• PAX8 • PAX2 • CD10 • RCC • Vimentin • pVHL • KIM-1 (kidney injury molecule 1) • CEA negative

81.1 General Aspects

Table 81.12 (continued)

Primary tumor	Marker
RCC papillary	• P504S • RCCma • pVHL • PAX8 • KIM-1
Bladder	• P63 • Thrombomodulin • Uroplakin • GATA3 • CDX2 variable
Urothelial carcinoma	• GATA3 • Uroplakin II (UPII) • S100P • CK903 • p63 • CK5/6
Female gynecological tract	• PAX8 • ER/PR • WT1 (serous carcinoma)
Endometrium carcinoma	• ER • PAX8 • Vimentin • CEA negative
Endocervical carcinoma	• PAX8 • p16 • Human papilloma virus (HPV) • CEA • Vimentin negative • ER/PR negative
Ovarian serous carcinoma	• PAX8 • Wilms tumor 1 (WT1) • Inhibin • ß-catenin • ER/PR • Mesothelin • CEA negative
Ovarian mucinous carcinoma	• PAX8 • Mucin 5AC (MUC5AC) • ß-catenin/MUC2 negative • CDX2 variable
Intestine	• CDX2 • Villin • Special AT-rich sequence binding protein 2 (SATB2)
Hepatocellular carcinoma	• HepPar-1 • Canalicular CD10 • CEA • Glypican-3 • Arginase-1 • CD34 • Alpha Fetoprotein • Albumin • MOC-31 negative • CK-19 negative

Table 81.12 (continued)

Cholangiocarcinoma	• CEA • CK19 • MOC-31 • CA19-9 • CDX2 variable • HepPar negative
Pancreas	• Loss of DPC4 expression • CK17 • Mucin 5AC (MUC5AC) • CEA • CA19-9 • MUC2 negative • CDX2 variable
Colorectal carcinoma	• CDX-2 • CEA • MUC2 • MUC5AC negative
Merkel cell carcinoma	• Synaptophysin • Chromogranin • CD56
Non-seminoma germ cell tumor	• PLAP • EMA negative
Yolk sac tumor	• SALL4 • LIN28 • Glypican-3 • AFP
Embryonal carcinoma	• Oct3/4 • CD30

Table 81.13 Antibodies used to immunophenotype sarcomas, modified after Bhargava and Dabbs (2018) reproduced with kind permission by Elsevier

Sarcoma type	IHC
Ewing sarcoma/PNET	• CD99 • FLI1
Rhabdomyosarcoma	• MSA • Desmin • Myoglobin • Myogenin • MyoD1
Desmoplastic round cell tumor	• Vimentin • Cytokeratin • EMA • Desmin • WT1
Synovial sarcoma	• EMA • Keratin • D99 • Bcl2 • TLE1
Clear cell sarcoma	• S-100 • HMB-45 • Melan-A

(continued)

Table 81.13 (continued)

Sarcoma type	IHC
Alveolar soft-part sarcoma	• PASD • TFE3
PEComas	• HMB-45 • Melan-A • S-100 negative
Epithelioid sarcoma	• Keratin • EMA • Vimentin • CD34 • CF5/6 negative • P63 negative
Vascular tumors	• Factor Viii • CD32 • CD34 • FLI1 • Thrombomodulin • Keratin (patchy)
Leiomyosarcoma	• SMA • HHF.35 • Desmin • Caldesmon • Keratin (patchy)
Malignant peripheral nerve sheath tumor	• S-100 • CD56 • CD57 • PGP9.5 • CD99
Chordoma	• Brachyury (nuclear) • S-100 • Keratin • EMA • CK7 negative • CK20 negative
Extraskeletal myxoid chondrosarcoma	• S-100 • NSE • Synaptophysin • Keratin negative • Chromogranin negative
Endometrial stromal sarcoma	• CD10 • ER • SMA • Desmin • Bcl-2 negative • CD34 negative
Gastrointestinal stromal tumor (GIST)	• DOG1 • CD117 • CD34 • S-100 negative • Actin negative • Desmin negative

Table 81.14 Staining patterns of various tumor markers

Marker	Staining pattern	Tumor site
Calretinin	Nuclear/cytoplasmic	• Mesothelioma • Sex cord-stroma • Adrenocortical
Calponin	Cytoplasm	• Breast
CDX-2	Nuclear	• Colorectal/duodenal
D2-40	Membranous	• Mesothelioma • Lymphatic endothelial cell marker
Estrogen receptor	Nuclear	• Breast • Ovary • Endometrium
Gross cystic disease fluid protein 15 (GCDFP15)	Cytoplasmic	• Breast
HepPar1	Cytoplasmic	• Hepatocellular
Inhibin	Cytoplasmic	• Sex cord-stromal • Adrenocortical
Mammaglobin	Cytoplasmic	• Breast
Melan-A	Cytoplasmic	• Adrenocortical • Melanoma
Mesothelin	Cytoplasmic/membranous	• Mesothelioma
P63	Nuclear	• Squamous cell carcinoma
Progesterone receptor	Nuclear	• Breast • Ovary • Endometrium
Prostate acid phosphatase	Cytoplasmic	• Prostate
Prostate-specific antigen (PSA)	Cytoplasmic	• Prostate
Renal cell carcinoma (RCC)	Membranous	• Renal
S-100	Cytoplasm	
Smooth muscle actin (SMA)	Cytoplasm	
Smooth muscle myosin heavy chain	Cytoplasm	
Thyroglobulin	Cytoplasmic	• Thyroid
Thyroid transcription factor 1 (TTF1)	Nuclear	• Lung • Thyroid
Uroplakin III	Membranous	• Urothelial
Villin	Apical	• Gastrointestinal
Wilms tumor 1 (WT1)	Nuclear	• Ovarian serous • Mesothelioma • Wilms • Desmoplastic, small round cell

81.2 Lung Tumors

The various lung tumors as distinguished by the WHO classification (see Appendix B).

81.2.1 General Aspects

The *malignant* tumors affecting the lung with the potential for brain metastasis can roughly be grouped into:
- Adenocarcinoma
- Squamous cell carcinoma
- Small cell carcinoma
- Large cell undifferentiated carcinoma
- Adenosquamous carcinoma
- Carcinoid tumor

Basically two groups of lung carcinomas are distinguished:
- Small cell lung carcinoma (SCLC)
- Non-small cell lung carcinoma (NSCLC)
  - Adenocarcinoma
  - Squamous cell carcinoma
  - Large cell carcinoma

81.2.2 Neuropathology Findings

Histologic features of brain metastases from primary *lung tumors* include:
- Squamous cell carcinoma (Fig. 81.6g, h)
  - Keratinization
    - Squamous keratin pearls
    - Individual tumor cells with markedly eosinophilic dense cytoplasm
  - Intercellular bridges
  - Keratin pearls
- Adenocarcinoma (Fig. 81.6a–d)
  - Growth patterns:
    - Lepidic
    - Acinar
    - Papillary
    - Solid
  - Cuboidal or columnar cells
  - Glandular differentiation/structures
  - Mucin production (Fig. 81.6m–t)
  - Prominent nucleoli
- Small cell carcinoma (Fig. 81.6i, l)
  - Small, round, oval, or spindle-shaped cells with scant cytoplasm
  - Nuclei with finely granular chromatin and absent or inconspicuous nucleoli
  - Nuclear molding
- Large cell carcinoma
  - Poorly differentiated tumor lacking squamous or glandular differentiation
  - Large cells with ample cytoplasm
  - Prominent nucleoli and vesicular chromatin

81.2.3 Immunophenotype (Fig. 81.7)

The immunophenotype of various lung cancers is given in Tables 81.15 and 81.16.

81.3 Breast Tumors

The various lung tumors as distinguished by the WHO classification (see Appendix B).

81.3.1 General Aspects

The *malignant* tumors affecting the breast with the potential for brain metastasis can roughly be grouped into:
- Invasive ductal carcinoma
- Invasive lobular carcinoma
- Additional types
  - Colloid
  - Medullary
  - Tubular

81.3.2 Neuropathology Findings

Histologic features of brain metastases from primary *breast tumors* include (Fig. 81.8):
- Large pleomorphic cells
  - Variable in size and shape
  - Abundant cytoplasm
  - Irregular nuclei with prominent nucleoli

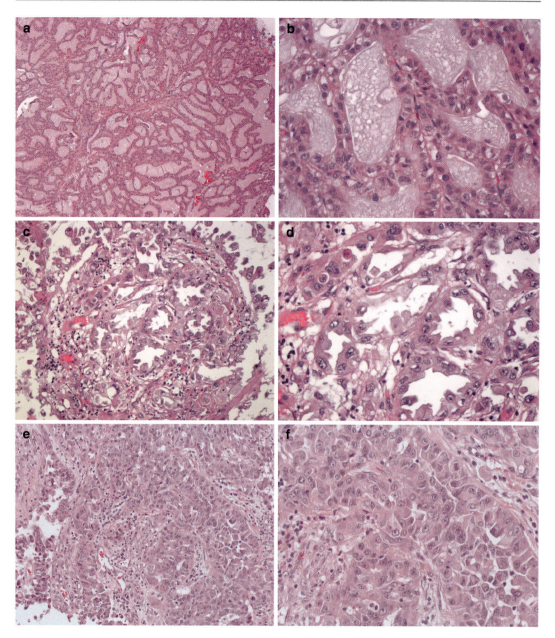

Fig. 81.6 Lung: The tumor shows adenoid architecture (**a–d**), acinar appearance (**e, f**), squamous differentiation (**g, h**), solid growth in neuroendocrine carcinoma (**i–l**), with secretion of mucoid substances (**m–t**; **o, p** stain: PAS, **q, r** stain: Alcian blue)

81.3 Breast Tumors

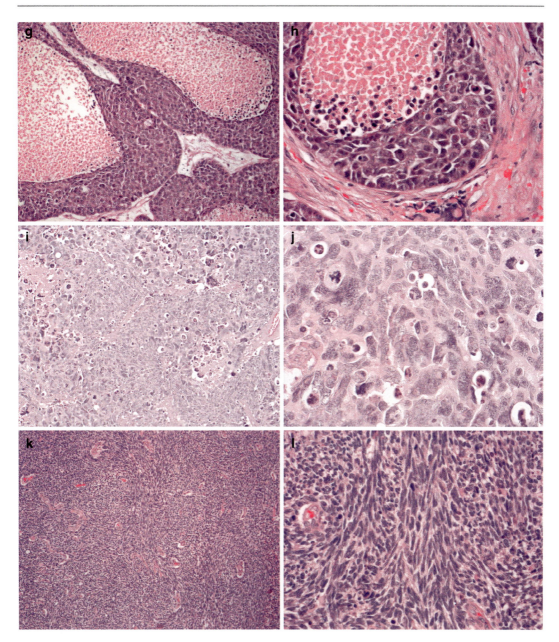

Fig. 81.6 (continued)

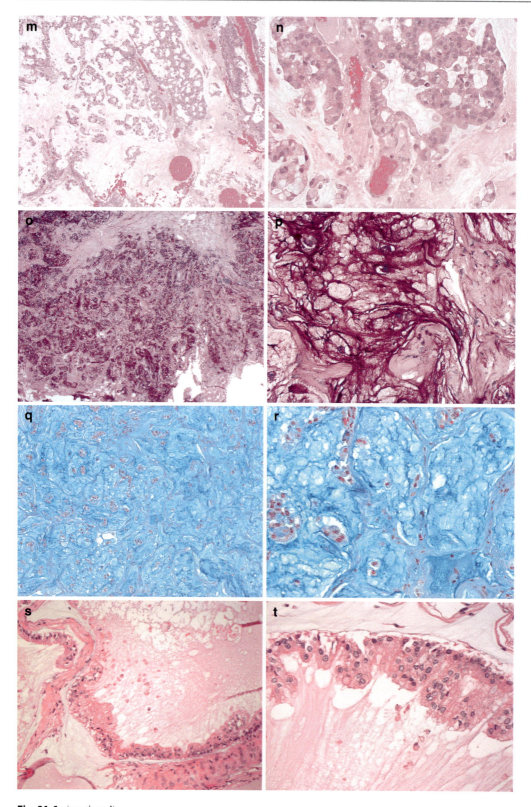

Fig. 81.6 (continued)

81.3 Breast Tumors

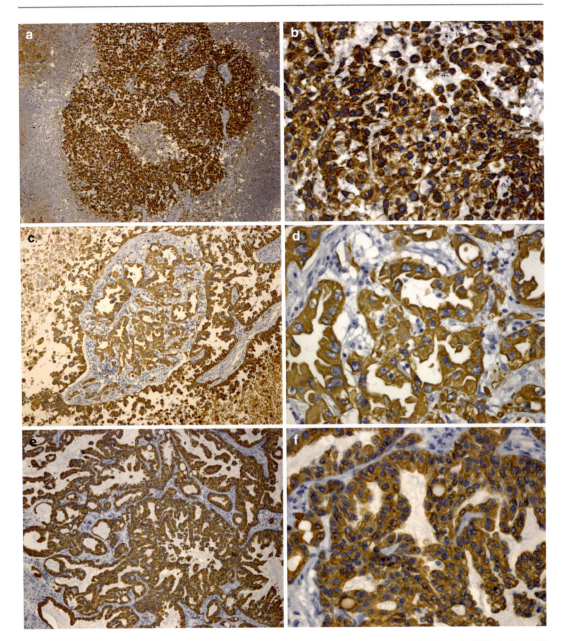

Fig. 81.7 Lung: Immunophenotype: the tumor cells are positive for pancytokeratin AE1/AE3 (**a–d**), CK7 (**e–j**), TTF1 (**k**), CD56 (in neuroendocrine carcinoma) (**l**), napsin A (**m, n**), and p63 (in squamous carcinoma) (**o, p**)

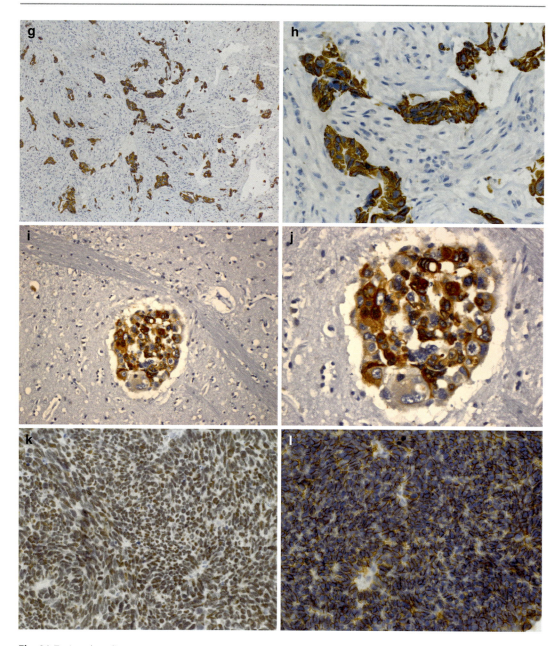

Fig. 81.7 (continued)

- Growth pattern
  - Cribriform
  - Micropapillary
  - Papillary
  - Solid
  - Comedo
- Invasive ductal carcinoma
  - Neoplastic glands to sheets of neoplastic cells
- Invasive lobular carcinoma
  - Neoplastic cells in single-file "Indian file"
  - Signet ring cells with intracytoplasmic mucin droplets
- Medullary
  - Sheets of anaplastic cells associated with lymphocytic infiltrates
- Colloid
  - Production of abundant mucin

81.3 Breast Tumors

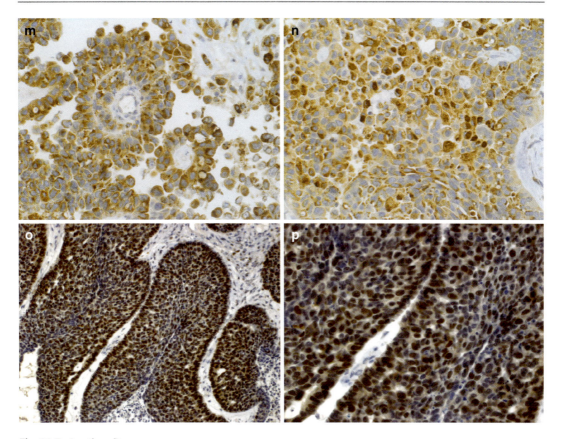

Fig. 81.7 (continued)

Table 81.15 Summary of useful markers in lung carcinoma

	Positivity	Negativity
Squamous cell carcinoma	• CK5/6 • CK5 • p40 • p63 • Desmoglein3	• TTF1 • NapsinA
Adenocarcinoma	• TTF1 • NapsinA	• CK5/6 • CK5 • p40 • p63 • Desmoglein3
Adenocarcinoma non-mucinous	• CK7 • CK20 • TTF1 • Napsin A	• CDX2 • Hepatocyte nuclear factor 4 α (HNF4α)
Invasive mucinous adenocarcinoma	• Hepatocyte nuclear factor 4 α (HNF4α)	

Table 81.16 Markers for primary lung carcinoma modified after Zhang et al. (2015) reproduced with kind permission by Springer Nature

Antibodies	AdenoCA	Squamous cell carcinoma	Adenosquamous carcinoma	Large cell carcinoma (LCC)	Large cell neuroendocrine carcinoma (LCNEC)	Small cell lung carcinoma (SCLC)
CK7	+	−	+	+	+	− or + (focal)
CK20	−/+	−		−	−	−
TTF-1	+	−	+	− or +	− or +	+ (>90% of cases)
NapsinA	+	−	+	+		
CDX2	+					
CK5/6	−	+	+	−		
p63	−	+	+	− or +		−
CK5	−	+	+			
p40	−	+	+			
SP-A	−/+ (46%+)					
SP-B	−/+ (52%+)					
GCDFP-15	−/+ (5%+)					
ER	Variable					
PR	variable					
Villin	+ (6–68%)					
DC-LAMP	+ (Clara cell)					
Inhibin-α	−/+					
CD56		− or +			+ or −	+
CK903			+	UK		
CEA			+			
CK19			+	UK		
CA19-9			+			
CK17				UK		
Synaptophysin					+	+ or −
Chromogranin					+ or −	− or +
Ki-67					high	High (>90%)
MASH1					+ or −	+
NeuroD					+ or −	− or +
P16					+ or −	+
PTEN					− or +	− or +
p63					− or +	
CK1/3						+ (weak to moderate)
CAM5.2						+

81.3 Breast Tumors

- Tubular
  - Well-formed tubules
- Comedo
  - Tumor cells with pleomorphic high-grade nuclei
  - Areas of central necrosis

Possible prognostic factors in metastases from breast carcinoma
- Estrogen receptor positivity
- Progesterone receptor positivity
- Her-2-Neu positivity

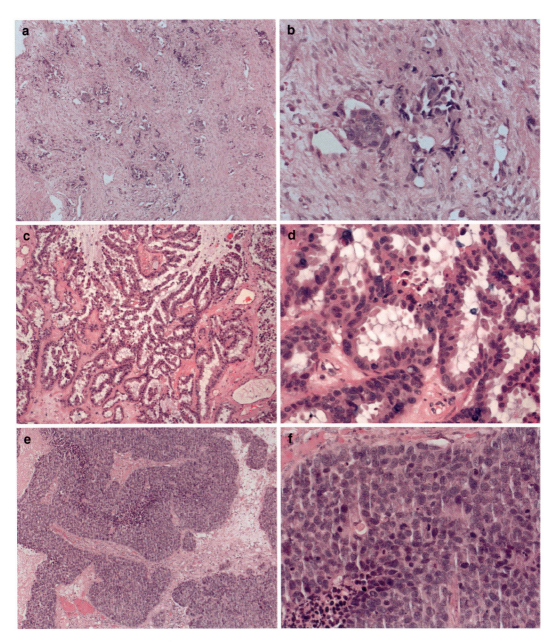

Fig. 81.8 Breast: The tumor cells can be seen grouped in small nests (**a, b**), with adenoid architecture (**c, d**), with solid growth pattern (**e–h**), with comedo-structures (**i, j**). In meningeosis carcinomatosa, the tumor cells are found in the subarachnoidal space (**k, l**)

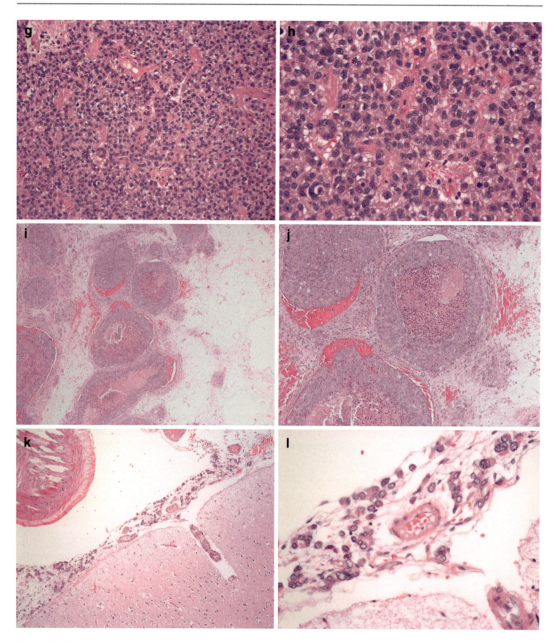

Fig. 81.8 (continued)

81.3.3 Immunophenotype (Fig. 81.9)

The immunophenotype of various breast cancers is given in Tables 81.17, 81.18, and 81.19.

81.4 Skin Tumors: Melanoma

The various tumors affecting the skin as distinguished by the WHO classification are listed in Appendix B.

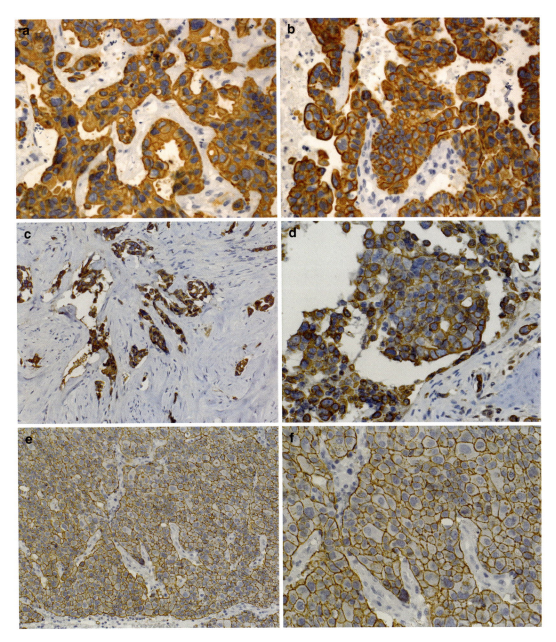

Fig. 81.9 Breast: Immunophenotype: The tumor cells are positive for pancytokeratin AE1/AE3 (**a–c**), CK7 (**d**), her2 (**e, f**), estrogen receptor (**g, h**), progesterone receptor (**i, j**), mammoglobin (**k, l**), and GATA3 (**m, n**)

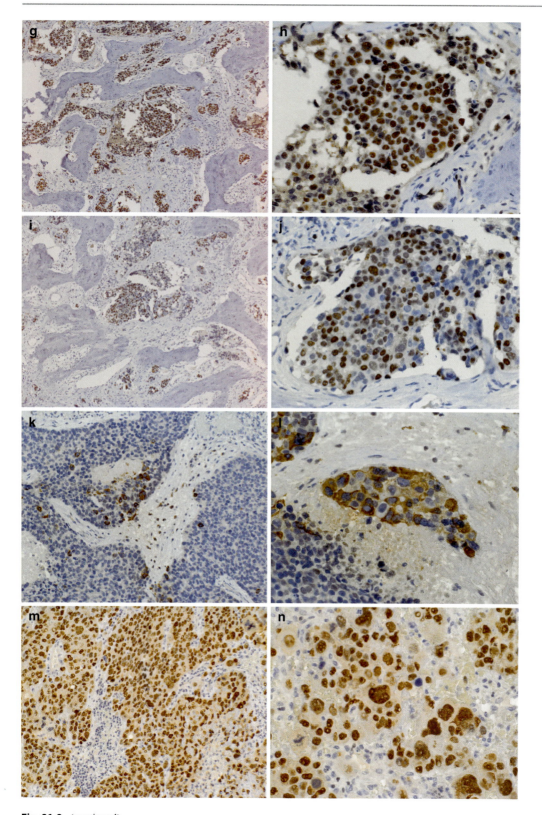

Fig. 81.9 (continued)

81.4 Skin Tumors: Melanoma

Table 81.17 Markers used in the evaluation of metastatic breast carcinoma

Marker	Pattern
CK7	+
CK20	−
GATA-3	+
Mammaglobin	+ or −
GCDFP-15	− or +
ER, PR	+ or −
NY-BR-1	+
Her-2/neu	− or +
P120-catenin	+

Table 81.18 Markers used in the differentiation between ductal carcinoma and lobular carcinoma

Marker	Ductal CA	Lobular CA
E-cadherin	+	−
P 120 catenin	+, Membranous	+, Cytoplasmic
CK903	−	+
CK8	+, Peripheral-predominant membranous pattern	+, Perinuclear, ring-like, cytoplasmic pattern

Table 81.19 Immunophenotype of various types of breast carcinoma, modified after Liu (2015) and Zhang et al. (2015) reproduced with kind permission by Springer Nature

Marker	Ductal carcinoma	Lobular carcinoma	Medullary carcinoma of breast	Metaplastic carcinoma
GATA-3	+, N 94.0%	+, N 100%	− or +	− or +
E-cadherin	+, M		+	
CK7	+ 91.7%	+ 90%	+ or −	+
ER	+ or − 59.1%	+ 83.7%	−	−
PR			−	−
Her-2			−	−
Mammaglobin	− or + 42.2%	+ or − 69.5%	−	
GCDFP-15	− or + 31.4%	− or + 28.3%		
NY-BR-1	+	+		
P 120 catenin	+, M 94.6%, M	+, C 100%		
CK8	+, peripheral-predominant membranous pattern 98.8%	+, perinuclear, ring-like, cytoplasmic pattern 100%		
CK903	−	+ 96.3%	+ or −	+
TFF1	+, C 72%	+, C 87%		
TFF3	+, C84%	+, C 94%		
MUC1	+, C97%	+ 100%		
MUC2	− or +, C 3%	−0		
MUC4,	− 0	−0		
MUC5AC	0	−0		
MUC6	− or +, C 8.4%	− or + 16.2%		
p53			+ or	
MIB-1			High	
CK5/6, CK14			+ or −	+
P-cadherin			+ or −	
EMA			+	
AE1/AE3, CAM5.2			+	+ or −
S100 protein			+	
Vimentin			+ or −	+
Pan-CK (MNF-116)				+
MEC markers (p63, CD10, Calponin, SMA)				+
EGFR				+
CD34				−
SOX10				+ or −

81.4.1 General Aspects

The tumors affecting the skin are divided into the following groups:
- Melanocytic tumors
  - Melanocytic skin tumors include a large variety of benign and malignant neoplasms with distinct clinical, morphological, and genetic profiles.
- Keratinocytic tumors
  - Keratinocytic tumors are derived from epidermal and adnexal keratinocytes and comprise a large spectrum of lesions ranging from benign proliferations (acanthomas) to malignant squamous cell carcinomas which occasionally show aggressive growth and even metastatic potential.
- Appendageal tumors
  - Appendageal tumors are neoplasms whose differentiation is towards one or more of the adnexal structures of the skin. While mesenchymal tumors of various kinds are technically in this category, conventionally, the term refers to those with origin from, or differentiation toward epithelial adnexal neoplasms.
- Hematolymphoid tumors
  - Lymphoma may involve the skin as the primary and only site of involvement, or may spread to the skin as a secondary site of disease. Some cutaneous lymphomas morphologically resemble their counterparts in lymph node, but differ in terms of phenotype, genotype, and clinical behavior, suggesting that they represent an independent entity.
- Soft tissue tumors
- Neural tumors
  - Cutaneous neural tumors represent a small but important part of the cutaneous soft tissue neoplasms. Their histogenesis is conceptually analogous to their deep soft tissue or visceral counterpart, i.e., they recapitulate to variable extent the architectural and cytologic constituents of normal peripheral or autonomic nerves.

The *malignant* tumors affecting the skin with the potential to metastasize to the brain can roughly be grouped into:
- Melanocytic tumors (Fig. 81.10)
  - Melanomas
- Keratinocytic tumors
  - Basal cell carcinomas

81.4.2 Neuropathology Findings

Histologic features of brain metastases from *melanoma* include (Fig. 81.11):
- Large cells most often without melanin pigment
- Prominent nucleoli
- Scant cytoplasm
- Partly well demarcated from brain tissue

Metastases from melanoma can occur within a few years from excision of the primary tumor. However, it is important to remember that late metastases (>10 years, sometimes even over 25 years after excision of the primary tumor) are not uncommon.

Histologic features of brain metastases from *basal cell carcinoma* include:
- Neoplastic cells resembling basal cells of the epidermis
- Peripheral palisading and separation clefts
- Mucoid matrix

Additional testing:
- Braf mutation-specific antibody
- Braf mutation

81.4 Skin Tumors: Melanoma

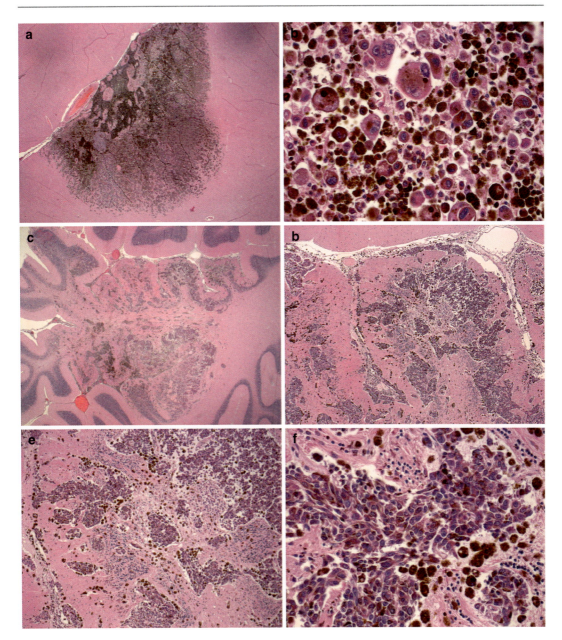

Fig. 81.10 Skin: Growth pattern of melanoma in the cerebral cortex (**a**, **b**), cerebellum (**c–f**), diffuse infiltration into the brain tissue (**g**, **h**). Not all tumor cells contain pigment (**i–n**)

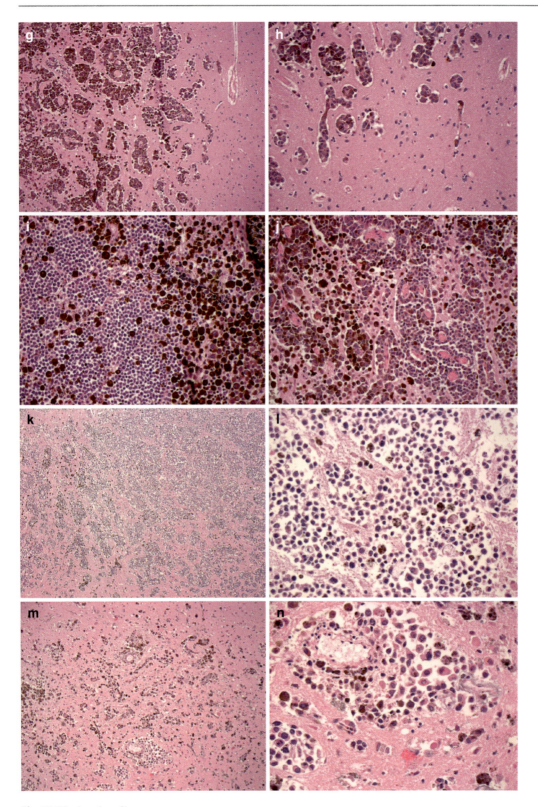

Fig. 81.10 (continued)

81.4 Skin Tumors: Melanoma

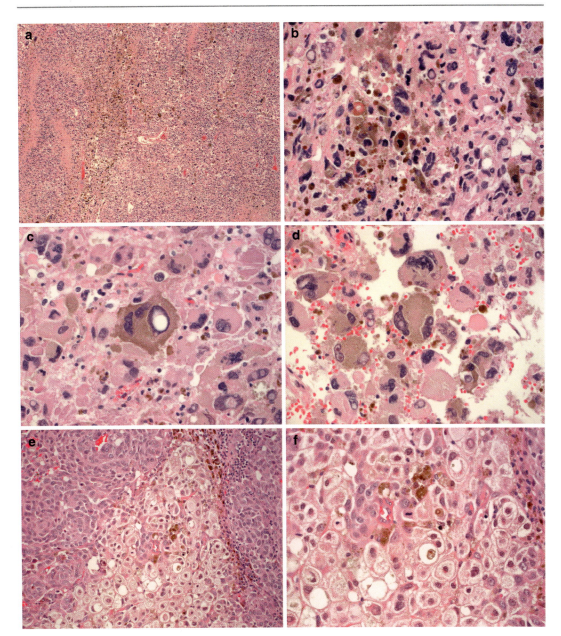

Fig. 81.11 Skin: The tumor cells of melanoma show a variegated appearance and mimick growth pattern and cell type of other carcinomas ("Melanoma is the great mimicker") (**a–r**)

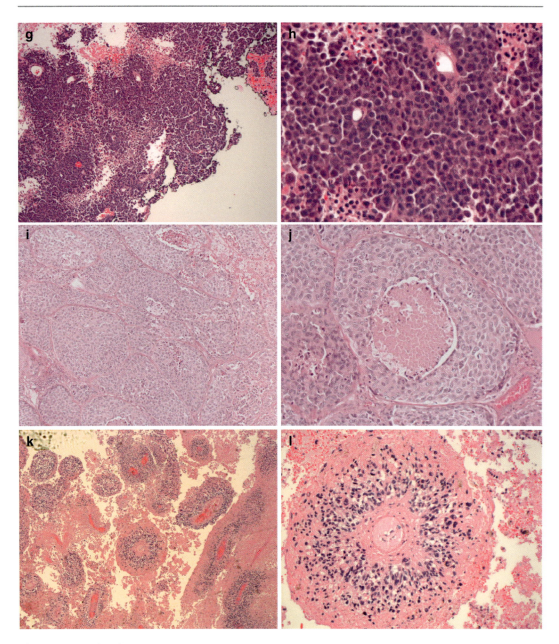

Fig. 81.11 (continued)

81.4 Skin Tumors: Melanoma

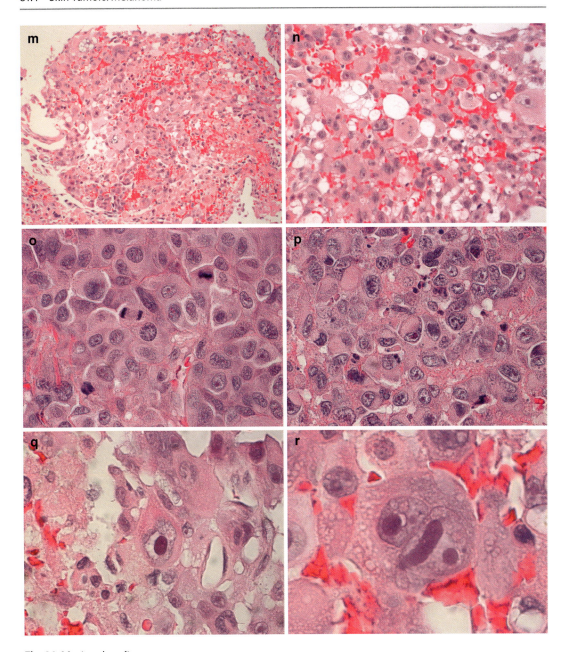

Fig. 81.11 (continued)

81.4.3 Immunophenotype (Fig. 81.12)

The immunophenotype of various skin cancers is given in Table 81.20, while specific markers for differentiation, proliferation, signaling, transcription, and adhesion in melanoma are listed in Table 81.21.

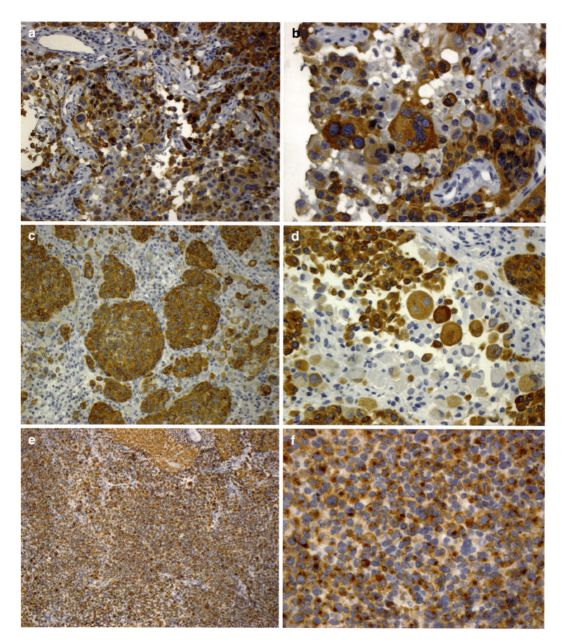

Fig. 81.12 Skin: Immunophenotype : The tumor cells are positive for melan-A (**a–d**), HMB45 (**e, f**), S-100 (**g, h**). The Braf V600 mutation can be shown with a mutation-specific antibody (**i, j**)

81.4 Skin Tumors: Melanoma

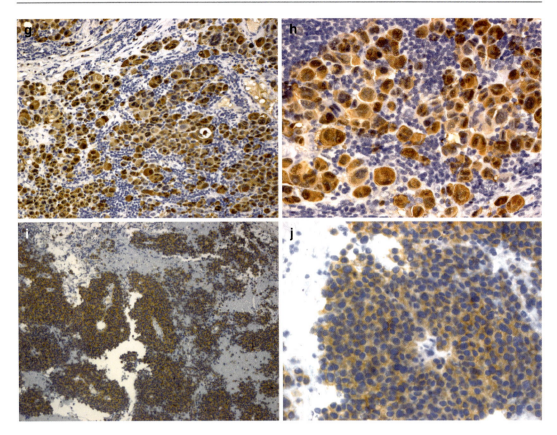

Fig. 81.12 (continued)

Table 81.20 Markers for primary cutaneous melanoma, cutaneous spindle cell squamous cell carcinoma, and Merkel cell carcinoma, modified after Ferringer (2015) and Zhang et al. (2015), reproduced with kind permission by Springer Nature

Antibodies	Cutaneous melanoma	Cutaneous spindle cell squamous cell carcinoma (sSCC)	Merkel cell carcinoma (MCC)
S100	+ 93.4%	−	−/+
HMB-45	+ 75%		
MART1	+ 88.8%		
MITF	+ 79.8%		
Tyrosinase	+ 94.3%		
NKI-C3	+ 95.5%		
MUM-1	+ 75.6%		
SOX-10	+		
AE1/AE3		+	
CAM5.2		+/−	
CK903		+	
CK5/6		+	
MNF116		+	
p63		+	
Desmin		−	
NSE			+

(continued)

Table 81.20 (continued)

Antibodies	Cutaneous melanoma	Cutaneous spindle cell squamous cell carcinoma (sSCC)	Merkel cell carcinoma (MCC)
Chromogranin			+/−
Synaptophysin			+/−
CK20			+
TTF-1			−
Ber-EP4			+
CD56			+
LCA			−
CD99			−/+
NFP			+/−
CK7			−/+
FLI1			−/+
PAX-5			+
Bcl-2			+
TdT			+/−
CD117			+/−

Table 81.21 Specific markers for differentiation, proliferation, signaling, transcription, and adhesion in melanoma. (↑Upregulation with tumor progression; ↓downregulation with tumor progression)

Type of marker	Marker
Differentiation	• Tyrosinase • TRP-1 • AIM-1 Mitf • gp100 • TRP-2 • S-100 • HMW-MAA • Melan-A/MART-1 • MC1R
Proliferation	• Cyclin A ↑ • Cdk2 ↑ • PCNA ↑ • Cyclin B1 ↑ • p15 ↓ • p27 ↓ • mdm-2 ↑ • Cyclin D1/D3 ↑ • p16 ↓ • Ki67 ↑ • Telomerase ↑ • Cyclin E ↑
Signaling	• c-Kit ↓ • N-ras ↑ • EGFR ↑ • PTEN ↓ • c-Myc ↑ • ß-catenin ↓ • Transferrin receptor ↑

Table 81.21 (continued)

Transcription	• ATF-1 ↑ • AP-2 ↓
Adhesion	• E-Cadherin ↓ • ICAM-1 ↑ • ALCAM ↑ • N-Cadherin ↑ • MCAM ↑ • vß3 ↑ • CD44 v6 ↑ • VCAM-1 ↓
Proteases	• MMP-1 ↑ • MMP-13 ↑ • TIMP-3 ↑ • PA-system ↑ • MMP-2 ↑ • MT1-MMP ↑ • EMMPRIN ↑ • Cathepsin B • MMP-9 ↑ • TIMP-1 ↑ • D, H, L ↑
Other	• ME491/CD63 ↓ • HLA class I ↓ • Osteonectin ↑ • Fas/Fas ligand • HLA Class II ↑ • CTAs ↑

81.5 Renal Tumors

The various tumors affecting the kidney as distinguished by the WHO classification are listed in Appendix B.

81.5.1 General Aspects

The *malignant* tumors affecting the *kidney* with the potential for brain metastasis can roughly be grouped into:
- Renal cell tumors
  - Clear cell renal cell carcinoma
  - Chromophobe renal cell carcinoma
  - Papillary renal cell carcinoma
- Metanephric tumors
- Nephroblastic tumors

81.5.2 Neuropathology Findings

Histologic features of brain metastases from primary *renal cell carcinomas* include:
- Clear cell renal cell carcinoma (Fig. 81.13)
  - Tumor cells with small round nuclei and abundant clear or granular cytoplasm (containing glycogen and lipids)
  - Arranged in nests, partly showing alveolar pattern with delicate intervening stroma
  - Delicate branching vasculature
- Chromophobe renal cell carcinoma
  - Tumor cells with abundant pale eosinophilic cytoplasm
  - Perinuclear halo
- Papillary renal cell carcinoma
  - Fibrovascular papillae lined with neoplastic cells
  - Cuboidal or low columnar cells
  - Foamy macrophages within the papillae

81.5.3 Immunophenotype

The immunophenotype of various renal carcinomas is given in Tables 81.22 and 81.23.

81.6 Urinary Tract Tumors

The various tumors affecting the urinary tract as distinguished by the WHO classification are listed in Appendix B.

81.6.1 General Aspects

The *malignant* tumors affecting the urinary tract (urinary bladder) with the potential for brain metastasis can roughly be grouped into:
- Urothelial carcinoma (transitional cell carcinoma) (Fig. 81.14)
- Squamous cell carcinoma
- Adenocarcinoma

81.6.2 Neuroimaging Findings

Histologic features of brain metastases from primary *urothelial carcinomas* include:
- Urothelial carcinoma (transitional cell carcinoma) (Fig. 81.15)
  - Dyscohesive cells with large hyperchromatic nuclei
  - Papillary front
  - Fibrovascular core
- Squamous cell carcinoma
  - Squamous differentiation
  - Squamous cells with keratinization
  - Intercellular bridges
- Adenocarcinoma
  - Papillary architecture
  - Resemblance to mucinous adenocarcinoma of the colon

81.6.3 Immunophenotype

The immunophenotype of urothelial carcinoma and squamous lesions of the bladder is given in Table 81.24.

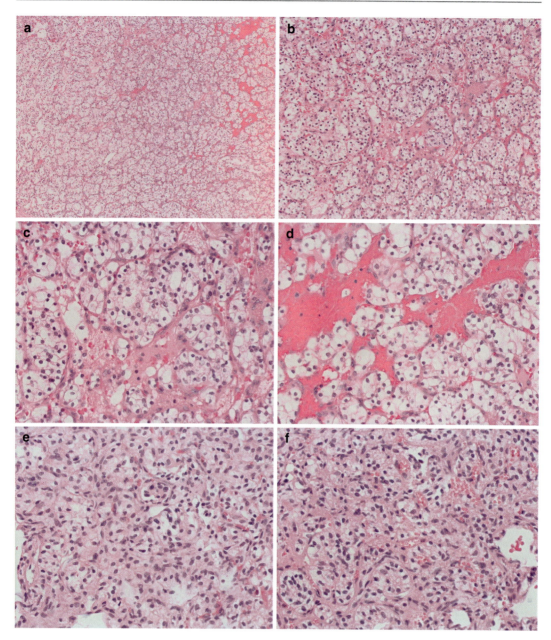

Fig. 81.13 Kidney: The tumor solid growth pattern (**a–d**). The tumor cells display a typical clear-cell cytoplasm (**a–d**); this pattern might be lost (**e, f**). The growth pattern can also be adenoid (**g, h**). Immunophenotype: The tumor cells are positive for pancytokeratin AE1/AE3 (**I–l**), CK7 (**m**), and CD10 (**n**)

81.6 Urinary Tract Tumors

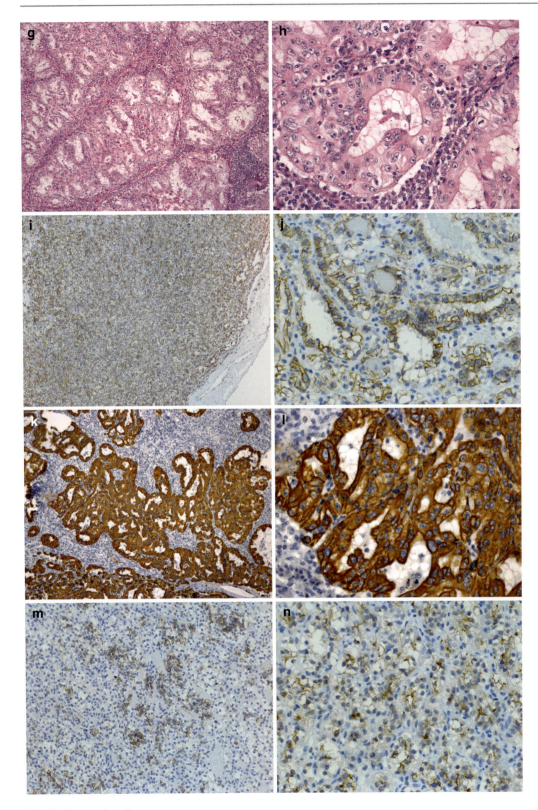

Fig. 81.13 (continued)

Table 81.22 Markers for clear cell renal cell carcinoma, modified after (Lin and Yang 2015) and Zhang et al. (2015) reproduced with kind permission by Springer Nature

Antibodies	Literature	Frequencies
CD10	+	90%
PAX8	+	95%
RCCMa	+	89%
Vimentin	+	86%
EMA	+	85%
KIM-1	+	75%
CA IX	+	91%
pVHL	V	99%
PAX2	+	84%
P504S	− or +	44%
S100	+	85%
S100A1	+	80%
GST-alpha	+	ND
CK7	−	11%
CK20	−	0
CK19	+ or −	58%
CD117	−	5%
Ksp-cad	− or +	40%
Parvalbumin	−	2.5%

81.7 Prostate Tumors

The various tumors affecting the prostate as distinguished by the WHO classification are listed in Appendix B.

81.7.1 General Aspects

The *malignant* tumors affecting the prostate with the potential for brain metastasis can roughly be grouped into:
- Prostatic adenocarcinoma

81.7.2 Neuropathology Findings

Histologic features of brain metastases from primary *prostate* tumors include:
- Prostatic adenocarcinoma (Fig. 81.16)
  - Small glands, back to back
  - Single cell layer of cuboidal or low columnar epithelium (no basal cell layer)

Table 81.23 Summary of common immunostaining markers in renal epithelial neoplasms, modified after (Lin and Yang 2015) reproduced with kind permission by Springer Nature

Antibodies	Clear cell renal cell carcinoma (CRCC)	Papillary renal cell carcinoma (PRCC)	Chromophobe renal cell carcinoma (ChRCC)	Oncocytoma	Collecting duct carcinoma (CDC)	Mucinous tubular and spindle cell carcinoma (MTSCC)	Urothelial carcinoma (UC)
EMA	+	+	+	+	+	+	+
CK7	−	+	+	−	+	+	+
CK20	−	−	−	−	−	−	+ or −
CK903	−	−	−	−	+	−	+
p63	−	−	−	−	−	+	−
CD10	+	+	− or +	− or +	−	−	−
KIM-1 a	+	+	−	−	−	ND	−
PAX2/PAX8	+	+	+ or −	+	+	−	−
RCCMa	+	+	− or +	−	−	−	−
CD117	−	−	+	+	+	−	−
S100A1	+	+ or −	−	+	−	−	−
S100P	−	−	−	−	−	−	+
CD15	−	−	−	+ or −	−	−	+ or −
GST-alpha	+	− or +	−	− or +	ND	−	ND
Vimentin	+	+ or −	−	−	+	−	−
Ksp-cad	− or +	−	+	+	−	−	−
P504S (AMACR)	− or +	+	−	−	−	+ or −	−
CA IX	+	− or +	−	−	− or +	ND	− or +
pVHL	+	+	+	+	ND	ND	−

81.7 Prostate Tumors

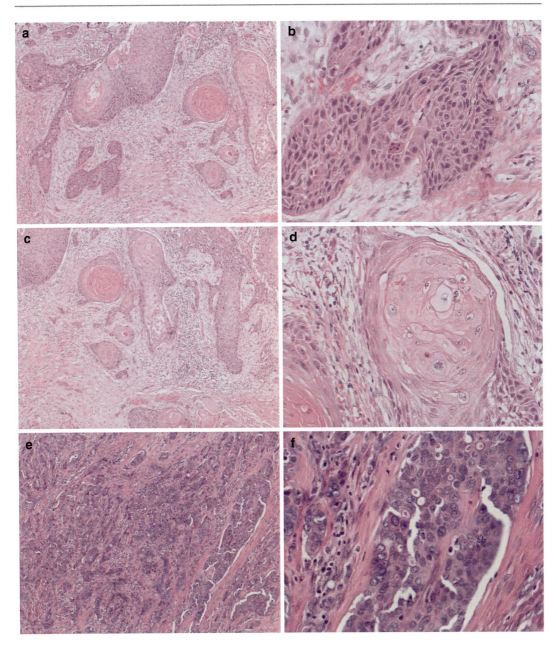

Fig. 81.14 Urinary bladder: The tumor shows squamous differentiation (**a–d**) with formation of keratinized structures (**c, d**) and strongly diffuse infiltrative growth (**e–h**). Immunophenotype: The tumor cells are positive for pan-cytokeratin AE1/AE3 (**i, j**), and p63 (**k, l**)

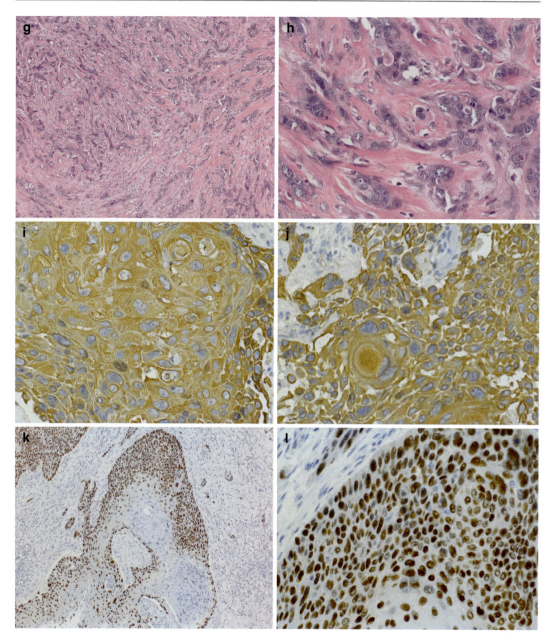

Fig. 81.14 (continued)

81.7 Prostate Tumors

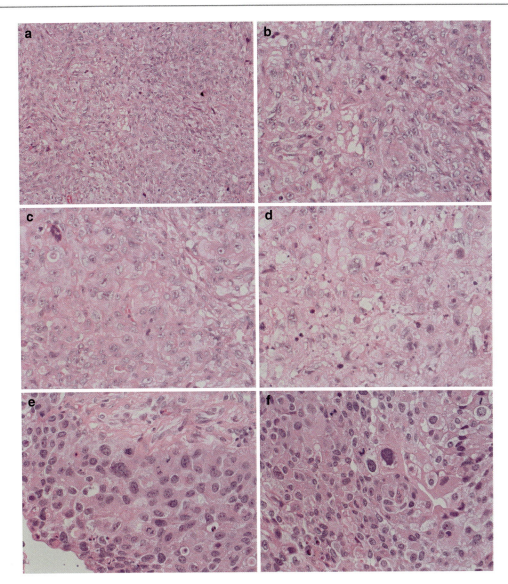

Fig. 81.15 Urothelial carcinoma: The tumor shows a solid growth pattern (**a–d**) with partial squamous differentiation (**e, f**). Immunophenotype: The tumor cells are positive for CK7 (**g**), CK18/19 (**h**), thrombomodulin (**i**), GATA3 (**j**), and p63 (**k**). High proliferative activity (**l**, stain: Ki-67)

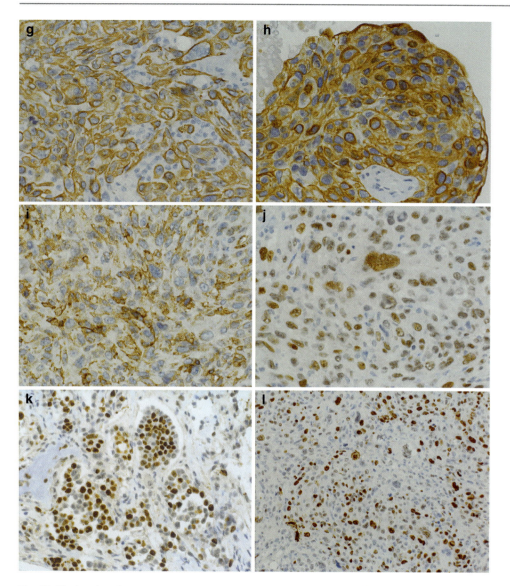

Fig. 81.15 (continued)

Table 81.24 Markers for urothelial carcinoma vs. squamous lesions in the bladder, modified after Wilkerson and Cheng (2015b) reproduced with kind permission by Springer Nature

Antibodies	Urothelial carcinoma (UC)	Urothelial carcinoma with squamous differentiation (UCSq)	Squamous cell carcinoma, bladder primary (SqCBl)
S100P	+	+	− or +
GATA3	+	− or +	−
CK14	− or +	+	+
Desmoglein	−	+ or −	+
UPIII	+ or −	− or +	−
p16		− or +	− or +
TM	+ or −	ND	+
CK20	+ or −	ND	ND
CK7	+	ND	ND
TRIM29	ND	+	+
MAC387	ND	+	+

81.7 Prostate Tumors

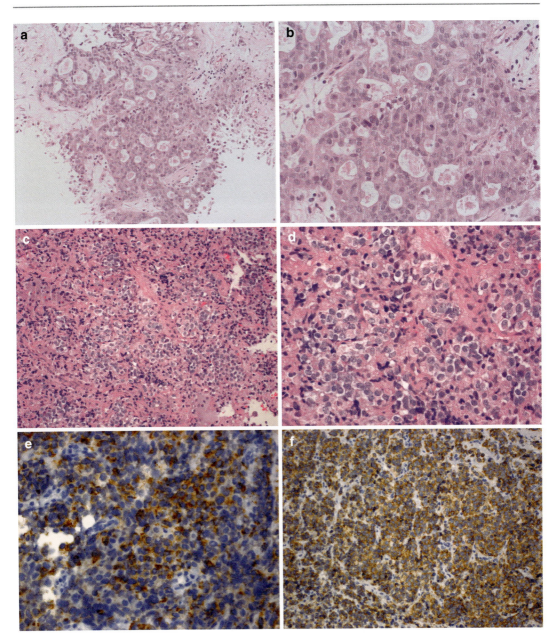

Fig. 81.16 Prostate: The tumor shows adenoid architecture (**a**, **b**) or a solid growth pattern (**c**, **d**). Immunophenotype: The tumor cells are positive for prostate-specific antigen (PSA) (**e**), p504s (**f**), prostate-specific membrane antigen (PSMA) (**g**), molecular high weight cytokeratin (**h**), and pancytokeratin AE1/AE3 (**i**)

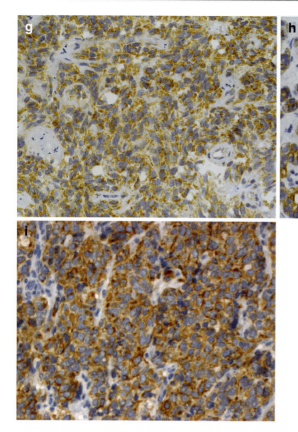

Fig. 81.16 (continued)

- Prominent nucleoli
- No recognizable glandular structures
- Infiltration in rows
- Mucin production possible

81.7.3 Immunophenotype

The immunophenotype of prostate carcinoma and its various types is given in Tables 81.25 and 81.26.

81.8 Testicular Tumors

The various testicular tumors as distinguished by the WHO classification are listed in Appendix B.

81.8.1 General Aspects

The *malignant* tumors affecting the testis with the potential for brain metastasis can roughly be grouped into:

- Germ cell tumor
  - Seminoma
  - Embryonal carcinoma
  - Yolk sac tumor
  - Choriocarcinoma
  - Teratoma
- Non-germ cell tumor
  - Sex cord-stromal tumor
  - Leydig cell tumor

81.8.2 Neuropathology Findings

Histologic features of brain metastases from primary *testicular tumors* include:
- Seminoma
  - Large mononuclear cells with clear cytoplasm
  - Fibrous septae with lymphocytes
- Embryonal carcinoma
  - Alveolar or tubular architecture

81.8 Testicular Tumors

Table 81.25 Markers for prostatic adenocarcinoma, modified after Liu et al. (2015), reproduced with kind permission by Springer Nature

Antibody	Pattern	Frequencies
P504S	+	97.8%
p63	–	–
PSA	+	100%
CK7	–	3.7%
ERG	– or +	38.1%
NKX3.1	+	100%
CK5/6	–	–
CK903	–	–
CAM 5.2	+	100%
AE1/AE3	+	88.4%
CK20	–	2.9%
MUC1	+	63%

- Pleomorphic, primitive looking cells
- Abundant mitotic figures
- Yolk sac tumor
  - Various histologic patterns
  - Schiller-Duval bodies
    - Capillary at the core surrounded by a visceral and a parietal layer
    - Resemble endodermal sinuses
- Choriocarcinoma
  - Syncytiotrophoblasts (multinucleated cells)
  - Cytotrophoblasts
- Teratoma
  - Mature teratoma
    - Fully differentiated tissue from all three germlines

Table 81.26 Markers for the differentiation between various types of prostate carcinoma, modified after Liu et al. (2015), reproduced with kind permission by Springer Nature

Antibody	Basal cell carcinoma	Mucinous adenocarcinoma	Ductal adenocarcinoma	Signet ring cell carcinoma	Small cell carcinoma	Squamous cell carcinoma
p63	+		–		– or +	+
CK903	+	–	–	–	– or +	+
Bcl 2	+					
P504S	–		+ or –			
CK7	+	–			+ or –	–
CK5/6	+		–			+
PSA	–	+	+ or –	+ or –	– or +	–
PSAP	–	+	+ or –	+ or –	– or +	–
P501S					– or +	
AE1/AE3	+			+	+	
CK20	–	–			–	–
CEA		–				
CDX-2		–				
PAS-D				+		
Mucicarmine				+ or –		
Alcian Blue				+ or –		
CAM 5.2				+	+ or –	
Chromogranin					+	
CD 56					+	
TTF-1					+ or –	
CD44					+	
Synaptophysin					+	
AR					– or +	
C-kit (CD117)					+	
Bcl2					+	
EGFR					+ or –	

- Immature teratoma
  - Areas of tumor appear as fetal or embryonic tissue

Seminoma is radiosensitive
Choriocarcinoma responsive to chemotherapy

81.8.3 Immunophenotype

The immunophenotype of germ cell tumors is given in Table 81.27.

81.9 Gastro-Intestinal Tumors

The various gastro-intestinal tumors as distinguished by the WHO classification are listed in Appendix B.

81.9.1 General Aspects

Based on the WHO Classification of tumors of the digestive system, the following organs are separated:
- Esophagus

Table 81.27 Markers for germ cell tumors, modified after Wilkerson and Cheng (2015a) reproduced with kind permission by Springer Nature

Antibodies	Intratubular germ cell neoplasia	Classic seminoma	Spermatocytic seminoma	Embryonal carcinoma	Yolk sac tumor	Choriocarcinoma	Teratoma
PLAP	+	+	−	+	− or +	+ or −	−
SALL4	+	+	+	+	+	+	− or +
OCT4	+	+	−	+	−	−	−
CD30	−	−	−	+	−	−	ND
SOX17	+	+ or −	−	−	− or +	−	ND
AFP	−	−	−	− or +	+	−	−
GPC3	−	−	−	− or +	+	− or +	ND
GATA3	ND	−	−	− or +	+	+	ND
c-kit		+	− or +	− or +	− or +	−	− or +
NANOG	+	+	−	+	−	−	−
LIN28	+	+	− or +	+	+	+ or −	− or +
D2-40	+	+	−	− or +	−	−	−
CD44	+	+	ND	ND	ND	ND	ND
AE1/AE3	−	− or +	−	+	+	+	+
SP1	ND	−	−	−	ND	+	ND
HPL	ND	−	−	− or +	−	+	ND
CD10	ND	+	ND	ND	ND	+	ND
EMA	ND	−	ND	−	−	− or +	ND
INHA	−	−	−	−	−	+	ND
Vim	ND	− or +	− or +	−	− or +	−	ND
NSE	+	+	−	+ or −	+ or −	− or +	ND
CK18	ND	ND	+	+	+	+	ND
p53	+	+	+	+	−	−	ND
CEA	ND	−	−	− or +	− or +	+ or −	ND
hCG	−	−	−	−	−	+	−
A-AT	ND	− or +	ND	− or +	+	− or +	−
CD99	−	−	ND	−	− or +	−	ND
CAM 5.2	−	− or +	− or +	+	+	+	+
Chrom	−	−	−	−	− or +	−	− or +
S100	−	−	−	− or +	−	−	ND
Desmin	ND	− or +	−	−	ND	ND	ND
SOX2	−	−	−	+	−	−	ND
CDX2	−	−	−	− or +	− or +	+	+ or −
SF-1	−	−	ND	−	− or +	−	ND

- Stomach
- Ampullary region
- Small intestine
- Appendix
- Colon and rectum
- Anal canal
- Liver and intrahepatic bile duct
- Gallbladder and extrahepatic bile ducts
- Pancreas

The *malignant* tumors affecting the GI tract with the potential for brain metastasis can roughly be grouped into:
- Adenocarcinoma of the colon
- Hepatocellular carcinoma
- Cholangiocarcinoma

81.10 Colon Carcinoma

81.10.1 Neuropathology Findings

Histologic features of brain metastases from primary *colon carcinoma* include:
- Adenocarcinoma (Fig. 81.17)
  - Tall columnar cells
  - Gland formation
  - Mucin production
  - Signet ring cells

81.10.2 Immunophenotype

The immunophenotype of colorectal cancers is given in Tables 81.28, 81.29, and 81.30.

81.11 Esophageal Carcinoma

81.11.1 Neuropathology Findings

Histologic features of brain metastases from primary *esophageal carcinoma* include:
- Squamous cell carcinoma
  - Solid nests of neoplastic cells
  - Abundant pink cytoplasm
  - Distinct cell borders
- Adenocarcinoma
  - Intestinal-type tubular neoplasm
  - Glandular structures with central lumen
  - Papillary, mucinous, and signet ring cell

81.12 Gastric Carcinoma

81.12.1 Neuropathology Findings

Histologic features of brain metastases from primary *gastric* include:
- Gastric adenocarcinoma (Fig. 81.18)
- Increased nuclear to cytoplasm ratio
- Nuclear hyperchromatism
- Gland formation possible
- Marked pleomorphism
- Cytoplasm filled with clear vacuoles of mucin with nucleus displaced to the periphery "signet ring"

81.12.2 Immunophenotype

The immunophenotype of esophageal and gastric carcinomas is given in Table 81.31.

81.13 Liver Carcinoma

81.13.1 Neuropathology Findings

Histologic features of brain metastases from primary *liver carcinoma* include:
- Hepatocellular carcinoma (Fig. 81.19)
  - Large, hyperchromatic and irregular nuclei
  - Breakdown in architecture (can form cords)
  - Areas of necrosis
- Cholangiocarcinoma
  - Glandular appearance
  - Mucin production possible

81.13.2 Immunophenotype

The immunophenotype of hepatocellular carcinoma and cholangiocarcinoma is given in Tables 81.32 and 81.33.

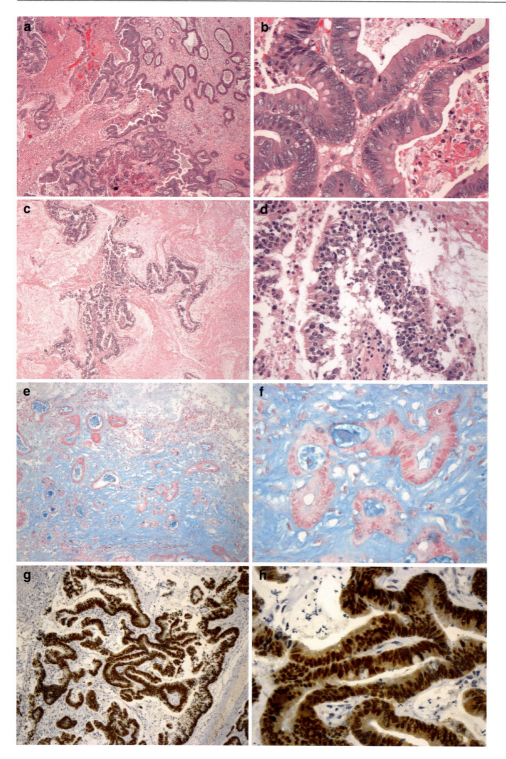

Fig. 81.17 Colon Rectum: The tumor shows a papillary architecture (**a–d**) with secretion of mucinous substances (**e–f**, stain: Alcian blue). Immunophenotype: The tumor cells are positive for CDX2 (**g, h**)

81.13 Liver Carcinoma

Table 81.28 Staining patterns of commonly used markers in usual colorectal adenocarcinoma, modified after Chen et al. (2015a) reproduced with kind permission by Springer Nature

Markers	Frequencies
AE1/3	97%
CK7	3%
CK20	97%
CDH17	97%
SATB2	97%
CK17	0
CK19	16%
CAM5.2	100%
MUC1	16%
MUC2	55%
MUC4	74%
MUC5AC	26%
MUC	68%
ER	0
PR	0
GCDFP-15	0
S100P	55
IMP3 (KOC)	50%
Maspin	89%
pVHL	16%
CA19-9	55%
CDX2	95%
TTF-1	0
CEA	100%
MOC31	100%
BerEP4	100%
CD10	16%
Vimentin	0
Beta-catenin	63%
Villin	82%
Napsin A	29%
Hep Par1	11%
P504S	90%

Table 81.29 Different staining patterns between usual colonic adenocarcinoma and some of its unique variants, modified after Chen et al. (2015a) reproduced with kind permission by Springer Nature

Markers	Usual colonic adenocarcinoma	Mucinous/signet ring cell carcinoma	Medullary carcinoma Literature	Medullary carcinoma GML	Micropapillary carcinoma
CDH17	+	+ or −	+ or −	89%	+
SATB2	+	+ or −	+ or −	89%	+
CDX2	+	− or +	− or +	67%	+
CK7	−	− or +	− or +	6%	−
CK20	+	+ or −	− or +	28%	+
MSI	Absent	Present in about 50% of cases	Present in >80% of cases	83%	Usually absent
Calretinin	−	− or +	+ or −	67%	−
MUC1	− or +	"−" in signet ring cell carcinoma	− or +	N/D	Positive in basal-lateral aspects of the tumor cells at the tumor-stromal interface

Table 81.30 Markers to differentiate common mesenchymal tumors of the colon and rectum, modified after Chen et al. (2015a) reproduced with kind permission by Springer Nature

Marker	Gastrointestinal stromal tumor (GIST)	Leiomyosarcoma	Schwannoma	Kaposi sarcoma	Solitary fibrous tumor (SFT)	Granular cell tumor
Desmin	− or +	+	−	−	−	−
SMA	− or +	+	−	+ or −	−	−
CD117	+	−	−	− or +	−	−
CD34	+ or −	−	−	+	+	−
S100	−	−	+	−	−	+
NSE	−	−	+ or −	−	−	−
HHV8	−	+	−	+	−	−
CD99	−	−	−	−	+	−
Bcl2	−	−	−	+/−	+ or −	−

81.13 Liver Carcinoma

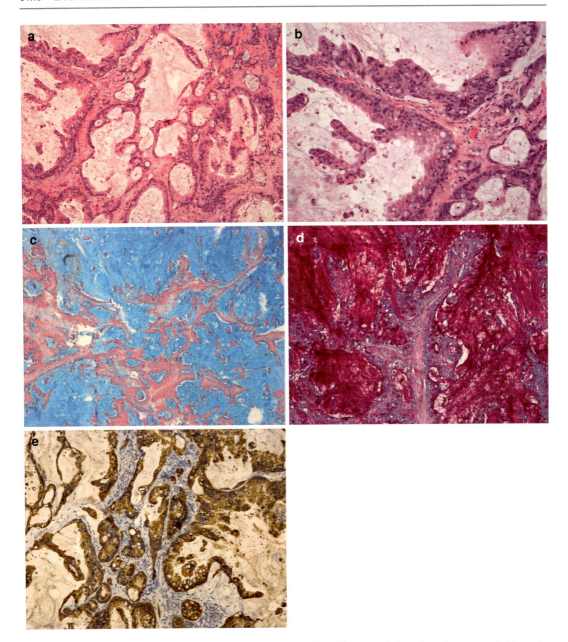

Fig. 81.18 Stomach: The tumor shows a papillary structure (**a, b**) with accumulation of mucinous material (**c**: stain: Alcian blue; **d**: stain: PAS). Immunophenotype: The tumor cells are positive for AE1/AE3 (**e**)

Table 81.31 Markers for esophageal and gastric adenocarcinoma, modified after Li and Lin (2015), reproduced with kind permission by Springer Nature

Antibodies	Esophageal adenocarcinoma	Gastric adenocarcinoma
AE1/AE3	100%	100%
CK7	83%	83%
CK20	37%	61%
CK5/6		0
CK903		6%
CAM 5.2	100%	
MUC1	27%	13%
MUC2	7% focal	17%
MUC4	37%	22%
MUC5AC	43%	0
MUC6	40%	0
ER/PR	0	0
GCDFP-15	0	0
S100P	73%	67%
IMP-3 (KOC) 5	7%	56%
Maspin	100%	67%
CDX-2	43%	39%
TTF1	0	0
CEA	83%	ND
MOC-31	100%	67%
Ber-EP4	100%	67%
TAG 7	2 (B72.3) 30%	
Napsin A	17%	
Hep Par1	33%	
P504S	73%	
SATB-2	7%	
CDH-17	66%	25%
VHL		0
CA19-9		39%
CD10		28%

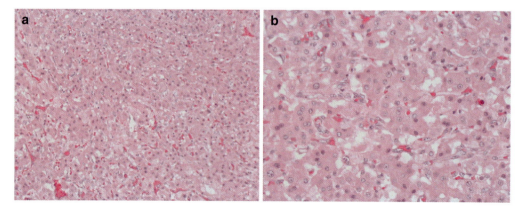

Fig. 81.19 Liver: The tumor cells have cuboidal shape and round pale nuclei (**a, b**); bile may be seen in the canaliculi (**c, d**). Immunophenotype: The tumor cells are positive for AE1/AE3 (**e, f**), hepatocyte marker (**g, h**), and CK18 (**i, j**)

81.13 Liver Carcinoma

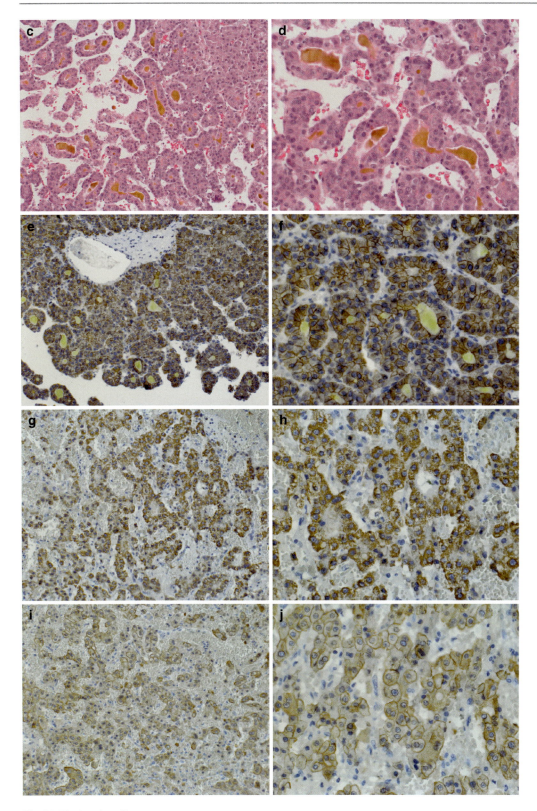

Fig. 81.19 (continued)

Table 81.32 Marker for the differentiation between hepatocellular carcinoma and cholangiocarcinoma, modified after Chen et al. (2015b), reproduced with kind permission by Springer Nature

Markers	Hepatocellular carcinoma	Cholangiocarcinoma
Arginase 1	+	−
HepPar 1	+	−
AFP	− or +	−
pCEA	+ (canalicular)	+ (non-canalicular)
Glypican-3	+	−
CD10	+ (canalicular)	− or + (cytoplasmic or brushing border)
MOC-31	− or +	+
CK7	− or +	+
CK19	−	+

Table 81.33 Summary of common markers in common lesions, modified after Chen et al. (2015b), reproduced with kind permission by Springer Nature

Markers or antibodies	Hepatocellular carcinoma (HCC)	Cholangiocarcinoma (CC) intrahepatic	Cholangiocarcinoma (CC) extrahepatic
Arginase 1	+	−	−
HepPar 1	+	−	−
AFP	+ or −	−	−
Glypican-3	+ or −	−	−
pCEA	+ (canalicular)	+ or −	+ or −
mCEA	−	+ or −	+ or −
CD10	+ or − (canalicular)	− or +	−
Villin	− or + (canalicular)	− or +	− or +
CD34	+ (sinusoidal)	−	−
MOC-31	− or +	+	+
CD56	−	+ or −	−
CK7	− or +	+	+
CK19	−	+	+
CK20	−	− or +	− or +
CAM 5.2	+	+	+
CK AE1/3	− or +	+	+
S100	−	−	−
HMB-45	−	−	−
Vimentin	−	− or +	− or +
ER	−	−	−
PR	− or +	−	−
S100P	− or +	− or +	+ or −
pVHL	− or +	+ or −	−
IMP3 (KOC)	− or +	− or +	+
Maspin	−	− or +	+

81.14 Pancreas

81.14.1 Neuropathology Findings

Histologic features of brain metastases from primary *pancreatic carcinoma* include:
- Pancreatic adenocarcinoma (Fig. 81.20)
- Irregular gland formation
- Intracytoplasmic mucin production

81.14.2 Immunophenotype

The immunophenotype of pancreatic carcinomas is given in Tables 81.34 and 81.35.

81.15 Female Genital Tract

The various tumors affecting the female genital tract as distinguished by the WHO classification are listed in Appendix B.

81.15.1 General Aspects

Tumors affecting the female genital tract can be divided by organ in tumors of:
- Ovary
- Peritoneum
- Fallopian tube
- Broad ligament and other uterine ligaments
- Uterine corpus
- Gestational trophoblastic disease
- Uterine cervix
- Vagina
- Vulva

81.16 Ovarian Carcinoma

The *malignant* tumors affecting the ovary with the potential for brain metastasis can roughly be grouped into:
- Surface epithelial tumors
    - Serous carcinoma
    - Mucinous

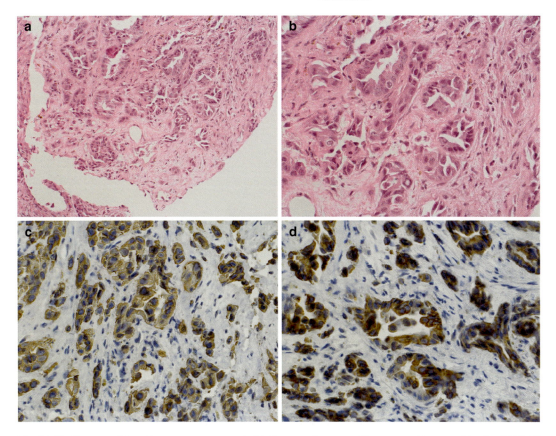

Fig. 81.20 Pancreas: Adenoid structures are seen (**a**, **b**). Immunophenotype: The tumor cells are positive for AE1/AE3 (**c**) and CK18 (**d**)

Table 81.34 Markers for ductal adenocarcinoma of the pancreas, modified after Lin and Wang (2015), reproduced with kind permission by Springer Nature

Antibodies	Literature	Frequency
pVHL	−	100
Maspin	+	100
IMP-3	+	90
S100P	+	96
S100A6	+	96
CAM5.2	+	75
CK7	+	96
CK20	− or focally +	15
CK17	+	60
CK19	+	75
Mesothelin	+	57
mCEA	+	85
MOC-31	+	97
CA19-9	+	84
Annexin A8	+	ND
MUC1	+	95
MUC2	−	4
MUC4	+	50
MUC5AC	+	67
MUC6	− or +	17
Claudin 4	+	94
Claudin 18	+	80
PSCA	+ or −	56
DPC4/SMAD4	+ or −	41
p53	+ or −	60
CDX-2	− or +	5
Fascin	+	85
CDH17	+ or −	18
Annexin A10	+	ND
AKR1B10	+	ND
Plectin-1	+	ND

Table 81.35 Markers for various types of pancreatic carcinoma, modified after Lin and Wang (2015), reproduced with kind permission by Springer Nature

Antibodies	Adenosquamous carcinoma of the pancreas	Colloid carcinoma	Medullary carcinoma	Undifferentiated carcinoma	Signet ring cell carcinoma	Hepatoid carcinoma
CK7	+	+	+	+ or −	+	+ or −
CK19	+			+ or −		
CEA	+	+	+ or −	+ or −	+	
CA19-9	+	+	+ or −	+ or −	+ or −	
CK5/6	+					
CK903	+					
p63	+					
MUC1		− or +		+ or −		
MUC2		+				
CDX-2		+			+ or −	
CK20		+ or −	−	−	+ or −	

81.16 Ovarian Carcinoma

Table 81.35 (continued)

Antibodies	Adenosquamous carcinoma of the pancreas	Colloid carcinoma	Medullary carcinoma	Undifferentiated carcinoma	Signet ring cell carcinoma	Hepatoid carcinoma
pVHL		−				
S100P		+				
IMP-3		+				
Maspin		+				
MLH1			+ or −			
MSH2			+ or −			
MSH6			+ or −			
PMS2			+ or −			
E-cadherin			+	−		
Vimentin				+ or −		
MSI markers				+		
MOC-31					+	
Hep Par 1						+
Polyclonal CEA Canalicular						+
CD10 Canalicular						+
AFP						+ or −
Bile stain						+ or −

- Endometrioid
- Clear cell
- Brenner or transitional
- Germ cell tumors
  - Teratoma
- Sex cord-stromal
  - Thecoma
  - Granulosa cell tumor

81.16.1 Neuropathology Findings

Histologic features of brain metastases from primary *ovarian carcinoma* include:
- Surface epithelial tumors (Fig. 81.21)
  - Serous carcinoma
    ○ Micropapillary serous carcinoma: medusa-head pattern, flower-like shaped tumor nests, nuclei point outwards
    ○ High-grade serous carcinoma: mitotically active, apoptotic, pleomorphic blue nuclei, papillary, micropapillary, solid architecture or in nests with slit-like spaces
  - Mucinous
    ○ Cystadenocarcinoma: well-differentiated to poorly differentiated carcinoma. G1: epithelial stratification, cytological atypia stromal invasion, G2: complex and small glands, greater stratification, areas of solid growth, G3: large sheets if solid tumor growth without glands, marked cytologic atypia, multinucleated tumor cells.
  - Endometrioid
    ○ Carcinoma: tubular to cribriform glands, villous structures
  - Clear cell
    ○ Carcinoma: clear cells in papillary, glandular, nested or trabecular patterns, hobnailed layer of cells outlining nests
  - Brenner or transitional
    ○ Very atypical cells
- Germ cell tumors
  - Teratoma
    ○ Composed of at least two of the three embryonic derivatives, often cystic, elements include squamous epithelium, skin adnexal structures, hair, fat, cartilage, thyroid, brain, etc.

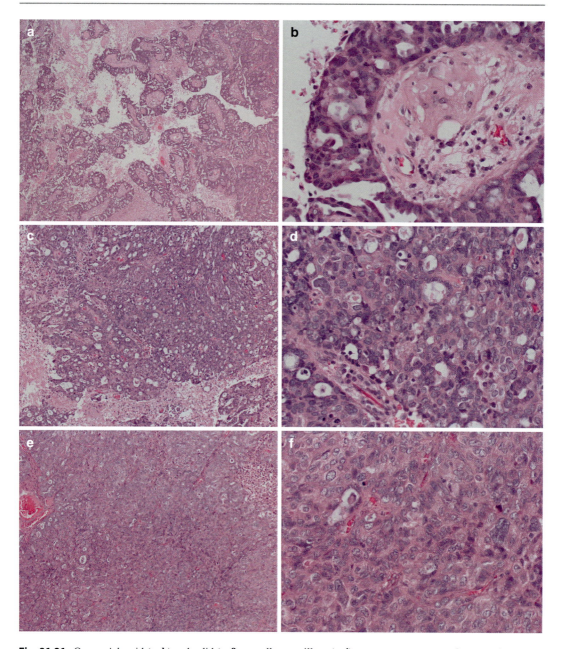

Fig. 81.21 Ovary: Adenoid (**a**, **b**) and solid (**c**–**f**) as well as papillary (**g**–**j**) structures are present. Immunophenotype: The tumor cells are positive for AE1/AE3 (**k**, **l**), CK7 (**m**, **n**), WT1 (**o**, **p**), p16 (**q**, **r**), PAX 8 (**s**, **t**), and p53 (**u**, **v**)

81.16 Ovarian Carcinoma

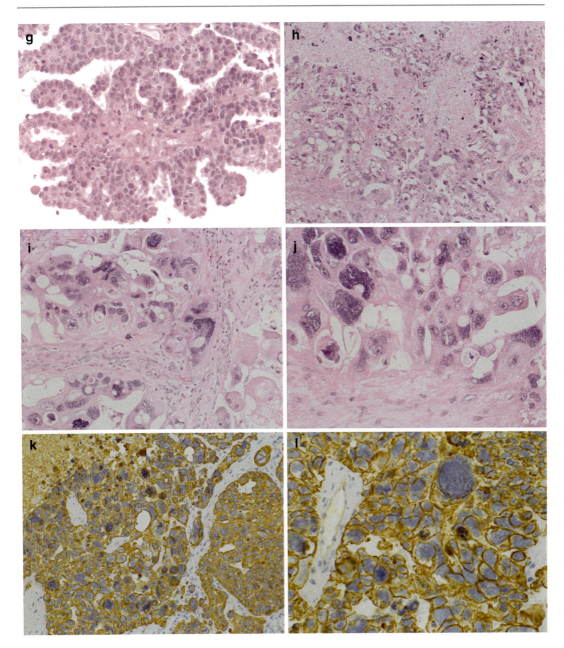

Fig. 81.21 (continued)

2098　81　Metastatic Tumors

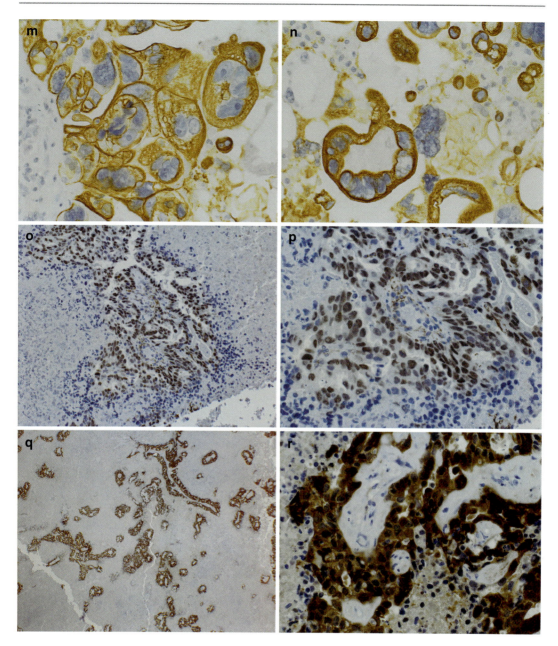

Fig. 81.21 (continued)

81.17 Carcinoma of the Vagina and Cervix

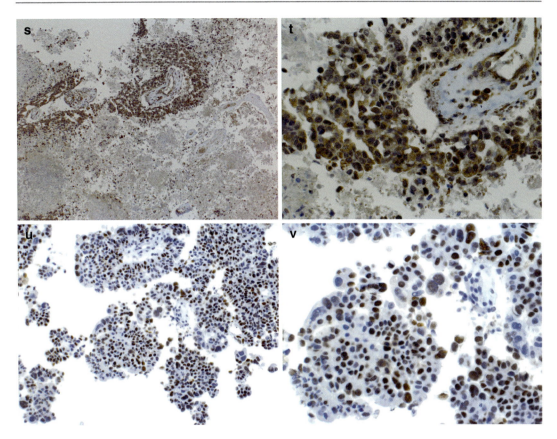

Fig. 81.21 (continued)

- Sex cord-stromal
  - Thecoma
    - Sheet-like pattern with bland, spindled cells
  - Granulosa cell tumor
    - Closely packed uniform appearing cells arranged in sheets with a zigzag "watered silk" pattern

81.16.2 Immunophenotype

The immunophenotype of ovarian cancers is given in Tables 81.36 and 81.37.

81.17 Carcinoma of the Vagina and Cervix

The *malignant* tumors affecting the *vagina and cervix* with the potential for brain metastasis can roughly be grouped into:

- Invasive squamous cell carcinoma
- Invasive adenocarcinoma

81.17.1 Neuropathology Findings

Histologic features of brain metastases from primary *cervical carcinoma* include:
- Invasive squamous cell carcinoma
  - Deep keratinization
  - Large nucleoli
  - Blurred or sawtooth interface between epithelium and stroma
  - Loss of palisading basal layer
  - Desmoplastic response within stroma
- Invasive adenocarcinoma
  - Close clusters of dark glands
  - Nuclei are tall, pseudostratified, enlarged and hyperchromatic
  - Luminal mitoses
  - Papillary or cribriform architecture

Table 81.36 Screening panel for common ovarian epithelial tumors, modified after Prichard and Kaspar (2015), reproduced with kind permission by Springer Nature

Antibodies	Serous	Clear cell	Intestinal type mucinous	Endometrioid	Transitional
WT1	+	−	−	−	+
p53	+	+	−/+	−/+	+
ER	+/−	−/+	−	+	−

Table 81.37 Markers for various types of ovarian tumors, modified after Prichard and Kaspar (2015), reproduced with kind permission by Springer Nature

Antibody	Serous	Mucinous	Clear cell	Endometrioid
AE1/AE3	+	+		+
AFP			−/+	
ARID1A				−/+
BerEP4	+	+		
CA125	+	−/+	−/+	
CAM5.2				+
Calretinin	−/+	−/+		−/+
CD15			+	
CD56	−			−/+
CD59				−/+
CDX2	−	−/+		
CEA	−	+/−		
Chromogranin				−/+
CK5/6	−	−		
CK7	+	+	+	+
CK19		+		
CK20	−	−/+		
D2-40	−	−		
EMA			+	+
ER	+/−	−/+	−/+	+
GCDFP-15	−	−		
Glypican-3	−	−	−/+	−/+
HepPar1	−	−		
HNF-1-ß			−	
HPV-IS				−
IMP(KOC)	−	ND		
INHA	−	−		
KIM-1	−	ND	+	
MOC31	+	+		
MUC1	ND	+		
MUC2	ND	+/−		
MUC4	ND	+/−		
MUC5AC	ND	+		
NapsinA	ND	ND		

(continued)

81.18 Uterine Carcinoma

Table 81.37 (continued)

Antibody	Serous	Mucinous	Clear cell	Endometrioid
OCT4	−	−		
p16	−	−/+		+
P504S	−	ND		
p53	−/+	−/+	−/+	−/+
PAX2	+	ND		
PAX8	+	−	+	
PR	+/−			+
RCC	−	−	−/+	
S100	−	−		
SALL-4			−/+	
Synaptophysin				−/+
TAG72	+			
TTF1	−	−	−/+	
VHL	ND	ND	+	
Vimentin	+	−		+
WT1	+	−		−/+

- Cell clusters diving off into the stroma
- Desmoplastic response

81.17.2 Immunophenotype

The immunophenotype of cervical carcinoma is given in Table 81.38.

81.18 Uterine Carcinoma

The *malignant* tumors affecting the *uterus* with the potential for brain metastasis can roughly be grouped into:
- Endometrioid carcinoma
- Serous carcinoma
- Clear cell carcinoma
- Endometrial stromal carcinoma

81.18.1 Neuropathology Findings

Histologic features of brain metastases from primary *uterine carcinoma* include:
- Endometrioid carcinoma
  - Cribriform or villoglandular pattern
  - Nuclear atypia
- Serous carcinoma
  - Papillary architecture
  - Extreme atypia, cherry-red nuclei, bizarre mitoses, multinucleated cells
- Clear cell carcinoma
  - Glycogen-rich and clear cytoplasm
  - Tubular, papillary, or solid architecture
- Endometrial stromal carcinoma
  - Minimal atypia, few mitoses
  - Prominent plexiform vascular proliferation

81.18.2 Immunophenotype

The immunophenotype of uterine carcinomas is given in Table 81.39.

Table 81.38 Markers for cervix carcinoma, modified after Kaspar and Crum (2015), reproduced with kind permission by Springer Nature

Antibodies	Invasive squamous cell carcinoma of the cervix	Invasive endocervical (mucinous) and endometrioid adenocarcinoma of cervix	In-situ and invasive intestinal-type endocervical adenocarcinoma
p63	+	−/+	
p16	+	+	+
CK (AE1, AE3)	+	+	+
CK5/6	+		
CK7	+	+	+
CK20			−
Bcl-2	+/−		
P53	+/−		
GATA3	−/+		
CEA-P	−/+	+	+
CEA-M		+	+
Bcl2	−/+		
PAX-8	−	+	
EMA		+	+
HepPar1		+	
ProEx C		+/−	
WT1		+/−	+/−
CA125		+/−	+/−
p53		+/−	−/+
MUC2		−/+	
MUC6		−/+	−/+
MUC1			+
MUC5AC			+
CDX-2		−/+	+
Vimentin		−/+	
PAX-2		−	
pRB			+
CD19-9			−/+

81.18 Uterine Carcinoma

Table 81.39 Summary of useful markers in common tumors of the uterus, modified after Kaspar and Crum (2015), reproduced with kind permission by Springer Nature

Antibodies	Cervical squamous cell carcinoma (SCCx)	Cervical Adenocarcinoma (AdenoCx)	Endometrial endometrioid adenocarcinoma (AdenoEM)	Endometrial serous carcinoma (SerEM)	Endometrial clear cell carcinoma (CCEM)	Endometrial stromal sarcoma (ESS)	Leiomyosarcoma (LMS)
P16	+	+	– or +	+ or –	+ or –	–	+ or –
P53	–	– or +	– or +	+	+ or –	– or +	– or +
P63	+	– or +	– or +	– or +	– or +	–	–
WT1	ND	+ or –	– or +	– or +	–	ND	– or +
CD10	–	–	–	–	–	+	– or +
ER	–	– or +	+	– or +	– or +	+	– or +
Vimentin	–	–	+	+	+	+	+
Desmin	–	–	–	–	–	– or +	+
PAX-8	–	–	+	+	ND	–	–
PR	–	– or +	+	– or +	– or +	+	+ or –
EMA	+	+	+	+	+	–	– or +
CK(AE1,AE3)	+	+	+	+	+	– or +	– or +
CK7	+	+	+	+	+	– or +	– or +
CK20	–	– or +	– or +	–	–	–	–
Calponin	–	–	–	–	–	+ or –	+
SMA	–	–	–	–	–	+ or –	+
S100	–	–	–	–	–	–	– or +
HMB45	–	–	–	–	–	–	– or +
MART-1	–	–	–	–	–	– or +	–

Selected References

Abate-Daga D, Ramello MC, Smalley I, Forsyth PA, Smalley KSM (2018) The biology and therapeutic management of melanoma brain metastases. Biochem Pharmacol 153:35–45. https://doi.org/10.1016/j.bcp.2017.12.019

Alexander BM, Brown PD, Ahluwalia MS, Aoyama H, Baumert BG, Chang SM, Gaspar LE, Kalkanis SN, Macdonald DR, Mehta MP, Soffietti R, Suh JH, van den Bent MJ, Vogelbaum MA, Wefel JS, Lee EQ, Wen PY (2018) Clinical trial design for local therapies for brain metastases: a guideline by the Response Assessment in Neuro-Oncology Brain Metastases working group. Lancet Oncol 19(1):e33–e42. https://doi.org/10.1016/s1470-2045(17)30692-7

Berghoff AS, Preusser M (2017) Targeted therapies for melanoma brain metastases. Curr Treat Options Neurol 19(4):13. https://doi.org/10.1007/s11940-017-0449-2

Bhargava R, Dabbs DJ (2018) Immunohistology of carcinoma of unknown primary site. In: Dabbs DJ (ed) Diagnostic immunohistochemistry. theranostic and genomic applications, 5th edn. Elsevier, Amsterdam, pp 219–260

Bohn JP, Pall G, Stockhammer G, Steurer M (2016) Targeted therapies for the treatment of brain metastases in solid tumors. Target Oncol 11(3):263–275. https://doi.org/10.1007/s11523-015-0414-5

Camidge DR, Lee EQ, Lin NU, Margolin K, Ahluwalia MS, Bendszus M, Chang SM, Dancey J, de Vries EGE, Harris GJ, Hodi FS, Lassman AB, Macdonald DR, Peereboom DM, Schiff D, Soffietti R, van den Bent MJ, Wefel JS, Wen PY (2018) Clinical trial design for systemic agents in patients with brain metastases from solid tumours: a guideline by the Response Assessment in Neuro-Oncology Brain Metastases working group. Lancet Oncol 19(1):e20–e32. https://doi.org/10.1016/s1470-2045(17)30693-9

Castro BA, Kuang R, Brastianos PK (2016) Novel approaches in genetic characterization and targeted therapy for brain metastases. Discov Med 22(122):237–250

Chamberlain MC, Baik CS, Gadi VK, Bhatia S, Chow LQ (2017) Systemic therapy of brain metastases: non-small cell lung cancer, breast cancer, and melanoma. Neuro Oncol 19(1):i1–i24. https://doi.org/10.1093/neuonc/now197

Chen ZE, Li J, Lin F (2015a) Lower gastrointestinal tract. In: Lin F, Prichard J (eds) Handbook of practical immunohistochemistry. Springer, Berlin, pp 543–555

Chen ZE, Prichard J, Lin F (2015b) Liver, bile ducts and gallbladder. In: Lin F, Prichard J (eds) Handbook of practical immunohistochemistry. Springer, Berlin, pp 503–523

Christensen TD, Spindler KL, Palshof JA, Nielsen DL (2016) Systematic review: brain metastases from colorectal cancer—incidence and patient characteristics. BMC Cancer 16:260. https://doi.org/10.1186/s12885-016-2290-5

Chukwueke UN, Brastianos PK (2017) Sequencing brain metastases and opportunities for targeted therapies. Pharmacogenomics 18(6):585–594. https://doi.org/10.2217/pgs-2016-0170

Ciminera AK, Jandial R, Termini J (2017) Metabolic advantages and vulnerabilities in brain metastases. Clin Exp Metastasis 34(6-7):401–410. https://doi.org/10.1007/s10585-017-9864-8

Devoid HM, McTyre ER, Page BR, Metheny-Barlow L, Ruiz J, Chan MD (2016) Recent advances in radiosurgical management of brain metastases. Front Biosci 8:203–214

Ferguson SD, Wagner KM, Prabhu SS, McAleer MF, McCutcheon IE, Sawaya R (2017) Neurosurgical management of brain metastases. Clin Exp Metastasis 34(6-7):377–389. https://doi.org/10.1007/s10585-017-9860-z

Ferringer T (2015) Skin. In: Lin F, Prichard J (eds) Handbook of practical immunohistochemistry. Springer, Berlin, pp 665–688

Fink KR, Fink JR (2013) Imaging of brain metastases. Surg Neurol Int 4(Suppl 4):S209–S219. https://doi.org/10.4103/2152-7806.111298

Garrett MD, Wu CC, Yanagihara TK, Jani A, Wang TJ (2016) Radiation therapy for the management of brain metastases. Am J Clin Oncol 39(4):416–422. https://doi.org/10.1097/coc.0000000000000296

Han CH, Brastianos PK (2017) Genetic characterization of brain metastases in the era of targeted therapy. Front Oncol 7:230. https://doi.org/10.3389/fonc.2017.00230

Hardesty DA, Nakaji P (2016) The current and future treatment of brain metastases. Front Surg 3:30. https://doi.org/10.3389/fsurg.2016.00030

Jandial R, Hoshide R, Waters JD, Somlo G (2018) Operative and therapeutic advancements in breast cancer metastases to the brain. Clin Breast Cancer 18(4):e455–e467. https://doi.org/10.1016/j.clbc.2017.10.002

Kaspar HG, Crum CP (2015) Uterus. In: Lin F, Prichard J (eds) Handbook of practical immunohistochemistry. Springer, Berlin, pp 343–369

Khalifa J, Amini A, Popat S, Gaspar LE, Faivre-Finn C (2016) Brain metastases from NSCLC: radiation therapy in the era of targeted therapies. J Thorac Oncol 11(10):1627–1643. https://doi.org/10.1016/j.jtho.2016.06.002

Kleihues P, Burger PC, Scheithauer BW (1993) Histological typing of tumours of the central nervous system, 2nd edn. Springer-Verlag, Berlin

Li J, Lin F (2015) Upper gastrointestinal tract. In: Lin F, Prichard J (eds) Handbook of practical immunohistochemistry. Springer, Berlin, pp 525–541

Lin X, DeAngelis LM (2015) Treatment of brain metastases. J Clin Oncol 33(30):3475–3484. https://doi.org/10.1200/jco.2015.60.9503

Lin F, Wang HL (2015) Pancreas and ampulla. In: Lin F, Prichard J (eds) Handbook of practical immunohistochemistry. Springer, Berlin, pp 481–502

Lin F, Yang XL (2015) Kidney. In: Lin F, Prichard J (eds) Handbook of practical immunohistochemistry. Springer, Berlin, pp 439–463

Lin J, Jandial R, Nesbit A, Badie B, Chen M (2015) Current and emerging treatments for brain metastases. Oncology 29(4):250–257

Liu H (2015) Breast. In: Lin F, Prichard J (eds) Handbook of practical immunohistochemistry. Springer, Berlin, pp 183–215

Liu H, Lin F, Zhai QJ (2015) Prostate gland. In: Lin F, Prichard J (eds) Handbook of practical immunohistochemistry. Springer, Berlin, pp 397–420

Lukas RV, Gondi V, Kamson DO, Kumthekar P, Salgia R (2017) State-of-the-art considerations in small cell lung cancer brain metastases. Oncotarget 8(41):71223–71233. https://doi.org/10.18632/oncotarget.19333

Matzenauer M, Vrana D, Melichar B (2016) Treatment of brain metastases. Biomed Papers 160(4):484–490. https://doi.org/10.5507/bp.2016.058

McGranahan T, Nagpal S (2017) A neuro-oncologist's perspective on management of brain metastases in patients with EGFR mutant non-small cell lung cancer. Curr Treat Options Oncol 18(4):22. https://doi.org/10.1007/s11864-017-0466-0

Mege D, Sans A, Ouaissi M, Iannelli A, Sielezneff I (2017) Brain metastases from colorectal cancer: characteristics and management. ANZ J Surg. https://doi.org/10.1111/ans.14107

Nam JY, O'Brien BJ (2017) Current chemotherapeutic regimens for brain metastases treatment. Clin Exp Metastasis 34(6-7):391–399. https://doi.org/10.1007/s10585-017-9861-y

Nelson JS, von Deimling A, Petersen I, Janzer RC (2000) Metastatic tumours of the CNS. In: Kleihues P, Cavenee WK (eds) Pathology and genetics of tumours of the nervous system, 3rd edn. IARC, Lyon, pp 250–253

Patil CG, Pricola K, Sarmiento JM, Garg SK, Bryant A, Black KL (2017) Whole brain radiation therapy (WBRT) alone versus WBRT and radiosurgery for the treatment of brain metastases. Cochrane Database Syst Rev 9:Cd006121. https://doi.org/10.1002/14651858.CD006121.pub4

Prichard J, Kaspar HG (2015) Ovary. In: Lin F, Prichard J (eds) Handbook of practical immunohistochemistry. Springer, Berlin, pp 371–395

Rancoule C, Vallard A, Guy JB, Espenel S, Diao P, Chargari C, Magne N (2017) Brain metastases from non-small cell lung carcinoma: changing concepts for improving patients' outcome. Crit Rev Oncol Hematol 116:32–37. https://doi.org/10.1016/j.critrevonc.2017.05.007

Schneider G, Schmidt-Supprian M, Rad R, Saur D (2017) Tissue-specific tumorigenesis: context matters. Nat Rev Cancer 17(4):239–253. https://doi.org/10.1038/nrc.2017.5

Shonka N, Venur VA, Ahluwalia MS (2017) Targeted treatment of brain metastases. Curr Neurol Neurosci Rep 17(4):37. https://doi.org/10.1007/s11910-017-0741-2

Specht HM, Combs SE (2016) Stereotactic radiosurgery of brain metastases. J Neurosurg Sci 60(3):357–366

Tan AC, Heimberger AB, Menzies AM, Pavlakis N, Khasraw M (2017) Immune checkpoint inhibitors for brain metastases. Curr Oncol Rep 19(6):38. https://doi.org/10.1007/s11912-017-0596-3

Thiagarajan A, Yamada Y (2017) Radiobiology and radiotherapy of brain metastases. Clin Exp Metastasis 34(6-7):411–419. https://doi.org/10.1007/s10585-017-9865-7

Tsao MN (2015) Brain metastases: advances over the decades. Ann Palliat Med 4(4):225–232. https://doi.org/10.3978/j.issn.2224-5820.2015.09.01

Vargo MM (2017) Brain tumors and metastases. Phys Med Rehabil Clin N Am 28(1):115–141. https://doi.org/10.1016/j.pmr.2016.08.005

Venur VA, Ahluwalia MS (2017) Novel therapeutic agents in the management of brain metastases. Curr Opin Oncol 29(5):395–399. https://doi.org/10.1097/cco.0000000000000393

Venur VA, Leone JP (2016) Targeted therapies for brain metastases from breast cancer. Int J Mol Sci 17(9):1543. https://doi.org/10.3390/ijms17091543

Wang S, Kim SJ, Poptani H, Woo JH, Mohan S, Jin R, Voluck MR, O'Rourke DM, Wolf RL, Melhem ER, Kim S (2014) Diagnostic utility of diffusion tensor imaging in differentiating glioblastomas from brain metastases. Am J Neuroradiol 35(5):928–934. https://doi.org/10.3174/ajnr.A3871

Waqar SN, Morgensztern D, Govindan R (2017) Systemic treatment of brain metastases. Hematol Oncol Clin North Am 31(1):157–176. https://doi.org/10.1016/j.hoc.2016.08.007

Wesseling P, von Deimling A, Aldape KD (2007) Metastatic tumours of the CNS. In: Louis DN, Ohgaki H, Wiestler OD, Cavenee WK (eds) WHO classification of tumours of the central nervous system, 4th edn. International Agency for Research on Cancer, Lyon, pp 248–251

Wesseling P, von Deimling A, Aldape KD, Preusser M, Rosenblum MK, Mittelbronn M, Tanaka S (2016) Metastatic tumours of the CNS. In: Louis DN, Ohgaki H, Wiestler OD, Cavenee WK (eds) WHO classification of tumours of the central nervous system, Revised 4th edn. IARC, Lyon, pp 338–341

Wilkerson ML, Cheng L (2015a) Testis and paratesticular tissues. In: Lin F, Prichard J (eds) Handbook of practical immunohistochemistry. Springer, Berlin, pp 465–480

Wilkerson ML, Cheng L (2015b) Urinary bladder and urachus. In: Lin F, Prichard J (eds) Handbook of practical immunohistochemistry. Springer, Berlin, pp 421–437

Wong A (2017) The emerging role of targeted therapy and immunotherapy in the management of brain metastases in non-small cell lung cancer. Front Oncol 7:33. https://doi.org/10.3389/fonc.2017.00033

Zhang K, Deng H, Cagle PT (2015) Pleuropulmonary and mediastinal neoplasms. In: Lin F, Prichard J (eds) Handbook of practical immunohistochemistry. Springer, Berlin, pp 313–341

Therapy-Induced Lesions

82.1 Introduction

The following therapy-associated neuropathologic changes are encountered:

- Radiation necrosis and fibrosis
- Therapy-induced leukoencephalopathies
- Therapy-induced vasculopathies
- Therapy-induced secondary neoplasms

Surgical complications include:
- Hemorrhage
- Vascular damage
- Infarcts
- Coagulopathies
- Malignant cerebral edema with herniation
- Postoperative infection

Tumor embolization complications include:
- Infarcts
- Hemorrhages
- Intratumoral necrosis
- Reactive changes

82.2 General Imaging Findings

- Phases
  - Acute: (1–6 weeks)
    - Edema
  - Early-delayed: (3 weeks–several months)
    - Periventricular, reversible white matter lesions +/− enhancement
  - Late-delayed: (months–years)
    - Necrosis
    - Demyelination
    - Gliosis
    - Vasculopathies
    - Calcifications
    - Atrophy
- Manifestations
  - Focal
    - Focal edema
    - Focal radiation necrosis
  - Diffuse
    - Leukoencephalopathy, necrotizing leukoencephalopathy
    - Mineralizing microangiopathies
    - Radiation-induced neoplasms
    - Radiation-induced vascular malformations (cavernomas and capillary telangiectasias
    - Radiation-induced vasculopathy

82.3 Radiation Necrosis

The following types of radiation necrosis can be distinguished:

- Acute
- Early-delayed
- Late-delayed

© Springer-Verlag GmbH Austria, part of Springer Nature 2019
S. Weis et al., *Imaging Brain Diseases*, https://doi.org/10.1007/978-3-7091-1544-2_82

82.3.1 Epidemiology

Incidence
- 5–25% of cases after conventional doses

Localization
- Area of primary site of brain tumor

82.3.2 Neuroimaging Findings

General
Irregular, peripheral enhancing lesion; mimicking tumor

CT non-contrast-enhanced
- Hypodense lesion

CT contrast-enhanced
- Irregular, ring enhancement around former tumor

MRI-T2 (Fig. 82.1a, g)
- Hyperintense

MRI-FLAIR (Fig. 82.1b, h)
- Hyperintense
- Surrounding edema

MRI-T1 (Fig. 82.1c, i)
- Hypointense

MRI-T1 contrast-enhanced (Fig. 82.1d, j)
- Peripheral accentuated, irregular, reticular enhancement

MR-Diffusion Imaging (Fig. 82.1e, k)
- Facilitated diffusion

MRI-Perfusion (Fig. 82.1f, l)
- rCBV decreased

MR-Diffusion Tensor Imaging
- Fractional anisotropy lower than in recurrent tumor

MR-Spectroscopy
- Reduced NAA, Cho, Cr peaks
- Lactate and lipid peaks possible

Differences between radiation injury and glioblastoma based on neuroradiology features have been published (Shah et al. 2012) and are summarized in Table 82.1.

Nuclear Medicine Imaging Findings (Fig. 82.2)
- FDG, MET, FET, FLT, and other radiotracers are used to differentiate brain tumors from radiation injury.
- Lower or even lacking uptake in radiation injury.
- Amino acid tracers are superior to FDG-PET in differentiating tumor from radiation injury.
- PET is known to demonstrate hypometabolism in acute to chronic brain radiation injury with a sensitivity of about 90% and a specificity of 40–94% in FDG-PET.
- Inflammatory processes have to be taken into account, which can show an uptake in FDG, MET and rarely in FET.
- Disrupted blood-brain barrier can result in false positive findings.
- Ideally the patient is screened 3 months after radiotherapy.
- Automated analysis can result in false negative or positive findings, depending on the reference region. Thus, visual interpretation should be done in every patient.

Differences between radiation injury and glioblastoma based on nuclear medicine features are shown in Table 82.2.

82.3.3 Neuropathology Findings

Macroscopic Features (Fig. 82.3)
- Firm
- Ill-defined
- Glioma-like (GBM)
- Hemorrhages
- Necroses (yellow to tan-brown)
- Cyst formation

82.3 Radiation Necrosis

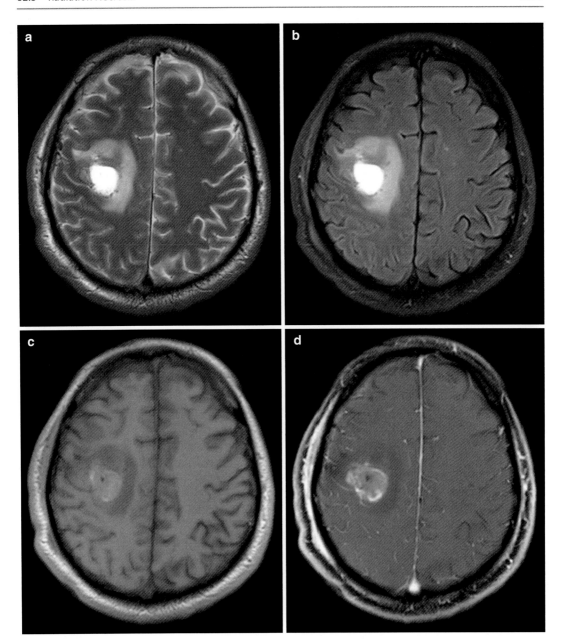

Fig. 82.1 Lesion in the right precentral gyrus after resection of a glioblastoma multiforme in T2 (**a**), FLAIR (**b**), T1 (**c**), T1 contrast (**d**), DWI (**e**), rCBV (**f**) and 4 months after radiation in T2 (**g**), FLAIR (**h**), T1 (**i**), T1 contrast (**j**), DWI (**k**), rCBV (**l**)

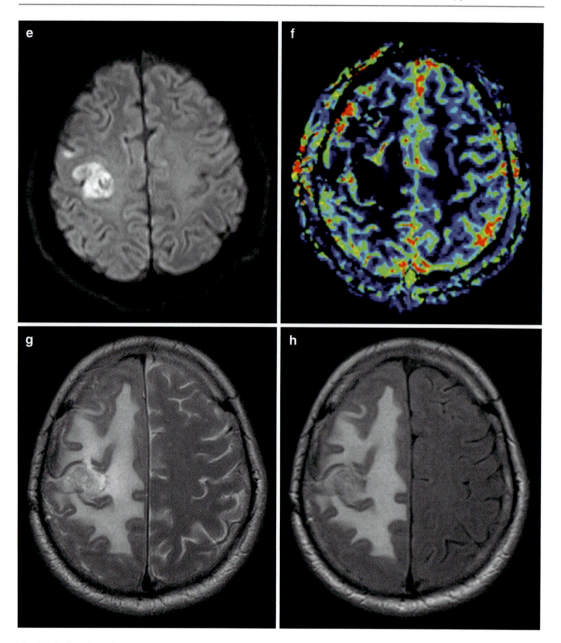

Fig. 82.1 (continued)

82.3 Radiation Necrosis

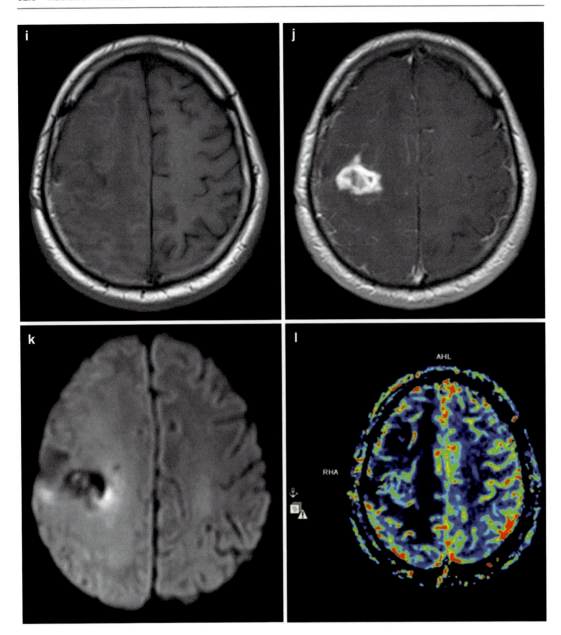

Fig. 82.1 (continued)

Table 82.1 Summary of differing features between radiation injury and glioblastoma

Radiology features	Radiation injury	Glioma recurrence/progression
CT	• Calcification • Mineralizing microangiopathy	• Rare calcifications
T1 contrast-enhanced	• Rim-enhancing • "Soap bubble" or "swiss cheese" interior	• Rim-enhancing • Homogeneous hypointense center
Diffusion imaging	• Heterogeneous • Hypointense	• Hyperintense
Perfusion MRI	• Decreased rCBV	• Increased rCBV
MR Spectroscopy	• Decreased peaks • No change in lactate peak • No change in lipid peak	• Increased choline peak

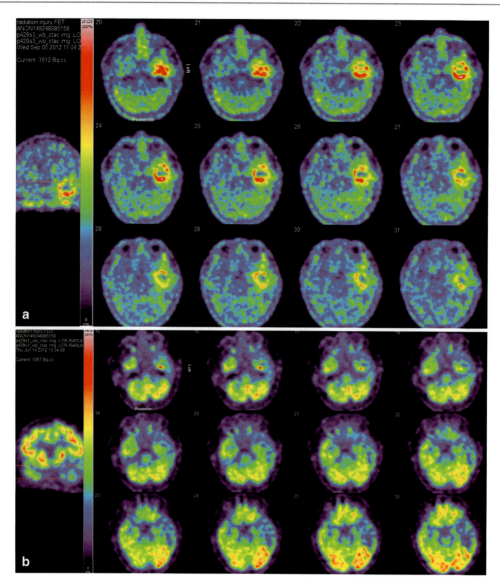

Fig. 82.2 Patient with a metastasis of a primary lung cancer after LINAC radiosurgery. The FET-PET scan shows a central necrosis most probably radiation-induced surrounded by vital tumor tissue (**a**). A corresponding FDG-PET scan with increased uptake (and higher background) as well as surrounding hypometabolism (resulting primarily from edema) is shown in (**b**)

Table 82.2 Differences between radiation injury and glioblastoma

Nuclear Medicine features	Radiation injury	Glioma recurrence/progression
FDG-PET	• Hypometabolism	• Hyper/Hypometabolism
FET-PET	• Hypometabolism	• Hypermetabolism

82.3 Radiation Necrosis

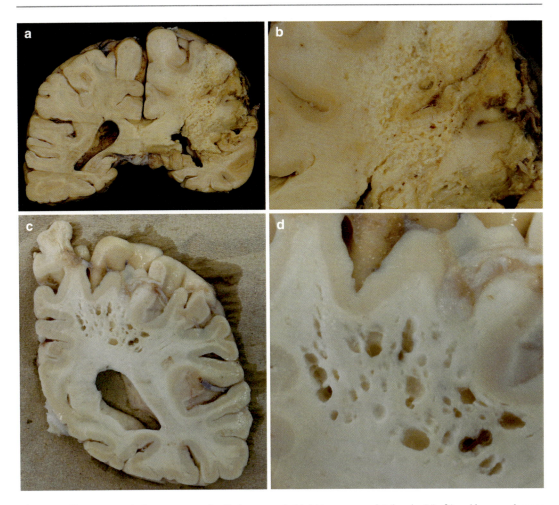

Fig. 82.3 Gross-anatomical appearance of radiation necrosis (right temporo-parietal region) (**a**, **b**) and lacunar changes in radiation injury (right parietal lobe) (**c**, **d**)

Microscopic Features (Figs. 82.4 and 82.5)
- Coagulative or fibrinoid necrosis (Fig. 82.4a, b)
- Vascular hyalinization with luminal stenosis (Fig. 82.4e, f)
- Fibrinoid vascular necrosis
- Rosenthal fibers (Fig. 82.4c, d)
- Hemorrhage
- Thrombosis
- Capillary telangiectasias
- Fibrosis
- Dystrophic calcifications
- Histiocytic infiltrates
- Myelin damage with myelin loss and reactive astrogliosis (Fig. 82.5a–d)

Radiation-induced cytologic atypia is characterized by:
- Increased nuclear polymorphism
- Accumulation of eosinophilic cytoplasm
- Cytomegalic cells with bizarre nuclei

Grading of glial tumors after radiation therapy should be avoided.

Differential Diagnosis
- Glioma recurrence/progression (see Table 82.3)

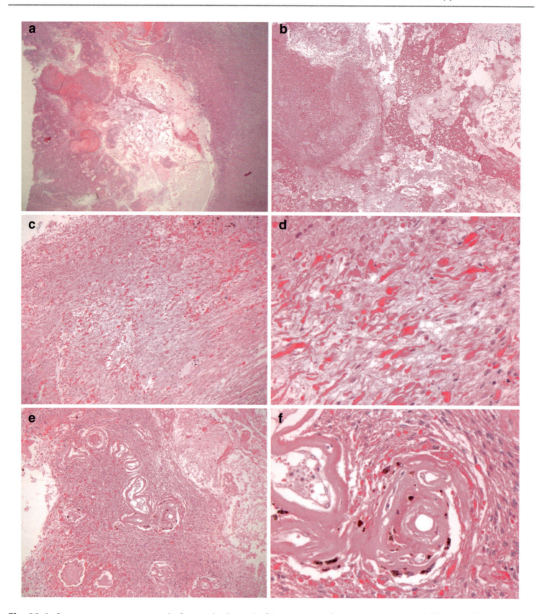

Fig. 82.4 Large areas are composed of necrotic tissue (**a**, **b**), presence of numerous Rosenthal fibers (**c**, **d**), hyalinized vessels (**e**, **f**) with perivascular hemosiderinophages (**f**)

82.3.4 Molecular Neuropathology

- Developing brain (infants, young children) is particularly vulnerable.
- Blood-brain barrier disruption and cerebral edema in acute and early-delayed.
- White matter is very susceptible.
  - U-fibers usually spared
  - Small to medium-sized vessels with susceptible endothelium
- Oligodendrocyte toxicity.
- Coagulopathies.
- Autoimmune vasculitis.

82.3 Radiation Necrosis

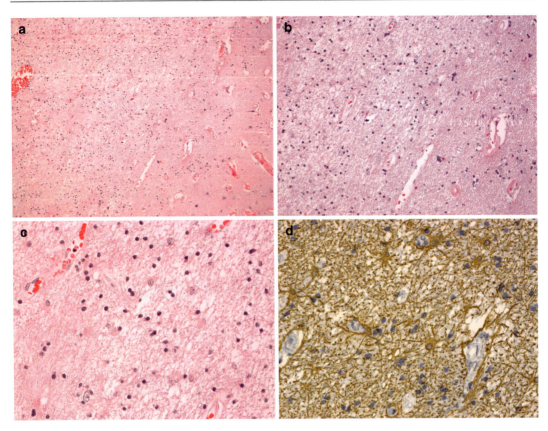

Fig. 82.5 White matter is rarefied (**a**, **b**) homing numerous reactive astrocytes (**c**, **d**) which stain positive for GFAP (**f**)

Table 82.3 Differences between radiation injury and glioblastoma

Histology features	Radiation injury	Glioma recurrence/progression
Necrosis	• Coagulative necrosis • Hypocellular edges • Dystrophic calcifications	• Large or microscopic foci • Hypercellular edges • Pseudopalisading edges
Blood vessels	• Telangiectatic • Hyalinized • Angionecrotic	• Microvascular proliferation
Mitoses	• Rare	• Frequent
Cytologic atypia	• Bizarre nuclei • Abundant cytoplasm	• High nuclear-to-cytoplasmic ratio
Adjacent brain	• Rarefied or vacuolated • Pale • Gliotic	• Nearly normal • Infiltrated by tumor cells

82.3.5 Treatment and Prognosis

Treatment
- Conservative therapy
  - Observation
  - Supportive care
- Apparent mass effect
  - Steroids
  - Debulking surgery
  - Hyperbaric oxygen

Biologic Behavior–Prognosis–Prognostic Factors
- Children long-term survivors develop:
  - Cognitive deficits
  - Low IQ
  - Learning disabilities
  - Hormonal deficits
  - Stunted growth
  - Psychomotor retardation
- Individual susceptibility.
- Predisposing factors are unknown.
- Neurofibromatosis type I patients at greater risk.

82.4 Therapy-Induced Leukoencephalopathy

Therapy-induced leukoencephalopathies can be subdivided as follows:

- Radiation leukoencephalopathy
- Chemotherapy-induced leukoencephalopathy
  - Methotrexate leukoencephalopathy
  - White matter based neurotoxic condition
  - Military, small rounded to large confluent areas of non-inflammatory demyelination
  - White matter necrosis
- Diffuse necrotizing leukoencephalopathy
  - Widespread and severe form
- Reversible posterior leukoencephalopathy
  - Milder and often reversible form

82.4.1 Clinical Signs

- Irritability
- Somnolence
- Ataxia
- Memory deficits
- Apathy
- Psychiatric disturbances

82.4.2 Neuroimaging Findings

General
Diffuse, symmetric white matter lesions, sparing U-fibers

CT non-contrast-enhanced
- Hypodense

CT contrast-enhanced
- No enhancement

MRI-T2
- Hyperintense

MRI-FLAIR
- Hyperintense

MRI-T1
- Hypointense

MRI-T1 contrast-enhanced
- No enhancement

MR-Diffusion Imaging
- No restricted diffusion

82.4.3 Neuropathology Findings

Microscopic Features
- Coagulative or fibrinoid necrosis
- Vascular hyalinization with luminal stenosis
- Fibrinoid vascular necrosis
- Hemorrhage
- Thrombosis
- Capillary telangiectasias
- Fibrosis
- Dystrophic calcifications
- Histiocytic infiltrates
- Myelin damage with myelin pallor and myelin loss

- Oligodendrocyte loss
- Axonal swelling
- Astrogliosis

Risk factor
- Hypertension

82.4.4 Molecular Neuropathology

- Toxic effects on
  - Axons
  - Oligodendrocytes
  - Myelin
  - Progenitor cells
- Secondary immunologic reactions
- Oxidative stress
- Microvascular injury

82.5 Therapy-Induced Secondary Neoplasms

Radiation-associated neoplasms should fulfill the following criteria (Cahan et al. 1998):

- Histologically different from the treated tumor
- Arise within the irradiation field
  - over a sufficient latency period (years)

Secondary, radiation-associated neoplasms affecting the brain include:

- Meningioma
- Nerve sheath tumors (benign and malignant)
- Pituitary adenomas
- Gliomas
- Sarcomas
- Embryonal neoplasms

82.5.1 Molecular Neuropathology

- Radiation-induced DNA mutations
- Predisposing genetic syndromes
  - Neurofibromatosis type I and II
  - Li–Fraumeni syndrome
- Childhood susceptibility
  - Radiation for ALL

Selected References

Alexiou GA, Tsiouris S, Kyritsis AP, Voulgaris S, Argyropoulou MI, Fotopoulos AD (2009) Glioma recurrence versus radiation necrosis: accuracy of current imaging modalities. J Neurooncol 95(1):1–11. https://doi.org/10.1007/s11060-009-9897-1

Cahan WG, Woodard HQ, Higinbotham NL, Stewart FW, Coley BL (1998) Sarcoma arising in irradiated bone: report of eleven cases. 1948. Cancer 82(1):8–34

Chao ST, Ahluwalia MS, Barnett GH, Stevens GH, Murphy ES, Stockham AL, Shiue K, Suh JH (2013) Challenges with the diagnosis and treatment of cerebral radiation necrosis. Int J Radiat Oncol Biol Phys 87(3):449–457. https://doi.org/10.1016/j.ijrobp.2013.05.015

Eisele SC, Dietrich J (2015) Cerebral radiation necrosis: diagnostic challenge and clinical management. Rev Neurol 61(5):225–232

Fink J, Born D, Chamberlain MC (2012) Radiation necrosis: relevance with respect to treatment of primary and secondary brain tumors. Curr Neurol Neurosci Rep 12(3):276–285. https://doi.org/10.1007/s11910-012-0258-7

Furuse M, Nonoguchi N, Kawabata S, Miyatake S, Kuroiwa T (2015) Delayed brain radiation necrosis: pathological review and new molecular targets for treatment. Med Mol Morphol 48(4):183–190. https://doi.org/10.1007/s00795-015-0123-2

Giglio P, Gilbert MR (2003) Cerebral radiation necrosis. Neurologist 9(4):180–188. https://doi.org/10.1097/01.nrl.0000080951.78533.c4

Hustinx R, Pourdehnad M, Kaschten B, Alavi A (2005) PET imaging for differentiating recurrent brain tumor from radiation necrosis. Radiol Clin North Am 43(1):35–47

Jandial R, Duenas VJ, Chen BT (2011) Molecular imaging based on differential protein content in differentiating glioma from radiation necrosis. Neurosurgery 68(6):N16–N17. https://doi.org/10.1227/01.neu.0000398208.56326.19

Lubelski D, Abdullah KG, Weil RJ, Marko NF (2013) Bevacizumab for radiation necrosis following treatment of high grade glioma: a systematic review of the literature. J Neurooncol 115(3):317–322. https://doi.org/10.1007/s11060-013-1233-0

Miyatake S, Nonoguchi N, Furuse M, Yoritsune E, Miyata T, Kawabata S, Kuroiwa T (2015) Pathophysiology, diagnosis, and treatment of radiation necrosis in the brain. Neurol Med Chir 55(1):50–59. https://doi.org/10.2176/nmc.ra.2014-0188

Na A, Haghigi N, Drummond KJ (2014) Cerebral radiation necrosis. Asia Pac J Clin Oncol 10(1):11–21. https://doi.org/10.1111/ajco.12124

Parvez K, Parvez A, Zadeh G (2014) The diagnosis and treatment of pseudoprogression, radiation necrosis and brain tumor recurrence. Int J Mol Sci 15(7):11832–11846. https://doi.org/10.3390/ijms150711832

Perry A (2010) Therapy-associated neuropathology. In: Perry A, Brat DJ (eds) Practical surgical neuropathology. Churchill Livingstone Elsevier, Philadelphia, PA, pp 417–425

Perry A, Schmidt RE (2006) Cancer therapy-associated CNS neuropathology: an update and review of the literature. Acta Neuropathol 111(3):197–212. https://doi.org/10.1007/s00401-005-0023-y

Rahmathulla G, Marko NF, Weil RJ (2013) Cerebral radiation necrosis: a review of the pathobiology, diagnosis and management considerations. J Clin Neurosci 20(4):485–502. https://doi.org/10.1016/j.jocn.2012.09.011

Shah R, Vattoth S, Jacob R, Manzil FF, O'Malley JP, Borghei P, Patel BN, Cure JK (2012) Radiation necrosis in the brain: imaging features and differentiation from tumor recurrence. Radiographics 32(5):1343–1359. https://doi.org/10.1148/rg.325125002

Shah AH, Snelling B, Bregy A, Patel PR, Tememe D, Bhatia R, Sklar E, Komotar RJ (2013) Discriminating radiation necrosis from tumor progression in gliomas: a systematic review what is the best imaging modality? J Neurooncol 112(2):141–152. https://doi.org/10.1007/s11060-013-1059-9

Zhang H, Ma L, Wang Q, Zheng X, Wu C, Xu BN (2014) Role of magnetic resonance spectroscopy for the differentiation of recurrent glioma from radiation necrosis: a systematic review and meta-analysis. Eur J Radiol 83(12):2181–2189. https://doi.org/10.1016/j.ejrad.2014.09.018

Tumor Progression–Pseudoprogression

83.1 Introduction

The following lines in the treatment of malignant brain tumors are followed:

- First line
  - Surgery–radiotherapy–chemotherapy (Temodal)
- Second line
  - Bevacizumab (Avastin)
- Tertiary line
  - Other chemotherapeutics, e.g., CCNU, PVC, BCNU

The **therapeutic response** can be defined as:
- Complete remission/response (CR)
  - The disappearance of all signs of cancer in response to treatment. This does not always mean the cancer has been cured. Also called complete response.
- Partial remission/response (PR)
  - A decrease in the size of a tumor or in the extent of cancer in the body, in response to treatment. Also called partial response.
- Stable disease
  - Cancer that is neither decreasing nor increasing in extent or severity.
- Progressive disease
  - Cancer that is growing, spreading, or getting worse.

83.2 Neuroimaging Findings

General imaging findings
- *Tumor progression*: growing tumor according to mentioned criteria
- *Pseudoprogression*: paradoxical increase of contrast enhancement within 12 weeks of chemo-radiation therapy
- *Pseudoresponse*: paradoxical decrease in the enhancing area in patients treated with anti-angiogenic agents

CT non-contrast-enhanced
- Increase of tumor

CT contrast-enhanced
- Growth of tumor

MRI-T2/ FLAIR (Fig. 83.1a, b, f, g)
- Increase of hyperintensities

MRI-T1 (Fig. 83.1c, h)
- Progressing inhomogeneous hypointensities

MRI-T2∗/SWI
- Increase of hyperintensities
- Hemorrhages possible

MRI-T1 contrast-enhanced (Fig. 83.1d, i)
- Enhancement is not a measure of tumor activity but rather reflects a disturbed blood-brain barrier.
- Tumor progression: ≥ 25% increase in sum of the products of perpendicular diameters of all measurable enhancing lesions (RANO).
- Pseudoprogression: increase of contrast enhancement.
- Pseudoresponse: reduced contrast enhancement, even when the tumor is progressing.

MR-Diffusion Imaging
- Tumor progression: restricted diffusion, lower ADC values than pseudoprogression
- Pseudoresponse: restricted diffusion possible, low ADC values described

MRI-Perfusion (Fig. 83.1e, j)
- Elevated rCBV in tumor progression.
- Decreased rCBV indicates pseudoprogression.

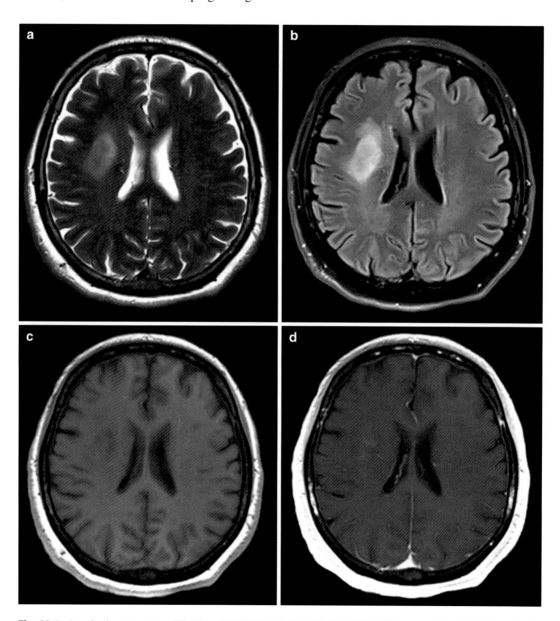

Fig. 83.1 Anaplastic astrocytoma III right with MR T2 (**a**), FLAIR (**b**), T1 (**c**), T1 contrast (**d**), rCBV (**e**) and after 6 month T2 (**f**), Flair (**g**), T1 (**h**), T1 contrast (**i**), rCBV (**j**)

83.2 Neuroimaging Findings

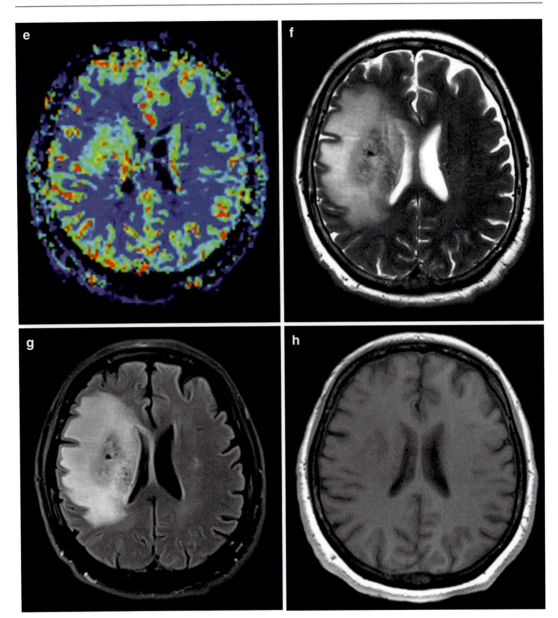

Fig. 83.1 (continued)

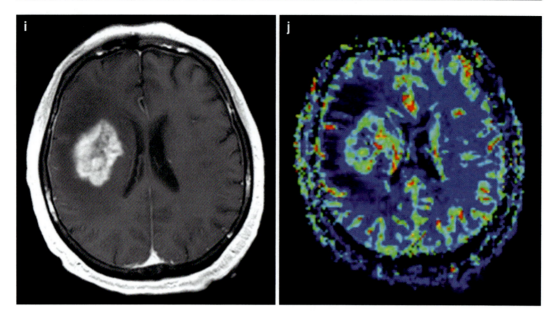

Fig. 83.1 (continued)

MR-Diffusion Tensor Imaging
- No sufficient information for differential diagnosis between pseudoprogression and tumor progression

MR-Spectroscopy
- Tumor progression and pseudoprogression similar, low NAA, high Cho, lactate/lipids peaks

83.3 Neuroimaging Criteria for Therapeutic Outcome

Neuroimaging criteria used to assess more reliably therapeutic outcome among patients with high-grade gliomas, low-grade gliomas, or brain metastases are given in Table 83.1.

83.3.1 RANO Response Criteria for *Low-Grade Glioma* (van den Bent et al. 2011)

- **Complete response**
  - Complete disappearance of the lesion on T2 or FLAIR imaging (if enhancement had been present, it must have resolved completely).
  - No new lesions, no new T2 or FLAIR abnormalities apart from those consistent with radiation effects, and no new or increased enhancement.
  - Patients must be off corticosteroids or only on physiological replacement doses.
  - Patients should be stable or improved clinically.

- **Partial response**
  - Greater than or equal to 50% decrease in the product of perpendicular diameters of the lesion on T2 or FLAIR imaging sustained for at least 4 weeks compared with baseline.
  - No new lesions, no new T2 or FLAIR abnormalities apart from those consistent with radiation effects, and no new or increased enhancement.
  - Patients should be on a corticosteroid dose that should not be greater than the dose at time of baseline scan, and should be stable or improved clinically.

- **Minor response**
  - Minor response requires the following criteria compared with baseline:

83.3 Neuroimaging Criteria for Therapeutic Outcome

Table 83.1 Neuroimaging criteria, i.e., standardized critical radiographic parameters, are used to assess more reliably therapeutic outcome among patients with high-grade gliomas (Macdonald et al. 1990; Wen et al. 2010), low-grade gliomas (van den Bent et al. 2011), or brain metastases (Lin et al. 2015)

	MacDonald	RANO (Response Assessment in Neuro-Oncology)
Complete response	• Complete disappearance of all enhancing measurable and non-measurable disease sustained for at least 4 weeks • No new lesions • No corticosteroids • Stable or improved clinically	• Disappearance of all enhancing measurable and non-measurable disease sustained for a minimum of 4 weeks • Stable or improved FLAIR/T2 lesions • No new lesion • Stable or improved clinically • Patients cannot be receiving corticosteroids (physiologic doses are acceptable)
Partial response	• ≥50% decrease compared with baseline in the sum of products of perpendicular diameters of all measurable enhancing lesions sustained for at least 4 weeks • No new lesions • Stable or reduced corticosteroid dose • Stable or improved clinically	• ≥50% decrease (compared with baseline) in the sum of products of perpendicular diameters of all measurable enhancing lesions sustained for a minimum of 4 weeks • No progression of non-measurable disease • No new lesions • Stable or improved FLAIR/T2 lesions • Stable or improved clinically • Corticosteroid dosage at the time of the scan should be no greater than the dosage at the time of the baseline scan
Stable disease	• Does not qualify for CR, PR, or PD • Stable clinically	• Patient does not qualify for CFR, PR, or PD • Stable FLAIR/T2 lesions on a corticosteroid dose no greater than at baseline • Stable clinically
Progressive disease	• ≥25% increase in sum of the products of perpendicular diameters of enhancing lesions relative to best previous scan • Any new lesion • Clinical deterioration	• ≥25% increase in sum of the products of perpendicular diameters of all measurable enhancing lesions compared with the smallest tumor measurement obtained either at baseline or best response following the initiation of therapy, while on a stable or increasing dose of corticosteroids • Significant increase in FLAIR/T2 lesions compared with baseline or best response following initiation of therapy, not caused by comorbid events (e.g., radiation therapy, ischemic injury, seizures, postoperative changes, other treatment effects), while on a stable or increasing dose of corticosteroids • New lesions • Clinical deterioration not attributable to other causes apart from the tumor (e.g., seizures, medication side effects, complications of therapy, cerebrovascular events, or infection) or decreases in corticosteroid dose • Failure to return for evaluation owing to death or deteriorating condition • Clear progression of non-measurable disease

- A decrease of the area of non-enhancing lesion on T2 or FLAIR MR imaging between 25 and 50% compared with baseline.
- No new lesions, no new T2 or FLAIR abnormalities apart from those consistent with radiation effect, and no new or increased enhancement.
- Patients should be on a corticosteroid dose that should not be greater than the dose at time of baseline scan, and should be stable or improved clinically.

- **Stable disease**
  - Stable area of non-enhancing abnormalities on T2 or FLAIR imaging.
  - No new lesions, no new T2 or FLAIR abnormalities apart from those consistent with radiation effect, and no new or increased enhancement.
  - Patients should be on a corticosteroid dose that should not be greater than the dose at time of baseline scan, and should be stable or improved clinically.

- **Progression** (Tables 83.2 and 83.3)
  - Development of new lesions or increase of enhancement (radiological evidence of malignant transformation)
  - A 25% increase of the T2 or FLAIR non-enhancing lesion on stable or increasing doses of corticosteroids compared with baseline scan or best response after initiation of therapy, not attributable to radiation effect or to comorbid events
  - Definite clinical deterioration not attributable to other causes apart from the tumor, or decrease in corticosteroid dose; or failure to return for evaluation because of death or deteriorating condition, unless caused by documented non-related disorders

Table 83.2 Progression types after *anti-angiogenic therapy* in recurrent glioblastoma, (Nowosielski et al. 2014), reproduced with kind permission by Wolters Kluwer Health

Type I: T2-diffuse	• Complete decrease in CE or • Only a few faintly speckled CE lesions on cT1 images • At progression, these patients show a signal increase exclusively on T2-weighted images with a homogeneous signal pattern, signs of mass effect, exceeding of anatomical structures and poorly defined borders on MRI • Hypointensity seen on T1-weighted images is faint and disproportionally smaller than T2-hyperintensity or even not present at all
Type II: cT1 flare-up	• This PT is characterized by an initial decrease in CE on T1-weighted sequences (cT1) at first follow-up imaging after treatment initiation. This CE, however, increases again ("flare-up") at tumor progression • T2 signal stays stable or increases
Type III: Primary non-responder	• This PT is defined by stable, increased, or new CE lesions distant from the original tumor site at first follow-up imaging after commencement of therapy • T2 signal remains stable or increases
Type IV: T2-circumscribed	• This PT is characterized at tumor progression by either a complete decrease in CE on T1-weighted images or only a few faintly speckled CE lesions are visible on cT1 images • This T2-hyperintense tumor progression is characterized by a bulky and inhomogeneous structure with sharp borders that correspond to a T1-hypointense signal seen on T1-weighted images

83.5 Molecular Neuropathology

Table 83.3 Summary of progression types (Nowosielski et al. 2014), reproduced with kind permission by Wolters Kluwer Health

Progression type	MRI appearance at first follow-up		MRI appearance at tumor progression		
	T1 contrast	T2	T1 contrast	T2	T1 hypointense area
Type I: T2-diffuse	↓	↔ or ↓	• No or • Speckled contrast enhancement	• ↑ • Homogeneous • Poorly defined borders	Disproportionally smaller
Type II: cT1 flare-up	↓	↔ or ↑			
Type III: primary non-responder	↔ or ↑	↔ or ↑			
Type IV: T2-circumscribed	↓	↔ or ↓	• No or • Speckled contrast enhancement	• ↑ • Inhomogeneous • Bulky • Sharp borders	Corresponding to T2

83.3.2 The Immunotherapy Response Assessment in Neuro-Oncology (iRANO) Criteria

The *immunotherapy Response Assessment in Neuro-Oncology* (iRANO) criteria integrate into the existing RANO criteria for malignant glioma, low-grade glioma, and brain metastases by providing recommendations for the interpretation of progressive imaging changes (Okada et al. 2015) (Tables 83.4 and 83.5).

- iRANO recommends confirmation of disease progression on follow-up imaging 3 months after initial radiographic progression if there is no new or substantially worsened neurological deficits that are not due to comorbid events or concurrent medication, and it is 6 months or less from starting immunotherapy.
- If follow-up imaging confirms disease progression, the date of actual progression should be back-dated to the date of initial radiographic progression. The appearance of new lesions 6 months or less from the initiation of immunotherapy alone does not define progressive disease. *FLAIR* fluid attenuated inversion recovery. *iRANO* immunotherapy Response Assessment in Neuro-Oncology.

83.4 Nuclear Medicine Findings

Nuclear Medicine Imaging Findings (Figs. 83.2, 83.3, 83.4 and 83.5)

- Metabolic images of the tumor lesion can give insight to changed biological behavior of the tumor.
- Increasing uptake of FDG, MET, or FET represent altered metabolism and thereby progression or even changed tumor grading.
- Tumor extent can be assessed as well by 3-dimensional ROI analysis and thereby representing viable tumor volume.
- PET is able to detect tumor progression earlier than was MRI.
- It has been shown that PET is able to detect tumor progression earlier (especially by calculating the biological tumor volume) than MRI not only but especially in patients with anti-angiogenic treatment, although influences of anti-angiogenic treatment on PET images have been shown.

83.5 Molecular Neuropathology

Possible mechanisms for avastin resistance include:

- Proneuronal to mesenchymal transition of tumor cells
- Pro-inflammatory factors

Table 83.4 The immunotherapy Response Assessment in Neuro-Oncology (iRANO) criteria, after Okada et al. (2015), reproduced with kind permission by Elsevier

	Low-grade glioma	Malignant glioma	Metastases
Complete response	• Disappearance of all enhancing disease for ≥4 weeks • No new lesions; stable or improved T2/FLAIR • No more than physiological steroids • Clinically stable or improved	• Disappearance of all enhancing and T2/FLAIR disease for ≥4 weeks • No new lesions • No more than physiological steroids • Clinically stable or improved	• Disappearance of all enhancing target and non-target lesions for ≥4 weeks • No new lesions • No steroids • Clinically stable or improved
Partial response	• ≥50% decrease in the sum of biperpendicular diameter of T2/FLAIR disease for ≥4 weeks • No new lesions • Stable or decreased steroid dose • Clinically stable or improved	• ≥50% decrease in the sum of biperpendicular diameters of enhancing disease for ≥4 weeks • No new lesions • Stable or improved T2/FLAIR • Stable or decreased steroid dose • Clinically stable or improved	• ≥30% decrease in sum of longest diameters of target lesions for ≥4 weeks • No new lesions • Stable or decreased steroid dose • Clinically stable or improved
Minor response	• 25–49% decrease in the sum of biperpendicular diameters of T2/FLAIR disease for ≥4 weeks • No new lesions • Clinically stable or improved	Not Applicable	Not Applicable
Stable disease	• Does not qualify for complete response • Partial response, or progressive disease • No new lesions • Stable or improved T2/FLAIR • Stable or decreased steroid dose • Clinically stable or improved	• Does not qualify for complete response, partial response, or progressive disease • No new lesions • Stable or improved T2/FLAIR • Stable or decreased steroid dose • Clinically stable or improved	• Does not qualify for complete response • Partial response, or progressive disease
Progressive disease	• ≥25% decrease in the sum of biperpendicular diameters of T2/FLAIR disease • or new lesions; • or substantial clinical decline	• ≥25% decrease in the sum of biperpendicular diameters of enhancing disease • or new lesions; • or substantial worsened T2/FLAIR; • or substantial clinical decline	• ≥20% decrease in the sum of longest diameters of target lesions; or unequivocal progression of enhancing non-target lesions; • or new lesions • or substantial clinical decline

83.5 Molecular Neuropathology

Table 83.5 Key considerations for RANO criteria, immune-related response criteria, and iRANO criteria, after Okada et al. (2015), reproduced with kind permission by Elsevier

	RANO16	Immune-related response criteria	iRANO (if ≤6 months after start of immunotherapy)	iRANO (if >6 months after start of immunotherapy)
Is a repeat scan needed to confirm radiographic progressive disease for patients without significant clinical decline?	No	Yes	Yes	No
Minimum time interval for confirmation of disease progression for patients without significant clinical decline	N/A	≥4 weeks	≥3 months	N/A
Is further immunotherapy treatment allowed after initial radiographic progressive disease (if clinically stable) pending disease progression confirmation?	N/A	Yes	Yes	N/A
Does a new lesion define progressive disease?	Yes	No	No	Yes

N/A not applicable

- Increased infiltration by CD11b granulocyte
- Increased infiltration by Gr1 granulocyte
- → Tumors develop aggressive mesenchymal features and increased stem cell marker expression.
- Upregulation of ß1-integrin and its downstream effector kinase FAK
- Activated MET signaling induced by inhibition of VEGF signaling
- Tyrosine kinase c-Met receptor upregulation, increased c-Met phosphorylation, and increased phosphorylation of c-Met-activated focal adhesion kinase
- Upregulation of the STAT3 pathway with increase of p-STAT3 expressing cells
- Myeloid cell infiltration
- Stem cell accumulation
- Tumor-derived endothelial cell-induced angiogenesis and vasculogenic mimicry
- Hypoxia
  - Increased hypoxia induces tumor cell autophagy as a cytoprotective adaptive response, thereby promoting treatment resistance.
  - Hypoxia-inducible factor-1alpha (HIF-1alpha)/AMPK pathway.
  - Hypoxia-mediated autophagy promotes tumor cell survival.
- Differences between glycolysis and mitochondrial respiration
- Inhibition of VEGF signaling through a variety of mechanisms
- Hepatocyte growth factor
- Increased expression of genes associated with a mesenchymal origin, cellular migration/invasion, and inflammation

Fig. 83.2 FET-PET of an oligo-astrocytoma II frontal right after surgery with viable tumor tissue (**a**) and with a slight progression after 6 months (tumor volume) (**b**) and a clear progression after 2 years (volume and uptake) (**c**)

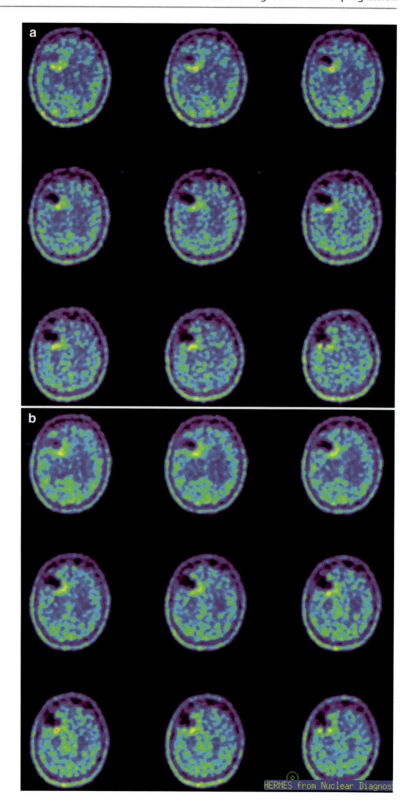

83.5 Molecular Neuropathology

Fig. 83.2 (continued)

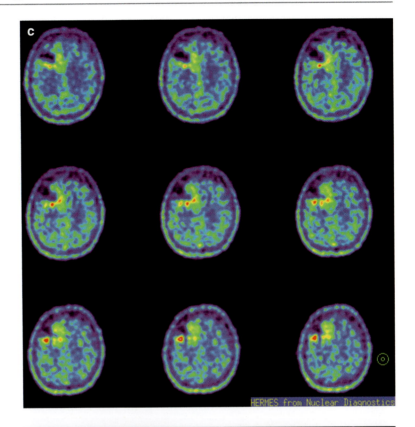

Fig. 83.3 FET-PET of an oligo-astrocytoma II frontal right after surgery with clear visible tumor (**a**) and a progression of the tumor volume after 3 months (with lower uptake due to chemotherapy) (**b**), progression of the tumor volume and uptake after 6 months (**c**) and again progression of the tumor volume and uptake after 1 year (**d**)

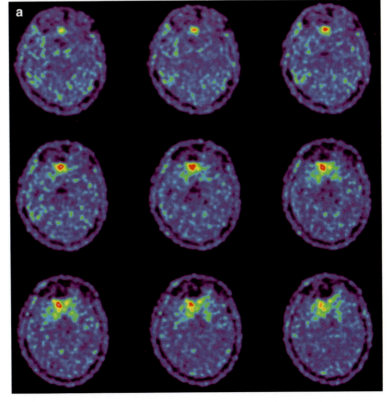

Fig. 83.3 (continued)

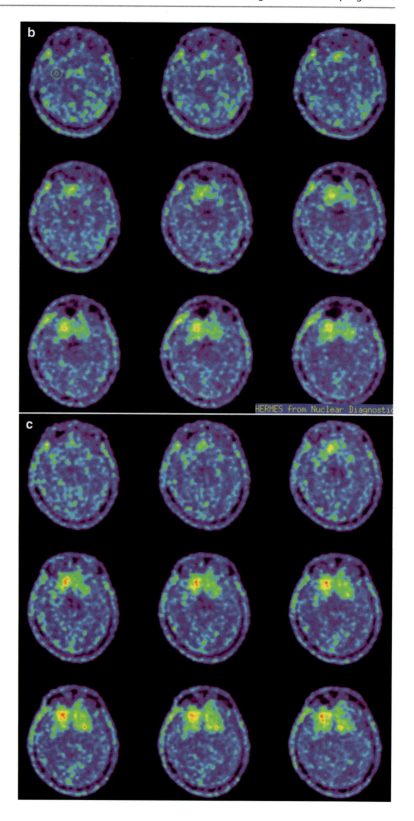

83.5 Molecular Neuropathology

Fig. 83.3 (continued)

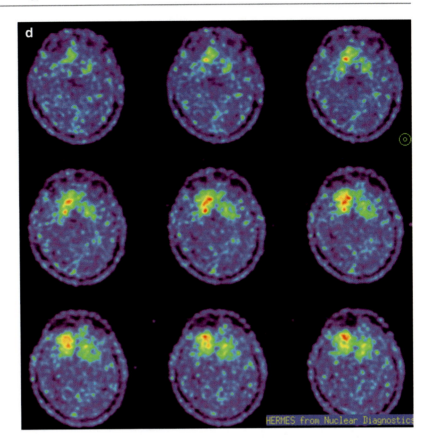

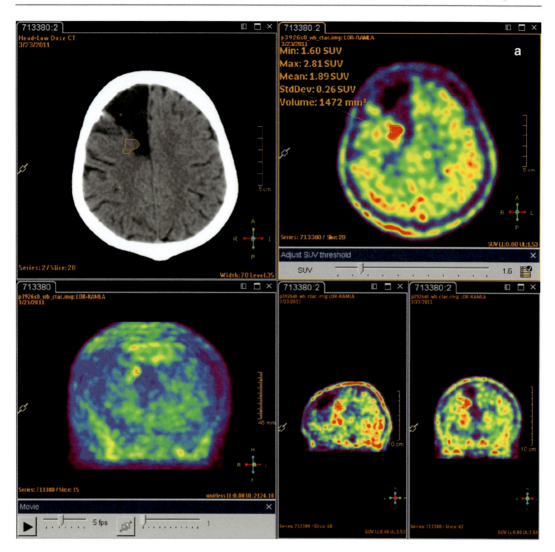

Fig. 83.4 FET-PET with a calculated 3D-ROI with an iso-SUV of 1.6 of a glioblastoma after surgery with a progression of the tumor volume and the maximum SUV from March to December 2011 (transversal, coronal and sagittal slice, 3D PET image, CT)

83.5 Molecular Neuropathology

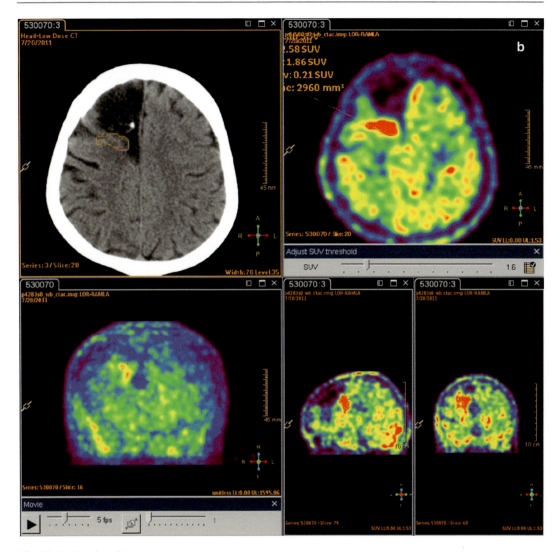

Fig. 83.4 (continued)

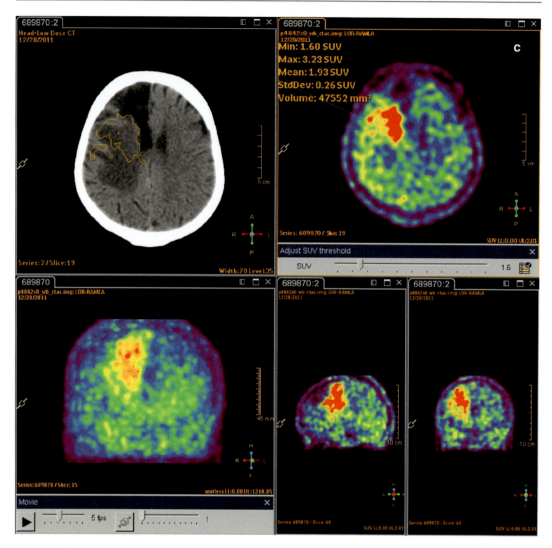

Fig. 83.4 (continued)

83.5 Molecular Neuropathology

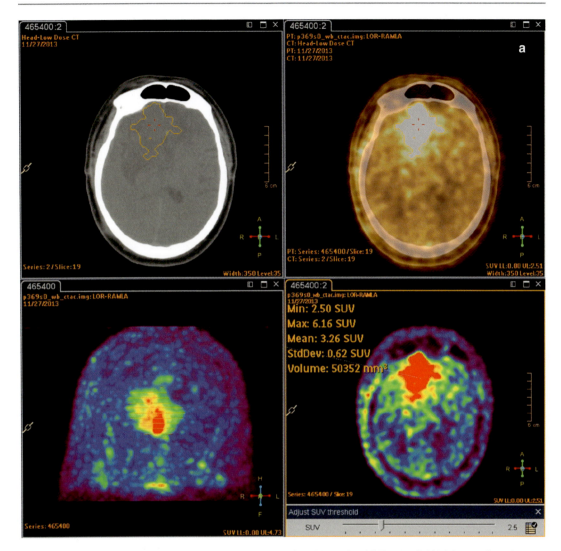

Fig. 83.5 FET-PET with 3D-ROI with an iso-SUV of 2.5 of an astrocytoma III frontal right with a progression of the tumor volume and nearly identical maximum SUV from November 2013 to April 2014 due to a flare phenomenon after radiation

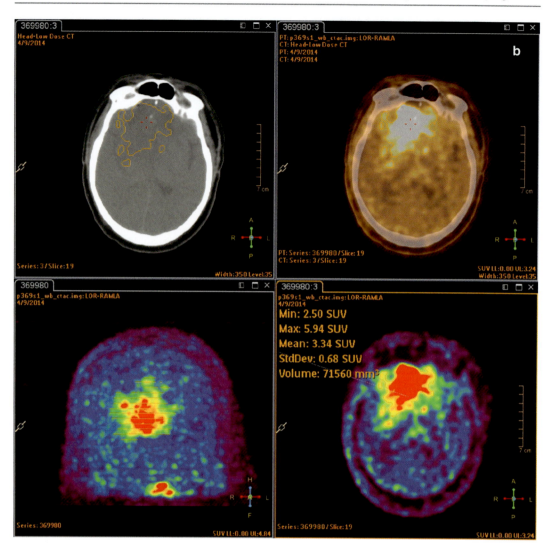

Fig. 83.5 (continued)

Selected References

Barone A, Rubin JB (2013) Opportunities and challenges for successful use of bevacizumab in pediatrics. Front Oncol 3:92. https://doi.org/10.3389/fonc.2013.00092

Carbonell WS, DeLay M, Jahangiri A, Park CC, Aghi MK (2013) Beta1 integrin targeting potentiates antiangiogenic therapy and inhibits the growth of bevacizumab-resistant glioblastoma. Cancer Res 73(10):3145–3154. https://doi.org/10.1158/0008-5472.can-13-0011

Chamberlain MC (2012) Role for cytotoxic chemotherapy in patients with recurrent glioblastoma progressing on bevacizumab: a retrospective case series. Expert Rev Neurother 12(8):929–936. https://doi.org/10.1586/ern.12.84

de Groot J, Liang J, Kong LY, Wei J, Piao Y, Fuller G, Qiao W, Heimberger AB (2012) Modulating antiangiogenic resistance by inhibiting the signal transducer and activator of transcription 3 pathway in glioblastoma. Oncotarget 3(9):1036–1048

Gahramanov S, Muldoon LL, Varallyay CG, Li X, Kraemer DF, Fu R, Hamilton BE, Rooney WD, Neuwelt EA (2013) Pseudoprogression of glioblastoma after chemo- and radiation therapy: diagnosis by using dynamic susceptibility-weighted contrast-enhanced perfusion MR imaging with ferumoxytol versus gadoteridol and correlation with survival. Radiology 266(3):842–852. https://doi.org/10.1148/radiol.12111472

Gatson NN, Chiocca EA, Kaur B (2012) Anti-angiogenic gene therapy in the treatment of malignant gliomas. Neurosci Lett 527(2):62–70. https://doi.org/10.1016/j.neulet.2012.08.001

Hu YL, DeLay M, Jahangiri A, Molinaro AM, Rose SD, Carbonell WS, Aghi MK (2012) Hypoxia-induced autophagy promotes tumor cell survival and adaptation to antiangiogenic treatment in glioblastoma. Cancer Res 72(7):1773–1783. https://doi.org/10.1158/0008-5472.can-11-3831

Hutterer M, Nowosielski M, Putzer D, Waitz D, Tinkhauser G, Kostron H, Muigg A, Virgolini IJ, Staffen W, Trinka E, Gotwald T, Jacobs AH, Stockhammer G (2011) O-(2-18F-fluoroethyl)-L-tyrosine PET predicts failure of antiangiogenic treatment in patients with recurrent high-grade glioma. J Nucl Med 52(6):856–864. https://doi.org/10.2967/jnumed.110.086645

Hygino da Cruz LC Jr, Rodriguez I, Domingues RC, Gasparetto EL, Sorensen AG (2011) Pseudoprogression and pseudoresponse: imaging challenges in the assessment of posttreatment glioma. Am J Neuroradiol 32(11):1978–1985. https://doi.org/10.3174/ajnr.A2397

Jahangiri A, De Lay M, Miller LM, Carbonell WS, Hu YL, Lu K, Tom MW, Paquette J, Tokuyasu TA, Tsao S, Marshall R, Perry A, Bjorgan KM, Chaumeil MM, Ronen SM, Bergers G, Aghi MK (2013) Gene expression profile identifies tyrosine kinase c-Met as a targetable mediator of antiangiogenic therapy resistance. Clin Cancer Res 19(7):1773–1783. https://doi.org/10.1158/1078-0432.ccr-12-1281

Kumar K, Wigfield S, Gee HE, Devlin CM, Singleton D, Li JL, Buffa F, Huffman M, Sinn AL, Silver J, Turley H, Leek R, Harris AL, Ivan M (2013) Dichloroacetate reverses the hypoxic adaptation to bevacizumab and enhances its antitumor effects in mouse xenografts. J Mol Med 91(6):749–758. https://doi.org/10.1007/s00109-013-0996-2

Lin NU, Lee EQ, Aoyama H, Barani IJ, Barboriak DP, Baumert BG, Bendszus M, Brown PD, Camidge DR, Chang SM, Dancey J, de Vries EG, Gaspar LE, Harris GJ, Hodi FS, Kalkanis SN, Linskey ME, Macdonald DR, Margolin K, Mehta MP, Schiff D, Soffietti R, Suh JH, van den Bent MJ, Vogelbaum MA, Wen PY (2015) Response assessment criteria for brain metastases: proposal from the RANO group. Lancet Oncol 16(6):e270–e278. https://doi.org/10.1016/s1470-2045(15)70057-4

Lu KV, Bergers G (2013) Mechanisms of evasive resistance to anti-VEGF therapy in glioblastoma. CNS Oncol 2(1):49–65. https://doi.org/10.2217/cns.12.36

Lutz K, Radbruch A, Wiestler B, Baumer P, Wick W, Bendszus M (2011) Neuroradiological response criteria for high-grade gliomas. Clin Neuroradiol 21(4):199–205. https://doi.org/10.1007/s00062-011-0080-7

Macdonald DR, Cascino TL, Schold SC Jr, Cairncross JG (1990) Response criteria for phase II studies of supratentorial malignant glioma. J Clin Oncol 8(7):1277–1280. https://doi.org/10.1200/jco.1990.8.7.1277

McCarty JH (2013) Glioblastoma resistance to anti-VEGF therapy: has the challenge been MET? Clin Cancer Res 19(7):1631–1633. https://doi.org/10.1158/1078-0432.ccr-13-0051

Moreno Garcia V, Basu B, Molife LR, Kaye SB (2012) Combining antiangiogenics to overcome resistance: rationale and clinical experience. Clin Cancer Res 18(14):3750–3761. https://doi.org/10.1158/1078-0432.ccr-11-1275

Nowosielski M, Wiestler B, Goebel G, Hutterer M, Schlemmer HP, Stockhammer G, Wick W, Bendszus M, Radbruch A (2014) Progression types after antiangiogenic therapy are related to outcome in recurrent glioblastoma. Neurology 82(19):1684–1692. https://doi.org/10.1212/wnl.0000000000000402

Okada H, Weller M, Huang R, Finocchiaro G, Gilbert MR, Wick W, Ellingson BM, Hashimoto N, Pollack IF, Brandes AA, Franceschi E, Herold-Mende C, Nayak L, Panigrahy A, Pope WB, Prins R, Sampson JH, Wen PY, Reardon DA (2015) Immunotherapy response assessment in neuro-oncology: a report of the RANO working group. Lancet Oncol 16(15):e534–e542. https://doi.org/10.1016/s1470-2045(15)00088-1

Piao Y, Liang J, Holmes L, Zurita AJ, Henry V, Heymach JV, de Groot JF (2012) Glioblastoma resistance to anti-VEGF therapy is associated with myeloid cell infiltration, stem cell accumulation, and a mesenchymal phenotype. Neuro Oncol 14(11):1379–1392. https://doi.org/10.1093/neuonc/nos158

Piao Y, Liang J, Holmes L, Henry V, Sulman E, de Groot JF (2013) Acquired resistance to anti-VEGF therapy in glioblastoma is associated with a mesenchymal transition. Clin Cancer Res 19(16):4392–4403. https://doi.org/10.1158/1078-0432.ccr-12-1557

Shah AH, Snelling B, Bregy A, Patel PR, Tememe D, Bhatia R, Sklar E, Komotar RJ (2013) Discriminating radiation necrosis from tumor progression in gliomas: a systematic review what is the best imaging modality? J Neurooncol 112(2):141–152. https://doi.org/10.1007/s11060-013-1059-9

Soda Y, Myskiw C, Rommel A, Verma IM (2013) Mechanisms of neovascularization and resistance to anti-angiogenic therapies in glioblastoma multiforme. J Mol Med 91(4):439–448. https://doi.org/10.1007/s00109-013-1019-z

Spasic M, Chow F, Tu C, Nagasawa DT, Yang I (2012) Molecular characteristics and pathways of Avastin for the treatment of glioblastoma multiforme. Neurosurg Clin N Am 23(3):417–427. https://doi.org/10.1016/j.nec.2012.05.002

van den Bent MJ, Wefel JS, Schiff D, Taphoorn MJ, Jaeckle K, Junck L, Armstrong T, Choucair A, Waldman AD, Gorlia T, Chamberlain M, Baumert BG, Vogelbaum MA, Macdonald DR, Reardon DA, Wen PY, Chang SM, Jacobs AH (2011) Response assessment in neuro-oncology (a report of the RANO group): assessment of outcome in trials of diffuse low-grade gliomas. Lancet Oncol 12(6):583–593. https://doi.org/10.1016/s1470-2045(11)70057-2

Weller M, Cloughesy T, Perry JR, Wick W (2013) Standards of care for treatment of recurrent glioblastoma—are we there yet? Neuro Oncol 15(1):4–27. https://doi.org/10.1093/neuonc/nos273

Wen PY, Macdonald DR, Reardon DA, Cloughesy TF, Sorensen AG, Galanis E, Degroot J, Wick W, Gilbert MR, Lassman AB, Tsien C, Mikkelsen T, Wong ET, Chamberlain MC, Stupp R, Lamborn KR, Vogelbaum MA, van den Bent MJ, Chang SM (2010) Updated response assessment criteria for high-grade gliomas: response assessment in neuro-oncology working group. J Clin Oncol 28(11):1963–1972. https://doi.org/10.1200/jco.2009.26.3541

Autoimmune Encephalitis: Paraneoplastic Syndromes

84.1 Definitions

Autoimmune diseases are related by the fact that host-directed immune responses play a significant role in their etiology and pathogenesis (Rose and Mackay 2014). Diseases characterized by activation of the immune system in the absence of an external threat to the organism are distinguished from diseases characterized by an activation of the adaptive immune response with T- and B-lymphocytes responding to self-antigen in the absence of any detectable microbial assault or tumor invasion (Davidson and Diamond 2014).

Paraneoplastic disorders are caused by cancer but not by a direct result of cancer invasion of the affected tissue or organ. Neurologic signs and symptoms result from either direct or indirect damage to the nervous system. Any part of the nervous system can be involved including the cerebral cortex, neuromuscular junction, and autonomic nervous system (Darnell and Posner 2011; Graus and Dalmau 2012).

Autoimmune encephalitis (AE) is a diverse group of neuropsychiatric disorders associated with systemic autoimmune disorders, CNS autoimmune disorders, and paraneoplastic syndromes. AE is mediated by antibodies (Abs) directed against membrane receptors (e.g., N-methyl D-aspartate receptors) and ion channel-associated CNS proteins (e.g., voltage-gated potassium channels) (Dalmau et al. 2017; Leypoldt et al. 2015). The diseases are usually not related to cancer.

84.2 Epidemiology

Incidence
- Rare
- 20% of cancer patients suffer one or more neurologic signs and symptoms

Age Incidence
- Mainly adults
- Rarely children

Sex Incidence
- Male/Female: depends on associated tumor

Localization
- Supratentorial cerebrum
- Brain stem
- Cerebellum
- Cranial verves
- Spinal cord
- Dorsal root ganglia
- Peripheral nervous system
- Neuromuscular junction and muscle

84.3 Clinical Signs

- Usually no evidence of cancer
- Cognitive impairment
- Seizures
- Extrapyramidal symptoms
- Autonomic changes

- Myoclonus
- Psychiatric symptoms (hallucinations, depression, anxiety)

Clues to an autoimmune etiology include:
- Change in baseline neurologic function
- Subacute onset (days to weeks)
- Fluctuating course
- Personal or family history of organ- or non-organ-specific autoimmune disorder
- Systemic markers of autoimmunity: e.g., elevated antinuclear (ANA) or antithyroperoxidase (TPO) antibodies
- History of or concurrent malignancy
- CSF studies: elevated white blood cell count (<100 cells/μL), protein (<100 mg/dL), IgG index, oligoclonal bands, synthesis rate
- EEG: focal abnormalities
- MRI: T2/FLAIR hyperintensities, rarely enhancement
- PET brain: areas of hyper/hypometabolism

- Response to immunosuppression
- Identification of a neural autoantibody

Paraneoplastic nervous system syndromes based on their topographical brain involvement are listed in Table 84.1 while clinical clues in the recognition of particular types of autoimmune encephalitis are given in Table 84.2.

Table 84.1 The following paraneoplastic nervous system syndromes based on their topographical brain involvement are distinguished

Region involved	Disease entity
Brain (supratentorial)	• Encephalomyelitis • Limbic encephalitis • Demyelinating encephalopathy • Chorea • Parkinsonism
Brain stem and cerebellum	• Brain stem encephalitis • Cerebellar degeneration • Opsoclonus/myoclonus
Cranial nerves	• Cancer-associated retinopathy • Melanoma-associated retinopathy • Optic neuropathy
Spinal cord	• Inflammatory myelitis • Stiff-person syndrome • Subacute motor neuronopathy
Dorsal root ganglia and peripheral nervous system	• Sensory neuronopathy • Autonomic neuropathy • Polyradiculopathy (Guillain–Barré)
Neuromuscular junction and muscle	• Lambert–Eaton myasthenic syndrome (LEMS) • Myasthenia gravis • Dermatomyositis

Table 84.2 Clinical clues in the recognition of particular types of autoimmune encephalitis modified after Lancaster (2016), reproduced with kind permission by Kamje Press, open access

Clinical finding	Associated autoantibody disorders
Psychosis	• NMDAR • AMPAR • GABA-B-R
Dystonia, chorea	• NMDAR
Sydenham chorea	• D2R
Hyperekplexia	• GlyR
Status epilepticus	• Most characteristic of GABA-B-R and GABA-A-R • NMDAR is much more common • May occur in other types as well
New onset type 1 diabetes	• GAD65
Fasciobrachial dystonic seizures	• LGI1
Neuromyotonia, muscle spasms, fasciculations	• Caspr2
Stiff-person syndrome and/or exaggerated startle	• GAD65 • GlyR • Amphiphysin (with GAD65 being most common in stiff person/stiff limb and GlyR in PERM, and amphiphysin in women with breast cancer)
CNS (myoclonus, startle, delirium) and gastrointestinal hyperexcitability	• DPPX
Cranial neuropathies	• Ma2, Hu, Miller-Fisher, Bickerstaff (but also infections like Sarcoidosis, Lyme, TB)
Cerebellitis	• GAD65 • PCA-1 (Yo) • ANNA-1 (Hu) • DNER (Tr) • mGluR1 • VGCC

84.3 Clinical Signs

Diagnostic criteria for paraneoplastic neurologic syndromes are given as follows (Graus et al. 2004) (Table 84.3):

- **Definite paraneoplastic neurologic syndromes**
  - A classical syndrome and cancer that develops within 5 years of the diagnosis of the neurological disorder
  - A non-classical syndrome that resolves or significantly improves after cancer treatment without concomitant immunotherapy, provided that the syndrome is not susceptible to spontaneous remission
  - A non-classical syndrome with onconeural antibodies (well characterized or not) and cancer that develops within 5 years of diagnosis of the neurological disorder
  - A neurological syndrome (classical or not) with well-characterized onconeural antibodies (anti-Hu, Yo, CV2, Ri, Ma-2, or amphiphysin), and cancer
- **Possible paraneoplastic neurologic syndromes**
  - A classical syndrome, no onconeural antibodies, no cancer but at high risk to have an underlying tumor

Table 84.3 Diagnostic criteria for possible autoimmune encephalitis modified after Graus et al. (2016a), reproduced with kind permission by Elsevier

Possible AE	1. Subacute onset (rapid progression of less than 3 months) of working memory deficits (short-term memory loss), altered mental status, or psychiatric symptoms 2. At least one of the following: • New focal CNS findings • Seizures not explained by a previously known seizure disorder • CSF pleocytosis (white blood cell count of more than 5 cells per mm^3) • MRI features suggestive of encephalitis 3. Reasonable exclusion of alternative causes
Definite AE	1. Subacute onset (rapid progression of less than 3 months) of working memory deficits, seizures, or psychiatric symptoms suggesting involvement of the limbic system 2. Bilateral brain abnormalities on T2-weighted fluid-attenuated inversion recovery MRI highly restricted to the medial temporal lobes 3. At least one of the following: • CSF pleocytosis (white blood cell count of more than five cells per mm^3) • EEG with epileptic or slow-wave activity involving the temporal lobes 4. Reasonable exclusion of alternative causes
Definite acute disseminated encephalomyelitis	1. A first multifocal, clinical CNS event of presumed inflammatory demyelinating cause 2. Encephalopathy that cannot be explained by fever 3. Abnormal brain MRI: • Diffuse, poorly demarcated, large (>1–2 cm) lesions predominantly involving the cerebral white matter. • T1-hypointense lesions in the white matter in rare cases. • Deep gray matter abnormalities (e.g., thalamus or basal ganglia) can be present. 4. No new clinical or MRI findings after 3 months of symptom onset 5. Reasonable exclusion of alternative causes
Autoantibody-negative but probable Autoimmune encephalitis	1. Rapid progression (less than 3 months) of working memory deficits (short-term memory loss), altered mental status, or psychiatric symptoms 2. Exclusion of well-defined syndromes of autoimmune encephalitis (e.g., typical limbic encephalitis, Bickerstaff's brain stem encephalitis, acute disseminated encephalomyelitis) 3. Absence of well-characterized autoantibodies in serum and CSF, and at least two of the following criteria: • MRI abnormalities suggestive of autoimmune encephalitis • CSF pleocytosis, CSF-specific oligoclonal bands or elevated CSF IgG index, or both • Brain biopsy showing inflammatory infiltrates and excluding other disorders (e.g., tumor) 4. Reasonable exclusion of alternative causes

- A neurologic syndrome (classical or not) with partially characterized onconeural antibodies and no cancer
- A non-classical syndrome, no onconeural antibodies, and cancer present within 2 years of diagnosis

84.4 Autoimmune Encephalitides

84.4.1 Limbic Encephalitis (LE)

- Coined by Corsellis in 1968
- Seizures (temporal lobe, psychomotor or generalized, or mixed)
- Loss of short-term memory
- Episodic memory impairment
- Acute confusional stage
- Disorientation and agitation
- Behavioral abnormalities (affective changes, hallucinations, disinhibition, and personality changes)
- Sleep disturbances
- Hallmark of the syndrome:
  - anterograde memory deficit for people, places, objects, facts, and events
  - failure of declarative or explicit memory mechanisms
- Improvement after treatment of the primary tumor
- Poor prognosis
- Regions involved:
  - medial temporal lobes
  - hippocampus
  - amygdala
  - frontobasal cortex
  - cingulate cortex
- Histological evidence of medial temporal lobe inflammation
- Associated with lung cancer (Hu antibody), Ma2 with testicular tumors (Ma2 antibodies), and thymoma (CRMP5/CV2 antibodies)

84.4.2 Paraneoplastic Limbic Encephalitis (PLE)

- Personality changes
- Irritability
- Depression
- Seizures
- Memory loss
- Loss of ability to form new memories
- Sometimes dementia
- Diagnosis of PLE requires
  - neuropathological examination or
  - the presence of the four following criteria:
    - a compatible clinical picture
    - an interval of <4 years between the development of neurological symptoms and tumor diagnosis
    - exclusion of other neuro-oncological complications
    - at least one of the following:
      - CSF with inflammatory changes but negative cytology
      - MRI demonstrating temporal lobe abnormalities
      - EEG showing epileptic activity in the temporal lobes

84.4.3 NMDA-R Encephalitis

- Ionotropic glutamate receptor
  - subunits: GluN1, GluN2, GluN3
  - GluN1 and GluN3 bind glycine, GluN2 binds glutamate
  - GluN1/GluN2B extrasynaptic receptors of hippocampal neurons
  - GluN1/GluN2A/GluN2B major synaptic receptors in hippocampus and forebrain
- The most common Ab-mediated autoimmune encephalopathy.
- First described in 2005 as a paraneoplastic syndrome associated with ovarian teratomas in young women.
- Antigenic target was determined in 2007.
- Age:
  - frequently 5–76 years.
  - Median age of patients was 23 years.
  - 40% of patients younger than 18 years.
- Sex: 80% Female.
- IgG antibodies against GluNR1 or GluNR2 subunits of the NMDA receptor (main epitope targeted is in the extracellular N-terminal domain of the GluNR1 subunit).

- Disrupt interaction of the receptor with EphB2.
- Associated with:
  - teratomas of the ovary
  - rarely other tumors and Herpes simplex encephalitis
  - no trigger found in 55–60% of patients
- Prodrome (70% of patients)
  - Headache
  - Fever
  - Nausea
  - Vomiting
  - Diarrhea
  - Upper respiratory tract symptoms
- Within a few days, usually less than 2 weeks patients develop:
  - Behavioral disturbance: agitation
  - Auditory and visual hallucinations
  - Delusions
  - Psychosis
  - Amnesia
  - Seizures
  - Dyskinesias, catatonia, orolingual dyskinesias, and stereotypic movement
  - Autonomic dysfunction
  - Decreased level of consciousness often requiring ventilatory support
  - Viral-like syndrome
  - Behavioral disorders
  - Cognitive disorder
  - Various seizure types including status epilepticus
  - Movement disorders (orofacial dyskinesias, dystonia)
  - Eye-movement disorders (nystagmus, ocular dipping, opsoclonus/myoclonus)
  - Autonomic dysfunction
  - Coma

The diagnostic criteria for anti-NMDA receptor encephalitis are shown in Table 84.4.

84.4.4 Voltage-Gated Potassium Antibody Syndromes

The clinical spectrum includes both central and peripheral nervous system disorders.

Clinical features
- Age: Adult and Elderly
- Sex: Both
- Onset: Subacute
- Behavior change
- Memory loss, confabulation
- Confusion and disorientation
- Hallucinations
- Dyssomnia
- Seizures focal and generalized, myoclonic
- Extrapyramidal dysfunction
- Brain stem/cranial nerve dysfunction
- Dysautonomia
- Neuromyotonia

Table 84.4 Diagnostic criteria for anti-NMDA receptor encephalitis (Graus et al. 2016a), reproduced with kind permission by Elsevier

Probable anti-NMDA receptor encephalitis	1. Rapid onset (less than 3 months) of at least four of the six following major groups of symptoms: • Abnormal (psychiatric) behavior or cognitive dysfunction • Speech dysfunction (pressured speech, verbal reduction, mutism) • Seizures • Movement disorder, dyskinesias, or rigidity/abnormal postures • Decreased level of consciousness • Autonomic dysfunction or central hypoventilation 2. At least one of the following laboratory study results: • Abnormal EEG (focal or diffuse slow or disorganized activity, epileptic activity, or extreme delta brush) • CSF with pleocytosis or oligoclonal bands 3. Reasonable exclusion of other disorders
Definite anti-NMDA receptor encephalitis	Diagnosis can be made in the presence of one or more of the six major groups of symptoms and IgG anti-GluN1 antibodies,[†] after reasonable exclusion of other disorders

- Peripheral nerve dysfunction
- Hyponatremia

Clinical features of anti-*LGI1 (leucine-rich glioma-inactivated 1) encephalitis*

- Patient demographics
  - 67% male
  - Age 50–70 years (can be younger)
- Clinical syndrome: limbic encephalitis (90%)
  - Seizures (90%)
    ○ Faciobrachial dystonic seizures (50%)
    ○ Subtle focal seizures (65%)
    ○ Tonic-clonic seizures (65%)
  - Cognitive decline
    ○ Memory disturbance (97%)
    ○ Behavioral disturbance (90%)
    ○ Spatial disorientation (50%)
- Insomnia (65%)
- Ancillary testing
  - Hyponatremia (65%)
  - Brain MRI: mesial temporal lobe hyperintensity (75%)
  - Cerebrospinal fluid: normal (75%)
  - Tumor (<10%)

Clinical features of *Caspr2 (contactin-associated protein-like 2) disease*

- Patient demographics
  - 90% male
  - Age 60–70 years
- Caspr2 core symptoms
  - Cerebral symptoms (cognition 80%, epilepsy 50%)
  - Cerebellar symptoms (35%)
  - Peripheral nerve hyperexcitability (55%)
  - Autonomic dysfunction (45%)
  - Insomnia (55%)
  - Neuropathic pain (60%)
  - Weight loss (60%)
- Ancillary testing
  - Brain MRI: normal (70%)
  - Cerebrospinal fluid: normal (75%)
  - Tumor (20%, mostly thymoma)

Anti-voltage-gated potassium channel (VGKC) antibodies against:

- LIG1
- CASPR2 (contactin-associated protein 2)
- Contactin 2
- Potassium channel (KIR4.1)

VGKC complex Abs were first described in association with *acquired neuromyotonia (NMT) or Isaacs' syndrome*

- painful muscle cramps
- slow muscle relaxation after contraction
- hyperhidrosis
- myokymic and neuromyotonic discharges on EMG
- associated with thymoma

Pathogenesis

The voltage-gated potassium channel (VGKC) complex is composed of

- Kv1 subunits and other proteins.
- They are tightly complexed with the Kv1 subunits in the nerve membrane.
- They are widely expressed in the nervous system, particularly
  - at the juxtaparanodes of the nodes of Ranvier
  - at peripheral motor nerve
  - perhaps sensory terminals
  - in central synapses
- VGKCs regulate neuronal activity throughout the nervous system as their opening following each action potential leads to repolarization of the membrane.
- It is possible that Abs bind to intracellular targets on the solubilized VGKC complex.

VGKC antibodies spectrum

- LGI1
  - The main targets for the Abs are LGI1.
  - Typically associated with LE, and faciobrachial dystonic seizures (FBDS).
  - In around 20–40% of patients with LGI1 Abs, a specific seizure type can precede the occurrence of full-blown limbic encephalitis: "tonic seizures," or FBDS.

84.4 Autoimmune Encephalitides

- brief and very frequent involuntary movement with dystonic features involving mainly the arm, the ipsilateral side of the face, and, less frequently, the leg.
  - The response to anticonvulsant drugs is usually poor.
  - A dramatic reduction or complete resolution of the FBDS can be obtained with oral steroids.
  - Cognitive impairment might be present in patients who did not receive immunotherapy.
  - Early treatment can result in a better recovery and sometimes prevent progression to encephalopathy.
- Contactin-associated protein like (CASPR2)
  - associated with a broader spectrum of central and peripheral nervous system disorders such as LE, NMT, or a combination of the two (MoS).
- Contactin 2
  - has been identified, usually in patients with concomitant anti-LGI1 or anti-CASPR2 Abs and with no specific phenotype, suggesting an unclear clinical relevance.
- Potassium channel (KIR4.1)
  - Abs to dipeptidyl-peptidase-like protein-6 were identified
    - in patients with a form of LE associated with gastrointestinal dysmotility (due to the involvement of the myenteric plexus), sleep disturbances, cognitive and psychiatric manifestations, and dysautonomic features
    - in a disease presenting with hyperekplexia, trunk rigidity, and cerebellar ataxia

84.4.5 Morvan Syndrome

Clinical features
- Described by Morvan in 1890
- Male (93%)
- Neuromyotonia (100%)
  - myokymia (muscle twitching) associated with muscle pain, excessive sweating, and disordered sleep
- Fluctuating delirium
- Neuropsychiatric features (insomnia 89.7%, confusion 65.5%, amnesia 55.6%, and hallucinations 51.9%)
- Dysautonomia (hyperhidrosis 86.2%, cardiovascular 48.3%)
- Neuropathic pain (62.1%)
- Associated tumors: thymoma in (41.4%)
- Some similarities to Isaacs' syndrome

84.4.6 AMPAR (GluR1, GluR2) Antibody Syndrome

Clinical features
- Age: Median age was 62 years (range 23–81; 64% female).
- Common
  - Limbic encephalitis (LE) (55%)
  - Limbic dysfunction along with multifocal/diffuse encephalopathy (36%)
- Rare
  - LE preceded by motor deficits
  - Psychosis with bipolar features
  - Progressive dementia

Associated tumors
- lung, thymoma, breast, ovarian teratoma (64%)

AMPA (α-amino-3-hydroxy-5-methyl-4-isoxazolepropionic acid):
- Anti-α-amino-3-hydroxy-5-methyl-4-isoxazolepropionic acid receptor (AMPAR)
- A subgroup of ionotropic glutamate receptor
- Mainly present in excitatory synapses of the CNS
- Abs against the extracellular domains of AMPA subunits GluRA1 and GluRA2 were associated originally with a particularly aggressive form of LE, often accompanied by the presence of a tumor.

84.4.7 Glycine Receptor Antibody Syndrome

Clinical features
- Variants of Stiff-person syndrome:
- Progressive encephalomyelitis
- Rigidity
- Myoclonus
- Stimulus-sensitive spasms
- Hyperekplexia
- Autonomic disturbances
- Brain stem disorders
- Isolated optic neuritis
- Focal seizure in adult

Pathogenesis
- Abs directed against the α1 subunit of the glycine receptor (GlyR)

84.4.8 Dopamine 2 Receptor Antibody Syndrome (D2RA)

Clinical features
- Movement disorder
  - Dystonia
  - Parkinsonism
  - Chorea
  - Ocular flutter
  - Motor tics
- Psychiatric symptoms
- Agitation
- Emotional lability
- Psychosis
- Depression

Associated symptoms
- Encephalopathy
- Sleep disorder
- Reduced consciousness
- Mutism

Possible autoimmune mechanism for
- Sydenham's chorea
- Encephalitis lethargica with Parkinsonian syndrome
- Pediatric autoimmune neuropsychiatric disorders associated with streptococcal infection (PANDAS)
- Autoimmune subgroup in Tourette's syndrome
- Autoimmune movement disorder with basal ganglia encephalitis associated with D2RA

Pathogenesis
- D1- and D2-class receptors have high expression in:
  - basal ganglia, for example striatum (caudate–putamen)
  - cortex
  - hippocampus
  - substantia nigra
- Modulation of D2R expression in the basal ganglia has been associated with schizophrenia, depression, and movement disorders.
- D2R is intimately linked to the control of movement and behavior.
  - Myoclonus dystonia is associated with *D2R* gene mutations.
  - Movement and psychiatric disorders associated with D2R antibody are biologically plausible as D2R is intimately linked to the control of movement and behavior.

84.4.9 GABA Receptor Ab Syndrome

Clinical features
- Clinical triad of
  - Seizures (47%)
  - Memory impairment (47%) with confusion or disorientation (27%)
  - Psychiatric features (33%) with hallucinations (33%) or anxiety (27%)
  - Refractory status epilepticus
- Rarely
  - Ataxia
  - Status epilepticus
  - Opsoclonus-myoclonus syndrome (OMS)
- Tumor association
  - Small cell lung cancer in 50% of GABAb Ab syndrome
  - Lymphoma in few cases of GABAa Ab syndrome
- MRI were normal or nonspecific in most cases.

- CSF examination was also not informative.
- Treatment
  - The administration of immunotherapy, in association with chemotherapy or tumor removal
- Prognosis
  - Complete recovery following immunotherapy and tumor removal.
  - Untreated cases died within few months of onset.
  - Some patients have a poor outcome despite sustained immunosuppression.
    ○ often related to tumor progression
    ○ associated with the presence of Abs directed against intracellular Ags such as GAD Abs or amphiphysin Abs
    ○ reflect the involvement of an additional cytotoxic T-cell mechanism in the progression of the disease

GABA$_B$ receptor
- is a protein widely distributed in the brain.
- located both pre- and postsynaptically.
- Genetic alterations of the receptor are associated with epilepsy and cognitive impairment.
- Abs against the B1 subunit are found in patients with LE and, rarely, ataxia, 50% of whom will have a small cell lung carcinoma.

84.4.10 Metabotropic Glutamate Receptor Antibody Syndrome

Clinical features:
- mGluR1 Subacute cerebellar ataxia
  - rare syndrome
  - associated with Hodgkin lymphoma
- mGluR5 encephalitis named Ophelia syndrome
- mGluR5 Abs were identified in 2 patients with limbic encephalopathy and Hodgkin lymphoma, i.e., as Ophelia syndrome
- Ophelia syndrome was characterized by:
  - Confusion
  - Agitation
  - Memory loss
  - Delusions
  - Paranoid ideation
  - Hallucinations
  - Psychosis
  - Seizures
- Pathogenesis:
  - Metabotropic glutamate receptors belong to a large family of cell surface receptors.
  - Transmit signals into the cell by coupling to guanine nucleotide-binding proteins (G-proteins) in the cytoplasm.
  - The epitopes are in the extracellular domain of the receptor.
  - The antibodies specifically react with mGluR5.
- The neurologic disorder is reversible.
  - tumor treatment (excision or chemotherapy)
  - steroids

84.4.11 IgLON5 Ab Syndrome

- First described in 2014
- Syndrome with
  - Sleep disorders (parasomnia and breathing dysfunction)
  - Gait instability
  - Brain stem symptoms
- Isolated dysphagia as initial sign
- Further clinical symptoms
  - negative in progressive supranuclear palsy
  - negative in cortico-basal syndrome
  - associated with chorea
  - associated with parkinsonism
- Surface Abs to the neuronal cell adhesion protein IgLON5
- Neuropathological changes:
  - tau aggregates in the tegmentum of the brain stem and in the hypothalamus
  - not classifiable within any known tauopathy
  - possible neurodegenerative etiology of the disease
- Immunosuppressive treatments including steroids, IVIg, cyclophosphamide, and rituximab
  - poor response
  - some improvement

- Whether the Abs are a primary or secondary element in the disease development needs to be clarified.

84.5 Neuroimaging Findings

84.5.1 General Imaging Findings

Initial edema, later atrophy of affected region (limbic encephalitis, rhombencephalitis).

Imaging without pathological findings does not exclude paraneoplastic syndromes.

CT non-contrast-enhanced
- Hypodense

CT contrast-enhanced
- Usually no enhancement

MRI-T2 (Fig. 84.1a, b)
- Hyperintense

MRI-FLAIR (Fig. 84.1c)
- Hyperintense

MRI-T1 (Fig. 84.1d)
- Hypointense

MRI-T2∗/SWI
- Hemorrhages rare

MRI-T1 contrast-enhanced (Fig. 84.1e)
- Enhancement described but not typical, in cases of laminar necrosis

MR-Diffusion Imaging (Fig. 84.1f)
- Restricted diffusion rare

A summary of imaging characteristics associated with established neuronal surface antibody syndromes is shown in Table 84.5.

Nuclear Medicine Imaging Findings (Figs. 84.2, 84.3 and 84.4)
- In patients with limbic encephalitis, hypermetabolism in FDG-PET in the temporal (especially temporo-mesial—also bilaterally) and orbitofrontal cortex with occipital hypometabolism is described.
- Another pattern, especially in older patients can mimic neurodegenerative disease.
- In patients with limbic encephalitis, FDG-PET/CT can be used as a screening tool for malignancy by covering the whole torso of the patient in a one-stop-shop study and excluding (or revealing) many possible malignancies.
- FDG-PET/CT has a higher sensitivity for detecting malignancy in these patients than CT alone.

84.6 Neuropathology Findings

Macroscopic Features (Fig. 84.5a)
- No gross-anatomical changes
- Atrophy of the hippocampal formation
- Atrophy of the cerebellum
- No changes in consistency of the tissue to light softening

Microscopic Features (Figs. 84.5b and 84.6a–h)
- Variable loss of neurons in the hippocampal formation
- Gliomesenchymal nodules
- Neuronal damage
- Softening of the tissue
- Perivascular lymphocytic infiltrates

Immunophenotype (Figs. 84.5c–j and 84.7a–n)
- CD3
- CD4
- CD8
- Granzyme B
- Increases in
  - GFAP-positive astrocyte
  - HLA-DRII positive microglia
  - CD86 positive macrophages

Proliferation Markers
- Ki-67 positive lymphocytes and macrophages/microglia

Differential Diagnosis
- Inflammatory disorder
- Infectious disease
- Hippocampal sclerosis

84.6 Neuropathology Findings

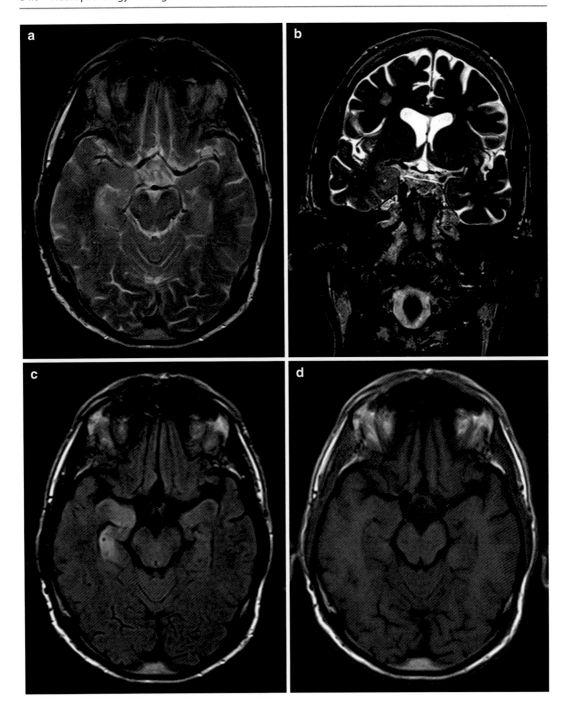

Fig. 84.1 LIG1-positive limbic encephalitis. T2 (**a**), T2 cor (**b**), FLAIR (**c**), T1 (**d**), T1 contrast (**e**), DWI (**f**)

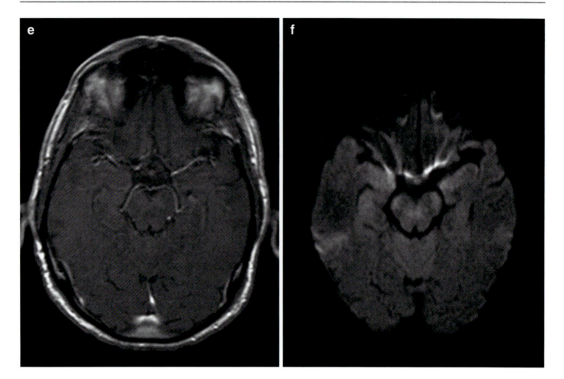

Fig. 84.1 (continued)

Table 84.5 Summary of imaging characteristics associated with established neuronal surface antibody syndromes, modified after Ramanathan et al. (2014), reproduced with kind permission by Elsevier

Autoantibody	MRI findings
NMDAR	• Up to 50% abnormal • Medial temporal lobe hyperintensity • Focal cortical T2-weighted/FLAIR hyperintensity
LGI1	• 85% medial temporal lobe FLAIR high signal
Caspr2	• 40% abnormal, medial temporal lobe FLAIR high signal
AMPAR	• 90% abnormal • Medial temporal lobe FLAIR high signal
GABABR	• 65% medial temporal lobe FLAIR high signal
Glycine R	• Frequently normal

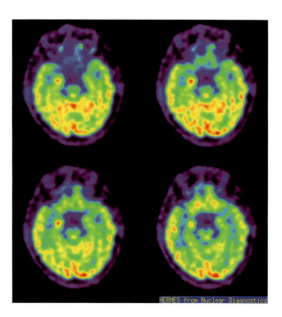

Fig. 84.2 Patient after resuscitation (thereby with a low FDG uptake in the cortex) with hypermetabolism of the left temporo-mesial region corresponding to limbic encephalitis

84.7 Molecular Neuropathology

Paraneoplastic (Table 84.6)
- Immune responses against intraneuronal proteins.
- Ectopic expression of neuronal proteins triggers immune response misdirected against the nervous system.
- Antigens released by apoptotic tumor cells are taken up and processed by antigen-presenting cells at the regional lymph node, presented to immunological system eliciting an anti-tumor immune response.
- Prominent cytotoxic T-cell responses.
- Neuronal degeneration via perforin or granzyme-related mechanisms.

Neuronal
- Antibodies access cell surface targets and alter their structure and function.
- Cross-linking and internalization of the receptors.
- Functional blocking of receptors.
- Complement-mediated changes in the neuromuscular junction.
- Priming B-cell immune responses leading to production of autoantibodies with functional and reversible rather than structural and irreversible neuronal alteration.
- Tumor (teratoma) contains itself immature neuronal tissue.
- Loss of self-tolerance produced by alterations in the mechanisms of positive and negative T-cell selection production of autoregulatory T-cells affecting B-cell function.

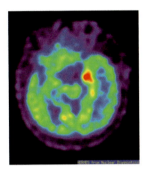

Fig. 84.3 Slices of an FDG-PET of a patient with limbic encephalitis with hypermetabolism of the right temporomesial region

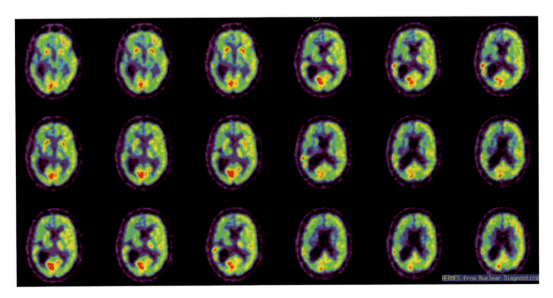

Fig. 84.4 FDG-PET of a patient with Rasmussen encephalitis demonstrating the loss of glucose metabolism due to neuronal loss

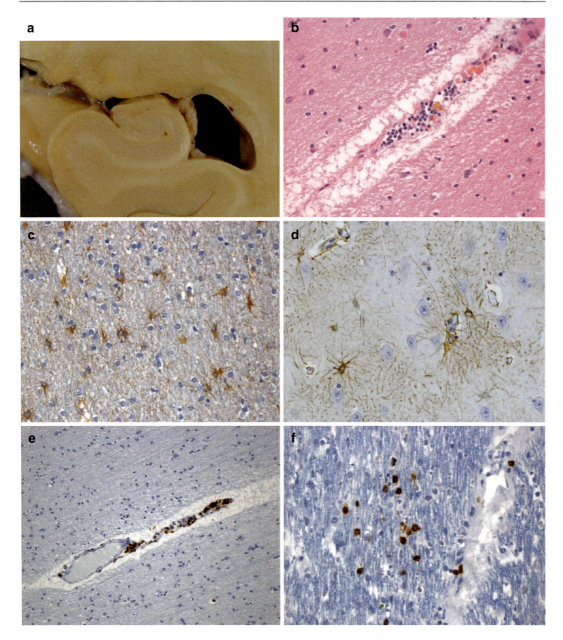

Fig. 84.5 GABA-B receptor encephalitis: The hippocampal formation does not show any abnormalities, i.e., atrophy at the gross-anatomical level (**a**). Scant lymphocytic infiltrates are seen predominantly in a perivascular location (**b**); mild reactive astrogliosis (**c**, **d**; IHC: GFAP); scant presence of CD3-positive lymphocytes (**e**, **f**); mild to moderate reactive microgliosis in the cerebellar white matter (**g**), hippocampal formation (**h**), and cerebral white matter (**i**, **j**)

84.7 Molecular Neuropathology

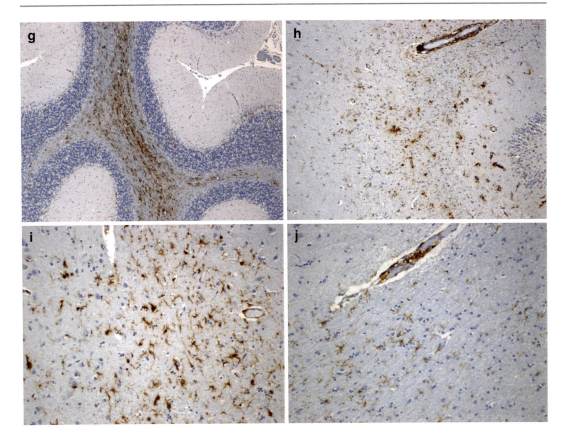

Fig. 84.5 (continued)

- Virus-induced inflammatory disorder triggers autoantibodies against cell surface and synaptic receptors.

84.7.1 Predisposition to Autoimmunity

Genetic susceptibility
- HLA associations with LGI1 and IgLON5 antibodies

Three ways for affection of the nervous system by non-metastatic disorders:

- Cancer damages non-neural issues:
  – Directly by metastases
  – Indirectly by:
    ○ Vascular disorders
    ○ Infections
    ○ Nutritional disorders
    ○ Side effects of therapy
    ○ Remote or paraneoplastic syndromes
- Non-neural organ causes structural damage to the nervous system.
  – Hypercoagulation associated with cancer
- Directly affects the nervous system via immune mediation.
  – Paraneoplastic disorders

IgG antibodies
- Cytotoxic T-cells in
  – Intracellular-onconeural
  – Intracellular-synaptic
- Antibodies
  – Cell surface or synaptic receptors

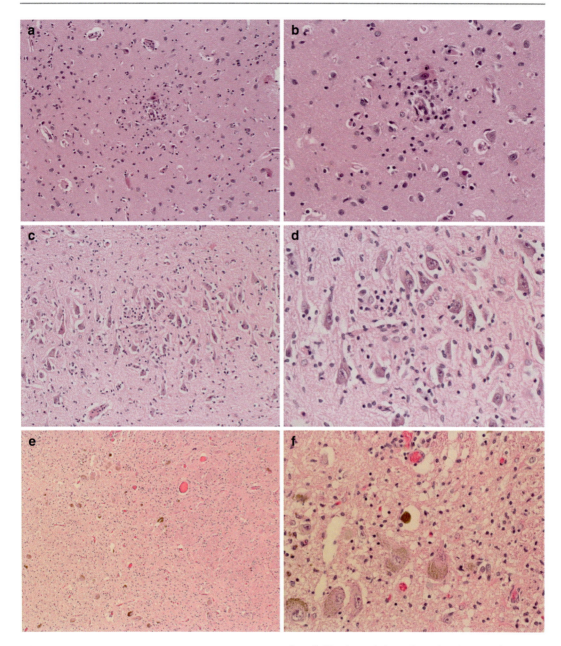

Fig. 84.6 mGluR5-Encephalitis: Accumulation of inflammatory cells (T-lymphocytes in the form of gliomesenchymal nodules in the cerebral cortex, (**a–d**), as diffuse infiltration of the substantia nigra (**e, f**), and as perivascular vascular lymphocytic cuffing (**g, h**) (**a–h**: HE)

84.8 Treatment and Prognosis

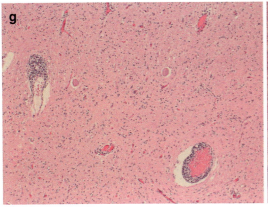
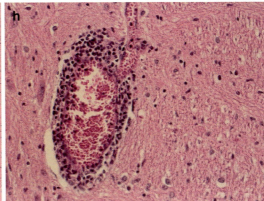

Fig. 84.6 (continued)

N-methyl-D-aspartate receptors-antibody cases
- no evidence of antibody-mediated tissue injury
- no evidence of complement-mediated tissue injury
- absence of clear neuronal pathology and a low density of inflammatory cells

Voltage-gated potassium channel complex encephalitis
- antibody-mediated immune response
- complement-mediated immune
- responsible for neuronal loss and cerebral atrophy

The following categories of autoantibodies are defined (Shoenfeld et al. 2014) (Tables 84.7, 84.8, 84.9 and 84.10):

- Paraneoplastic antinuclear and antinucleolar antibodies
  - Anti-Hu (ANNA-1), Anti-Ri (ANNA-2), Anti-Ma1, Ma2, ANNA3, Zic-4, SOX1 (antiglial nuclear antibody)
- Cytoplasmic antibodies
  - Anti-Yo, anti-Tr, Anti.CV2 (CRMP5), Anti-PCA-2, anti-kinase antibodies, anti-ubiquitin conjugating enzyme (UBE2E1), Anti-NB (beta-NAP), anti-proteasome, anti-CARP VIII
- Synaptic and channel antibodies
  - Intracellular synaptic antibodies (AB)
    - Anti-amphiphysin AB, anti-glutamic acid decarboxylase AB, anti-gephyrin AB, anti-synaptotagmin AB, anti-synaptophysin AB
  - Synaptic receptor antibodies
    - Anti-GABA receptor AB, anti-glutamate receptor AB, anti-glycine receptor AB, anti-ganglionic neuronal acetylcholine receptor AB
  - Ion channel antibodies
    - Anti-P/Q type voltage-gated calcium channel AB, anti-voltage-gated potassium channels (VGKC)
  - Postsynaptic receptor antibodies
    - Anti-acetylcholine receptor AB, anti-muscle AB, antineuronal surface antigen AB
- Anti-retinal and optic nerve antibodies
  - Carcinoma-associated retinopathy, isolated cone dysfunction, melanoma-associated retinopathy, bilateral diffuse uveal melanocytic proliferation

84.8 Treatment and Prognosis

Treatment
- Find and treat cancer
  - Surgery
  - Radiation
  - chemotherapy

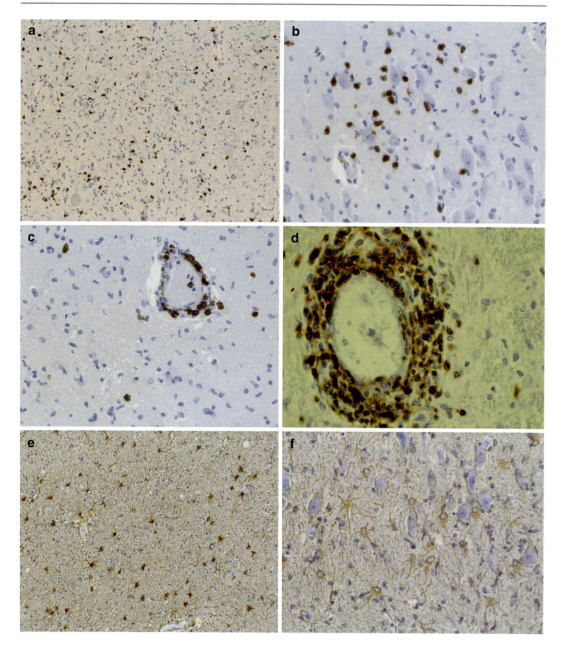

Fig. 84.7 mGluR5-Encephalitis: The lymphocytes are CD3-positive T-lymphocytes (**a–d**), moderate reactive astrogliosis (**e, f**), and severe reactive microgliosis in the cerebral cortex (**g, h**), spinal cord (**i**), cerebellar dentate nucleus (**j**), and hippocampal formation (**k–n**)

84.8 Treatment and Prognosis

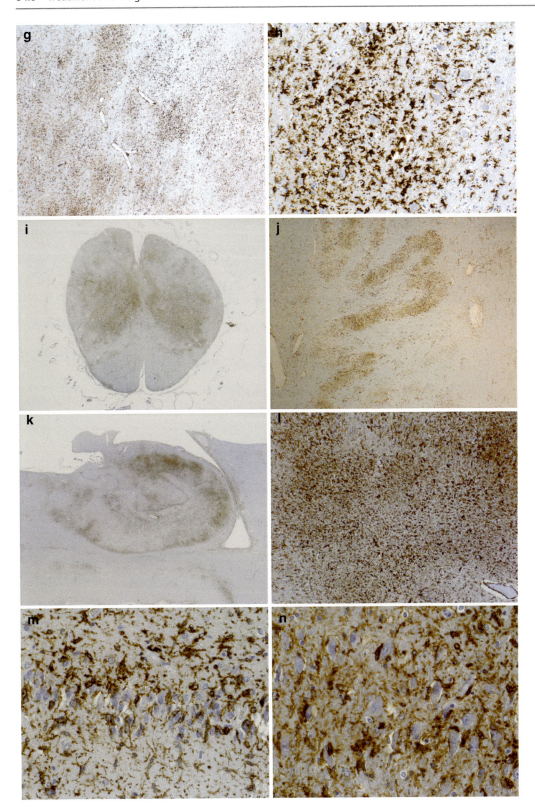

Fig. 84.7 (continued)

Table 84.6 Summary of neurologic manifestation/syndrome according to the nervous system level with neural antibodies and their associated neoplasms, modified after Pittock and Vincent (2016), reproduced with kind permission by Elsevier

Level	Syndrome/disorder	Neural antibody (IgG) associations	Neoplasm: frequency
Cerebral cortex	Encephalitis (limbic)/encephalopathy	VGKC complex (LGI1)	Thymoma, SCLC, other: <10%
		VGKC complex (CASPR2)	Thymoma: <40%
	Autoimmune epilepsy	NMDAR	Ovarian teratoma: 50%
	Autoimmune cognitive disorder/dementia	CRMP-5 (CV2)	SCLC>thymoma: >90%
		ANNA-1 (Hu)	SCLC>neuroblastoma: >80%
		GABA R	Lung, neuroendocrine: 50%
		Ma2	Testicular, lung: >90%
		Ma1	Breast, colon, parotid, lung: >90%
		Amphiphysin	Breast, SCLC: >90%
		IgLON 5 (cognitive disorder/dementia)	No tumor association known
		AMPAR	Lung, breast, thymoma: 70%
		GAD65	Lung, neuroendocrine, thymoma: <10%
Diencephalon	Hypothalamic dysfunction Ehlers–Danlos syndrome (EDS), narcolepsy/cataplexy, syndrome of inappropriate antidiuretic hormone (SIADH)	Ma1, Ma2 (EDS, cataplexy)	Testicular, lung: >90% Breast, colon, parotid, lung: >90%
		VGKC complex (LGI1, CASPR2, other), AQP4	Breast/lung/thymoma/carcinoid: <5%
Basal ganglia	Chorea/dystonia/dyskinesia	CRMP-5 (CV2)	SCLC>thymoma: >90%
		GAD65	Lung, neuroendocrine, thymoma: <10%
		ANNA-1 (Hu)	SCLC>neuroblastoma: >80%
		VGKC complex (LGI1, CASPR2, other)	Breast/lung/thymoma/carcinoid: <5%
		Amphiphysin	Breast, SCLC: >90%
Cerebellum	Cerebellar ataxia Cerebellar degeneration	PCA-1 (Yo)	Ovarian, breast, mullerian duct: >90%
		PCA-Tr (DNER)	Hodgkin lymphoma: >80%
		ANNA-1 (Hu)	SCLC>neuroblastoma: >80%
		CRMP-5 (CV2)	SCLC>thymoma: >90%
		mGluR-1	Hodgkin lymphoma: few cases
		GAD65	Lung, neuroendocrine, thymoma: <10%
		VGCC (PQ and N type)	SCLC, other: 50%
Brainstem	Brainstem encephalitis/encephalopathy	CRMP-5 (CV2)	SCLC>thymoma: >90%
		ANNA-1 (Hu), OMS	SCLC>neuroblastoma: >80%
	Opsoclonus myoclonus (OMS)	ANNA-2 (Ri), OMS	
	Stiff-person syndrome (SPS)	Amphiphysin	Breast, SCLC: >90%
	PERM (progressive encephalomyelitis with rigidity and myoclonus)	Ma2	Testicular, lung: >90%
		Ma1	Breast, colon, parotid, lung: >90%
		GlyαR (SPS, PERM)	Thymoma, lymphoma: 20%
		AQP4	
		GAD65 (SPS)	Lung, neuroendocrine, thymoma: <10%

84.8 Treatment and Prognosis

Table 84.6 (continued)

Level	Syndrome/disorder	Neural antibody (IgG) associations	Neoplasm: frequency
Spinal cord	Myelopathy and myoclonus	AQP4	
		CRMP5 (CV2)	SCLC>thymoma: >90%
		Amphiphysin	Breast, SCLC: >90%
Peripheral nerves and ganglia	Sensory neuronopathy and sensorimotor neuropathies Peripheral nerve hyperexcitability	ANNA-1 (Hu	SCLC>neuroblastoma: >80%
		CRMP-5 (CV2)	SCLC>thymoma: >90%
		Amphiphysin	Breast, SCLC: >90%
		Ganglionic AChR	Breast, prostate, lung, gastrointestinal: <15%
	Autonomic neuropathies (pandysautonomia or limited)	VGKC antibodies (CASPR2)	Breast/lung/thymoma/carcinoid: <5%
Neuromuscular junction	Myasthenia gravis	Muscle AChR	Thymoma: <20%
	Lambert–Eaton syndrome	VGCC (PQ type>N type)	SCLC: 50%
		SOX1	SCLC: >90%
Muscle	Acute necrotizing myositis	SRP54	Low risk
	Dermatomyositis	Anti TIF1g or NXP2	Adenocarcinoma: >70%

AChR acetylcholine receptor; *AMPAR* alpha-amino-3-hydroxy-5-methyl-4-isoxazolepropionic acid receptor; *ANNA* antineuronal nuclear antibody; *AQP4* aquaporin-4; *CASPR2* contactin-associated protein-like 2; *CRMP-5 (CV2)* collapsin response mediator protein 5; *DNER* delta/notch-like epidermal growth factor receptor; *GABAR* gamma-aminobutyric acid receptor; *GAD-65* glutamic acid decarboxylase; *GlyaR* glycine alpha receptor; *IgLON5* immunoglobulin-like family member 5; *LGI1* leucine-rich, glioma-inactivated 1; *mGluR* metabotropic glutamate receptor; *NMDAR* N-methyl-D-aspartic acid receptor; *NXP* nuclear matrix protein; *PCA* Purkinje cell cytoplasmic antibody; *SIADH* secretion; *SOX1* sex determining region Y box 1 transcription factor; *SRP* signal recognition particle; *TIF* transcription intermediary factor; *VGCC* voltage-gated calcium channel; *VGKC* voltage-gated potassium channel. Lung cancer includes both small cell lung cancer (SCLC) and non-small cell lung cancer, unless otherwise specified

- Immunity suppression
  - Predominantly T-cell suppression
    Corticosteroids
    Cyclophosphamide
    Tacrolimus
    Stem cell transplantation
  - Predominantly B-cell suppression
    Plasma exchange
    Intravenous immunoglobulin (IVIG)
    Antibodies (e.g., rituximab)
- Control of symptoms
  - Ataxia
  - Stiff muscle
  - Weakness
  - Pain
  - Cognitive dysfunction
  - seizures

Table 84.7 Examples of intracellular and cell surface antigens

	Antigens
Intracellular-onconeural	• HU • CRMP5 • Ri • Yo • Ma2
Intracellular-synaptic	• GAD • Amphiphysin
Cell surface or synaptic receptor	• NMDA-R • AMPA-R • GABA-B-R • LGI1 • Caspr2 • Gly-R

Table 84.8 Intracellularly targeted (neuronal nucleus, cytoplasm, nucleolus) antibodies

Autoantibodies	Associated diseases	Associated tumors
Anti-HU (antineuronal nuclear antibody ANNA-1, Antineuronal nuclear antibodies)	• Encephalomyelitis • Limbic encephalitis • Extra-limbic encephalitis • Subacute sensory neuronopathy (Denny-Brown syndrome) • Autonomic neuropathy	• Small cell lung cancer • Neuroblastoma
Anti-Ri (antineuronal nuclear antibody ANNA-2, Antineuronal nuclear antibodies)	• Opsoclonus-myoclonus syndrome • Cerebellar degeneration • Brain stem encephalitis • Dementia • Limbic encephalitis Nova-1: cerebellar degeneration, encephalitis, myelitis, opsoclonus myoclonus Nova-2: paraneoplastic opsoclonus-myoclonus ataxia, myoclonus, encephalitis, cerebellar degeneration and myelitis	• Small cell lung cancer • Breast carcinoma
ANNA-3 (antineuronal nuclear antibody)	• Cerebellar degeneration • Encephalomyelitis, sensory neuropathy	• Lung cancer (60%)
Anti-SOX1 (sex determining region Y box 1 transcription factor) [antiglial nuclear antibody (AGNA)]	• Lambert–Eaton myasthenic syndrome • Cerebellar degeneration • Sensory neuropathy	• Small cell lung cancer
Anti-CV-2/CRMP5 (collapsin response mediator protein 5)	• Encephalitis • Extrapyramidal-motoric syndromes • Chorea • Cerebellar degeneration • Sensory and autonomic neuropathy • Optic neuritis and retinitis • Myelopathy • Neuropathy • Lambert–Eaton myasthenic syndrome	• Small cell lung cancer • Thymoma
Anti-GAD65	• Stiff-person syndrome • Diabetes mellitus Type I • Limbic encephalitis	• Breast carcinoma • Thyroid carcinoma • Other
Anti-Ma1	• Brain stem encephalitis • Limbic encephalitis	• Bronchial carcinoma • Testicular carcinoma • Breast carcinoma
Anti-Ma2	• Brain stem encephalitis • Limbic encephalitis • Hypothalamic	• Testicular carcinoma
Anti-PCA-1 (Anti-Yo)	• Paraneoplastic cerebellar syndrome: Ataxia, dysarthria, nystagmus, peripheral neuropathy	• Breast • Gynecologic • Lung cancer
Anti-PCA-2 (Purkinje cell autoantibodies)	• Limbic/Brain stem encephalitis • Cerebellar ataxia • Lambert–Eaton myasthenic syndrome (LEMS) • Autonomic neuropathy • Motor neuropathy	• Small cell lung cancer • Gynecological tumors
Anti-MAG	• Paraneoplastic neuropathy • Monoclonal IgM-gammopathy, i.e., monoclonal gammopathy of unknown significance (MGUS) and Waldenström disease	• Waldenström macroglobulinemia
Anti-Myelin	• Diagnostic significance controversial	
Anti-Recoverin	• Retinopathy	• Small cell lung cancer • Ovarian carcinoma

84.8 Treatment and Prognosis

Table 84.8 (continued)

Autoantibodies	Associated diseases	Associated tumors
Anti-TRPM-1	• Retinopathy	• Melanoma
Amphiphysin	• Paraneoplastic Stiff-person syndrome • Myelitis	• Breast carcinoma • Small cell lung cancer
Retinal [cancer-associated retinopathy (CAR), melanoma-associated retinopathy (MAR)]	• Retinopathy	• Uncertain incidence (small cell lung cancer, breast, gynecologic, melanoma)
Striational	• Myasthenia gravis • Common with muscle AChR • Considered marker of autoimmunity when occurring in isolation	• Thymoma (30%)
ZIC (zinc finger protein)	• Encephalomyelitis • Cerebellar degeneration • Opsoclonus	• Small cell lung cancer

Table 84.9 Antibodies to neuronal cell surface proteins and synaptic receptors

Antigen	Associated diseases	Associated tumors

AchR	• Muscle:
	  – Myasthenia gravis
	• Ganglionic:
	  – Autonomic dysfunction
	  – Encephalopathy
	  – Peripheral neuropathy
		• Muscle: thymoma (10%)
		• Ganglionic: breast, prostate
		• Lung
		• Gastrointestinal cancer

Aquaporin 4	• Neuromyelitis optica (NMO) Devic disease • Longitudinal extensive transverse myelitis (LETM) • Recurrent optic neuritis • Encepalopathy • Vomiting	• Lung carcinoma • Breast carcinoma • Thymoma • Carcinoid • B-cell lymphoma

NMDA Receptor (GluN1)	• Anti-Glutamate-Receptor-(Typ NMDA)—Encephalitis:
	  – Psychiatric manifestations
	  – Insomnia
	  – Reduced verbal output
	  – Seizures
	  – Amnesia
	  – Movement disorders
	  – Catatonia
	  – Autonomic instability
	  – Coma
		• Ovarial teratoma
		• Testicular teratoma

AMPA-Receptor (GluA1 or GluA2)	• Limbic encephalitis • Psychosis	• Bronchial carcinoma • Breast carcinoma • Malignant thymoma
GABA$_A$ Receptor	• Refactory seizures • Status epilepticus	• Infrequent
GABA$_B$ Receptor (B1 subunit)	• Limbic encephalitis • Seizures • Status epilepticus	• Small cell lung cancer • Neuroendocrine carcinoma

(continued)

Table 84.9 (continued)

Antigen	Associated diseases	Associated tumors
Glycine α-Receptor	• Stiff-person syndrome • PERM (progressive encephalomyelitis with rigidity and myoclonus • Limbic encephalitis • Cerebellar degeneration • Optic neuritis	• Infrequent
mGluR1	• Cerebellar ataxia	• Hodgkin lymphoma

mGluR5	• Ophelia syndrome
	  – Limbic encephalitis
	  – Myoclonus
		• Hodgkin lymphoma

MOG (myelin oligodendrocyte glycoprotein)	• NMO-like phenotype:
	  – Optic neuritis
	  – Longitudinally extensive transverse myelitis
	  – ADEM
		• Infrequent

DNER (delta/notch-like epidermal growth factor related receptor (PCA-Tr), Purkinje cell cytoplasmic antibody	• Cerebellar degeneration	• Hodgkin lymphoma

DPPX (dipeptidyl-peptidase-like protein-6)	• Encephalitis with CNS hyperexcitability
	  – Confusion
	  – Tremor
	  – Myoclonus
	  – Nystagmus
	  – Hyperekplexia
	  – PERM-like symptoms
	  – Ataxia
		• B-cell neoplasms (rare)

Dopamine-2 receptor	• Basal ganglia encephalitis • Lethargy • Psychiatric symptoms • Abnormal movements • Gait disturbance	• Not applicable
Neurexin-3α	• Encephalitis • Confusion • Seizures	• Not applicable
IgLON5 (immunoglobulin-like family members 5	• Abnormal sleep movements and behaviors • Obstructive sleep apnea • Stridor • Dysarthria • Dysphagia • Ataxia • Chorea • Refractory to immunotherapy	• None reported
VGCC (voltage-gated calcium channel) P/Q type, N-type	• P/Q & N : Lambert–Eaton myasthenic syndrome • P/Q : cerebellar degeneration, seizures • N : encephalopathy, seizures	• LEMS small cell lung cancer
VGKC (voltage-gated potassium channel complex)	• Includes LGI-1 • Includes CASPR2 • Dementia • Pain syndromes	• Small cell lung cancer • Thymoma
LGI1 (voltage-gated potassium channels (VGKC))	• Limbic encephalitis • Myoclonus • Seizures • Hyponatremia	• Thyroid carcinoma
CASPR2 (voltage-gated potassium channels (VGKC))	• Limbic encephalitis • Neuromyotonia • Morvan syndrome	• Thymoma • Uterine carcinoma

Table 84.10 Involved antigens with their function and pathogenic mechanism (Lancaster and Dalmau 2012), reproduced with kind permission by Springer Nature

Antigen	Antigen function	Mechanisms
Neuronal nonsynaptic autoantibody targets		
Hu proteins (primarily HuD, but also HuC, Hel-N1, and Hel-N2)	HuD is important for neuronal RNA handling, cell cycle regulation, and cell development	Antibodies are not directly pathogenic; possibly T-cell-mediated
Collapsin response mediator protein 5	Regulation of neurite outgrowth, and neurogenesis	Possibly T-cell-mediated
Ma1	Promotion of apoptosis	Probably T-cell-mediated rather than antibody-mediated
Ma2 (also known as Ta)	Not known	Not known
Yo proteins (also known CDR1 and CDR2)	• CDR1 is strongly expressed in Purkinje cells; function unknown • CDR2 may be involved in cell cycle regulation, mitosis, and transcriptional regulation	• Conflicting data in patients regarding a role for T-cells • Antibodies trigger neuronal cell death in slice culture
Ri proteins (also known as Nova-1 and Nova-2)	Nova-1 is an RNA-binding protein expressed by subcortical neurons Function of Nova-2 is not known	Antibodies may prevent binding of Nova-1 to RNA126 Unclear whether antibodies are pathogenic; comorbid antibodies are common and can occur in asymptomatic cancer patients
Tr	Found in Purkinje neurons; Function not known	Not known
Zinc finger protein ZIC 4	Important for brain development	Antibodies may not be pathogenic; 80% of patients have other antibodies as well
Gephyrin and GABARAP	Associated with GABA-ergic transmission	Not known
Synaptic autoantibody targets—Intracellular antigens		
65 kDa glutamic acid decarboxylase	Crucial for synthesis of GABA	Evidence for both T-cell-mediated and antibody-mediated mechanisms Pathogenic role in other syndromes is not clear
Amphiphysin	Important for recycling of synaptic vesicles	Antibodies are directly pathogenic
Synaptic autoantibody targets—Extracellular antigens		
NMDAR	Crucial for learning and memory	Antibodies disrupt NMDAR function by cross-linking and internalization of receptors
Leucine-rich glioma-inactivated protein 1 (LGI1)	Secreted protein that regulates presynaptic Kv1 channels and postsynaptic AMPARs	Unknown
Contactin-associated protein-like 2 (CASPR2)	Organizes Kv1 channels on myelinated axons	Unknown
GABAB receptor	Mediates inhibitory synaptic transmission	Unknown
AMPAR	Crucial for learning and memory	Antibodies cause cross-linking and internalization of AMPARs
P/Q-type voltage-gated calcium channels	Crucial for calcium influx into presynaptic terminals	Antibodies block channels at presynaptic terminal of neuromuscular junction; possibly also pathogenic in CNS
Metabotropic glutamate receptor 1	Crucial for cerebellar function	Unknown
Metabotropic glutamate receptor 5	Crucial for hippocampal function	Unknown

Biologic Behavior–Prognosis–Prognostic Factors

- Intracellular-onconeural
  - 10–30% of patients with mild response
  - Infrequent relapses, usually monophasic and irreversible
- Intracellular-synaptic
  - About 60% of patients have partial improvement.
  - Infrequent relapses.
  - Symptoms may fluctuate.
- Cell surface or synaptic receptor
  - Substantial or full recoveries (75–80%).
  - Relapses vary with antigen (10–25%).

Selected References

Armangue T, Leypoldt F, Dalmau J (2014) Autoimmune encephalitis as differential diagnosis of infectious encephalitis. Curr Opin Neurol 27(3):361–368. https://doi.org/10.1055/s-0034-1390394

Bauer J, Bien CG (2016) Neuropathology of autoimmune encephalitides. Handb Clin Neurol 133:107–120. https://doi.org/10.1016/b978-0-444-63432-0.00007-4

Bruggemann N, Wandinger KP, Gaig C, Sprenger A, Junghanns K, Helmchen C, Munchau A (2016) Dystonia, lower limb stiffness, and upward gaze palsy in a patient with IgLON5 antibodies. Mov Disord 31(5):762–764. https://doi.org/10.1002/mds.26608

Chastain EM, Miller SD (2012) Molecular mimicry as an inducing trigger for CNS autoimmune demyelinating disease. Immunol Rev 245(1):227–238. https://doi.org/10.1111/j.1600-065X.2011.01076.x

Corrigan JJ, Crisp SJ, Kullmann DM, Vincent A (2016) Autoimmune synaptopathies. Nat Rev Neurosci 17(2):103–117. https://doi.org/10.1038/nrn.2015.27

Dale RC, Merheb V, Pillai S, Wang D, Cantrill L, Murphy TK, Ben-Pazi H, Varadkar S, Aumann TD, Horne MK, Church AJ, Fath T, Brilot F (2012) Antibodies to surface dopamine-2 receptor in autoimmune movement and psychiatric disorders. Brain 135(Pt 11):3453–3468. https://doi.org/10.1093/brain/aws256

Dalmau J, Rosenfeld MR (2014) Autoimmune encephalitis update. Neuro Oncol 16(6):771–778. https://doi.org/10.1093/neuonc/nou030

Dalmau J, Geis C, Graus F (2017) Autoantibodies to synaptic receptors and neuronal cell surface proteins in autoimmune diseases of the central nervous system. Physiol Rev 97(2):839–887. https://doi.org/10.1152/physrev.00010.2016

Darnell RB, Posner JB (2011) Paraneoplastic syndromes. Oxford University Press, Oxford

Davidson A, Diamond B (2014) General features of autoimmune disease. In: Rose NR, Mackay IR (eds) The autoimmune diseases, 5th edn. Elsevier, Amsterdam, pp 19–37

Dubey D, Blackburn K, Greenberg B, Stuve O, Vernino S (2016) Diagnostic and therapeutic strategies for management of autoimmune encephalopathies. Expert Rev Neurother 16(8):937–949. https://doi.org/10.1080/14737175.2016.1189328

Fukata M, Yokoi N, Fukata Y (2017) Neurobiology of autoimmune encephalitis. Curr Opin Neurobiol 48:1–8. https://doi.org/10.1016/j.conb.2017.07.012

Gaspard N (2016) Autoimmune epilepsy. Continuum 22(1 Epilepsy):227–245. https://doi.org/10.1212/con.0000000000000272

Gastaldi M, Thouin A, Vincent A (2016) Antibody-mediated autoimmune encephalopathies and immunotherapies. Neurotherapeutics 13(1):147–162. https://doi.org/10.1007/s13311-015-0410-6

Gelpi E, Hoftberger R, Graus F, Ling H, Holton JL, Dawson T, Popovic M, Pretnar-Oblak J, Hogl B, Schmutzhard E, Poewe W, Ricken G, Santamaria J, Dalmau J, Budka H, Revesz T, Kovacs GG (2016) Neuropathological criteria of anti-IgLON5-related tauopathy. Acta Neuropathol 132(4):531–543. https://doi.org/10.1007/s00401-016-1591-8

Graus F, Dalmau J (2012) Paraneoplastic neurological syndromes. Curr Opin Neurol 25(6):795–801. https://doi.org/10.1097/WCO.0b013e328359da15

Graus F, Delattre JY, Antoine JC, Dalmau J, Giometto B, Grisold W, Honnorat J, Smitt PS, Vedeler C, Verschuuren JJ, Vincent A, Voltz R (2004) Recommended diagnostic criteria for paraneoplastic neurological syndromes. J Neurol Neurosurg Psychiatry 75(8):1135–1140. https://doi.org/10.1136/jnnp.2003.034447

Graus F, Titulaer MJ, Balu R, Benseler S, Bien CG, Cellucci T, Cortese I, Dale RC, Gelfand JM, Geschwind M, Glaser CA, Honnorat J, Hoftberger R, Iizuka T, Irani SR, Lancaster E, Leypoldt F, Pruss H, Rae-Grant A, Reindl M, Rosenfeld MR, Rostasy K, Saiz A, Venkatesan A, Vincent A, Wandinger KP, Waters P, Dalmau J (2016a) A clinical approach to diagnosis of autoimmune encephalitis. Lancet Neurol 15(4):391–404. https://doi.org/10.1016/s1474-4422(15)00401-9

Graus F, Titulaer MJ, Balu R, Benseler S, Bien CG, Cellucci T, Cortese I, Dale RC, Gelfand JM, Geschwind M, Glaser CA, Honnorat J, Hoftberger R, Iizuka T, Irani SR, Lancaster E, Leypoldt F, Pruss H, Rae-Grant A, Reindl M, Rosenfeld MR, Rostasy K, Saiz A, Venkatesan A, Vincent A, Wandinger KP, Waters P, Dalmau J (2016b) A clinical approach to diagnosis of autoimmune encephalitis. Am J Neuroradiol 15(4):391–404. https://doi.org/10.1016/s1474-4422(15)00401-9

Griffith B, Haitao R, Yingmai Y, Yan H, Fei H, Xia L, Honglin H, Chaiyan L, Stocker W, Liying C, Hongzhi G (2016) Chorea and parkinsonism associated with autoantibodies to IgLON5 and responsive to immunotherapy. J Neuroimmunol 300:9–10. https://doi.org/10.1016/j.jneuroim.2016.09.012

Heine J, Pruss H, Bartsch T, Ploner CJ, Paul F, Finke C (2015) Imaging of autoimmune encephalitis—relevance for clinical practice and hippocampal function. Neuroscience 309:68–83. https://doi.org/10.1016/j.neuroscience.2015.05.037

Hogl B, Heidbreder A, Santamaria J, Graus F, Poewe W (2015) IgLON5 autoimmunity and abnormal behaviours during sleep. Lancet 385(9977):1590. https://doi.org/10.1016/s0140-6736(15)60445-7

Iorio R, Lennon VA (2012) Neural antigen-specific autoimmune disorders. Immunol Rev 248(1):104–121. https://doi.org/10.1111/j.1600-065X.2012.01144.x

Kalman B (2017) Autoimmune encephalitides: a broadening field of treatable conditions. Am J Neuroradiol 22(1):1–13. https://doi.org/10.3174/ajnr.A5086

Kawakami N (2016) In vivo imaging in autoimmune diseases in the central nervous system. Allergol Int 65(3):235–242. https://doi.org/10.1016/j.alit.2016.02.001

Kelley BP, Patel SC (2017) Autoimmune encephalitis: pathophysiology and imaging review of an overlooked diagnosis. Am J Neuroradiol 38(6):1070–1078. https://doi.org/10.3174/ajnr.A5086

Lancaster E (2016) The diagnosis and treatment of autoimmune encephalitis. J Clin Neurol 12(1):1–13. https://doi.org/10.3988/jcn.2016.12.1.1

Lancaster E, Dalmau J (2012) Neuronal autoantigens—pathogenesis, associated disorders and antibody testing. Nat Rev Neurol 8(7):380–390. https://doi.org/10.1038/nrneurol.2012.99

Leypoldt F, Armangue T, Dalmau J (2015) Autoimmune encephalopathies. Ann N Y Acad Sci 1338:94–114. https://doi.org/10.1111/nyas.12553

Linnoila J, Pittock SJ (2016) Autoantibody-associated central nervous system neurologic disorders. Semin Neurol 36(4):382–396. https://doi.org/10.1055/s-0036-1585453

Linnoila JJ, Rosenfeld MR, Dalmau J (2014) Neuronal surface antibody-mediated autoimmune encephalitis. Semin Neurol 34(4):458–466. https://doi.org/10.1055/s-0034-1390394

Mangesius S, Sprenger F, Hoftberger R, Seppi K, Reindl M, Poewe W (2017) IgLON5 autoimmunity tested negative in patients with progressive supranuclear palsy and corticobasal syndrome. Parkinsonism Relat Disord 38:102–103. https://doi.org/10.1016/j.parkreldis.2017.03.002

Marin HL, McKeon A (2016) Autoimmune encephalopathies and dementias. Continuum 22(2 Dementia):538–558. https://doi.org/10.1212/con.0000000000000299

McKeon A, Pittock SJ (2011) Paraneoplastic encephalomyelopathies: pathology and mechanisms. Acta Neuropathol 122(4):381–400. https://doi.org/10.10007/s00401-011-0876-1

Mitsias PD, Pittock SJ, Vincent A (2016) Introduction to autoimmune neurology. Handb Clin Neurol 133:3–14. https://doi.org/10.1016/b978-0-444-63432-0.00001-3

Pittock SJ, Vincent A (2016) Introduction to autoimmune neurology. Handb Clin Neurol. 133:3-14. https://doi.org/10.1016/B978-0-444-63432-0.00001-3

Ramanathan S, Mohammad SS, Brilot F, Dale RC (2014) Autoimmune encephalitis: recent updates and emerging challenges. J Clin Neurosci 21(5):722–730. https://doi.org/10.1016/j.jocn.2013.07.017

Rose NR, Mackay IR (2014) The autoimmune diseases, 5th edn. Elsevier-Academic Press, Amsterdam

Rosenfeld MR, Dalmau JO (2012) Paraneoplastic disorders of the CNS and autoimmune synaptic encephalitis. Continuum 18(2):366–383. https://doi.org/10.1212/01.CON.0000413664.42798.aa

Sabater L, Gaig C, Gelpi E, Bataller L, Lewerenz J, Torres-Vega E, Contreras A, Giometto B, Compta Y, Embid C, Vilaseca I, Iranzo A, Santamaria J, Dalmau J, Graus F (2014) A novel non-rapid-eye movement and rapid-eye-movement parasomnia with sleep breathing disorder associated with antibodies to IgLON5: a case series, characterisation of the antigen, and post-mortem study. Lancet Neurol 13(6):575–586. https://doi.org/10.1016/s1474-4422(14)70051-1

Sabater L, Planaguma J, Dalmau J, Graus F (2016) Cellular investigations with human antibodies associated with the anti-IgLON5 syndrome. J Neuroinflammation 13(1):226. https://doi.org/10.1186/s12974-016-0689-1

Schroder JB, Melzer N, Ruck T, Heidbreder A, Kleffner I, Dittrich R, Muhle P, Warnecke T, Dziewas R (2017) Isolated dysphagia as initial sign of anti-IgLON5 syndrome. Neurol Neuroimmunol Neuroinflamm 4(1):e302. https://doi.org/10.1212/nxi.0000000000000302

Shoenfeld Y, Meroni PL, Gershwin ME (2014) Autoantibodies, 3rd edn. Elsevier, Amsterdam

Simabukuro MM, Sabater L, Adoni T, Cury RG, Haddad MS, Moreira CH, Oliveira L, Boaventura M, Alves RC, Azevedo Soster L, Nitrini R, Gaig C, Santamaria J, Dalmau J, Graus F (2015) Sleep disorder, chorea, and dementia associated with IgLON5 antibodies. Neurol Neuroimmunol Neuroinflamm 2(4):e136. https://doi.org/10.1212/nxi.0000000000000136

van Sonderen A, Petit-Pedrol M, Dalmau J, Titulaer MJ (2017) The value of LGI1, Caspr2 and voltage-gated potassium channel antibodies in encephalitis. Nat Rev Neurol 13(5):290–301. https://doi.org/10.1038/nrneurol.2017.43

Appendix A: WHO Classification of Tumors of the Central Nervous System

WHO Classification 1979

Zülch KJ (1979) Histological typing of tumours of the central nervous system. 1st ed. World Health Organization, Geneva

Tumours of Neuroepithelial tissue
- Astrocytic tumours
- Astrocytoma
  - fibrillary
  - protoplasmic
  - gemistocytic
- Pilocytic astrocytoma
- Subependymal giant cell astrocytoma [ventricular tumour of tuberous sclerosis]
- Astroblastoma
- Anaplastic [malignant] astrocytoma
- Oligodendroglial tumours
- Oligodendroglioma
- Mixed-oligo-astrocytoma
- Anaplastic [malignant] oligodendroglioma
- Ependymal and choroid plexus tumours
- Ependymoma
  - Myxopapillary
  - Papillary
  - Subependymoma
- Anaplastic [malignant] ependymoma
- Choroid plexus papilloma
- Anaplastic [malignant] choroid plexus papilloma
- Pineal cell tumour
- Pineocytoma [pinealocytoma]
- Pineoblastoma [pinealoblastoma]
- Neuronal tumour
- Gangliocytoma
- Ganglioglioma
- Ganglioneuroblastoma
- Anaplastic [malignant] gangliocytoma and ganglioglioma
- Neuroblastoma
- Poorly differentiated and embryonal tumours
- Glioblastoma
  - Variants:
  - Glioblastoma with sarcomatous component [mixed glioblastoma and sarcoma]
  - Giant cell glioblastoma
- Medulloblastoma
  - Variants:
  - desmoplastic medulloblastoma
  - medullomyoblastoma
- Medulloepithelioma
- Primitive polar spongioblastoma
- Gliomatosis cerebri

Tumours of nerve sheath cells
- Neurilemmoma [Schwannoma, neurinoma]
- Anaplastic [malignant] neurilemmoma [schwannoma, neurinoma]
- Neurofibroma
- Anaplastic [malignant] neurofibroma [neurofibrosarcoma, neurogenic sarcoma]

Tumours of meningeal and related tissues
- Meningioma
  - meningotheliomatous [endotheliomatous, syncytial, arachnotheliomatous]
  - fibrous [fibroblastic]
  - transitional [mixed]
  - psammomatous
  - Angiomatous
  - haemangioblastic
  - haemangiopericytic

© Springer-Verlag GmbH Austria, part of Springer Nature 2019
S. Weis et al., *Imaging Brain Diseases*, https://doi.org/10.1007/978-3-7091-1544-2

- papillary
- anaplastic [malignant] meningioma
• Meningeal sarcomas
  - Fibrosarcoma
  - Polymorphic cell sarcoma
  - Primary meningeal sarcomatosis
• Xanthomatous tumours
  - Fibroxanthoma
  - Xanthosarcoma [malignant fibroxanthoma]
• Primary melanotic tumours
  - Melanoma
  - Meningeal melanomatosis
• others

Primary Malignant Lymphomas

Tumours of blood vessel origin
• Haemangioblastoma [capillary haemangioblastoma]
• Monstrocellular sarcoma

Germ Cell Tumours
• Germinoma
• Embryonal carcinoma
• Choriocarcinoma
• Teratoma

Other malformative tumours and tumour-like lesions
• Craniopharyngioma
• Rathke' cleft cyst
• Epidermoid cyst
• Dermoid cyst
• Colloid cyst of the third ventricle
• Enterogenous cyst
• Other cysts
• Lipoma
• Choristoma [pituicytoma, granular cell "myoblastoma"]
• Hypothalamic neuronal hamartoma
• Nasal glial heterotopia [nasal glioma]

Vascular malformations
• Capillary telangiectasia
• Cavernous angioma
• Arteriovenous malformation
• Venous malformation
• Sturge-Weber disease [cerebrofacial or cerebrotrigeminal angiomatosis]

Tumours of the anterior pituitary
• Pituitary adenoma
• acidophil
• basophil [mucoid cell]
• mixed acidophil-basophil
• chromophobe
• Pituitary adenocarcinoma

Local extensions from regional tumours
• Glomus jugulare tumour [chemodectoma, paragnglioma]
• Chordoma
• Chondroma
• Chondrosarcoma
• Olfactory neuroblastoma [esthesioneuroblastoma]
• Adenoid cystic carcinoma [cylindroma]
• others

Metastatic tumours
Unclassified tumours

WHO Classification 1993

Kleihues P, Burger PC, Scheithauer BW: Histological Typing of Tumours of the Central Nervous System. Springer Verlag, 1993, 2nd edition

Tumours of Neuroepithelial tissue
• Astrocytic tumours
  - Astrocytoma
    ○ Fibrillary
    ○ Protoplasmic
    ○ Gemistocytic
  - Anaplastic (malignant) astrocytoma
  - Glioblastoma
    ○ Giant cell glioblastoma
    ○ Gliosarcoma
  - Pilocytic astrocytoma
  - Pleomorphic xanthoastrocytoma
  - Subependymal giant cell astrocytoma (Tuberous sclerosis)
• Oligodendroglial tumours
  - Oligodendroglioma
  - Anaplastic (malignant) oligodendroglioma
• Ependymal and choroid plexus tumours
  - Ependymoma

- o Cellular
- o Papillary
- o Clear cell
- – Anaplastic (malignant) ependymoma
- – Myxopapillary ependymoma
- – Subependymoma
- Mixed gliomas
  - – Oligo-astrocytoma
  - – Anaplastic (malignant) oligo-astrocytoma
  - – Others
- Chororid plexus tumours
  - – Choroid plexus papilloma
  - – Choroid plexus carcinoma
- Neuroepithelial tumours of uncertain origin
  - – Astroblastoma
  - – Polar spongioblastoma
  - – Gliomatosis cerebri
- Neuronal and mixed neuronal-glial tumours
  - – Gangliocytoma
  - – Dysplastic gangliocytoma of cerebellum (Lhermitte-Duclos)
  - – Desmoplastic infantile ganglioglioma
  - – Ganglioglioma
  - – Anaplastic (malignant) ganglioglioma
  - – Central neuroblastoma
  - – Paraganglioma of the filum terminale
  - – Olfactory neuroblastoma (Aesthesioneuro-blastoma)
    - o Olfactory neuroepithelioma
- Pineal parenchymal tumours
  - – Pineocytoma
  - – Pineoblastoma
  - – Mixed/transitional pineal tumours
- Embryonal tumours
  - – Medulloepithelioma
  - – Neuroblastoma
    - o Ganglioneuroblastoma
  - – Ependymoblastoma
  - – Primitive neuroectodermal tumours (PNET)
  - – Medulloblastoma
    - o Desmoplastic medulloblastoma
    - o Medullomyoblastoma
    - o Melanotic medulloblastoma

Tumours of Cranial and Spinal Nerves
- Schwannoma
  - – Cellular
  - – Plexiform
  - – Melanotic
- Neurofibroma
  - – Circumscribed (solitary)
  - – Plexiform
- Malignant peripheral nerve sheath tumour (MPNST)
  - – Epitheloid
  - – MPNST with divergent mesenchymal and/or epithelial differentiation
  - – Melanotic

Tumours of the Meninges
- Tumours of meningothelial cells
  - – Meningioma
    - o Meningothelial]
    - o Fibrous (fibroblastic)
    - o Transitional (mixed)
    - o Psammomatous
    - o Angiomatous
    - o Microcystic
    - o Secretory
    - o Clear cell
    - o Chordoid
    - o Lymphoplasma-cyte rich
    - o Metaplastic
  - – Atypical meningioma
  - – Papillary meningioma
  - – Anaplastic (malignant) meningioma
- Mesenchymal, non-meningothelial tumours
  - – Benign neoplasm
    - o Osteocartilaginous tumours
    - o Lipoma
    - o Fibrous histiocytoma
    - o Others
  - – Malignant neoplasms
    - o Hemangiopericytoma
    - o Chondrosarcoma
    - o Mesenchymal chondrosarcoma
    - o Rhabdomyosarcoma
    - o Meningeal sarcomas
    - o Others
  - – Primary melanocytic lesions
    - o Diffuse melanosis
    - o Melanocytoma
    - o Malignant melanoma
    - o Meningeal melanomatosis
  - – Tumours of uncertain histogenesis
    - o Haemangioblastoma (capillary haemangioblastoma)

Lymphomas and Haemopoietic Neoplasms
- Malignant lymphoma
- Plasmacytoma
- Granulocytic sarcoma
- Others

Germ Cell Tumours
- Germinoma
- Embryonal carcinoma
- Yolk sac tumour (endodermal sinus tumour)
- Choriocarcinoma
- Teratoma
  - Immature
  - Mature
  - Teratoma with malignant transformation
- Mixed germ cell tumours

Cysts and tumour-like lesions
- Rathke cleft cyst
- Epidermoid cyst
- Dermoid cyst
- Colloid cyst of the third ventricle
- Enterogenous cyst
- Neuroglial cyst
- Granular cell tumour (Choristoma, Pituicytoma)
- Hypothalamic neuronal hamartoma
- Nasal glial heterotopias
- Plasma cell granuloma

Tumours of the Sellar Region
- Pituitary adenoma
- Pituitary carcinoma
- Craniopharyngioma
  - Adamantinomatous
  - Papillary

Local extensions from regional tumours
- Paraganglioma (chemodectoma)
- Chordoma
- Chondroma
- Chondrosarcoma
- Carcinoma

Metastatic tumours
Unclassified tumours

WHO Classification 2000

Kleihues P, Cavenee WK: World Health Organization Classification of Tumours. Pathology & Genetics. Tumours of the Nervous System. IARC Press, 2000, 3rd edition

Tumours of Neuroepithelial tissue
- Astrocytic tumours
  - Diffuse astrocytoma
    - Fibrillary
    - Protoplasmic
    - Gemistocytic
  - Anaplastic astrocytoma
  - Glioblastoma
    - Giant cell glioblastoma
  - Gliosarcoma
  - Pilocytic astrocytoma
  - Pleomorphic xanthoastrocytoma
  - Subependymal giant cell astrocytoma (Tuberous sclerosis)
- Oligodendroglial tumours
  - Oligodendroglioma
  - Anaplastic oligodendroglioma
- Mixed gliomas
  - Oligo-astrocytoma
  - Anaplastic oligo-astrocytoma
- Ependymal and choroid plexus tumours
  - Ependymoma
    - Cellular
    - Papillary
    - Clear cell
    - Tanycytic
  - Anaplastic ependymoma
  - Myxopapillary ependymoma
  - Subependymoma
- Choroid plexus tumours
  - Choroid plexus papilloma
  - Choroid plexus carcinoma
- Glial tumours of uncertain origin
  - Astroblastoma
  - Gliomatosis cerebri
  - Chordoid glioma of the 3rd ventricle
- Neuronal and mixed neuronal-glial tumours
  - Gangliocytoma

- Dysplastic gangliocytoma of cerebellum (Lhermitte-Duclos)
- Desmoplastic infantile astrocytoma/ganglioglioma
- Dysembryoplastic neuroepithelial tumour
- Ganglioglioma
- Anaplastic ganglioglioma
- Central neurocytoma
- Cerebellar liponeurocytoma
- Paraganglioma of the filum terminale
- Neuroblastic tumours
  - Olfactory neuroblastoma (Aesthesioneuroblastoma)
  - Olfactory neuroepithelioma
  - Neuroblastoma of the adrenal gland and sympathetic nervous system
- Pineal parenchymal tumours
  - Pineocytoma
  - Pineoblastoma
  - Pineal parenchymal tumour of intermediate differentiation
- Embryonal tumours
  - Medulloepithelioma
  - Ependymoblastoma
  - Medulloblastoma
    ○ Desmoplastic medulloblastoma
    ○ Large cell medulloblastoma
    ○ Medullomyoblastoma
    ○ Melanotic medulloblastoma
  - Supratentorial primitive neuroectodermal tumour (PNET)
    ○ Neuroblastoma
    ○ Ganglioneuroblastoma
  - Atypical teratoid/rhabdoid tumour

Tumours of Cranial and Spinal Nerves
- Schwannoma (Neurilemmoma, Neurinoma)
  - Cellular
  - Plexiform
  - Melanotic
- Neurofibroma
  - Plexiform
- Perineurioma
  - Intraneural perineurinoma
  - Soft tissue perineurinoma
- Malignant peripheral nerve sheath tumour (MPNST)
  - Epitheloid
  - MPNST with divergent mesenchymal and/or epithelial differentiation
  - Melanotic
  - Melanotic psammomatous

Tumours of the Meninges
- Tumours of meningothelial cells
  - Meningioma
    ○ Meningothelial
    ○ Fibrous (fibroblastic)
    ○ Transitional (mixed)
    ○ Psammomatous
    ○ Angiomatous
    ○ Microcystic
    ○ Secretory
    ○ Lymphoplasma-cyte rich
    ○ Metaplastic
    ○ Clear cell
    ○ Chordoid
    ○ Atypical
    ○ Papillary
    ○ Anaplastic meningioma
- Mesenchymal, non-meningothelial tumours
  - Lipoma
  - Angiolipoma
  - Hibernoma
  - Liposarcoma
  - Solitary fibrous tumour
  - Fibrosarcoma
  - Malignant fibrous histiocytoma
  - Leiomyoma
  - Leiomyosarcoma
  - Rhabdomyoma
  - Rhabdomyosarcoma
  - Chondroma
  - Chondrosarcoma
  - Osteoma
  - Osteosarcoma
  - Osteochondroma
  - Haemangioma
  - Epitheloid haemangioendothelioma
  - Hemangiopericytoma
  - Angiosarcoma
  - Kaposi sarcoma
- Primary melanocytic lesions
  - Diffuse melanosis

- Melanocytoma
- Malignant melanoma
- Meningeal melanomatosis
• Tumours of uncertain histogenesis
  - Haemangioblastoma

Lymphomas and Haemopoietic Neoplasms
• Malignant lymphoma
• Plasmacytoma
• Granulocytic sarcoma

Germ Cell Tumours
• Germinoma
• Embryonal carcinoma
• Yolk sac tumour
• Choriocarcinoma
• Teratoma
  - Immature
  - Mature
  - Teratoma with malignant transformation
• Mixed germ cell tumours

Tumours of the Sellar Region
• Craniopharyngioma
  - Adamantinomatous
  - Papillary
• Granular cell tumour

Metastatic tumours

WHO Classification 2007

Louis DN, Ohgaki H, Wiestler OD, Cavenee WK: WHO Classification of Tumours of the Central Nervous System. IARC Press, 2007, 4th edition

Tumours of Neuroepithelial tissue
• Astrocytic tumours
  - Pilocytic astrocytoma
    ○ Pilomyxoid astrocytoma
  - Subependymal giant cell astrocytoma
  - Pleomorphic xanthoastrocytoma
  - Diffuse astrocytoma
    ○ Fibrillary astrocytoma
    ○ Gemistocytic astrocytoma
    ○ Protoplasmic astrocytoma
  - Anaplastic astrocytoma
  - Glioblastoma
    ○ Giant cell glioblastoma
    ○ Gliosarcoma
  - Gliomatosis cerebri
• Oligodendroglial tumours
  - Oligodendroglioma
  - Anaplastic oligodendroglioma
• Oligoastrocytic tumours
  - Oligoastrocytoma
  - Anaplastic oligoastrocytoma
• Ependymal and choroid plexus tumours
  - Subependymoma
  - Myxopapillary ependymoma
  - Ependymoma
    ○ Cellular
    ○ Papillary
    ○ Clear cell
    ○ Tanycytic
  - Anaplastic ependymoma
• Chororid plexus tumours
  - Choroid plexus papilloma
  - Atypical choroid plexus papilloma
  - Choroid plexus carcinoma
• Other neuroepithelial tumours
  - Astroblastoma
  - Chordoid glioma of the third ventricle
  - Angiocentric glioma
• Neuronal and mixed neuronal-glial tumours
  - Dysplastic gangliocytoma of cerebellum (Lhermitte-Duclos)
  - Desmoplastic infantile astrocytoma/ganglioglioma
  - Dysembryoplastic neuroepithelial tumour
  - Gangliocytoma
  - Ganglioglioma
  - Anaplastic ganglioglioma
  - Central neurocytoma
  - Extraventricular neurocytoma
  - Cerebellar liponeurocytoma
  - Papillary glioneuronal tumour
  - Rosette-forming glioneuronal tumour of the fourth ventricle
  - Paraganglioma
• Tumours of the pineal region
  - Pineocytoma
  - Pineal parenchymal tumour of intermediate differentiation
  - Pineoblastoma

- Papillary tumour of the pineal region
- Embryonal tumours
  - Medulloblastoma
    - Desmoplastic/nodular medulloblastoma
    - Medulloblastoma with extensive nodularity
    - Anaplastic medulloblastoma
    - Large cell medulloblastoma
  - CNS primitive neuroectodermal tumour
    - CNS Neuroblastoma
    - CNS Ganglioneuroblastoma
    - Medulloepithelioma
    - Ependymoblastoma
  - Atypical teratoid/rhabdoid tumour

Tumours of Cranial and Spinal Nerves
- Schwannoma (Neurilemmoma, Neurinoma)
  - Cellular
  - Plexiform
  - Melanotic
- Neurofibroma
  - Plexiform
- Perineurioma
  - Perineurinoma, NOS
  - Malignant perineurinoma
- Malignant peripheral nerve sheath tumour (MPNST)
  - Epithelioid MPNST
  - MPNST with divergent mesenchymal differentiation
  - Melanotic MPNST
  - MPNST with glandular differentiation

Tumours of the Meninges
- Tumours of meningothelial cells
  - Meningioma
    - Meningothelial
    - Fibrous (fibroblastic)
    - Transitional (mixed)
    - Psammomatous
    - Angiomatous
    - Microcystic
    - Secretory
    - Lymphoplasma-cyte rich
    - Metaplastic
    - Chordoid
    - Clear cell
    - Atypical
    - Papillary
    - Rhabdoid
    - Anaplastic (malignant)
- Mesenchymal, non-meningothelial tumours
  - Lipoma
  - Angiolipoma
  - Hibernoma
  - Liposarcoma
  - Solitary fibrous tumour
  - Fibrosarcoma
  - Malignant fibrous histiocytoma
  - Leiomyoma
  - Leiomyosarcoma
  - Rhabdomyoma
  - Rhabdomyosarcoma
  - Chondroma
  - Chondrosarcoma
  - Osteoma
  - Osteosarcoma
  - Osteochondroma
  - Haemangioma
  - Epithelioid haemangioendothelioma
  - Haemangiopericytoma
  - Anaplastic haemangiopericytoma
  - Angiosarcoma
  - Kaposi sarcoma
  - Ewing sarcoma - PNET
- Primary melanocytic lesions
  - Diffuse melanocytosis
  - Melanocytoma
  - Malignant melanoma
  - Meningeal melanomatosis
- Other neoplasma related to the meninges
  - Haemangioblastoma

Lymphomas and Haemopoietic Neoplasms
- Malignant lymphoma
- Plasmacytoma
- Granulocytic sarcoma

Germ Cell Tumours
- Germinoma
- Embryonal carcinoma
- Yolk sac tumour
- Choriocarcinoma
- Teratoma
  - Immature
  - Mature
  - Teratoma with malignant transformation
- Mixed germ cell tumours

Tumours of the Sellar Region
- Craniopharyngioma
  - Adamantinomatous
  - Papillary
- Granular cell tumour
- Pituicytoma
- Spindle cell oncocytoma of the adenohypophysis

Metastatic tumours

WHO Classification 2016

Louis DN, Ohgaki H, Wiestler OD, Cavenee WK, Ellison DW, Figarella-Branger D, Perry A, Reifenberger G, von Deimling A (2016) WHO classification of tumours of the central nervous system. Revised 4th ed. IARC, Lyon
Italic: provisional tumour entities

Diffuse astrocytic and oligodendroglial tumours
- Diffuse astrocytoma, IDH-mutant
- Gemistocytic astrocytoma, IDH-mutant
  - *Diffuse astrocytoma, IDH-wildtype*
- Diffuse astrocytoma, NOS
- Anaplastic astrocytoma, IDH-mutant
- *Anaplastic astrocytoma, IDH-wildtype*
- Anaplastic astrocytoma, NOS
- Glioblastoma, IDH-wildtype
  - Giant cell glioblastoma
  - Gliosarcoma
  - *Epithelioid glioblastoma*
- Glioblastoma, IDH-mutant
- Glioblastoma, NOS
- Diffuse midline glioma, H3 K27M–mutant
- Oligodendroglioma, IDH-mutant and 1p/19q-codeleted
- Oligodendroglioma, NOS
- Anaplastic oligodendroglioma, IDH-mutant and 1p/19q-codeleted
- *Anaplastic oligodendroglioma, NOS*
- *Oligoastrocytoma, NOS*
- *Anaplastic oligoastrocytoma, NOS*

Other astrocytic tumours
- Pilocytic astrocytoma
  - Pilomyxoid astrocytoma
- Subependymal giant cell astrocytoma
- Pleomorphic xanthoastrocytoma
- Anaplastic pleomorphic xanthoastrocytoma

Ependymal tumours
- Subependymoma
- Myxopapillary ependymoma
- Ependymoma
  - Papillary ependymoma
  - Clear cell ependymoma
  - Tanycytic ependymoma
- Ependymoma, RELA fusion–positive
- Anaplastic ependymoma

Other gliomas
- Chordoid glioma of the third ventricle
- Angiocentric glioma
- Astroblastoma

Choroid plexus tumours
- Choroid plexus papilloma
- Atypical choroid plexus papilloma
- Choroid plexus carcinoma

Neuronal and mixed neuronal–glial tumours
- Dysembryoplastic neuroepithelial tumour
- Gangliocytoma
- Ganglioglioma
- Anaplastic ganglioglioma
- Dysplastic cerebellar gangliocytoma (Lhermitte–Duclos disease)
- Desmoplastic infantile astrocytoma and ganglioglioma
- Papillary glioneuronal tumour
- Rosette-forming glioneuronal tumour
- *Diffuse leptomeningeal glioneuronal tumour*
- Central neurocytoma
- Extraventricular neurocytoma
- Cerebellar liponeurocytoma
- Paraganglioma

Tumours of the pineal region
- Pineocytoma
- Pineal parenchymal tumour of intermediate differentiation
- Pineoblastoma
- Papillary tumour of the pineal region

Embryonal tumours
- Medulloblastoma, genetically defined
  - Medulloblastoma, WNT-activated
  - Medulloblastoma, SHH-activated and *TP53*-mutant
  - Medulloblastoma, SHH-activated and *TP53*-wildtype
  - Medulloblastoma, non-WNT/non-SHH
    - *Medulloblastoma, group 3*
    - *Medulloblastoma, group 4*
- Medulloblastoma, histologically defined
  - Medulloblastoma, classic
  - Desmoplastic/nodular medulloblastoma
  - Medulloblastoma with extensive nodularity
  - Large cell/anaplastic medulloblastoma
- Medulloblastoma, NOS
- Embryonal tumour with multilayered rosettes, C19MC-altered
- *Embryonal tumour with multilayered rosettes, NOS*
- Medulloepithelioma
- CNS neuroblastoma
- CNS ganglioneuroblastoma
- CNS embryonal tumour, NOS
- Atypical teratoid/rhabdoid tumour
- *CNS embryonal tumour with rhabdoid features*

Tumours of the cranial and paraspinal nerves
- Schwannoma
  - Cellular schwannoma
  - Plexiform schwannoma
- Melanotic schwannoma
- Neurofibroma
  - Atypical neurofibroma
  - Plexiform neurofibroma
- Perineurioma
- Hybrid nerve sheath tumours
- Malignant peripheral nerve sheath tumour
  - Epithelioid MPNST
  - MPNST with perineurial differentiation

Meningiomas
- Meningioma
- Meningothelial meningioma
- Fibrous meningioma
- Transitional meningioma
- Psammomatous meningioma
- Angiomatous meningioma
- Microcystic meningioma
- Secretory meningioma
- Lymphoplasmacyte-rich meningioma
- Metaplastic meningioma
- Chordoid meningioma
- Clear cell meningioma
- Atypical meningioma
- Papillary meningioma
- Rhabdoid meningioma
- Anaplastic (malignant) meningioma

Mesenchymal, non-meningothelial tumours
- Solitary fibrous tumour/haemangiopericytoma
  - Grade 1
  - Grade 2
  - Grade 3
- Haemangioblastoma
- Haemangioma
- Epithelioid haemangioendothelioma
- Angiosarcoma
- Kaposi sarcoma
- Ewing sarcoma/PNET
- Lipoma
- Angiolipoma
- Hibernoma
- Liposarcoma
- Desmoid-type fibromatosis
- Myofibroblastoma
- Inflammatory myofibroblastic tumour
- Benign fibrous histiocytoma
- Fibrosarcoma, NOS
- Undifferentiated pleomorphic sarcoma/malignant fibrous histiocytoma
- Leiomyoma
- Leiomyosarcoma
- Rhabdomyoma
- Rhabdomyosarcoma
- Chondroma
- Chondrosarcoma
- Osteoma
- Osteochondroma
- Osteosarcoma

Melanocytic tumours
- Meningeal melanocytosis
- Meningeal melanocytoma
- Meningeal melanoma
- Meningeal melanomatosis

Lymphomas
- Diffuse large B-cell lymphoma of the CNS
- Immunodeficiency-associated CNS lymphoma
  - AIDS-related diffuse large B-cell lymphoma
  - EBV-positive diffuse large B-cell lymphoma
  - Lymphomatoid granulomatosis
- Intravascular large B-cell lymphoma
- Low-grade B-cell lymphoma of the CNS
- T-cell and NK/T-cell lymphoma of the CNS
- Anaplastic large cell lymphoma, ALK-positive
- Anaplastic large cell lymphoma, ALK-negative
- MALT lymphoma of the dura

Histiocytic tumours
- Langerhans cell histiocytosis
- Erdheim–Chester disease
- Rosai–Dorfman disease
- Juvenile xanthogranuloma
- Histiocytic sarcoma

Germ cell tumours
- Germinoma
- Embryonal carcinoma
- Yolk sac tumour
- Choriocarcinoma
- Teratoma
  - Teratoma, mature
  - Teratoma, immature
- Teratoma with malignant transformation
- Mixed germ cell tumour

Tumours of the sellar region
- Craniopharyngioma
  - Adamantinomatous craniopharyngioma
  - Papillary craniopharyngioma
- Granular cell tumour of the sellar region
- Pituicytoma
- Spindle cell oncocytoma

Metastatic tumours

Changes in the Various WHO Classification Editions

A summary of changes from the 1979 baseline through the 1993, 2000, 2007, and 2016 editions patterned after Scheithauer (2009) (Table A.1).

Table A.1 Changes in the classification of brain tumors as given in the WHO classification systems from 1979 until 2016, modified after Scheithauer (2009)

Astrocytic tumors	
1979	• The category includes astrocytoma and anaplastic astrocytoma (but not glioblastoma), astroblastoma, pilocytic astrocytoma and subependymal giant cell astrocytoma • Note—Glioblastoma is defined as "An anaplastic, highly cellular tumor consisting of fusiform cells, small, poorly differentiated round cells or pleomorphic cells alone or in varying combinations. Necrosis, pseudopalisading, fistulous vessels and vascular endothelial proliferation, hemorrhage and invasive growth and usually prominent features" • "Some typical glioblastomas show no evidence of a more differentiated tumor, whereas others are predominantly glioblastomas with focal areas of recognizable astrocytoma, less commonly oligodendroglioma, or exceptionally, ependymoma. Any of these gliomas may, in fact, terminate as a glioblastoma" • Giant cell glioblastoma was considered both a glioblastoma variant and an entity among Tumours of Blood Vessel Origin ("monstrocellular sarcoma")
1993	• Pleomorphic xanthoastrocytoma added • Glioblastoma removed from "Poorly Differentiated and Embryonal Tumours" and included in the spectrum of "Astrocytic Tumours" • Astroblastoma moved to "Tumours of Uncertain Histogenesis" • The four parameters of the Ste. Anne Mayo method of classifying infiltrative astrocytic tumors into grades II-IV are adopted by the World Health Organization; these include nuclear abnormalities, mitotic activity, endothelial proliferation and necrosis not limited to the pseudopalisading variety
2000	• No substantial changes

Table A.1 (continued)

2007	• Pilomyxoid astrocytoma added as a subset of pilocytic astrocytoma • Glioneuronal tumor with neuropil-like islands included in anaplastic astrocytoma category
2016	• Protoplasmatic astrocytoma (→ diffuse astrocytoma) deleted • Fibrillary astrocytoma (→ diffuse astrocytoma) deleted • Glioblastoma subtypes: PNET-like, small cell, granular are defined as growth pattern • GBM with oligodendroglial component: if IDH1/2 and 1p 19q → either anaplastic Oligodendroglioma with necroses or Glioblastoma • Gliomatosis cerebri deleted • Diffuse midline glioma H3 K27M-mutation (pontine glioma) added • Anaplastic pleomorphic xanthoastrocytoma added • Diffuse gliomas with incorporation of genetically defined entities

Oligoastrocytomas and mixed gliomas

1979	• Variants include oligodendroglioma and mixed oligo-astrocytoma, as well as anaplastic oligodendroglioma
1993	• Anaplastic oligoastrocytoma recognized
2000	• No substantial change
2007	• High-grade oligo-astrocytic tumors with necrosis are included under the pattern designation "glioblastoma with oligodendroglial component"
2016	• Oligoastrocytoma only recognized as NOS

Ependymomas

1979	• Variants include myxopapillary and papillary ependymoma as well as subependymoma
1993	• Clear cell variant added
2000	• Tanycytic variant added
2007	• No substantial change
2016	• Cellular ependymoma deleted • Ependymoma, RELA fusion–positive added

Pineal tumors

1979	• Variants include pineocytoma and pineoblastoma
1993	• Mixed/transitional pineal tumors added
2000	• Mixed/transitional category deleted • Pineal parenchymal tumor of intermediate differentiation added
2007	• Consideration given to splitting pineal parenchymal tumor of intermediate differentiation into low (grade II) and high (grade III) forms • Papillary tumor of the pineal region added
2016	

Choroid plexus tumors

1979	• Variants include choroid plexus papilloma and anaplastic choroid plexus papilloma
1993	• No substantial change
2000	• No substantial change
2007	• Atypical choroid plexus papilloma added
2016	

Neuroepithelial tumors of uncertain origin (glial tumors of uncertain origin)

1993	• Polar spongioblastoma and gliomatosis cerebri moved to this category from "Poorly Differentiated and Embryonal Tumours category" • Astroblastoma moved to this category from "Astrocytic Tumours"
2000	• Chordoid glioma added • Polar spongioblastoma deleted
2007	• Angiocentric glioma added
2016	

Neuronal (mixed neuronal-glial) tumors

1979	• Variants include gangliocytoma and ganglioglioma, anaplastic gangliocytoma and ganglioglioma, neuroblastoma and ganglioneuroblastoma

(continued)

Table A.1 (continued)

Year	Changes
1993	• Dysplastic gangliocytoma of cerebellum (Lhermitte–Duclos disease) added • Desmoplastic infantile ganglioglioma added • Dysembryoplastic neuroepithelial tumor added • Central neurocytoma added • Paraganglioma of filum terminale added • Olfactory neuroblastoma added • Neuroblastoma and ganglioneuroblastoma deleted and moved to "Embryonal Tumours" category
2000	• Cerebellar liponeurocytoma added • Olfactory neuroblastoma and neuroblastoma of adrenal/sympathetic nervous system moved to new category "Neuroblastic Tumours"
2007	• Extraventricular neurocytoma added • Papillary glioneuronal tumor added • Rosette-forming glioneuronal tumor added
2016	• diffuse leptomeningeal glioneuronal tumor (disseminated oligodendroglia-leptomeningeal neoplasm (DOLN)) added

Poorly differentiated and embryonal tumors (embryonal tumors)

Year	Changes
1979	• Category includes glioblastoma, gliosarcoma, giant cell glioblastoma (considered synonymous with "monstrocellular sarcoma") and gliomatosis. Category also includes medulloblastoma and its desmoplastic and medullomyoblastic variants, as well as medulloepithelioma and primitive polar spongioblastoma
1993	• Central nervous system neuroblastoma and ganglioneuroblastoma added • Note—Olfactory neuroblastoma as well as neuroblastic tumors of the adrenal gland and sympathetic nervous system entered into the classification under a new category of "Peripheral Neuroblastic Tumours" • Ependymoblastoma added • Primitive neuroectodermal tumor (PNET) added as a category for medulloblastoma-like tumors outside the cerebellum • Melanotic medulloblastoma added as a medulloblastoma variant
2000	• Desmoplastic and large cell medulloblastoma variants added • Atypical teratoid rhabdoid tumor added
2007	• Extensively nodular and anaplastic variants added to "Medulloblastoma" category • PNET category expanded to include not only small cell-containing tumors including ependymoblastoma, but medulloepithelioma, a patently epithelial phenotype, as well
2016	• Embryonal tumour with multilayered rosettes, C19MC-altered • Embryonal tumour with multilayered rosettes, NOS • Medulloepithelioma • CNS neuroblastoma • CNS ganglioneuroblastoma • CNS embryonal tumour, NOS • Atypical teratoid/rhabdoid tumour • CNS embryonal tumour with rhabdoid features • Primitive neuroectodermal tumour" terminology deleted ***Medulloblastoma, genetically defined*** • Medulloblastoma, WNT-activated • Medulloblastoma, SHH-activated and *TP53*-mutant • Medulloblastoma, SHH-activated and *TP53*-wildtype • Medulloblastoma, non-WNT/non-SHH • *Medulloblastoma, group 3* • *Medulloblastoma, group 4* ***Medulloblastoma, histologically defined*** • Medulloblastoma, classic • Desmoplastic/nodular medulloblastoma • Medulloblastoma with extensive nodularity • Large cell/anaplastic medulloblastoma ***Medulloblastoma, NOS***

Table A.1 (continued)

Meningiomas	
1979	• Category includes meningotheliomatous, fibrous, transitional, psammomatous, angiomatous, hemangioblastic, hemangiopericytic, papillary and anaplastic meningioma
1993	• Microcystic, secretory, clear cell, chordoid, lymphoplasmacytic and metaplastic meningioma added • Atypical meningioma introduced as a category, but not clearly defined • Hemangioblastic category deleted • Hemangiopericytoma moved to "Mesenchymal, Non-Meningothelial Tumours" category
2000	• Rhabdoid meningioma added • Atypical and anaplastic meningioma categories clearly defined in terms of histologic criteria
2007	• No substantial change
2016	• Addition of brain invasion as a criterion for atypical meningioma
Tumors of nerve sheath cells (tumors of cranial and spinal nerves)	
1979	• Category included schwannoma, anaplastic schwannoma, neurofibroma and anaplastic neurofibroma
1993	• Cellular schwannoma added • Plexiform schwannoma added • Melanotic schwannoma added • Malignant peripheral nerve sheath tumor (MPNST) with divergent differentiation added • Melanotic MPNST added
2000	• Intraneural and soft tissue perineurioma added • Malignant melanotic schwannoma and its psammomatous variant added
2007	• No substantial change
2016	• Plexiform neurofibroma deleted • Separation of melanotic schwannoma from other schwannomas • Hybrid nerve sheath tumors added
Primary melanocytic tumors	
1979	• Category included melanoma and meningeal melanomatosis
1993	• Diffuse melanosis added • Melanocytoma added
2000	• No substantial change
2007	• No substantial change
2016	
Tumors of the anterior pituitary (tumors of the sellar region)	
1979	• Category included pituitary adenoma and pituitary adenocarcinoma
1993	• Adamantinomatous craniopharyngioma added • Papillary craniopharyngioma added
2000	• Granular cell tumor added
2007	• Pituicytoma added • Spindle cell oncocytoma added
2016	
Hematopoetic	
2016	• Expansion of entities included in hematopoietic/lymphoid tumors of the CNS (lymphomas and histiocytic tumors)
Soft Tissue tumors	
2016	• Restructuring of solitary fibrous tumor and hemangiopericytoma (SFT/HPC) as one entity and adapting a grading system to accommodate this change

Scheithauer BW (2009) Development of the WHO classification of tumors of the central nervous system: a historical perspective. Brain pathology (Zurich, Switzerland) 19 (4):551-564. doi:10.1111/j.1750-3639.2008.00192.x

Appendix B: WHO Classification of Tumors

Breast
- Lakhani SR, Ellis IO, Schnitt SJ, Tan PH, van de Vijver MJ (eds.): WHO Classification of Tumours of the Breast. IARC Press, 2012, 4th ed.

Digestive Tract
- Bosman FT, Carneiro F, Hruban RH, Theise (eds): WHO Classification of Tumours of the Digestive System. IARC Press, 2010, 4th ed.

Endocrine Organs
- Lloyd RV, Osamura RY, Klöppel G, Rosai J (eds.): WHO Classification of Tumours of Endocrine Organs. IARC Press, 2017, 4th ed.

Female reproductive organs
- Kurman RJ, Carcangiu ML, Herrington CS, Young RF (eds.): WHO Classification of Tumours of Female Reproductive Organs. IARC Press, 2014, 4th ed.

Haematopoietic System
- Swerdlow SH, Campo E, Harris NL, Jaffe ES, Pileri SA, Stein H, Thiele (eds.): WHO Classification of Tumours of Haematopoietic and Lymphoid tissues, IARC Press, 2017, revised 4th edition

Lung—Pleura—Thymus—Heart
- Travis WD, Brambilla E, Burke AP, Marx A, Nicholson AG (eds.): WHO Classification of Tumours of the Lung, Pleura, Thymus and Heart. IARC Press, 2015, 4th ed.

Skin
- LeBoit PE, Burg G, Weedon D, Sarasin A (eds.): Pathology and Genetics of Skin Tumours. IARC *Press,* Lyon, 2005, 3rd ed.

Soft Tissue and Bone
- Fletcher CDM, Bridge JA, Hagendoorn PCW, Mertens F (eds.): WHO Classification of Tumours of Soft Tissue and Bone. IARC Press, 2013, 4th edition

Urinary System and Male Genital Organs
- Moch H, Humphrey PA, Ulbright TM, Reuter VE (ed.s): WHO Classification of Tumours of the Urinary System and Male Genital Organs. IARC Press, 2016, 4th ed.

Lung Tumors

Epithelial tumours
- Adenocarcinoma
    - Lepidic adenocarcinoma
    - Acinar adenocarcinoma
    - Papillary adenocarcinoma
    - Micropapillary adenocarcinoma
    - Solid adenocarcinoma
    - Invasive mucinous adenocarcinoma (mixed invasive mucinous and non-mucinous adenocarcinoma)
    - Colloid adenocarcinoma
    - Fetal adenocarcinoma
    - Enteric adenocarcinoma
    - Minimally invasive adenocarcinoma
    - Preinvasive lesions

- Squamous cell carcinoma
  - Keratinizing squamous cell carcinoma
  - Non-keratinizing squamous cell carcinoma
  - Basaloid squamous cell carcinoma
  - Preinvasive lesion (squamous cell carcinoma in situ)
- Neuroendocrine tumours
- Large cell carcinoma
- Adenosquamous carcinoma
- Pleomorphic carcinoma
- Spindle cell carcinoma
- Giant cell carcinoma
- Carcinosarcoma
- Pulmonary blastoma
- Other and unclassified carcinomas
- Salivary gland tumours
  - Mucoepidermoid carcinoma
  - Adenoid cystic carcinoma
  - Epithelial-myoepithelial carcinoma
    - Pleomorphic adenoma
- Papillomas
  - Squamous cell papilloma
    - Exophytic
    - Inverted
  - Glandular papilloma
  - Mixed squamous cell and glandular papilloma
- Adenomas
  - Sclerosing pneumocytoma
  - Alveolar adenoma
  - Papillary adenoma
  - Mucinous cystadenoma
  - Mucous gland adenoma

Mesenchymal tumours
- Pulmonary hamartoma
- Chondroma
- PEComatous tumours
- Lymphangioleiomyomatosis
- PEComa, benign (clear cell tumour)
- PEComa, malignant
- Congenital peribronchial myofibroblastic tumour
- Diffuse pulmonary lymphangiomatosis
- Inflammatory myofibroblastic tumour
- Epithelioid haemangioendothelioma
- Pleuropulmonary blastoma
- Synovial sarcoma
- Pulmonary artery intimal sarcoma
- Pulmonary myxoid sarcoma with *EWSR1-CREB1* translocation

Lymphohistiocytic tumours
- Extranodal marginal zone lymphoma of mucosa-associated lymphoid tissue (MALT lymphoma)
- Diffuse large B-cell lymphoma
- Lymphomatoid granulomatosis
- Intravasal large B-cell lymphoma
- Pulmonary Langerhans cell histiocytosis
- Erdheim-Chester disease

Tumors of ectopic origin
- Germ cell tumours
  - Teratoma, mature
  - Immature
  - Other germ cell tumours
- Intrapulmonary thymoma
- Melanoma
- Meningioma, NOS

Metastatic tumours

Breast Tumors

Epithelial tumours
- Invasive breast carcinoma
  - Invasive carcinoma of no special type (NST)
    - Pleomorphic carcinoma
    - Carcinoma with osteoclast-like stromal giant cells
    - Carcinoma with choriocarcinomatous features
    - Carcinoma with melanotic features
  - Invasive lobular carcinoma
    - Classic lobular carcinoma
    - Solid lobular carcinoma
    - Alveolar lobular carcinoma
    - Pleomorphic lobular carcinoma
    - Tubulolobular carcinoma
    - Mixed lobular carcinoma
  - Tubular carcinoma
  - Cribriform carcinoma
  - Mucinous carcinoma

- Carcinoma with medullary features
  - Medullary carcinoma
  - Atypical medullary carcinoma
  - Invasive carcinoma NST with medullary features
- Carcinoma with apocrine differentiation
- Carcinoma with signet-ring-cell differentiation
- Invasive micropapillary carcinoma
- Metaplastic carcinoma of no specific type
  - Low-grade adenosquamous carcinoma
  - Fibromatosis-like metaplastic carcinoma
  - Squamous cell carcinoma
  - Metaplastic carcinoma with mesenchymal differentiation
  - Chondroid differentiation
  - Osseous differentiation
  - Other types of mesenchymal differentiation
  - Mixed metaplastic carcinoma
  - Myoepithelial carcinoma
- Carcinoma with neuroendocrine features
  - Neuroendocrine tumor, well differentiated
  - Neuroendocrine carcinoma, poorly differentiated (small cell carcinoma)
  - Carcinoma with neurorndocrine differentiation
- Secretory carcinoma
- Invasive papillary carcinoma
- Acinic cell carcinoma
- Mucoepidermoid carcinoma
- Polymorphous carcinoma
- Oncocytic carcinoma
- Lipid-rich carcinoma
- Glycogen-rich clear cell carcinoma
- Sebaceous carcinoma
- Salivary gland/skin adnexal type tumours
  - Cylindroma
  - Clear cell hidradenoma
- Epithelial-myoepithelial tumours
  - Pleopmorphic adenoma
  - Adenomyoepithelioma
    - Adenomyoepithelioma with carcinoma
  - Adenoid cystic carcinoma
- Precursor lesions
  - Ductal carcinoma in situ
  - Lobular neoplasia
    - Lobular carcinoma in situ
    - Classic lobular carcinoma in situ
    - Pleomorphic lobular carcinoma in situ
    - Atypical lobular hyperplasia
- Intraductal proliferative lesions
  - Usual ductal hyperplasia
  - Columnar cell lesions including flat epithelial atypia
  - Atypical ductal hyperplasia
- Papillary lesions
  - Intraductal papilloma
    - Intraductal papilloma with atypical hyperplasia
    - Intraductal papilloma with ductal carcinoma in situ
    - Intraductal papilloma with lobular carcinoma in situ
  - Intraductal papillary carcinoma
  - Encapsulated papillary carcinoma
    - Encapsulated papillary carcinoma with invasion
  - Solid papillary carcinoma
    - In situ
    - invasive
- Benign epithelial proliferations
  - Sclerosing adenosis
  - Apocrine adenosis
  - Microglandular adenosis
  - Radial scar/complex sclerosing lesion
  - Adenomas
    - Tubular adenoma
    - Lactating adenoma
    - Apocrine adenoma
    - Ductal adenoma

Mesenchymal tumours
- Nodular fasciitis
- Myofibroblastoma
- Desmoid-type fibromatosis
- Inflammatory myofibroblastic tumour
- Benign vascular lesions
  - Haemangioma
  - Angiomatosis
  - Atypical vascular lesions
- Pseudoangiomatous stromal hyperplasia
- Granular cell tumour

- Benign peripheral nerve-sheath tumours
  - Neurofibroma
  - Schwannoma
- Lipoma
  - Angiolipoma
- Liposarcoma
- Angiosarcoma
- Rhabdomyosarcoma
- Osteosarcoma
- Leiomyoma
- Leiomyosarcoma

Fibroepithelial tumours
- Fibroadenoma
- Phyllodes tumour
  - Benign
  - Borderline
  - Malignant
  - Periductal stromal sarcoma, low grade
- Hamartoma

Tumours of the nipple
- Nipple adenoma
- Syringomatous tumor
- Paget disease of the nipple

Malignant lymphoma
- Diffuse large B-cell lymphoma
- Burkitt lymphoma
- T-cell lymphoma
  - Anaplasric large cell lymphoma, ALK-negative
- Extranodal marginal-zone B-cell lymphoma of MALT type
- Follicular lymphoma

Metastatic tumours

Tumours of the male breast
- Gynaecomastia
- Carcinoma
  - Invasive
  - In

Skin Tumors

Keratinocytic tumours
- Basal cell carcinoma
- Superficial basal cell carcinoma
- Nodular (solid) basal cell carcinoma
- Micronodular basal cell carcinoma
- Infiltrating basal cell carcinoma
- Fibroepithelial basal cell carcinoma
- Basal cell carcinoma with adnexal differentiation
- Basosquamous carcinoma
- Keratotic basal cell carcinoma
- Squamous cell carcinoma
- Acantholytic squamous cell carcinoma
- Spindle-cell squamous cell carcinoma
- Verrucous squamous cell carcinoma
- Pseudovascular squamous cell carcinoma
- Adenosquamous carcinoma
- Bowen disease
- Bowenoid papulosis
- Actinic keratosis
- Arsenical keratosis
- PUVA keratosis
- Verrucas
- Verruca vulgaris
- Verruca plantaris
- Verruca plana
- Acanthomas
- Epidermolytic acanthoma
- Warty dyskeratoma
- Acantholytic acanthoma
- Lentigo simplex
- Seborrhoeic keratosis
- Melanoacanthoma
- Clear cell acanthoma
- Large cell acanthoma
- Keratoacanthoma
- Lichen planus-like keratosis

Melanocytic tumours
- Malignant melanoma
  - Superficial spreading melanoma
  - Nodular melanoma
  - Lentigo maligna
  - Acral-lentiginous melanoma
  - Desmoplastic melanoma
  - Melanoma arising from blue naevus
  - Melanoma arising in a giant congenital naevus
  - Melanoma of childhood
  - Naevoid melanoma
  - Persistent melanoma

- Benign melanocytic tumours
  - Congenital melanocytic naevi
  - Superficial type
  - Proliferative nodules in congenital melanocytic naevi
  - Dermal melanocytic lesions
  - Mongolian spot
  - Naevus of Ito and Ota
  - Blue naevus
  - Cellular blue naevus
  - Combined naevus
  - Melanotic macules, simple lentigo and lentiginous naevus
  - Dysplastic naevus
  - Site-specific naevi
  - Acral
  - Genital
  - Meyerson naevus
  - Persistent (recurrent) melanocytic naevus
  - Spitz naevus
  - Pigmented spindle cell naevus (Reed)
  - Halo naevus

Tumours with apocrine and eccrine differentiation
- *Malignant tumours*
  - Tubular carcinoma
  - Microcystic adnexal carcinoma
  - Porocarcinoma
  - Spiradenocarcinoma
  - Malignant mixed tumour
  - Hidradenocarcinoma
  - Mucinous carcinoma
  - Digital papillary carcinoma
  - Adenoid cystic carcinoma
  - Apocrine carcinoma
  - Paget disease of breast
  - Extramammary Paget disease
- *Benign tumours*
  - Hidrocystoma
  - Syringoma
  - Poroma
  - Syringofibroadenoma
  - Hidradenoma
  - Spiradenoma
  - Cylindroma
  - Tubular adenoma
  - Tubular papillary adenoma
  - Syringocystadenoma papilliferum
  - Hidradenoma papilliferum
  - Mixed tumour (chondroid syringoma)

Tumours with follicular differentiation
- *Malignant tumours*
  - Pilomatrical carcinoma
  - Proliferating tricholemmal tumour
- *Benign tumours*
  - Trichoblastoma
  - Pilomatricoma
  - Tricholemmoma
  - Multiple tricholemmomas
  - Trichofolliculoma
  - Fibrofolliculoma/trichodiscoma

Tumours with sebaceous differentiation
- Sebaceous carcinoma
- Sebaceous adenoma
- Sebaceoma
- Cystic sebaceous tumour

Vascular tumour
- Haemangioma of infancy
- Cherry haemangioma
- Sinusoidal haemangioma
- Hobnail haemangioma
- Glomeruloid haemangioma
- Microvenular haemangioma
- Angiolymphoid hyperplasia with eosinophilia
- Spindle cell haemangioma
- Tufted angioma
- Arteriovenous haemangioma
- Cutaneous angiosarcoma

Lymphatic tumours
- Lymphangioma circumscriptum
- Progressive lymphangioma

Smooth and skeletal muscle tumours
- Pilar leiomyoma
- Cutaneous leiomyosarcoma

Fibrous, fibrohistiocytic and histiocytic tumours
- Dermatomyofibroma
- Infantile myofibromatosis
- Sclerotic fibroma

- Pleomorphic fibroma
- Giant cell fibroblastoma
- Dermatofibrosarcoma protuberans
- Dermatofibroma (fibrous histiocytoma)

Neuronal tumours
- Primitive neuroectodermal tumour (PNET)
- Ewing sarcoma
- Nerve sheath myxoma
- Merkel cell carcinoma
- Granular cell tumour

Kidney Tumors

Renal cell tumours
- Clear cell renal cell carcinoma
- Multilocular clear cell renal cell carcinoma
- Papillary renal cell carcinoma
- Hereditary leiomyomatosis and renal cell carcinoma-associate renal cell carcinoma
- Chromophobe renal cell carcinoma
- Collecting duct carcinoma
- Renal medullary carcinoma
- MiT family translocation renal cell carcinoma
- Succinate dehydrogenase-deficient renal cell carcinoma
- Mucinous tubular and spindle cell carcinoma
- Tubulocystic renal cell carcinoma
- Acquired cystic disease-associated renal cell carcinoma
- Clear cell papillary renal cell carcinoma
- Renal cell carcinoma, unclassified
- Papillary adenoma
- Oncocytoma

Metanephric tumours
- Metanephric adenoma
- Metanephric adenofibroma
- Metanephric stromal tumour

Nephroblastic and cystic tumours occurring mainly in children
- Nephrogenic rests
- Nephroblastoma
- Cystic partially differentiated nephroblastoma
- Paediatric cystic nephroma

Mesenchymal tumours
Mesenchymal tumours occurring mainly in Children
- Clear cell sarcoma
- Rhabdoid tumour
- Congenital mesoblastic nephroma
- Ossifying renal tumour of infants

Mesenchymal tumours occurring mainly in adults
- Leiomyosarcoma
- Angiosarcoma
- Rhabdomyosarcoma
- Osteosarcoma
- Synovial sarcoma
- Ewing sarcoma
- Angiomyolipoma
- Epithelioid angiomyolipoma
- Leiomyoma
- Haemangioma
- Lymphangioma
- Haemangioblastoma
- Juxtaglomerular cell tumour
- Renomedullary interstitial cell tumour
- Schwannoma
- Solitary fibrous tumour

Mixed epithelial and stromal tumour family
- Adult cystic nephroma
- Mixed epithelial and stromal tumour

Neuroendocrine tumours
- Well-differentiated neuroendocrine tumour
- Large cell neuroendocrine carcinoma
- Small cell neuroendocrine carcinoma
- Paraganglioma

Miscellaneous tumours
- Renal haematopoietic neoplasms
- Germ cell tumours

Metastatic tumours

Urinary Tract Tumors

Urothelial tumours
- Infiltrating urothelial carcinoma

- Nested, including large nested
- Microcystic
- Micropapillary
- Lymphoepithelioma-like
- Plasmacytoid/signet ring/diffuse
- Sarcomatoid
- Giant cell
- Poorly differentiated
- Lipid-rich
- Clear cell
• Non-invasive urothelial neoplasias
  - Urothelial carcinoma in situ
  - Non-invasive papillary urothelial carcinoma, low grade
  - Non-invasive papillary urothelial carcinoma, high grade
  - Papillary urothelial neoplasm of low malignant potential
  - Urothelial papilloma
  - Inverted urothelial papilloma
  - Urothelial proliferation of uncertain malignant potential
  - Urothelial dysplasia

Squamous neoplasms
• Pure squamous cell carcinoma
• Verrucous carcinoma
• Squamous cell papilloma

Glandular neoplasms
• Adenocarcinoma
  - Enteric
  - Mucinous
  - Mixed
• Villous adenoma

Urachal carcinoma

Tumours of Müllerian type
• Clear cell carcinoma
• Endometroid carcinoma

Neuroendocrine tumours
• Small cell neuroendocrine carcinoma
• Large cell neuroendocrine carcinoma
• Well-differentiated neuroendocrine tumour
• Paraganglioma

Melanocytic tumours
• Malignant melanoma
• Naevus
• Melanosis

Mesenchymal tumours
• Rhabdomyosarcoma
• Leiomyosarcoma
• Angiosarcoma
• Inflammatory myofibroblastic tumour
• Perivascular epitheloid cell tumour
  - Benign
  - Malignant
• Solitary fibrous tumour
• Leiomyoma
• Haemangioma
• Granular cell tumour
• Neurofibroma

Urothelial tract haematopoietic and lymphoid tumours
• **Miscellaneous tumours**
  - Carcinoma of Skene, Cowper and Littre glands
  - Metastatic tumours and tumours extending from other organs
  - Epithelial tumours of the upper urinary tract
  - Tumour araising in a bladder diverticulum
  - Urothelial tumours of the urethra

Prostate Tumors

Epithelial tumours
• Glandular neoplasms
  - Acinar adenocarcinoma
    ○ Atrophic
    ○ Pseudohyperplastic
    ○ Microcystic
    ○ Foamy gland
    ○ Mucinous (colloid)
    ○ Signet ring-like cell
    ○ Pleomorphic giant cell
    ○ Sarcomatoid
  - Prostatic intraepithelial neoplasia, high grade
  - Intraductal carcinoma
  - Ductal adenocarcinoma
    ○ Cribriform
    ○ Papillary
    ○ Solid
  - Urothelial carcinoma

- Squamous neoplasms
  - Adenosquamous carcinoma
  - Squamous cell carcinoma
- Basal cell carcinoma

Neuroendocrine tumours
- Adenocarcinoma with neuroendocrine differentiation
- Well-differentiated neuroendocrine tumour
- Small cell neuroendocrine carcinoma
- Large cell neuroendocrine carcinoma

Mesenchymal tumours
- Stromal tumour of uncertain malignant potential
- Stromal sarcoma
- Leiomyosarcoma
- Rhabdomyosarcoma
- Leiomyoma
- Angiosarcoma
- Synovial sarcoma
- Inflammatory myofibroblastic tumour
- Osteosarcoma
- Undifferentiated pleomorphic sarcoma
- Solitary fibrous tumour
- Solitary fibrous tumour, malignant
- Haemangioma
- Granular cell tumour

Haematolymphoid tumours
- Diffuse large B-cell lymphoma
- Chronic lymphocytic leukaemia/small lymphocytic lymphoma
- Follicular lymphoma
- Mantle cell lymphoma
- Acute myeloid leukaemia
- B lymphoblastic leukaemia/lymphoma

Miscellaneous tumours
- Cystadenoma
- Nephroblastoma
- Rhabdoid tumour
- Germ cell tumours
- Clear cell adenocarcinoma
- Melanoma
- Paraganglioma
- Neuroblastoma

Metastatic tumours

Tumours of the Seminal Vesicles

Epithelial tumours
- Adenocarcinoma
- Squamous cell carcinoma

Mixed epithelial and stromal tumours
- Cystadenoma

Mesenchymal tumours
- Leiomyoma
- Schwannoma
- Mammry-type myofibroblastoma
- Gastrointestinal stromal tumour, NOS
- Leiomyosarcoma
- Angiosarcoma
- Liposarcoma
- Solitary fibrous tumour
- Haemangiopericytoma

Miscellaneous tumours
- Choriocarcinoma
- Seminoma
- Well-differentiated neuroendocrine tumour
- Lymphomas
- Ewing sarcoma

Metastatic tumours

Testicular Tumors

Germ cell tumours derived from germ cell neoplasia in situ
- Non-invasive germ cell neoplasia
  - Germ cell neoplasia in situ
  - Specific forms of intratubular germ cell neoplasia
- Tumours of one histological type (pure forms)
  - Seminoma
  - Seminoma with syncytiotrophoblastic cells
  - Non-seminomatous germ cell tumours
  - Embryonal carcinoma
  - Yolk sac tumour, postpubertal type
  - Trophoblastic tumours
    - Choriocarcinoma
    - Non-choriocarcinomatous trophoblastic tumours

- - Placental site trophoblastic tumour
  - - Epitheloid trophoblastic tumour
  - - Cystic trophoblastic tumour
  - Teratoma, postpubertal-type
  - Teratoma with somatic type malignancies
- Non-seminomatous germ cell tumour of more than one histological type
  - Mixed germ cell tumours
- Germ cell tumours of unknown type
  - regressed germ cell tumours

Germ cell tumours unrelated to germ cell neoplasia in situ
- Spermatocytic tumour
- Teratoma, prepubertal type
  - Dermoid cyst
  - Epidermoid cyst
  - Well-differentiated neuroendocrine tumour (monodermal teratoma)
- Mixed teratoma and yolk sac tumour, prepubertal type
- Yolk sac tumour, prebubertal type

Sex cord/gonadal stromal tumours
- Pure tumours
  - Leydig cell tumour
    - Malignant Leydig cell tumour
  - Sertoli cell tumour
    - Malignant Sertoli cell tumour
    - Large cell calcifying Sertoli cell tumour
    - Intratubular large cell hyalizing Sertoli cell neoplasia
  - Granulosa cell tumour
    - Adult type granulosa cell tumour
    - Juvenile type granulosa cell tumour
  - Tumours in the thecoma-fibroma group
- Mixed and unclassified sex cord-stromal tumours
- Mixed sex cord-stromal tumour
- Unclassified sex cord-stromal tumour

Tumours containing both germ cell and sex cord/gonadal stromal elements
- Gonadoblastoma

Miscellaneous tumours of the testis
- Ovarian epithelial-type tumors
  - Serous cystadenoma
  - Serous tumour of borderline malignancy
  - Serous cystadenocarcinoma
  - Mucinous cystadenoma
  - Mucinous borderline tumour
  - Mucinous cystadenocarcinoma
  - Endometrioid adenocarcinoma
  - Clear cell adenocarcinoma
  - Brenner tumour
- Juvenile xanthogranuloma
- Haemangioma

Haematolymphoid tumours
- Diffuse large B-cell lymphoma
- Follicular lymphoma, NOS
- Extranodal NK/T-cell lymphoma, nasal type
- Plasmacytoma
- Myeloid sarcoma
- Rosai-Dorfman disease

Tumours of collecting ducts and rete
- Adenoma
- Adenocarcinoma

Tumours of paratesticular structures
- Adenomatoid tumour
- Malignant mesothelioma
  - Well differentiated papillary mesothelioma
- Epididymal tumours
  - Cystadenoma of the epididymis
  - Papillary cystadenoma
  - Adenocarcinoma of the epididymis
- Squamous cell carcinoma
- Melanotic neuroectodermal tumour
- Nephroblastoma
- Paraganglioma

Mesenchymal tumours of the spermatic cord and testicular adnexae
- Adipocytic tumours
  - Lipoma
  - Well-differentiated liposarcoma
  - Dedifferentiated liposarcoma
  - Myxoid liposarcoma
  - Pleomorphic liposarcoma
- Smooth muscle tumours
  - Leiomyoma
  - Leiomyosarcoma
- Skeletal muscle tumours

- Rhabdomyoma
- Rhabdomyosarcoma
  - Embryonal type
  - Alveolar type
  - Pleomorphic type
  - Spindle cell/sclerosing type
- Fibroblastic/myofibroblastic tumours
  - Cellular angiofibroma
  - Mammary-type myofibroblastoma
  - Deep ("aggressive") angiomyxoma
  - Nerve sheath tumours
- Other mesenchymal tumours of the spermatic cord and testicular adnexa
  - Haemangioma
  - Desmoplastic small round cell tumour

Metastatic tumours

Tumors of the Digestive System: Oesophagus

Epithelial tumours
- Premalignant lesions
  - Squamous
    - Intraepithelial neoplasia (dysplasia), low grade
    - Intraepithelial neoplasia (dysplasia), high grade
  - Glandular
    - Dysplasia (intraepithelial neoplasia), low grade
    - Dysplasia (intraepithelial neoplasia), low grade
- Carcinoma
  - Squamous cell carcinoma
  - Adenocarcinoma
  - Adenoid cystic carcinoma
  - Adenosquamous carcinoma
  - Basaloid squamous cell carcinoma
  - Mucoepidermoid carcinoma
  - Spindle cell (squamous) carcinoma
  - Verrucous (squamous) carcinoma
  - Undifferentiated carcinoma
- Neuroendocrine neoplasms
  - Neuroendocrine tumour (NET)
    - NET G1 (carcinoid)
    - NET G2

- Neuroendocrine carcinoma
  - Large cell NEC
  - Small cell NEC
- Mixed adenoneuroendocrine carcinoma

Mesenchymal tumours
- Granular cell tumour
- Haemangioma
- Leiomyoma
- Lipoma
- Gastrointestinal stromal tumour
- Kaposi sarcoma
- Leiomyosarcoma
- Melanoma
- Rhabdomyosarcoma

Lymphoma
Secondary tumours

Tumors of the Digestive System: Stomach

Epithelial tumours
- Premalignant lesions
  - Adenoma
  - Intraepithelial neoplasia (dysplasia), low grade
  - Intraepithelial neoplasia (dysplasia), high grade
- Carcinoma
  - Adenocarcinoma
    - Papillary adenocarcinoma
    - Tubular adenocarcinoma
    - Mucinous adenocarcinoma
    - Poorly cohesive carcinoma (including signet ring cell carcinoma and their variants)
  - Adenosquamous carcinoma
  - Carcinoma with lymphoid stroma (medullary carcinoma)
  - Hepatoid adenocaecinoma
  - Squamous cell carcinoma
  - Undifferentiated carcinoma
- Neuroendocrine neoplasms
  - Neuroendocrine tumour (NET)
    - NET G1 (carcinoid)
    - NET G2
  - Neuroendocrine carcinoma

- Large cell NEC
- Small cell NEC
- Mixed adenoneuroendocrine carcinoma
- EC cell, serotonin-producing NET
- Gastrin-producing NET (gastrinoma)

Mesenchymal tumours
- Glomus tumour
- Granular cell tumour
- Leiomyoma
- Plexiform fibromyxoma
- Schwannoma
- Inflammatory myofibroblastic tumor
- Gastrointestinal stromal tumour
- Kaposi sarcoma
- Leiomyosarcoma
- Synovial sarcoma

Lymphoma
Secondary tumours

Tumors of the Digestive System: Small Intestines

Epithelial tumours
- Premalignant lesions
  - Adenoma
    - Tubular
    - Villous
    - Tubulovillous
  - Dysplasia (intraepithelial neoplasia), low grade
  - Dysplasia (intraepithelial neoplasia), low grade
- Hamartomas
  - Juvenile polyp
  - Peutz-Jeghers polyp
- Carcinoma
  - Adenocarcinoma
    - Mucinous adenocarcinoma
    - Signet-ring cell carcinoma
  - Adenosquamous carcinoma
  - Medullary carcinoma
  - Squamous cell carcinoma
  - Undifferentiated carcinoma
- Neuroendocrine neoplasms
  - Neuroendocrine tumour (NET)
    - NET G1 (carcinoid)
    - NET G2
  - Neuroendocrine carcinoma
    - Large cell NEC
    - Small cell NEC
- Mixed adenoneuroendocrine carcinoma
- EC cell, serotonin-producing NET
- Gangliocytic paraganglioma
- Gastrinoma
- L-cell, glucagon-like peptide and PP/PYY producing tumour
- Somatostatin cell tumour

Mesenchymal tumours
- Leiomyoma
- Lipoma
- Angiosarcoma
- Gastrointestinal stromal tumour
- Kaposi sarcoma
- Leiomyosarcoma

Lymphomas
Secondary tumours

Tumors of the Digestive System: Colon and Rectum

Epithelial tumours
- Premalignant lesions
  - Adenoma
    - Tubular
    - Villous
    - Tubulovillous
  - Dysplasia (intraepithelial neoplasia), low grade
  - Dysplasia (intraepithelial neoplasia), low grade
- Serrated lesions
  - Hyperplastic polyp
  - Sessile serrated adenoma/polyp
  - Traditional serrated adenoma
- Hamartomas
  - Cowden-associated polyp
  - Juvenile polyp
  - Peutz-Jeghers polyp

- Carcinoma
  - Adenocarcinoma
    - Cribriform comedo-type adenocarcionoma
    - Medullary carcinoma
    - Micropapillary carcinoma
    - Mucinous adenocarcinoma
    - Serrated adenocarcinoma
    - Signet-ring cell carcinoma
  - Adenosquamous carcinoma
  - Spindle cell carcinoma
  - Squamous cell carcinoma
  - Undifferentiated carcinoma
- Neuroendocrine neoplasms
  - Neuroendocrine tumour (NET)
    - NET G1 (carcinoid)
    - NET G2
  - Neuroendocrine carcinoma
    - Large cell NEC
    - Small cell NEC
- Mixed adenoneuroendocrine carcinoma
- EC cell, serotonin-producing NET
- L-cell, glucagon-like peptide and PP/PYY producing tumour

Mesenchymal tumours
- Leiomyoma
- Lipoma
- Angiosarcoma
- Gastrointestinal stromal tumour
- Kaposi sarcoma
- Leiomyosarcoma

Lymphomas
Secondary tumours

Tumors of the Digestive System: Liver and Intrahepatic Bile Ducts

Epithelial tumours: hepatocellular
- Benign
  - Hepatocellular adenoma
  - Focal nodular hyperplasia
- Malignancy-associated and premalignant lesions
  - Large cell change (formerly "dysplasia")
  - Small cell change (formerly "dysplasia")
  - Dysplastic nodules
    - Low grade
    - High grade
- Malignant
  - Hepatocellular carcinoma
  - Hepatocellular carcinoma, fibrolamellar variant
  - Hepatoblastoma, epithelial variants
  - Undifferentiated carcinoma

Epithelial tumours: biliary
- Benign
  - Bile duct adenoma (peribiliary gland hamartoma and others)
  - Microcystic adenoma
  - Biliary adenofibroma
- Premalignant lesions
  - Biliary intraepithelial neoplasia, grade III (BilN-3)
  - Intraductal papillary neoplasm with low- or intermediate-grade intraepithelial neoplasia
  - Intraductal papillary neoplasm with high-grade intraepithelial neoplasm
  - Mucinous cystic neoplasm with low- or intermediate-grade intraepithelial neoplasia
  - Mucinous cystic neoplasm with high-grade intraepithelial neoplasis
- Malignant
  - Intrahepatic cholangiocarcinoma
  - Intraductal papillary neoplasm with an associated invasive carcinoma
  - Mucinous cystic neoplasm with an associated invasive carcinoma

Malignancies of mixed or uncertain origin
- Calcifying nested epithelial stromal tumour
- Carcinosarcoma
- Combined hepatocellular-cholangiocarcinoma
- Hepatoblastoma, mixed epithelail-mesenchymal
- Malignant rhabdoid tumour

Mesenchymal tumours
- Benign
  - Angiomyolipoma (PEComa)
  - Cavernous haemangioma
  - Infantile haemangioma
  - Inflammatory pseudotumour

- Lymphangioma
- Lymphangiomatosis
- Mesenchymal hamartoma
- Solitary fibrous tumour
- Malignant
  - Angiosarcoma
  - Embryonal sarcoma (undifferentiated sarcoma)
  - Epithelioid haemangioendothelioma
  - Kaposi sarcoma
  - Leiomyosarcoma
  - Rhabdomyosarcoma
  - Synovial sarcoma

Germ cell tumours
- Teratoma
- Yolk sac tumour (endodermal sinus tumour)

Lymphomas
Secondary tumours

Tumors of the Digestive System: Pancreas

Epithelial tumours
- Benign
  - Acinar cell cystadenoma
  - Serous cystadenoma
- Premalignant lesions
  - Pancreatic intraepithelial neoplasia, grade 3 (PanIN-3)
  - Intraductal papillary mucinous neoplasm with low- or intermediate-grade dysplasia
  - Intraductal papillary mucinous neoplasm with high-grade dysplasia
  - Intraductal tubulopapillary neoplasm
  - Mucinous cystic neoplasm with low- or intermediate-grade dysplasia
  - Mucinous cystic neoplasm with high-grade dysplasia
- Malignant
  - Ductal adenocarcinoma
    - Adenosquamous carcinoma
    - Colloid carcinoma (mucinous noncystic carcinoma)
    - Hepatoid carcinoma
    - Medullary carcinoma
    - Signet ring cell carcinoma
    - Undifferentiated carcinoma
    - Undifferentiated carcinoma with osteoclast-like giant cells
  - Acinar cell carcinoma
  - Acinar cystadenocarcinoma
  - Intraductal papillary mucinous neoplasm with an associated invasive carcinoma
  - Mixed acinar-ductal carcinoma
  - Mixed acinar-neuroendocrine carcinoma
  - Mixed acinar-neuroendocrine-ductal carcinoma
  - Mixed ductal-neuroendocrine carcinoma
  - Mucinous cystic neoplasm with an associated invasive carcinoma
  - Pancreatoblastoma
  - Serous cystadenocarcinoma
  - Solid-papillary neoplasm
- Neuroendocrine neoplasms
  - Pancreatic neuroendocrine microadenoma
  - Neuroendocrine tumour (NET)
    - Nonfunctional pancreatic NET, G1, G2
    - NET G1
    - NET G2
  - Neuroendocrine carcinoma (NEC)
    - Large cell NEC
    - Small cell NEC
- EC cell, serotonin-producing NET (carcinoid)
- Gastrinoma
- Glucagonoma
- Insulinoma
- Somatostatinoma
- VIPoma

Mature teratoma
Mesenchymal tumours
Lymphomas
Secondary tumours

Female Genital tract Tumors: Ovary

Epithelial tumours
- Serous tumours
  - Benign
    - Serous cystadenoma
    - Serous Adenofibroma
    - Serous surface papilloma

- Borderline
  - Serous borderline tumour/Atypical proliferative serous tumour
  - Serous borderline tumour - micropapillary variant/Non-invasive low-grade
- Malignant
  - Low-grade serous carcinoma
  - High-grade serous carcinoma
- Mucinous tumours
  - Benign
    - Mucinous cystadenoma
    - Mucinous adenofibroma
  - Borderline
    - Mucinous borderline tumour/Atypical proliferative mucinous tumor
  - Malignant
    - Mucinous carcinoma
- Endometrioid tumours
  - Benign
    - Endometriotic cyst
    - Endometriotic cystadenoma
    - Endometriotic adenofibroma
  - Borderline
    - Endometriotic borderline tumour/ Atypical proliferative endometrioid tumor
  - Malignant
    - Endometriotic carcinoma
- Clear cell tumours
  - Benign
    - Clear cell cystadenoma
    - Clear cell adenofibroma
  - Borderline
    - Clear cell borderline tumour/Atypical proliferative clear cell tumor
  - Malignant
    - Clear cell carcinoma
- Brenner tumours
  - Benign
    - Brenner tumour
  - Borderline
    - Borderline Brenner tumour/Atypical proliferative Brenner tumour
  - Malignant
    - Malignant Brenner tumour
- Seromucinous tumour
  - Benign
    - Seromucinous cystadenoma
    - Seromucinous adenofibroma
  - Borderline
    - Seromucinous borderline tumour/Atypical proliferative seromucinous tumour
  - Malignant
    - Seromucinous carcinoma
- Undifferentiated carcinoma

Mesenchymal tumours
- Low-grade endometrioid stromal sarcoma
- High-grade endometrioid stromal sarcoma

Mixed epithelial and mesenchymal tumours
- Adenosarcoma
- Carcinosarcoma

Sex cord-stromal tumours
- Pure stromal tumors
  - Fibroma
  - Cellular fibroma
  - Thecoma
  - Luteinized thecoma associated with sclerosing peritonitis
  - Fibrosarcoma
  - Sclerosing stromal tumour
  - Signet-ring stromal tumour
  - Microcystic stromal tumour
  - Leydig cell tumour
  - Steroid cell tumour
  - Steroid cell tumour, malignant
- Pure sex cord tumours
  - Adult granulosa cell tumour
  - Juvenile granulosa cell tumour
  - Sertoli cell tumour
  - Sex cord tumour with annular tubules

Mixed sex cord-stromal tumours
- Sertoli-Leydig cell tumours
  - Well differentiated
  - Moderately differentiated
    - With heterologous elements
  - Poorly differentiated
    - With heterologous elements
  - Retiform
    - With heterologous elements
- Sex cord-stromal tumours, NOS

Germ cell tumours
- Dysgerminoma
- Yolk say tumour
- Embryonal carcinoma

- Non-gestational choriocarcinoma
- Mature teratoma
- Immature teratoma
- Mixed germ cell tumour

Monodermal teratoma and somatic-type tumours arising from a dermoid cyst
- Struma ovarii, benign
- Struma ovarii, malignant
- Carcinoid
  - Struma carcinoid
  - Mucinous carcinoid
- Neuroectodermal-type tumours
- Sebaceous tumours
  - Sebaceous adenoma
  - Sebaceous carcinoma
- Other rare monodermal tumours
- Carcinomas
  - Squamous cell carcinoma
  - Others

Germ cell: sex cord-stromal tumours
- Gonadoblastoma, including gonadoblastoma with malignant germ cell tumour
- Mixed germ cell-sex cord-stromal tumour unclassified

Miscellaneous tumours
- Tumours of rete ovarii
  - Adenoma of rete ovarii
  - Adenocarcinoma of rete ovarii
- Wolffian tumour
- Small cell carcinoma, hypercalcaemic type
- Small cell carcinoma, pulmonary type
- Wilms tumour
- Paraganglioma
- Solid pseudopapillary neoplasm

Mesothelial tumours
- Adenomatoid tumour
- Mesothelioma

Soft tissue tumours
- Myxoma
- Others

Tumour-like lesions
- Follicle cyst
- Corpus luteum cyst
- Large solitary luteinized follicle cyst
- Hyperreactio luteinalis
- Preganancy luteoma
- Stromal hyperplasia
- Stromal hyperthecosis
- Fibromatosis
- Massive oedema
- Leydig cell hyperplasia
- Others

Lymphoid and myeloid tumours
- Lymphomas
- Plasmacytoma
- Myeloid neoplasms

Secondary tumours

Female Genital Tract Tumors: Uterine Corpus

Epithelial tumours and precursors
- Precursors
  - Hyperplasia without atypia
  - Atypical hyperplasia/Endometrioid intraepithelial neoplasia
- Endometrial carcinomas
  - Endometrioid carcinoma
    - Squamous infiltration
    - Villoglandular
    - Secretory
  - Mucinous carcinoma
  - Serous endometrial intraepithelial carcinoma
  - Serous carcinoma
  - Clear cell carcinoma
  - Neuroendocrine tumours
    - Low-grade neuroendocrine tumour
    - Carcinoid
    - High-grade neuroendocrine carcinoma
    - Small cell neuroendocrine carcinoma
    - Large cell neuroendocrine carcinoma
  - Mixed cell adenocarcinoma
  - Undifferentiated carcinoma
  - Dedifferentiated carcinoma
- Tumor-like lesions
  - Polyp
  - Metaplasia
  - Arias-Stella reaction
  - Lymphoma-like lesion

Mesenchymal tumours
- Leiomyoma
  - Cellular leiomyoma
  - Leiomyoma with bizarre nuclei
  - Mitotically active leiomyoma
  - Hydropic leiomyoma
  - Apoplectic leiomyoma
  - Lipomatous leiomyoma (Lipoleiomyoma)
  - Epitheloid leiomyoma
  - Myxoid leiomyoma
  - Dissecting (cotyledonoid) leiomyoma
  - Diffuse leiomyoma
  - Intravenous leiomyomatosis
  - Metastasizing leiomyoma
- Smooth muscle tumour of uncertain malignant potential
- Leiomyosarcoma
  - Epitheloid leiomyosarcoma
  - Myxoid leiomyosarcoma
- Endometrial stromal and related tumours
  - Endometrial stromal nodule
  - Low-grade endometrial stromal sarcoma
  - High-grade endometrial stromal sarcoma
  - Undifferentiated uterine sarcoma
  - Uterine tumour resembling ovarian sex cord tumour
- Miscellaneous mesenchymal tumours
  - Rhabdomyosarcoma
  - Perivascular epithelioid tumour
    - Benign
    - Malignant
- Others

Mixed epithelial and mesenchymal tumours
- Adenomyoma
- Atypical polypoid adenomyoma
- Adenofibroma
- Adenosarcoma
- Carcinosarcoma

Miscellaneaous tumours
- Adenomatoid tumour
- Neuroectodermal tumours
- Germ cell tumours

Lymphoid and myeloid tumours
- Lymphomas
- Myeloid neoplasms

Secondary tumours

Female Genital Tract Tumors: Uterine Cervix

Epithelial tumours
- Squamous cell tumours and precursors
  - Squamous intraepithelial lesions
    - Low-grade squamous intraepithelial lesion
    - High-grade squamous intraepithelial lesion
  - Squamous cell carcinoma, NOS
    - Keratinizing
    - Non-keratinizing
    - Papillary
    - Basaloid
    - Warty
    - Verrucous
    - Squamotransitional
    - Lymphoepithelioma-like
  - Benign squamous cell lesions
    - Squamous metaplasia
    - Condyloma acuminatum
    - Squamous papilloma
    - Transitional metaplasia
- Glandular tumours and precursors
  - Adenocarcinoma in situ
  - Adenocarcinoma
    - Endocervical adenocarcinoma, usual type
    - Mucinous carcinoma, NOS
    - Gastric type
    - Intestinal type
    - Signet-ring cell type
    - Villoglandular carcinoma
    - Endometrioid carcinoma
    - Clear cell carcinoma
    - Serous carcinoma
    - Mesonephric carcinoma
    - Adenocarcinoma admixed with neuroendocrine carcinoma
- Benign glandular tumours and tumour-like lesions
  - Endocervical polyp
  - Müllerian papilloma
  - Nabothian cyst
  - Tunnel clusters
  - Microglandular hyperplasia
  - Lobular endocervical glandular hyperplasia
  - Diffuse laminar endocervical hyperplasia

- Mesonephric remnants and hyperplasia
- Arias Stella reaction
- Endocervicosis
- Endometriosis
- Tuboendemetrioid metaplasia
- Ectopic prostate tissue
• Other epithelial tumours
  - Adenosquamous carcinoma
    ○ Glassy cell carcinoma
  - Adenoid basal cell carcinoma
  - Adenoid cystic carcinoma
  - Undifferentiated carcinoma
• Neuroendocrine tumours
  - Low-grade neuroendocrine tumour
    ○ Carcinoid tumour
    ○ Atypical carcinoid tumour
  - High-grade neuroendocrine carcinoma
    ○ Small cell neuroendocrine carcinoma
    ○ Large cell neuroendocrine carcinoma

Mesenchymal tumours and tumour-like lesions
• Benign
  - Leiomyoma
  - Rhabdomyoma
  - Others
• Malignant
  - Leiomyosarcoma
  - Rhabdomyosarcoma
  - Alveolar soft-part sarcoma
  - Angiosarcoma
  - Malignant peripheral nerve sheath tumour
  - Other sarcomas
    ○ Liosarcoma
    ○ Undifferentiated endocervical sarcoma
    ○ Ewing sarcoma
  - Tumour-like lesions
    ○ Postoperative spindle-cell nodule
    ○ Lymphoma-like lesions

Mixed epithelial and mesenchymal tumours
• Adenomyoma
• Adeonsarcoma
• Carcinosarcoma

Melanocytic tumours
• Blue naevus
• Malignant melanoma

Germ cell tumours
• Yolk sac tumour

Lymphoid and myeloid tumours
• Lymphomas
• Myeloid neoplasms

Secondary tumours

Female Genital Tract Tumors: Vagina

Epithelial tumours
• Squamous cell tumours and precursors
  - Squamous intraepithelial lesions
    ○ Low-grade squamous intraepithelial lesion
    ○ High-grade squamous intraepithelial lesion
  - Squamous cell carcinoma, NOS
    ○ Keratinizing
    ○ Non-keratinizing
    ○ Papillary
    ○ Basaloid
    ○ Warty
    ○ Verrucous
  - Benign squamous cell lesions
    ○ Condyloma acuminatum
    ○ Squamous papilloma
    ○ Fibroepithelial polyp
    ○ Tubulosquamous polyp
    ○ Transitional cell metaplasia
• Glandular tumours and precursors
  - Adenocarcinomas
    ○ Endometrioid carcinoma
    ○ Clear cell carcinoma
    ○ Mucinous carcinoma
    ○ Mesonephric carcinoma
  - Benign glandular lesions
    ○ Tubulivillous adenoma
    ○ Villous adenoma
    ○ Müllerian papilloma
    ○ Adenosis
    ○ Endometriosis
    ○ Endocervicosis
    ○ Cysts
• Other epithelial tumours
  - Mixed tumour

- Adenosquamous carcinoma
- Adenoid basal carcinoma
- High-grade neuroendocrine carcinoma
  - Small cell neuroendocrine carcinoma
  - Large cell neuroendocrine carcinoma

Mesenchymal tumours
- Leiomyoma
- Rhabdomyoma
- Leiomyosarcoma
- Rhabdomyosarcoma, NOS
  - Embryonal rhabdomyosarcoma
- Undifferentiated sarcoma
- Angiomyofibroblastoma
- Aggressive angiomyxoma
- Myofibroblastoma

Tumour-like lesions
- Postoperative spindle-cell nodule

Mixed epithelial and mesenchymal tumours
- Adenosarcoma
- Carcinosarcoma

Lymphoid and myeloid tumours
- Lymphomas
- Myeloid neoplasms

Melanocytic tumours
- Naevi
  - Melanocytic naevus
  - Blue naevus
- Malignant melanoma

Miscellaneous tumours
- Germ cell tumours
  - Mature teratoma
  - Yolk sac tumour
- Others
  - Ewing sarcoma
  - Paraganglioma

Secondary tumours

Female Genital Tract Tumors: Vulva

Epithelial tumours
- Squamous cell tumours and precursors
  - Squamous intraepithelial lesions
    - Low-grade squamous intraepithelial lesion
    - High-grade squamous intraepithelial lesion
    - Dedifferentiated-type vulvar intraepithelial neoplasia
  - Squamous cell carcinoma
    - Keratinizing
    - Non-keratinizing
    - Basaloid
    - Warty
    - Verrucous
  - Basal cell carcinoma
  - Benign squamous lesions
    - Condyloma acuminatum
    - Vestibular papilloma
    - Seborrheic keratosis
    - Keratoacanthoma
- Glandular tumours
  - Paget disease
  - Tumours arising from Bartholin and other specialized anogenital glands
    - Bartholin gland carcinoma
    - Adenocarcinoma
    - Squamous cell carcinoma
    - Adenosquamous carcinoma
    - Adnpid cystic carcinoma
    - Transitional cell carcinoma
    - Adenocarcinoma of mammary gland type
    - Adenocarcinoma of Skene gland origin
    - Phylloides tumour, malignant
  - Adenocarcinomas of other types
    - Adenocarcinoma of sweat gland type
    - Adenocarcinoma of intestinal type
  - Benign tumours and cysts
    - Papillary hidradenoma
    - Mixed tumour
    - Fibroadenoma
    - Adenoma
    - Adenomyoma
    - Bartholin gland cyst
    - Nodular Bartholin gland hyperplasia
    - Other vestibular gland cysts
    - Other cysts
- Neuroendocrine tumours
  - High-grade neuroendocrine carcinoma
    - Small cell neuroendocrine carcinoma
    - Large cell neuroendocrine carcinoma
  - Merkel cell tumour

Neuroectodermal tumours
- Ewing sarcoma

Soft tissue tumours
- Benign
  - Lipoma
  - Fibroepithelial stromal polyp
  - Superficial angiomyxoma
  - Superficial myofibroblastoma
  - Cellular angiofibroma
  - Angiomyofibroblastoma
  - Aggressive angiomyxoma
  - Leiomyoma
  - Granular cell tumor
  - Other benign tumours
- Malignant tumours
  - Rhabdomyosarcoma
    - Embryonal
    - Alveolar
  - Leiomyosarcoma
  - Epitheloid sarcoma
  - Alveolar soft part sarcoma
  - Other sarcomas
    - Liposarcoma
    - Malignant peripheral nerve sheath tumour
    - Kaposi sarcoma
    - Fibrosarcoma
    - Dermatofibrosarcoma protuberans

Melanocytic tumours
- Melanocytic naevi
  - Congenital melanocytic naevus
  - Acquired melanocytic naevus
  - Blue naevus
  - Atypical melnocytic naevus of genital type
  - Dysplastic meloncytic naevus
- Malignant melanoma

Germ cell tumours
- Yolk sac tumour

Lymphoid and myeloid tumours
- Lymphomas
- Myeloid neoplasms

Secondary tumours

Endocrine Tumors: Pituitary

Pituitary adenomas
- Pituitary adenoma
- Somatotroph adenoma
- Lactotroph adenoma
- Thyrotroph adenoma
- Corticotroph adenoma
- Gonadotroph adenoma
- Null cell adenoma
- Plurihormonal and double adenomas

Pituitary carcinoma

Pituitary blastoma

Craniopharyngioma
- Adamantinomatous craniopharyngioma
- Papillary craniopharyngioma

Neuronal and paraneuronal tumours
- Gangliocytoma and mixed gangliocytoma-adenoma
- Neurocytoma
- Paraganglioma
- Neuroblastoma

Tumours of the posterior pituitary
- Pituicytoma
- Granular cell tumour of the sellar region
- Spindle cell ancocytoma
- Sellar ependymoma

Mesenchymal and stromal tumours
- Meningioma
- Schwannoma
- Chordoma, NOS
  - Chondroid chordoma
  - Dedifferentiated chordoma
- Haemangiopericytoma/Solitary fibrous tumour
  - Grade 1 HPC/SFT
  - Grade 2 HPC/SFT
  - Grade 3 HPC/SFT

Haematolymphoid tumours

Germ cell tumours
- Germinoma
- Yolk sac tumour

- Embryonal carcinoma
- Choriocarcinoma
- Teratoma, NOS
- Mature teratoma
- Immature teratoma
- Teratoma with malignant transformation
- Mixed germ cell tumour

Secondary tumours

Endocrine Tumors: Thyroid Gland

Follicular adenoma
Hyalinizing trabecular tumour

Other encapsulated follicular-patterned thyroid tumours
- Follicular tumour of uncertain malignant potential
- Well-differentiated tumour of uncertain malignant potential
- Non-invasive follicular thyroid neoplasm with papillary-like nuclear features

Papillary thyroid carcinoma (PTC)
- Papillary carcinoma
- Follicular variant of PTC
- Encapsulated variant of PTC
- Papillary microcarcinoma
- Columnar call variant of PTC
- Oncocytic variant of PTC

Follicular thyroid carcinoma (FTC), NOS
- FTC, minimally invasive
- FTC, encapsulated angioinvasive
- FTC, widely invasive

Hürthle (oncocytic) cell tumours
- Hürthle cell adenoma
- Hürthle cell carcinoma

Poorly differentiated thyroid carcinoma
Anaplastic thyroid carcinoma
Squamous cell carcinoma
Medullary thyroid carcinoma
Mixed medullary and follicular thyroid carcinoma
Mucoepidermoid carcinoma
Sclerosing mucoepidermoid carcinoma with eosinophilia
Mucinous carcinoma
Ectopic thymoma
Spindle epithelial tumour with thymus-like differentiation
Intrathyroid thymic carcinoma

Paraganglioma and mesenchymal/stromal tumours
- Paraganglioma
- Peripheral nerve sheath tumours (PNSTs), Schwannoma, Malignant PNST
- Benign vascular tumours, Haemangioma, Cavernous haemangioma, Lymphangioma
- Angiosarcoma
- Smooth muscle tumours, Leiomyoma, Leiomyosarcoma
- Solitary fibrous tumour

Haematolymphoid tumours
- Langerhans cell histiocytosis
- Rosai-Dorfman disease
- Follicular dentritic cell sarcoma
- Primary thyroid lymphoma

Germ cell tumours
- Benign teratoma (grade 0 or 1)
- Immature teratoma (grade 2)
- Malignant teratoma (grade 3)

Secondary tumours

Endocrine Tumors: Parathyroid Glands

Parathyroid carcinoma
Parathyroid adenoma
Secondary, mesenchymal and other tumours

Endocrine Tumors: Adrenal Cortex

Adrenal cortical carcinoma
Adrenal cortical adenoma
Sex cord-stromal tumours
Adenomatoid tumour

Mesenchymal and stromal tumours
- Myelolipoma
- Schwannoma

Haematolymphoid tumours
Secondary tumours

Endocrine Tumors: Adrenal Medulla and Extra-adrenal Paraganglia

Phaeochromocytoma

Extra-adrenal paragangliomas
- Head and neck paragangliomas
- Carotid body paraganglioma
- Jugulotympanic paraganglioma
- Vagal paraganglioma
- Laryngeal paraganglioma

Sympathetic paragangliomas

Neuroblastic tumours of the adrenal gland
- Neuroblastoma
- Ganglioneuroblastoma, nodular
- Ganglioneuroblastoma, intermixed
- Ganglioneuroma

Composite phaeochromocytoma
Composite paraganglioma

Endocrine Tumors: Neuroendocrine Pancreas

Non-functioning (non-syndromic) neuroendocrine tumours
- Pancreatic neuroendocrine microadenoma
- Non-functioning pancreatic neuroendocrine tumour

Insulinoma
Glucagonoma
Somatostatinoma
Gastrinoma
VIPoma

Serotonin-producing tumours with and without carcinoid syndrome
- Serotonin-producing tumour

ACTH-producing tumour with Cushing syndrome
- ACTH-producing tumour

Pancreatic neuroendocrine carcinoma (poorly differentiated neuroendocrine neoplasm)
- Neuroendocrine carcinoma (poorly differentiated neuroendocrine neoplasm)
- Small cell neuroendocrine carcinoma
- Large cell neuroendocrine carcinoma

Mixed neuroendocrine-non-neuroendocrine neoplasms
- Mixed ductal-neuroendocrine carcinomas
- Mixed acinar-neuroendocrine carcinomas

Soft tissue Tumors

Adipocytic
- Benign
- Lipoma
- Lipomatosis
- Lipomatosis of nerve
- Lipoblastoma/lipoblastmatosis
- Angiolipoma
- Myolipoma
- Chondroid lipoma
- Extra-renal angiomyolipoma
- Extra-adrenal myelolipoma
- Spindle cell/pleomorphic lipoma
- Hibernoma
- Intermediate
- Atypical lipomatous tumor/well differentiated liposarcoma
- Malignant
- Dedifferentiated liposarcoma
- Myxoid liposarcoma
- Pleomorphic liposarcoma
- Liposarcoma NOS

Fibroblastic/Myofibroblastic
- Benign
- Nodular fasciitis
- Proliferative fasciitis
- Proliferative myositis
- Myositis ossificans
- Fibro-osseous pseudotumour of digits
- Ischaemic fasciitis

- Elastofibroma
- Fibrous hamartoma of infancy
- Fibromatosis colli
- Juvenile hyaline fibromatosis
- Inclusion body fibromatosis
- Fibroma of tendon sheath
- Desmoplastic fibroblastoma
- Mammary-type myofibroblastoma
- Calcifying aponeurotic fibroma
- Angiomyofibroblastoma
- Cellular angiofibroma
- Nuchal-type fibroma
- Gardner fibroma
- Calcifying fibrous tumour
- Intermediate (locally aggressive)
- Palmar/plantar fibromatosis
- Desmoids-type fibromatosis
- Lipofromatosis
- Giant cell fibroblastoma
- Intermediate (rarely metastasizing)
- Dermatofibrosarcoma protuberans
- Solitary fibrous tumor
- Inflammatory myofibroblastic tumour
- Low-grade myofibroblastic sarcoma
- Myxoinflammatory fibroblastic sarcoma/atypical myxoinflammatory fibroblastic tumour
- Infantile fibrosarcoma
- Malignant
- Adult fibrossarcoma
- Myxofibrosarcoma
- Low-grade fibromyxoid sarcoma
- Sclerosing epithelioid fibrosarcoma

So-called fibrohistiocytic
- Benign
- Tenosynovial giant cell tumour
- Deep benign fibrous histiocytoma
- Intermediate
- Plexiform fibrohistiocytic tumor
- Giant cell tumor of soft tissues

Smooth muscle
- Benign
- Deep leiomyoma
- Malignant
- Leiomyosarcoma

Pericytic
- Glomus tumor
- Myopericytoma
- Angioleiomyoma

Skeletal muscle
- Benign
- Rhabdomyoma
- Malignant
- Embryonal rhabdomyosarcoma
- Alveolar rhabdomyosarcoma
- Pleomorphic rhabdomyosarcoma
- Spindle cell/sclerosing rhabdomyosarcoma

Vascular
- Benign
- Hemangioma
- Epithelioid hemangioma
- Angiomatosis
- Lymphangioma
- Intermediate (locally aggressive)
- Kaposiform haemangioendothelioma
- Intermediate (rarely metastasizing)
- Retiform hemangioendothelioma
- Papillary intralymphatic angioendothelioma
- Composite haemangioendothelioma
- Pseudomyogenic haemangioendothelioma
- Kaposi sarcoma
- Malignant
- Epithelioid hemangioendothelioma
- Angiosarcoma of soft tissue

Chondro-osseous
- Benign
- Soft tissue chondroma
- Extraskeletal mesenchymal chondrosarcoma
- Extraskeletal ostersarcoma

Gastrointestinal stromal
- Benign gastrointestinal stromal tumour
- Gastrointestinal stromal tumor, uncertain malignant potential
- Gastrointestinal stromal tumour, malignant

Nerve sheath
- Benign

- Schwannoma
- Melanotic schwannoma
- Neurofibroma
- Perineurioma
- Granular cell tumpr
- Dermal nerve sheath myxoma
- Solitary circumscribed neuroma
- Ectopic meningioma
- Nasal glial hetertopia
- Benign Triton tumor
- Hybrid nerve sheath tumours
- Malignant
- Malignant peripheral nerve sheath tumour
- Epithelioid malignant peripheral nerve sheath tumour
- Malignant Triton tumour
- Malignant granular cell tumour
- Ectomesenchymoma

Uncertain differentiation
- Benign
- Acral fibromyxoma
- Intramuscular myxoma
- Juxta-articular myxoma
- Deep angiomyxoma
- Pleomorphic hyalinising angiectatic tumour
- Ecopic hamartomatous thymoma
- Intermediate (locally aggressive)
- Haemosiderotic fibrolipomatous tumour
- Intermediate (rarely metastasizing)
- Atypical fibroxanthoma
- Angiomatoid fibrous histiocytoma
- Ossifying fibromyxoid tumor
- Mixed tumour NOS
- Mixed tumour NOS, malignant
- Myoepithelioma
- Myoepithelial carcinoma
- Phosphaturic mesenchymal tumour, benign
- Phosphaturic mesenchymal tumour, malignant
- Malignant
- Synovial sarcoma NOS
- Epitheloid sarcoma
- Alveolar soft-part sarcoma
- Clear cell sarcoma of soft tissue
- Extraskeletal myxoid chondrosarcoma
- Extraskeletal Ewing sarcoma
- Desmoplastic small round tumor
- Extra-renal rhabdoid tumor

- Neoplasms with perivascular epithelioid cell differentiation (PEComa)
- Intimal sarcoma

Undifferentiated/unclassified sarcomas
- Undifferentiated spindle cell sarcoma
- Undifferentiated pleomorphic sarcoma
- Undifferentiated round cell sarcoma
- Undifferentiated epitheloid sarcoma
- Undifferentiated sarcoma NOS

Bone Tumors

Chondrogenic
- Benign
- Osteochondroma
- Chondroma
- Osteochondromyxoma
- Subungual exostosis
- Intermediate
- Chondroblastoma
- Malignant
- Chondrosarcoma (grade II, III)
- Dedifferentiated chondrosarcoma
- Mesenchymal chondrosarcoma
- Clear cell chondrosarcoma

Osteogenic
- Benign
- Osteoma
- Osteoid osteoma
- Intermediate
- Osteoblastoma
- Malignant
- Low-grade central osteosarcoma
- Conventional osteosarcoma
- Osteosarcoma subtypes (see WHO)

Fibrogenic
- Intermediate
- Desmoplastic fibroma of bone
- Malignant
- Fibrosarcoma of bone

Fibrohystiocytic
- Benign fibrous histiocytoma/non-ossifying fibroma

Hematopoietic
- Malignant
- Plasma cell myeloma
- Solitary plasmacytoma of bone
- Primary non-Hodgkin lymphoma of bone

Osteoclastic giant cell rich
- Benign
- Giant cell lesion of the small bones
- Intermediate
- Giant cell tumor of bone
- Malignant
- Malignancy in giant cell tumor of bone

Notochordal
- Benign
- Benign notochordal tumor
- Malignant
- Chordoma

Vascular
- Benign
- Hemangioma
- Intermediate
- Epithelioid hemangioma
- Malignant
- Epithelioid hemangioendothelioma
- Angiosarcoma

Myogenic
- Benign
- Leiomyoma of bone
- Malignant
- Leiomyosarcoma of bone

Lipogenic
- Benign
- Lipoma of bone
- Malignant
- Liposarcoma of bone

Undefined neoplastic nature
- Benign
- Simple bone cyst
- Fibrous dysplasia
- Osteofibrous dysplasia
- Chondromesenchymal hamartoma
- Rosai-Dorfman disease
- Intermediate
- Aneurysmal bone cyst
- Langerhans cell histiocytosis
- Erdheim-Chester disease

Miscellaneous
- Ewing sarcoma (PNET)
- Adamantinoma
- Undifferentiated high-grade pleomorphic sarcoma of bone

Hematopoetic System Tumors

Myeloproliferative neoplasms (MPN)
- Chronic myeloid leukemia (CML), BCR-ABL1-positive
- Chronic neutrophilic leukemia (CNL)
- Polycythemia vera (PV)
- Primary myelofibrosis (PMF)
- Essential thrombocythaemia (ET)
- Chronic eosinophilic leukemia, not otherwise specified (NOS)
- Myeloproliferative neoplasm, unclassifiable

Mastocytosis
- Cutaneous mastocytosis
- Indolent systemic mastocytosis
- Systemic mastocytosis with an associated haematological neoplasm
- Aggressive systemic mastocytosis
- Mast cell leukemia
- Mast cell sarcoma

Myeloid/lymphoid neoplasms with eosinophilia and gene rearrangement
- Myeloid/lymphoid neoplasms with *PDGFRA* rearrangement
- Myeloid/lymphoid neoplasms with **PDGFRB** rearrangement
- Myeloid/lymphoid neoplasms with **FGFR1** rearrangement
- Myeloid/lymphoid neoplasms with *PCM1-JAK2*

Myelodysplastic/myeloproliferative neoplasms (MDS/MPN)
- Chronic myelomonocytic leukemia (CMML)

- Atypical chronic myeloid leukemia (aCML), BCR-ABL1-negative
- Juvenile myelomonocytic leukemia (JMML)
- Myelodysplastic/myeloproliferative neoplasm with ring sideroblasts and thrombocytosis (MDS/MPN-RS-T)
- Myelodysplastic/myeloproliferative, unclassifiable

Myelodysplastic syndromes (MDS)
- Myelodysplastic syndrome with single lineage dysplasia
- Myelodysplastic syndrome with ring sideroblasts (MDS-RS) and single lineage dysplasia
- Myelodysplastic syndrome with ring sideroblasts and multilineage dysplasia
- Myelodysplastic syndrome with multilineage dysplasia
- Myelodysplastic syndrome with excess blasts
- Myelodysplastic syndrome with isolated del(5q)
- Myelodysplastic syndrome, unclassifiable
- Refractory cytopenia of childhood

Myeloid neoplasms with germ line predisposition
- Acute myeloid leukemia with germline *CEBPA* mutation
- Myeloid neoplasms with germline *DDX41* mutation
- Myeloid neoplasms with germline *RUNX1* mutation
- Myeloid neoplasms with germline *ANKRD26* mutation
- Myeloid neoplasms with germline *ETV6* mutation
- Myeloid neoplasms with germline *GATA2* mutation

Acute myeloid leukemia (AML) and related neoplasms

AML with recurrent genetic abnormalities
- AML with t(8;21)(q22;q22.1); *RUNX1-RUNX1T1*
- AML with inv(16)(p13.1q22) or t(16,16)(p13.1;q22); *CBFB-MYH11*
- Acute promyelocytic leukemia with *PML-RARA*
- AML with t(9,11)(p21.3;q23.3); *MLLT3-KMT2A*
- AML with t(6,9)(p23;q34.1); *DEK-NUP214*
- AML with inv(3)(q21.3q26.2) or t(3,3)(q21.3;q26.2); *GATA2, MECOM*
- AML (megakaryoblastic) with t(1,22)(p13.3;q13.3); *RBM15-MKL1*
- AML with *BCR-ABL1*
- AML with mutated *NPM1*
- AML with biallelic mutations of *CEBPA*
- AML with mutated *RUNX1*

AML with myelodysplasia-related changes
Therapy-related myeloid neoplasms

Acute myeloid leukemia, NOS
- AML with minimal differentiation
- AML without maturation
- AML with maturation
- Acute myelomonocytic leukemia
- Acute monoblastic and monocytic leukemia
- Pure erythroid leukemia
- Acute megakaryoblastic leukemia
- Acute basophilic leukemia
- Acute panmyelosis with myelofibrosis

Myeloid sarcoma

Myeloid proliferations associated with Down syndrome
- Transient abnormal myelopoiesis (TAM) associated with Down syndrome
- Myeloid leukemia associated with Down syndrome

Blastic plasmacytoid dendritic cell neoplasm

Acute leukemias of ambiguous lineage
- Acute undifferentiated leukemia
- Mixed-phenotype acute leukemia (MPAL) with t(9,22)(q34.1;q11.2); *BCR-ABL1*
- Mixed-phenotype acute leukemia with t(v;11q23.3); *KMT2A* rearranged
- Mixed-phenotype acute leukemia, B/myeloid, NOS

- Mixed-phenotype acute leukemia, T/myeloid, NOS
- Mixed-phenotype acute leukemia, NOS, rare types
- Acute leukemias of ambiguous lineage, NOS

Precursor lymphoid neoplasms
- B-lymphoblastic leukemia/lymphoma, NOS
- B-lymphoblastic leukemia/lymphoma with t(9,22)(q34.1;q11.2); *BCR-ABL1*
- B-lymphoblastic leukemia/lymphoma with t(v;11q23.3); *KMT2A* rearranged
- B-lymphoblastic leukemia/lymphoma with t(12,21)(p13.2;q22.1); *ETV6-RUNX1*
- B-lymphoblastic leukemia/lymphoma with hyperdiploidy
- B-lymphoblastic leukemia/lymphoma with hypodiploidy (hypodiploid ALL)
- B-lymphoblastic leukemia/lymphoma with t(5,14)(q31.1;q32.3); *IGH/IL3*
- B-lymphoblastic leukemia/lymphoma with t(1,19)(q23;p13.3); *TCF3-PBX1*
- Provisional entity: B-lymphoblastic leukemia/lymphoma, *BCR-ABL1*–like
- Provisional entity: B-lymphoblastic leukemia/lymphoma with *iAMP21*
- T-lymphoblastic leukemia/lymphoma
- Early T-cell precursor lymphoblastic leukemia
- NK-lymphoblastic leukemia/lymphoma

Mature B-cell neoplasms
- Chronic lymphocytic leukemia (CLL)/small lymphocytic lymphoma
- Monoclonal B-cell lymphocytosis, CLL-type
- Monoclonal B-cell lymphocytosis, non-CLL-type
- B-cell prolymphocytic leukemia
- Splenic marginal zone lymphoma
- Hairy cell leukemia
- Splenic B-cell lymphoma/leukemia, unclassifiable
  - Splenic diffuse red pulp small B-cell lymphoma
  - Hairy cell leukemia-variant
- Lymphoplasmacytic lymphoma
  - Waldenström macroglobulinemia
- IgM Monoclonal gammopathy of undetermined significance (MGUS)
- Heavy chain diseases
  - Mu heavy-chain disease
  - Gamma heavy-chain disease
  - Alpha heavy-chain disease
- Plasma cell neoplasms
  - Non-IgM monoclonal gammopathy of undetermined significance
  - Plasma cell myeloma
  - Solitary plasmacytoma of bone
  - Extraosseous plasmacytoma
  - Monoclonal immunoglobulin deposition diseases
    - Primary amyloidosi
    - Light chain and heavy chain deposition diseases
- Extranodal marginal zone lymphoma of mucosa-associated lymphoid tissue (MALT lymphoma)
- Nodal marginal zone lymphoma
  - Pediatric nodal marginal zone lymphoma
- Follicular lymphoma
  - In situ follicular neoplasia
  - Duodenal-type follicular lymphoma
  - Testicular follicular lymphoma
- Pediatric-type follicular lymphoma
- Large B-cell lymphoma with *IRF4* rearrangement
- Primary cutaneous follicle center lymphoma
- Mantle cell lymphoma
  - In situ mantle cell neoplasia
- Diffuse large B-cell lymphoma (DLBCL), NOS
  - Germinal center B-cell type
  - Activated B-cell type
- T-cell/histiocyte-rich large B-cell lymphoma
- Primary DLBCL of the central nervous system (CNS)
- Primary cutaneous DLBCL, leg type
- EBV-positive DLBCL, NOS
- EBV-positive mucocutaneous ulcer
- DLBCL associated with chronic inflammation
  - Fibrin-associated diffuse large B-cell lymphoma
- Lymphomatoid granulomatosis, grade 1, 2
- Lymphomatoid granulomatosis, grade 3
- Primary mediastinal (thymic) large B-cell lymphoma
- Intravascular large B-cell lymphoma

- ALK-positive large B-cell lymphoma
- Plasmablastic lymphoma
- Primary effusion lymphoma
- HHV8-positive DLBCL, NOS
- HHV8-positive germinotropic lymphoproliferative disorder
- Burkitt lymphoma
- Burkitt-like lymphoma with 11q aberration
- High-grade B-cell lymphoma
  - High-grade B-cell lymphoma with *MYC* and *BCL2* and/or *BCL6* rearrangements
  - High-grade B-cell lymphoma, NOS*
- B-cell lymphoma, unclassifiable, with features intermediate between DLBCL and
  - Hodgkin lymphoma

Mature T and NK neoplasms
- T-cell prolymphocytic leukemia
- T-cell large granular lymphocytic leukemia
- Chronic lymphoproliferative disorder of NK cells
- Aggressive NK-cell leukemia
- Systemic EBV1 T-cell lymphoma of childhood
- Chronic active EBV infection of T- and NK-cell type, systemic form
- Hydroa vacciniforme–like lymphoproliferative disorder
- Severe mosquito bite allergy
- Adult T-cell leukemia/lymphoma
- Extranodal NK-/T-cell lymphoma, nasal type
- Enteropathy-associated T-cell lymphoma
- Monomorphic epitheliotropic intestinal T-cell lymphoma
- Intestinal T-cell lymphoma, NOS
- Indolent T-cell lymphoproliferative disorder of the gastrointestinal tract
- Hepatosplenic T-cell lymphoma
- Subcutaneous panniculitis-like T-cell lymphoma
- Mycosis fungoides
- Sézary syndrome
- Primary cutaneous CD30-positive T-cell lymphoproliferative disorders
  - Lymphomatoid papulosis
  - Primary cutaneous anaplastic large cell lymphoma
- Primary cutaneous gamma delta T-cell lymphoma
- Primary cutaneous CD8-positive aggressive epidermotropic cytotoxic T-cell lymphoma
- Primary cutaneous acral CD8-positive T-cell lymphoma
- Primary cutaneous CD4-positive small/medium T-cell lymphoproliferative disorder
- Peripheral T-cell lymphoma, NOS
- Angioimmunoblastic T-cell lymphoma
- Follicular T-cell lymphoma
- Nodal peripheral T-cell lymphoma with T follicular helper phenotype
- Anaplastic large-cell lymphoma, ALK-positive
- Anaplastic large-cell lymphoma, ALK-negative
- Breast implant–associated anaplastic large-cell lymphoma

Hodgkin lymphoma
- Nodular lymphocyte predominant Hodgkin lymphoma
- Classical Hodgkin lymphoma
  - Nodular sclerosis classical Hodgkin lymphoma
  - Lymphocyte-rich classical Hodgkin lymphoma
  - Mixed cellularity classical Hodgkin lymphoma
  - Lymphocyte-depleted classical Hodgkin lymphoma

Immunodeficiency-associated lymphoproliferative disorders
- Post-transplant lymphoproliferative disorders (PTLD)
  - Non-destructive PTLD
  Plasmacytic hyperplasia PTLD
  Infectious mononucleosis PTLD
  Florid follicular hyperplasia PTLD
  - Polymorphic PTLD
  - Monomorphic PTLD (B- and T-/NK-cell types)
  - Classical Hodgkin lymphoma PTLD
- Other iatrogenic immunodeficiency-associated lymphoproliferative disorders

Histiocytic and dendritic cell neoplasms
- Histiocytic sarcoma
- Langerhans cell histiocytosis, NOS
- Langerhans cell histiocytosis, monostotic
- Langerhans cell histiocytosis, polystotic
- Langerhans cell histiocytosis, disseminated
- Langerhans cell sarcoma
- Indeterminate dendritic cell tumour
- Interdigitating dendritic cell sarcoma
- Follicular dendritic cell sarcoma
- Fibroblastic reticular cell tumor
- Disseminated juvenile xanthogranuloma
- Erdheim-Chester disease

References

Neuroanatomy—Neurohistology—Neurochemistry

Albertstone CD, Benzel EC, Najm IM, Steinmetz MP (2009) Anatomic basis of neurologic diagnosis. Thieme, New York, Stuttgart

Andersen P, Morris R, Amaral D, Bliss T, O'Keefe J The hippocampus book. Oxford University Press, Oxford, p 2007

Armati PJ, Mathey EK (eds) (2010) The biology of oligodendrocytes. Cambridge University Press, Cambridge

Arslan OE (2015) Neuroanatomical basis of clinical neurology, 2nd edn. CRC, Boca Raton, FL

Augustine JR (2017) Human neuroanatomy, 2nd edn. Wiley Blackwell, Hoboken, NJ

Brady ST, Siegel GJ, Albers RW, Price DL (2012) Basic neurochemistry, 8th edn. Academic, New York

Davies RW, Morris BJ (eds) (2004) Molecular biology of the neuron, 2nd edn. Oxford University Press, Oxford

Felten DL, Shetty AN (2010) Netter's atlas of neuroscience, 2nd edn. Elsevier-Saunders, Philadelphia

Haines DE (2008) Neuroanatomy. An atlas of structures, sections, and systems, 7th edn. Wolters Kluwer—Lippincott Williams & Wilkins, Philadelphia

Hammond C (ed) (2008) Cellular and molecular neurophysiology, 3rd edn. Elsevier-Academic, New York

Heimer L (1983) The human brain and spinal cord. Functional neuroanatomy and dissection guide. Springer, Berlin

Kettenmann H, Ransom BR (eds) (2013) Neuroglia, 3rd edn. Oxford University Press, Oxford

Kierszenbaum AAL, Tres LL (2012) Histology and cell biology. An introduction to pathology, 3rd edn. Elsevier, Amsterdam

Levitan IB, Kaczmarek LK (1991) The neuron. Cell and molecular biology. Oxford University Press, Oxford

Mescher AL (2013) Junqueira's basic histology. Text & Atlas, 13th edn. McGraw Hill, New York

Mills SE (ed) (2012) Histology for pathologists, 4th edn. Wolter Kluwer Lippincott Williams & Wilkins, Philadelphia

Nieuwenhuys R, Puelles L (2016) Towards a new neuromorphology. Springer, Berlin

Nieuwenhuys R, Voogd J, van Huijzen C (1988) The human central nervous system, 3rd edn. Springer, Berlin

Ovalle WK, Nahirney PC (2013) Netter's essential histology, 2nd edn. Elsevier, Amsterdam

Parpura V, Haydon PG (eds) (2009) Astrocytes in (patho) physiology of the nervous system. Springer, Berlin

Schmahmann JD, Pandya DN (2006) Fiber pathways of the brain. Oxford University Press, Oxford

Shepard GM, Grillner S (eds) (2010) Handbook of brain microcircuits. Oxford University Press, Oxford

Smith CUM (2002) Elements of molecular neurobiology, 3rd edn. Wiley, New York

Steiner H, Tseng KY (eds) (2017) Handbook of basal ganglia structure and function, 2nd edn. Academic, New York

Verkhratsky A, Butt A (2007) Glial neurobiology. Wiley, New York

Verkhratsky A, Butt A (2013) Glial physiology and pathophysiology. Wiley-Blackwell, Hoboken, NJ

Neuropathology

Armstrong D, Halliday W, Hawkins C, Takashima S (2007) Pediatric neuropathology. A text-atlas. Springer, Berlin

Badaut J, Plesnila N (2017) Brain edema. From molecular mechanisms to clinical practice. Academic, New York

Burger PC, Scheithauer BW, Kleinschmidt-DeMasters BK, Ersen A, Rodriguez FJ, Tihan T, Rushing EJ (2012) Diagnsotic pathology: neuropathology. AMIRSYS, Salt Lake City, UT

Caplan LR, Biller J, Leary MC, Lo EH, Thomas AJ, Yenari M, Zhang JH (eds) (2017a) Primer on cerebrovascular diseases, 2nd edn. Academic

Chu P, Weiss L (2009) Modern immunohistochemistry. Cambridge University Press, Cambridge

Dawson TP, Neal JW, Llewellyn L, Thomas C (2003) Neuropathology techniques. Arnold, London

Esiri M, Perl D (2006) Oppenheimer's diagnostic neuropathology. A practical manual, 3rd edn. Hodder Arnold, London

Fuller GN, Goodman JC (2001) Practical review of neuropathology. Lippincott Williams & Wilkins, Philadelphia

Garcia JH (ed) (1997) Neuropathology. The diagnostic approach. Mosby, Maryland Heights, MO

Gray F, Duyckaerts C, De Girolami U (eds) (2014) Escourolle and Poirier's manual of basic neuropathology. In: Oxford University Press, Oxford

Gokden M, Kumar M (eds) (2017) Neuropathologic and neuroradiologic correlations. A differential diagnostic text and atlas. Cambridge University Press, Cambridge

Haberland C (2007) Clinical neuropathology. Text and color atlas. Demos Medical, New York

Josef JT (2007) Diagnostic neuropathology smears. Lippincott Williams & Wilkins, Philadelphia

Louis DN, Frosch MP, Mena H, Rushing EJ, Judkins AR (2009) Non-neoplastic diseases of the central nervous system. AFIP atlas of nontumor pathology. ARP, Washington, DC

Love S, Budka H, Ironside JW, Perry A (eds) (2015) Greenfield's neuropathology, 9th edn. CRC, Boca Raton, FL

Mallucci C, Sgouros S (2010) Cerebrospinal fluid disorders. Informa Healthcare, London

Perry A, Brat DJ (2010) Practical surgical neuropathology. A diagnostic approach. Churchill Livingstone Elsevier, London

Prayson RA (ed) (2011) Neuropathology, 2nd edn. Elsevier-Churchill Livingstone, London

Prayson RA, Cohen ML (2000) Practical differential diagnosis in surgical neuropathology. Humana Press, New York

Vogel H (2009) Illustrated surgical pathology: nervous system. Cambridge University Press, Cambridge

Yachnis A, Rivera-Zengotita M (eds) (2013) Neuropathology. Elsevier–Saunders, Philadelphia

Forensic Neuropathology

Dolinak D, Matshes E (2002) Medicolegal neuropathology. A color atlas. CRC, Boca Raton, FL

Itabashi HH, Andrews JM, Tomiyasu U, Erlich SS, Sathyavagiswaran L (2007) Forensic neuropathology. A practical review of the fundamentals. Elsevier-Academic Press, New York

Leestma JE (2014) Forensic neuropathology, 3rd edn. Talyor & Francis Inc, Abingdon

Oehmichen M, Auer RN, König HG (2006) Forensic neuropathology and neurology. Springer, Berlin

Troncoso JC, Rubio A, Fowler D (eds) (2010) Essential forensic neuropathology. Wolters-Kluver & Lippincott Williams & Wilkins, Philadelphia

Whitwell HL (2005) Forensic neuropathology. CRC, Boca Raton, FL

Molecular (Neuro)Biology

Fain GL (2014) Molecular and cellular physiology of neurons, 2nd edn. Harvard University Press, Cambridge, MA

Johnston MV, Adams HP, Fatemi A (eds) (2016) Neurobiology of disease, 2nd edn. Oxford University Press, Oxford

Neidhart M (2016) DNA methylation and complex human disease. Elsevier, Amsterdam

Rosenberg RN, Pascual JM (eds) (2015) Rosenberg's molecular and genetic basis of neurological and psychiatric disease, 5th edn. Academic, New York

Sweatt JD, Meaney MJ, Nestler EJ, Akbarian S (eds) (2013) Epigenetic regulation in the nervous system. basic mechanisms and clinical impact. Elsevier-Academic, New York

Thompkins JRL Understanding stem cell research.

Tost J (ed) (2008) Epigenetics. Caister Academic Press, Poole

Tost J (ed) (2009) DNA methylation. Methods and protocols. Humana Press, New York

Waxman SG (ed) (2007) Molecular neurology. Elsevier-Academic Press, New York

Cognitive Neurosciences

Baars BJ, Gage NM (eds) (2010) Cognition, brain, and consciousness. Introduction to cognitive neuroscience, 2nd edn. Elsevier-Academic Press, New York

Bear M, Paradiso M, Barry W, Connors BW (2015) Neuroscience: exploring the brain, 4th edn. Lippincott Williams& Wilkins, Philadelphia

Eagleman D, Downar J (2015) Brain and behavior: a cognitive neuroscience perspective. Oxford Univ Press, Oxford

Filley CM (2012) The behavioral neurology of white matter, 2nd edn. Oxford University Press, Oxford

Galizia G, Lledo PM (2013) Neurosciences—from molecule to behavior: a university textbook. Springer, Berlin

Gazzaniga M, Ivry RB, Mangun GR (2016) Cognitive neuroscience: the biology of the mind, Revised 4th edn. WW Norton, New York

Gazzaniga MS (2014) Cognitive Neurosciences (The Cognitive Neurosciences), 5th edn. Mit University Press Group, Cambridge, MA

Kolb B, Whishaw IQ (2004) An introduction to brain and behavior, 2nd edn. Worth, New York

Kolb B, Whishaw IQ (2015) Fundamentals of human neuropsychology, 7th edn. Worth, New York

Lezak MD, Howieson DB, DB EDBED, Daniel Tranel D (2012) Neuropsychological assessment, 5th edn. Oxford University Press, Oxford

Neuro Infections

Ball GV, Bridges SL (eds) (2008) Vasculitis. Oxford University Press, Oxford

Boos J, Esiri M (2003) Viral encephalitis in humans. ASM, Washington, DC

Johnson RT (1998) Viral infections of the nervous system, 2nd edn. Lippincott-Raven, Philadelphia

Levy JA (2007) HIV and the Pathogenesis of AIDS, 3rd edn. ASM, Washington, DC

Murray PR, Rosenthal KS, Pfaller MA (2013) Medical microbiology, 7th edn. Elsevier Saunders, Amsterdam

Neuro-Oncology

Ali-Osman F (ed) (2005) Brain tumors. Humana Press, New York

Barnett GH (ed) (2007) High-grade gliomas: diagnosis and treatment. Human Press, New York

Batchelor T (ed) (2004) Lymphoma of the nervous system. Butterworth-Heinemann, Oxford

Berger MS, Prados MD (eds) (2005) Textbook of neuro-oncology. Elsevier-Saunders, Amsterdam

Burger PC, Scheithauer BW (2007) Tumors of the Central Nervous System. AFIP Atlas of Tumor Pathology, Series 4. ARP, Washington, DC

Dellaire G, Berman J, Arceci R (2014) Cancer genomics: from bench to personalized medicine. Academic Press, New York

DeMonte F, Gilbert MR, Mahajan A, McCutcheon IE (eds) (2007) Tumors of the brain and spine. Springer, Berlin

DeVita VT, Lawrence TS, Rosenberg SA (eds) (2011) Primer of the molecular biology of cancer. Wolters Kluwer, Lippincott, Williams & Wilkins, Philadelphia

Erdmann VA, Reifenberger G, Barciszewski J (eds) (2009) Therapeutic ribonucleic acids in brain tumors. Springer, Berlin

Figg WD, Folkman J (eds) (2008) Angiogenesis. An integrative approach from science to medicine. Springer, Berlin

Gupta N, Banerjee A, Haas-Kogan D (eds) (2004) Pediatric CNS tumors. Springer, Berlin

Harvey A (ed) (2013) Cancer cell signalling. Wiley Blackwell, Hoboken, NJ

Ironside JW, Moss TH, Louis DN, Low JS, Weller RO (2002) Diagnostic Pathology of nervous system tumours. Churchill Livingstone, London

McLendon RE, Bigner DD, Bigner SH, Provenzale JM (2000) Pathology of tumors of the central nervous system. A guide to histologic diagnosis. Arnold, London

Mendelsohn J, Gray JW, Howley PM, Israel MA, Thompson CB (2015) The molecular basis of cancer. Elsevier, Amsterdam

Pecorino L (2016) Molecular biology of cancer. Mechanisms, targets, and therapeutics, 4th edn. Oxford University Press, Oxford

Pelengaris S, Khan M (eds) (2013) The molecular biology of cancer. A bridge from bench to bedside, 2nd edn. Wiley-Blackwell, Hoboken, NJ

Perry MC, Doll DC, Freter CE (eds) (2012) Perry's the chemotherapy source book, 5th edn. Wolter Kluwer Lippincott Williams & Wilkins, Philadelphia

Prayson R, Kleinschmidt-DeMasters BK, Cohen ML (2010) Brain tumors. DemosMedical, New York

Sandberg AA, Stone JF (2008) The genetics and molecular biology of neural tumors. Humana Press, New York

Schulz WA (2007) Molecular biology of human cancers. Springer, Berlin

Stein GS, Pardee AB (eds) (2004) Cell cycle and growth control. Biomolecular regulation and cancer, 2nd edn. Wiley-Liss, Wilmington, DE

Wagener C, Stocking C, Müller O (2017) Cancer signaling. From molecular biology to targeted therapy. Wiley-VCH, Hoboken, NJ

Weinberg RA (2014) The biology of cancer, 2nd edn. Garland Science, New York

Neurodegeneration

Beal MF, Land AE, Ludolph A (eds) (2005) Neurodegenerative diseases. Neurobiology, pathogenesis, therapeutics. Cambridge University Press, Cambridge, MA

Budson AE, Kowall NW (eds) (2011) The handbook of Alzheimer's disease and other dementias. Wiley-Blackwell, Hoboken, NJ

Calne DB (ed) (1994) Neurodegenerative diseases. Saunders, Philadelphia

Dawbarn D, Allen SJ (eds) (2007) Neurobiology of Alzheimer's disease, 3rd edn. Oxford University Press, Oxford

Dening T, Thomas A (eds) (2013) Oxford textbook old age psychiatry, 2nd edn. Oxford University Press, Oxford

Dickerson BC (ed) (2016) Hodges' frontotemporal dementia, 2nd edn. Cambridge University Press, Cambridge, MA

Dickson DW, Weller RO (eds) (2011) Neurodegenration. The molecular pathology of dementia and movement disorders, 2nd edn. Wiley-Blackwell, Hoboken, NJ

Donaldson I, Marsden CD, Schneider SA, Bhatia KP (2012) Marsden's Book of Movement Disorders. Oxford University Press, Oxford

Duckett S (1991) The pathology of the aging human nervous system. Lea & Febiger, Philadelphia

Duyckaerts C, Levitan I (eds) (2008) Dementias. handbook of clinical neurology, vol 89. Elsevier, Amsterdam

Hardiman O, Doherty CP (eds) (2011) Neurodegenerative disorders. Springer, Berlin

Hodges JR (ed) (2007) Frontotemporal dementia syndromes. Cambridge University Press, Cambridge, MA

Kovacs GG (ed) (2015) Neuropathology of neurodegenerative diseases. A pratical guide. Cambridge University Press, Cambridge, MA

Mann DMA, Neary D, Testa H (1994) Color atlas and text of adult dementias. Mosby-Wolfe, London

Markesbery WR (ed) (1998) Neuropathology of dementing disorders. Arnold, London

O'Brien J, McKeith I, Ames D, Chiu E (eds) (2006) Dementia with Lewy bodies and Parkinson's disease dementia. Taylor & Francis, Abingdon

Olanow CW, Stocchi F, Lang AE (eds) (2011) Parkinson's disease. Non-motor and non-dopaminergic features. Wiley-Blackwell, Hoboken, NJ
Riddle DR (ed) (2007) Brain aging. Models, methods, and mechanisms. CRC, Boca Raton, FL
Saba L (ed) (2015) Imaging in neurodegenerative disorders. Oxford University Press, Oxford
Schapira A, Wszolek Z, Dawson TM, Wood N (eds) (2017) Neurodegeneration. Wiley-Blackwell, Hoboken, NJ
Selkoe DJ, Mandelkow E, Holtzman DM (eds) (2012) The biology of Alzheimer disease. Cold Spring Harbor Laboratory Press, New York
Strong MJ (ed) (2012) Amyotrophic lateral sclerosis and the frontotemporal dementias. Oxford University Press, Oxford
Watts RL, Standaert D, Obeso JA (eds) (2012) Movement disorders, 3rd edn. McGraw Hill, New York

Epilepsy

Blümcke I, Sarnat HB, Coras R (2015) Surgical neuropathology of focal epilepsies: textbook and atlas. John Libbey Eurotext, Montrouge
Chugani HT (2010) Neuroimaging in epilepsy. Oxford University Press, Oxford
Engel J (2012) Seizures and epilepsy, 2nd edn. Oxford University Press, Oxford
Engel J, Pedley TA, Aicardi J, Dichter MA, Moshe S (eds) (2007) Epilepsy: a comprehensive textbook. Lippincott Williams & Wilkinson, Philadelphia
Hubbard JA, Binder DK (2016) Astrocytes and epilepsy. Academic, New York
Kuzniecky R, Jackson GD (eds) (2005) Magnetic resonance in epilepsy. Academic, New York
Lahl R, Villagran R, Teixeira W (2003) Neuropathology of focal epilepsies: an atlas. John Libbey, Montrouge
Luders Hans O (ed) (2008) Textbook of epilepsy surgery. Informa Healthcare, London
Noebels J, Avoli M, Rogawski M (eds) (2012) Jasper's basic mechanisms of the epilepsies, 4th edn. Oxford University Press, Oxford
Olivier A (2012) Techniques in epilepsy surgery. Cambridge University Press, Cambridge, MA
Panayiotopoulos CP (2007) A clinical guide to epileptic syndromes and their treatment, 2nd edn. Springer, Berlin
Schwartzkroin PA (ed) (2007) Epilepsy: models, mechanisms and concepts. Cambridge University Press, Cambridge, MA
Shorvon SD (2010) Handbook of epilepsy treatment, 3rd edn. Wiley, New York
Shorvon SD, Andermann F, Guerrini R (eds) (2011) The causes of epilepsy: common and uncommon causes in adults and children. Cambridge University Press, Cambridge, MA
Shorvon SD, Guerrini RE, Cook M, Lhatoo SD (eds) (2012) Oxford textbook of epilepsy and epileptic seizures. Oxford University Press, Oxford
Stefan H (2012a) Epilepsy: basic principles and diagnosis part I (handbook of clinical neurology). Elsevier Science, Amsterdam
Stefan H (2012b) Epilepsy: treatment part II (handbook of clinical neurology): handbook of clinical neurology, vol 108. Elsevier Science, Amsterdam
Urbach H (2013) MRI in epilepsy. Springer Verlag, Berlin
Werz MA (2011) Epilepsy syndromes. Elsevier Saunders, Philadelphia
Wyllie E, Cascino G, Gidal B (eds) (2010) Wyllie's treatment of epilepsy: principles and practice, 5th edn. Lippencott Williams & Wilkins, Philadelphia

Neuroradiology

Bottomley PA, Griffiths JR (eds) (2016) Handbook of magnetic resonance spectroscopy in vivo: MRS theory, practice and applications. Wiley, New York
Brown RW, Cheng YCN, Haacke EM (2014) Magnetic resonance imaging: physical principles and sequence design, 2nd edn. Wiley-Blackwell, Hoboken, NJ
Bushong SC (2014) Magnetic resonance Imaging: physical and biological principles, 4th edn. Mosby, London
Buxton RB (2009) Introduction to functional magnetic resonance imaging: principles and techniques, 2nd edn. Cambridge University Press, Cambridge, MA
Constantinides C (2014) Magnetic resonance imaging. Routledge, New York
Huettel SA, Song AW, McCarthy G (2014) Functional magnetic resonance imaging, 3rd edn. Sinauer, Sunderland, MA
Jackson A (ed) (2015) Magnetic resonance spectroscopy. MI Books International
Johansen-Berg H, TEJ B (eds) (2013) Diffusion MRI. From quantitative measurement to in vivo neuroanatomy, 2nd edn. Elseveier-Academic, New York
Leite C, Castillo M (eds) (2015) Diffusion weighted and diffusion tensor imaging: a clinical guide. Thieme, Stuttgart
Mettler FA (2013) Essentials of radiology. Elsevier, Amsterdam
Mori S, Tournier JD (2013) Introduction to diffusion tensor imaging, 2nd edn. Elsevier, Amsterdam
Newton HB, Jolesz FA (eds) (2008) Handbook of neuro-oncology neuroimaging. Elsevier-Academic, New York
Rinck PA (ed) (2018) Magnetic resonance in medicine: a critical introduction. Books on Demand, New York
Osborn AG, Blaser SI, Salzman KL, Katzman GL, Provenzale J, Castillo M, Hedlund GL, Illner A, Harnsberger HR, Cooper JA, Kones BV, Hamilton BE (2007) Diagnostic imaging: brain. Amirsys, Salt Lake City, UT
Stagg C (2014) Magnetic resonance spectroscopy: tools for neuroscience research and emerging clinical applications. Elsevier, Amsterdam
Stieltjes B, Brunner RM, Fritzsche K, Laun P (2012) Diffusion tensor imaging: introduction and atlas. Springer, Berlin

van Hecke W, Emsell L, Sunaert S (eds) (2016) Diffusion tensor imaging: a practical handbook. In: Springer, Berlin

Wang Y (2012) Principles of magnetic resonance imaging: physics concepts, pulse sequences, & biomedical applications. CreateSpace Independent Publishing Platform, Scotts Valley, CA

Weishaupt D, Kochli VD, Marincek B (2008) How does MRI work? An introduction to the physics and function of magnetic resonance imaging, 2nd edn. Springer, Berlin

Pathology

The following books series are to be recommended:

- Diagnostic Pathology, Elsevier
- Differential Diagnoses in Surgical Pathology, Lippincott Williams & Wilkinson
- A Volume in the Pattern Recognition Series, Elsevier
- Foundations in Diagnostic Pathology, Elsevier
- Armed Forces Institute of Pathology (AFIP) Atlas of Tumor Pathology, American Registry of Pathology
- Armed Forces Institute of Pathology (AFIP) Atlas of Nontumor Pathology, American Registry of Pathology

Burt AD, Ferrell LD, Hubscher SG (eds) (2017) MacSween's pathology of the liver, 7th edn. Elsevier, Amsterdam

Cagle PT (ed) (2018) Pulmonary pathology: an atlas and text, 3rd edn. Lippincott Williams & Wilkinson, Philadelphia

Czerniak B (2015) Dorfman and Czerniak's bone tumors, 2nd edn. Elsevier, Amsterdam

Dabbs DJ (ed) (2016) Breast pathology, 2nd edn. Elsevier, Amsterdam

Fletcher CDM (ed) (2013) Diagnostic histopathology of tumors, 4th edn. Churchill Livingstone, Philadelphia

Goldblum JR, Lamps LW, McKenney JK, Myers JL (2017) Rosai and Ackerman's surgical pathology, 11th edn. Elsevier, Amsterdam

Kumar V, Abbas AK, Aster JC (eds) (2014) Robbins and Cotran pathologic basis of disease, 9th edn. Saunders, Philadelphia

Kurman RJ, Lora HE, Ronnett BM (eds) (2011) Blaustein's pathology of the female genital tract, 6th edn. Springer, Berlin

Lager DJ, Abrahams N (eds) (2013) Practical renal pathology, a diagnostic approach. Elsevier, Amsterdam

Mills SE, Greenson JK, Hornick JL, Longacre TA, Reuter VE (eds) (2015) Sternberg's diagnostic surgical pathology, 6th revised edn. Lippincott Williams & Wilkins, Philadelphia

Noffsinger AE (ed) (2017) Fenoglio-Preiser's gastrointestinal pathology, 4th edn. Lippincott Williams & Wilkins, Philadelphia

Patterson JW (2015) Weedon's skin pathology, 4th edn. Elsevier, Amsterdam

Suster S, Zynger D, Parwani A (eds) (2014) Prostate pathology. Demos Health, New York

Zhou M, Magi-Galluzzi C (eds) (2015) Genitourinary pathology, 2nd edn. Saunders, Philadelphia

Neuroimmunology

Darnell RB, Posner JB (2011) Paraneoplastic syndromes. Oxford University Press, Oxford

Pollard KM (2006) Autoantibodies and autoimmunity. Wiley-VCH, New York, p 608

Rose NR, Mackay IR (2014) The autoimmune diseases, 5th edn. Elsevier, Amsterdam

Shoenfeld Y, Meroni PL, Gershwin ME (2014) Autoantibodies, 3rd edn. Elsevier, Amsterdam

Woodroofe N, Amor S (2014) Neuroinflammation and CNS disorders. Wiley Blackwell, Hoboken, NJ

Neurovascular

Caplan LR, van Gjin J (eds) (2012) Stroke syndromes, 3rd edn. Cambridge University Press, Cambridge, MA

Caplan LE (ed) (2016) Caplan's stroke: a clinical approach, 5th edn. Cambridge University Press, Cambridge, MA

Caplan LR, Biller J, Leary MC, Lo EH, Thomas AJ, Yenari M, Zhang JH (eds) (2017b) Cerebrovascular diseases, 2nd edn. Academic, New York

Caplan L, Biller J (eds) (2018) Uncommon causes of stroke, 3rd edn. Cambridge University Press, Cambridge, MA

Chen J, Zhang JH, Hu X (eds) (2018) Non-neuronal mechanisms of brain damage and repair after stroke. Springer, Berlin

Grotta JC, Albers GW, Broderick JP, Kasner SE, Lo EH, Mendelow AD, Sacco RL, LKS W (eds) (2016) Stroke. Pathophysiology, diagnosis and management, 6th edn. Elsevier, Amsterdam

Harrigan MR, Deveiklis JP (eds) (2018) Handbook of cerebrovascular disease and neurointerventional technique, 3rd edn. Humana Press, New York

Laakso A, Hernesniemi J, Yonekawa Y, Tsukahara T (eds) (2012) Surgical management of cerebrovascular disease. Springer, Berlin

Lau GKK, Pendlebury ST, Rothwill PM (2018) Transient ischemic attack and stroke, 2nd edn. Cambridge University Press, Cambridge, MA

Lawton MT, Su H (eds) (2018) Molecular, genetic, and cellular advances in cerebrovascular diseases. World Scientific, Singapore

Norrving B (ed) (2014) Oxford textbook of stroke and cerebrovascular disease. Oxford University Press, Oxford

Rangel-Castilla L, Nakaji P, Siddiqui AH, Spetzler RF, Levy EI (eds) (2018) Decision making in neurovascular disease. Thieme, Stuttgart

Runge VM (2016) Imaging of cerebrovascular disease: a practical guide, 3rd edn. Thieme, Stuttgart

Saba L, Raz E (eds) (2016) Neurovascular imaging: from basics to advanced concepts. Springer, Berlin

Seshadri S, Debette S (eds) (2016) Risk factors for cerebrovascular disease. Oxford University Press, Oxford

Index

A

Abdominal dyskinesia, 416
Abducens nucleus, 158
ABL, 1289, 1290, 1331
Abnormal head posture, 420
Abscesses, 428, 656, 658, 665, 666, 673, 680, 690, 752, 775–777, 783
Absence seizures, 1121
Abulia, 207, 208, 405, 475
Acalculia, 406, 407
Acceleration-deceleration injury, 1185, 1188
Accumbens nucleus, 76
Acentric fragment lagging, 1271
Acetazolamide, 9, 52, 632
Acetazolamide challenge, 9
Acetylation, 648, 925, 1017, 1309
Acetylcholine, 111, 236, 300, 370, 372–376, 632, 699, 815, 836, 863, 895, 926, 934, 935, 941, 942, 1134, 1135, 1243, 1256, 2171, 2176
AchR, 2171, 2173
Achromatopia, 209
Acquired toxoplasmosis, 749, 751, 755
Acromegaly, 418, 1671, 1781, 1785, 1793, 1794, 1806
ACTH, *see* Adrenocorticotropic hormone
Actin
  binding proteins, 1405
  filaments, 228, 1135
Actinomyces, 655, 657
Action tremor, 209, 417
Activated microglia, 99, 225, 247, 665, 690, 718, 732, 752, 879, 881, 1215
Activation pathways, 247
Active plaque, 1082, 1088
Acute
  bacterial meningitis, 653
  confusional stage, 2154
Acute disseminated encephalomyelitis (ADEM), 641, 1072, 1105–1115, 2154, 2174
Acute hemorrhagic leukoencephalopathy (AHL), 1072, 1105, 1106, 1113, 1115, 1914
"Adam," "XTC" 4-MTA (4-methylthioamphetamine, "Flatliners"), 1259
Adaptive immune response, 690, 1934, 2152
ADC maps, 477, 802, 1370, 1375
ADEM, *see* Acute disseminated encephalomyelitis

Adenocarcinoma, 83, 85, 103, 1289, 1290, 1510, 1748, 1875, 1882, 1885, 2022, 2050, 2055, 2058–2060, 2063, 2069, 2085, 2088, 2095, 2097, 2099, 2102, 2105, 2107, 2111, 2114, 2115, 2171
Adenocarcinoma of the colon, 2085, 2097
Adenoid GBM, 1386
Adenosine triphosphatase (ATP), 44, 110, 372, 441, 455, 471, 720, 883, 895, 923–925, 1093, 1254, 1288, 1294, 1295, 1313, 1405, 1654, 1792
Adenosquamous carcinoma, 2063, 2070, 2106, 2107
Adipocytes, 1312, 1979, 1983, 1984
Adjuvant therapy, 1265, 1269
ADP, 293, 441, 884, 1017, 1178, 1285, 1286, 1293, 1296, 1301
Adrenaline, 370, 376, 384–385
Adrenergic receptor family, 385
Adrenocorticotropic hormone (ACTH), 108, 371, 1754, 1780, 1781, 1787, 1789, 1791, 1794, 1800, 1802, 1803, 1810, 1812
Adrenoleukodystrophy, 827, 864, 865, 1035, 1072, 1089
Adult polyglucosan body disease (APBD), 825, 828, 838, 861
Advanced Fast Marching (aFM), 20
Adventitia, 254–256, 258, 260, 585, 607, 613, 641, 644
AE1/AE3, 103, 104, 108, 255, 322, 1499, 1527, 1557, 1738, 1764, 1829, 1837, 1838, 1844, 1851, 1855, 1867, 1874, 1878, 2025, 2058, 2060, 2067, 2073, 2075, 2083, 2086, 2089, 2093, 2095, 2101, 2102, 2105, 2108, 2112
Affective aspects of motor behavior, 404
Afferent pathway, 121, 325, 342
AFP, 1866, 1867, 1873, 1875, 2061, 2096, 2104, 2107, 2112
Age-related wisdom, 870
Aging, 228, 244, 326, 367, 836, 846, 849, 856, 869–890, 895, 896, 915–917, 924, 925, 999, 1007, 1011, 1092, 1132, 1304
Agitated delirium, 208, 409, 476
Agitation, 79, 417, 419, 859, 895, 896, 1060, 1258, 2154, 2155, 2158, 2160
Agnosia visual, 401, 407, 409, 413
Agranular cortex:, 267, 290
Agraphia, 208, 209, 401, 404, 407, 408, 413–415, 476, 946

© Springer-Verlag GmbH Austria, part of Springer Nature 2019
S. Weis et al., *Imaging Brain Diseases*, https://doi.org/10.1007/978-3-7091-1544-2

AHL, *see* Acute hemorrhagic leukoencephalopathy
AICA syndrome (lateral pontine syndrome), 191, 208
AIDS dementia complex (ADC), 19, 430, 432, 447, 461,
    477, 659, 661, 664, 701, 714, 725, 726, 733,
    734, 737, 738, 753, 766, 778, 783, 799, 801,
    802, 975, 980, 1004, 1022, 1024, 1074, 1076,
    1078, 1106, 1107, 1109, 1126, 1144, 1234,
    1235, 1238, 1246, 1354, 1370, 1375, 1426,
    1429, 1493, 1511, 1576, 1615, 1697, 1709,
    1755, 1825, 1827, 1834, 1895, 2039, 2040,
    2132
AIDS-related PML, 722
AIF1-allograft inflammatory factor 1, 249
Akathisia, 416, 1245, 1255
Akinesia, 405, 417, 946, 947, 974
Akinesia (bilateral akinetic mutism), 405
Akinetic mutism, 208, 405, 797, 816, 818, 857, 945, 968
Akinetopsia, 361, 422
Alcian blue, 57, 84, 85, 1508, 1510, 1514, 1679, 1776,
    1853, 2025, 2064, 2095, 2098, 2101
Alcohol abuse, 517, 1223–1225, 1228
Alcoholism, 76, 388, 533, 1224–1228, 1237
Aldh1, 97
Alexander disease, 243, 864, 1072
Alexia
    with agraphia, 408
    without agraphia, 208, 401, 407, 413, 415, 476
Algorithm of filtered back-projection, 7
Alien hand sign, 405
Alien limb phenomenon, 980
Allesthesia, 406, 408
Allocortex (Hippocampal formation and olfactory
    system), 269, 295, 299, 837, 1012
α-amino-3-hydroxy-5-methyl-4-isoxazole propionic acid
    (AMPA) receptor, 392, 886, 1138, 1157, 1168,
    1216, 2173
α-1 antichymotrypsin, 615, 1438
α-1 antitrypsin, 517, 1438, 1775
Alpha fetoprotein, 108, 1873, 2061
Alpha radiation, 31
Alpha synuclein, 100, 101, 844, 1028
Altered level of consciousness, 1267
Altitudinal field defect, 207, 475
Alzheimer dementia, 448, 826, 933
Alzheimer II, 1228
Alzheimer's disease, 87, 100, 101, 244, 248, 249, 420,
    615, 818, 826, 827, 835–839, 842, 845, 846,
    849, 851, 852, 859, 865, 879, 881, 882, 884,
    885, 895–926, 933–935, 937, 960, 987, 988,
    996, 999, 1017, 1212, 1213, 1297
Amebiasis, 750
Aminergic fibers from locus coeruleus, 351
Aminergic fibers from the raphe nuclei, 350
Amino acid PET, 29, 32, 39, 44, 48–49, 1542, 1554,
    1563, 1576, 1615, 1961
Amino acids, 32, 39, 44, 48–49, 95, 100, 370, 376, 381,
    384, 385, 388–395, 520, 605, 612, 641, 663,
    666, 839, 848, 849, 873, 940, 954, 959, 1067,
    1090, 1101, 1214, 1219, 1295, 1304, 1305,
    1307, 1320, 1337, 1340, 1348, 1354, 1412,
    1419, 1435, 1444, 1450, 1451, 1458, 1462,
    1466, 1470, 1477, 1490, 1522, 1529, 1530,
    1542, 1554, 1563, 1573, 1576, 1615, 1652,
    1899, 1961, 2042, 2120
Ammonia, 1233
Amnesia (impaired storage), 409, 417, 418, 422, 626,
    859, 946, 947, 1187, 1216, 2155, 2158, 2173
Amoebic meningoencephalitis, 750
AMP, 369, 441
AMPA (α-amino-3-hydroxy-5-methyl-4-
    isoxazolepropionic acid), 392, 395, 886, 1138,
    1139, 1157, 1168, 1216, 2158, 2171, 2173
AMPAR, 2151, 2153, 2158, 2162, 2170, 2171, 2175
AMPAR (GluR1, GluR2) antibody syndrome, 2158
AMPA-receptor (GluA1 or GluA2), 2173
Amphetamine, 50, 371, 503, 1085, 1244, 1245,
    1258–1259
Amphiphysin, 236, 2153, 2154, 2159, 2170, 2171, 2173,
    2175
Amusia sensory, 410
Amygdala, 76, 138, 142, 144, 167, 204, 205, 244, 267,
    300–301, 305, 326, 343, 350–352, 357, 375,
    380, 381, 387, 401, 409, 410, 414, 422, 607,
    838, 856, 859, 861, 914, 919, 920, 941, 954,
    960, 962, 964–966, 982, 1040, 1064, 1134,
    1138, 1143, 1154, 1213, 1214, 1245, 1254,
    1342, 1934, 1936, 2155
Amygdalar System, 326, 350
Amyloid beta (A4) precursor protein APP, 844
Amyloid cascade hypothesis, 825, 845–847
Amyloid deposits, 605, 606, 629, 641, 825, 830,
    834–836, 839–841, 846, 855, 856, 873, 895,
    901, 908, 917, 918, 920, 921, 937, 996, 1064,
    1215
Amyloid imaging, 29, 53–54, 947
Amyloid-plaques, 629, 802, 812, 818–820, 830, 840,
    844–847, 852, 855, 856, 865, 901, 907, 908,
    917, 965, 967
Amyotrophic lateral sclerosis (ALS), 101, 245, 818, 835,
    838, 845, 849, 850, 957, 968, 1037–1039,
    1053, 1297
Anaphase, 1271, 1282, 1284
Anaphase-promoting, 1284
Anaphase-telophase poles, 1271
Anaplasia, 1265, 1268, 1270, 1353, 1354, 1391, 1398,
    1444, 1447, 1459, 1469, 1476, 1500, 1534,
    1565, 1572
Aneurysm
    age incidence, 551
    biologic behavior-prognosis-prognostic factors, 576
    CTA, 552
    CT-contrast-enhanced, 552
    CT-non contrast-enhanced, 552
    differential diagnosis, 558
    dissecting aneurysms (arterial dissections), 551, 552
    dolichoectasia, 551, 552
    DSA, 552
    false aneurysm "pseudoaneurysm," 551
    fusiform aneurysms, 551, 552
    general imaging findings, 552–576

Index

immunophenotype, 552
incidence, 551
inflammatory/infective "mycotic" (septic) aneurysms, 551, 552
localization, 552
macroscopic features, 552
microscopic features, 552
molecular neuropathology, 558–576
MRA, 552, 553
MRI-FLAIR, 552
MRI-T1, 552
MRI-T2, 552
MRI-T1 contrast-enhanced, 2029
MRI-T2∗/SWI, 552
mycotic aneurysm, 552, 565
nuclear medicine imaging findings, 552
pathogenesis, 558–575
saccular (berry) aneurysms, 551, 552
sex incidence, 551–552
treatment, 551, 570–576
ultrastructural features, 558
Aneurysmal bone cyst
CT-non contrast-enhanced, 2029
differential diagnosis, 2029
general imaging findings, 2029
localization, 2029
macroscopic features, 2029
microscopic features, 2029
MRI-T1, 2029
MRI-T2, 2029
MRI-T1 contrast-enhanced, 2029
WHO definition, 2029
Angiocentric infiltration, 1901
Angiogenesis, 257, 1056, 1265, 1266, 1272, 1280, 1291, 1303, 1306, 1307, 1309–1314, 1331, 1491, 1702, 1997, 1998, 2139
Angiogram, 4, 9, 191, 194–199
Angiography, 3, 4, 7–9, 11, 14, 16–17, 477, 478, 501, 578, 585, 601, 640, 1255, 1714, 1716, 1970
Angiolipoma, 1956, 1984
Angiosarcoma, 1656, 1690, 1982, 1991, 1992
Anhidrosis, 418
Animalia (Metazoa), 749
ANNA-1 (Hu), 2153, 2170–2172
ANNA-3, 2172
Annihilation radiation, 29, 30, 42, 43
Anosognosia, 405–407, 413
Anoxia, 456, 849, 1313
Ansa lenticularis, 150, 334, 416
Anterior approach, 65
Anterior cerebral artery, 63, 155, 192, 193, 196, 198, 200, 202, 203, 205, 573
Anterior cerebral artery syndrome, 202–208
Anterior commissure, 77, 127, 150, 151, 167, 205, 300, 307, 347, 348, 358, 420, 875, 1237
Anterior cranial fossa, 136, 193
Anterior external arcuate fibers, 160
Anterior limb of the internal capsule, 127, 147, 203
Anterior perforated substance, 155, 205
Anterior pituitary gland, 355

Anterior roots, 1042
Anterior thalamic nucleus, 347, 348, 352
Anterior-to-middle fossa herniation, 427, 436
Anterograde amnesia, 417
Anterograde memory deficit, 2155
Antiangiogenic therapy, 1266
Antibodies, 89–91, 95, 105, 108, 111–113, 235, 244, 257, 270, 388, 636–639, 641, 687, 698, 699, 725, 776, 812, 999, 1092, 1097–1098, 1101, 1103, 1210, 1269, 1302, 1311, 1312, 1329, 1341, 1362, 1391, 1396, 1453, 1462, 1475, 1479, 1499, 1646, 1652, 1685, 1689, 1767, 1771, 1776, 1787, 1812, 1850, 1866, 1875, 1879, 1904, 1905, 1916, 1924, 1928, 1938, 1948, 1964, 1969, 2057, 2061, 2070, 2076, 2082–2084, 2088, 2092, 2095, 2096, 2102, 2104, 2106, 2107, 2112–2115, 2151–2162, 2165, 2167, 2170–2176
Anti-CARP VIII, 2171
Anticoagulation therapy, 473, 496
Anti-CV-2/CRMP5 (collapsin response mediator protein 5), 2172
Anti-GAD65, 2172
Anti-HU, 1579, 2154, 2171, 2172
Anti-Ma1, 2171, 2172
Anti-Ma2, 2172
Anti-MAG, 2172
Anti-myelin, 2173
Anti-NB (beta-NAP), 2171
Antiparallel state, 10
Anti-PCA-1 (Anti-Yo), 2172
Anti-PCA-2 (Purkinje cell autoantibodies), 2171, 2172
Antiplatelet therapy, 473, 496, 987, 995
Anti-proteasome, 2171
Anti-recoverin, 2173
Anti-Ri, 2171, 2172
Anti-TRPM-1, 2173
Anti-ubiquitin conjugating enzyme (UBE2E1), 2171
Antoni A pattern, 1661, 1669
Antoni B pattern, 1661, 1669
Anton's syndrome, 208, 401, 407, 413, 421, 476
Anton syndrome, 208, 401, 407, 413, 421, 476
Apallic syndrome, 458, 466, 468, 470, 857
Apathy, 405, 417–419, 626, 843, 858, 859, 897, 932, 966, 988, 1002, 1060, 1212, 2128
APBD, see Adult Polyglucosan Body Disease
Aperceptive agnosia, 421
Aphasia
anomic, 413
broca, 133, 401, 405, 413, 414, 420
conduction, 401, 406, 414, 420
global, 207, 401, 413, 420, 475, 626, 843
sensory, 401, 407, 409, 414, 859
transcortical motor, 207, 401, 405, 413, 414, 420, 475
transcortical sensory, 401, 407, 409, 413, 414, 420, 859
wernicke, 134, 401, 406, 409, 414, 420
Apical cilia, 249, 1530, 1843, 1844
Apnea, 456, 2174

Apoptosis, 97, 245, 484, 517, 569, 718, 814, 843, 849, 850, 879, 880, 887, 923, 925, 1086, 1089, 1214, 1217, 1219, 1235, 1258, 1266, 1281, 1285, 1288, 1291, 1293–1303, 1310, 1313, 1317, 1367, 1398, 1400, 1403, 1489–1491, 1622, 1646, 1701, 1749, 1789, 1790, 1795, 1913, 1995, 1997, 2175
Apraxia ideational, 401, 413
Aprosodia sensory, 410
Aquaporin-1, 1979
Aquaporin 4, 243, 249, 259, 294, 1097, 1101, 1103, 1215, 2171, 2173
Aquaporin(s), 243, 249, 259, 294, 427, 441, 1097, 1101, 1103, 1215, 1979, 2171, 2173
Aqueductal flow void sign, 444, 445, 447
Aqueductal stenosis, 443–445, 449, 451, 1694
Arachidonic acid, 441, 718
Arachnoidal cyst
    age incidence, 1856
    biologic behavior-prognosis-prognostic factors, 1860
    CT-contrast-enhanced, 1856
    CT-non contrast-enhanced, 1856
    differential diagnosis, 1859–1860
    general imaging findings, 1856
    immunophenotype, 1859
    incidence, 1856
    localization, 1856
    macroscopic features, 1858
    microscopic features, 1858–1859
    MRI-diffusion imaging, 1857
    MRI-FLAIR, 1856
    MRI-perfusion, 1857
    MRI-T1, 1856
    MRI-T2, 1856
    MRI-T1 contrast-enhanced, 1857
    MRI-T2∗/SWI, 1857
    pathogenesis, 1860
    proliferation markers, 1859
    sex incidence, 1856
    treatment, 1860
    ultrastructural features, 1859
Arachnoidal granulations, 188–189
Arachnoidal villi, 176, 188, 451
Arachnoid membrane, 213, 252, 1823, 1860
Architectonics
    angioarchitectonics, 278, 282
    anterior and posterior temporal arteries, 202
    anterior cerebral artery (ACA)
        A1 segment, 196
        A2 segment, 196, 202
        A3 segment (callosal segment), 196
    anterior choroidal artery, 193, 196, 203, 205
    anterior circulation, 191, 474
    anterior communicating artery, 196, 200, 203, 205, 510, 552, 559, 561, 570, 573
    anterior inferior cerebellar artery (AICA), 192, 198, 202, 204, 208, 881
    anterior meningeal branches, 181
    anterior spinal arteries, 199
    anterior temporal artery, 196
    arteries, 191–209
    artery of the foramen rotundum, 193
    artery of the pterygoid canal (vidian artery), 193
    ascending pharyngeal artery, 191, 203
    basilar artery, 202
    basilar perforating arteries, 202
    basilary artery, 538
    calcarine artery, 192, 202
    capsular branches, 193
    caroticotympanic artery, 193
    carotid system, 191–199, 215
    chemoarchitectonics, 269, 278
    common carotid artery, 191, 254
    cytoarchitectonics, 269, 270, 273–278, 281, 332
    dendrite architectonics, 269, 278
    external carotid artery, 191, 203, 1716, 1959
    facial artery, 191, 203
    frontobasal arteries, 197, 204
    frontopolar artery, 192, 196
    glia architectonics, 269, 278
    inferolateral trunk, 193, 207, 475
    insular arteries, 197, 204
    internal carotid artery (ICA)
        C1: cervical segment (extracranial portion), 193
        C2: petrous segment, 193, 198, 203
        C3: lacerum segment, 193, 198, 203
        C4: cavernous segment, 193, 198, 203
        C5: clinoid segmen, 193, 198, 203
        C6: ophthalmic segment, 193, 198, 203
        C7: communicating (terminal) segment, 193, 198, 203
    labyrinthine artery, 202, 204
    lateral lenticulostriate arteries, 196
    lateral occipital artery, 202, 204
    lateral posterior coroidal artery, 202
    lingual artery, 191, 203
    maxillary artery, 181, 191, 203
    medial lenticulostriate arteries, 196
    medial posterior choroidal artery, 202
    medullary perforating branches, 199
    meningohypophyseal trunk, 193
    middle cerebral artery (a terminal branch), 196
    middle cerebral artery (MCA)
        M1 segment (sphenoidal/horizontal segment), 196
        M2 segment (insular segment), 197
        M3 segment (opercular segment), 197
        M4 segment (terminal segment), 197
    middle meningeal artery, 191, 192, 203, 522, 530, 533, 1959
    myeloarchitectonics, 269, 273, 274, 278, 279, 281
    occipital artery, 181, 191, 192, 202–204
    ophthalmic artery, 181, 193
    parietooccipital artery, 135
    peduncular perforating arteries, 202
    pigmentarchitectonics, 269, 278, 279, 281
    posterior cerebral artery (PCA)
        P1 precommunicating segment, 198, 202
        P2 ambient segment, 198, 202
        P3 quadrigeminal, 202
        P4 calcarine segment, 202

posterior circulation, 191, 474, 552
posterior communicating artery, 192, 193, 205, 561
posterior inferior cerebellar artery (PICA), 192,
    198–200, 204, 208–209, 559, 561
posterior meningeal artery, 199
posterior spinal arteries, 199
posterior splenial arteries, 202
posterior thalamoperforating arteries, 202
receptor architectonics, 269, 278, 283
recurrent artery of heubner (medial striate
    artery), 196
superficial temporal artery, 191, 203
superior cerebellar artery (SCA), 192, 198, 202, 204,
    207, 476
superior hypophyseal artery, 193, 358
superior thyroid artery, 191, 203
temporal arteries, 197, 202, 204, 641
terminates as two branches, 191
thalamogeniculate arteries, 202
thalamostriate arteries, 196, 203
vertebral artery
    extracranial portion, 199, 204
    intracranial segment, 199
    V0, 199, 204
    V1, 199, 204, 291, 328, 332, 333, 358, 360, 361,
        408, 915, 1317
    V2, 199, 204, 294, 328, 333, 915
    V3, 199, 204, 294, 328, 333, 915
    V4 intradural segment, 199
vertebro-basilar system, 191, 192, 199–202, 215, 552
in vivo architectonics, 282, 288
Arcuate fascicle, 148
Area postrema, 158, 267, 312, 1098
Argyrophilic grain-disease, 825, 837, 848, 849, 859–861,
    953, 956, 957, 962, 963, 965
Arterial dissection, 499, 514, 551, 552, 997
Arterial feeders, 578
Arterial oxygen concentration, 456
Arterial spin-labeling methods, 19, 22
Arterial supply, 191–209
Arteriole, 225, 254–257, 259, 312, 537, 605–607, 613,
    616, 629, 630, 638, 639, 990, 996
Arteriolosclerosis, 489, 537, 614, 629, 879, 996, 997
Arteriosclerosis
    age incidence, 538
    biologic behavior-prognosis-prognostic factors, 542
    CTA/MRA/DSA, 538
    CT-contrast-enhanced, 552
    CT-non contrast-enhanced, 552
    differential diagnosis, 540
    general imaging findings, 538
    immunophenotype, 540
    incidence, 537
    localization, 538
    macroscopic features, 538
    microscopic features, 538–540
    molecular neuropathology, 570, 573
    nuclear medicine imaging findings, 538
    pathogenesis, 542
    prognosis, 542
    prognostic factors, 542
    sex incidence, 538
    treatment, 542
    ultrastructural features, 540
Arteriovenous malformations, 499, 503, 514, 522,
    577–585, 1131, 1132, 1255
Arteritis, 496, 540, 635, 636, 638–641, 648, 694, 751,
    763, 774, 827, 987, 990, 1253
Artery, (AU: Whole book deals on this topic please
    check.)
Ascending ramus, 132
Aspartate, 370, 388, 392, 395, 814, 1233, 1247, 1286,
    1293, 2151, 2152, 2167
Aspergillosis, 775–778
Aspergillus fumigatus, 702, 777–790
Aspergillus spp., 774, 775
Aspiny non-pyramidal cells, 268
Aß-related angiitis, 636
Assessment of regional blood flow, 29
Association fibers, 20, 147, 148, 289, 296, 343, 402
Associationist models, 401, 403
Astrocytes, 85, 86, 97, 225, 235, 239–245, 250, 258, 294,
    301, 302, 369, 370, 372, 458, 484, 492, 493,
    510, 518, 680, 684, 690, 700, 717–719, 728,
    730, 732, 752, 757, 795, 814, 816, 835–837,
    844–846, 860, 861, 865, 878, 880–882, 926,
    960, 976, 979, 981, 984, 990, 992, 1040, 1082,
    1088, 1092, 1101, 1143, 1153, 1162, 1164,
    1205, 1217, 1224, 1228, 1233, 1235, 1237,
    1243, 1250, 1253, 1254, 1275, 1309, 1337,
    1338, 1341, 1343, 1344, 1368, 1387, 1398,
    1433, 1434, 1438, 1470, 1511, 1518, 1541,
    1543, 1548, 1553, 1554, 1557, 1559,
    1561–1563, 1573, 1626, 1766, 1771, 1888,
    1977, 2127, 2165
Astrocytic plaque, 813, 837, 844, 983
Astrocytoma
    age incidence, 1338
    biologic behavior-prognosis-prognostic factors,
        1349–1350
    CT-contrast-enhanced, 1338
    CT-non contrast-enhanced, 1338
    differential diagnosis, 1343
    DNA methylation, 1340, 1354
    epigenetics, 1349
    gene expression, 1349
    general imaging findings, 1338
    genetics, 1348–1349
    immunophenotype, 1341
    incidence, 1338
    localization, 1369
    macroscopic features, 1341
    microRNAs, 1341
    microscopic features, 1341
    molecular neuropathology, 1348–1350
    MRI-diffusion imaging, 1338
    MRI-diffusion tensor imaging, 1338
    MRI-FLAIR, 1338
    MRI-perfusion, 1338
    MRI-T1, 1338

Astrocytoma (cont.)
    MRI-T2, 1338
    MRI-T1 contrast-enhanced, 1338
    MRI-T2∗/SWI, 1338
    MR-spectroscopy, 1338
    nuclear medicine imaging findings, 1340–1341
    pathogenesis, 1343
    proliferation markers, 1341
    sex incidence, 1338
    treatment, 1349
    ultrastructural features, 1343
    WHO definition, 1337–1348
    WHO grade, 1338
Astrocytoma anaplastic
    age incidence, 1354
    biologic behavior-prognosis-prognostic factors, 1365
    CT-contrast-enhanced, 1354
    CT-non contrast-enhanced, 1354
    differential diagnosis, 1364
    DNA methylation, 1360–1361
    epigenetics, 1403
    gene expression, 1365
    general imaging findings, 1354
    genetics, 1364
    immunophenotype, 1362–1364
    incidence, 1354
    localization, 1354
    macroscopic features, 1358–1360
    microRNAs, 1362
    microscopic features, 1360
    molecular neuropathology, 1364–1365
    MRI-diffusion imaging, 1354
    MRI-diffusion tensor imaging, 1354
    MRI-FLAIR, 1354
    MRI-perfusion, 1354
    MRI-T1, 1354
    MRI-T2, 1354
    MRI-T1 contrast-enhanced, 1354
    MRI-T2∗/SWI, 1354
    MR-spectroscopy, 1354
    nuclear medicine imaging findings, 1354–1360
    pathogenesis, 1364
    proliferation markers, 1364
    sex incidence, 1354
    treatment, 1365
    ultrastructural features, 1364
    WHO definition, 1353
    WHO grade, 1353–1365
Astrocytoma pilocytic
    age incidence, 1434
    biologic behavior-prognosis-prognostic factors, 1444
    CT-contrast-enhanced, 1434
    CT-non contrast-enhanced, 1434
    differential diagnosis, 1438
    DNA methylation, 1450
    epigenetics, 1444
    gene expression, 1459
    general imaging findings, 1434
    genetics, 1443
    immunophenotype, 1438
    incidence, 1434
    localization, 1434
    macroscopic features, 1435
    microRNAs, 1444
    microscopic features, 1438
    molecular neuropathology, 1443–1444
    MRI-diffusion imaging, 1434
    MRI-FLAIR, 1434
    MRI-perfusion, 1434
    MRI-T1, 1434
    MRI-T2, 1434
    MRI-T1 contrast-enhanced, 1434
    MRI-T2∗/SWI, 1434
    MR-spectroscopy, 1434–1435
    nuclear medicine imaging findings, 1435
    pathogenesis, 1438
    proliferation markers, 1438
    sex incidence, 1434
    treatment, 1444
    ultrastructural features, 1438
    WHO definition, 1433–1443
    WHO grade, 1434
Astrogliosis, 241, 244, 245, 458, 470, 484, 489, 495, 496, 516, 616, 685, 698, 706, 718, 728, 732, 740, 791, 797, 802, 805, 810, 818, 820, 844, 854–859, 862–864, 878, 958–960, 965–967, 982, 1008, 1028, 1037, 1042, 1059, 1063, 1064, 1066, 1085, 1093, 1111, 1113, 1151, 1152, 1162, 1164, 1166, 1214, 1223, 1227, 1229, 1231, 1233, 1236, 1243, 1253, 1260, 1265, 1271, 1275, 1341, 1343, 1364, 1453, 1464, 1475, 1479, 1569, 1920, 1947, 2126, 2129, 2164, 2168
Asymbolia for pain, 406
Asymptomatic neurocognitive impairment (ANI), 693, 701
α-synuclein, 100, 101, 108, 245, 833, 838, 844, 845, 847–848, 938, 941, 967, 1001, 1003, 1007, 1010, 1012–1014, 1017, 1018, 1028, 1256
Ataxia, 207, 209, 243, 332, 361, 415, 419, 420, 423, 475, 476, 505, 622, 658, 818–820, 826, 828, 838, 845, 848, 851, 857, 858, 861, 862, 864, 1021, 1022, 1034, 1035, 1054, 1055, 1093, 1105, 1212, 1223, 1224, 1229, 1233, 1267, 1285, 1288, 1490, 1824, 1935, 2054, 2055, 2128, 2152, 2158–2160, 2170, 2172, 2174, 2176
Atherosclerosis, 473, 489, 537, 558, 567, 639, 656, 869, 888, 988, 995–997, 999
Atherosclerotic plaque, 538
Athetosis, 416
Atom, 15, 30
Atomic force miscrocopy (AFM), 57, 114
Atomic shell, 30
Atonic seizures, 1122
Atrophy of superior vermis, 1225
Attenuation, 4–6, 33, 34, 40, 42, 44, 48–53, 552, 661, 977
Attenuation correction, 33, 34, 40, 42, 44, 48–53
Atypical AD, 896, 897

Atypical Fronto-temporal lobar degeneration with ubiquitin-positive inclusions, 954, 957, 967
Atypical mitoses, 1265, 1270, 1367, 1386, 1396, 1420, 1979
Atypical parkinsonism, 54, 1001
Atypical teratoid/rhabdoid tumor (ATRT)
   age incidence, 1651
   biologic behavior-prognosis-prognostic factors, 1654
   CT-contrast-enhanced, 1652
   CT-non contrast-enhanced, 1652
   differential diagnosis, 1652–1654
   general imaging findings, 1652
   immunophenotype, 1652
   incidence, 1651
   localization, 1652
   macroscopic features, 1652
   microscopic features, 1652
   molecular neuropathology, 1654
   MRI-diffusion imaging, 1652
   MRI-FLAIR, 1652
   MRI-perfusion, 1652
   MRI-T1, 1652
   MRI-T2, 1652
   MRI-T1 contrast-enhanced, 1652
   MRI-T2∗/SWI, 1652
   MR-spectroscopy, 1652
   nuclear medicine imaging findings, 1652
   pathogenesis, 1654
   proliferation markers, 1652
   sex incidence, 1651
   treatment, 1654
   ultrastructural features, 1652
   WHO definition, 1651–1657
   WHO grade, 1651
Autoimmune diseases, 731, 827, 1097, 1103, 1297, 1301, 2152
Autoimmune encephalitis (AE), 2151–2176
Automated analysis, 32, 2125
Autonomic changes, 1223, 1229, 2152
Autonomic dysfunction, 932, 1002, 1013, 1021, 1054, 2156, 2157, 2173
Autonomic dysregulation (Shy-Drager-Syndrome), 1021, 1022, 1028
Autonomic nervous system, 95, 122–123, 2152
Autonomic system, 123, 326
Autophagy, 720, 825, 842, 850, 880–882, 1013, 1051–1053, 1059, 1067, 1266, 1293–1300, 2139
Autotopagnosia, 406
Avoiding immune destruction (emerging hallmark), 1265, 1280, 1281
Axial skeleton, 1990, 2005, 2018
Axin, 1049, 1052, 1056, 1306, 1320, 2054
Axonal
   collaterals, 226, 227
   disconnection, 1207, 1214, 1217
   guidance molecules, 1267, 1316
   swelling, 484, 864, 966, 1042, 1209, 2129
   terminals, 227, 859
   transport, 100, 228, 736, 839, 845, 847, 895, 924, 1012, 1037, 1045, 1051, 1056, 1093, 1209, 1214, 1217
Axon hillock, 226, 228
Azathioprine, 635, 642, 731, 1072, 1093, 1103

B

Bag of worms, 1679, 1680
Balint syndrome, 208, 423, 476, 896
Ballismus, 416
Balloon cells, 1157, 1158, 1160, 1163, 1164, 1166, 1168
Ballooned Neurons, 839, 854, 860, 861, 960, 973, 982
Balós disease, 244
Band heterotopia, 1132, 1135, 1171, 1174, 1178, 1179
Basal cell carcinomas, 1291, 1326, 2076, 2095
Basal ganglia, 5, 9, 13, 48, 76, 77, 86, 126, 129, 143–146, 151, 153, 155, 203, 211, 267, 301–305, 334, 339, 350, 357, 377, 385, 387, 401, 416, 417, 450, 457, 459, 461, 468, 482, 489, 490, 501, 502, 506, 507, 538, 541, 586, 605, 607, 614, 616, 622, 625, 627, 629, 640, 658, 666, 673, 697, 698, 703, 715, 737, 738, 752, 755, 775, 782, 795, 797, 798, 800, 802, 805, 817, 818, 820, 838, 848, 850, 856, 863, 865, 871, 873, 901, 914, 932, 960, 966, 977, 979, 987, 989, 990, 992, 995, 996, 1012, 1025, 1028, 1060, 1106, 1213, 1227, 1233, 1245, 1257, 1259, 1342, 1434, 1448, 1761, 1895, 1898, 1899, 1934, 1936, 2154, 2159, 2170, 2174
Basal ganglionic system, 326, 334
Basal lamina, 176, 249, 252, 254–258, 267, 321, 322, 717, 1311, 1553, 1559, 1648, 1675, 1768
Base excision repair (BER), 1286, 1287
Basidiomycetes, 774
Basilar fissure, 157
Basket, 94, 233, 267, 292, 296, 314, 344, 347, 349, 353
Basolateral nuclear group (deep nuclei), 301
Basophilic inclusion body disease (BIBD), 849, 954, 956, 957, 966–967
Basophilic inclusions, 849, 954, 956, 957, 966–967, 973, 983, 1037, 1042
B-cell suppression, 2152, 2176
β-CIT, 49, 54, 573, 975, 1004, 1023, 1226
BCNU, 2131
Behavioral impairment, 1038
Benign fibrous histiocytoma, 1956, 1985, 1991–1993
Bequerel, 39
Ber-EP4, 103, 2058, 2060, 2084, 2102
Bergmann astrocytes, 1224, 1233
Beta-amyloid, 100, 101, 839, 1404
Beta-catenin, 1759, 2099
Beta radiation, 31
Betz giant pyramidal cells, 294
Bevacizumab (Avastin), 49, 1329–1331, 1406, 1414, 1420, 2056, 2131, 2139
Bielschowsky, 84–87, 839, 841, 908, 914, 916
Bi-hemispheric syndromes, 401, 413
Bilateral homonymous hemianopia, 209

Bilateral ideomotor apraxia, 405
Bilateral leukoaraiosis, 996
Bilateral, symmetrical ischemic lesions/necrosis of the globus pallidus, 1247
Binswanger disease, 605, 606, 615–621, 827, 987
Biological therapy, 1269
Biphasic pattern, 1433, 1434, 1438, 1439, 1637, 1646
Birbeck granules, 1938
Bizarre astrocytes, 728, 730, 732
"Black-and-white mixed" pattern, 1958
Blast induced trauma (bTBI), 1189, 1218
Blast injury, 1185, 1188, 1211, 1218
Blastomycosis, 777
Blast wave, 1189, 1218
Blepharoplasts, 1496, 1501, 1648
Block design, 21
Blood-brain-barrier BBB, 176
Blood-fluid levels, 1584
Blood-liquor-barrier, 176, 177
Blood oxygenated level-dependent (BOLD) response, 3, 20, 21
Blooming, 477, 586, 1448, 1461, 1477, 1597
Blunted affect (apathetic, indifferent), 404, 966
B-lymphocyte, 105, 106, 641, 647, 690, 1920, 1923, 2152
Body of the caudate nucleus (corpus nuclei caudati), 144
Bone invasion, 1958
Bone matrix, 1998, 2005
Bone tumors
  age incidence, 1990
  biologic behavior-prognosis-prognostic factors, 1995–1998
  classification, 1990
  molecular pathogenesis, 1994–1998
  nuclear medicine imaging findings, 1990–1994
  treatment, 1995
Borrelia burgdorferi, 655, 657
Boutons terminaux, 227
Bovine spongiform encephalopathy (BSE), 796, 797
Bowel, bladder, and/or sexual dysfunction, 1093, 1267
Braak stages, 918
Brachium colliculi inferioris, 150
Brachium colliculi superioris, 150
Brachyury, 1979, 1996, 1997, 2022, 2062
Bradykinesia/hypokinesia, 843, 932, 988, 1001, 1002, 1022, 1060
Bradykinin, 371, 441
Bradyzoites, 752, 756, 759, 761
BRAF, 1305, 1306, 1323–1325, 1328, 1329, 1433, 1443, 1444, 1561, 1565, 1573, 1759, 2054, 2055, 2057
BRAF V600E, 1323–1325, 1328, 1396, 1402, 1444, 1561, 1565, 1573, 1591, 1759, 1907, 1911
Brain
  abscess, 49, 653, 654, 656–658, 661–663, 665, 666, 675, 690, 751, 773, 774, 776, 1247
  atrophy, 60, 696, 698, 703, 712, 870, 871, 882, 933, 937, 980, 990, 996, 1003, 1039, 1061, 1074, 1192, 1193, 1225, 1227
  cancer stem cells, 1267, 1319–130
  death, 30, 52, 54, 432, 436, 456, 465

Brain edema
  age incidence, 428
  biologic behavior-prognosis-prognostic factors, 441
  CT-contrast-enhanced, 429
  CT-non contrast-enhanced, 428–429
  cytotoxic edema, 428
  differential diagnosis, 471
  general imaging findings, 428–434
  immunophenotype, 687
  interstitial edema, 427
  localization, 428
  macroscopic features, 434–439
  microscopic features, 439
  molecular neuropathology, 440–441
  MRI-diffusion imaging, 432
  MRI-diffusion tensor imaging, 432
  MRI-FLAIR, 429
  MRI-perfusion, 432
  MRI-T1, 429
  MRI-T2, 429
  MRI-T1 contrast-enhanced, 429
  MRI-T2∗/SWI, 429
  MR-spectroscopy, 432
  nuclear medicine imaging findings, 432
  osmotic edema, 428
  pathogenesis, 427
  proliferation markers, 1341
  sex incidence, 428
  treatment, 441
  ultrastructural features, 440
  vasogenic edema, 427–428
Brain-liquor-barrier (BLB), 176
Brain perfusion SPECT, 29, 51–53, 697, 901, 1119, 1125, 1576, 1866
Brain stem
  cranial nerves, 326
  encephalitis, 2170
Brain swelling, 427, 428, 715, 1185, 1187, 1188, 1207
Bremsstrahlung, 31
Broca's area, 401, 410, 413
Broca's speech area, 132, 278, 405
Brodmann area, 76, 273, 278, 283, 331–335, 404–407, 409, 410, 1228, 1253
4-bromo-2,5-dimethoxyamphetamine (DOB), 1244, 1259
Brownian motion of water molecules, 3, 19
Bulbar atrophy, 1037, 1038
Bunina bodies, 1037, 1042, 1045
Bunyaviridae, 695, 696, 736

C

^{13}C (carbon), 10, 15
Café-au-lait macules, 1694
Cajal-Retzius cells, 1143, 1151, 1153, 1179
Calbindin, 95, 1153
Calcarine fissure, 134–137, 407
Calcifications, 457, 484, 529, 537, 538, 540, 552, 578, 585, 586, 596, 605, 609, 622, 625, 698, 720, 721, 751, 752, 760, 763, 768, 825, 836, 837,

Index

857, 865, 1338, 1354, 1369, 1434, 1435, 1438, 1447, 1448, 1451, 1452, 1460–1463, 1470, 1474, 1475, 1477, 1493, 1511, 1516, 1523, 1534, 1542, 1545, 1554, 1563, 1566, 1568, 1573, 1575–1577, 1584, 1597, 1598, 1606, 1615, 1639, 1642, 1643, 1646, 1648, 1652, 1666, 1667, 1699, 1709, 1720, 1735, 1753, 1755, 1757, 1759, 1766, 1782, 1824, 1827, 1833, 1836, 1841, 1843, 1846, 1853, 1868, 1882–1884, 1958, 1962, 1979, 1989, 1998, 2011, 2020, 2026, 2119, 2120, 2124, 2126–2128
Calcium channels, 236, 427, 441, 605, 616, 1134, 1135, 1219, 1404, 1405, 2171, 2174–2176
Calponin, 102, 2058, 2062, 2075, 2115
Calretinin (CR), 92, 95, 233, 292, 1143, 1153, 1176, 1675, 2060, 2062, 2099, 2112
Calvarium, 60, 61, 1924, 1958, 2018
Cam5.2, 103, 2058, 2060, 2070, 2075, 2083, 2099, 2106, 2112
Canavan disease, 864, 1072
Cancer stem cell (CSC), 1267, 1300, 1313, 1319–1320, 1867
Candida albicans, 702, 790–792
Candida glabrata, 774
Candidiasis, 777, 792
Cannabinoid (CB)-receptors, 1244, 1245, 1257
Cannabis, 1243–1245, 1255–1258
Cannabis-induced hypotension, 1256
Cannabis-induced vasospasm, 1256
Cannibalism, 796, 820
Capgras syndrome, 422
Capillary
 hemangioma, 577
 telangiectasias, 577, 593, 596–598, 2120, 2126, 2128
 telangiectasis, 577
Ca2+ pump, 455, 471
CARASAL Cathepsin A-related arteriopathy with strokes and leukoencephalopathy, 606
CARASIL Cerebral recessive dominant arteriopathy with subcortical infarcts and leukoencephalopathy, 606
Carbonic anhydrase, 97, 252, 293, 717, 1979
Carbon monoxide, 370, 457
Carcinogens, 1267, 1303, 1321, 1322
Carcinoid tumor, 1694, 2063
Cardiac arrest, 457, 461, 996, 999
Cardiac arrest encephalopathy, 457
Cardiac arrhythmias, 457, 1229
Cardiac embolism, 489
Cardiac output (CO), 191, 456
Cardioembolism, 474
Caseous necrosis, 687
Caspase-independent cell death, 1301
Caspases, 1209, 1293–1296, 1301, 1302
CASPR2, 2153, 2157, 2162, 2171
CASPR2 (voltage-gated Potassium channels (VGKC)), 2157, 2170, 2171, 2174, 2175
CASPR2 (contactin-associated protein-like 2) disease, 2153, 2157, 2162, 2171, 2175

Catecholamines, 370, 376–387, 519, 1007, 1220
Catenin, 92, 719, 815, 1291, 1306, 1320, 1613, 1624, 1626, 1628, 1629, 1753, 1759, 1765, 1966, 1989, 1995, 2054, 2055, 2061, 2075, 2084, 2099
Cauda equina, 65, 166, 186, 436, 637, 1280, 1490, 1506, 1507, 1648, 1679
Cauda equina syndrome, 637
Caudal ganglionic eminence (CGE), 232, 291
Caudate nucleus, 50, 51, 76, 125–127, 143–147, 150, 153, 167, 168, 174, 175, 203, 204, 267, 301–304, 334, 357, 388, 458, 475, 478, 501, 538, 629, 698, 818, 819, 856, 858, 873, 966, 967, 980, 989, 1003, 1007, 1059–1066, 1254–1256, 1415, 1542, 1944
Cavernous hemangioma, 505, 577, 578, 586–595, 997, 1131, 1132
CBF-scans, 32
CBF SPECT, 448, 449, 458, 478, 501, 510, 521, 538, 616, 622, 802, 804, 899, 947, 976, 990, 1007, 1028, 1106, 1192, 1226, 1245
CCNU, 1329, 1447, 1466, 2131
C3d complement receptor CR2 (CD21), 699
Cell body, 95, 99, 226, 228, 251, 252, 268, 283, 304, 455, 458, 1212, 1316, 1341, 1344, 1433, 1438
Cell cycle, 107, 843, 849, 879, 925, 959, 1265, 1266, 1281–1285, 1288, 1290, 1291, 1293, 1304, 1308, 1323, 1367, 1398, 1400, 1491, 1789, 1790, 1792, 1913, 2175
Cell membrane, 19, 95, 97, 105, 111, 226, 228, 371, 427, 441, 717, 815, 1254, 1307, 1530, 1701, 1871, 1872, 1880
Cells of Martinotti, 268, 269
Cellularity, 585, 1083, 1265, 1268, 1270, 1272, 1344, 1353, 1354, 1360, 1375, 1433, 1438, 1439, 1444, 1447, 1452, 1459, 1469, 1472, 1476, 1477, 1483, 1489, 1496, 1500, 1501, 1503, 1527, 1530, 1531, 1561, 1568, 1573, 1595, 1597, 1601, 1604–1606, 1609, 1618, 1623, 1661, 1669, 1677, 1679, 1681, 1682, 1690, 1707, 1740, 1762, 1773, 1894, 1920, 1927, 1947, 1955, 1962, 1965, 1975, 1985, 1989, 2009
Cellular prion protein (PrPC), 795, 796, 814–816, 820
Cellulifugal transport, 228
Cellulipetal transport, 228
Central Brain Tumor Registry of the United states (CBTRUS), 1279
Central canal, 169, 318–321
Central motor system, 326, 334
Central nervous system (CNS), (AU: Whole book deals on this topic please check)
Central nuclear group, 301
Central photophobia, 209
Central pontine myelinolysis (CPM), 1072, 1223, 1224, 1233–1236
Central volume principle, 9
Cerebellar ataxia, 209, 505, 828, 862, 1021, 1035, 1054, 1055, 1224, 1233, 1490, 2158, 2160, 2170, 2172, 2174

Cerebellar degeneration, 1035, 1223, 1224, 1233, 2153, 2170, 2172–2174
Cerebellar tentorium, 62, 136, 137, 180, 181, 434
Cerebellar tonsillar herniation, 436
Cerebelloreticular fibers, 350
Cerebellorubral fibers, 350
Cerebellothalamic fibers, 350
Cerebellum
    ala lobuli centralis, 162, 164
    anterior lobe, 162, 166, 419, 1810
    basket cells, 314
    cerebellar cortex, 76, 79, 230, 232, 267, 313, 314, 316, 325, 350, 352, 353, 385, 387, 392, 817, 819, 820, 914, 1071, 1086
    cerebellar foliae, 162
    cerebellar hemispheres, 71, 72, 74, 162–164, 181, 204, 507, 1437, 1613, 1615, 1652, 1967
    dentate nucleus, 315
    emboliform nucleus, 315
    fastigial nucleus, 163
    fissura prima, 162
    flocculus, 162, 164, 174
    fusiform nucleus, 267, 315
    globose nucleus, 163
    golgi cells, 267, 313–315, 351, 353
    gracile lobule, 162
    granular cells, 313
    granular cell layer, 314–316, 1233
    horizontal fissure, 162
    inferior cerebellar peduncles, 72, 74, 163, 204, 312
    inferior semilunar lobule, 162
    lobulus biventer, 162, 164
    lobulus gracilis, 162, 164
    lobulus quadrangularis anterior, 162, 164
    lobulus quadrangularis posterior, 162, 164
    lobulus semilunaris inferior, 162, 164
    lobulus semilunaris superior, 162, 164
    middle cerebellar peduncles, 1022, 1023, 1028
    molecular layer, 281, 282, 287, 289, 314–316, 346, 351, 818, 819, 1150, 1151, 1223, 1224, 1227, 1233
    posterior lobe, 162, 1754, 1771
    posterior quadrangular lobule, 162
    purkinje cell layer, 314, 1028, 1224, 1233, 1243, 1247, 1253
    purkinje cells, 314
    stellate cells, 267, 269, 279, 287, 289, 300, 314, 342, 344, 353
    superior anterior fissure, 162
    superior cerebellar peduncles, 174, 311, 381, 476, 863, 973–975
    superior posterior fissure, 162
    superior semilunar lobule, 162
    tonsil, 62, 162, 203, 204, 436, 816, 819
    vermis
        "arbor vitae," 163
        culmen, 163, 164
        declive, 163, 164
        folium, 163, 164
        lingula, 163
        lobulus centralis, 163, 164
        nodulus, 163, 164
        pyramis, 161, 163, 164
        tuber, 163, 164
        uvula, 163, 164
Cerebral activation paradigm, 21
Cerebral amyloid (congophilic) angiopathy (CAA), 53, 489, 499, 503, 505, 514, 521, 605–615, 797, 827, 841, 845, 899, 908, 987, 988, 995, 996, 999
Cerebral aqueduct, 71, 156, 169, 171, 174, 175, 435, 677, 755, 1596, 1618, 1899
Cerebral blood dynamics, 20
Cerebral blood flow (CBF), 9, 11, 18–20, 22, 32, 52, 54, 257, 432, 448, 449, 451, 458, 477–479, 501, 510, 521, 538, 607, 616, 622, 641, 666, 802, 804, 872, 873, 899, 933, 947, 976, 990, 1007, 1028, 1060, 1106, 1126, 1147, 1192, 1217, 1226, 1227, 1243, 1245, 1246, 1255, 1257, 1716
Cerebral blood volume (CBV), 9, 18, 21, 22, 477, 479, 1126, 1525, 1534, 1585, 1619, 1640
Cerebral cortex and limbic system, 326
Cerebral falx, 180
Cerebral hemisphere, 129, 137, 163, 186, 223, 732, 752, 773, 856, 1353, 1354, 1368, 1412, 1425, 1426, 1448, 1470, 1477, 1576, 1632, 1638, 1646, 1648, 1652, 1824, 1833, 1856, 2038
Cerebral hemorrhage, 499–505, 507, 511, 551, 558, 576, 607, 615, 640, 897, 987, 989, 999, 1131, 1207, 1244, 1258, 1914
Cerebral infarction, 19, 473, 496, 640, 666, 1131, 1244, 1256, 1260, 1914
Cerebral ischemia, 3, 9, 19, 428, 471, 518, 519, 814, 987, 1245
Cerebral malaria, 750, 751
Cerebral peduncles, 156, 186, 204, 205, 209, 334, 1237
Cerebral rate of oxygen metabolism ($CMRO_2$), 20
Cerebro-ocular muscular syndromes, 1132
Cerebroretinal vasculopathy, 606
Cerebrospinal fluid (CSF), 6, 12–14, 58, 61, 158, 169–177, 186, 188, 243, 249, 250, 260, 321, 441, 443, 444, 451, 510, 517–519, 522, 653, 654, 658, 660, 664, 715, 718, 730, 731, 763, 766, 790, 851, 852, 854, 862, 870, 896, 897, 899, 926, 1002, 1090–1092, 1186, 1216, 1218, 1407, 1434, 1523, 1559, 1595, 1606, 1614–1616, 1618, 1631, 1639, 1648, 1652, 1666, 1755, 1824, 1825, 1846, 1853, 1856, 1858, 1865, 1868, 1998, 2152, 2154–2157, 2159
Cerebrospinal fluid (CSF)-barriers, 169–177
Cerebrospinal nervous system, 122–123
Cerebrovascular disease, 52, 54, 615, 702, 896, 897, 932, 987, 989, 990, 999, 1243, 1245, 1253
Cerebrovascular occlusive disease with retinal involvement, 988
Cerebrovascular reserve, 9, 52

Cerebrovestibular fibers, 350
Cerebrum, 205, 213, 533, 776, 1073, 1280, 1639, 1642, 1666, 1885, 2152
Cestodes, 750, 771
Chandelier, 233, 269, 292, 342, 344, 1153
Changes in behaviour or personality, 410, 622, 640, 722, 736, 857, 859, 962, 966, 988, 1755, 1895, 2154, 2155
Changes of muscle tone, 456
Chaperone proteins, 455, 471, 931, 941
Charcot type, 1071, 1072, 1093
Charged multivesicular body protein 2B (CHMP2B), 849, 850, 956, 960, 1049, 1052
Chemical shift selective (CHESS), 15
Chemotherapy, 32, 48, 773, 776, 778, 792, 1269, 1277, 1310, 1320, 1326, 1330, 1337, 1349, 1353, 1365, 1382, 1403, 1407, 1411, 1417, 1420, 1425, 1431, 1447, 1466, 1469, 1484, 1489, 1501, 1521, 1522, 1561, 1573, 1614, 1631, 1637, 1646, 1647, 1865, 1868, 1891, 1913, 1918, 1929, 1938, 1955, 1967, 1989, 1990, 1995, 2037, 2053, 2095, 2119, 2128, 2131, 2141, 2159, 2160, 2176
Chemotherapy-induced leukoencephalopathy, 2119, 2128
Chiari type I malformation, 1592
Chicken-wire pattern, 1453, 1456, 1462, 1463
Childhood ataxia with central nervous system hypomyelination (CACH), 243
Cho/Cr, 1226
Cholangiocarcinoma, 2059, 2061, 2097, 2104
Cholecystokinin (CCK), 95, 233, 234, 292, 293, 349, 370, 371, 836
Choline, 16, 17, 293, 300, 372, 373, 432, 766, 863, 1077, 1192, 1207, 1338, 1340, 1354, 1373, 1376, 1377, 1430, 1434, 1448, 1449, 1460, 1462, 1470, 1471, 1477, 1478, 1525, 1534, 1535, 1554, 1563, 1573, 1576, 1584, 1615, 1642, 1897, 2124
Choline acetyltransferase (ChAT), 233, 292, 373
cholinergic receptor nicotinic alpha 4 subunit (CHRNA4), 236, 1136
Chondrocytes, 1989, 2009, 2012, 2013, 2016
Chondroitin sulfate proteoglycans, 92, 97, 1093, 1267, 1316
Chondroma
  differential diagnosis, 2009
  localization, 2009
  macroscopic features, 2009
  microscopic features, 2009
  WHO definition, 2009
Chondrosarcoma
  CT-non contrast-enhanced, 2011
  differential diagnosis, 2013
  general imaging findings, 2011
  localization, 2011
  macroscopic features, 2011
  microscopic features, 2013
  MRI-T1, 2011
  MRI-T2, 2011
  MRI-T1 contrast-enhanced, 2011
  WHO definition, 2011
CHOP, 1891, 1913, 1918
Chordoma
  CT-contrast-enhanced, 2018
  CT-non contrast-enhanced, 2018
  differential diagnosis, 2022
  general imaging findings, 2018
  localization, 2018
  macroscopic features, 2020
  microscopic features, 2020–2022
  MRI-T1, 2018
  MRI-T2, 2018
  MRI-T2∗, 2020
  MRI-T1 contrast-enhanced, 2020
  WHO definition, 2018
Chorea, 416, 818, 828, 1054, 1059, 1060, 1068, 2153, 2158–2160, 2170, 2172, 2174
Choreoathetosis, 209, 417, 858, 1245, 1255
Choriocarcinoma
  general imaging findings, 1880
  immunophenotype, 1880
  macroscopic features, 1880
  microscopic features, 1880
  ultrastructural features, 1880
  WHO definition, 1880
Choroid epithelium, 225, 240
Choroid plexus, 7, 97, 174, 176, 177, 203, 204, 211, 225, 254, 255, 267, 321–322, 387, 443, 449, 475, 499, 500, 718, 1275, 1276, 1323, 1500, 1501, 1521–1539, 1823, 1824, 1843, 1885, 1935, 1956, 1974
Choroid plexus carcinoma
  age incidence, 1522
  biologic behavior-prognosis-prognostic factors, 1522
  CT-contrast-enhanced, 1534
  CT-non contrast-enhanced, 1534
  differential diagnosis, 1522
  general imaging findings, 1534
  immunophenotype, 1539
  incidence, 1522
  localization, 1522
  macroscopic features, 1534
  microscopic features, 1534
  MRI-diffusion imaging, 1534
  MRI-FLAIR, 1534
  MRI-perfusion, 1534
  MRI-T1, 1534
  MRI-T2, 1534
  MRI-T1 contrast-enhanced, 1534
  MRI-T2∗/SWI, 1534
  MR-spectroscopy, 1534
  pathogenesis, 1522
  proliferation markers, 1539
  sex incidence, 1539
  treatment, 1522
  ultrastructural features, 1530
  WHO definition, 1534
  WHO grade, 1534

Choroid plexus hemorrhage, 499, 500
Choroid plexus papilloma
  age incidence, 1522
  biologic behavior-prognosis-prognostic factors, 1522
  CT-contrast-enhanced, 1523
  differential diagnosis, 1522
  general imaging findings, 1523
  immunophenotype, 1527, 1529
  incidence, 1522
  localization, 1522
  macroscopic features, 1525
  microscopic features, 1527–1529
  MRI-diffusion imaging, 1525
  MRI-FLAIR, 1523
  MRI-perfusion, 1525
  MRI-T1, 1523
  MRI-T2, 1523
  MRI-T1 contrast-enhanced, 1523
  MRI-T2*/SWI, 1523
  MR-spectroscopy, 1525
  nuclear medicine imaging findings, 1522
  proliferation markers, 1530
  sex incidence, 1522
  treatment, 1522
  ultrastructural features, 1530
  WHO definition, 1523–1530
  WHO grade, 1523
Choroid plexus papilloma atypical
  age incidence, 1522
  biologic behavior-prognosis-prognostic factors, 1522
  differential diagnosis, 1522
  general imaging findings, 1530
  immunophenotype, 1530
  incidence, 1522
  localization, 1522
  macroscopic features, 1530
  microscopic features, 1530
  proliferation markers, 1530
  sex incidence, 1522
  treatment, 1522
  ultrastructural features, 1530
  WHO definition, 1530
  WHO grade, 1530
Chromatid bridges, 1271
Chromatin, 227, 648, 889, 890, 925, 1049, 1052, 1056, 1228, 1268, 1278, 1284, 1293, 1295, 1296, 1301, 1337, 1341, 1343, 1344, 1353, 1360, 1400, 1405, 1454, 1477, 1493, 1497, 1575, 1577, 1579, 1580, 1584, 1588, 1591, 1595, 1597, 1601, 1613, 1614, 1618, 1631–1634, 1637, 1643, 1644, 1648, 1651, 1652, 1654, 1655, 1663, 1700, 1702, 1707, 1729, 1742, 1748, 1754, 1776, 1779, 1794, 1796, 1871, 1903, 1904, 1955, 1962, 1965, 1984, 1989, 2009, 2012, 2013, 2055, 2063
Chromatin condensation, 1293, 1295
Chromogranin, 96, 1600, 1604, 1608, 1770, 1776, 1810, 2060–2062, 2070, 2084, 2095, 2112
Chromogranin A, 102, 236, 841, 1579, 1601, 1765, 1775, 2058, 2060

Chromophobe renal cell carcinoma, 2085, 2088
Chromosomal imbalances, 1324, 1325, 1596
Chromosomal instability (CIN), 1266, 1284, 1304, 1328
Chromosomal translocations, 1171, 1178, 1891, 1913
Chromosome
  2, 1765
  7, 568, 1306, 1322–1324, 1348, 1353, 1364, 1399, 1401, 1402, 1561, 1565
  11, 1325, 1596
  13, 1692, 1703
  14, 1325
  17, 825, 828, 855–856, 1325, 1630, 1662, 1692, 1703
  18, 1521, 1522, 1662, 1692, 1703
  22, 1306, 1325, 1326, 1596, 1662, 1686, 1702
  10 loss, 1322, 1403, 1466
  1p, 1469, 1476, 1484, 1661, 1675, 1747
  1p32, 1290, 1747, 1748
  1p36.12, 1014, 1015, 1748
  2p, 1575, 1582, 1996
  3p, 1521, 1522, 1553, 1559, 1749, 1787, 1996
  3p21, 1291, 1629
  8p11.21, 1747
  9p, 957, 958, 1326, 1401, 1403, 1748
  9p21, 569, 1055, 1291, 1323, 1364, 1399, 1662, 1692, 1703, 1748
  11p, 1364
  11p15.5, 1290, 1747
  12p13, 1747
  16p13.3, 1135, 1138, 1747
  17p, 1348, 1349, 1353, 1364, 1401, 1458, 1466, 1469, 1476, 1484
  17p13.1, 1337, 1349, 1399, 1629, 1630
  1p/19q, 1459, 1466, 1476, 1575, 1582
  1p/19q co-deletion, 1322, 1324, 1326, 1327, 1337, 1349, 1353, 1364, 1447, 1448, 1458, 1459, 1464, 1466, 1469, 1476, 1484, 1541, 1550
  2q14, 923, 1053, 1289, 1324, 1399, 1401, 1613, 1630, 1747
  3q, 1553, 1559, 1630, 1632
  3q26.3, 1399
  4q, 1325, 1596, 1996
  4q12, 1324, 1399, 1401
  4q22.1, 1013, 1014, 1747
  5q, 1521, 1522, 1553, 1559, 1632
  5q13.1, 1399
  6q, 1326
  7q, 1326, 1327, 1553, 1559, 1647
  7q32.3, 1137, 1630, 1747
  9q22.3, 1291, 1629, 1747
  9q34, 1051, 1054, 1135, 1137, 1289, 1661, 1675
  10q, 1401, 1630
  10q23.3, 1399
  11q, 1326, 1328, 1553, 1559, 1647, 1893
  12q, 1325, 1326, 1596
  12q14, 1053, 1289, 1324, 1399, 1401
  12q14-15, 1399, 1401
  13q, 1401, 1521, 1522, 1575, 1582, 1996
  13q14.2, 1399
  14q, 1326, 1553, 1559, 1630, 1632, 1748, 1749, 1996
  14q11.2, 1054, 1748

14q32, 569, 1179, 1747, 1748
16q22.1, 1291, 1747, 1997
17q, 1324–1326, 1541, 1550, 1630, 1632, 1661, 1675
17q11.2, 1399, 1401, 1403, 1443, 1662, 1693, 1697, 1700
17q23, 569, 1747, 1748
18q, 1326, 1521, 1522, 1575, 1585, 1632
19q, 1364, 1401, 1448, 1476, 1484, 1565
21q, 856, 1553, 1559, 1996
22q, 1326, 1328, 1364, 1521, 1522, 1553, 1559, 1657, 1662, 1675, 1686, 1700
22q11.2, 1053, 1135, 1326, 1651, 1654, 1663, 1700, 1702, 1747
22q11.23, 1053, 1663, 1700, 1747
5q21-q22, 1629, 1747
12q13.2-q13.3, 1613, 1630, 1747
Chromosome 17-associated Dementia, 825, 855–856
Chromosome bridges, 1271
Chromosome lagging, 1271
Chromosome segregation errors, 1271
Chronic
    endothelial injury, 542
    hypoperfusion, 987
    traumatic brain injury, 1192, 1193
Chronic traumatic encephalopathy (CTE), 837, 1185, 1211–1214
Chronic wasting disease of mule, elk, and deer (CWD), 797
Chronic Wernicke-Korsakoff encephalopathy, 1229–1233
Chymotrypsin, 102, 2058
Cilia, 249, 1496, 1501, 1510, 1518, 1530, 1646, 1648, 1843, 1844, 1850, 1853
Cingulate gyrus, 76, 135–138, 143, 148, 150, 167, 168, 325, 343, 350, 357, 405, 436, 437, 734, 838, 855, 861, 901, 916, 937, 965, 2052
Cingulum, 148, 343, 422, 901
Circadian abnormalities, 418
Circuit, 325, 326, 334, 339, 344, 346, 347, 349–356, 364, 376, 388, 858, 859, 1012, 1119, 1134, 1154, 1217, 1227, 1279
Circular insular fissure, 134
CJD types, 818
Claude's syndrome, 209
Clear cell carcinoma, 1458, 1500, 2113, 2115
Clear cell renal cell carcinoma, 2059, 2085, 2088
Clearing, 79, 847, 1125, 1216, 1492, 1742, 1868
Climbing fibers, 325, 351, 353, 355
Clinical PD, 1002
Clipping, 499, 514, 551, 570, 582
Clot, 63, 477, 510, 521, 552, 610
Clot retrieval, 4
Clumsiness, 404, 945, 1059, 1073
CNS embryonal tumors, NOS
    age incidence, 1639
    biologic behavior-prognosis-prognostic factors, 1646
    CT-contrast-enhanced, 1639
    CT-non contrast-enhanced, 1639
    differential diagnosis, 1643
    general imaging findings, 1639

    immunophenotype, 1643
    incidence, 1639
    localization, 1642
    macroscopic features, 1642
    microscopic features, 1643
    MRI-diffusion imaging, 1642
    MRI-FLAIR, 1642
    MRI-perfusion, 1642
    MRI-T1, 1642
    MRI-T2, 1639
    MRI-T1 contrast-enhanced, 1642
    MRI-T2∗/SWI, 1642
    MR-spectroscopy, 1642
    nuclear medicine imaging findings, 1642
    pathogenesis, 1646
    proliferation markers, 1643
    sex incidence, 1639
    treatment, 1646
    ultrastructural features, 1643
    WHO definition, 1639–1646
    WHO grade, 1639
Coagulative or fibrinoid necrosis, 2126, 2128
Cocaine, 49, 371, 503, 514, 517, 636, 1243–1245, 1255–1258
Cocci, 655, 656
Coccidioidomycosis, 777
Coenurosis, 749, 750, 762–771
Cognitive dysfunction, 885, 974, 1093, 1224, 2152, 2156, 2176
Cognitive impairment, 53, 444, 456, 614, 622, 693, 701, 702, 817–819, 848, 885, 896, 901, 914, 917, 933, 956, 988, 989, 995–999, 1002, 1013, 1038, 1073, 1185, 1211, 1212, 1237, 1267, 1631, 1755, 2152, 2157, 2159
Cognitive processes, 21, 122, 416, 870
Coherent anti-Stokes Raman scattering (CARS) microscopy, 114
Coiled bodies, 837, 844, 849, 860–862, 965, 977, 979, 982, 983
Coiling, 499, 514, 551, 553, 570, 997
Collagen
    fibers, 252, 255, 258, 521, 768, 1614, 1661, 1677, 1679, 1682, 1983
    IV, 103, 717, 1675, 1686
Collimators, 31, 40
Colloid, 90, 763–765, 1823, 1824, 1829, 1837, 1843–1852, 2063, 2070, 2106, 2107
Colloid cyst of the third ventricle
    age incidence, 1846
    biologic behavior-prognosis-prognostic factors, 1850
    CT-contrast-enhanced, 1846
    CT-non contrast-enhanced, 1846
    differential diagnosis, 1850
    general imaging findings, 1846
    immunophenotype, 1850
    incidence, 1843
    localization, 1846
    macroscopic features, 1846
    microscopic features, 1846
    MRI-diffusion imaging, 1846

Colloid cyst of the third ventricle (*cont.*)
  MRI-FLAIR, 1846
  MRI-perfusion, 1846
  MRI-T1, 1846
  MRI-T2, 1846
  MRI-T1 contrast-enhanced, 1846
  MRI-T2*/SWI, 1846
  pathogenesis, 1850
  proliferation markers, 1850
  sex incidence, 1846
  treatment, 1850
  ultrastructural features, 1850
  WHO definition, 1843–1850
Color agnosia, 401, 413, 420
Color anomia, 209, 415
Color blindness, 209, 401, 413
Color dysnomia, 208, 476
Columnar disorganization, 1159
Coma, 417, 418, 456, 524, 606, 626, 694, 731, 736, 820, 1186, 1187, 1218, 1224, 1229, 1779, 1813, 2156, 2173
Commensals, 775
Commissural fibers, 20, 147–150, 289, 296, 347, 349, 350
Common fragile sites (CFSs), 1288
Communicative abilities, 134, 409
Compacted myelin, 99, 251
Compact plaque, 834, 836
Complement system, 689
Complete remission/response (CR), 1269, 2131
Complex partial seizures, 1121, 1123, 1124
Complex visual hallucinations, 407, 410
Comprehension, 10, 21, 403, 410, 413, 414, 420, 946
Computed tomography (CT), 4–7, 9, 29, 30, 39–42, 615, 1246
Computerized tomography angiography (CTA)/ magnetic resonance angiography (MRA), 538, 1716
Concentric type Balo, 1072
Concomitant therapy, 1265, 1269
Concussion, 1187
Conditioned reflex., 122
Conduction aphasia, 401, 406, 414, 420
Cones, 228, 312, 326, 331, 436, 2176
Confocal laser scanning microscopy, 57, 114
Confusion, 407, 456, 474, 520, 626, 694, 749, 752, 773, 1186, 2154, 2156, 2158–2160, 2174
Congenital, 451, 496, 558, 577, 585, 694, 699, 751, 755, 760, 836, 1072, 1157, 1179, 1824, 1829, 1841, 1974
Congenital toxoplasmosis, 749, 751, 755
Congestion, 599, 675, 734, 737, 1105, 1106, 1247
Congo red, 89, 90, 607, 839, 914
Conjunction design, 21
Connectional methods, 402
Connectional neuroanatomy, 361
Connectionism, 364
Connective tissue growth factor (CTGF), 291

Connectome, 325, 361–365
Connectopathies, 325, 364
Consistency, 60, 434, 521, 1229, 1359, 1360, 1383, 1420, 1477, 1542, 1555, 1652, 1670, 1671, 1680, 1690, 1730, 1771, 1798, 1802, 1816, 1979, 2018, 2021, 2050, 2163
Consortium to Establish a Registry for Alzheimer's Disease CERAD criteria, 915–916
Constructional apraxia, 401, 406, 407, 413, 414
Continuous capillary, 257
Contralateral central facial weakness, 207, 475
Contralateral decreased sensation, 207, 476
Contralateral foot and leg weakness, 207, 475
Contralateral gaze paresis, 207, 475
Contralateral grasp reflex, 208
Contralateral hemianesthesia, 417
Contralateral hemianopia, 209
Contralateral hemianopsia, 417
Contralateral hemiparesis, 207, 209, 475
Contralateral hemisensory/motor syndrome, 207, 475
Contralateral homonymous hemianopia, 207, 208, 475, 476
Contralateral IVth nerve palsy, 207
Contralateral pure motor hemiparesis, 207, 475
Contralateral weakness, 404
Contrast medium, 7, 14, 15
Contusion, 428, 521, 522, 530, 533, 1185, 1187, 1192, 1193, 1196, 1201, 1207
Conus medullaris, 163, 164, 166, 187, 1490, 1506, 1507
Copper-binding protein, 814
Copper-binding sialoglycoprotein, 814
Corona radiata, 19, 147, 204, 334, 475, 1074, 1218
Corpora amylacea, 83, 873–875
Corpora mamillaria, (AU: Not found)
Corpus callosum
  genu, 148–150
  knee, 148–150
  rostrum, 148–150
  splenium, 148–150
  truncus, 148–150
  trunk, 148–150
Correlational methods, 402
Cortical-basal ganglionic degeneration, 416
Cortical blindness, 208, 209, 413, 421
Cortical dysplasia, 85, 94, 1119, 1121, 1130, 1132, 1157–1161, 1168, 1175, 1541, 1542, 1545, 1550, 1554, 1563
Cortical laminar necrosis, 457, 996
Cortical laminar pan-necrosis, 458
Cortical sensory loss, 208
Cortical tubers in tuberous sclerosis complex (TSC), 1157
Cortico-basal degeneration (CBD), 826–828, 837–839, 842, 848, 849, 852, 933, 953, 956, 957, 962, 973–984, 1004
Corticobulbar tract, 308, 310, 334
Corticomedial nuclear group (superficial nuclei), 300

Corticonigral degeneration with neuronal achromasia, 380
Corticospinal decussation, 311
Corticospinal tract, 312, 314, 334, 335, 858, 1037, 1039, 1040, 1101
Corticosteroids, 441, 642, 741, 778, 1097, 1103, 1105, 1115, 1933, 1948, 2132, 2135, 2136, 2176
Corticotropin, 349, 352, 370, 371
Corticotropin-releasing factor, 349, 370, 372
Cotton whool and inflammatory plaques, 835, 844
Covalent inter/intrastrand crosslinks, 186, 1285
11C-Pittsburgh-Compound-B (11C-PIB), 29, 53, 899
C1Q (complement C1q A chain), 236, 242, 249, 886
Cr3/43 (HLA-DR II), 99, 100, 248, 471
11C-raclopride, 29, 50, 51, 449, 976, 1007, 1028
Cranial nerve palsies, 505, 637, 640, 658, 1663
Cranial nerves, 27, 61, 74, 122, 137, 158, 162, 230, 312, 325, 326, 435, 505, 576, 637, 640, 654, 658, 666, 675, 694, 751, 763, 774, 1106, 1186, 1280, 1662, 1663, 1666, 1685, 1690, 1699, 1700, 1750, 1824, 2153, 2156
Cranial neuropathies, 640, 1267, 2153
Craniopharyngeal duct, 1753, 1754, 1765
Craniopharyngioma
  adamantinomatous, 1754–1760, 1765
  age incidence, 1755
  biologic behavior-prognosis-prognostic factors, 1766
  clinical signs and symptoms, 1754–1755
  CT-contrast-enhanced, 1755
  CT-non contrast-enhanced, 1755
  differential diagnosis, 1765
  DNA methylation, 1748
  epigenetics, 1748
  gene expression, 1749
  general imaging findings, 1755
  genetics, 1748
  immunophenotype, 1759, 1764
  incidence, 1755
  localization, 1755
  macroscopic features, 1755, 1760
  microRNAs, 1748–1749
  microscopic features, 1755, 1762, 1763
  molecular neuropathology, 1765
  MRI-diffusion imaging, 1755
  MRI–FLAIR, 1755–1757
  MRI-T1, 1755
  MRI-T2, 1755
  MRI-T1 contrast-enhanced, 1755
  MRI-T2∗/ SWI, 1755
  MR–spectroscopy, 1755
  nuclear medicine imaging findings, 1755, 1760
  papillary, 1754, 1759
  pathogenesis, 1756
  prognosis, 1768
  prognostic factors, 1766
  proliferation markers, 1764
  sex incidence, 1755
  treatment, 1749
  ultrastructural features, 1764–1765
  WHO definition, 1754
  WHO grade, 1754
Craniospinal dissemination, 1582
Craniospinal radiotherapy, 1631
Creatine, 17, 520, 800, 1060
Cresyl violet (Nissl stain), 57, 84–86, 268, 270, 289, 295, 309, 314, 315, 707, 709, 759, 787, 1065, 1546
Creutzfeldt-Jakob-Disease (CJD), 84, 96, 795–798, 800–803, 812, 815–819, 827, 839, 852, 853, 857, 859
Criblures, 990
Crista galli, 180
Crura cerebri, 156
Crus cerebri, 205, 307
Cryo-electron tomography, 114
Cryptococcosis, 775, 777, 783, 786, 790
Cryptococcus neoformans, 702, 774–776, 782–790
Cryptogenic stroke, 496
CSF dissemination, 1595, 1606, 1615, 1616
CT-angiography, 7–9, 477, 501, 640, 643
CT-perfusion, 9, 477
Cuneate fascicle, 162
Cuneate nucleus, 162, 313, 335, 343
Cuneate tubercle, 162
Cuneus, 135–137, 150, 204, 205, 401, 407, 476
Curettage, 1989, 1990, 1995
Cushing syndrome, 418, 1671, 1781
Cyberknife, 1661, 1675
Cyclic limbic pathway, 325, 343
2'-3'-Cyclic nucleotide 3'-phosphatase (CNP), 99
2',3'-cyclic nucleotide 3'-phosphodiesterase (CNP), 225, 251, 717, 1089, 1093
Cyclophosphamide, 642, 731, 1891, 1913, 2152, 2160, 2176
Cyclotron, 30, 36–38, 48
Cyst(s), 13, 78, 177, 243, 522, 749, 750, 756, 759, 763–765, 767, 770, 1133, 1343, 1383, 1412, 1448, 1460, 1461, 1477, 1493, 1516, 1554, 1555, 1639, 1646, 1652, 1666, 1667, 1690, 1755, 1782, 1824, 1853, 1859, 1871, 1875, 1883–1885, 1935, 1958, 2029
Cystatin C, 615, 845, 998, 1037, 1042
Cysticercosis, 750, 762, 764, 768
Cytokeratins, 92, 102, 103, 322, 795, 1396, 1398, 1458, 1510, 1529, 1530, 1539, 1647, 1648, 1775, 1776, 1802, 1829, 1837, 1843, 1852, 1853, 1879, 1908, 1984, 1997, 2057, 2058, 2061, 2093
Cytokines, 243, 247, 248, 441, 517, 567–569, 641, 649, 689, 690, 710, 718, 719, 786, 816, 843, 869, 881, 885, 1089, 1092, 1215–1217, 1219, 1256, 1257, 1269, 1272, 1282, 1284, 1294, 1296, 1306, 1311–1313, 1317, 1492, 1788–1791, 1924
Cytomegalovirus, 107, 414, 451, 693, 695, 697, 700, 702, 715, 720, 721, 723

Cytoplasm, 19, 54, 84, 95, 99, 103, 194, 226–228, 245, 247, 250, 258, 385, 699, 701, 703, 717, 728, 732, 837, 839, 844, 851, 860, 865, 1034, 1157, 1158, 1273, 1275, 1284, 1297, 1300, 1341, 1343, 1344, 1346, 1353, 1354, 1362, 1364, 1386, 1397, 1456, 1475, 1479, 1506, 1534, 1556, 1579, 1584, 1588, 1589, 1591, 1597, 1601, 1605, 1606, 1609, 1613, 1615, 1618, 1621, 1622, 1629, 1646, 1652, 1655, 1661, 1662, 1669, 1679, 1682, 1689–1691, 1740, 1742, 1753, 1754, 1770, 1771, 1773, 1776, 1794, 1796, 1798, 1799, 1804, 1806, 1807, 1812, 1843, 1850, 1853, 1855, 1868, 1871, 1872, 1875, 1878–1881, 1903, 1927, 1933, 1938, 1939, 1944, 1945, 1958, 1962, 1965, 1967, 1969, 1979, 1982, 1985, 1989, 1990, 2009, 2012, 2013, 2016, 2020, 2025, 2027, 2028, 2057, 2062, 2063, 2076, 2085, 2086, 2094, 2097, 2113, 2127, 2160, 2172
Cytoplasmic dense bodies, 241, 249
Cytotoxic activities, 1934
Cytotoxic T-cells, 1297, 1894, 2151, 2159, 2165, 2167

D

D2-40, 102, 105, 1867, 2058, 2060, 2062, 2096, 2112
DAO, 1050
Dark neurons, 458
Data analysis, 21, 32, 33
Death receptors, 1294–1296, 1302, 1303
Death signals, 1294–1296, 1302, 1303
Declarative/explicit memory, 2155
Decussation of the medial lemniscus, 312
Decussatio pyramidum, 160
Definite CJD, 797, 816
Dehydration, 76, 79, 1235
Delayed tumor blushing, 1958
Deletion, 111, 113, 114, 250, 629, 632, 881, 882, 925, 1014–1016, 1092, 1135, 1137, 1178, 1179, 1219, 1266, 1284, 1285, 1287, 1288, 1290, 1304, 1305, 1307, 1308, 1322–1328, 1337, 1349, 1350, 1353, 1364, 1399, 1402, 1411, 1417, 1420, 1443, 1447, 1448, 1458, 1459, 1464, 1466, 1476, 1484, 1491, 1541, 1550, 1561, 1565, 1575, 1582, 1596, 1630, 1657, 1662, 1686, 1692, 1701–1703, 2054
Dementia
 in Parkinson disease, 826
 pugilistica, 826, 828, 836, 846, 865
Dementia lacking distinctive histopathology (DLDH), 825, 855
Dementia with Lewy bodies (DLB), 843, 848, 932, 933, 935, 990, 1002, 1007, 1892, 1893, 1913
Demyelinating encephalopathy, 2153
Dendrites, 93–95, 226–228, 230, 233, 235, 268, 269, 278, 287, 289, 292, 293, 296, 299, 301, 302, 304, 313, 316, 326, 342, 344, 346–349, 351, 353, 458, 693, 716, 818, 836, 837, 844, 859, 873, 918–920, 1154, 1161, 1212, 1247

Dendritic cells, 342, 344, 816, 819, 909, 1300, 1894, 1934, 1945
Dendritic spines, 28, 226, 268, 305, 342, 394, 1134
Denial of blindness, 208, 209, 413, 476
Density, 3, 5–7, 9, 11–13, 106, 233, 235, 241, 246, 269, 273, 278, 292, 298, 305, 461, 542, 615, 715–719, 843, 863, 877, 886, 901, 914, 916, 918, 920, 937, 1042, 1086, 1129, 1134, 1213, 1217, 1218, 1233, 1253–1257, 1268, 1270, 1278, 1279, 1300, 1367, 1386, 1397, 1489, 1492, 1504, 1521, 1534, 1538, 1618, 1624, 1743, 1804, 1841, 1998, 2167
Dentate gyrus, 138, 267, 294, 295, 297, 298, 325, 346, 347, 350, 387, 850, 855, 856, 861, 875, 960, 965, 966, 1042, 1134, 1147–1152, 1159, 1257
Dentate nucleus, 72, 74, 76, 163, 165, 267, 319, 355, 622, 625, 858, 859, 863, 865, 964, 976, 977, 1935, 1943, 2168, 716857
Dentate-rubro-pallido-lysian atrophy, 851
Dentato-rubro-pallido-luysii degeneration, 825, 828, 858–859
Dentato-rubro-pallido-nigral degeneration, 828, 858
Deoxyhemoglobin (dHBO2), 20, 1215
Dependence, 11, 1224, 1260, 1294, 1295, 1317
Dephasing, 11
Depression or anxiety, 942
Depurination, 1266, 1285
Depyrimidination, 1266, 1285
Dermoid cyst
 age incidence, 1833
 biologic behavior-prognosis-prognostic factors, 1841
 CT-contrast-enhanced, 1833
 CT-non contrast-enhanced, 1833
 differential diagnosis, 1837, 1841
 general imaging findings, 1833
 immunophenotype, 1837–1840
 incidence, 1833
 localization, 1833
 macroscopic features, 1836–1837
 microscopic features, 1836–1837
 MRI-diffusion imaging, 1834–1836
 MRI-FLAIR, 1833–1836
 MRI-perfusion, 1834–1836
 MRI-T1, 1833–1836
 MRI-T2, 1833–1836
 MRI-T1 contrast-enhanced, 1834–1836
 MRI-T2∗/ SWI, 1836
 MR-spectroscopy, 1834–1836
 pathogenesis, 1837
 proliferation markers, 1837
 sex incidence, 1833
 treatment, 1837
 ultrastructural features, 1837
 WHO definition, 1833
Descending limbic pathways, 325, 343, 346
Desinhibition-Dementia-Parkinsonism-amyotrophy-complex, 825
Desmin, 102, 108, 113, 1396, 1624, 1775, 1776, 1985, 1986, 2058, 2061, 2062, 2084, 2096, 2100, 2115

Desmoglein, 2092
Desmoid-type fibromatosis, 1956, 1985
Desmoplasia, 87, 1265, 1274, 1275, 1557, 1618
Desmoplastic astrocytoma/ganglioglioma
    age incidence, 1554
    biologic behavior-prognosis-prognostic factors, 1559
    CT-contrast-enhanced, 1554
    CT-non contrast-enhanced, 1554
    desmoplastic infantile astrocytoma (DIA), 1553
    desmoplastic infantile ganglioglioma (DIG), 1553
    differential diagnosis, 1559
    general imaging findings, 1554–1559
    immunophenotype, 1557–1558
    incidence, 1554
    localization, 1554
    macroscopic features, 1554–1555
    microscopic features, 1555–1557
    molecular neuropathology, 1559
    MRI–FLAIR, 1554
    MRI-T1, 1554
    MRI-T2, 1554
    MRI-T1 contrast-enhanced, 1554
    MRI-T2∗/SWI, 1554
    MR–spectroscopy, 1554
    nuclear medicine imaging findings, 1554
    pathogenesis, 1559
    proliferation markers, 1558
    sex incidence, 1554
    treatment, 1559
    ultrastructural features, 1558–1559
    WHO definition, 1553–1554
    WHO grade, 1554
Deterministic effects, 38
Devic disease, 1072, 1097, 2173
Diagnostic neuroradiology, 4, 27
Diaphragma sellae, 166, 180, 224, 252
Diastase-sensitive PAS/PAS with diastase digestion, 83–84
Diencephalon, 76, 129, 150–156, 169, 174, 267, 305–306, 376, 380, 381, 385, 820, 1223, 1227, 2170
Diethylenetriaminepentaacetate (DTPA), 15, 39, 1664, 1969
Difficulty with initiating contralateral arm movements, 405
Diffuse axonal injury (DAI), 828, 1185, 1207–1211, 1217, 1218
Diffuse large B-cell lymphoma of the CNS
    age incidence, 1895
    biologic behavior-prognosis-prognostic factors, 1913
    CT-contrast-enhanced, 1895–1897
    CT-non contrast-enhanced, 1895–1897
    differential diagnosis, 1904, 1909
    DNA methylation, (AU: Not found)
    epigenetics, (AU: Not found)
    gene expression, (AU: Not found)
    general imaging findings, 1895
    genetics, (AU: Not found)
    immunophenotype, 1902–1912
    incidence, 1895
    localization, 1895
    macroscopic features, 1899–1900
    microRNAs, (AU: Not found)
    microscopic features, 1901–1904
    molecular neuropathology, 1913
    MRI-diffusion imaging, 1895–1897
    MRI-diffusion tensor imaging, 1895–1897
    MRI–FLAIR, 1895–1897
    MRI–perfusion, 1895–1897
    MRI–T1, 1895–1897
    MRI–T2, 1895–1897
    MRI–T1 contrast-enhanced, 1895–1897
    MRI–T2∗/ SWI, 1895
    MR-spectroscopy, 1897
    nuclear medicine imaging findings, 1897–1899
    pathogenesis, 1909, 1913
    proliferation markers, 1901–1904
    sex incidence, 1895
    treatment, 1913
    ultrastructural features, 1904
    WHO definition, 1892, 1895
    WHO grade, 1892, 1895
Diffuse/multifocal TBI, 1187
Diffuse necrotizing leukoencephalopathy, 2119, 2128
Diffuse neurofibrillary tangles with calcifications (DNTC), 825, 857
Digital subtractive angiography (DSA), 479, 510, 513, 538, 539, 552, 553, 556, 559, 579, 586, 596, 640, 642, 1716, 1958, 1959, 1970
Diplopia, 418, 640, 725, 988, 1073, 1267
Direct pathway, 339, 346, 347, 349, 1012
Discogram, 4
Discontinuous capillary, 257
Disease-free survival (DFS), 1265, 1270
Disinterest, 417
Disorientation, 209, 406, 413, 520, 1186, 2154, 2156, 2159
Disrupted axonal transport, 845
Dissection of large arteries, 845
Disturbed sleep/wake rhythm, 820
Disturbed speech understanding, 134, 409
Dizziness, 9, 474, 520, 658, 1071, 1073, 1186, 1490
D1-like receptors, 50
D2-like receptors, 50
DNA damage
    recognition, 1285–1286
    repair, 1266, 1286–1287
DNA damage responses (DDR), 1265, 1266, 1281, 1285–1288, 1304
DNA-dependent protein kinase (DNA-PK), 1285–1288
DNA integrity, 1281, 1283
DNA methylation, 642, 648, 889, 925, 1001, 1017, 1067, 1068, 1090, 1266, 1309, 1310, 1323, 1328, 1368, 1403, 1707, 1748
DNA probe, 111
DNA repair pathways, 1281
DNA replication, 107, 1280, 1282, 1283, 1285, 1288, 1304
DNA replication errors, 1266, 1285
DNAses, 471, 648, 1296, 1298

DNA viruses, 694, 699, 720–722
Dominant hemisphere syndromes, 401, 413
Dopamine
    receptors, 50, 304, 305, 339, 380, 873, 1001, 1012, 1018
    transporter, 29, 33, 49, 54, 377, 897, 932, 935, 975, 1004, 1023, 1220, 1256, 1258
Dopamine b-hydroxylase (DBH), 376, 381, 384, 1220
Dopamine-2 receptor, 2174, 2176
Dopamine 2 receptor antibody syndrome (D2RA), 2151, 2158–2159
Dopaminergic system, 50, 506, 864, 935, 1226, 1244, 1256–1258
Dopamine transporter (DAT), 29, 49, 50, 372, 373, 1220, 1226, 1245, 1256, 1258
Dorsal columns-medial lemniscus system, 342
Dorsal longitudinal fasciculus, 343, 355
Dorsal, parieto-frontal network, 291
Dorsal stream, 328, 332, 333, 357–359, 361, 409
Dorso-dorsal (d-d) stream, 332
Dorsomedial and midline thalamic nuclei, 352
Dorsomedial area, 333
Dosimeters, 38, 39
Dot blot, 57, 112, 113
Double-strand break repair (DSBR), 1266, 1286–1287
Double-strand breaks (DSBs), 1285, 1286, 1288
Down syndrome, 825, 836–838, 846, 856, 897, 921, 1130
DPD, 1990
D2R, 2153, 2159
Draining veins, 213, 219, 254, 578
D2 receptor, 29, 50–51, 54, 449, 976, 1007, 1025, 1027, 1060, 1220, 1226, 1245, 1785, 1786, 1811
D2 receptor ligands, 29, 50–51
D3 receptors, 50, 1256
Dressing apraxia, 401, 406, 413
Δ^9-tetrahydrocannabinol (THC), 1244, 1256–1258
Dural AV-fistula, 599–602
Dural sinuses
    cavernous sinus, 183–185
    inferior sagittal sinus, 182–184
    occipital sinus, 184, 185
    sigmoid sinus, 182–185
    sphenoparietal sinus, 182–185
    straight sinus, 182, 184
    superior and inferior petrosal sinuses, 184, 185
    superior sagittal sinus, 182–186
    transverse sinus, 182–185
"Dural tail," 1666, 1709, 1714, 1783, 1958
Dura mater, 60, 65, 67, 166, 179–186, 188, 203, 211, 218, 221, 225, 252, 253, 520, 521, 525, 529, 530, 796, 862, 1187, 1269, 1554, 1654, 1679, 1718, 1730, 1810, 1934, 1935, 1941, 1944
Dynein, 229, 1093
Dynorphin, 301, 349, 370, 371, 1256
Dysarthria, 207, 208, 404, 420, 475, 622, 654, 694, 751, 774, 819, 820, 858, 865, 945, 967, 974, 988, 1022, 1038, 1039, 1073, 1212, 1224, 1233, 1239, 1935, 2172, 2174

Dysautonomia, 1022, 1034, 2156, 2158
Dysembryoplastic neuroepithelial tumor (DNT)
    age incidence, 1542
    biologic behavior-prognosis-prognostic factors, 1550
    CT-contrast-enhanced, 1542
    CT-non contrast-enhanced, 1542
    differential diagnosis, 1545, 1550
    DNT-complex form, 1543
    DNT-simple form, 1543
    general imaging findings, 1542–1550
    immunophenotype, 1545, 1548–1550
    incidence, 1542
    localization, 1542
    macroscopic features, 1542
    microscopic features, 1543, 1545–1547
    molecular neuropathology, 1550
    MRI-diffusion imaging, 1542
    MRI-FLAIR, 1542–1545
    MRI-perfusion, 1542
    MRI-T1, 1542–1545
    MRI-T2, 1542, 1543
    MRI-T1 contrast-enhanced, 1542–1545
    MRI-T2∗/ SWI, 1542
    MR-spectroscopy, 1542, 1544
    nuclear medicine imaging findings, 1542
    pathogenesis, 1550
    proliferation markers, 1545
    sex incidence, 1542
    treatment, 1550
    ultrastructural features, 1545
    WHO definition, 1541–1542
    WHO grade, 1542
Dysesthesias, 209
Dyskinesia (Hyperkinesia-Hypotonia syndrome), 207, 388, 416, 476, 1001, 1002, 1018, 1136, 2155, 2156, 2170
Dyslamination, 1159, 1164, 1166, 1168
Dysmorphic neurons, 1157, 1158, 1160, 1163, 1164, 1168, 1562
Dysmyelination, 1072
Dysnomic aphasia, 208, 476
Dysphagia, 207, 404, 475, 731, 820, 865, 945, 946, 967, 974, 980, 988, 1002, 1022, 1038, 1039, 1060, 1073, 1224, 1233, 1935, 2160, 2174
Dysphoric angiopathy, 607
Dysplasia, 85, 94, 606, 997, 1119, 1121, 1130, 1132, 1157–1161, 1168, 1175, 1541, 1542, 1545, 1550, 1554, 1563, 1694, 1990–1993, 1995, 2018, 2019, 2021
Dysplastic ganglion cells, 1561, 1562, 1572
Dyspnoea, (AU: Not found)
Dystonia, 416, 818, 828, 838, 858, 973, 974, 980, 984, 1014, 1016, 1060, 1245, 1255, 1914, 2153, 2156, 2158, 2159, 2170
Dystroglycan 1 (DAG1), 236
Dystrophic calcifications, 484, 2126–2128
Dystrophic neuritis, 836, 837, 954, 958, 959

E

Early onset AD (EOAD), 898, 899, 901, 923
Early subacute, 500, 501
Eastern equine encephalitis, 696, 737
Echo time (TE), 12
Ecstasy, 1244, 1259, 1260
Ectonucleoside triphosphate diphosphohydrolase 2 (ENTPD2), 241, 887
Ectopia, 1771
Edema
    cytotoxic edema, 427–430, 432, 439–441, 457, 477
    interstitial edema, 427, 1338, 1354
    osmotic edema, 427, 428
    vasogenic edema, 427–429, 432, 439–441, 1369
EEG epileptic discharges, 1120
Efferent pathway, 121, 295, 325, 342
EGF family, 370
EGFR amplification, 1322, 1323, 1329, 1353, 1365, 1401, 1402, 1417, 1420, 1575, 1582
EGFR/ERBB1, 1289
EGFRvIII expression, 1329
Elastic artery, 254, 255
Elastica van Gieson, 87, 511, 1393, 1734
Elastic fibers, 87, 88, 252, 255, 256, 538, 540, 585, 1393
Electroencephalography, 402, 862, 1144
Electromagnetic field, 37
Electron microscopy, 57, 58, 77, 108, 109, 237, 241, 632, 717, 797, 816
Electrons, 15, 30, 31, 41–43, 57, 58, 77, 108, 109, 111, 114, 227–229, 237, 241, 257, 321, 629, 630, 632, 703, 717, 797, 816, 838, 845, 879, 924, 1016, 1045, 1343, 1438, 1444, 1454, 1771, 1850, 1969
Elephantiasis neuromatosa, 1677
Elevated intracranial pressure (ICP), 465, 1218, 1267
EMA dot-like reactivities, 1496, 1501
Embedding, 79, 80, 91
Embolization, 585, 589, 1716, 2119
Embryonal carcinoma
    CT-contrast-enhanced, 1875
    CT-non contrast-enhanced, 1875
    differential diagnosis, 1879
    general imaging findings, 1875–1879
    immunophenotype, 1877–1879
    macroscopic features, 1877
    microscopic features, 1877–1879
    MRI-diffusion imaging, 1877
    MRI-FLAIR, 1876, 1877
    MRI-T1, 1877
    MRI-T2, 1876, 1877
    MRI-T1 contrast-enhanced, 1877
    MRI-T2*/ SWI, 1877
    MR-spectroscopy, 1877
    ultrastructural features, 1879
    WHO definition, 1875
Embryonal tumors
    CNS embryonal tumor (NOS), 1638
    CNS embryonal tumor with rhabdoid features, 1638
    CNS Ewing sarcoma family tumor with CIC alteration (CNS EFT-CIC), 1638
    CNS ganglioneuroblastoma, 1638
    CNS high-grade neuroepithelial tumor with BCOR alterations (CNS HGNET-BCOR), 1638
    CNS high-grade neuroepithelial tumor with MN1 alteration (CNS HGNET-MN1), 1638
    CNS neuroblastoma, 1638
    CNS neuroblastoma with FOXR2 activation (CNS NB-FOXR2), 1638
    medulloepithelioma, 1638
    with multilayered rosettes (ETMR), C19MC-altered, 1638
    with multilayered rosettes, NOS, 1638
Embryonal tumour with multilayered rosettes, C19MC-altered
    age incidence, 1646
    biologic behavior-prognosis-prognostic factors, 1647
    differential diagnosis, 1647
    immunophenotype, 1646–1647
    incidence, 1646
    localization, 1646
    macroscopic features, 1646
    microscopic features, 1646
    molecular neuropathology, 1647
    pathogenesis, 1647
    proliferation markers, 1647
    sex incidence, 1646
    treatment, 1647
    WHO definition, 1646
    WHO grade, 1646
Embryonic stem cells (ECS), 259, 1311–1314, 1319, 1867
Emotional lability, 722, 1073, 1224, 1233, 2159
Emotion and memory, 291
Emperipolesis, 1933, 1944, 1945
Encapsulation, 523, 1265, 1273, 1563, 1573, 1690
Encephalin, 301, 370, 836
Encephalitis, 54, 105, 653, 654, 657, 661, 666, 675, 683, 693, 694, 696–698, 700, 702, 703, 707, 714, 715, 718, 731–741, 750, 751, 760, 774, 777, 791, 827, 828, 1072, 1131, 1132, 1157, 1158, 1333, 1909, 2151–2176
Encephalitis lethargica, 2159
Encephalomyelitis, 641, 697, 1072, 1093, 1105–1115, 1918, 2153, 2154, 2170–2174
Enchondroma, 1990, 1992, 1993, 2009, 2013
Endarteritis obliterans, 687
Endfeet of glial cells, 235
Endocannabinoid (2-AG), 236
Endometrial stromal carcinoma, 2113
Endometrioid carcinoma, 2113
Endomucin (EMCN), 259
Endoneurium, 238, 1661, 1685, 1686
Endonucleases, 471, 1287, 1288
Endoplasmic reticulum (ER), 226–228, 258, 321, 471, 720, 882–883, 1013, 1045, 1051, 1052, 1178, 1299, 1343, 1454, 1510, 1559, 1787, 1793, 1871, 1879, 1880, 1904, 2060–2062, 2070, 2075, 2099, 2102, 2104, 2112, 2115
Endothelial cell adhesion molecule (ESAM), 254, 259

Endothelial cells, 97, 103, 105, 176, 225, 255–259, 294, 440, 521, 540, 542, 567, 577, 583, 593, 693, 717, 718, 863, 1092, 1229, 1244, 1256, 1259, 1272, 1278, 1309, 1311–1313, 1341, 1367, 1386, 1397, 1545, 1672, 1962, 1982, 2062, 2139
Endothelial dysfunction, 542, 551, 567, 568
Endothelial layer, 254, 255
Endothelial proliferation, 484, 493, 858, 1231, 1265, 1272, 1278, 1279, 1369, 1391, 1392, 1397, 1398, 1444, 1618
Endothelial selective adhesion molecule (ESAM), 254, 259
Endothelin-1, 517, 568, 569
Endpoints on clinical trials, 1269–1270
Energy of emission, 29, 31
Enkephalins and dynorphins, 349, 370
Enterococcus, 655–657
Enterogeneous cyst
  age incidence, 1853
  biologic behavior-prognosis-prognostic factors, 1854
  CT-contrast-enhanced, 1853
  CT-non contrast-enhanced, 1853
  differential diagnosis, 1853
  general imaging findings, 1853
  immunophenotype, 1853, 1855–1856
  incidence, 1853
  localization, 1853
  macroscopic features, 1853
  microscopic features, 1853
  MRI-diffusion imaging, 1853–1855
  MRI-FLAIR, 1853–1855
  MRI-perfusion, 1853
  MRI-T1, 1853–1855
  MRI-T2, 1853
  MRI-T1 contrast-enhanced, 1853–1855
  MRI-T2∗/ SWI, 1853
  pathogenesis, 1854
  proliferation markers, 1853
  sex incidence, 1853
  treatment, 1854
  ultrastructural features, 1853
  WHO definition, 1853
Entorhinal area, 138, 300, 325, 346–350
Entorhinal cortex, 138, 267, 300, 346, 347, 349, 351, 817, 836, 852, 855, 859, 861, 873, 918, 921, 937, 962, 965, 979, 1011, 1154, 1213, 1214
Env, 701
Environmental dependency syndrome, 405
Enzyme histochemistry, 57, 108–111
Eosinophilic granular bodies (EGB), 1433, 1438, 1439, 1584
Ependymal cell, 240, 249, 250, 255, 267, 321, 1492, 1496, 1501, 1506, 1511, 1518, 1888
Ependymoma
  age incidence, 1492
  biologic behavior-prognosis-prognostic factors, 1500
  clear cell ependymoma, 1455, 1489, 1492, 1493, 1500
  CT-contrast-enhanced, 1493
  CT-non contrast-enhanced, 1493
  differential diagnosis, 1496
  ependymoma, RELA fusion-positive, 1491, 1492
  general imaging findings, 1493
  immunophenotype, 1496
  incidence, 1492
  infratentorial ependymomas, 1490–1492
  localization, 1492
  macroscopic features, 1493, 1495, 1496
  microscopic features, 1493, 1497–1498
  molecular neuropathology, 1490–1492
  MRI-diffusion imaging, 1493
  MRI-diffusion tensor imaging, 1493
  MRI-FLAIR, 1493, 1494
  MRI-perfusion, 1493
  MRI-T1, 1493, 1494
  MRI-T2, 1493–1494
  MRI-T1 contrast-enhanced, 1493, 1494
  MRI-T2∗/ SWI, 1493
  MR-spectroscopy, 1493
  nuclear medicine imaging findings, 1493
  papillary ependymoma, 85, 1492, 1493, 1500
  pathogenesis, 1492
  proliferation markers, 1491, 1492
  sex incidence, 1492
  supratentorial ependymomas, 1490
  tanycytic ependymoma, 1489, 1492, 1493
  treatment, 1500
  ultrastructural features, 1496
  WHO definition, 1492
  WHO grade, 1492
Ependymoma anaplastic
  age incidence, 1501
  biologic behavior-prognosis-prognostic factors, 1504
  differential diagnosis, 1501
  general imaging findings, 1501
  immunophenotype, 1501
  incidence, 1501
  localization, 1501
  macroscopic features, 1501
  microscopic features, 1501, 1503–1504
  pathogenesis, 1501
  proliferation markers, 1501, 1505–1506
  sex incidence, 1501
  treatment, 1501
  ultrastructural features, 1501
  WHO definition, 1500
  WHO grade, 1500
Ependymoma myxopapillary
  age incidence, 1506
  biologic behavior-prognosis-prognostic factors, 1511
  CT-contrast-enhanced, 1507
  CT-non contrast-enhanced, 1507
  differential diagnosis, 1510
  general imaging findings, 1507
  immunophenotype, 1508–1510
  incidence, 1506
  localization, 1507
  macroscopic features, 1508
  microscopic features, 1508–1510

Index

MRI-FLAIR, (AU: Not found)
MRI-T1, 1507
MRI-T2, 1507
MRI-T1 contrast-enhanced, 1507, 1508
  pathogenesis, 1510
  proliferation markers, 1508–1510
  sex incidence, 1507
  treatment, 1510
  ultrastructural features, 1510
  WHO definition, 1506
  WHO grade, 1506
Epidermal growth factor (EGF), 241, 629, 816, 1289, 1306, 1313, 1315, 1349, 1399, 1400, 1405, 1469, 1476, 1484, 2055, 2057, 2171, 2174
Epidermal growth factor receptor (EGFR), 92, 241, 629, 630, 632, 1289, 1305–1039, 1313, 1322–1324, 1326, 1327, 1329, 1331, 1349, 1350, 1353, 1365, 1368, 1395, 1399–1403, 1408, 1417, 1420, 1476, 1484, 1575, 1582, 1591, 1789, 1979, 1996, 1997, 2055–2057, 2075, 2084, 2095
Epidermoid cyst
  age incidence, 1824
  biologic behavior-prognosis-prognostic factors, 1831
  CT-contrast-enhanced, 1824
  CT-non contrast-enhanced, 1824–1827
  differential diagnosis, 1829
  general imaging findings, 1824
  immunophenotype, 1829
  incidence, 1824
  localization, 1824
  macroscopic features, 1827, 1829, 1831
  microscopic features, 1829, 1832–1833
  MRI-diffusion imaging, 1824–1828
  MRI-FLAIR, 1824–1827
  MRI-perfusion, 1827
  MRI-T1, 1825–1827
  MRI-T2, 1824–1827
  MRI-T1 contrast-enhanced, 1825–1827
  MRI-T2*/ SWI, 1827
  pathogenesis, 1829
  proliferation markers, 1829
  sex incidence, 1824
  treatment, 1834
  ultrastructural features, 1829
  WHO definition, 1824
Epidural hemorrhage, 60, 499, 500, 529–533, 1196
Epidural injection, 4
Epigenetics, 880, 889, 890, 895, 925–926, 1001, 1017–1018, 1034, 1067–1068, 1266, 1267, 1309–1310, 1326–1328, 1337, 1349, 1403, 1417, 1420, 1444, 1459, 1466, 1491, 1631–1634, 1654, 1657, 1703, 1707, 1748–1749, 1929
Epilepsies, 1119–1139, 1143–1154, 1157–1169, 1171–1179
  genes, 1119, 1135
Epileptic seizure, 858, 1120–1122, 1124, 1139
Epileptic spike focus, 1120

Epileptogenesis, 1120, 1134, 1135
Epileptogenicity, 1120
Epileptogenic lesion, 401, 410, 1120, 1121
Epileptogenic zone or region, 1120–1121
Epineurium, 238, 239, 1689, 1690
Epiretinal membrane, 1662, 1699, 1700
Epithalamus, 138, 155–156, 381
Epithelial membrane antigen (EMA), 102–104, 108, 1137, 1338, 1396, 1398, 1455, 1458, 1496, 1499, 1501, 1505, 1508, 1516, 1529, 1530, 1539, 1557, 1647, 1648, 1654, 1681, 1684, 1686, 1689, 1734, 1742, 1744–1746, 1750, 1770, 1776, 1823, 1829, 1837, 1843, 1852, 1853, 1859, 1861, 1867, 1908, 1966, 1997, 2022, 2058–2061, 2075, 2088, 2096, 2112, 2114, 2115
Epithelioid hemangioendothelioma, 1956, 1982, 1991, 1992
Epithelium, 177, 225, 240, 249, 254, 267, 321, 322, 1297, 1522, 1523, 1530, 1534, 1637–1639, 1647, 1648, 1690, 1692, 1754, 1757, 1759, 1762, 1765, 1810, 1813, 1823, 1824, 1829, 1832, 1833, 1836–1838, 1841, 1843, 1844, 1850, 1853, 1855, 1866, 1887, 1889, 1934, 2088, 2107, 2111
Epitheloid GBM, 1386, 1396, 1402
Epitheloid macrophages, 687
Epstein-Barr virus (EBV), 107, 636, 697, 698, 1092, 1322, 1892–1894, 1907–1909, 1912, 1914, 1919, 1920, 1923, 1924, 1986
Erdheim chester disease
  CT-contrast-enhanced, 1943
  CT-non contrast-enhanced, 1943
  general imaging findings, 1943–1948
  MRI-FLAIR, 1943
  MRI-T1, 943
  MRI-T2, 1943
  nuclear medicine imaging findings, 1943
ERG, 105, 1090, 1982, 1984, 2060, 2095
Erosion of calvaria, 1958
ER/PR (tamoxifen for breast cancer), 91
Escherichia coli, 655, 657, 702
Estrogen receptor, 104, 1459, 1466, 1759, 1787, 2054, 2060, 2062, 2070, 2073
Ethanol, 77, 79, 91, 1224–1228, 1240
Ethyl cysteine dimer (ECD), 39, 51, 52, 54, 697, 802, 901, 1125
Euascomycetes, 774
Evasion of cell death, 1281
Evasion of growth inhibitory signals, 1265, 1279, 1281
Event-free survival (EFS), 1270, 1940
Event-related design, 21
Ewing sarcoma/peripheral primitive neuroectodermal tumour, 1956, 1984
Ewing's saroma RNA-binding protein1 (EWSR1), 844, 1049, 1984
Excessive daytime sleepiness, 942, 1002
Excitatory transmitters, 369
Excitotoxicity, 845
Execution of movement, 404

Executive function, 291, 402–404, 417, 626, 826, 843, 878, 899, 932, 1239
Executive function and comportment, 291
Exophytic growth, 1542
Exotic ruminant spongiform encephalopathy, 797
External band of Baillarger, 289
External magnetic field, 10, 11, 15
External regulatory circuits, 325, 349–350
Extracellular lipid (cholesterol and cholesterol esters), 538, 542, 558
Extracellular matrix, 235, 255, 519, 538, 540, 542, 567, 569, 815, 1267, 1313, 1314, 1491, 1990, 2025
Extra-pyramidal symptoms, 819, 2152
Extrapyramidal system, 334, 921
Extrastriate visual cortex, 294, 333
Extrinsic death receptor pathway, 1296
Ezrin, 1701, 1702, 1977, 1979

F

FA, 1101, 1370, 1375, 1709, 1895
Fabry disease, 496, 998
Face and object recognition, 291, 946
Facetiousness ("Witzelsucht" or moria), 405
Facial, 24, 123, 158, 182, 191, 203, 207–209, 213, 215, 219, 220, 310, 311, 361, 405, 409, 416, 475, 476, 862, 998, 1186, 1237, 1239, 1240, 1671
Facial nerve, 158, 209, 310
Factor VIII, 102, 103, 717, 1948, 2058, 2062
Factor XIIIa, 1966
Fahr disease, 605, 606, 622–626, 857
Falling to the side of the lesion, 208
Falx cerebri, 129, 180–185, 188, 219–223, 252, 436
Familial ALS, 965, 1050, 1051, 1053, 1054
Familial amyloidosis-finnish type, 615
Familial amyloidotic polyneuropathy/meningovascular amyloidosis, 615
Familial British dementia, 615, 837, 845
Familial (genetic) Creutzfeldt-Jakob-Disease (fCJD), 795, 803
Familial Danish dementia, 615, 837
Familial idiopathic basal ganglia calcification, 605, 622
Familial myotrophic lateral sclerosis, 1037
Familial presenile dementia with tangles (FPDT), 825, 856
Fascicles, 125, 127, 147, 148, 160, 162, 239, 677, 963, 1492, 1510, 1556, 1557, 1671, 1681, 1685, 1690, 1729, 1753, 1754, 1771, 1773, 1776, 1905, 1955, 1962, 1985
Fascicular atrophy, 1042
Fasciculus gracilis, fasciculus cuneatus, 342
Fascin, 105, 1908, 2106
Fast axoplasmic flow, 228
Fatal familial Insomnia (FFI), 795, 797, 820
Fatty streak, 538
18F-desmethoxyfallypride (DMFP), 29, 50
Feline spongiform encephalopathy (FSE), 796, 797
Fenestrated capillary, 257, 1765
Ferroptosis, 1266, 1293, 1300
Ferruginated neurons, 458

Fetal alcohol spectrum disorders (FASD), 1224, 1237–1240
FET-PET, 48, 665, 667, 1341, 1358, 1378, 1414, 1420, 1437, 1452–1455, 1473, 1481, 1579, 1598, 1664, 1760, 1785, 1811, 1969, 2042, 2124, 2125, 2140, 2141, 2144, 2147
FET proteins, 844
18F-fallypride, 29, 50, 51, 976, 1007, 1028
18F-fluorodeoxyglucose-positron emission tomography (FDG-PET), 34, 44–48, 50, 54, 434, 458, 464, 478, 482, 483, 501, 506, 510, 521, 538, 541, 607, 609, 616, 622, 629, 640, 641, 665, 667, 697, 767, 802–804, 851–853, 872, 873, 899, 901, 902, 932, 935, 947, 949, 976, 990, 992, 1005, 1007, 1022, 1025, 1028, 1040–1042, 1060, 1062, 1063, 1077, 1128, 1144, 1146, 1147, 1158, 1161, 1192, 1194, 1226, 1227, 1245, 1340, 1412, 1454, 1455, 1563, 1652, 1663, 1665, 1824, 1832, 1858, 1859, 1897–1899, 1914, 1925, 1926, 1934, 1961, 2042, 2120, 2124, 2125, 2162, 2163
[18F]fluoroethyl)-L-tyrosine (FET), 48, 54, 665, 667, 849, 899, 1077, 1340, 1341, 1354, 1356, 1380, 1381, 1412, 1419, 1430, 1450, 1451, 1462, 1470, 1473, 1477, 1490, 1596, 1663, 1716, 1717, 1722, 1755, 1811, 1866, 1898, 1938, 2042, 2050, 2120, 2125, 2137
18F-FMISO, 1381
F18-FMISO, 1969
Fiber type grouping, 1042
Fibrae corticonucleares, 156
Fibrae parietotemporopontinae, 156
Fibrae pontinae, 156
Fibrillary astrocytes, 240, 1341, 1344
Fibrinoid necrosis, 609, 614, 1113, 2126, 2128
Fibrinoid vascular necrosis, 2126, 2128
Fibroatheroma, 538, 540
Fibroblasts, 97, 241, 248, 252, 255, 257, 521, 529, 568, 585, 684, 1093, 1274, 1289, 1311, 1313, 1431, 1555–1557, 1559, 1648, 1661, 1677, 1679, 1682, 1789, 1985, 1990, 2029, 2032
Fibromuscular dysplasia, 606, 997
Fibromuscular dysplasia/hyperplasia, 1694
Fibrosarcoma, 1414, 1683, 1692, 1701, 1956, 1964, 1979, 1985, 1991, 1992, 2007
Fibrosis, 60, 87, 607, 641, 687, 768, 849, 861, 862, 1101, 1559, 1795, 1798, 1800, 1933, 1944, 1951, 1962, 1984, 2119, 2126, 2128
Fibrous cap, 538, 540
Fibrous dysplasia
  CT-non contrast-enhanced, 2018
  differential diagnosis, 2018
  general imaging findings, 2018
  localization, 2018
  macroscopic features, 2018, 2021–2022
  microscopic features, 2018, 2021–2022
  MRI-T1, 2018–2020
  MRI-T2, 2018–2020
  MRI-T1 contrast-enhanced, 2018
  WHO definition, 2018

Fiducial coordinate system, 23
Filaments, 95–97, 103, 839, 849, 954, 956, 966, 1084, 1624, 2057
Filariasis, 750
Filtered back projection, 5, 7, 40, 42, 50, 52
Filtering methods, 33
Filum teminale, 1507
Finger agnosia, 406, 413
Fixation, 58–79, 91, 185, 841, 1793
Flair sign, 477, 1153
Flaviviridae, 695, 696, 736
Fleecy, lake-like deposits, 834, 836, 844
Flexner-Wintersteiner rosette, 1274, 1606, 1609
Florbetaben, 53, 854
Florbetapir, 53, 854
Florid plaques, 812, 818, 819
Flow
　compensation techniques, 13
　voids, 444, 445, 447, 552, 578, 1370, 1523, 1576, 1958, 1969
Flow-sensitive pulse sequences, 11
Fluency, 133, 403, 405, 413, 419, 420
Fluid attenuated inversion recovery (FLAIR) sequence, 12, 126, 132, 429, 444, 457, 477, 499, 501, 552, 578, 607, 640, 659, 696, 752, 775, 795, 870, 896, 947, 974, 990, 1022, 1039, 1060, 1074, 1098, 1106, 1125, 1144, 1158, 1172, 1192, 1225, 1246, 1338, 1354, 1370, 1412, 1428, 1434, 1448, 1470, 1493, 1523, 1542, 1563, 1576, 1584, 1597, 1615, 1640, 1652, 1666, 1709, 1755, 1782, 1824, 1869, 1895, 1935, 1958, 2000, 2038, 2120, 2132, 2153 (AU: More than 350 instances. We have picked the first instance page numbers from each chapter and where the term is explained in detail)
Fluorescence microscopy, 57, 108, 111, 114, 840
Fluoride-18, 30
Fluorine-18 fluoro-2-deoxyglucose (FDG), 29, 31, 32, 44, 48, 50, 52, 54, 432, 458, 541, 641, 665, 697, 735, 739, 767, 872, 873, 935, 980, 1023, 1060, 1077, 1101, 1106, 1128, 1193, 1354, 1380, 1412, 1419, 1435, 1450, 1454, 1462, 1470, 1477, 1490, 1522, 1542, 1554, 1563, 1576, 1615, 1642, 1664, 1716, 1719, 1755, 1897, 1899, 1925, 1934, 1936, 1938, 1961, 1994, 2005, 2042, 2050, 2120, 2125, 2137
Fluoroscopy, 3, 4
Flutemetamol, 53, 54, 609, 854
Foam cells, 538, 540, 2018
Focal cerebral ischemia, 987
Focal cortical dysplasia (FCD), 94, 1119, 1130, 1132, 1157–1169, 1175, 1550
Focal epilepsy, 52, 606, 637, 1124, 1125, 1138
Focal neurologic deficit, 653, 654, 694, 715, 749, 751, 762, 774, 988, 1267
Focal TBI, 1187
Follicle-stimulating hormone (FSH), 108, 371, 1087, 1754, 1780, 1781, 1787, 1791, 1794, 1796, 1803, 1804, 1806, 1812
Follicular dendritic cells (FDC), 816, 1934
Foramen magnum, 61, 160, 182, 223, 224, 436
Fore population, 820
Foresight, 404
Forkhead box P2 (FOXP2), 291, 925
Formaldehyde, 64, 77, 91
Formalin-fixed, paraffin-embedded (FFPE), 79
Fornix, 148, 152, 155, 167, 205, 307, 343, 347, 348, 350, 352, 358, 375, 449, 1144
Fossa interpeduncularis, 156
Fourth ventricle
　lateral aperture, 174
　medial aperture, 174
Fovea centralis, 326
FPCIT, 933, 935, 1226
Freckling, 1662, 1663, 1693, 1694
Free induction decay (FID), 10
Free radicals, 883, 1216
Free ribosomes, 226, 258, 1591
Fregoli phenomenon, 423
Frenulum veli medullare, 174
Friedreich ataxia, 826, 851, 857, 1035
Frontal
　cortical release reflexes, 208
　lobes
　　dysfunction, 443
　　syndrome, 1237
　medial gyrus, 76
　poles, 60, 62, 130, 135, 404–405, 1196
　release signs, 207, 475
Fronto-temporal dementia (FTD), 826–828, 835, 837, 838, 842, 845, 847, 849, 850–855, 859, 901, 945–947, 950, 954, 957–959, 964, 966, 968, 974, 990, 1042, 1050–1055
Fronto-temporal dementia complex, 826
Fronto-temporal lobar degeneration
　with C9ORF mutation, 953, 959
　with FUS proteinopathy, 954, 965–966
　with GRN mutation, 953, 958–959
　with MAPT mutation, 954, 965
　with motor neuron disease type inclusions, 953, 956–958
　with no inclusions, 954, 967–968
　with tauopathy, 953, 960
　with TDP-43 proteinopathy, 953–956
　with ubiquitin-positive inclusions, 849, 954, 960, 966, 967
　with VCP mutation, 953, 959
Fronto-temporal lobe dementia (FTLD), 849, 850, 854, 945, 954–968
FTD-behavioral variant, 945, 947
FTD with motor neuron disease/ALS, 945
Full-field optical coherence microscopy, 114
Functional deficit zone, 1121
Functional genomics microarray, 111, 114
Functional MRI (fMRI), 3, 20–22, 123, 328, 336, 402, 411, 1121
Fungi, 89, 90, 657, 702, 749, 773–792
Fungus cerebri, 427, 436, 438
Fusiform cells, 268, 269, 287, 289, 1369, 1420, 1434

G

GABA$_A$ receptors, 242, 283, 391, 458, 478, 501, 510, 521, 538, 1134, 1135, 1138, 1139, 1146, 1168, 2159, 2173
GABA-B-R, 2153, 2171
GABA$_B$-receptor (B1 subunit), 391, 2159, 2173, 2175
GABA-ergic interneurons, 95
GABA receptor Ab syndrome, 2151, 2159
GABA receptors, 305, 388, 391, 886, 1153, 1233, 2151, 2159, 2176
Gadolinium, 14, 15, 1074, 1098, 1107, 1782
Gag, 701
Gait apraxia, 208, 404
Gait difficulties, 419
Gait disorders, 443, 444, 817, 1002
Gait disturbance, 443, 896, 1002, 1018, 1935, 2174
Galactocerebrosides (GalC), 97, 250
Galactolipids, 250
Galea aponeurotica, 500
Gallyas, 57, 84–87, 832, 839, 840, 859, 911, 962, 963, 1028, 1030
γ-aminobutyric acid (GABA), 236, 283, 370, 372, 373, 386, 388–391, 886, 1138, 1139, 1143, 1153, 1154, 1168, 1228, 1233, 1243, 1256, 2175
Gamma-aminobutyric acid (GABA) A receptor, subunit alpha 1 (GABRA1), 236, 1136
Gamma-aminobutyric acid type A receptor beta3 subunit (GABRB3), 236, 886
Gamma-aminobutyric acid type A receptor gamma2 subunit (GABRG2), 236, 1136
Gamma camera, 38, 40–42
Gamma-knife, 1661, 1662, 1675, 1692, 1793
Gamma radiation, 31
Gamma rays, 30, 1269
Ganglia, 5, 9, 13, 48, 55, 65, 76, 77, 86, 125, 126, 129, 143–146, 151, 153, 164, 203, 211, 257, 267, 301–305, 334, 339, 350, 357, 359, 373, 377, 385, 387, 401, 416, 417, 450, 455, 457, 459, 461, 468, 482, 489, 490, 501, 502, 506, 507, 538, 541, 586, 605, 607, 614, 616, 622, 625, 627, 629, 640, 658, 666, 673, 697, 698, 703, 715, 737, 738, 752, 755, 775, 782, 795, 797, 798, 800, 802, 805, 817–820, 838, 848, 850, 856, 863, 865, 871, 873, 901, 914, 932, 960, 966, 977, 979, 989, 990, 992, 995, 996, 1012, 1025, 1028, 1060, 1106, 1213, 1227, 1233, 1245, 1259, 1342, 1434, 1448, 1669, 1761, 1895, 1898, 1899, 1934, 1936, 2152–2154, 2159, 2170, 2171, 2174
Gangliocytoma, 1132, 1276, 1324, 1561–1573, 1754
Ganglioglioma
    age incidence, 1562
    biologic behavior-prognosis-prognostic factors, 1565
    CT-contrast-enhanced, 1563
    CT-non contrast-enhanced, 1563
    differential diagnosis, 1563
    general imaging findings, 1563
    immunophenotype, 1563, 1569–1572
    incidence, 1562
    localization, 1562–1563
    macroscopic features, 1563
    microscopic features, 1563, 1568
    molecular neuropathology, 1565
    MRI-diffusion imaging, 1563–1565
    MRI-FLAIR, 1563–1567
    MRI-perfusion, 1563–1565
    MRI-T1, 1563–1567
    MRI-T2, 1563
    MRI-T1 contrast-enhanced, 1563–1567
    MRI-T2∗/SWI, 1563
    MR-spectroscopy, 1563
    nuclear medicine imaging findings, 1563
    pathogenesis, 1563, 1565
    proliferation markers, 1563, 1569–1572
    sex incidence, 1562
    treatment, 1565
    ultrastructural features, (AU: Not found)
    WHO definition, 1561–1563
    WHO grade, 1562
Ganglioglioma anaplastic
    age incidence, 1572
    biologic behavior-prognosis-prognostic factors, 1573
    CT-contrast-enhanced, 1572
    CT-non contrast-enhanced, 1572
    differential diagnosis, 1573
    general imaging findings, 1572
    immunophenotype, 1573
    incidence, 1572
    localization, 1572
    macroscopic features, 1573
    microscopic features, 1573
    molecular neuropathology, 1573
    MRI-diffusion tensor imaging, 1563–1565
    MRI-FLAIR, 1572
    MRI-perfusion, 1572
    MRI-T1, 1572
    MRI-T2, 1572
    MRI-T1 contrast-enhanced, 1572
    nuclear medicine imaging findings, 1573
    pathogenesis, 1573
    proliferation markers, 1573
    sex incidence, 1572
    treatment, 1573
    WHO definition, 1572
    WHO grade, 1572
Ganglioid cells, 1578
Gangliosides, 250
GAP-43, 236
Gap junction protein beta 1 (GJB1), 247
Gap junctions, 235, 241, 244, 245, 247, 249, 259, 1153, 1964
Gastric adenocarcinoma, 1290, 2059, 2097, 2102
GATA3, 1305, 2054, 2060, 2061, 2073, 2091, 2092, 2096, 2114
Gaze paresis, 207, 475
GBM multiforme type or classical type, 1386
GBM with oligodendroglioma component, 1386
GBM with primitive neuronal component, 1386
Gelastic seizures, 418, 1125
Gelsolin (GSN), 247, 615, 998

Gemistocytic, 458, 484, 1275, 1329, 1337, 1341, 1343, 1346, 1349, 1364, 1387, 1472
Generalized (non-focal) cortical dysplasias, 1157
Generalized seizures of non-focal origin (convulsive/non-convulsive), 1121–1122
General linear model, 21
Gene silencing, 925, 1017, 1280, 1290, 1310
Genome instability and mutation, 1265, 1281
Genomic instability, 889, 1266, 1281, 1304–1305, 1400
Genu corporis callosi, 76, 148
Germ cell tumor
    age incidence, 1866
    biologic behavior-prognosis-prognostic factors, 1868
    differential diagnosis, 1867
    immunophenotype, 1866–1867
    incidence, 1866
    localization, 1866
    nuclear medicine imaging findings, 1866
    pathogenesis, 1867–1868
    sex incidence, 1866
    treatment, 1868
    WHO definition, 1866
Germinal matrix hemorrhage, 499, 500
Germinoma
    CT-contrast-enhanced, 1868
    CT-non contrast-enhanced, 1868–1871
    general imaging findings, 1868
    immunophenotype, 1871–1873
    macroscopic features, 1871
    microscopic features, 1871–1873
    MRI-diffusion imaging, 1869–1871
    MRI-FLAIR, 1869–1871
    MRI-T1, 1869–1871
    MRI-T2, 1869–1871
    MRI-T1 contrast-enhanced, 1869–1871
    MRI-T2∗/SWI, 1871
    MR-spectroscopy, 1871
    nuclear medicine imaging findings, 1871
    proliferation markers, 1871
    ultrastructural features, 1871
    WHO definition, 1868
Gerstmann's syndrome, 401, 413
Gerstmann–Sträussler–Scheinker syndrome (GSSS), 797
Ghost neurons, 455, 458
Giant cell glioblastoma
    age incidence, 1412
    biologic behavior-prognosis-prognostic factors, 1417
    differential diagnosis, 1417
    general imaging findings, 1412
    immunophenotype, 1417–1419
    incidence, 1412
    localization, 1412
    macroscopic features, 1414, 1415
    microscopic features, 1414, 1416–1417
    molecular neuropathology, 1417
    nuclear medicine imaging findings, 1412
    pathogenesis, 1417
    proliferation markers, 1417–1419
    sex incidence, 1412
    treatment, 1417
    ultrastructural features, 1417
    WHO definition, 1411–1412
    WHO grade, 1412
Giant cell/temporal arteritis (GCA), 636, 638, 648
Giant cell tumor
    CT-non contrast-enhanced, 2026
    differential diagnosis, 2029
    general imaging findings, 2026
    localisation, 2026
    macroscopic features, 2027
    microscopic features, 207, 2028
    MRI-T1, 2026, 2027
    MRI-T2, 2026, 2027
    MRI-T1 contrast-enhanced, 2026, 2027
    WHO definition, 2026
Giemsa stain, 776
Gigantism, 418, 1677, 1781, 1785, 1791, 1794
Glasgow coma scale (GCS), 518, 519, 1186, 1187
Glial cells, 17, 85, 97, 125, 158, 234, 235, 239–240, 243, 252, 278, 301, 303, 314, 326, 370, 371, 388, 391, 392, 394, 441, 484, 510, 690, 722, 814, 840, 865, 911, 920, 979, 1045, 1171, 1178, 1217, 1228, 1306, 1426, 1430, 1472, 1474, 1510, 1513, 1514, 1562, 1568, 1645, 1699
Glial fibrillary acidic protein (GFAP), 91, 92, 96, 102, 108, 240, 241, 243, 244, 249, 470, 471, 489, 516, 518, 680, 685, 687, 717, 728, 740, 810, 856, 887, 992, 1066, 1113, 1151, 1152, 1158, 1162, 1164–1166, 1168, 1205, 1223, 1228, 1231, 1236, 1243, 1248, 1250, 1253, 1275, 1320, 1341, 1346, 1347, 1362, 1364, 1391, 1394, 1396, 1398, 1417–1420, 1422, 1431, 1433, 1438, 1439, 1442, 1452, 1454, 1457, 1464, 1465, 1475, 1476, 1479, 1480, 1485, 1493, 1496, 1497, 1499, 1501, 1505, 1508, 1510, 1516, 1527, 1529–1531, 1539, 1541, 1543, 1545, 1548, 1557, 1558, 1563, 1569, 1573, 1589, 1590, 1609, 1624, 1626, 1645, 1648, 1654, 1656, 1675, 1770, 1773, 1775, 1776, 1843, 1852, 1886, 1920, 1977, 2058, 2127, 2164, 2165
Glial inclusions, 855, 953, 954, 964, 966, 973, 983, 1042
Glial intermediate filaments, 1343, 1364
Glial nodules, 1541, 1543
Glioblastoma
    age incidence, 1369
    biologic behavior-prognosis-prognostic factors, 1407–1408
    CT-contrast-enhanced, 1369–1370
    CT-non contrast-enhanced, 1369–1371
    differential diagnosis, 1397–1398
    DNA methylation, 1403
    epigenetics, 1403
    gene expression, 1403–1405
    general imaging findings, 1369–1386
    genetics, 1400–1402
    immunophenotype, 1382, 1394–1396
    incidence, 1369
    localization, 1369
    macroscopic features, 1382–1384

Glioblastoma (cont.)
  microRNAs, 1403
  microscopic features, 1386–1394
  molecular neuropathology, 1398–1405
  MRI-diffusion imaging, 1370, 1375–1376
  MRI-diffusion tensor imaging, 1370, 1375–1376
  MRI-FLAIR, 1370, 1372–1377
  MRI-perfusion, 1370, 1372
  MRI-T1, 1370–1372
  MRI-T2, 1370–1371
  MRI-T1 contrast-enhanced, 1370–1377
  MRI-T2∗/ SWI, 1370
  MR-spectroscopy, 1373, 1374, 1376, 1377
  nuclear medicine imaging findings, 1376, 1378–1383
  pathogenesis, 1397–1398
  primary GBM, 1367, 1401
  proliferation markers, 1396, 1397
  secondary GBM, 1367, 1401
  sex incidence, 1369
  treatment, 1406–1407
  ultrastructural features, 1397
  WHO definition, 1368–1369
  WHO grade, 1369
Glioma invasion, 1266, 1314–1319
Glioma stem-like cells, 1320
Gliomatosis cerebri
  age incidence, 1426
  biologic behavior-prognosis-prognostic factors, 1431
  CT-contrast-enhanced, 1429
  CT-non contrast-enhanced, 1426–1428
  differential diagnosis, 1431
  DNA methylation, (AU: Not found)
  epigenetics, (AU: Not found)
  gene expression, (AU: Not found)
  general imaging findings, 1426
  genetics, (AU: Not found)
  immunophenotype, 1431
  incidence, 1426
  localization, 1426
  macroscopic features, 1430
  microRNAs, (AU: Not found)
  microscopic features, 1430–1431
  molecular neuropathology, 1431
  MRI-diffusion imaging, 1426–1430
  MRI-diffusion tensor imaging, 1427, 1430
  MRI-FLAIR, 1426–1430
  MRI-perfusion, 1427, 1430
  MRI-T1, 1426–1430
  MRI-T2, 1426–1430
  MRI-T1 contrast-enhanced, 1426–1430
  MRI-T2∗/SWI, 1430
  MR-spectroscopy, 1428, 1430
  nuclear medicine imaging findings, 1430
  pathogenesis, 1431
  proliferation markers, 1431
  sex incidence, 1426
  treatment, 1431
  ultrastructural features, 1431
  WHO definition, 1425–1426

Gliomesenchymal nodules, 683, 698, 700, 706, 707, 740, 757, 759, 2151, 2163, 2166
Glioneuronal element, 1541, 1543
Gliosarcoma
  age incidence, 1412
  biologic behavior-prognosis-prognostic factors, 1417
  CT-contrast-enhanced, 1412
  CT-non contrast-enhanced, 1412
  differential diagnosis, 1417
  general imaging findings, 1412
  immunophenotype, 1417–1419
  incidence, 1412
  localization, 1412
  macroscopic features, 1414, 1415
  microscopic features, 1414, 1416–1417
  molecular neuropathology, 1417
  MRI-diffusion imaging, 1412
  MRI-FLAIR, 1412, 1413
  MRI-perfusion, 1412, 1413
  MRI-T1, 1412, 1413
  MRI-T2, 1412–1414
  MRI-T1 contrast-enhanced, 1412, 1413
  MRI-T2∗/ SWI, 1412
  MR-spectroscopy, 1412
  nuclear medicine imaging findings, 1412
  pathogenesis, 1417
  proliferation markers, 1417–1419
  sex incidence, 1412
  treatment, 1417
  ultrastructural features, 1417
  WHO definition, 1411–1412
  WHO grade, 1412
Global aphasia, 207, 401, 413, 420, 475
Global cerebral ischemia, 987
Globular astroglial inclusions (GAIs), 837
Globular oligodendroglial inclusions (GOI), 837
Globus pallidus, 76, 125, 126, 143, 145–147, 150, 167, 168, 204, 231, 300, 303–305, 334, 338, 339, 357, 475, 798, 818, 857–859, 863, 864, 871, 947, 964, 967, 976, 982, 983, 989, 1011, 1012, 1060, 1062, 1063, 1243, 1247, 1260
Globus pallidus pars externa, 145
Globus pallidus pars interna, 145
Glucose transporter (GLUT1), 1689, 1982
Glutamate
  excitotoxicity, 244, 1092, 1093, 1185, 1214
  receptors, 392, 395, 814, 815, 1134, 1214, 2151, 2155, 2158, 2160, 2171, 2173, 2175, 2176
Glutamate transporter-1 (GLT-1), 97, 372, 392, 1214
Glutamic acid decarboxylase (GAD65), 2153, 2170, 2172
Glutaraldehyde, 77, 91
Glut transporters, 392
Glycine
  α-receptor, 2174
  receptor antibody syndrome, 2151, 2158
Glycine receptor (GlyR), 2153, 2158
Glycolipids, 97, 250
Glycolysis, 242, 1281, 1313, 2139
Glycophorin A, 105, 2058

Glycoprotein, 95, 96, 98–100, 105, 236, 252, 258, 293, 690, 701, 717, 720, 731, 1089, 1093, 1267, 1315, 1316, 1702, 1759, 1795, 1806, 1808, 1813, 1866, 1867, 2174
Glycosphingolipids, 250
'Glymphatic' system, 225, 243, 259
G2/M transition (= DNA replication checkpoint), 1282, 1283
Golgi-apparatus, 226–228, 1579, 1591, 1797, 1804, 1879
Golgi Cox silver impregnation, 85
Gomori methenamine silver (GMS), 89, 776
G1 phase (gap 1), 1281–1283
G2 phase (gap 2), 1281, 1283, 1287
G protein-coupled, 95, 392
G-protein coupled receptors, 392, 1254, 1289, 1405
Gracile fascicle, 160, 162
Gracile nucleus, 162, 335, 343
Gracile tubercle, 160
Gradient coils, 9
Gradient-echo imaging, 14
Gradient moment rephrasing, 13
Grains, 87, 825, 828, 837, 844, 848, 849, 859–861, 953, 956, 957, 962, 963, 965, 968
Gram-negative, 89, 655, 657
Gram-positive, 89, 655, 776
Gram stain, 89, 655, 656, 776
Granular cell glioblastoma, 1386
Granular cell tumor of the sellar region
    age incidence, 1771
    biologic behavior-prognosis-prognostic factors, 1775
    CT-contrast-enhanced, 1771
    CT-non contrast-enhanced, 1771
    differential diagnosis, 1771
    general imaging findings, 1771
    immunophenotype, 1771, 1774–1775
    incidence, 1771
    localization, 1771
    macroscopic features, 1771
    microscopic features, 1771, 1773–1775
    molecular neuropathology, (AU: Not found)
    MRI-FLAIR, 1771, 1772
    MRI-T1, 1771, 1772
    MRI-T2, 1771, 1772
    MRI-T1 contrast-enhanced, 1771, 1772
    pathogenesis, 1771, 1775
    proliferation markers, 1771
    sex incidence, 1771
    treatment, 1775
    ultrastructural features, 1771
    WHO definition, 1770–1771
    WHO grade, 1771
Granular cortex, 290
Granularity, 1360, 1477
Granular osmiophilic material (GOM), 605–606, 629, 630, 996
Granule cell dispersion (GCD), 1148, 1150
Granulocyte, 83, 666, 678, 1092, 1933, 1944, 1947, 2139
Granulosa cell tumor, 2107, 2111
Granulovacuolar degeneration, 838–839, 901, 913
Granzyme B, 1908, 2163
Grasp reflexes, 207, 208, 475, 988

Gray matter, 6, 86, 125, 145, 155, 212, 230, 240, 245, 246, 267, 318–320, 334, 352, 429, 432, 456, 458, 607, 616, 693, 703, 717, 732, 797, 802, 803, 813, 837, 852, 853, 863, 933, 1043, 1044, 1060, 1061, 1078, 1087, 1101, 1106, 1109, 1132, 1133, 1158, 1162, 1164, 1166, 1171, 1172, 1175, 1207, 1223, 1229, 1243, 1253, 1338, 1354, 1378, 1380, 1412, 1419, 1425, 1426, 1694, 1935, 2154
Grocott, 89, 90, 776, 781, 787, 791
Growth factors, 92, 97, 241, 248, 291, 294, 441, 568, 605, 614, 622, 629, 816, 878, 885, 1056, 1093, 1134, 1266, 1279–1283, 1289, 1306, 1311, 1313, 1315, 1324, 1331, 1337, 1349, 1365, 1395, 1399, 1400, 1405, 1431, 1447, 1459, 1466, 1469, 1476, 1484, 1648, 1747, 1749, 1789, 1979, 2055, 2057, 2131, 2148, 2171, 2174
Growth factor signaling, 1279
Growth inhibitory signals, 1265, 1279–1281
Growth signal autonomy, 1265, 1279, 1281
GSK-3ß/NF-κB, 1989, 1995
GSS with neurofibrillary tangles, 819, 820
G1/S transition (= restriction checkpoint), 1282
Gut-brain peptides, 370
Gyrus
    ambient gyrus, 138, 965
    angular gyrus, 133, 401, 407, 413
    cingulate gyrus, 68, 76, 135–138, 143, 148, 150, 167, 168, 325, 343, 350, 356, 357, 405, 436, 437, 734, 837, 838, 855, 861, 901, 916, 937, 965, 2052
    dentate gyrus, 138, 267, 294, 295, 297, 298, 346, 347, 350, 387, 850, 855, 856, 861, 875, 960
    inferior frontal gyrus
        anterior ramus, 132
        orbital part, 136, 137
        triangular part, 132
    inferior temporal gyrus, 134, 135, 167, 168, 853, 1201
    isthmus of the cingulate gyrus, 135
    lateral occipito-temporal gyrus, 137
    lingual gyrus, 137, 205, 209
    medial frontal gyrus, 132, 135–137, 167, 168, 916
    medial occipito-temporal gyrus, 137
    middle frontal gyrus, 76, 131, 132, 150, 167, 168, 404, 405, 800
    middle temporal gyrus, 134, 135, 167, 168, 918
    orbital gyri, 137, 148, 168, 204
    parahippocampal gyrus, 137, 138, 148, 167, 168, 205, 299, 300, 343, 347, 348, 434, 435, 856, 864
    postcentral gyrus, 131–133, 167, 168, 406, 980
    precentral gyrus, 123, 131–133, 150, 160, 167, 168, 204, 232, 294, 295, 328, 334, 336, 801, 976, 980, 1039, 1042, 1043, 1944, 2121
    straight gyrus, 76, 137, 901, 1196
    superior frontal gyrus, 76, 77, 131, 132, 167, 168, 328, 405, 901
    superior temporal gyrus, 133–135, 167, 168, 351, 409, 410, 853, 857, 901, 916, 960
    supramarginal gyrus, 133, 406, 414
    transverse gyri, 134, 204

H

¹H, 10, 15, 16, 889
Habenula, 155
Habenulopeduncular tract, 343
Haemorrhage, 1369
Half-life, 30–32, 38, 48–51, 1255, 1341, 1356, 1380, 1381, 1414, 1420, 1451, 1462, 1470, 1477, 1716, 2050
Hallervorden-Spatz disease, 826, 836, 838, 864
The Hallmarks of cancer, 1265, 1279–1281
Hallucinations
   auditory, 410
   complex visual, 407, 410
Hand and foot grasp, 405
Hanning and Shepp-Logan filters, 33, 51
H-caldesmon, 102, 2058
Headache, 418, 419, 443, 456, 500, 505, 520, 622, 640, 653, 654, 658, 694, 731, 736, 749, 751, 763, 773, 774, 862, 1073, 1105, 1186, 1267, 1490, 1708, 1804, 1813, 1824, 2155
Head injury, 1131, 1153
Head of the caudate nucleus (caput nuclei caudate), 144, 147, 174, 175
Hearing loss, 14, 208, 639, 862, 1073, 1663
Heat fixation, 76
Heavy metal (lead, manganese mercury, aluminum)-induced encephalopathies, 244
Hedgehog (Hh), 925, 1291, 1746–1747, 1749, 1990, 1995
Hedgehog signaling, 1266, 1306, 1320–1321, 1325
Helical path, 37
Hemangioblastoma
   age incidence, 1967
   biologic behavior-prognosis-prognostic factors, 1974
   CT-contrast-enhanced, 1969
   CT-non contrast-enhanced, 1969
   differential diagnosis, 1969
   general imaging findings, 1967–1969
   immunophenotype, 1969–1974
   incidence, 1967
   localization, 1967
   macroscopic features, 1969
   microscopic features, 1969
   MRI-diffusion imaging, 1969
   MRI-FLAIR, 1969
   MRI-perfusion, 1969
   MRI-T1, 1969
   MRI-T2, 1969
   MRI-T1 contrast-enhanced, 1969
   MRI-T2∗/SWI, 1969
   nuclear medicine imaging findings, 1969
   proliferation markers, 1969
   sex incidence, 1967
   treatment, 1966–1967, 1974
   ultrastructural features, 1969
   WHO definition, 1967
Hemangioma, 1956, 1979, 1982, 1991
Hemangiopericytoma, 1957–1968, 1992, 1993
Hemangiopericytoma phenotype, 1955, 1962, 1964, 1967

Hematoma, 6, 11, 500, 510, 521–524, 529, 530, 533, 1207
Hematoxylin and eosin stain (H&E), 79, 83, 84, 239, 247, 249, 268, 295–297, 306, 309, 310, 700, 707, 709, 711, 713, 756, 757, 759, 768, 781, 787, 791, 830, 832, 836, 907, 916, 1029, 1042, 1065, 1082, 1149, 1152, 1162–1164, 1166, 1207, 1231, 1236, 1248, 1387, 1580, 1963
Hemiakinesia, 404
Hemiascomycetes, 774
Hemiasomatognosia, 406
Hemiataxia, 208, 417
Hemicraniectomy, 496
Hemimegalencephaly, 1125, 1130, 1132, 1157, 1168
Hemineglect/apraxia, 404
Hemiparesis, 207, 209, 475, 505, 658, 722, 731, 752, 763, 862, 988, 1105, 1267
Hemisensory deficits, 208, 476
Hemisensory loss, 207, 475
Hemispatial neglect, 361, 406, 415, 423
Hemisphere, 63, 65, 71, 72, 74, 129, 130, 146–148, 180, 208, 213, 288, 345, 410, 415, 421, 436, 482, 728, 876, 947, 948, 1120, 1127, 1233, 1382, 1481, 1825
Hemivisual neglect, 209
Hemorrhage
   age incidence, 500, 505, 520
   biologic behavior-prognosis-prognostic factors, 505, 517, 524, 532
   choroid plexus hemorrhage, 499, 500
   clinical signs and symptoms, 500, 505, 520, 529
   CT-angiography, 501
   CT-contrast-enhanced, 501, 510, 520, 529
   CT-non contrast-enhanced, 501, 510, 520, 529
   differential diagnosis, 503, 514, 521
   epidural hemorrhage, 499, 500, 529–533
   general imaging findings, 501, 510, 520, 529
   germinal matrix hemorrhage, 500
   immunophenotype, (AU: Not found)
   incidence, 500, 505, 520, 529
   intracerebral hemorrhage, 499–505, 507, 510, 607, 987, 989, 999
   intramedullary hemorrhage, 499, 500
   localization, 500, 501, 510, 520, 529
   macroscopic features, 501, 507–510, 515, 521, 530
   microscopic features, 501, 511–512, 521, 527–529
   MRI-diffusion imaging, 501, 521
   MRI-FLAIR, 501–505, 510, 513–514, 520, 523–524, 529, 531–532
   MRI-T1, 501–504, 510, 513–514, 520, 523, 529
   MRI-T2, 501–505, 510, 520, 523–524, 529, 531, 532
   MRI-T1 contrast-enhanced, 501–505, 510, 513–514, 521, 523, 530–531
   MRI-T2∗/SWI, 501–505, 510, 521, 523–524, 530–532
   nuclear medicine imaging findings, 501, 510, 521
   pathogenesis, 503, 514, 522–524, 530
   sex incidence, 500, 505, 520
   subarachnoid hemorrhage, 9, 499, 500, 505–520, 715, 775–777, 997, 999

Index

subcutaneous hemorrhage, 499
subdural hemorrhage, 60, 188, 499, 500, 520–529, 1196
subgaleal hemorrhage, 499, 500
treatment, 505, 514, 524, 532
Hemorrhagic conversion of cerebral infarct, 503
Hemorrhagic dementia, 988, 989, 997
Hemorrhagic stroke, 473, 474, 1258
Hemosensitive sequences, 501, 596
Hemosiderin, 89, 90, 501, 510, 585, 586, 594, 607, 1028, 1232, 1371, 1435, 1438, 1507, 1584, 1765, 2026, 2028
Hemosiderinophages, 495, 552, 565, 992, 1202, 1439, 2126
Hemostatic drug therapy, 505
Hepatic encephalopathy, 244
Hepatocellular carcinoma, 1302, 2054, 2059, 2061, 2097, 2104
Hereditary Aβ CAA (Dutch and Flemish types, familial AD), 615
(Non) Hereditary bilateral striatal necrosis, 825, 828, 858
Hereditary cerebral hemorrhage with amyloid angiopathy–Icelandic type, 615
Hereditary endotheliopathy with retinopathy, nephropathy, and stroke (HERNS), 606
Hereditary hemorrhagic telangiectasia (Rendu-Osler-Weber syndrome), 585, 596
Hereditary vascular retinopathy, 606
Herniation
 anterior-to-middle fossa herniation, 436
 cerebellar tonsillar herniation, 436
 fungus cerebri, 436, 438–439
 spinal cord herniation, 436–437
 subarachnoid cerebellar tissue emboli, 436
 subfalcial herniation-supracallosal (subfalcine/cingulate) herniation, 436, 437
 transtentorial herniation, 430, 434, 435
 upward transtentorial herniation, 436
Herpes simplex virus (HSV), 107, 696, 697, 699, 731–736, 2155
 HSV-1, 107, 695, 697
 HSV-2, 107, 695, 697
Herringbone, 1662, 1690, 1691, 1985
Heterogeneous enhancement, 1412, 1434, 1502, 1534, 1572, 1576, 1597, 1615, 1639, 1642, 1652, 1666, 1677, 1690, 1755, 1776, 1783, 1877, 1958, 2011, 2018, 2020, 2026
Heterotopia(s), 1125, 1130, 1132, 1171–1179, 1986
Heterotypic cortex, 291
Hexamethyl propylene amine oxime (HMPAO), 51, 52, 54, 697, 802, 901, 1125
Hibernoma, 1956, 1984
Higher nuclear:cytoplasmic ratio, 1268, 1270
Highly active anti-retroviral therapies (HAART), 703, 712–715
High-resolution-CT, 7
Hippocampal body, 138
Hippocampal dysplasia, 1132
Hippocampal formation, 76, 86, 93, 138–141, 231, 269, 343, 381, 434, 468, 487, 813, 818, 899, 901, 911, 913, 914, 918–920, 1113, 1147, 1151, 1152, 1247, 1253, 1342, 1830, 2163, 2164, 2168
Hippocampal head, 138
Hippocampal sclerosis, 108, 849, 988, 999, 1125, 1129, 1131–1133, 1143, 1148, 1152–1154, 1158, 1165, 2165
Hippocampal sclerosis ILAE type, 1148–1151
Hippocampal system, 326, 346–350
Hippocampal tail, 138
Hippocampus
 alveus, 295–297, 347, 348
 cornu ammonis (hippocampus proper), 295–299
 dentate gyrus (fascia dentata), 295, 297, 299–300
 polymorphic layer, 295, 299, 346, 347
 stratum granulosum, 295, 299, 347
 stratum lacunosum, 295, 298, 347
 stratum moleculare, 295, 297–299, 346, 347
 stratum oriens, 295–298, 347, 349
 stratum pyramidale with CA1, CA2, CA3, CA4, 295, 296, 298, 347
 stratum radiatum, 295, 296, 299, 347
Hippocampus (proper), 138, 295–299
Histamine, 370, 441
Histiocytes, 103, 105, 675, 703, 752, 1934, 1941, 1944, 1945, 1947, 1949, 1979
Histiocytic infiltrates, 2126, 2128
Histiocytic sarcoma, 1894, 1934, 1941, 1944, 1945
Histiocytic tumors
 age incidence, 1934, 1935, 1941
 incidence, 1934, 1935, 1941
 localization, 1934, 1935, 1941
 nuclear medicine imaging findings, 1934, 1936, 1938, 1943
 sex incidence, 1934, 1935, 1941
 WHO definition, 1934–1935, 1941
Histone modifications, 642, 648, 889, 925, 1017, 1266, 1309, 1310
Histoplasmosis, 777
HIV-associated dementia (HAD), 702, 703, 715, 720
HIV-associated neurocognitive disorders (HAND), 701
HIV-1 encephalitis (HIVE), 702–703, 707, 710, 714, 715
HIV-1 leukoencephalopathy (HIVL), 702, 706, 714
HIV-1 myelitis, 702
HMB-45, 102, 104, 1669, 2058, 2061, 2062, 2082, 2083, 2104, 2115
^{1}H MRS, 15, 16
Hockey stick sign, 798, 853
Holistic models, 402
Homer Wright rosette, 1274, 1562, 1578, 1606, 1609, 1615, 1643, 1984
Homologous recombination (HR), 1286–1288
Homonymous hemianopia, 207, 209, 408, 475, 658, 722
Homonymous hemianopsia with macular sparing, 207, 208, 407, 475, 476
Homotypic cortex, 291
Homunculus, 123, 124
Honeycomb appearance, 1452, 1456, 1577
Horizontal cells of Cajal, 268, 269
Hormesis theory, 38

Hormone therapy, 1138, 1269
"Hot cross bun" sign, 1022, 1023
Hounsfield, 4
Hu, 2153, 2155, 2170, 2175
Human alveolar macrophage 56 (HAM56), 103, 248, 2058
Human chorionic gonadotropin (HCG), 108, 1765, 1880, 1881, 2096
Human herpesvirus, 695, 697
    HHV8, 1984, 2100
Human immunodeficiency virus (HIV)-1, 248, 700–720, 1247, 1256, 1984
Human immunodeficiency virus (HIV), 107, 693, 696–698, 701, 703, 704, 706, 708, 710, 715, 755, 767, 786, 792
Hummingbird/penguin sign, 853, 974, 975
Huntingtin, 1052, 1066, 1067
Huntington disease (HD), 50, 54, 245, 388, 392, 818, 826, 827, 835, 845, 849, 851, 854, 881, 882, 1035, 1059–1068
Hyaline arteriosclerosis, 540
Hybrid nerve sheath tumors
    biologic behavior-prognosis-prognostic factors, 1689
    hybrid neurofibroma/perineurioma, 1689
    hybrid schwannoma/neurofibroma, 1689
    hybrid schwannoma/perineurioma, 1687–1689
    immunophenotype, 1689
    macroscopic features, 1687
    microscopic features, 1687–1689
    treatment, 1689
    WHO definition, 1686–1687
Hydrocephalus
    age incidence, 444
    aqueductal stenosis, 444–445, 447, 449, 451
    biologic behavior-prognosis-prognostic factors, 451
    clinical signs and symptoms, 443–444
    communicating hydrocephalus, 443–444, 449, 451
    CT-contrast-enhanced, 444
    CT-non contrast-enhanced, 444
    definition, 443–444
    general imaging findings, 444–450
    incidence, 444
    localization, 444
    macroscopic features, 449–450
    microscopic features, 449
    molecular neuropathology, 451
    MRI-CISS, 444–448
    MRI-FLAIR, 444
    MRI-T1, 444
    MRI-T2, 444
    MRI-T1 contrast-enhanced, 444
    MRI-T2∗/SWI, 444
    MR-spectroscopy, 444
    non-communicating hydrocephalus, 443
    normal pressure hydrocephalus, 451
    nuclear medicine imaging findings, 448–449
    sex incidence, 444
    treatment, 451
Hyperacute, 500, 501, 520, 1105

Hyperdense, 477, 501, 520, 529, 552, 578, 586, 622, 720, 752, 763, 1192, 1369, 1523, 1534, 1554, 1576, 1615, 1617, 1652, 1666, 1709, 1710, 1824, 1846, 1853, 1868, 1882, 1895, 1941, 1958, 1969, 1999
Hyperintense
    lesion, 752, 799, 1106, 1207, 1237, 1260, 1370, 1924, 1943
    leukencephalopathy, 607
Hyperintensities, 444, 457, 614, 616, 627, 628, 661, 696, 703, 720, 797, 798, 802, 853, 870, 875–878, 980, 1022, 1039, 1040, 1060, 1074, 1098, 1144, 1158, 1229, 1233, 1666, 1755, 1914, 1935, 1943, 2132, 2156, 2162
Hyperplastic arteriosclerosis, 540
Hyperprolactinemia, 418, 1781, 1793, 1794, 1798, 1804
Hypersensitivity vasculitis, 1260
Hypersomnia, 418, 932
Hypertensive angiopathy, 606, 988
Hyperthermia, 418, 1229, 1259, 1260
Hypodense, 477, 501, 520, 529, 616, 627, 639, 664, 696, 720, 731, 752, 1074, 1106, 1192, 1237, 1369, 1434, 1542, 1554, 1584, 1597, 1639, 1666, 1677, 1685, 1755, 1782, 1824, 1846, 1882, 1919, 1969, 1979, 1999, 2038, 2120, 2128, 2160
Hypointense, 429, 477, 501, 510, 520, 521, 529, 530, 552, 578, 586, 593, 596, 600, 628, 661, 696, 720, 725, 731, 732, 734, 752, 775, 777, 783, 990, 1075, 1101, 1106, 1158, 1192, 1207, 1235, 1237, 1338, 1354, 1370, 1372, 1412, 1426, 1430, 1434, 1470, 1493, 1507, 1511, 1523, 1534, 1542, 1572, 1576, 1584, 1597, 1606, 1615, 1617, 1642, 1652, 1666, 1685, 1690, 1709, 1755, 1776, 1782, 1783, 1785, 1813, 1836, 1883, 1895, 1919, 1924, 1935, 1943, 1969, 2000, 2005, 2018, 2026, 2029, 2038, 2040, 2120, 2124, 2128, 2160
Hyponatremia, 418, 428, 1233, 1235, 1260, 2156, 2174
Hypoperfusion dementia, 988, 989, 996
Hypophysiotropic peptides, 370, 371
Hypophysis, 155, 164, 1777, 1841
Hypothalamic sulcus, 150, 153
Hypothalamus, 95, 138, 150, 153–155, 166, 174, 300, 305–307, 326, 348, 350–352, 355–357, 375, 376, 380, 381, 387, 388, 402, 418, 449, 607, 853, 856, 861, 920, 921, 965, 1213, 1214, 1229, 1254, 1259, 1434, 1438, 1444, 1562, 1782, 1944, 2160
    and hypophyseal system, 326, 352–356, 358
Hypothermia, 418, 441, 1253
Hypotonia, 416, 419, 420
Hypoxia
    age incidence, 457
    anemic hypoxia, 457
    biologic behavior-prognosis-prognostic factors, 471–472
    clinical signs and symptoms, 456
    CT-contrast-enhanced, 457, 459–460
    CT-non contrast-enhanced, 457

differential diagnosis, 471
general imaging findings, 457–471
histotoxic hypoxia, 457
hypoxic hypoxia, 456
immunophenotype, 470
incidence, 457
ischemic/stagnant hypoxia, 457
localization, 457
macroscopic features, 458
microscopic features, 458, 467–471
molecular neuropathology, 471
MRI-diffusion imaging, 457, 459–460
MRI-FLAIR, 457, 459–463
MRI-T1, 457, 461–463
MRI-T2, 457, 459–463
MRI-T1 contrast-enhanced, 457, 461–463
MRI-T2∗/SWI, 457
nuclear medicine imaging findings, 458, 464–465
sex incidence, 457
treatment, 471
Hypoxia-inducible factor (HIF), 879, 1266, 1306, 1318
Hypoxic and ischemic encephalopathy, 456
Hypoxic-ischemic leukoencephalopathy, 458, 1247, 1253

I
Iatrogenic Creutzfeldt–Jakob disease, 795
[123I]β-CIT, 49
IBZM, 54, 976, 1007, 1025, 1027, 1060
Ictus and ictal event, 1120
Ideomotor apraxia, 405, 413, 980
IDH-mutant, 1327, 1329, 1330, 1337, 1338, 1353, 1365, 1368, 1448, 1459, 1575
123I-epidepride, 29, 50, 51
123I-FP-CIT, 29, 49–50
IgG antibodies, 2155, 2167
IgL-and IgH-chain genes, 1929
IgLON5 Ab Syndrome, 2160
123I-IBZM, 29, 50, 51
Illusory visual spread, 209, 422
123I-MIBG, 933, 976, 1007, 1028
Immediate early genes (IGE), 441, 471, 1134, 1259
Immune reconstitution inflammatory syndrome (IRIS), 712–715, 725
Immune surveillance, 248, 880, 1280
Immunoexcitotoxicity, 1215
Immunoglobulin-like family members 5 (IgLON5), 2151, 2160, 2167, 2174
Immunohistochemistry, 79, 83, 89–108, 110, 111, 240, 703, 706, 707, 710, 723, 735, 797, 812, 816, 830, 832–835, 861, 875, 908, 911, 1082, 1084, 1087, 1205, 1247, 1398, 1458, 1577, 1804, 1927, 1966, 1985
Immunotherapy Response Assessment in Neuro-Oncology (iRANO) criteria, 2136–2139
Impact injury, 1188
Impaired ability to multitask, 405, 415
Impaired appreciation of social nuances, 404
Impaired check and excessive rebound, 420
Impaired conflict resolution, 404
Impaired contralateral saccades, 404
Impaired emotion regulation (changes in affect, euphoria, emotional instability), 405
Impaired goal-directed behavior, 405
Impaired ipsilateral scanning, 408
Impaired optokinetic nystagmus, 408
Impairment of discriminative sensation, 405
Impotence, 405
Impotence erectile dysfunction, 1021, 1073
Inactive plaque, 1082, 1088
Incidental white matter changes, 875–880
Inclusion bodies, 698, 700, 720, 723, 732, 844, 845, 849–851, 959, 1051, 1052, 1054
Incontinence, 207, 474, 475, 615, 820, 947, 980, 988
Increased intracranial pressure, 428, 443, 524, 1490, 1755, 1813, 1895
Indusium griseum, 136, 138
Infarct
  acute infarct, 484, 616, 640, 988, 992
  chronic infarct, 484
  lacunar infarcts, 474, 489, 616, 626, 897, 990, 995–997
  subacute infarct, 484
Infarction, 9, 17, 245, 428, 429, 434, 436, 458, 473–496, 666, 878, 990, 997, 1245, 1259, 1914, 1918
Infections, 17, 247, 428, 451, 552, 653–691, 693–741, 749–771, 773–792, 815, 820, 857, 1105, 1106, 1115, 1125, 1247, 1269, 1271, 1294, 1295, 1867, 1924, 1929, 1938, 1951, 2136, 2153, 2167
Inferior colliculi/colliculus, 74, 150, 156, 158, 306, 357, 381
Inferior horn of the lateral ventricle, 142, 171, 303
Inferior longitudinal fascicle, 148, 422, 423
Inferior medullary velum, 174
Inferior olivary complex, 312, 313, 384
Inferior olivary nucleus, 76, 86, 161, 231, 313, 351, 381, 716, 856, 1233
Inferior parietal lobule, 133, 150, 294, 406, 410, 853, 916, 1042
Infiltration, 568, 641, 644, 684, 685, 714, 1266, 1300, 1314, 1317, 1338, 1354, 1358, 1360, 1370, 1375, 1383, 1386, 1420, 1425, 1431, 1438, 1451, 1456, 1462, 1477, 1508, 1584, 1606, 1618, 1643, 1648, 1655, 1708, 1710, 1726, 1730, 1743, 1755, 1924, 1927, 1928, 1939, 1945, 1962, 2050, 2077, 2088, 2139, 2166
Inflammatory myofibroblastic tumour, 1956, 1985
Infratentorial, 213, 214, 505, 1075, 1077, 1208, 1267, 1426, 1490–1492, 1591, 1646, 1647, 1657
Infundibulum, 71, 153, 155, 181, 418, 1766, 1768, 1770, 1771, 1943
Inhibitory signals, 1279, 1280
Inhibitory transmitters, 369, 388
Inhomogeneous, 478, 538, 541, 616, 990, 992, 1128, 1357, 1412, 1430, 1451, 1473, 1481, 1534, 1584, 1606, 1782, 1813, 1883, 1895, 1994, 2132, 2137
Insertion, 629, 632, 1219, 1287, 1288, 1304, 1305, 1701, 2054

In situ hybridization (ISH), 111, 112, 703, 706, 714, 1927
Insomnia, 418, 820, 1212, 2156–2158, 2173
Instrumental reaction, 122
Insula, 130, 131, 134, 136, 143, 145, 150, 167, 168, 351, 367, 731, 734, 802, 920, 937, 1144, 1245, 1342
Integrins, 517, 1267, 1315–1316, 1331, 1701
Intellectual and emotional aspects of behavior, 404
Intensity, 4–6, 11, 13, 36, 113, 1039, 1339, 1375, 1827, 1998
Intention tremor, 209, 419, 420
Interanular segment, 237
Interdigitating dendritic cells (IDC), 1894, 1934
Interfascicular oligodendrocytes, 245
Interferon alpha, 1948
Interhemispheric disconnection syndrome, 1237
Interictal period, 1120, 1121
Interleukins, 248, 370, 441, 517, 1313
Intermediate fields, 278, 290
Intermediate filament proteins, 97, 103, 839, 2057
Intermediate filaments, 91, 92, 228, 241, 321, 349, 815, 838, 941, 1296, 1545, 1558, 1629, 1652, 1746, 1768, 1792, 1797, 1798, 1802, 1889, 1964
Internal capsule, 125, 127, 143, 145–147, 150, 155, 167, 168, 203, 204, 334, 475, 476, 501, 626, 666, 715, 873, 875, 1039, 1066, 1207
Internal carotid artery (ICA), 60, 62, 63, 191–196, 198, 203, 215, 216, 224, 510, 538, 543, 552, 559, 1716, 1782, 1795
Internal elastic lamina, 255, 256, 552, 567, 578, 609, 629, 641
Internal occipital protuberans, 180
Internal regulatory circuits, 349
Internodium, 237
Interpeduncular fossa, 71
Interphase, 1281–1283
Interthalamic adhesion, 150, 171, 175
Interventional neuroradiology, 4, 570
Interventricular foramen, 150, 169, 174–176, 213
Intima (tunica intima), 186, 254, 255, 538, 542
Intimal fibrosis, 641
Intimal proliferation, 641
Intracellular deposits, 835, 836
Intracerebral hemorrhage, 499–505, 507, 511, 558, 576, 607, 637, 987, 989, 999, 1207, 1258
Intramedullary hemorrhage, 499, 500
Intraneuronal processes, 369
Intraoperative MR imaging (iMRI), 27
Intravascular lymphoma
   age incidence, 1914
   biologic behavior-prognosis-prognostic factors, 1919
   clinical signs and symptoms, 1914
   CT-contrast-enhanced, 1914–1915
   CT-non contrast-enhanced, 1914–1915
   differential diagnosis, 1918
   general imaging findings, 1914–1916
   immunophenotype, 1916–1919
   incidence, 1914
   localization, 1914
   macroscopic features, 1914
   microscopic features, 1916–1918
   MRI-diffusion imaging, 1914, 1916
   MRI-FLAIR, 1914–1915
   MRI-T1, 1914–1915
   MRI-T2, 1914–1915
   MRI-T1 contrast-enhanced, 1914, 1916
   MRI-T2∗/SWI, 1914
   nuclear medicine imaging findings, 1914
   pathogenesis-molecular biology findings, 1918
   proliferation markers, 1916, 1918
   sex incidence, 1914
   treatment, 1918–1919
   WHO definition, 1914
Intravenous immunoglobulin (IVIG), 2160, 2176
Intrinsic mitochondrial apoptosis pathway, 1297–1298
Invasion, 91, 97, 635, 718, 778, 1266, 1273, 1274, 1302, 1303, 1314, 1316–1318, 1320, 1383, 1501, 1523, 1527, 1534, 1597, 1606, 1711, 1716, 1720, 1740, 1749–1751, 1766, 1776, 1782, 1793, 1794, 1810, 1901, 1956, 1958, 1962, 1997, 2037, 2050, 2148, 2152
   and metastasis, 1280, 1318, 1997
Invasive adenocarcinoma, 2111
Invasive ductal carcinoma, 2063
Invasive lobular carcinoma, 2063
Invasive squamous cell carcinoma, 2111, 2114
Inversion recovery (IR), 15, 1160, 1173
Iodine-131, 31
Ion channel, 883, 1092, 1134, 1138, 1168, 1404, 1405, 2176
Ionic channels, 369
Ionotropic GABAA receptor, 391
Ionotropic glutamate receptor, 2155, 2158
Ipsilateral ataxia, 207, 476, 658
Ipsilateral deafness, 207, 476
Ipsilateral facial anesthesia, 207, 476
Ipsilateral facial sensory loss, 207, 475, 476
Ipsilateral Horner syndrome, 207, 418, 475, 476
Ipsilateral limb ataxia, 207, 476
Ipsilateral nuclear facial and abducens palsy, 207, 476
Ipsilateral tremor/dyskinesia, 207, 476
Iron, 99, 228, 252, 257, 308, 458, 814, 837, 838, 864, 871, 884–885, 974, 975, 990, 1003, 1004, 1016, 1022, 1024, 1039, 1056
Irreversible coma, 456
Irritability, 419, 859, 898, 1060, 1212, 1800, 2128, 2155
Irritative zone, 1121
Ischemia, 9, 17, 19, 71, 74, 76, 245, 367, 456, 457, 473–496, 510, 637, 827, 865, 881, 882, 1192, 1207, 1217, 1295, 1297
Ischemic/stagnant hypoxia, 457
Ischemic stroke, 473, 474, 542, 568, 614, 626, 996, 1258–1260
Ischemic 'tolerance,' 471
Isocitrate dehydrogenase 1 (IDH1), 91, 108, 1271, 1305, 1322–1324, 1327, 1329, 1337, 1341, 1348, 1349, 1364, 1367, 1368, 1391, 1398, 1400–1403, 1408, 1448, 1458, 1466, 1496, 1501, 1510, 1793

Isocortical, 290, 918–921
Isodense, 501, 520, 1172, 1507, 1652, 1666, 1755, 1782, 1833, 1856, 1895
Iterative reconstructions, 33, 40, 50, 52, 53

J

John Cunningham Virus (JCV), 695, 698, 722, 730, 731, 1072, 1093
Judgment, 404, 898
Juvenile Huntington's disease, 1060
Juvenile xanthogranuloma and xanthoma disseminatum, 1934, 1941, 1948

K

^{39}K (potassium), 15
Kainate receptor, 392, 814, 1139
Kaposi sarcoma, 702, 1322, 1956, 1984, 2100
Karnofsky performance score (KPS), 1407, 1408, 1431, 2053, 2057
Karnofsky score, 1459
Karyorrhexis, 1618
Kawasaki's arteritis, 636
KCNA2 (potassium voltage-gated channel subfamily A member 2), 236
Kearns-Sayre syndrome (KSS), 828, 862, 863
Kennedy disease, 851, 1045
Kernel, 6, 7
Kernohan, J.W., 1277
Ki-67, 91, 92, 105, 106, 108, 1341, 1346, 1347, 1349, 1362, 1364, 1396, 1397, 1418, 1422, 1431, 1442, 1457, 1465, 1475, 1476, 1485, 1505, 1508, 1516, 1531, 1538, 1569, 1573, 1581, 1625, 1626, 1645, 1656, 1675, 1676, 1692, 1742, 1743, 1764, 1771, 1787, 1796, 1801, 1901, 1914, 1916, 1920, 1927, 1945, 1949, 1968, 1977, 2010, 2070, 2084, 2091, 2165
Ki-67 LI, 1341, 1349, 1364, 1417, 1431, 1438, 1454, 1459, 1476, 1480, 1496, 1500, 1501, 1510, 1518, 1530, 1539, 1545, 1579, 1582, 1590, 1600, 1604, 1608, 1624, 1643, 1647, 1648, 1652, 1764, 1767, 1776, 1793, 1796, 1798, 1804, 1806, 1810, 1813, 1904, 1938, 1964, 1969
Ki67/MIB1, 91, 105, 106, 1742
Kleine–Levin syndrome, 417
Klüver–Bucy syndrome, 409
Knee of the internal capsule, 127, 147
Korsakoff amnestic syndrome, 1229
Krabbe disease, 864, 1072
Kuru, 796, 797, 820, 827
Kuru-type plaques, 812, 817
Kyphoplasty, 4

L

Laboratory transmission of scrapie, 797
Laceration, 60, 521, 522, 530, 1187, 1196, 1201–1205
Lack of spontaneity, 208
Lactate, 17, 242, 444, 478, 520, 661, 663, 666, 752, 766, 814, 815, 828, 862, 947, 1125, 1214–1216, 1311, 1313, 1376, 1377, 1412, 1434, 1493, 1525, 1534, 1615, 1642, 1652, 1834, 1871, 1877, 1897, 2042, 2120, 2124, 2132
Lactate storm, 1214–1215
Lactic acid, 471
Lacunar infarcts including temporopolar white matter and internal/ external capsule, 626
Lacunar lesions, 616, 627, 628, 876
Lacunar state, 987, 992
Lacunar syndromes, 207, 474, 476, 614
Lacunes, 614, 990, 995–999
Lambert–Eaton myasthenic syndrome, 2153, 2171, 2172, 2174
Lamina affixa, 150
Lamina medullaris medialis, 145
Laminin receptor, 814, 815
Landmarks, 23–25, 51, 74, 130, 409
Langerhans cell histiocytosis (LCH)
    age incidence, 1935
    biologic behavior-prognosis-prognostic factors, 1940
    clinical signs and symptoms, 1935
    CT-non contrast-enhanced, 1935–1936
    differential diagnosis, 1938
    general imaging findings, 1935–1938
    immunophenotype, 1938–1940
    incidence, 1935
    localization, 1935
    macroscopic features, 1938
    microscopic features, 1938–1940
    MRI-FLAIR, 1935, 1937
    MRI-T1, 1935–1936
    MRI-T2, 1935, 1937
    MRI-T1 contrast-enhanced, 1935–1937
    nuclear medicine imaging findings, 1936, 1938
    pathogenesis, 1938
    proliferation markers, 1938
    sex incidence, 1935
    treatment, 1938
    ultrastructural features, 1938
    WHO definition, 1934–1935
Langerhans cells (LC), 1934, 1938, 1939
Langerin (CD207), 1934, 1940
Language, 21, 148, 291, 403, 406, 410–413, 415, 417, 420, 422, 474, 701, 725, 817, 853, 896, 945–947, 988, 989, 1212, 1239
Large cell undifferentiated carcinoma, 2063
Larmor equation, 10
Late onset AD (LOAD), 883, 898–899, 901, 922–925
Lateral geniculate body, 150, 305, 326, 328, 331, 333, 351, 356, 357, 408, 417, 1235
Lateral hypothalamic region, 306
Lateral longitudinal striae, 136, 150
Lateral medullary syndrome, 208
Lateral ventricle, 14, 136, 138, 142, 144, 150, 167–177, 303, 321, 435, 444, 449, 450, 715, 876–878, 960, 1060–1062, 1066, 1075, 1100, 1144, 1171, 1212, 1492, 1501, 1507, 1511, 1522, 1534, 1542, 1575, 1576, 1581, 1824, 1833

Late subacute, 457, 500–502, 529
Layer II: external granular layer, 282, 287
Layer III: external pyramidal cell layer, 282, 289
Layer I: molecular layer, 281, 282, 287, 314
Layer IV: internal granular layer, 282, 289
Layer V: internal pyramidal cell layer, 282, 289
Layer VI: plexiform (multiform) layer, 282, 289–290
Lead collimators, 40
Lectins, 89, 100, 690, 1316, 1365
Left-hand apraxia, 207, 414, 415, 475
Leiomyoma, 1956, 1985, 1991
Leiomyosarcoma, 1956, 1979, 1985–1986, 1991, 1992, 2062, 2100, 2115
Lesion models, 402
Lethargy to deep coma, 456
Leucine-rich glioma-inactivated protein 1 (LGI1), 1136, 1137, 2153, 2156, 2157, 2162, 2167, 2170, 2171, 2174, 2175
Leukoaraiosis, 615, 875, 877, 995, 996
Leukodystrophies, 243, 826, 864–865, 1072, 1089
Leukoencephalopathy, 606, 607, 616, 626, 629, 714, 862, 1244, 1260, 2120
Leukotrienes, 441
Levodopa-resistance, 974
Lewy body
　dementia, 416, 813, 826, 827, 838, 839, 842, 851, 931–942
　disease, 100, 102, 818, 859, 897, 916, 931, 933
Lewy body-like hyaline inclusions, 1042
Leydig cell tumor, 2094
Li-Fraumeni syndrome, 2129
Ligand-gated channels, 373, 387, 392, 1134
Limb ataxia, 207, 419, 420, 1022
Limbic
　network, 291, 1135
　system, 137–142, 155, 326, 333, 343–346, 352, 358, 380, 414, 417, 696, 698, 731, 733, 856, 1245, 1256, 2154
Limbic encephalitis (LE), 827, 2153–2158, 2160–2163, 2170, 2172–2174
Limen insulae, 134, 148
Limiting basal lamina, 1559
LINAC, 1662, 1675, 1692, 1793, 2124
Linear attenuation coefficients
　of the voxel, 5
　of water, 5
　of x-rays, 5
Lipidized GBM, 1386
Lipids, 17, 89, 237, 238, 250, 538, 542, 655, 666, 752, 815, 843, 848, 884, 885, 887, 888, 922–924, 1056, 1216, 1257, 1258, 1300, 1309, 1313, 1322, 1376, 1412, 1642, 1652, 1755, 1836, 1871, 1877, 1884, 1969, 2085, 2120, 2124, 2132
Lipofuscin, 83, 89, 228, 279, 865, 1011
Lipoma
　CT-contrast-enhanced, 1979
　CT-non contrast-enhanced, 1979–1980
　general imaging findings, 1979
　macroscopic features, 1979, 1983
　microscopic features, 1979, 1983
　MRI-FLAIR, 1979, 1981
　MRI-T1, 1979, 1981
　MRI-T2, 1979, 1981
　MRI-T1 contrast-enhanced, 1979, 1981–1982
Liposarcoma, 1050, 1956, 1984, 1991
Lisch nodules, 1662, 1693, 1694
Lissencephaly, 1132, 1135
Listeriosis, 665, 666
Lobar hematomas, 607
Lobe
　frontal lobe, 60, 63, 71, 76, 130–133, 136, 137, 147, 148, 150, 167, 169, 203, 204, 279, 290, 294, 380, 405, 436, 443, 475, 487, 515, 610, 658, 661, 667, 725, 733, 756, 764, 817, 838, 853, 856, 873, 875, 933, 945, 947, 954, 959, 967, 996, 1064, 1080, 1144, 1160, 1213, 1226, 1227, 1237, 1257, 1280, 1385, 1436, 1448, 1460, 1477, 1576, 1646, 1648, 1859
　occipital lobe, 71, 75, 76, 130, 131, 133–134, 137, 148, 150, 167–169, 204, 209, 274, 294, 332, 333, 356, 357, 361, 407–409, 413, 434, 476, 485, 609, 802, 817, 856, 873, 920, 934, 935, 960, 967, 1080, 1280, 1375, 1448, 1482, 1898, 1899
　parietal lobe, 76, 130–133, 135–136, 147, 148, 150, 154, 167, 168, 203, 204, 209, 294, 328, 332, 334, 351, 361, 407, 413, 422, 475, 487, 490, 507, 658, 803, 851, 853, 901, 958, 962, 966, 977, 980, 1042, 1201, 1280, 1378, 1415, 1419, 1448, 1482, 1899, 2052, 2125
　temporal lobe, 13, 14, 76, 130, 131, 133–138, 142, 144, 148, 154, 169, 204, 214, 223, 290, 294, 332, 361, 392, 410, 413, 598, 658, 696–698, 715, 731, 734, 735, 854, 855, 863, 873, 933, 947, 949, 950, 954, 955, 960, 962, 964–967, 1042, 1080, 1124, 1125, 1134, 1158, 1165, 1175, 1193, 1212, 1214, 1257, 1338, 1385, 1419, 1482, 1541, 1542, 1562, 1572, 1830, 2154, 2155
Localizationist models, 403
Locked-in syndrome, 1224, 1233
Locus coeruleus, 159, 228, 311–312, 333, 350–352, 381, 382, 384, 387, 937, 976, 982, 1007, 1028, 1213, 1214, 1227, 1254, 1260
Long association fibers, 147
Longitudinal fissure, 129, 167
Longitudinal magnetization (Mz), 10, 11
Long-spacing collagen, 1675
Lower motor neuron (LMN), 334, 835, 1037–1039, 1042, 1054
Low-pass filter, 33, 50–53
Lung cancer, 2063, 2155, 2172
Luse body, 1675
Luteinizing hormone (LH), 371, 1754, 1781, 1787, 1803–1804, 1806, 1812
Luteinizing hormone-releasing hormone, 370
Lutetium-177, 31, 1716

Index

Luxol fast blue (LFB), 84–86, 310, 314, 320, 619, 685, 709, 713, 876, 1044, 1065, 1082, 1083, 1085, 1089, 1102, 1112, 1166, 1176, 1231, 1236, 1248
Lymphocytes, 83, 105, 540, 542, 644, 675, 678, 684, 685, 687, 714, 728, 736, 752, 757, 768, 1078, 1082, 1088, 1106, 1133, 1275, 1556, 1739, 1945, 1979, 2059, 2094, 2168
Lymphocytic meningitis (LM), 702, 706, 711–712, 1247
Lymphoma, 39, 88, 89, 641, 702, 752, 1279, 1663, 1867, 1929, 1938, 2170
Lysosomes, 226, 228, 881, 1297, 1300, 1795, 1880
Lytic skull lesions, 1935

M

Ma2, 2153–2155, 2170, 2171, 2175
MAC 387, 103, 1948, 2058, 2092
Macrocephaly, 1694
Macrophages, 83, 100, 247, 248, 441, 458, 484, 492, 493, 510, 511, 517, 521, 529, 538, 540, 542, 567, 568, 665, 675, 680, 684, 685, 687, 688, 690, 700, 701, 703, 706, 708, 714, 717, 718, 732, 736, 737, 786, 787, 864, 865, 881, 886, 937, 990, 995, 1007, 1078, 1082, 1086–1089, 1101, 1106, 1114, 1205, 1250, 1272, 1278, 1293, 1312, 1765, 1851, 1938, 1941, 1945, 2026
Macular sparing, 208, 209, 407, 408, 476
Magnet, 9
Magnetic resonance imaging (MRI), 4, 5, 9, 14, 15, 18, 23, 32, 33, 35, 36, 40, 44, 45, 48, 49, 51–54, 132, 402, 875, 974, 990, 995, 1003, 1022, 1077, 1098, 1208, 1372, 1373, 1378, 2137, 2139, 2153–2155, 2159
Magnetoencephalography (MEG), 402, 1121
Major dense line, 99, 250, 251
Malformations of cortical development (MCD), 1125, 1133, 1138, 1157–1169, 1171–1179
Malignancy, 48, 91, 636, 637, 646, 1268, 1270, 1277, 1438, 1459, 1476, 1501, 1534, 1604, 1631, 1742, 1841, 1957, 1991, 2152, 2162
Malignant peripheral nerve sheath tumor (MPNST)
  age incidence, 1689
  biologic behavior-prognosis-prognostic factors, 1692
  CT-contrast-enhanced, 1690
  CT-non contrast-enhanced, 1690
  differential diagnosis, 1692
  epithelioid MPNST, 1692
  general imaging findings, 1690
  glandular MPNST, 1690, 1692
  immunophenotype, 1692–1693
  incidence, 1689
  localization, 1690
  macroscopic features, 1690
  malignant triton tumor, 1692
  microscopic features, 1690–1691
  molecular neuropathology, 1692
  MPNST with divergent differentiation, 1690, 1692
  MPNST with perineurial differentiation, 1692
  MRI-diffusion imaging, 1690
  MRI-FLAIR, 1690
  MRI-T1, 1690
  MRI-T2, 1690
  MRI-T1 contrast-enhanced, 1690
  MRI-T2∗/SWI, 1690
  pathogenesis, (AU: Not found)
  proliferation markers, 1692
  sex incidence, 1689
  treatment, 1692
  ultrastructural features, 1692
  WHO definition, 1689
  WHO grade, 1689
Mamillotegmental tract, 346, 358
Mammillary bodies, 71, 137, 153, 155, 156, 204, 306, 343, 347, 348, 352, 414, 476, 861, 1144, 1213, 1214, 1229–1231
Mammillary region, 306
Marburg type, 1072, 1093
Marchiafava-Bignami disease (MBD), 1072, 1089, 1224, 1237, 1238
Marfan syndrome, 606, 998
Margin
  inferior, 130, 133, 134, 184, 223
  lateral, 130, 974
  superior, 123, 130, 131, 133, 184, 222
MART1, 2060, 2083, 2115
Martinotti, 95, 233, 268, 269, 287, 289, 292
Matrix, 12, 13, 79, 1341, 1614, 1631, 1990, 2026
Matrix metalloproteinases (MMPs), 441, 567, 568, 1267, 1303, 1311, 1312, 1315, 1431, 1990, 1995
Maxillary artery, 181, 191
MDE (3,4-methylenedioxyethylamphetamine, "Eve"), 1259
MDEA, 1244, 1259
MDMA (3,4-methylenedioxymethamphetamine, "Ecstasy"), 1244, 1259, 1260
MDP, 1990
Mean transit time (MTT), 9, 18, 477, 479, 1035
Measles virus, 696, 697
Mechanoporation, 1207
Media (tunica media), 254
Medial eminence, 157, 158
Medial forebrain bundle, 352
Medial ganglionic eminence (MGE), 232, 291
Medial geniculate body, 150, 204, 306, 351, 357, 417, 476, 838
Medial hypothalamic region, 306
Medial longitudinal stria, 136
Medial meningeal artery, 181
Median fissure, 157, 160
Medulla oblongata, 68, 71, 76, 86, 129, 130, 137, 157, 160–163, 169, 186, 204, 224, 246, 267, 311–315, 334, 381, 385, 386, 436, 666, 698, 737, 779, 785, 855, 1012, 1042, 1257–1258, 1563, 1944
Medullary, 199, 212, 214, 290, 312, 352, 381, 1928, 1990, 1998, 2063, 2070

Medullary carcinoma of breast, 2075
Medulloblastoma
    age incidence, 1615
    biologic behavior-prognosis-prognostic factors, 1631, 1634
    classic, 1614, 1618, 1631, 1632
    CT-contrast-enhanced, 1615
    CT-non contrast-enhanced, 1615, 1617
    desmoplastic/nodular medulloblastoma, 1615–1629
    differential diagnosis, 1629
    DNA methylation, (AU: Not found)
    epigenetics, 1631–1634
    with extensive nodularity, 1614, 1618
    gene expression, 1629–1630
    general imaging findings, 1615
    genetics, 1629–1631
    immunophenotype, 1624, 1626, 1628
    incidence, 1615
    large cell/anaplastic medulloblastoma, 1622, 1631, 1632
    localization, 1615
    macroscopic features, 1616, 1618, 1620
    microRNAs, 1630
    microscopic features, 1618, 1621–1625
    molecular neuropathology, 1629–1633
    MRI-diffusion imaging, 1615
    MRI-FLAIR, 1615–1617, 1619
    MRI-perfusion, 1615, 1619
    MRI-T1, 1615–1617, 1619
    MRI-T2, 1615–1617, 1619
    MRI-T1 contrast-enhanced, 1615–1617, 1619
    MRI-T2∗/ SWI, 1615
    MR-spectroscopy, 1615
    non-WNT/non-SHH, 1614, 1628, 1629, 1632
    NOS, 1614
    nuclear medicine imaging findings, 1615–1616
    pathogenesis, 1629
    proliferation markers, 1624, 1626
    sex incidence, 1615
    SHH-activated and TP53-wildtype, 1614, 1628
    SHH-activated-medulloblastoma, SHH-activated and TP53-mutant, 1614, 1626, 1628, 1631, 1634
    treatment, 1631
    ultrastructural features, 1624, 1628–1629
    WHO definition, 1614–1615
    WHO grade, 1615
    WNT-activated, 1614, 1626, 1628
Medulloepithelioma
    age incidence, 1647
    biologic behavior-prognosis-prognostic factors, 1648
    differential diagnosis, 1648
    immunophenotype, 1648
    incidence, 1647
    localization, 1647–1648
    macroscopic features, 1648
    microscopic features, 1648
    pathogenesis, 1648
    proliferation markers, 1648
    sex incidence, 1647
    treatment, 1648
    ultrastructural features, 1648
    WHO definition, 1647–1648
    WHO grade, 1647
Medullomyoblastoma, 1618, 1622, 1986
Megakaryocyte, 105
Megalencephalic leukoencephalopathy with subcortical cysts (MLC), 243
Melan-A, 102, 108, 1396, 2058, 2060–2062, 2082, 2084
Melanin, 89, 228, 308, 311, 716, 937, 1007, 1618, 1629, 2076
Melanocyte stimulating hormone, 370
Melanocytic medulloblastoma, 1618, 1622
Melanomas, 91, 104, 1289, 1291, 1297, 1302, 1742, 1979, 2038, 2042, 2051, 2052, 2055–2057, 2060, 2062, 2073, 2076–2084, 2173
Melatonin synthesis, 1325, 1596
Membrane
    blebbing, 1293–1295
    budding, 1293
    leakage, 1214
Memory and cognitive impairment, 456
Memory deficits, 420, 422, 847, 878, 882, 988, 1239, 2128, 2154, 2155
Memory disturbance, 208, 418, 476, 2156
Memory impairment, 443, 896, 932, 1212, 2154, 2159
Meningeal lymphocytic infiltration (MLI), 702, 710, 711
Meningeal spaces
    epidural space, 182, 188, 658, 666, 1986
    subarachnoidal space, 176, 186, 188, 436, 449, 451, 510, 658, 1268, 2071
    subdural space, 188, 213
    subpial space, 188
Meninges
    arachnoidea, 186–188, 252, 253, 500, 1679
    dura mater
        inner meningeal layer, 179
        outer periosteal layer, 179
        stratum meningeale, 179
        stratum periostale, 179
    leptomeninges, 14, 60, 67, 68, 254, 282, 444, 500, 578, 639, 641, 660, 666, 669, 687, 688, 706, 736, 773, 784, 785, 787, 861, 862, 960, 998, 1106, 1171, 1269, 1383, 1437, 1438, 1451, 1462, 1553, 1554, 1606, 1618, 1749, 1934, 1935, 1941, 1944, 1967, 1973, 1986, 2038, 2050
    pachymeninx, 179, 763, 777
    pia mater, 177, 179, 186–188, 252–253, 321
Meningioma
    age incidence, 1708
    anaplastic meningioma, 1708, 1719, 1742, 1743, 1746, 1749–1751
    angiography, 1715, 1716
    angiomatous, 1720
    atypical meningioma, 1722–1724, 1740–1742
    biologic behavior-prognosis-prognostic factors, 1749–1751
    chordoid, 1720, 1740
    clear cell, 1740–1742
    CT-contrast-enhanced, 1709–1710

CT-non contrast-enhanced, 1709–1712
differential diagnosis, 1746
DNA methylation, 1748
epigenetics, 1748–1749
fibroblastic, 1729, 1734
gene expression, 1749–1751
general imaging findings, 1708–1724
genetics, 1746–1747
immunophenotype, 1742, 1745
incidence, 1748
localization, 1708
lymphoplasmacyte-rich, 1708, 1720, 1733, 1739
macroscopic features, 1720, 1725–1726
meningothelial, 1720, 1729, 1732, 1745, 1746
metaplastic, 1708, 1720, 1733
microcystic, 1720, 1733, 1737, 1749
microRNAs, 1748–1749
microscopic features, 1742–1744
modified Shinshu grade, 1750
molecular neuropathology, 1746–1747
MRI-diffusion imaging, 1709
MRI-diffusion tensor imaging, 1709, 1713
MRI-FLAIR, 1709–1710, 1712–1714, 1716
MRI-perfusion, 1709, 1713
MRI-T1, 1709, 1714
MRI-T2, 1709–1710, 1712–1714, 1716
MRI-T1 contrast-enhanced, 1709–1714
MRI-T2∗/SWI, 1709
MR-spectroscopy, 1714, 1716
nuclear medicine imaging findings, 1716–1724
papillary, 1708, 1742, 1751
pathogenesis, 1746
proliferation markers, 1742, 1746
psammomatous, 1708, 1720, 1731, 1735
rhabdoid, 1742, 1744
secretory, 85, 1720, 1733, 1738, 1742
sex incidence, 1708
Simpson grading, 1750
transitional, 1731, 1735
treatment, 1749
ultrastructural features, 1746
WHO definition, 1718–1720
WHO grade, 1720
Meningism, 637, 749, 773, 1105, 1267
Mesaxon, 236
Mesencephalon, 68, 71, 72, 129, 130, 150, 155–158, 169, 174, 186, 306–311, 376, 381, 385, 559, 671, 863, 916, 976, 1028, 1615, 1620
Mesenchymal, 97, 102, 540, 990, 1274, 1275, 1277, 1368, 1402, 1403, 1411, 1414, 1417, 1562, 1648, 1651, 1652, 1663, 1690, 1733, 1780, 1955–1986, 2005, 2011, 2058, 2076, 2100, 2139, 2148
Mesial temporal lobe epilepsy in adults with drug-resistant TLE, 1143
Meso-limbo-cortical dementia, 856
Metabolic disorders, 428, 896, 897, 989, 1125
Metabolism, 11, 29, 30, 32, 153, 227, 391–392, 418, 852, 853, 872, 879, 884, 899, 1072, 1255, 1257, 1313, 1716, 1824, 2050, 2137

Metabolites, 14–17, 1101, 1245, 1255, 1313
Metabotropic GABA$_B$ receptor, 391
Metabotropic glutamate receptor antibody syndrome, 2160
Metabotropic glutamate receptors, 815, 2160, 2175
Metachromatic leukodystrophy, 864, 1072
Metamorphopsia, 209
Metanephric tumors, 2085
Metaphase, 1281, 1284, 1288
Metaphase/anaphase transition (= spindle apparatus checkpoint), 1282
Metaplasia, 1270, 1765
Metastases, 14, 78, 85, 102, 104, 687, 698, 776, 828, 1267–1269, 1291, 1300, 1302, 1303, 1318, 1397, 1398, 1407, 1444, 1490, 1511, 1559, 1604, 1608, 1618, 1631, 1632, 1675, 1686, 1750, 1780, 1810, 1967, 1994, 1997, 2038, 2042, 2050–2053, 2057, 2070, 2076, 2085, 2088, 2094, 2097, 2105, 2111, 2113, 2124, 2132, 2135, 2136, 2138, 2167
Metastatic disease, 1269
Metastatic tumors
    age incidence, 2038
    biologic behavior-prognosis-prognostic factors, 2053
    breast tumor, 2063, 2071–2072
    colorectal tumor, 2096–2098
    CT-contrast-enhanced, 2038
    CT-non contrast-enhanced, 2038–2039, 2041
    female genital tract tumor, 2105, 2107–2111
    general imaging findings, 2038
    immunohistochemical approach, 2057–2062
    incidence, 2037
    localization, 2038
    lung tumor, 2063–2064
    melanoma, 2073, 2076–2081
    microscopic features, 2050
    molecular neuropathology, 2053
    MRI-diffusion imaging, 2040
    MRI-diffusion tensor imaging, 2040
    MRI-FLAIR, 2038–2039, 2041
    MRI-perfusion, 2040
    MRI-T1, 2038–2039, 2041
    MRI-T2, 2038–2039, 2041
    MRI-T1 contrast-enhanced, 2040–2041
    MRI-T2∗/SWI, 2040
    MR-spectroscopy, 2042
    nuclear medicine imaging findings, 2042–2050
    pathogenesis, 2050
    proliferation markers, 2050
    prostate tumor, 2088, 2093–2094
    renal tumor, 2050, 2085
    sex incidence, 2038
    testicular tumor, 2094–2096, 2155
    treatment, 2053, 2056–2057
    ultrastructural features, (AU: Not found)
    urinary tract tumor, 2085, 2089–2092
    WHO definition, 2037–2038
Metencephalon, 129
Methamphetamine, 720, 1244, 1245, 1258–1259
Methotrexate leukoencephalopathy, 2128

Methylation, 925, 1017, 1090, 1266, 1285, 1309, 1657, 1748, 1766
Methylation-mediated gene silencing, 1290
[Methyl-11C]-L-methionine (MET), 29, 48, 49, 54, 665, 1324, 1327, 1328, 1340, 1341, 1356, 1380, 1381, 1402, 1412, 1414, 1419, 1420, 1451, 1462, 1470, 1477, 1591, 1755, 1961, 1996, 2050, 2120, 2125, 2137, 2139
4-Methyl-2,5-dimethoxyamphetamine (DOM), 1244, 1259
3,4-Methylenedioxyamphetamine (MDA), 1244, 1259
3,4-Methylenedioxymethamphetamine (MDMA), 1244, 1259, 1260
mGluR1, 2153, 2160, 2170, 2174
mGluR5, 2160, 2174
MGMT promoter methylation, 1310, 1322, 1323, 1326, 1327, 1403, 1431
MIB-1, 105, 1742, 1808, 1809, 2075
Microarray techniques, 114
Microcircuit, 326, 342
Microdialysis (MD), 402, 520
Microdysgenesis, 1132
Microelectrodes, 402
Microenvironment, 247, 248, 881, 1266, 1314–1319
Microglia, 85, 99, 100, 239, 240, 247–249, 301, 458, 665, 685, 687, 690, 700, 703, 717–720, 732, 790, 816, 835, 836, 846, 878–882, 1040, 1082, 1088, 1089, 1092, 1217, 1253, 1315, 1888, 2165
Microglial activation, 843, 845, 880, 887, 1040, 1077, 1275
Microplaques, 812
MicroRNAs (miRNAs)
  miR-7, 1018, 1403
  miR-17, 886, 1403
  miR-21, 649, 1403, 1703
  miR-93, 1403, 1444
  miR-128, 1403
  miR-137, 925, 1403
  miR-204, 1703
  miR-214, 1703, 1787
  miR-221, 1403
  miR-222, 1403
  miR-34a, 1403, 1444, 1703
  miR-10b, 1403, 1703, 1996
  miR-29c, 1703
Microsatellite instability (MSI), 1304, 2099, 2107
Microtubuli-associated protein (MAP2), 228, 878, 1007, 1176, 1431, 1454, 1589, 1656
Microtubuli-associated proteins (MAPs), 228, 626, 1645, 1648
Microtubule-associated proteins tau (MAPT), 814, 844, 847, 850, 851, 954, 956, 957, 965, 968, 979, 984, 1001, 1016, 1017
Microtubule disruption, 1214
Microtubules, 93, 228, 229, 249, 251, 815, 847, 1012, 1209, 1214, 1217, 1284, 1404, 1510, 1579, 1591, 1629, 1806
Microvilli, 321, 322, 1496, 1501, 1518, 1530, 1648, 1692, 1843, 1850, 1853, 1875, 1880

Microwave fixation, 76
Midbrain tegmentum, 307, 853, 980
Midbrain tegmentum (reticular formation), 352
Middle cerebral artery syndrome, 208
Middle cranial fossa, 137, 185, 214, 223, 436
Middle frontal gyrus, 76, 131, 132, 150, 167, 168, 404, 405, 800
Middle temporal visual cortex, 333
Mild malformation of cortical development (mMCD), 1157
Mild neurocognitive disorder (MND), 701, 933
MILD surgery, 4
Mild traumatic brain injury, 1186
Milk fat globule epidermal growth factor 8 (MFGE8), 816
Miller Dieker, 1132
Mineralization, 712, 862, 863, 1178, 1990
Mineralizing microangiopathy, 2120, 2124
Minichromosome maintenance complex component 2 (MCM2), 92, 107
Minicolumns, 290
Minigemistocytes, 1452, 1454, 1456, 1462
Mismatched bases, 1266, 1285, 1288
Mismatch repair (MMR), 1266, 1288, 1291
MITF, 102, 1657, 2058, 2060, 2083
Mitochondria, 54, 226, 227, 236, 243, 258, 321, 456, 862, 883, 1011, 1015, 1016, 1258, 1297, 1300, 1397, 1417, 1420, 1454, 1559, 1579, 1591, 1776, 1871, 1879, 1904
Mitochondrial DNA (mtDNA), 888, 924–925, 1016, 1092, 1266, 1285
Mitochondrial dysfunction, 845, 883, 1011, 1015, 1016, 1034, 1045, 1049, 1216
Mitochondrial encephalomyopathies, 825, 828, 862–864, 1035
Mitochondrial encephalopathy, lactate, acidosis and stroke-like episodes (MELAS), 825, 828, 862, 863, 998, 1035
Mitochondrial neurogastrointestinal encephalopathy (MNGIE), 826, 862
Mitogen-activated protein kinase (MAPK) signaling, 880, 1090, 1091, 1257, 1266, 1306, 1309, 1324, 1443, 1444, 1492, 1701, 1747, 1996
Mitoses, 959, 1049, 1268, 1270–1272, 1278, 1281, 1283, 1284, 1301, 1362, 1386, 1396, 1397, 1438, 1444, 1496, 1501, 1516, 1518, 1523, 1530, 1534, 1538, 1545, 1573, 1584, 1589, 1597, 1600, 1604, 1618, 1622, 1624, 1646, 1648, 1740, 1742, 1767, 1771, 1776, 1794, 1871, 1882, 1957, 1962, 1964, 1968, 1979, 1982, 1985, 2013, 2111, 2113, 2127, 2175
  M phase, 1281, 1283–1284
Mitotic activity, 1268, 1277, 1341, 1354, 1360, 1362, 1364, 1368, 1414, 1416, 1453, 1454, 1476, 1510, 1523, 1530, 1534, 1558, 1572, 1686, 1690, 1692, 1740, 1771, 1875, 1881, 1882, 1904, 1962, 1985
Mixed AD, 842, 897, 915, 996
Mixed dementia, 988
Modified Bielschowsky, 84–87, 916

Moesin-ezrin-radixin-like-protein, 1663, 1700
Molds, 79, 774, 775
Molecular biology technique, 111
Molecular imaging, 15, 113–114, 854
Molecular pathways genes
 ACT (α1 antichymotrypsin), 615, 1438
 activator protein-2γ (Ap-2γ), 1867
 acute, 2119
 acyl-coenzyme A oxidase 1 gene (ACOX1), 879
 ADAM metallopeptidase domain 22-ADAM metallopeptidase domain 23 (ADAM22-ADAM23), 236
 adenomatous polyposis coli (APC), 1306, 1320, 1613, 1629, 1747, 2054
 ADP, 441
 advanced glycation end-product (AGE), 883
 AFP-α-fetoprotein, 1866
 AIP, 409, 846, 1788, 1789, 1791
 AKT1, 1324, 1326, 1591
 AKT2, 1324, 1591
 AKT3, 1324, 1591
 Akt pathway, 1399, 1747, 1989
 alarin, 1496, 1501, 1510, 1516, 1529, 1530, 1539
 aldehyde dehydrogenase 1 family member L1 (ALDH1L1), 241
 alkaline phosphatase, liver/bone/kidney (ALPL), 1748
 alpha-internexin, 1431, 1452, 1493
 alpha-subunit, 293, 1787, 1803, 1812, 1990, 1995, 2055
 alsin ALS2, 1049, 1050
 amino acid transporter 2 (EEAT2), 1101
 AMP, 369, 441
 amplicon at 19q13.42, 1647
 amplification, 91, 113, 114, 1285, 1289, 1305–1307, 1322, 1324, 1326, 1327, 1329, 1349, 1350, 1399, 1401, 1402, 1417, 1476, 1484, 1630, 1637, 1638, 1646, 1747, 1748
 amyloid precursor protein (APP), 99, 100, 605, 612, 615, 839, 841, 1089, 1115, 1185, 1207, 1210
 angiogenin (ANG), 1049–1051
 angiopoietins, 1311, 1313, 1315
 angiotensin 1 converting enzyme (ACE), 615
 angiotensin converting enzyme gene, 1219
 angiotensin II, 370, 567, 568
 Annexin-A1, 1770
 α-1-antichimotrypsin, 1775
 anti-Hu, 1579, 2154, 2171, 2172
 α-1-antitrypsin, 1775
 APOE ε4 genotype, 879
 APOE gene, 249, 518, 614, 879, 885, 895, 899, 922, 924
 AQP4-IgG, 1098, 1103
 aquaporin, 4, 243, 249, 259, 441, 1067, 1068, 1101, 1103, 1215, 2171, 2173
 arachidonic acid, 441
 ARF, 1337, 1349
 ARFGEF2, 1178
 arginase 1, 2061, 2104
 ataxia telangiectasia (A-T) mutated (ATM), 1285–1286
 ATM-and Rad3-related (ATR), 1286
 ATP, 44, 110, 372, 441, 455, 471, 883, 1093, 1254, 1295
 ATP13A2 ATPase 13A2, 1014
 ATP-binding cassette, sub-family A (ABC1), member 7 ABCA7, 93, 895
 ATRX, 108, 1341, 1349, 1350, 1353, 1364, 1367, 1400, 1401, 1442, 1453, 1464
 AURKB, 142
 autophagy, 720, 850, 880–882, 1051, 1053, 1059, 1067, 1266, 1293–1297, 1300, 2139
 basal/stem cell factor (p63), 102, 104, 1303, 2058, 2060, 2067, 2069, 2075, 2083, 2088, 2089, 2091, 2095, 2106, 2114, 2115
 basic fibroblast growth factor, 241, 248, 568, 1648
 BCL1, 1289, 1906, 1907, 1929
 BCL-2, 1219, 1297, 1302, 1303, 1341, 1364, 1749, 1770, 1776, 1906–1908, 1913, 2084, 2114
 bcl6, 105, 887, 1893, 1905–1908, 1914
 Bcl-6, 1905–1908, 1913, 1914
 BCL11B (CTIP2) B-cell CLL/lymphoma 11B (zinc finger protein), 291
 BCOR-CCNB3 intrachromosomal inversion, 1984
 BMP-4, 1788, 1789
 bradykinin, 371, 441
 BRAF gene, 1306, 1433, 1443
 BRaf protein-BRAF gene, 1306
 BRAF V600E mutations, 1324, 1753, 1759, 1766
 brain-derived neurotrophic factor (BDNF), 248, 1219
 breakpoint cluster region (BCR), 1747
 breast carcinoma amplified sequence (BCAS1), 1, 247
 bridging integrator 1 BIN1, 895, 924
 cadherins, 1267, 1318
 calcineurin, 1563, 1573
 calcium channels, 236, 605, 1219
 calcium channel subunit gene (CACNA1A), 236, 1219
 calcium channel, voltage-dependent, gamma subunit 2 (CACNG2), 236
 calcium voltage-gated channel subunit alpha1 A (CACNA1A), 236, 1219
 calretinin, 92, 95, 233, 292, 1176, 1675, 2060, 2062, 2099, 2112
 cAMP response element binding-protein (CREB), 883, 885, 925, 1254, 1256, 1787, 1789
 Ca^{2+} pump, 455, 471
 carcinogen-metabolizing gene, 1368, 1408
 catechol-O-methyl transferase (COMT), 381, 1001, 1018, 1220
 catenin pathway, 1981, 1995
 cathepsin B, 1775, 2084
 cathepsins, 568, 869, 884, 1311, 1312
 CCND1, 1285, 1328, 1657, 1789, 1913
 CCT1 (KRIT1), 577, 593
 CCT2 (malcavernin, MG4707), 577, 593
 CCT3 (programmed cell death 10, PCD10), 577, 593

Molecular pathways genes (cont.)
  CD3, 92, 103, 105, 527, 641, 1114, 1907, 1908, 1912, 1917
  CD4, 105, 583, 641, 699, 701, 715, 718, 731, 786, 1082, 1088, 1733, 1982, 2163
  CD5, 105, 1905–1910, 1913, 1918
  CD8, 105, 1908, 1909, 1912, 2163
  CD9, 1349
  CD10, 105, 1905–1907, 1909–1911, 1914, 1918, 1929, 2060–2062, 2075, 2086, 2088, 2096, 2099, 2102, 2104, 2107, 2115
  CD19, 1905–1097, 1918, 1929
  CD20, 92, 103, 105, 106, 1901, 1907–1910, 1912, 1917, 1918, 1929, 2058
  CD23, 105, 1906, 1907, 1909, 1910
  CD24, 887, 1325, 1596, 1997
  CD30, 92, 1867, 1905, 1908, 1909, 1912, 1948, 2061, 2096
  CD31, 102, 103, 105, 578, 593, 594, 596, 1966, 1979, 1982, 2058
  CD34, 102, 103, 105, 108, 593, 596, 598, 1164, 1558, 1563, 1569, 1672, 1684, 1686, 1736, 1750, 1776, 1906, 1909, 1979, 1985, 2058, 2062, 2075, 2100, 2104
  CD38, 1906, 1907, 1929
  CD44 (hyaluronic acid receptor), 887, 1320, 1431, 1702, 1891, 1918, 1997, 2095, 2096
  CD56, 102, 108, 1624, 1626, 1912, 1977, 1979, 2058, 2060–2062, 2067, 2070, 2084, 2104, 2112
  CD57, 102, 1454, 1912, 2058, 2062
  CD61, 105, 2058
  CD99, 1647, 1906, 1909, 1965, 1966, 1984, 2061, 2062, 2084, 2096, 2100
  CD138, 103, 105, 1906, 1908, 1920, 1927, 1929, 2058
  CD141 (thrombomodulin), 102, 103, 2058
  CD163, 103, 248, 1909, 1948, 2027, 2058
  CD1a, 1909, 1934, 1939, 1940, 1948
  CD79a, 103, 105, 1905–1909, 1918, 2058
  CD2-associated protein CD2AP, 895, 923, 924
  CDC25, 1283, 1285
  CDH1 (cadherin 1), 1318, 1747, 1749, 1788, 1790, 2054
  CDH13, 293, 1788, 1790
  CD4-helper cells, 1082
  CD4-helper T-lymphocytes, 1082
  CDK1, 1265, 1282, 1283, 1285, 1788, 1790, 1791
  CDK2, 1265, 1282, 1283, 1285, 1788, 1790
  CDK4, 1350, 1788, 1789, 2056, 2057
  CDK6, 925, 1282, 1285, 1325, 1327, 1328, 1350, 1632, 1657, 1788, 1789, 1996, 2056, 2057
  CDKN1A, 1091, 1282, 1325, 1788, 1790
  CDKN2A, 568, 1285, 1305, 1322–1324, 1326, 1328, 1350, 1364, 1399, 1401, 1403, 1447, 1561, 1565, 1573, 1662, 1692, 1703, 1747, 1788, 1789, 1996, 2054, 2055
  CDKN1B, 1282, 1285, 1788, 1790, 1791, 1996
  CDKN2B, 568, 1324, 1350, 1561, 1573
  CDKN1C, 1282, 1285

CD45/LCA, 103, 2058
CD33 protein CD33, 895, 923
CD8-suppressor/cytotoxic cell, 1082
CD8-suppressor/cytotoxic T-lymphocytes, 1088, 1115
CD3 T-lymphocytes, 1088, 1113
CEA, 1522, 1692, 1733, 1738, 1742, 2059–2061, 2070, 2095, 2096, 2099, 2102, 2106, 2107, 2112
cerebral autosomal dominant arteriopathy with subcortical infarcts and leukoencephalopathy (CADASIL), 605, 606, 626, 627, 629, 630, 632, 854, 995, 996, 998, 999
channelopathies, 1134, 1135
chaperone proteins, 455, 471, 941
chemokine receptors, 248, 293, 816, 1313
chemokines, 247, 248, 370, 441, 719, 846, 1092, 1215, 1256
CHI3L1-chitinase 3-like 1, 1365, 1403
CHMP2B, 850, 956, 1050, 1052
chromogranin, 96, 102, 236, 841, 1600, 1604, 1608, 1765, 1810, 2060, 2061, 2070, 2084, 2095, 2112
chromosome 9 open reading frame 72 C9ORF72, 956, 1050
CIC (capicua transcriptional repressor), 1447, 1458, 1464, 1466, 1638
CIC-DUX4 inversion, 1984
CIMP-negative (CIMP-), 1491
CIMP-positive (CIMP+), 1491
Cip/Kip family (CDK interacting protein/Kinase inhibitory protein), 1282
CK5/6, 103, 258, 2060, 2069, 2070, 2075, 2083, 2095, 2102, 2106, 2112, 2114
CK7, 103, 108, 1529, 1530, 1539, 2060–2062, 2069, 2073, 2075, 2084, 2086, 2088, 2091, 2092, 2095, 2099, 2102, 2104, 2106, 2108, 2112, 2114, 2115
CK14, 2075, 2092
CK19, 2022, 2061, 2070, 2088, 2099, 2104, 2106, 2112
CK20, 103, 108, 2058, 2059, 2062, 2069, 2075, 2084, 2088, 2092, 2095, 2099, 2102, 2106, 2107, 2112, 2114, 2115
C-kit (CD117), 108, 1871, 1929, 1966, 2062, 2084, 2088, 2095, 2100
Class III ß-tubulin, 108, 1420, 1579
claudin +, 1681, 2106
claudin-3, 254
claudin-5, 254
CLDN5-claudin 5, 259
clusterin CLU, 924
cluster of microRNA, C19MC, 1647
c-Myc oncogene, 1459, 1466
CNTC6, 291
CNTF, 370
co-deletion, 1323, 1324, 1327, 1349, 1364, 1458, 1459, 1466, 1476, 1484, 1541, 1550
COL4A1 mutations (combined small vessel and large arterial disease), 606

Index 2255

COL4-collagen, type IV, 1365
collagen type IV, 83, 1365, 1557, 1648, 1681
complement component receptor 1 (CR1), 615
complement component (3b/4b) receptor 1 CR1, 895
connexins, 99, 242, 249, 252, 259
contactin, 2, 2157
contactin associated protein like 2 (CNTNAP2), 236, 2157, 2171, 2175
COQ2 gene, 1021, 1034
C6orf70, 1178
C11orf95, 1328, 1490
C9orf72 mutations, 1035
CpG island methylation, 1489, 1491
CRB3, 1325, 1596
CREB, 883, 885, 925, 1254, 1256, 1787, 1789
CSPG2, 568, 1337, 1349
CTNNB1, 925, 1324, 1325, 1613, 1629, 1632, 1766, 2054, 2055
Cut-like homeobox 1 (CUX1), 291
CU/Zn-superoxide dismutase SOD1, 245, 887, 1042, 1049–1051
CXCL12 (SDF-1), 1092, 1312, 1909
CXCL-13, IL-10, 1909
CXCR4, 248, 718, 1979, 1998
CX3CR1-C-X-3-C motif chemokine receptor 1, 249
cyclin D1, 105, 106, 1282, 1285, 1289, 1702, 1787, 1789, 1903, 1906, 1907, 1913, 1996, 2084
cyclin-dependent kinase 4 (CDK4), 2057
cyclin-dependent kinase inhibitor 3 (CDKN3), 1365
cyclin-dependent kinase inhibitor 2B (CDKN2B), 1285, 1365, 1399, 1401, 1459, 1466, 1692, 1703, 1747, 1748, 1788, 1789
cyclin-dependent kinase inhibitor 2C *(CDKN2C)*, 1282, 1748, 1788, 1789
cyclin-dependent kinases, 1265, 1282, 1989, 1995
cyclins, 1265, 1282, 1283, 1285, 1291
CYP46, 615
cystatin C/gamma trace, 615, 998, 1037
cytochrome P4502E1, 1228
cytokines, 243, 248, 441, 517, 567–570, 641, 649, 689, 690, 710, 718, 719, 786, 816, 843, 881, 885, 1092, 1215–1219, 1269, 1272, 1284, 1294, 1296, 1306, 1312, 1313, 1317, 1492, 1788–1791, 1924
DCHS1, 1178
DDX3X, 1325, 1326, 1613, 1629, 1630, 1632
death-associated protein kinase 1 (DAPK1), 1296, 1459, 1466
decorin (DCN), 1365
deleted in liver cancer 1 (DLC1 gene), 1749
deletion, 57, 111, 113, 250, 881, 882, 925, 1014–1016, 1092, 1137, 1171, 1179
delta/notch-like epidermal growth factor related receptor (PCA-Tr) Purkinje cell cytoplasmic antibody (DNER), 2174
DEPDC5, 1137, 1138, 1168
desert hedgehog (DHH), 1749
desmin, 102, 108, 113, 1396, 1624, 1775, 1776, 1966, 1986, 2058, 2061, 2062, 2084, 2096, 2100, 2115

DICER1, 925, 1090, 1791, 1813
Dickkopf homolog 1 (DKK1), 719
differentially expressed in adenocarcinoma of the lung-1 (DAL-1), 1748
DJ-1 DJ-1 (Parkinsonism associated deglycase), 1014, 1015, 1018
DLL3-delta-like 3 protein precursor; delta homolog, 1365
DLX1-distal-less homeobox 1, 234
DLX2-distal-less homeobox 2, 92, 234
DNAJC6 DnaJ heat shock protein family (Hsp40) member C6 (= auxilin), 1014
DNA repair, 851, 880, 888, 965, 1049, 1067, 1071, 1090, 1281, 1283, 1285, 1288, 1291, 1292, 1310, 1313, 1349, 1368, 1403, 1408, 1459, 1466, 1788, 1790, 2055
DNAses, 471
DNER (Tr), 2153
DNM-1KCNA1 (dynamin 1), 236
dopamine D2 receptor region DRD2 and ANKK1, 1220
dopamine transporter (DAT), 29, 49, 54, 377, 897, 932, 935, 975, 1004, 1023, 1220, 1256, 1258
doublecortin (DCX), 92, 1135, 1171, 1178, 1179
doublecortin (DCX) (XLIS) gene, 92, 1135, 1178, 1179
DPPX (dipeptidyl-peptidase-like protein), 6, 2157, 2174
DSG1, 1596
early-delayed, 2120
EIF4G1 eukaryotic translation initiation factor 4 gamma, 1, 1014, 1016
EML1, 1179
endonucleases, 471, 1287, 1288
endoplasmic reticulum stress, 882–883, 1045, 1051, 1052
endothelin-1, 517, 568, 569
EPH receptor A1 EPHA1, 895, 923, 924
ephrins, 370, 1093, 1267, 1316
epidermal growth factor receptor (EGFR), 92, 241, 629, 1289, 1307–1309, 1313, 1322–1324, 1326, 1327, 1331, 1348, 1349, 1368, 1400–1403, 1405, 1469, 1476, 1484, 1997, 2055, 2057, 2075, 2171
ER81, 95
ERα, 1780, 1787
ERBB2(NEU), 1289, 1305, 1307, 1657, 2055
ERBB3-erb-b2 receptor tyrosine kinase, 3, 247
ERGFRvIII, 1401
estrogen receptor 1 (ESR1), 1459, 1466, 2054
ETS family, 95
excitatory amino acid transporter-1 (EAAT1) molecular pathways–genes, 242, 372, 392, 394, 1522, 1530
expansion of CAG repeat, 1066
EZH2 gene, 1613, 1631
far upstream element binding protein 1 (FUBP1), 1447, 1458, 1466
Fas-binding factor 1 gene (FBF1), 879
FAT4, 1178, 2054, 2055

Molecular pathways genes (*cont.*)
fatty acid binding protein 7 *(FABP7),* 1365
fatty acid 2-hydroxylase (FA2H), 247
F-box only protein 7 (FBXO7), 1014
FGFR1, 1324, 1328, 1431, 1444, 1584, 1591
FGFR1-ITD/fusion, 1444
FGFR–TACC fusion, 1329
fibroblast growth factor receptor 1 (FGFR1), 1324, 1328, 1431, 1444, 1583, 1591, 1592
filamin A, 1135, 1171, 1178, 1628
Fli-1, 102, 105, 2058
fms related tyrosine kinase 1 (FLT1), 259
forkhead box protein M1 (FOXM1), 1321, 1747, 1749
frameshift mutations, 1178, 1179, 1305, 1675
free radicals, 441, 1216, 1217, 1244, 1258, 1260, 1313
FSH, 108, 371, 1781, 1787, 1791, 1803, 1806
fused in sarcoma (FUS), 101, 102, 108, 835, 845, 849, 851, 954, 956, 957, 960, 965, 1045, 1049–1051
fused in sarcoma/translated in liposarcoma FUS, 1050
GAB1, 1292, 1787
GADD45, 1292, 1787, 1790
GADD45B, 1788, 1790
GADD45G, 1788, 1790
gain of chromosome 7, 1324, 1399, 1401, 1565
gains of chromososmes, 1051
galactose-3-O-sulfotransferase 1 (GAL3ST1), 247
galectin 3, 1770, 1776, 1997
galectins, 1267, 1316
GATA-2, 1787
GDNF family, 370
genetic switch model of aging, 886
GH, 1779, 1781, 1787, 1789–1791, 1794, 1795
Ghrelin, 371, 869, 884–885
GLAST1, 97, 392
GLI, 1630
GLI1, 1613, 1630, 1747, 1996
glial cell line-derive growth factor (GDNF), 370, 1091, 1306
GLI1, GLI2 (GLI family zinc finger proteins), 1747
GLIS2 (GLI-similar zinc finger 2), 1747
Glut-1, 44, 54, 1134, 1686
glutamate, 97, 236, 242–245, 269, 370, 372, 388, 390, 392, 395, 427, 441, 455, 795, 814, 815, 1077, 1092, 1093, 1101, 1134, 1185, 1214, 1216, 1228, 1233, 2151, 2155, 2158, 2160, 2171
glutamate ionotropic receptor NMDA type subunit 2A (GRIN2A), 236, 2055
glutamate ionotropic receptor NMDA type subunit 2B (GRIN2B), 236
glutamate metabotropic receptor (GRM2), 2, 237, 815, 2151, 2160, 2175
glycerophosphodiester phosphodiesterase domain containing (GDPD2), 2, 241
glypican-3, 293, 2061, 2104, 2112
GNAQ, 1324, 1591

GNAS, 1324, 1591, 1789, 2055
GNAS1 gene, 1995
G protein-coupled receptor 84 (GPR84), 249
growth factors, 92, 241, 248, 294, 441, 568, 614, 629, 816, 878, 885, 1056, 1093, 1134, 1266, 1279–1283, 1289, 1306, 1311, 1313, 1315, 1331, 1337, 1349, 1365, 1395, 1399, 1400, 1405, 1459, 1466, 1476, 1648, 1749, 1789, 1979, 2057, 2131, 2148, 2171
GSP, 1787, 1789
haploinsufficiency of STXBP1, 1135
hepatocyte growth factor (HGF), 248, 1289, 1306, 1324, 2148
HepPar 1, 2061, 2062, 2104, 2112, 2114
HER2 (herceptin for breast cancer), 91, 92, 1331, 2056, 2057, 2060, 2075
high mobility group AT-hook 2 (HMGA2), 1703, 1789
HIOMT, 1596
Hippo pathway, 1701
Hist1H3D, 1596
Hist1H4E, 1596
2-hit hypothesis, 593
H3K27, 1631
H3 K27M-mutant, 1328
hnRNPA1, 1049, 1050, 1053
hnRNPA2B1, 1049, 1050
homeobox (HOX), 1657, 1748
HOXD13, 1325, 1596
HRAS1, 1290
HSTF1, 1289
human leukocyte antigen (HLA)-B∗51, 641
human placental lactogen (HPL), 1866, 1867, 1871, 1880, 2096
huntingtin, 845, 1052, 1059, 1066–1068
huntingtin gene (HTT), 1059, 1066, 1067
4-hydroxybenzoate polyprenyltransferase, 1021, 1034
hyperploidy, 1323, 1539
hypoplo, 1539
IDH1, 91, 108, 1271, 1305, 1323, 1337, 1341, 1348–1350, 1362, 1364, 1368, 1391, 1395, 1400–1403, 1448, 1475, 1793
IDH1/2, 1322, 1323, 1348, 1350, 1398, 1458, 1466, 1469, 1996
IDH2, 1323, 1327, 1333, 1341, 1348, 1353, 1364, 1367, 1368, 1398, 1402, 1447, 1448, 1458, 1466
immediate early genes, 441, 455, 471, 1119, 1134, 1259
immunoglobulin superfamiliy protein (ICAM-1), 699
immunoglobulin superfamily containing leucine rich repeat 2 (ISLR2), 234
inhibitors of kinase 4 (Ink4 family), 1282
INI, 1522, 1654, 1656
insulin, 44, 869, 885, 1492
insulin-like growth factor 1, 885, 1306, 1648
insulin-like growth factor 2 (IGF2), 1747, 1749
insulin-like growth factor binding protein 2 (IGFBP2), 1365

insulin-like growth factor binding protein 3 (IGFBP3), 1365
INT2, 1289
integrin α9β1, 585
integrins, 517, 1267, 1315, 1316, 1331, 1701
integrin subunit alpha 7 (ITGA7), 241
integrin subunit alpha M (ITGAM), 249
intercellular adhesion molecule (ICAM2), 2, 259, 568
interferon regulatory factor 8 (IRF8), 249
interleukin-1, 641
interleukin-4, 1368, 1408
interleukin-6, 641, 1217, 1219
interleukin-1 b, 1219
interleukins, 248, 370, 441, 517
interleukins IL-1α, IL-1β, IL-2, 441
INT1/WNT1, 1289
inward rectifier potassium channel Kir7.1, 1522, 1529, 1530
IQSEC2 (IQ motif and Sec7 domain 2), 236
iron, 85, 89, 99, 228, 252, 257, 308, 458, 529, 814, 837, 838, 864, 869, 871, 884, 885, 974, 975, 990, 1003, 1016, 1023, 1024, 1037, 1039, 1056
ischemic 'tolerance,' 471
ISG15, 622
isochromosome 17q, 1324, 1630, 1632
JAK-STAT, 1308–1309
KDM6A, 1325, 1613, 1631, 1632
KIAA1549, 1324, 1443
KIAA1549-BRAF, 1324, 1591, 1592
KIAA1161-KIAA1161 ortholog, 241
KIF2A, 1179
kinesin, 229, 1179
Kir4.1, 97, 242, 243, 245, 1153, 2157
klotho, 869, 884
KMT2D, 1325, 1630, 2054
KRAS, 1305, 1324, 1328, 1444, 1591, 1913, 2054, 2055
KRAS2, 1290
lactic acid, 471
laminin, 717, 795, 814, 815, 1315, 1317, 1365, 1686
laminin, beta 1 (LAMB1), 1365
late-delayed, 2120
lectin, galactoside-binding, soluble (LGALS1), 1, 1365
lectin, galactoside-binding, soluble, 3 (LGALS3), 1365, 1403
Leu-7, 1671, 1966
leucine rich repeat containing (LRRC25), 25
leukotrienes, 441
LH, 108, 371, 1781, 1787, 1804, 1806, 1812
lipolysis stimulated lipoprotein receptor (LSR), 259
LIS1, 1135, 1179
lissencephaly (LIS1) gene, 1135, 1179
LOH, 1327, 1349, 1364, 1400–1402, 1458, 1464, 1476, 1484, 1701, 1747, 1748
loss of chromosome 9q, 1561, 1565, 1630
loss of chromosomes, 1326, 1647

loss of heterozygosity, 1327, 1349, 1364, 1400, 1447, 1458, 1469, 1476, 1484, 1521, 1522, 1701, 1747
low density lipoprotein receptor 1 (LRP1), 615
LRRK2 leucine-rich repeat kinase 2, 1014
LZTR1, 1662, 1700
macrophage inflammatory protein-2 (MIP-2), 690
macrophage inflammatory proteins MIP-1, MIP-2, 441
major histocompatibility complex class I and II, 248, 1089, 1168
mammalian target of rapamycin (mTOR), 1168, 1169, 1307, 1308, 1331, 1701, 1989, 1995, 2054, 2057
MAP2, 2, 93–95, 878, 1007, 1161, 1165, 1166, 1168, 1176, 1569
maspin, 1302, 1996, 2099, 2102, 2104, 2106, 2107
maternally expressed gene 3 (MEG3), 1328, 1747, 1748, 1788, 1790
matrix metalloproteinases, 427, 441, 1267, 1303, 1311, 1315, 1431, 1995
MCP-1, 517, 567, 568, 1998
MDM2, 1289, 1293, 1305, 1308, 1323, 1324, 1350, 1399, 1411, 1417, 1539, 1788, 1789
MDM2 (E3 ubiquitin protein ligase), 1014, 1015, 1288, 1399
MDM2 SNP309 polymorphism, 1323, 1539
ME, 29, 39, 48, 49, 665, 1324, 1326–1328, 1340, 1341, 1350, 1356, 1380, 1381, 1412, 1414, 1419, 1451, 1462, 1470, 1477, 1755, 1961, 1996, 2050, 2120, 2125, 2131, 2137, 2139
membrane-spanning 4-domains, subfamily A MS4A4A MS4A6E, 895, 923, 924
MEN1, 1305, 1787, 1788, 1790, 1791
merlin, 1326, 1663, 1665, 1675, 1700–1702, 1747
MGMT gene, 1310, 1323, 1324, 1326, 1327, 1329, 1330, 1337, 1349, 1368, 1403, 1431, 1459, 1466, 1787
mitochondrial ribosomal protein L38 gene (MRPL38), 879
mitogen-activated protein kinase (MAPK), 1701, 1707, 1747
monoamine oxidase-A (MAO-A), 1220
monosomy, 1325–1327, 1596, 1629, 1662, 1686
MSH6, 1288, 1291, 1787, 2107
MTO, 1168–1169
mTOR pathway, 1168
MUC1, 2075, 2095, 2099, 2102, 2106, 2112, 2114
MUC2, 2061, 2075, 2099, 2102, 2106, 2112, 2114
MUC4, 2075, 2099, 2102, 2106, 2112
mutation, 111, 113, 245, 593, 632, 699, 815, 847, 955, 1035, 1168, 1179, 1265, 1266, 1290, 1322, 1326, 1328, 1348, 1355, 1365, 1368, 1400, 1402, 1453, 1654, 1700, 1813, 2057, 2060, 2076, 2082
MYB, 1289, 1323, 1328
MYC(c-MYC), 1290, 1321, 1459, 1466, 1749, 1907, 1913
MYC target 1 (MYCT1-), 259
NA/K+ pump, 471

Molecular pathways genes (*cont.*)
 NANOG, 1320, 1867, 2096
 NCAM, 699, 1516
 nestin, 92, 95, 1158, 1164, 1168, 1320, 1496, 1501, 1647, 1648
 neurexin 1 (NRXN1, 236, 1137
 neurexin-3α, 2174
 NeuroD1, 1787
 neurofibromin 1 (NF1), 1291, 1305, 1323, 1325–1328, 1350, 1399–1401, 1403, 1662, 1700, 2055
 neuron specific enolase, 92, 95, 102, 517, 854, 1176, 1516, 1589, 1600, 1604, 1608, 1645, 1662, 1663, 1669, 1677, 1687, 1690, 1693, 1694, 1701–1703, 1791, 1979, 1984, 2055, 2058
 neurotrophin, 3, 1349
 neutrophil cytosolic factor 1 (NCF1), 249
 NF2, 1291, 1323, 1326, 1328, 1489, 1491, 1662, 1665, 1669, 1675, 1687, 1699, 1700, 1702, 1747, 1748
 NF2 gene, 1326, 1491, 1662, 1665, 1699–1702, 1747
 NF-κB, 567, 568, 590, 1091, 1266, 1303, 1306, 1909, 1995
 NF-κB pathways, 1891, 1909
 nitric oxide, 233, 234, 292, 293, 370, 441, 451, 471, 568, 570, 1092, 1217, 1219, 1244, 1260, 1320
 nitric oxide synthase (NOS3), 1219
 N-Myc downstream-regulated gene 2 (NDRG2), 1748
 NOGO-A, 98, 252, 1454
 NOTCH1, 1353, 1365
 NOTCH2, 1353, 1365
 NOTCH3, 606, 629, 630, 632, 854, 996
 NOTCH4, 925, 1353, 1365
 NOTCH2NL, 1353, 1365
 notch pathway, 1320, 1353, 1365
 NPRL2, 1169
 NPRL3, 1169
 NRAS, 324, 1290, 1591, 1996, 2055, 11306
 N-terminal EF-hand calcium binding protein 1 (NECAB1), 291
 NTF3, 1337, 1349
 NTRK fusions, 1444
 Oct-4, 1867
 Olig 2, 1454, 1516
 O6-methylguanine-DNA methyltransferase, 1349, 1403, 1459, 1466
 OPN4, 1325, 1596
 Optineurin OPTN, 825, 844, 968, 1049, 1050, 1052, 1053
 P2, 99, 198, 202, 252, 291
 P16, 1282, 1285, 1411, 1417, 1420, 1692, 2061, 2070, 2084, 2092, 2112, 2114, 2115
 p27, 1282, 1285, 1308, 1331, 1692, 1906, 2084
 p53, 91, 108, 1071, 1090, 1283, 1285, 1288–1292, 1303, 1341, 1346, 1364, 1395, 1454, 1504, 1703, 1790, 1995, 2075, 2113, 2115
 P62 (p62/SQSTM1/A170), 102, 840
 p63, 102, 104, 1303, 2058, 2060, 2062, 2067, 2069, 2070, 2075, 2083, 2088, 2089, 2091, 2095, 2106, 2114, 2115, 2601
 p75, 1624, 1626, 1996
 parathyroid hormone 1 receptor (PTH1R), 1749, 1998
 p12ARF, 1662, 1692
 p14ARF, 1328, 1349, 1399, 1703, 1748, 1788, 1789
 PAX5, 103, 1906–1909, 2058, 2084
 PAX8, 2060, 2088, 2113–2115, 2601
 p16/CDKN2A, 1787
 PDGF-(the specific ligand of PDGFRβ), 622, 626, 1306, 1313, 1492, 1997
 PDGFR, 1306, 1307, 1318, 1331, 1395, 1459, 1466
 PDGFRA, 1305, 1324, 1326–1328, 1337, 1349, 1350, 1399, 1401–1403
 PDGFRβ autophosphorylation, 626
 PDGFRß (encodes a member of the platelet-derived growth factor receptor family type β), 605, 622
 PGP 9.5, 1600, 1604, 1608
 pH, 77, 110, 241–243, 471
 phosphate imbalance disorder, 605, 622
 phosphatidylinositol 3-kinase (PI3K), 1299, 1307, 1309, 1350, 1398, 1701, 1707, 1747, 2054–2057
 phospholipase A2, 441, 1014, 1016, 1256
 phospholipases, 471, 1093
 phospholipid phosphatase related 4 (PLPPR4), 236
 PI3K-AKT-mTOR signaling (phosphatidylinositol-4,5-biphosphate 3 kinase)-AKT-(mechanistic target of rapamycin), 1266, 1306
 PIK3CA, 1169, 1305, 1324, 1400, 1583, 1591, 2054, 2055
 PI3 kinase catalytic subunit α, 1399
 PIK3R1, 1305, 1327, 1399, 1400
 PI3K-related kinases, 1285
 p16INK4A, 1282, 1399, 1662, 1692, 1703, 1748
 p15INK4B, 1282, 1703
 p16INK4B, 1748
 p18INK4C, 1748, 1788, 1789
 PINK1 PTEN induced putative kinase 1, 1014–1016
 Pit-1, 1780, 1787
 PITX2, 1596
 PKC, 236, 1307, 1309, 1321
 p27/KIP1, 1787
 placenta-like alkaline phosphatase (PLAP), 108, 1866, 1867, 1872, 1878, 1879, 2061, 2096
 PLAGL1, 1789, 1790
 PLA2G6 phospholipase A2 group VI, 838, 1014, 1016
 plasminogen activator, tissue (PLAT), 1365
 plasmolipin (PLLP), 247
 platelet activating factor, 441, 1179
 platelet-derived growth factor, 1306
  platelet-derived growth factor receptor, alpha polypeptide (PDGFR-a), 97, 294, 1306, 1349, 1399, 1459, 1466
  platelet-derived growth factor receptor, beta polypeptide (PDGFR-b), 1306, 1459, 1466
 plexin B3 (PLXNB3), 247
 PMA (4-para-methoxyamphetamine), 1259
 podoplanin, 105, 1529, 1530, 1867

poly(ADP-ribose polymerase 1 (PARP1), 1219, 1285–1287, 1295, 1296, 1301
potassium channel (KIR4.1), 97, 242, 243, 245, 1134, 1136, 1153, 1154, 1404, 1522, 1529, 1530, 2157, 2171, 2174
POU3F2 (BRN2) (POU class 3 homeobox 2), 291
POU4F2, 1325, 1596
PRAME, 1325, 1596
p21-Ras, 1307, 1309
p16-Rb-E2F, 1654
pre-B-cell colony enhancing factor 1 (PBEF1), 1365
presenilin 1 PSEN1, 850, 851, 895–897, 922, 923
presenilin 2 PSEN2, 851, 895–897, 922, 923
PRKAR1A, 1661, 1675, 1791
PRKN parkin RBR E3 ubiquitin protein ligase, 1014–1016
PRL, 1782, 1787, 1793–1796, 1798, 1806, 1810
profilin PFN1, 1049, 1050, 1052
programmed cell death 4 (neoplastic transformation inhibitor) (PDCD4), 1403, 1703
prominin-1, 92, 1320
prominin-1 (CD33/PROM1), 92, 1320
prostaglandins, 243, 293, 441
proteases, 441, 471, 567, 884, 1209, 1293, 1299, 1990, 1995, 2084
protein kinase B (Akt (PKB)), 1316, 1701
protein kinase C (PKC), 236, 1254, 1286, 1306, 1307, 1309, 1321
P504S, 104, 2061, 2088, 2093, 2095, 2099, 2102, 2112
PTCH1, 1325, 1326, 1613, 1629, 1630, 1633, 1747, 1749, 1996
ptd-FGFR4, 1787
PTEN, 1014–1016, 1291, 1305–1308, 1322, 1324, 1402, 1403, 1417, 1420, 1431, 1703, 1913, 1996, 2054, 2055, 2070, 2084
PTTG, 1787, 1789
purine nucleotides, 441
purinergic receptor P2Y12 (P2RY12), 249
Rab 3, 236
Rac /PAK (rac GTPase / p21-activated kinase), 1701
RAF1 (c-RAF), 1290, 1328, 1444
RAS family, 236, 1290–1292, 1306, 1308, 1331, 1405, 1443, 1662, 1700, 1701, 1787
RAS gene-Ras protein, 1306
Ras pathway, 1399
RAS/PI3K, 1398, 1399
Ras protein-specific guanine nucleotide-releasing factor 2 (RASGFR2), 291
RASSF1, 1789, 1790
RASSF3, 1789, 1790, 1996
rat fibrosarcoma / extracellular signal-regulated kinase / mitogen-activated protein kinase (Raf/ERK/MAPK), 1701
reactive oxygen species (ROS), 883, 1092, 1217, 1266, 1285–1287, 1293, 1313, 1317, 1322
receptor activator of nuclear factor-κB ligand (RANKL), 1990, 1995, 1998
receptor for advanced glycation end products (RAGE), 1092, 1168

receptor protein tyrosine kinases, 1266, 1306, 1307
receptor tyrosine kinase (RTK), 247, 1367, 1398, 1399, 1405, 1458, 1466, 1867, 2055, 2057
receptor tyrosine kinases (RTK), 1289, 1308, 1398, 1399, 1458, 1466
Reelin (RELN), 232, 233, 291, 292, 1135
REL, 1290
RELA, 1323, 1489–1492
RELN (Reelin), 232, 233, 291, 292, 1135
RET, 1324, 1325, 1591, 1985
retinal S-antigen, 1600, 1604, 1608
retinoblastoma gene (RB1), 1353, 1365, 1399, 1400, 1466, 1499, 1748, 1789, 1994
RGS16, 1325, 1596
R132H, 1341, 1348, 1364, 1391, 1431, 1458, 1466
rho-associated, coiled-coil containing protein kinase 2 (ROCK2), 719
rhodopsin, 1600, 1604, 1608
ribosomal protein S6 kinase (RPS6K), 1747, 1748
R172K, 1458
robo receptor family proteins, 1317
S-100, 108, 1228, 1341, 1364, 1394, 1396, 1420, 1431, 1480, 1501, 1516, 1530, 1539, 1684, 1775, 1940, 1977, 1979, 2062, 2084
SALL4, 2061, 2096, 2113
SATB2, 2061, 2099, 2102
ß-catenin, 92, 1291, 1306, 1320, 1966, 2061, 2084
ßCIT, 49, 54, 873, 975, 1004, 1023, 1226
ß-crystallin, 1341, 1364
selectins, 517, 519, 568
senataxin SETX, 1049–1051
ß-endorphin, 370, 371
serotonin, 156, 370–373, 377, 385, 387, 441, 722, 836, 968, 1007, 1604
SF-1, 1780, 1787, 2096
SFRP1, 1291, 1320, 1613, 1624, 1629–1630
ß-HCG-human chorionic gonadotrophin, 1866
signal transducer and activator of transcription 3 (STAT3), 626, 1309, 1316, 1749, 1996, 2139
ß-III tubulin, 92
ß1-integrin, 2131, 2139
sirtuins, 869, 880, 883–884
SLC20A2, 622
Slit (Slit 1–3), 1317
SLUG, 1267, 1318
SMA, 102, 108, 291, 335, 336, 339, 540, 1012, 1054, 1624, 1654, 1986, 2058, 2062, 2075, 2100, 2115
SMARCA4, 1325, 1326, 1396, 1613, 1629, 1631, 1632, 1654, 2055
SMARCB1 (INI1), 1326, 1396, 1539, 1651, 1654, 1657, 1662, 1663, 1699, 1700, 1702, 1748, 1996
ß2-microglobulin, 1940
SMO, 925, 1326, 1613, 1630, 1632, 1747, 1749, 1913
SNAIL, 1267, 1318
SNAP, 25, 236, 886
SNCA G51D mutation, 1035
SOCS1, 1091, 1789, 1790, 1996

Molecular pathways genes (cont.)
  sodium, 15, 32, 49, 427, 441, 471, 883, 889, 1092, 1134–1136, 1138, 1139, 1214
  solute carrier family 12, member 5 (SLC12A5), 236
  solute carrier family 17 member 6 (SLC17A6), 234
  somatic copy number variations (SCNVs), 160, 1629
  sonic hedgehog (Shh), 1291, 1320, 1613, 1624, 1629, 1630
  sortilin-related receptor, L(DLR class) 1 SORL1, 923
  SOX1, 2171
  SOX10, 2060, 2075, 2083
  SOX17, 561, 568, 569, 2096
  SOX9-SRY-box 9, 241
  SOX10-SRY-box 10, 247
  spatacsin SPG11, 1049, 1050
  the specific ligand of PDGFRβ (PDGF), 622, 626, 1306, 1313, 1492, 1997
  SPI1—Spi-1 proto-oncogene, 249
  SPP1 (secreted phosphoprotein 1), 1747, 1749
  SQSTM1, 850, 1050, 1053, 1295
  SRGAP3, 1444
  SRPX (sushi repeat containing protein, X-linked), 236
  SSTR2, 1787
  SSTR5, 1787
  stanniocalcin-1, 1522, 1529, 1530
  STAT6, 1309, 1966
  stimulatory alpha subunit of G protein (Gs), 242, 244
  SUFU, 1321, 1325, 1326, 1630
  SV-2, 236
  SWI/SNF complex, 1654
  synaptic Ras GTPase activating protein 1 (SYNGAP1), 236, 1137
  synaptic vesicle glycoprotein 2A (SV2A), 236, 1138
  synaptosomal-associated protein 25kDa (SNP25), 236
  SYNs (synapsin), 236, 334, 886
  syntaxin 1B (STX1B), 236
  syntaxin binding protein 1 (STXBP1), 236
  tachykinin 1 (TAC), 233, 292
  TAF15: TATA-binding protein-associated factor 15, 844, 849, 1049, 1050
  TAR DANN-binding protein 43 TARDBP2, 1050
  T-box, brain 1 (TBR1), 234
  telomeres, 1017, 1280, 1304, 1310, 1400
  temozolomide (TMZ), 1329, 1330, 1368, 1402, 1403, 1408
  TERT, 1310, 1322, 1325–1327, 1400, 1401, 1596, 1632, 2055
  TERT promoter mutations, 1400, 1401
  TGFβ signaling, 1056, 1266, 1306
  thiamine transporters (SLC19A2 and SLC19A3), 1233
  thioflavin T, 607
  thrombin, 257, 441
  thrombospondin-1, 926
  thymine-DNA glycosylase (TDG), 1703
  thyrosine hydroxylase, 1563, 1573
  Tie-1, 1979
  TIMP3, 1315, 1349, 1748, 2084
  TIMP metallopeptidase inhibitor 3, 1349
  tissue inhibitor of metalloproteinase 1 (TIMP1), 1315, 1365, 1749, 2084
  TNF family death domain receptors, 1300
  toll like receptor 2 (TLR2), 249, 690, 886, 1168
  toll-like receptors 4, 568, 1168
  topoisomerase (DNA) II alpha (TOP2A), 1365, 1405
  TP53 gene, 1219, 1322, 1323, 1325–1327, 1349, 1350, 1364, 1398, 1399, 1417, 1419, 1420, 1431, 1466, 1476, 1484, 1541, 1550, 1632, 1634, 1692, 1702, 1994, 1996, 2054, 2055
  TPH1, 1325, 1596
  TP53-R72 variant, 1539
  transcription factor E2F, 1282, 1285
  transcription factors, 95, 97, 248, 293, 1018, 1052, 1254, 1256, 1285, 1303, 1787, 1792, 1867, 1995, 1998, 2062, 2171, 2172
  transducin-like enhancer of split 4 (TLE4), 95, 291
  transforming growth factor (TGF-α), 1306
  transforming growth factor ß1 (TGFß1), 568, 649, 1303, 1315–1318, 1998
  translocase of outer mitochondrial membrane 40 (TOMM40), 614, 895, 923
  translocator protein (TSPO), 884, 887
  transmembrane protein 119 (TMEM119), 249
  transthyretin, 615, 998, 1082, 1089, 1521, 1523, 1530, 1539
  TREM2, 249, 924, 926
  TRIM47, 879
  TRIM65, 879
  truncated protein products, 1675
  TSC2 gene, 1565
  TSC1/TSC2, 1169
  TSH, 108, 1754, 1779, 1781, 1787, 1791, 1793, 1799, 1812
  TTF1, 104, 108, 1753, 1767–1771, 1775–1777, 2060, 2062, 2069, 2070, 2084, 2102, 2113
  TUBA1A, 1179
  TUBG1, 1179
  tumor necrosis factors, 242, 248, 249, 816, 1217, 1311, 1313, 1315
  twist basic helix-loop-helix transcription factor 1 (TWIST1), 568, 1318, 1703
  TYRO3 protein tyrosine kinase, 1349
  ubiquilin-2 UBQLN2, 850, 1049, 1050, 1052
  UGT8-UDP glycosyltransferase 8, 247
  unfolded protein response (UPR), 882–8836
  valosin-containing protein VCP, 850, 851, 953, 956–959, 968, 1049, 1050, 1052
  vascular endothelial growth factor A (VEGF-A), 441
  vascular endothelial growth factor B (VEGF-B), 441
  vaso-active agents, 441
  versican, 1314, 1316, 1317, 1349
  vesicle-associated membrane protein B VAPB, 1049–1051
  villin, 2061, 2062, 2070, 2104
  VPS35 vacuolar protein sorting, 35, 1014, 1015
  WNT signaling pathway, 1266, 1306, 1320, 1321, 1324, 1614, 1629, 1981, 1995
  WT1, 2060–2062, 2108, 2112–2115

WW domain binding protein 2 gene (WBP2), 879
WWTR1-CAMTA1 fusion, 1982
XPR1, 622
YAP1, 1325, 1326, 1328, 1490, 1491, 1624, 1626, 1628
YAP1-MAMLD1 fusions, 1490
YAP1-TFE3 fusion, 1982
ZAC, 1787, 1789, 1790
ZEB, 925, 1267, 1318
Zic-4, 2171
zinc finger protein (ZIC), 1789, 1790, 2175
zink finge, 1613
Mönckeberg medial calcification (sclerosis) γ-enolase, 537
Monocular blindness, 207, 408, 475
Monocytes, 100, 248, 458, 517, 542, 567, 678, 684, 718, 719, 1215, 1934, 1995, 1998
Moon face, 1800
μ-opioid receptors, 1253, 1254, 1256
Morning glory sign, 974, 975
Morvan syndrome, 2158, 2174
MOSP (extracellular face of myelin), 99, 252
Mossy fibers, 298, 346, 347, 350, 351, 353
Motor and sensory deficits, 456
Motor aphasia, 207, 401, 404, 405, 414, 420, 475
Motor aprosodia, 404
Motor neglect, 417
Motor neuron disease, 701, 825, 826, 828, 838, 849, 851, 855, 945, 953, 956–958, 1038, 1338, 1373, 1376, 1377, 1412, 1426, 1430, 1434, 1448, 1449, 1460, 1462, 1470, 1471, 1477, 1493, 1513, 1525, 1534, 1542, 1550, 1563, 1573, 1576, 1584, 1615, 1640, 1642, 1652, 1716, 1836, 1877, 1878, 1884, 1897, 1958, 1959, 2042, 2120, 2132
Motor-neuron disease with dementia, 855, 1042
Motor/sensory deficits, 456, 1490
Motor system, 153, 156, 326, 334–337, 417, 1256
Movement planning/programming, 404, 405
Moyamoya angiopathy, 606, 997
Moyamoya disease, 496, 997, 998
MR angiography, 11, 14, 16–17, 478, 1255
MR-diffusion tensor imaging (DTI), 19–21, 127, 327, 335, 402, 1109, 1339, 1357, 1375
MR-diffusion weighted imaging (DWI), 3, 19, 432, 457, 459, 461, 477, 479, 502, 504, 523, 553, 597, 599, 661, 704, 726, 766, 802, 1024, 1074, 1076, 1126, 1230, 1234, 1235, 1825, 1834, 1857, 1883, 1896, 1915, 1942, 2121, 2161
MR-imaging, 9–27, 697, 698, 1037, 1059, 1071
MR-perfusion imaging, 18–19
MR spectroscopy, 11, 15–16, 432, 444, 663, 666, 752, 766, 1060, 1077, 1106, 1125, 1144, 1192, 1207, 1226
MR-spectroscopy, 432, 444, 478, 663, 752, 766, 899, 947, 990, 1004, 1039, 1060, 1077, 1101, 1106, 1125, 1144, 1175, 1192, 1207, 1226, 1338, 1354, 1373, 1412, 1426, 1430, 1434, 1448, 1460, 1462, 1470, 1471, 1477, 1493, 1513, 1525, 1534, 1535, 1563, 1573, 1576, 1584, 1585, 1615, 1640, 1642, 1652, 1716, 1755, 1836, 1871, 1877, 1884, 1897, 1961, 2042, 2120, 2132
MSA-C: predominantly cerebellar subtyp, 1034
MSA-P: predominantly parkinsonism subtype, 1022–1025, 1034, 1035
mtSOD1-mediated neurotoxicity, 1050
Mucicarmine, 776, 1853, 2095
Mucinous carcinoma, 2059, 2061
Mucin positive capsule, 784
Mucormycetes, 774, 775
Multicentric plaques, 812
Multicystic, 1542, 1543, 1584
Multi infarct dementia, 626, 818, 827, 914, 987, 988, 990, 995–997
Multinodular architecture, 1541, 1542
Multinucleated giant cells (MGC), 680, 688, 693, 698, 700, 703, 706, 709, 718, 740, 1278, 1360, 1367, 1368, 1386, 1419–1421, 1462, 1597, 1829, 1832, 1838, 1868, 1944, 1947, 1979, 2005, 2010
Multinucleated tumor cells, 1362, 1392, 2107
Multiphoton confocal fluorescence microscopy, 114
Multiple sclerosis (MS), 12, 30, 74, 732, 827, 1071–1093, 1101, 1106, 1131
Multiple-system-atrophy (MSA), 76, 87, 102, 416, 848, 854, 976, 980, 1021–1035, 2058, 2062
Multi-voxel MRS, 16
MUM1, 1901, 1907, 1918, 2083
Mumps virus, 451, 696, 697
Mural nodule, 1434, 1436, 1666, 1967
Muscarinic cholinergic receptors, 376
Muscle atrophy, 945, 1038
Muscle cramps, 998, 1038, 2157
Muscle-specific actin, 102, 2058
Muscle weakness, 862, 945, 959, 1038, 2152
Muscular arteries, 254, 537, 538
Mutation, 57, 111, 243, 250, 622, 626, 630, 632, 641, 642, 699, 796, 847, 896 (AU: More than 720 instances. We have picked the first instance page numbers from each chapter and where the term is explained in detail)
Mute/speech deficits, 404
Mutism, 207, 208, 405, 475, 797, 816, 818, 857, 946, 947, 968, 2156, 2159
Myasthenia gravis, 1103, 2153, 2171, 2173
Mycobacterium tuberculosis, 89, 655, 657, 690, 702
Mycotic aneurysm, 499, 514, 565, 684, 775, 777
Myelencephalon (medulla oblongata), 129, 384
Myelin-associated glycoprotein (MAG), 98, 99, 250, 251, 1086, 1089, 1093, 1250
Myelinated nerve fibers, 236–238, 1686
Myelin basic protein (MBP), 98, 99, 225, 250, 251, 274, 1087, 1089, 1250
Myelin damage with myelin loss and reactive astrogliosis, 2126
Myelin damage with myelin pallor and myelin loss, 2129
Myelin lamellae, 99, 250
Myelin oligodendrocyte basic protein (MOBP), 99, 251–252, 887

Myelin oligodendrocyte glycoprotein (MOG), 98, 99, 205, 251, 1089, 1250, 2174
Myelin/oligodendrocyte specific protein (MOSP), 99, 252
Myelin pallor, 85, 616, 619, 706, 709, 710, 712, 858, 865, 873, 875, 907, 992, 1042, 2129
Myelin regulatory factor (MYRF), 247
Myelin sheath, 99, 225–227, 229, 236–238, 245, 246, 250, 716, 864, 1034
Myelitis, 654, 694, 702, 736, 751, 774, 1072, 1097, 1098, 1245, 1247, 1914, 2172–2174
Myelopathy, 637, 697, 701, 702, 708, 713, 1089, 1245, 1247, 2171, 2172
Myeloperoxidase, 105, 567, 638, 2058
Myocloni, 797
Myoclonic epilepsy with ragged-red fibers (MERRF), 828, 862, 863, 998, 999
Myoclonic jerks, 456
Myoclonic seizures, 456, 1122, 1137
Myoclonus, 416, 456, 797, 816–818, 828, 858, 980, 984, 1068, 1124, 1130, 1135, 2152, 2153, 2158, 2159, 2170, 2172, 2174
MyoD, 102, 2058
Myofibroblastoma, 1956, 1985
Myogenin, 102, 1986, 2058
Myoglobin, 1396, 2061
Myoinositol, 17, 899, 1340, 1376, 1426, 1430, 1525, 1534, 1958
Myxoid matrix, 1508, 1510, 1873, 1875, 2013

N
^{23}Na, 10, 15
NAA/Cr, 947, 1023, 1039, 1060, 1144, 1175, 1226
NAB2, 1966
N-acetylaspartate (NAA), 16, 17, 432, 478, 766, 800, 899, 1004, 1023, 1077, 1106, 1144, 1175, 1192, 1354, 1428, 1430, 1525, 1534, 1554, 1615, 1897
   peak, 16, 1376
NACHT and WD repeat domain containing 1 (NWD1), 1, 241
Na-K-ATPase, 54
NA/K+ pump, 471
Naming, 209, 413, 422, 946, 1122
NANOG, 1320, 1867, 2096
Nano resolution optical imaging, 114
Narcolepsy, 418, 1098, 2170
Nasu–Hakola disease, 249, 849
Natalizumab, 725, 731, 1072, 1090, 1091, 1093
National Institute on Aging-Alzheimer's Association guidelines for the neuropathologic assessment of Alzheimer's disease, 896, 916, 917
Nausea and vomiting, 654, 736, 1490, 1813, 2155
Necroptosis, 1266, 1293, 1294, 1300
Necrosis, 48, 75, 248, 249, 434, 436, 457, 458, 461, 471, 484, 489, 493, 495, 503, 514, 521, 614, 685, 687, 698, 710, 752, 777, 778, 790, 865, 1101, 1188, 1248, 1272–1273, 1278, 1300, 1311, 1313, 1368, 1378, 1643, 1901, 1958, 2124, 2128 (AU: More than 310 instances. We have picked the first instance page numbers from each chapter and where the term is explained in detail)
Necrotizing leukoencephalopathy, 2120, 2128
Nef, 701
Neglect, 207–209, 361, 401, 406, 407, 413, 415, 417, 421, 423, 475, 496, 500, 896, 988, 1224
Neglect and denial, 413
Nelson syndrome, 1781
Nematodes, 750
Neocortex (=isocortex), 269, 300, 342, 350, 375, 381, 387, 468, 715, 801, 854–856, 861, 914, 915, 917, 921, 964, 965, 967, 968, 1011, 1012, 1185, 1212, 1245, 1257
Neologisms, 134, 409
Neoplasia, 1265, 1268, 1271, 1325, 1754, 1788, 1791, 1893
Neoplasm, 4, 9, 91, 103, 105, 702, 849, 914, 1266, 1268, 1314, 1338, 1490, 1511, 1523, 1530, 1534, 1575, 1595, 1597, 1685, 1718, 1766, 1780, 1803, 1882, 1891, 1892, 1894, 1923, 1933, 1985, 2005, 2029, 2058, 2059, 2119, 2129, 2170, 2171
Neoplastic stromal cells, 1955, 1967
Neovascularisation, 523, 1310
Neovascularity, 1272, 1360
Nephroblastic tumors, 2085
NER, *see* Nucleotide excision repair
Nerve cell, 94, 226, 227, 230, 888, 1132, 1247, 1253, 1260
Nerve fiber, 229, 236, 296, 865, 878, 1983
Nerve growth factor (NGF), 248, 249, 1306, 1996
Nerve sheath myxoma, 1663
Nervous system, 84, 89, 92, 95, 102, 121–127, 129–168, 216, 225–260, 267, 720, 881, 1265, 1275, 1629, 1703, 1893, 2156, (AU: More than 614 instances. We have picked the first instance page numbers from each chapter and where the term is explained in detail)
Nestin, 92, 95, 1158, 1164, 1168, 1320, 1496, 1647, 1648
NETosis, 1266, 1293, 1301
Netrins, 1267, 1316, 1317
NETs, *see* Neutrophil extracellular traps
Network, 185, 228, 241, 242, 288, 291, 308, 321, 326, 364–366, 402, 423, 552, 565, 875, 1135, 1139, 1341, 1416, 1419, 1420, 1453, 1556, 1601, 1609, 1615, 1962, 1965
NeuN, 92, 93, 95, 102, 108, 270, 1149, 1151, 1152, 1158, 1161, 1162, 1164, 1166, 1177, 1231, 1548, 1569, 1581, 1647, 2058
Neural, 20–22, 92, 95, 99, 102, 122, 123, 163, 166, 213, 241, 321, 326, 356, 364, 457, 719, 756, 815, 875, 1093, 1139, 1267, 1316, 1319, 1402, 1575, 1614, 1633, 1647, 1648, 1739, 1829, 1868, 1885, 2076, 2170, 2171
Neurite outgrowth, 814, 815, 845, 847, 2175
Neuritic plaque, 830, 834, 835, 917, 925
Neuroacanthocytosis, 825, 828, 858, 1130

Neuroaxis, 1615
Neuroborreliosis, 665, 666
Neurocysticercosis, 749, 750, 762, 764, 1131
Neurocytes, 1583, 1584, 1588
Neurocytic rosettes, 1274, 1584, 1588, 1589
Neurocytoma
    age incidence, 1576
    biologic behavior-prognosis-prognostic factors, 1582
    CT-contrast-enhanced, 1576
    CT-non contrast-enhanced, 1576
    differential diagnosis, 1580
    extraventricular neurocytoma, 1575
    general imaging findings, 1576–1579
    immunophenotype, 1579–1581
    incidence, 1576
    localisation, 1576
    macroscopic features, 1576
    microscopic features, 1576–1577, 1580
    molecular neuropathology, 1581–1582
    MRI-diffusion imaging, 1576
    MRI-flair, 1576
    MRI-T1, 1576, 1577
    MRI-T2, 1576
    MRI-T1 contrast-enhanced, 1576
    MRI-T2∗/ SWI, 1576
    MR-spectroscopy, 1576
    nuclear medicine imaging findings, 1576
    pathogenesis, 1580–1581
    proliferation Markers, 1579
    sex incidence, 1576
    treatment, 1582
    ultrastructural Features, 1579
    WHO definition, 1575–1576
    WHO grade, 1576
Neuroepithelial component, 1553, 1555, 1557, 1647
Neurofibrillary tangle (NFT), 101, 830, 836, 837, 840–844, 846, 860, 918–921, 957, 967, 973, 976, 977, 979, 1213, 1214
Neurofibrils, 228, 1563, 1573
Neurofibroma
    age incidence, 1677
    ancient neurofibroma, 1681
    atypical neurofibroma, 1681
    biologic behavior-prognosis-prognostic factors, 1683
    CT-contrast-enhanced, 1677
    CT-non contrast-enhanced, 1677
    differential diagnosis, 1683
    general imaging findings, 1677
    immunophenotype, 1681, 1684
    incidence, 1677
    localisation, 1677
    macroscopic features, 1679, 1680
    microscopic features, 1679, 1681
    MRI-diffusion imaging, 1679
    MRI-flair, 1677
    MRI-T1, 1677, 1678
    MRI-T2, 16777
    MRI-T1 contrast-enhanced, 1677
    MRI-T2∗/ SWI, 1677
    plexiform neurofibroma, 1681
    proliferation markers, 1681
    sex incidence, 1677
    treatment, 1683
    ultrastructural features, 1683
    WHO definition, 1677
    WHO grade, 1677
Neurofibromatosis type 1 (NF1)
    CT-non contrast-enhanced, 1694
    diagnostic criteria, 1694
    general imaging findings, 1694
    incidence, 1693
    macroscopic features, 1697
    molecular neuropathology, 1697
    MRI-diffusion imaging, 1697
    MRI-flair, 1694, 1695
    MRI-T1, 1694, 1695
    MRI-T2, 1694, 1695
    MRI-T1 contrast-enhanced, 1697
    WHO definition, 1693
    WHO grade, 1693
Neurofibromatosis type 2 (NF2)
    diagnostic criteria, 1699
    general imaging findings, 1699
    incidence, 1699
    molecular neuropathology, 1699
    WHO definition, 1699
    WHO grade, 1699
Neurofibromin, 1306, 1307, 1399, 1400, 1443, 1662, 1697, 1700, 1701, 1703, 1747, 2055
Neurofilament protein (NFP), 92, 518, 837, 839, 849, 1007, 1254, 1396, 1600, 1604, 1608, 1675, 2084
Neurofilaments, 92, 94, 95, 102, 108, 228, 229, 518, 837–839, 849, 856, 863, 937, 966, 967, 1011, 1035, 1037, 1042, 1045, 1077, 1082, 1158, 1159, 1163, 1209, 1214, 1254, 1557, 1559, 1569, 1573, 1579, 1600, 1601, 1604, 1608, 1647, 1654, 1675, 1686, 1775, 2058
Neurogranin, 926
Neurohypophyseal peptides, 370
Neurological Communicative Disorders and Stroke (NINCDS) Alzheimer's and Related Disorders Association (ADRDA) NINCDS-ADRA, 915
Neurologic deficit, 500, 518, 519, 653, 654, 694, 715, 725, 749, 751, 762, 774, 988, 1187, 1267, 1349, 1779, 1817
Neurolymphomatosis, 1892
Neuroma, 1644, 1663, 1677
Neuromodulators, 243, 278, 370, 371, 886
Neuromyelitis optica (NMO) (Dévic disease), 244, 1072, 1097–1103, 2173
Neuromyelitis optica spectrum disorder (NMOSD), 1097, 1098
Neuron
    bipolar neuron, 230, 331
    interneurons, 95, 230, 232–235, 268, 269, 289, 291–293, 296, 299, 302, 304, 315, 325, 331, 342, 349, 357, 388, 1063, 1153, 1178
    multipolar neuron, 230
    projection neurons, 95, 230–232, 268

Neuron (cont.)
  pseudounipolar neuron, 230
  type I neuron, 230, 232
  type II neuron, 230, 232, 301, 716, 1168
  unipolar neuron, 230, 313
Neuronal cytoplasmic inclusions (NCI), 954, 959, 966
Neuronal intermediate filament inclusion disease (NIFID), 954, 956, 957, 966
Neuronal intranuclear inclusions (NII), 954, 958, 959, 966, 967
Neuronal nitric oxide synthase (nNOS), 233, 292, 293
Neuronal polarity, 847
Neuronal progenitor cells, 1575, 1582
Neuronal programmed cell death, 249
Neuronavigation, 22–25, 27
Neuron-specific enolase (NSE), 92, 95, 102, 518, 852, 854, 1176, 1516, 1589, 1600, 1604, 1608, 1645, 1984, 2058
Neuro-oncology, 29, 44, 1268, 1289–1290, 1314–1319, 1329, 2135–2137
Neuropathic pain, 249, 2157, 2158
Neuropeptides, 95, 233, 292, 304, 350, 369–371, 1063, 1143, 1153, 1154
Neuropeptide Y (NPY), 95, 233, 292, 304, 349, 350, 371, 1063, 1143, 1153, 1154
Neuropil, 87, 125, 250, 260, 326, 484, 797, 802, 836, 837, 841, 861, 878, 901, 918, 962, 976, 979, 983, 1007, 1063, 1150, 1177, 1213, 1279, 1386, 1454, 1457, 1584, 1638, 1646, 1647
  threads, 87, 836, 837, 841, 861, 901, 918, 976, 979, 983
Neuroprotection, 245, 471, 496, 795, 814, 885, 888
Neurotensin, 301, 370, 371
Neurothekoma, 1663
Neurotransmitters, 49, 95, 234–236, 241–243, 278, 305, 349, 369–395, 471, 815, 836, 848, 884, 886, 887, 1012, 1056, 1133, 1134, 1168, 1228, 1253, 1255, 1260
  transporters, 371–372
Neurotrophic factors, 233, 234, 242, 243, 248, 292, 293, 370, 1219
Neurotrophins, 248, 370, 1215
Neurotubuli, 228
Neurovascular unit, 259–260, 720
Neutrons, 10, 31, 1269
Neutrophil extracellular traps (NETs), 242, 372, 373, 384, 1301
New variant Creutzfeldt-Jakob disease (vCJD), 795, 812, 818, 819
NF1, see Neurofibromatosis type 1
NF2, see Neurofibromatosis type 2
NFκB pathway, 1266, 1306, 1909
NFT, see Neurofibrillary tangle
NG2, 92, 97
NGB, 1219
NGF, see Nerve growth factor
Nicotinic acetylcholine receptor, 815, 1134, 1135
Nicotinic receptors, 236, 926
Nidus, 578, 585, 1999–2001, 2003
NIFID, see Neuronal intermediate filament inclusion disease

NIH criteria (Katchaturian), 914
NIH/Reagan, 916–918
NII, see Neuronal intranuclear inclusions
Ninjurin 2 (NINJ2), 247
Nissl substance, 84–85, 226–228, 1158, 1563, 1573, 1643
Nitric oxide, 233, 234, 259, 292–293, 370, 441, 451, 471, 568, 570, 1092, 1217, 1219, 1244, 1260, 1320
Nitric oxide synthase trafficking (NOSTRIN), 259
Nitrosourea, 1329, 1330
Nkx2.2, 97
NMDA Receptor (GluN1), 236, 392, 395, 719, 1139, 1168, 2055, 2155, 2156, 2171, 2173
NMDA-R encephalitis, 2155–2156
N-methyl-D-aspartate receptor (NMDAR), 392, 2153, 2155–2156, 2162, 2170, 2171, 2175
Node of Ranvier, 229, 237
Nodular Heterotopia, 1130, 1132, 1135, 1176–1178
Nogo-A (oligodendrocyte cell bodies), 98, 252, 1454
No hippocampal sclerosis, gliosis only (no-HS), 1148, 1150–1152
Non-germ cell tumor, 2094
Non-homologous end joining (NHEJ), 1286, 1287
Non-Langerhans cell histiocytosis
  age incidence, 1941
  biologic behavior-prognosis-prognostic factor, 1951
  differential diagnosis, 1948
  immunophenotype, 1948–1951
  incidence, 1941
  localisation, 1941
  macroscopic features, 1943–1944
  microscopic features, 1944–1948
  pathogenesis, 1948
  proliferation markers, 1948
  sex incidence, 1941
  treatment, 1948
  WHO definition, 1941
Non-Martinotti, 233, 292
Non-motor features of PD, 1002
Non-myelinated nerve fibers, 236–237, 301
Non-perfused brain, 457
Non-receptor membrane-associated tyrosine kinases (SRC, ABL, FGR), 1290
Noradrenaline, 242, 370, 376, 381–384
Normal Pressure Hydrocephalus (NPH), 444, 451, 861–862
Northern blot, 57, 111–113
Notch signaling, 925, 1266, 1306, 1317, 1747
NPY, see Neuropeptide Y
NSE, see Neuron-specific enolase
Nuclear atypia, 1268, 1270, 1277, 1278, 1354, 1360, 1368, 1414, 1416, 1476, 1477, 1500, 1534, 1545, 1604, 1605, 1692, 1733, 1962, 1968, 2022, 2113
Nuclear chromatin, 1268, 1454, 1962
Nuclear density, 1268, 1270
Nuclear medicine, 29–54, 273, 372, 373, 432, 448, 458, 478, 501, 521, 578, 586, 596, 606, 607, 616, 622, 629, 640, 665, 667, 766, 776, 872,

899–901, 933, 947, 975, 980, 990, 1004, 1023, 1040, 1060, 1077, 1106, 1125, 1128, 1129, 1142, 1158, 1192, 1226, 1245, 1247, 1255, 1340, 1412, 1419, 1450, 1573, 1615, 1716, 1755, 1914, 1961, 2005, 2120, 2125, 2137, 2162
Nuclear membrane, 227
Nuclear molding, 1618, 1621, 1625, 2063
Nuclear pores, 227
Nuclear size, 717, 1268, 1270, 1360, 1477, 1690, 1955, 1969
Nuclei, 9, 83, 125, 129, 204, 267, 325, 384, 401, 455, 468, 484, 622, 653, 690, 921, 1077, 1229, 1274, 1430, 1489, 1557, 1606, 1648, 1757, 1868, 1939, 1984, 2085, 2107, 2127 (AU: More than 442 instances. We have picked the first instance page numbers from each chapter and where the term is explained in detail)
Nucleolar organization, 847
Nucleolar prominence, 1360, 1477
Nucleolus, 226, 227, 1320, 1341, 1344, 1364, 1454, 1577, 1580, 1904, 1929, 2172
Nucleosidic reverse transcriptase inhibitors (NRTI), 712, 714
Nucleotide excision repair (NER), 1266, 1286, 1287
Nucleotide repeat disease, 851
Nucleus accumbens
　accumbens core, 145, 304
　accumbens shell, 145, 304, 416
Nucleus Basalis Meynert, 267, 300, 373, 966, 976, 982
Nucleus ruber, 156, 307–311, 982
Number of excitations (NEX), 12, 13
Nystagmus, 207–209, 408, 419, 475, 476, 640, 658, 1229, 1824, 2156, 2172, 2174

O
^{17}O (oxygen), 15
Occipital artery, 181, 191, 192, 202–204
Occipital lobe, 71, 75, 76, 130, 131, 133–134, 137, 148, 150, 167–169, 204, 209, 274, 294, 332, 333, 356, 357, 361, 407–409, 413, 434, 476, 485, 609, 698, 802, 817, 856, 920, 934, 935, 960, 967, 1080, 1126, 1280, 1375, 1482, 1898, 1899
Occlusion, 9, 14, 208, 209, 451, 478, 479, 538, 542, 640, 641, 865, 987, 996, 997, 1711, 1716, 1916, 1917
OCT4, 1867, 1871, 1875, 1879, 2096, 2112
Octreotide, 54
Ocular motor dysfunction, 420, 974
Oculomotor disorder, 420
O-(2-[18F]fluoroethyl)-L-tyrosine (FET), 48
15O-H$_2$O, 1381
Oil red O, 89
Olfactory and septal areas, 352
olfactory bulb, 93, 137, 150, 183, 220, 375, 381, 385, 388, 392, 420, 941
Olfactory tract, 137, 300
Olfactory tubercle, 155, 380, 381, 387
Olig1, 99
Olig2, 99
Olig3, 99
Oligo-astrocytoma
　age incidence, 1470
　biologic behavior-prognosis-prognostic factors, 1476
　CT-contrast-enhanced, 1470
　CT-non contrast-enhanced, 1470
　differential diagnosis, 1476
　general imaging findings, 1470
　immunophenotype, 1475
　incidence, 1470
　localisation, 1470
　macroscopic features, 1470, 1472
　microscopic features, 1472, 1475
　molecular neuropathology, 1476
　MRI, 1470, T2
　MRI-diffusion imaging, 1470
　MRI-flair, 1470, 1471
　MRI-perfusion, 1470
　MRI-T1, 1470, 1471
　MRI-T1 contrast-enhanced, 1470, 1472
　MRI-T2∗/SWI, 1470
　MR-spectroscopy, 1470, 1471
　nuclear medicine imaging findings, 1470, 1472, 1473
　pathogenesis, 1476
　proliferation markers, 1475
　sex incidence, 1470
　treatment, 1476
　ultrastructural features, 1476
　WHO definition, 1469–1470
　WHO grade, 1470
Oligo-astrocytoma anaplastic
　age incidence, 1477
　biologic behavior-prognosis-prognostic factors, 1484
　CT-contrast-enhanced, 1477
　CT-non contrast-enhanced, 1477
　differential diagnosis, 1482
　general imaging findings, 1477
　immunophenotype, 1479, 1485
　incidence, 1476
　localisation, 1477
　macroscopic features, 1477, 1482
　microscopic features, 1477, 1483
　molecular neuropathology, 1484
　MRI-diffusion imaging, 1477
　MRI-flair, 1477
　MRI-perfusion, 1477, 1478
　MRI-T1, 1477
　MRI-T2, 1477
　MRI-T1 contrast-enhanced, 1477, 1478
　MRI-T2∗/ SWI, 1477
　MR-spectroscopy, 1476, 1478
　nuclear medicine imaging findings, 1477
　pathogenesis, 1482
　proliferation markers, 1480, 1485
　sex incidence, 1477
　treatment, 1484
　ultrastructural features, 1480
　WHO definition, 1476
　WHO grade, 1476

Oligodendrocyte lineage transcription factor 2 (OLIG2), 92, 96, 98, 99, 108, 1403, 1442, 1548, 1590
Oligodendrocyte loss, 2129
Oligodendrocytes, 85, 92, 97–99, 225, 229, 236, 239, 240, 245–247, 250–252, 294, 301, 302, 449, 458, 616, 717, 728, 730, 732, 837, 844, 845, 863–865, 878, 884, 960, 964, 979, 983, 984, 1029, 1031, 1034, 1082, 1084, 1086, 1089, 1092, 1217, 1228, 1237, 1253, 1447, 1448, 1454, 1458, 1462, 1562, 1563, 1588, 2128, 2129, 2174
Oligodendroglia (oligodendrocytes), 57, 87, 97–99, 108, 243–247, 693, 717, 825, 834, 837, 842, 873, 965, 977, 979, 983, 1028, 1235, 1275, 1276, 1278, 1322, 1327, 1329, 1337–1350, 1353–1365, 1367–1408, 1411–1422, 1447–1466, 1469–1486, 1493, 1541, 1543, 1545, 1546, 1584
Oligodendroglioma
  age incidence, 1448
  biologic behavior-prognosis-prognostic factors, 1459
  CT-contrast-enhanced, 1448
  CT-non contrast-enhanced, 1448
  differential diagnosis, 1455, 1458
  DNA methylation, 1459
  epigenetics, 1459
  gene expression, 1459
  general imaging findings, 1448
  genetics, 1458
  immunophenotype, 1453–1454
  incidence, 1448
  localisation, 1448
  macroscopic features, 1451, 1452
  microRNAs, 1459
  microscopic features, 1452, 1453
  molecular neuropathology, 1458–1459
  MRI-diffusion imaging, 1448
  MRI-flair, 1448
  MRI-perfusion, 1448, 1449
  MRI-T1, 1448
  MRI-T2, 1448
  MRI-T1 contrast-enhanced, 1448
  MRI-T2*/ SWI, 1448
  MR-spectroscopy, 1448, 1449
  nuclear medicine imaging findings, 1450, 1451
  pathogenesis, 1458
  proliferation markers, 1454
  sex incidence, 1448
  treatment, 1459
  ultrastructural features, 1454–1455
  WHO definition, 1448
  WHO grade, 1448
Oligodendroglioma anaplastic
  age incidence, 1460
  biologic behavior-prognosis-prognostic factors, 1466
  CT-contrast-enhanced, 1461
  CT-non contrast-enhanced, 1460
  differential diagnosis, 1464
  DNA methylation, 1466
  epigenetics, 1466
  gene expression, 1466
  general imaging findings, 1460
  genetics, 1464, 1466
  immunophenotype, 1462, 1464
  incidence, 1459
  localisation, 1460
  macroscopic features, 1462
  microRNAs, 1466
  microscopic features, 1462
  molecular neuropathology, 1464–1466
  MRI-diffusion imaging, 1462
  MRI-flair, 1460, 1461
  MRI-perfusion, 1462
  MRI-T1, 1460, 1461
  MRI-T2, 1460, 1461
  MRI-T1 contrast-enhanced, 1460, 1461
  MRI-T2*/ SWI, 1461
  MR-spectroscopy, 1460, 1462
  nuclear medicine imaging findings, 1462
  pathogenesis, 1464
  proliferation markers, 1464
  sex incidence, 1460
  treatment, 1466
  ultrastructural features, 1464
  WHO definition, 1459
  WHO grade, 1459
Olivary nucleus, 76, 86, 160, 161, 231, 313, 315, 351, 381, 856, 1028, 1233
Olive, 160, 353, 355
Olivocerebellar fibers, 350
Olivo-Ponto-Cerebellar Atrophy (OPCA), 1021, 1022
OMgp (paranodal area), 99, 252
Oncogene, 1266, 1285, 1289–1290, 1319, 1324, 1367, 1399–1401, 1433, 1444, 1459, 1466, 1490, 1630, 1703, 1748, 1749, 1787
OncomiRs, 1267, 1319
Oocysts, 756
Opacity, 67, 1359, 1383, 1477, 1699
Opercula, 132, 134, 136, 150, 197, 198, 214, 413
15-O PET, 458, 478, 501, 510, 521, 538
Ophthalmic artery, 181, 193
Opiates, 1244–1249
Opsoclonus/myoclonus, 2156, 2159, 2170, 2172
Optic apraxia, 423
Optic ataxia, 332, 361, 415, 423
Optic chiasm, 60, 71, 153–155, 167, 175, 186, 200, 203, 223, 326, 331, 408, 671, 779, 1098, 1100, 1237, 1415, 1434, 1584, 1795
Optic nerves, 137, 180, 183, 203, 220, 246, 326, 331, 408, 475, 576, 716, 1073, 1077, 1098–1100, 1102, 1186, 1434, 1648, 1693, 1695, 1708, 1760, 2176
Optic neuritis (ON), 1072, 1097, 1098, 1105, 2158, 2172–2174
Optic radiation, 147, 150, 174, 203, 209, 296, 326, 331, 421, 1101
Optic tract, 150, 153, 213, 307, 326, 331, 408, 1100, 1218
Optineurin, 844, 968, 1049, 1050, 1052, 1053

Organelles, 19, 226, 370, 818, 881, 883, 960, 1067, 1282, 1294, 1343, 1364, 1643, 1646, 1648, 1764, 1850, 1879
Orofacial dyskinesia, 416
Orthostatic hypotension, 622, 932, 1003, 1021, 1022
Osmium tetroxide fixation, 77
Osmotic treatment with mannitol, 427, 441
Osp/claudin-11 (tight junctions of myelin sheaths), 99, 252
Osteoblastoma
    differential diagnosis, 2005
    localisation, 2005
    macroscopic features, 2005
    microscopic features, 2005–2007
    WHO definition, 2005
Osteoblasts, 1989, 1990, 1999, 2001, 2004–2006, 2018, 2021, 2029, 2032
Osteoclast, 1998, 1999, 2001, 2004–2006
Osteoid, 2005
Osteoid osteoma
    CT-contrast-enhanced, 2000
    CT-non contrast-enhanced, 1999, 2003
    differential diagnosis, 2005
    general imaging findings, 1999
    localisation, 1999
    macroscopic features, 2000–2001
    microscopic features, 2001, 2004
    MRI-T1, 2000
    MRI-T2, 2000
    MRI-T1 contrast-enhanced, 2000
    WHO definition, 1999
Osteoma
    CT-non contrast-enhanced, 1998–2000
    differential diagnosis, 1999
    general imaging findings, 1998
    localisation, 1998
    macroscopic features, 1999, 2001
    microscopic features, 1999, 2002–2003
    MRI-T1, 1998, 2000
    MRI-T2, 1998, 2000
    MRI-T1 contrast-enhanced, 1999, 2000
    WHO definition, 1998
Osteosarcoma
    CT-non contrast-enhanced, 2005, 2006
    differential diagnosis, 2007
    general imaging findings, 2005
    localisation, 2005
    macroscopic features, 2005
    microscopic features, 2005, 2007–2009
    MRI-T1, 2005
    MRI-T2, 2005, 2006
    MRI-T1 contrast-enhanced, 2005
    nuclear medicine imaging findings, 2005
    WHO definition, 2005
Osteosclerosis, 1943
Overall survival (OS), 1270, 1318, 1368, 1406–1408
Oxidation, 97, 843, 883, 885, 1266, 1285, 1287, 1313
Oxidative stress, 567, 649, 720, 795, 814, 843, 845, 880, 883, 886, 887, 1011, 1012, 1014–1016, 1045, 1049–1051, 1092, 1212, 1216, 1217, 1228, 1256, 1293, 1297, 1300, 2129
Oxygen
    consumption, 455
    delivery (DO$_2$), 455–456
    deprivation, 456
    extraction fraction, 458, 478, 501, 510, 521, 538
    uptake (VO$_2$), 455, 456
Oxygenation, 11, 455, 456
Oxyhemoglobin, 20
Oxytocin, 230, 370, 371, 384

P

^{31}P, 10, 15
Painful legs and moving toes, 416
Pain/temperature deficits, 207, 475
Palinopsia, 209, 408
Palisades, 1274, 1643, 1757, 1759, 1855
Pallidal degenerations, 828, 858
Pallido-luisy degeneration, 828, 858
Pallido-nigrale degeneration, 858
Pallido-nigro-luisy degeneration, 828, 858
Pallido-nigro-spinal degeneration, 828, 858
Pancreatic adenocarcinoma, 2105
Pantothenate kinase-associated neurodegeneration (PKAN), 864
Papillary renal cell carcinoma (PRCC), 2059, 2085, 2088
Papilledema, 653, 1267
Papp-Lantos body, 834
Papua and New Guinea, 820
Paracentral lobule, 135–137, 150
Paraganglioma, 1276, 1325, 1510, 1663, 1754, 1791
Paralysis, 208, 209, 404, 437, 697, 737, 1054, 1093, 1186, 1215
Paramagnetic contrast medium, 15
Paraneoplastic disorders, 2152, 2167
Paraneoplastic limbic encephalitis (PLE), 2155
Paraneoplastic movement disorders, 416
Paraparesis/paraplegia, 1245, 1267
Para-quadriparesis, 1224, 1233
Parasites, 657, 702, 749–771, 775, 787, 791
Parasubiculum, 138, 300, 919, 920
Paraterminal lobe, 135, 136
Paratonic rig, 208
Paravertebral soft tissue, 65
Paresthesias, 417
Parietal apraxia, 406
Parietal lobe, 76, 130–133, 135, 147, 148, 154, 167, 168, 203, 204, 209, 294, 328, 332, 334, 351, 361, 407, 413, 422, 475, 487, 490, 507, 658, 803, 851, 853, 901, 958, 962, 966, 977, 980, 1042, 1201, 1280, 1378, 1415, 1419, 1482, 1899, 2052, 2125
PARK, 1013
Parkinsonism, 49, 54, 416, 622, 626, 818, 828, 836, 837, 839, 848, 857, 858, 931–933, 942, 974, 980, 984, 988, 1001–1004, 1014, 1016–1018, 1021, 1022, 1034, 1035, 1054, 1055, 1212, 1245, 1255, 1258, 2153, 2160

Parkinson's disease (PD), 49, 50, 84, 100, 101, 245, 373, 381, 826–828, 835, 838, 842, 845, 848, 849, 881, 882, 915, 916, 931, 933, 942, 975, 976, 980, 1001–1018, 1027, 1034, 1035, 1053, 1054, 1196, 1297
Parkinson's disease dementia, 855, 933, 935, 937, 941, 1011
Paroxysmal dyskinesia, 416, 1136
Pars compacta (SNc), 307
Pars lateralis (SNl), 308
Pars reticulata (SNr), 308, 1062
Parthanatos, 1214, 1266, 1293–1296, 1301
Partial anterior circulation syndromes, 474
Partial remission/response (PR), 1270, 2131, 2132, 2135, 2138
Partial (focal) seizures, 731, 1120–1124, 1136, 1139, 1541, 2156, 2158
Partial volume effect, 6
Parvalbumin (PV), 95, 232, 233, 283, 291, 292, 304, 1176, 2088
Pathologic reflexes, 456
Pavlovian conditioning, 122
PCA-1 (Yo), 2153, 2170
PCNA, see Proliferating cell nuclear antigen
PCV regimen, 1466
PDGFRα, 92, 1306, 1318, 1349, 1996
Peduncular hallucinosis, 209
Pelizaeus-Merzbacher disease, 1072
Penetrating injury, 1188–1192
Pentanucleotide repeat disease, 851
Penumbra, 245, 477, 484
Periaqueductal gray, 308, 352, 384, 1212, 1229
Pericytes, 257, 629, 630, 717, 996, 1311, 1312, 1957
Pericytic differentiation, 1966
Perikaryon, 226, 230, 234, 235, 458, 836, 1228, 1343, 1364
Perineurial cells, 1661, 1662, 1677, 1685, 1686, 1689
Perineurioma
  age incidence, 1685
  biologic behavior-prognosis-prognostic factors, 1686
  CT-contrast-enhanced, 1685
  CT-non contrast-enhanced, 1685
  general imaging findings, 1685
  immunophenotype, 1685–1686
  incidence, 1685
  localisation, 1685
  macroscopic features, 1685
  microscopic features, 1685, 1686
  molecular neuropathology, 1686
  MRI-flair, 1685
  MRI-T1, 1685
  MRI-T2, 1685
  MRI-T1 contrast-enhanced, 1685
  pathogenesis, 1686
  proliferation markers, 1686
  sex incidence, 1685
  treatment, 1686
  ultrastructural features, 1686
  WHO definition, 1685
  WHO grade, 1685
Perineurium, 238, 239, 1690
Perineuronal satellite cells, 245, 246
Perinuclear halo, 1386, 1452, 1456, 1462, 1463, 1492, 1493, 1584, 2085
Periodic acid-Schiff (PAS), 83–85, 89, 102, 239, 611, 680, 756, 768, 776, 781, 787, 791, 830, 876, 907, 1386, 1648, 1762, 1771, 1773, 1776, 1796, 1844, 1853, 1855, 2058, 2064, 2101
Periosteal chondroma, 2009
Peripheral nervous system (PNS), 95, 98, 99, 121–122, 125, 236, 245, 251, 703, 1257, 1661–1703, 1956, 2152, 2153, 2156, 2157
Perisylvian dysplasia, 1132
Perisylvian network, 291
Perivascular lymphocytic cuffing, 484, 493, 698, 1085, 1275, 1947, 2050
Perivascular lymphocytic infiltration (PLI), 552, 565, 641, 702, 706, 710–712, 740, 865, 1112, 1341, 1771, 2163
Perivascular pseudorosette, 1274, 1489, 1492, 1493, 1497, 1501, 1503, 1577, 1583, 1584, 1588, 1589
Perivenous encephalomyelitis, 1105
Periventricular germinal matrix, 1591
Periventricular hypodensities, 444, 870
Periventricular nodular heterotopia, 1130, 1135, 1178
Perl's prussian blue, 89
Permanent global ischemia, 457
Perseveration, 405, 419, 422, 947
Persistent headache, 637
Personality, 132, 361, 404, 410, 419, 622, 640, 722, 736, 857, 859, 962, 966, 967, 988, 1194, 1224, 1267, 1755, 1895, 2154, 2155
PET/CT, 33, 41–43, 1376
Petechial hemorrhages, 449, 487, 585, 596, 619, 644, 684, 737, 998, 1111, 1202, 1229
PET/MR system, 42
PFS, see Progression-free survival
P-glycoprotein, 719, 720, 1313, 1759
pH, 77, 110, 241–243, 471, 776, 1215
Phagocytic microglia, 247
Phagocytosis, 248, 257, 510, 786, 816, 879–881, 1293, 1294, 1934
Pharmaceutical molecule, 29
Pharmacoresistant, 1139
Phase contrast MR-angiography, 17
Phonetic and/or semantic paraphasias, 134, 409
Phosphatidylinositol binding clathrin assembly protein (PICALM), 887, 923, 924
Phosphoinositide 3-kinase-related kinases, 1285, 1398–1400, 1701, 1995
Phospholipase A2, 441, 1014, 1016, 1256, 1792
Phospholipases, 471, 1093, 1404
Phospholipids, 250
Phosphorylated tau, 100, 101, 108, 813, 832, 837, 839, 844, 861, 982
Phosphorylation, 97, 227, 626, 814, 842, 884, 885, 924, 1283, 1286–1288, 1309, 1310, 1444, 1702, 1792, 2139
Phosphotungstic acid hematoxylin (PTAH), 85–86, 241, 1042, 1776

Index

Photomultiplier, 40, 41
Photons, 31, 40–42
Photophobia, 209, 654, 694, 751, 774, 974, 1895
Photosensitive crystals, 42
Physaliphorous cell, 1990, 2020, 2025
Pia mater intima, 186
Pick body, 830, 837, 960, 965
Pick disease (PiD), 813, 818, 826, 827, 837, 839, 842, 848–850, 852, 854, 857, 859, 914, 953, 956, 957, 960, 962, 967
Picornaviruses, 695, 697
Pigments, 228, 279, 308, 311, 529, 716, 958, 1007, 1028, 1232, 2076, 2077
Piloid cells, 1434, 1438
Pineal, 14, 204, 476, 1275, 1276, 1280, 1325, 1595–1610, 1824, 1868
Pineal gland, 148, 155, 156, 1325, 1438, 1563, 1584, 1595, 1596, 1604, 1606, 1652, 1866, 1868, 1935
Pineal parenchymal tumor of intermediate differentiation, 1325, 1595, 1596, 1604–1605
Pineoblastoma, 1273, 1274, 1276, 1325, 1595, 1596, 1604, 1606–1610, 1629
Pineocytoma
    age incidence, 1597
    biologic behavior-prognosis-prognostic factors, 1604
    CT-contrast-enhanced, 1597, 1598
    CT-non contrast-enhanced, 1597, 1598
    differential diagnosis, 1596
    general imaging findings, 1597
    immunophenotype, 1600–1603
    incidence, 1596
    localisation, 1596
    macroscopic features, 1597
    microscopic features, 1597, 1601
    molecular neuropathology, 1596
    MRI-flair, 1597, 1599
    MRI-T1, 1597, 1599
    MRI-T2, 1597, 1598
    MRI-T1 contrast-enhanced, 1597, 1599
    MRI-T2∗/ SWI, 1597
    nuclear medicine imaging findings, 1597, 1600
    pathogenesis, 1596
    proliferation markers, 1600, 1603
    sex incidence, 1596
    treatment, 1604
    ultrastructural features, 1604
    WHO definition, 1597
    WHO grade, 1597
Pineocytomatous rosettes, 1274, 1597, 1601, 1604, 1606, 1609
Pinocytotic vesicles, 1675, 1683
Piriform lobe, 138, 351
Pittsburgh compound B (PiB), 53, 54, 901
Pituicyte, 1753, 1754, 1768, 1771
Pituicytoma
    age incidence, 1766
    biologic behavior-prognosis-prognostic factors, 1768
    CT-contrast-enhanced, 1766
    CT-non contrast-enhanced, 1766
    differential diagnosis, 1768
    general imaging findings, 1766
    immunophenotype, 1767, 1769–1770
    incidence, 1766
    localisation, 1766
    macroscopic features, 1766
    microscopic features, 1767, 1769
    MRI-flair, 1766, 1767
    MRI-T1, 1766, 1767
    MRI-T2, 1766, 1767
    MRI-T1 contrast-enhanced, 1766–1768
    MRI-T2∗/ SWI, 1766
    pathogenesis, 1768
    sex incidence, 1766
    treatment, 1768
    WHO definition, 1766
    WHO grade, 1766
Pituitary, 91, 92, 108, 166, 223, 371, 1280, 1754, 1766, 1770, 1776, 1780–1790, 1793–1794, 1797, 1798, 1800, 1803–1806, 1810, 1813, 1817, 1824, 1841, 1843
Pituitary adenoma
    acidophilic adenoma, 1785
    acidophil stem cell adenomas, 1798
    age incidence, 1780
    atypical adenomas, 1808, 1809
    atypical pituitary adenoma, 1808–1809
    basophilic adenoma, 1787
    biologic behavior-prognosis-prognostic factors, 1798, 1804, 1806, 1808, 1810, 1813
    chromophobic adenoma, 1787
    corticotroph adenoma, 1800, 1802–1803
    Crooke's cell adenoma, 1802
    CT-contrast-enhanced, 1782
    CT-non contrast-enhanced, 1782
    differential diagnosis, 1787
    DNA methylation, 1792
    epigenetics, 1788–1789
    gene expression, 1788–1789
    general imaging findings, 1782
    genetics, 1788–1789
    giant adenoma, 1782
    gonadotroph adenoma, 1803–1805
    immunophenotype, 1795–1800, 1802–1807, 1810, 1812
    incidence, 1780
    lactotroph adenoma, 1798–1799
    localisation, 1794, 1798, 1800, 1802, 1804, 1806, 1810, 1811
    macroadenoma, 1782–1786
    macroscopic features, 1794, 1795, 1798, 1800, 1802, 1804, 1806, 1810, 1811
    microadenoma, 1782, 1783
    microRNAs, 1787, 1791
    microscopic features, 1794–1808, 1810, 1812
    molecular neuropathology, 1786–1793
    MRI-diffusion imaging, (AU: Not found)
    MRI-diffusion tensor imaging, (AU: Not found)
    MRI-flair, 1783, 1784
    MRI-perfusion, (AU: Not found)

Pituitary adenoma (*cont.*)
  MRI-T1, 1783, 1785
  MRI-T2, 1782–1784
  MRI-T1 contrast-enhanced, 1782–1785
  MRI-T2∗/ SWI, 1782, 1785
  MR-spectroscopy, (AU: Not found)
  nuclear medicine imaging findings, 1785, 1786
  null cell adenoma, 1804–1808
  pathogenesis, 1788–1790
  pituitary blastoma, 1810–1813
  pituitary carcinoma, 1809–1812
  pituitary hyperplasia, 1781
  plurihormonal adenomas, 1806–1808
  plurihormonal and double adenoma, 1806–1808
  proliferation markers, 1796–1798, 1800, 1802, 1804, 1806, 1810, 1813
  sex incidence, 1780
  somatotroph adenoma, 1794–1798
  thyrotroph adenoma, 1799–1802
  treatment, 1793
  ultrastructural features, 1797–1798, 1800, 1802, 1804, 1806, 1808, 1810, 1813
  WHO definition, 1780
  WHO grade, 1782
Pituitary apoplexy
  age incidence, 1813
  biologic behavior-prognosis-prognostic factors, 1817
  CT-contrast-enhanced, 1814
  CT-non contrast-enhanced, 1813, 1814
  differential diagnosis, 1816
  general imaging findings, 1813
  immunophenotype, 1818
  incidence, 1813
  localisation, 1813
  macroscopic features, 1816
  microscopic features, 1816, 1818–1819
  MRI-diffusion imaging, 1813
  MRI-diffusion tensor imaging, (AU: Not found)
  MRI-flair, 1813, 1814
  MRI-perfusion, (AU: Not found)
  MRI-T1, 1813–1815, 1817
  MRI-T2, 1813, 1814
  MRI-T1 contrast-enhanced, 1813, 1815, 1817
  MRI-T2∗/ SWI, 1813
  MR-spectroscopy, (AU: Not found)
  nuclear medicine imaging findings, 1816
  pathogenesis, 1816
  proliferation markers, 1816
  sex incidence, 1813
  treatment, 1817
  ultrastructural features, 1813
Pituitary gland
  adenohypophysis, 166
  anterior lobe of the pituitary, 166
  hypophyseal stalk, 166
  neurohypophysis, 166
  pituitary stalk, 166
Pituitary stalk, 60, 62, 137, 1766, 1770, 1771, 1935, 1937, 1941, 1943

Pixel, 4, 5, 37
Placenta-like alkaline phosphatase (PLAP), 108, 1866, 1867, 1871, 1872, 1878, 1879, 2061, 2096
Plain radiographs, 3, 4
Planum temporale, 294
Plasma cell, 103, 105, 641, 675, 684, 732, 752, 1086, 1101, 1106, 1892, 1893, 1923, 1924, 1927, 1929, 1944, 1945, 1991, 1992, 2058, 2059
Plasmacytoma, 105, 106, 112, 1277, 1891, 1892, 1923–1929, 1991, 1993
Plasma exchange, 2152, 2176
Platelet activating factor, 441, 1179
Pleomorphism, 1158, 1268, 1270, 1272, 1277, 1279, 1354, 1368, 1397, 1417, 1420, 1462, 1463, 1476, 1477, 1483, 1503, 1529–1531, 1534, 1573, 1614, 1618, 1625, 1671, 1690, 1691, 1743, 1754, 1776, 1795, 1798, 1800, 1801, 1810, 1904, 1985, 2013, 2097
PLP, *see* Proteolipid protein
PLS, *see* Primary lateral sclerosis
PML associated with monoclonal antibody therapy, 725
PML–IRIS immune reconstitution inflammatory syndrome, 725
Pneumocystidiomycetes, 774
Pogression types, 2131, 2137
Poikilothermia, 418
Point Resolved Excitation Spin-echo Sequence (PRESS), 16
Pol, 701, 1288
Pole
  pole-frontal pole, 60, 62, 130, 135, 404–405
  pole-occipital pole, 130, 204, 476
  pole-temporal pole, 63, 71, 130, 134, 137, 347, 349, 356, 965, 1192, 1196
Polioviruses, 697
Polydendrocytes, 97
Polymicrogyria, insscluding schizencephaly and opercular syndrome, 1157
Polyomaviridae family, 722
Polyradiculopathy, 2153
Polyribosomes, 1364, 1871
Polysynaptic pathway, 346, 347, 349
Pons, 68, 71, 72, 76, 129, 130, 137, 156–160, 162, 169, 175, 186, 204, 224, 308, 310–312, 334, 385, 386, 398, 436, 476, 490, 501, 586, 596, 614, 616, 627, 737, 785, 853, 990, 991, 1022, 1023, 1028, 1040, 1080, 1083, 1106, 1224, 1233, 1235, 1323, 1615, 1620
Pontocerebellar fibers, 350
Positron emission tomography (PET), 15, 30–34, 37–39, 41–44, 48–54, 402, 449, 458, 478, 501, 510, 521, 538, 607, 802, 851, 854, 896, 897, 901, 932, 934–941, 976, 1003, 1007, 1022, 1025, 1027, 1060, 1121, 1129, 1144, 1146, 1192, 1193, 1196, 1226, 1245, 1247, 1257, 1380–1383, 1542, 1554, 1563, 1576, 1615, 1664, 1716, 1718, 1720, 1722, 1755, 1785, 1811, 1961, 2050, 2125, 2139, 2144, 2153
Positrons, 30, 42

Possible CJD, 797, 816
Posterior approach, 65, 66
Posterior cerebral artery syndrome, 209
Posterior circulation syndromes, 474
Posterior column nuclei, 311
Posterior commissure, 150, 209, 307
Posterior cranial fossa posterior, 162
Posterior inferior cerebellar artery syndrome (PICA syndrome), 192, 198–200, 208–209, 559, 561
Posterior lens opacity, 1699
Posterior limb, 146, 147, 406, 475
Posterior limb of the internal capsule, 127, 147, 203, 204, 334
Posterior meningeal branches, 181
Posterior pituitary, 358, 1766, 1770, 1771
Posterior pituitary gland, 355
Posterior ramus, 132
Postictal period, 1120
Postictal phenomena, 1120
Postinfectious encephalomyelitis, 1105
Post-transplant lymphoproliferative disorders (PTLDs)
    age incidence, 1919
    biologic behavior-prognosis-prognostic factors, 1924
    CT-contrast-enhanced, 1919
    CT-non contrast-enhanced, 1919
    differential diagnosis, 1923
    general imaging findings, 1919–1923
    immunophenotype, 1921–1924
    incidence, 1919
    localisation, 1919
    macroscopic features, 1920
    microscopic features, 1920–1921, 1923
    molecular neuropathology, 1924
    MRI-diffusion imaging, 1919
    MRI-flair, 1919
    MRI-perfusion, 1919
    MRI-T1, 1919
    MRI-T2, 1919
    MRI-T1 contrast-enhanced, 1919
    MRI-T2∗/ SWI, 1919
    pathogenesis, 1924
    proliferation markers, 1923
    sex incidence, 1919
    treatment, 1924
    WHO definition, 1919
Postural hypotension, 942
Postural instability, 932, 974, 1002, 1018
Potassium channelopathies, 1135
PPA, see Primary progressive aphasia
Precession, 10
Precession frequency, 10
Preclinical PD, 1002
Preclinical states of AD, 897–901
Precuneus, 135–137, 150, 204, 476, 800, 852, 1042
Predictive biomarkers in clinical use, 1326
Prefrontal network, 291
Preganglionic autonomic neurons of the brainstem and spinal cord, 352, 373

Preoccipital incisure, 133, 134
Presenilin 1 (PSEN1), 850, 896–898, 922, 923
Prestriate cortex, 333
Presubiculum, 138, 300, 859, 861, 965
Presynaptic and postsynaptic SPECT and PET, 458, 478, 538
Pre-tangle, 837, 844, 1185, 1212, 1213
    neurons, 859
Primary angiitis of CNS (PACNS), 636
Primary axotomy, 1185, 1207
Primary CNS vasculitis (PCNSV), 637
Primary cortical areas, 123
Primary cortical motor area, 131
Primary lateral sclerosis (PLS), 849, 1035, 1037, 1038, 1053–1055
Primary progressive (PPMS), 1035, 1072, 1073, 1091, 1093
Primary progressive aphasia (PPA), 825, 826, 850, 852–854, 949, 974
Primary visual center, 134
Primary visual cortex, 20, 76, 278, 294, 326, 328, 331–333, 357, 360, 361, 407, 408, 421, 901
Primitive plaque, 819, 834, 836
Primordial fields, 278, 290
Primordial germ cells, 1865, 1867, 1868
Prion
    encephalopathies, 795–820
    strains, 795, 815
Prion protein (PrP^{res}) types, 812
PRKCQ—protein kinase C theta, 247
PRNP (gene), 795, 796, 814, 815, 817
PRNP codon 129 polymorphisms, 815, 817–819
Probable CJD, 797, 816
Procarbazine, 1329, 1330, 1431, 1447, 1466
Procaspase, 1296
Prodromal PD, 1002
Progesterone receptor, 1751, 1966, 2060, 2062, 2070, 2073
Progranulin, 249, 825, 845, 850, 956–959, 1056
Progression-free survival (PFS), 1270, 1406, 1476, 1561, 1573, 2056, 2057
Progressive bulbar palsy (PBP), 1037, 1038, 1054
Progressive disease (PD), 942, 968, 1073, 1093, 1270, 2132, 2136–2139
Progressive focal neurologic signs, 637
Progressive insomnia, 820
Progressive muscular atrophy (PMA), 1037, 1038, 1050, 1051, 1053–1055
Progressive non-fluent aphasia (PNFA), 945, 946, 949, 958
Progressive subcortical gliosis (PSG), 825, 855
Progressive supranuclear palsy (PSP), 49, 50, 416, 826–828, 836–839, 842, 848, 849, 852, 854, 859, 915, 933, 953, 956, 957, 962, 973–984, 1004, 1028, 1035, 1054, 2160
Proinflammatory factors, 2131
Projection fibers, 20, 147, 156, 289, 290
Proliferating cell nuclear antigen (PCNA), 105, 1288, 1396, 1675, 1788, 1790, 2084

Proliferation markers, 91, 92, 105–107, 1341, 1364, 1396, 1417, 1420, 1431, 1438, 1454, 1464, 1476, 1480, 1496, 1501, 1510, 1518, 1530, 1539, 1545, 1558, 1563, 1573, 1579, 1589, 1600, 1604, 1608, 1624, 1643, 1647, 1648, 1652, 1675, 1681, 1686, 1692, 1742, 1764, 1767, 1771, 1776, 1796, 1798, 1800, 1802, 1804, 1806, 1810, 1813, 1816, 1829, 1837, 1843, 1850, 1853, 1859, 1871, 1875, 1888, 1904, 1916, 1923, 1928, 1938, 1948, 1964, 1969, 2050, 2165
Proneural, 1368, 1402
Proopiomelanocortin derivatives, 370
Prophase, 1281, 1284
Prosencephalon, 129, 1012
Prosopagnosia, 209, 422, 946
Prosopoaffective agnosia, 417
Prostaglandins, 441
Prostate-specific antigen (PSA), 2060, 2062, 2093, 2095
Prostatic adenocarcinoma, 2088, 2095
Protease inhibitors (PI), 699, 712, 714, 719, 1302
Proteases, 441, 471, 567, 568, 701, 814, 884, 1093, 1209, 1293, 1990, 1995, 2084
14-3-3 protein, 815
Protein kinases, 884, 1266, 1306, 1492, 1702
Proteoglycans, 84, 255, 258, 538, 540, 1314, 1316
Proteolipid protein (PLP), 98, 99, 250, 255, 1087, 1089, 1093, 1250
Proton density (PD), 11–13
Protons, 9–11, 13–15, 17, 31, 372, 1269
Proto-oncogenes, 1266, 1284, 1285, 1289, 1490, 1630, 1792, 2054, 2055
Protoplasmic astrocytes, 240, 1341, 1344, 1438, 1439
Protozoa, 636, 749, 750, 1301
PrP cerebral amyloid angiopathy, 797
Pseudoarthrosis, 1694
Pseudoocclusion, 538
Pseudo-onion bulbs, 1685, 1686
Pseudopalisades, 1274
Pseudopalisading, 1273, 1278, 1390, 1397, 1398, 1420, 1500, 2127
Pseudo-progression, 1376, 2131–2148
Pseudoresponse, 2132
Pseudostratified epithelium, 1637, 1646, 1648
PSP, *see* Progressive supranuclear palsy
Psychiatric symptoms, 626, 629, 1245, 1256, 2152, 2154, 2158, 2174
Psychosis and hallucinations, 1002
PTLDs, *see* Post-transplant lymphoproliferative disorders
Pulvinar, 150, 305, 333, 357, 417, 819, 853, 857
Pulvinar sign, 798, 853
Pure agraphia, 404
Pure pallidal degeneration, 828, 858
Purine nucleotides, 441
Purkinje cell protein 4 (PCP4), 291
Putamen, 50, 51, 76, 125–127, 143, 145–147, 167, 168, 203, 204, 231, 301–305, 334, 357, 367, 380, 388, 449, 475, 501, 538, 542, 715, 795, 797, 818, 819, 858, 865, 873, 919, 933, 947, 966, 974–976, 980, 1003, 1004, 1007, 1022, 1024, 1027, 1028, 1060, 1062, 1063, 1066, 1194, 1248, 1255, 1256, 2159
Putaminal rim sign, 1022, 1024
PVC, 2131
Pyramid, 76, 160, 214
Pyramidal cells, 227, 230, 231, 268, 278, 282, 289, 290, 294, 342, 392, 918–920, 1148, 1161, 1171, 1178
Pyramidal decussation, 74
Pyramidal/extrapyramidal dysfunction, 797, 816, 864, 1022, 2156
Pyramidal system, 334
Pyramidal tract (PT), 125, 160, 293, 303, 334, 654, 694, 751, 774
Pyramis, 161, 163, 164, 267, 312, 314, 334
Pyrimidine dimers, 1285
Pyroptosis, 1266, 1293, 1294, 1300–1301

Q
Quadrantanopia contralateral superior, 410
Quadrigeminal bodies (lamina quadrigemina or tectum mesencephali), 156, 168

R
Rabies virus, 697–699
Raclopride, 54, 1060, 1226
Radial cortical lamination, 1158, 1161
Radial glia, 241, 250, 1178, 1179, 1492
Radiation
    fibrosis, 2119
    leukoencephalopathy, 2119, 2128
    necrosis, 48, 2119–2128
    protection, 38–39
Radiation-associated neoplasms, 2119, 2129
Radiation-induced DNA mutations, 2129
Radiation therapy (RT), 48, 1269, 1368, 1406, 1407, 1469, 1476, 1484, 1648, 1720, 1891, 1913, 1929, 1990, 1997, 2127, 2136
Radicular pain, 1267, 1663
Radioactive compound, 29, 30
Radioactive material, 1269
Radiofrequency (RF), 9, 10
Radiofrequency ablation, 1995
Radio frequency pulse, 9, 10
Radio frequency receiver coils, 10
Radioisotope, 19, 30–32, 37, 40, 41
Radiolabeled monoclonal antibody, 1269
Radiosensitivities, 38
Radiosurgery, 585, 1661, 1675, 1754, 1777, 1779, 1793, 2124
Radiotherapy, 48, 49, 585, 1269, 1320, 1329, 1330, 1365, 1406, 1407, 1414, 1417, 1420, 1447, 1451, 1462, 1466, 1470, 1477, 1521, 1522, 1561, 1573, 1575, 1582, 1595, 1608, 1614, 1616, 1631, 1637, 1638, 1642, 1646, 1647, 1652, 1654, 1661, 1675, 1779, 1793, 1865, 1868, 1891, 1924, 1938, 1955, 1967, 1990, 1995, 2053, 2125, 2131

Raised intracranial pressure, 500, 691, 1105, 1187, 1490
Ramified astrocyte, 837
RANK ligand inhibitors, 1990, 1997
Rapid eye movement sleep behavior disorder (RBD), 942
Rapid progressive dementia, 797
Rathke's cleft cyst
    age incidence, 1841
    biologic behavior-prognosis-prognostic factors, 1843
    CT-contrast-enhanced, 1841
    CT-non contrast-enhanced, 1841
    differential diagnosis, 1843
    general imaging findings, 1841
    immunophenotype, 1843, 1845–1846
    incidence, 1841
    localisation, 1841
    macroscopic features, 1843
    microscopic features, 1843–1846
    MRI-flair, 1841, 1842
    MRI-perfusion, 1843
    MRI-T1, 1842, 1843
    MRI-T2, 1841, 1842
    MRI-T1 contrast-enhanced, 1842, 1843
    MRI-T2∗/ SWI, 1843
    pathogenesis, 1843
    proliferation markers, 1843
    sex incidence, 1841
    treatment, 1843
    ultrastructural features, 1843
    WHO definition, 1841
Rathke's pouch, 1754, 1765
Ray intensity, 4, 5
rCBF, *see* Regional cerebral blood flow
rCBV, 661, 663, 899, 1077, 1106, 1109, 1125, 1338, 1339, 1354, 1355, 1357, 1370, 1372, 1412, 1413, 1423, 1429, 1430, 1434, 1448, 1449, 1462, 1470, 1471, 1477, 1478, 1493, 1542, 1563, 1564, 1566, 1572, 1584, 1606, 1615, 1642, 1652, 1666, 1667, 1709, 1713, 1825, 1827, 1834, 1836, 1846, 1853, 1857, 1895, 1896, 1915, 1919, 1925, 1943, 1958, 1959, 1969, 2039, 2120, 2121, 2124, 2132, 2133
RCCMa, 2061, 2088
Reactive astrogliosis, 245, 458, 470, 484, 495, 496, 516, 616, 685, 698, 706, 718, 728, 740, 791, 797, 802, 805, 810, 818, 820, 844, 854, 857–859, 863, 864, 959, 966, 982, 1008, 1059, 1063, 1064, 1066, 1085, 1093, 1111, 1113, 1151, 1152, 1162, 1164, 1166, 1223, 1227, 1229, 1231, 1233, 1236, 1271, 1275, 1341, 1343, 1364, 1453, 1464, 1475, 1479, 1569, 1920, 1947, 2126, 2164, 2168
Recanalization, 477, 496
Receptors
    binding, 29, 689, 885, 1060, 1128, 1245, 1256, 1405
    for growth factors, 1266, 1289
Recreational drugs, 503
Red nucleus, 71, 76, 307, 335, 858, 859
Reduced level of consciousness, 496, 1267
Reed–Sternberg cells, 105
Reference process, 25

Regional cerebral blood flow (rCBF), 11, 52, 54, 449, 1125
Region of interest (ROI), 34, 50, 51, 53, 113, 641
Registration process, 25
Regulated intramembrane proteolysis (RIP), 99
Reisberg Global Deterioration Scale, 898
Relapse-free survival (RFS), 1270, 1995
Relapsing progressive (PRMS), 1073, 1093
Relapsing remitting (RRMS), 1072, 1090, 1093, 1103
Renal cell tumors, 2085
Reoviridae, 695, 696, 736
Repetition, 332, 357, 413, 414, 420, 897, 898, 946
Repetition time (TR), 12, 13
Repetitive transcranial magnetic stimulation (rTMS), 402
Reprogramming energy metabolism, 1281
Resection, 23, 24, 582, 585, 592, 1119, 1138, 1143, 1154, 1287, 1342, 1349, 1359, 1382, 1407, 1431, 1452–1455, 1473, 1489, 1490, 1504, 1511, 1518, 1522, 1550, 1553, 1554, 1559, 1575, 1582, 1595, 1608, 1614, 1631, 1716, 1721, 1724, 1750, 1753, 1754, 1766, 1775, 1777, 1779, 1793, 1865, 1868, 1891, 1924, 1929, 1955, 1967, 1985, 1989, 1990, 1995, 2121
Resistin, 926
Respirator brain, 457, 458
Respiratory insufficiency, 1038
Response assessment in neuro-oncology (RANO), 2135, 2136
Resting microglia, 247
Restless legs syndrome and periodic limb movements of sleep, 416, 1003
Restriction checkpoint, 1282, 1283
Reticular formation (RF), 231, 307, 308, 311, 312, 326, 335, 350–352, 357, 373, 381, 859, 1028
Reticulin, 88–89, 1393, 1414, 1556, 1615, 1623, 1669, 1734, 1773, 1801, 1807, 1901, 1958, 1962, 1965, 1975
Reticulin network, 1416, 1419, 1420, 1621
Reticulocerebellar fibers, 350
Retina, 203, 230, 326, 331, 360, 372, 408, 475, 717, 1596
Retinal hamartoma, 1662, 1699, 1700
Retinal phototransduction, 1325, 1596
Retinopathy, 606, 2153, 2173
Retrograde transport, 228, 229, 1093
Retrolentiform part of the internal capsule, 147
Retroolivary sulcus, 160, 162
Rett syndrome, 249, 1130
Rev, 701
Reverse transcription PCR (RT-PCR), 111, 113, 114, 1984
Reversible posterior leukoencephalopathy, 2128
RGNT, *see* Rosette-forming glioneuronal tumor
Rhabdoid cells, 1368, 1386, 1651, 1742
Rhabdomyoma, 1956, 1986
Rhabdomyosarcoma, 1290, 1692–1694, 1882, 1885, 1956, 1986, 2061
Rhizotomies, 4
Rhombencephalon, 129, 373, 384

Rhomboid fossa, 157, 158, 174
Riboprobe, 111
Richardson/PSP syndrome, 974, 976, 980
Rich-club organization, 326, 364–367
Rich-club regions, 365, 366
Ricinus communis agglutinin (RCA), 100, 248
Right hemisphere syndromes, 146, 208, 288, 421
Rigidity, 79, 416, 537, 615, 653, 654, 843, 858, 864, 865, 932, 946, 947, 974, 980, 988, 1001, 1002, 1022, 1038, 1059, 1060, 1068, 1212, 2156, 2158, 2170, 2174
Ring enhancing mass, 1369
Ringertz, N., 1277–1278
Rituximab, 731, 1103, 1913, 1924, 2152, 2160, 2176
RNA-dependent DNA polymerase, 701
RNA viruses, 694, 698, 699, 701–720
Rods, 326, 331, 655, 656
RORß, 95
Rosai–Dorfman disease
    CT-contrast-enhanced, 1941
    CT-non contrast-enhanced, 1941
    MRI-flair, 1941, 1942
    MRI-perfusion, 1943
    MRI-T1, 1941, 1942
    MRI-T2, 1941, 1942
    MRI-T1 contrast-enhanced, 1941, 1942
Rosenthal fibers, 241, 1343, 1433, 1434, 1438, 1439, 1442, 1563, 1573, 1584, 1757, 1829, 1837, 1969, 2126
Rosette-forming glioneuronal tumor (RGNT)
    age incidence, 1583
    biologic behavior-prognosis-prognostic factors, 1592
    CT-contrast-enhanced, 1584
    CT-non contrast-enhanced, 1584
    differential diagnosis, 1591
    general imaging findings, 1584
    immunophenotype, 1589–1591
    incidence, 1583
    localisation, 1583–1584
    macroscopic features, 1584
    microscopic features, 1584, 1588–1589
    molecular neuropathology, 1591–1592
    MRI-diffusion imaging, 1584
    MRI-flair, 1584–1586
    MRI-perfusion, 1584, 1587
    MRI-T1, 1584, 1585
    MRI-T2, 1584–1586
    MRI-T1 contrast-enhanced, 1584–1586
    MRI-T2*/ SWI, 1584
    MR-spectroscopy, 1584, 1587
    nuclear medicine imaging findings, 1584
    pathogenesis, 1591–1592
    proliferation markers, 1589, 1591
    sex incidence, 1583
    treatment, 1592
    ultrastructural features, 1591
    WHO definition, 1583–1591
    WHO grade, 1583

Rosettes, 1273–1274, 1326, 1489, 1492, 1493, 1497, 1500, 1513, 1514, 1562, 1577, 1578, 1583, 1584, 1588, 1590, 1597, 1601, 1604, 1606, 1609, 1615, 1624, 1639, 1643, 1646, 1647, 1885, 1984
Ruptured aneurysm, 61, 503, 517, 533, 990

S
S-100, 92, 96, 97, 102, 108, 1164, 1223, 1228, 1341, 1347, 1362, 1364, 1394, 1396, 1420, 1431, 1442, 1454, 1476, 1480, 1485, 1496, 1501, 1505, 1508, 1510, 1516, 1521, 1523, 1527, 1529, 1530, 1539, 1589, 1624, 1643, 1645, 1656, 1671, 1672, 1676, 1681, 1684, 1686, 1687, 1689, 1692, 1693, 1742, 1745, 1746, 1769, 1770, 1773, 1775, 1776, 1843, 1909, 1920, 1934, 1939, 1940, 1945, 1948, 1949, 1966, 1977, 1979, 2016, 2022, 2058, 2061, 2062, 2075, 2082–2084, 2088, 2096, 2100, 2104, 2113, 2115
SAH, see Subarachnoid hemorrhage
"Salt and pepper," 1493, 1497
Saltatory impulse conduction, 237
"Salutatory" seizures, 405
Saprobes, 775
Satellitosis, 1269, 1453
Saturation (SAT) techniques, 13
Scalloping, 1507
Scanning electron microscopy, 108
Scavenger receptor family, 100
Scheltens-score, 899
Schizencephaly, 1130, 1132, 1135, 1157
Schmidt-Lanterman incisures, 238
Schwann cells, 99, 236, 237, 245, 251, 1661, 1662, 1665, 1669, 1677, 1679, 1683, 1686, 1689, 1699, 1702
Schwannoma
    age incidence, 1666
    ancient schwannoma, 1671
    biologic behavior-prognosis-prognostic factors, 1675
    cellular schwannoma, 1669, 1675
    conventional schwannoma, 1669
    CT-contrast-enhanced, 1666
    CT-non contrast-enhanced, 1666, 1667
    differential diagnosis, 1675
    general imaging findings, 1666
    immunophenotype, 1671, 1675, 1676
    incidence, 1666
    localisation, 1666
    macroscopic features, 1667, 1670, 1671
    melanotic schwannoma, 1669, 1671
    microscopic features, 1669, 1672–1675
    molecular neuropathology, 1675
    MRI-CISS, 1666, 1667, 1669
    MRI-diffusion imaging, 1666, 1667
    MRI-flair, 1666, 1668
    MRI-perfusion, 1666, 1667
    MRI-T1, 1666, 1668

MRI-T2, 1666–1668
MRI-T1 contrast-enhanced, 1666–1669
MRI-T2∗/ SWI, 1666, 1667
MR-spectroscopy, (AU: Not found)
nuclear medicine imaging findings, 1663–1665
pathogenesis, (AU: Not found)
plexiform schwannoma, 1669
proliferation markers, 1675, 1676
sex incidence, 1666
treatment, 1675
ultrastructural features, 1675
WHO definition, 1665
WHO grade, 1666
Schwannomatosis
diagnostic criteria, 1700
general imaging findings, 1702
incidence, 1700
localisation, 1702
sex incidence, 1700
WHO definition, 1699–1700
WHO grade, 1699–1700
Scintillating crystal, 40
Scintillation detectors, 4, 5
Scoliosis, 1694
Scrapie, 796, 797, 816, 852
Secondary auditory center, 134
Secondary cortical areas, 123–125
Secondary cortical motor area, 132
Secondary progressive (SPMS), 1073, 1090, 1093
Secondary visual cortex, 333
Secondary yolk sac, 1868
"Second-hit" model, 1701
Second messenger, 369, 1134, 1243, 1253, 1254
Secretogranin II, 236
Seeding, 1268–1269, 2038, 2050
Seizures
focus, 1120
onset zone, 1121, 1129, 1144, 1147
Selectins, 517, 519, 567, 568
Sellar diaphragm, 181
Sella turcica, 14, 164, 166, 1780, 1782, 1794
Semantic dementia (SD), 945–947, 949, 950, 958
Semaphorins, 1267, 1316, 1317, 1702
Semianular sulcus, 138
Semilunar gyrus, 138
Seminoma, 1868, 1871, 2094–2096
Senescent, 1280
Sensory loss/pain, 207–209, 406, 417, 475, 476, 725, 861, 1267
with sensory level, 1267
Sensory system, 326–343
Septic embolism, 657, 666, 684
Septum pellucidum, 136, 137, 167, 168, 174, 1511, 1542, 1576, 1577, 1584
Serine/threonine kinases, 1288, 1290, 1291, 1309, 2054, 2055
Serotonin, 156, 370, 372, 373, 376, 385–387, 441, 722, 836, 1243, 1244, 1254–1256, 1258, 1260, 1600, 1604, 1608

Serotonin receptors, 387, 722, 1154
Serous carcinoma, 2061, 2105, 2107, 2113, 2115
Sestamibi, 54
Sex cord stromal, 2062, 2107, 2111
tumor, 2094
Sex determining region Y-box 2 (SOX2), 92, 132, 887, 1867, 2096
Shadow plaque, 1071, 1082, 1084, 1086
Shim coils, 9
Short association fibers, 147, 343
Shunts, 4, 58, 388, 451, 489, 522, 599, 656, 1631
Signal transducers, 293, 626, 1266, 1290, 1315, 1404, 1405, 1749
Signal transduction, 369, 392, 814, 923, 1134, 1244, 1254, 1257, 1266, 1306–1309, 1315, 1320, 1321, 1492, 1791
Simple partial seizures, 1121, 1123, 1124, 1139
Simple visual hallucinations, 407
Simultanagnosia, 209, 361
Single photon emission computed tomography (SPECT), 30–34, 37, 39–44, 49–54, 458, 478, 538, 697, 852, 853, 901, 932–935, 975, 976, 1004, 1007, 1022, 1023, 1027, 1060, 1121, 1125, 1126, 1128, 1129, 1192–1194, 1196, 1226, 1247, 1257, 1576, 1716, 1824, 1866
acquisition, 39, 51, 52, 1126
Single-strand break repair (SSBR), 1266, 1287
Single-strand breaks (SSBs), 1285, 1287
Single-voxel spectroscopy (SVS), 16
Sinograms, 43
Sinus vein thrombosis, 1244, 1260
Sister chromatid segregation, 1271
Skinner's operant conditioning, 122
Skull, 22, 25, 27, 30, 40, 42, 58, 61, 62, 78, 182, 213, 436, 500, 522, 525, 529, 530, 533, 856, 1187, 1188, 1190, 1196, 1199, 1217, 1218, 1412, 1720, 1730, 1924, 1933, 1935, 1943, 1984, 1990, 1993, 1998, 1999, 2005, 2009
Skull base, 7, 1199, 1716, 1935, 1982, 1990, 1995, 2014, 2018
Slice thickness, 6, 12, 13
Slow axoplasmic flow, 228
Slowness, 208, 416, 932, 988
Small cell carcinoma, 1629, 1643, 1647, 1648, 2059, 2060, 2063, 2095
Small cell GBM, 1386
SMI-31, 93–95
SMI-32, 94, 95, 1163, 1176
Smith grading for oligodendroglioma, 1265, 1278–1279
Smooth muscle actin (SMA), 102, 540, 552, 578, 1775, 1776, 2058
Smooth muscle antigen, 1396
Smooth muscle cells (SMCs), 97, 255–258, 260, 294, 538, 540, 542, 567, 568, 612, 629, 630, 996, 1311
Smooth muscle myosin heavy chain (MHC), 102, 2058, 2062
SNCA, 887, 1013, 1014, 1016–1018, 1035
Sneddon syndrome, 606, 999

Sodium, 15, 49, 50, 62, 176, 293, 427, 441, 455, 471, 632, 883, 889, 1092, 1134–1136, 1138, 1139, 1214
Soft tissue tumors, 1277, 1685, 1955–1986, 2076
Solitary fibrous tumor (SFT)/hemangiopericytoma
    age incidence, 1958
    biologic behavior-prognosis-prognostic factors, 1967
    CT-contrast-enhanced, 1958, 1959
    CT-non contrast-enhanced, 1958
    DAS, 1958
    differential diagnosis, 1964
    general imaging findings, 1958–1964
    immunophenotype, 1964–1967
    incidence, 1958
    localisation, 1958
    macroscopic features, 1962
    microscopic features, 1962, 1963, 1965
    MRI-diffusion imaging, 1958
    MRI-flair, 1958, 1959, 1961
    MRI-perfusion, 1958, 1960
    MRI-T1, 1958, 1959, 1961
    MRI-T2, 1958, 1959, 1961
    MRI-T1 contrast-enhanced, 1958, 1960, 1962
    MRI-T2*/ SWI, 1958, 1962
    MR-spectroscopy, 1958, 1960
    nuclear medicine imaging findings, 1961
    pathogenesis, 1966
    proliferation markers, 1964
    sex incidence, 1958
    treatment, 1966–1967
    ultrastructural features, 1964
    WHO definition, 1957–1958
Solitary fibrous tumor (SFT) phenotype, 1955, 1962, 1964, 1967
Soma, 226–228, 233, 292, 296, 299, 920
Somatomotor, 122, 123
Somatosensory, 122, 123, 133, 283, 288, 290, 291, 335, 357, 361, 403, 405, 406, 420, 474, 1121
Somatosensory system, 326, 334–342
Somatostatin (SST), 95, 232, 233, 291, 292, 304, 349, 350, 370, 371, 373, 836, 1063, 1716, 1793, 1795
Somatostatin receptor (SSR), 39, 54, 95, 373, 1616, 1642, 1716, 1718–1722, 1759, 1785, 1786, 1961
Somatotopic organization, 123
Somnolence, 417, 736, 1003, 2128
Southern blot, 57, 111–113
Space-occupying effect, 510
Spasticity, 404, 505, 818, 850, 864, 945, 1038, 1039, 1073, 1093, 1212, 1935
Spastic paralysis, 404
Spatial disorientation, 406, 2156
Spatial orientation, 291
Spatial resolution, 6, 12, 17, 18, 22, 30, 37, 41, 43, 641, 1128, 1926
SPECT, *see* Single photon emission computed tomography
Spectrin, 236
Speech apraxia, 405, 974

S phase (DNA synthesis), 1281–1283, 1288, 1398
Sphenoid bone, 164, 185, 223, 224, 1694
Sphenoid wing dysplasia, 1694
Spin, 10, 19, 22
Spinal cord
    central canal, 319, 321
    Clarke's column, 318
    conus medullaris, 163, 166
    dorsal horn, 318
    dorso-lateral sulcus, 164
    dorso-median sulcus, 164
    filum terminale, 166
    herniation, 436–437
    lateral horn, 318
    nucleus propius (principal sensory nucleus), 318
    posteromarginal nucleus, 318
    Rexed laminae, 319
    substantia gelantinosa, 318
    ventral horn, 318, 319
    ventro-lateral sulcus, 164
    ventromedian fissure, 164
    vertebral canal, 163, 164
Spinal nerves, 122, 164, 181, 1663, 1666, 1669
Spin density, 9
Spindle apparatus checkpoint, 1282–1284
Spindle cell oncocytoma
    age incidence, 1776
    biologic behavior-prognosis-prognostic factors, 1776
    CT-contrast-enhanced, 1776
    CT-non contrast-enhanced, 1776
    differential diagnosis, 1776
    general imaging findings, 1776
    immunophenotype, 1776
    incidence, 1776
    localisation, 1776
    macroscopic features, 1776
    microscopic features, 1776
    molecular neuropathology, 1776
    MRI-flair, 1776
    MRI-T1, 1776
    MRI-T2, 1776
    MRI-T1 contrast-enhanced, 1776
    proliferation markers, 1776
    sex incidence, 1776
    treatment, 1776
    ultrastructural features, 1776
    WHO definition, 1775–1776
    WHO grade, 1776
Spindle multipolarity, 1271
Spindle symmetry, 1271
Spine, 3, 13, 66, 321, 687, 716, 1042, 1267, 1507, 1824, 1833, 1853, 1856, 1933, 1943, 1990, 1995, 2005, 2009, 2038, 2050
    and radicular pain, 1267
Spin-lattice-relaxation, 11
Spinocerebellar ataxia, 826, 845
Spinocerebellar tracts, 350
Spino-reticulo-thalamic tract, 342
Spinothalamic system, 342
Spiny non-pyramidal cells, 268

Spiral-CT, 7
Spongiform leukoencephalopathy (non-specific toxic demyelination), 1253
Sporadic Creutzfeldt–Jakob disease (sCJD), 795, 800, 802, 803, 812, 816, 818
Squamous cell carcinoma, 1289, 1302, 1303, 1885, 2059, 2060, 2062, 2063, 2069, 2070, 2076, 2085, 2095, 2097
SSR, *see* Somatostatin receptor; Somatostatin receptor (SSR)
SSR-PET, 1616, 1642, 1716, 1723, 1724, 1972
SSR-scintigraphy, 1663, 1664, 1724, 1934, 1936, 1961
Stabilisation of microtubules, 847
Stable disease, 1270, 2132, 2135, 2136, 2138
"Staghorn sinusoids," 1962
Staging of neurofibrillary tangle development, 918–921
Standardized acquisition protocols, 32, 44
Standardized uptake value (SUV), 32–34, 43, 44, 49, 641, 1356, 1381, 1383, 1412, 1419, 2050, 2144, 2147
St. Anne/Mayo, 1265, 1278
Staphylococcus spp., 656, 702
Static magnetic field, 9
Stationary detector array, 5
STAT3 pathway, 2139
Status cribrosus, 987
Stellate deposits, 834, 835
Stellate/granule cells, 95, 231, 268, 269, 279, 287, 289, 300, 314, 342, 344, 351, 353, 388, 468, 920, 960, 1150, 1153, 1154, 1233, 1633
Stem cell (SC)
  hypothesis, 1319–1321
  transplantation, 2152, 2176
Stem cell factor (SCF), 102, 1306, 2058
Stenting, 4, 539
Steroid hormone receptors, 91, 92
Stiff person syndrome (SPS), 388, 416, 828, 2153, 2158, 2170, 2172, 2174
STimulated Echo Acquisition Mode (STEAM) technique, 16
Stimulated emission depletion (STED) microscopy, 114
Stimulation methods, 402
Stochastic effects, 38
Stramenopila (formerly chromista), 749
Strategic infarct dementia, 988, 989, 995–997, 999
Street drugs, 1243–1260
Streptococcus spp., 636, 656, 657
Striae medullares, 157, 158
Stria medullaris, 153, 155, 375
Stria terminalis, 150, 351, 352, 380, 381, 401, 414
Striato-Nigral Degeneration (SND), 1021, 1022, 1028
Stroke
  age incidence, 474
  biologic behavior-prognosis-prognostic factors, 496
  cerebral infarction, 473
  clinical signs and symptoms, 474
  CT-angiography, 477
  CT-contrast-enhanced, 477
  CT-non contrast-enhanced, 477–479
  CT-perfusion, 477
  differential diagnosis, 489
  general imaging findings, 477–483
  hemorrhagic stroke, 473
  immunophenotype, 489
  incidence, 474–476
  infarct-acute infarct, 484, 487–489
  infarct-chronic infarct, 484, 490–491
  infarct-lacunar infarcts, 489
  infarct-subacute infarct, 484
  ischemic stroke, 473
  localisation, 474–476
  macroscopic features, 484–491
  microscopic features, 484, 489, 492–495
  MR-angiopgraphy, 478, 480
  MRI-diffusion imaging, 477, 479
  MRI-diffusion tensor imaging, (AU: Not found)
  MRI-flair, 477, 479
  MRI-perfusion, 477, 480–481
  MRI-T1, 477
  MRI-T2, 477
  MRI-T1 contrast-enhanced, 477, 479
  MRI-T2∗/ SWI, 479, 480
  nuclear medicine imaging findings, 478, 482, 483
  pathogenesis, 489, 496
  proliferation markers, (AU: Not found)
  race ethnicity, 474
  sex incidence, 474
  transient ischemic attack (TIA), 473
  treatment, 496
  ultrastructural features, (AU: Not found)
Stromal cells, 540, 1438, 1768, 1955, 1956, 1967, 1969, 1974, 1979, 1995, 1998, 2028
Stupor, 694, 736, 820, 1224
STUPP scheme, 1368, 1406
Sturge-Weber Syndrome, 1130, 1132
Subacute motor neuronopathy, 2153
Subarachnoidal cisterns
  ambiens cistern, 186
  cerebellomedullary cistern, 186
  chiasmatic cistern, 186
  cistern of the lateral fossa, 186
  interpeduncular cistern, 186
  lumbal cistern, 186
  pontine cistern, 186
Subarachnoidal hemorrhage, 637
Subarachnoidal space, 176, 186, 188, 436, 449, 451, 510, 658, 1268, 1525, 2071
Subarachnoid cerebellar tissue emboli, 436
Subarachnoid dissemination, 1511
Subarachnoid hemorrhage (SAH), 9, 499, 500, 505–520, 715, 775–777, 997, 999
Subcapsular cataract, 1662, 1699, 1700
Subcortical heterotopia, 1171, 1173, 1179
Subcortical laminar heterotopias, 1178, 1179
Subcutaneous hemorrhage, 499
Subdural empyema, 653, 657, 663–691
Subdural hemorrhage (SDH)
  acute, 521
  chronic, 521
  subacute, 521

Subendothelial layer, 254, 255
Subependymal heterotopia, 1171, 1172
Subependymal plate, 1518, 1580, 1581, 1591
Subependymoma
   age incidence, 1511
   biologic behavior-prognosis-prognostic factors, 1518
   CT-contrast-enhanced, 1511
   CT-non contrast-enhanced, 1511
   differential diagnosis, 1518
   general imaging findings, 1511
   immunophenotype, 1516–1517
   incidence, 1511
   localisation, 1511
   macroscopic features, 1513
   microscopic features, 1513–1516
   MRI-diffusion imaging, 1511
   MRI-flair, 1511, 1512
   MRI-perfusion, (AU: Not found)
   MRI-T1, 1511
   MRI-T2, 1511, 1512
   MRI-T1 contrast-enhanced, 1511, 1512
   MRI-T2∗/SWI, 1511
   MR-spectroscopy, 1513
   nuclear medicine imaging findings, 1490
   pathogenesis, 1518
   proliferation markers, 1518
   sex incidence, 1511
   treatment, 1518
   ultrastructural features, 1518
   WHO definition, 1511
   WHO grade, 1490, 1511–1518
Subgaleal hemorrhage, 499, 500
Subiculum, 138, 298–300, 346–349, 392, 818, 918, 919, 921, 961, 964, 965
Sublentiform part of the internal capsule, 147
Subpial deposits, 834, 836
Substance P, 349, 350, 370, 371, 836, 1151
Substantia centralis grisea, 156
Substantia nigra, 49, 71, 76, 156, 158, 228, 305, 307–309, 339, 376, 387, 388, 683, 716, 737, 755, 813, 855, 856, 858, 864, 914, 920, 921, 937, 958, 964, 966, 967, 976, 979–983, 1003, 1004, 1007, 1008, 1011, 1012, 1016, 1028, 1062, 1213, 1214, 1244, 1256–1258, 2159, 2166
Substantia reticularis degeneration, 828, 859
Substitution, 76, 1215, 1219, 1304, 1305, 1398
Subthalamus, 138, 155, 209, 982
Successful aging, 870, 880, 885–888
Sucking reflex, 208
Sudan black B, 89
Sulcus
   central sulcus, 130–133, 167, 168, 980
   cingulate sulcus, 135
   collateral sulcus, 137
   hippocampal sulcus, 138, 294, 296, 298, 299, 346, 347
   inferior frontal sulcus, 132
   inferior temporal sulcus, 134, 135
   intraparietal sulcus, 133, 134, 288, 409
   lateral sulcus, 130–135, 167, 168, 186, 205, 214, 409, 1859
   occipito-temporal sulcus, 137
   olfactory sulcus, 137
   orbital sulci, 137
   parieto-occipital sulcus, 131, 133, 135–137, 168
   postcentral sulcus, 133, 135
   precentral sulcus, 131, 132, 135
   superior frontal sulcus, 131, 132
   superior temporal sulcus, 134, 135, 409
   transverse occipital sulcus, 134
Sulcus corporis callosi, 135
Superficial epipial layer, 186
Superficial siderosis, 606, 607
Superior Alternating Syndrome, 209
Superior colliculi, 74, 150, 306
Superior colliculus, 150, 156, 158, 331, 357, 388, 976
Superior frontal gyrus, 76, 77, 131, 132, 167, 168, 328, 405, 901
Superior longitudinal fascicle, 127, 147, 148
Superior parietal lobule, 76, 133, 294
Superior sagittal sinus, 60, 182, 184–186, 212–215, 221–223, 254, 1711, 1730
Supero-lateral prefrontal cortex, 76
Superparamagnetic contrast medium, 15
Suppurative intracranial phlebitis, 657
Supraoptic region, 306
Supratentorial, 436, 505, 666, 752, 1107, 1267, 1323, 1444, 1470, 1490, 1491, 1493, 1500, 1501, 1541, 1542, 1554, 1563, 1638, 1646, 1657, 1856, 1895, 1958, 2152, 2153
Surface
   inferior surface, 129, 136–137, 224
   medial surface, 65, 129, 131, 133–137, 155, 204, 223, 345, 404, 407, 436, 476
   superolateral surface, 123, 129–133, 955
Surface receptors, 92, 248, 815, 1134, 1316, 2160
Surgical cranial decompression (large craniectomy), 441
Surgical evacuation, 505
SUV, see Standardized uptake value
Sydenham's chorea, 2153, 2159
Symbionts, 775
Symptomatogenic zone, 1121
Synapse
   asymmetric synapse, Gray type I, 235
   axo-axonal synapse, 235
   axo-dendritic synapse, 235
   axo-somatic synapse, 235
   chemical synapse, 235
   electrical synapse, 234–235
   excitatory postsynaptic potential (EPSP), 235
   excitatory synapses, 235
   inhibitory postsynaptic potential (IPSP), 235
   inhibitory synapses, 235
   interneuronal synapse, 235
   myoneuronal synapse, 235
   neuroglandular synapse, 235
   postsynaptic membrane, 234
   presynaptic membrane, 234
   symmetric synapse, Gray type II, 235

synapse à distance, 235
synapsins, 236
synaptic cleft, 234
synaptic plasticity, 249
synaptic proteins, 236
synaptic pruning, 249
"synaptic quadriga," 235
synaptobrevin, 236
synaptogamin, 236
synaptophysin, 236
synaptoporin, 236
synaptosomes, 235
tetrapartite synapse, 235
tripartite synapse, 235
Synaptophysin, 94, 95, 102, 108, 236, 716, 873, 1175–1176, 1396, 1454, 1458, 1527, 1529–1531, 1548, 1557, 1558, 1563, 1573, 1579, 1581, 1589, 1590, 1600, 1601, 1604, 1608, 1609, 1624, 1626, 1643, 1645, 1647, 1648, 1654, 1656, 1770, 1775, 1776, 1810, 1886, 1984, 2058, 2060–2062, 2070, 2084, 2095, 2113
Syncope, 456, 932
Syntaxin, 236, 1137
Synucleinopathies, 826, 828, 848
Syrinx formation, 1435

T

T1, 9–15, 23, 126, 134, 136, 145, 430, 432, 445, 447, 461, 479, 502, 504, 513, 523, 531, 553, 556, 579, 587, 590, 593, 597, 608, 617, 623, 627, 642, 659, 661, 664, 704, 721, 726, 732, 733, 738, 753, 764, 766, 778, 783, 798, 799, 900, 975, 991, 1023, 1024, 1074, 1076, 1078, 1100, 1107, 1109, 1126, 1145, 1172–1174, 1208, 1225, 1230, 1234, 1238, 1246, 1339, 1355, 1357, 1371, 1372, 1375, 1413, 1426, 1429, 1435, 1449, 1451, 1460, 1471, 1478, 1480, 1507, 1512, 1524, 1535, 1537, 1543, 1544, 1555, 1564, 1566, 1577, 1585, 1598, 1607, 1616, 1617, 1619, 1640, 1653, 1667, 1668, 1678.1695, 1711–1714, 1756, 1758, 1759, 1767, 1772, 1783, 1784, 1814, 1816, 1825, 1827, 1834, 1841, 1842, 1847, 1854, 1857, 1869, 1876, 1883, 1896, 1915, 1925, 1936, 1937, 1942, 1959, 1961, 1970, 1980, 2000, 2014, 2019, 2023, 2027, 2030, 2039, 2041, 2121, 2124, 2133, 2137, 2161

T2, 9, 11–15, 23, 126, 132, 133, 135, 136, 139, 142, 148, 162, 205, 430, 432, 445, 447, 459, 461, 501, 502, 504, 513, 531, 553, 556, 579, 587, 590, 593, 597, 599, 608, 617, 623, 627, 642, 659, 661, 664, 704, 721, 726, 733, 738, 753, 764, 766, 778, 783, 797–799, 871, 896, 900, 948, 975, 991, 1023, 1024, 1061, 1074, 1078, 1099, 1107, 1109, 1126, 1145, 1153, 1159–1161, 1172–1174, 1193, 1208, 1225, 1230, 1234, 1238, 1246, 1339, 1355, 1357, 1371, 1413, 1426, 1429, 1435, 1436, 1449, 1451, 1460, 1471, 1478, 1480, 1494, 1502, 1507, 1512, 1524, 1535, 1537, 1543, 1544, 1564, 1566, 1577, 1585, 1598, 1607, 1616, 1619, 1640, 1653, 1667, 1668, 1695, 1711, 1712, 1714, 1716, 1756, 1758, 1759, 1767, 1772, 1783, 1784, 1814, 1825, 1827, 1834, 1841, 1842, 1847, 1853, 1854, 1857, 1869, 1876, 1883, 1896, 1915, 1925, 1937, 1942, 1959, 1961, 1970, 1998, 2027, 2039, 2041, 2121, 2132, 2133, 2136, 2137, 2161

Tabes dorsalis, 1072
Tachyzoites, 752, 756, 759, 761
Tacrolimus, 731, 2152, 2176
Tactile examination, 68, 71, 74
Tactile naming, 209
Tactile representation of the body, 405
Taeniasis, 762–771
Taenia solium, 750, 751, 762, 763, 768, 770
Taenia thalami, 155
Tail of the caudate nucleus (cauda nuclei caudati), 144, 303
Takayasu's arteritis (TAK), 636, 638, 641
Tangential cortical lamination, 1158
Tangle-only dementia, 837, 849, 953, 956, 964
Tanycytes, 225, 240, 250, 1493
Tardive dyskinesia, 388, 416
Targeted therapy, 1269, 2053, 2056–2057
Tat, 701, 719
Tau
    tau 3 repeat (Tau 3R), 100, 108, 837, 839–840, 844, 956, 1212
    tau 4 repeat (Tau 4R), 100, 108, 837, 840, 844, 956, 1212
Tau-containing astrocytes, 860
Tauopathies include the following disease entities:, 837
Tauopathy/tauopathies, 828, 836–837, 847, 848, 853, 854, 917, 953, 956, 957, 960, 962–964, 973, 1215, 2160
Taurine, 370, 388
Tau-tracers, 901, 976, 980
T-cell suppression, 2151, 2176
Tc-99m, 1664, 1926, 1934, 1936, 1969, 1990
Tc99m-MIBI, 1899, 1926
TDP-43 proteinopathies, 849, 850, 953
Tectrotyd, 54
Tegmentospinal tract, 346
Tegmentum, 156, 204, 307, 311, 352, 381, 853, 974, 976, 980, 1012, 1229, 2160
Telencephalic GSS, 819
Telencephalon, 129–137, 143, 146, 150, 156, 158, 169, 181, 380, 381, 525, 863, 1369
Teleopsia, 209, 422
Telomerase, 1266, 1310, 1368, 1400, 1401, 1408, 1749, 2084
Telomeres, 880, 886, 1017, 1266, 1280, 1304, 1310, 1400
Telophase, 1282, 1284
Temodal, 2131
Temozolomide (TMZ), 1329, 1330, 1368, 1403, 1406, 1408

Temporal lobe, 13, 14, 76, 130, 131, 133–138, 142, 144, 148, 154, 169, 204, 214, 223, 290, 294, 332, 361, 392, 410, 413, 598, 658, 696–698, 715, 731, 734, 735, 854, 855, 863, 873, 933, 947, 949, 950, 954, 955, 960, 962, 964–967, 1042, 1080, 1124, 1125, 1134, 1158, 1165, 1175, 1193, 1212, 1214, 1257, 1338, 1385, 1419, 1482, 1541, 1542, 1562, 1572, 1830, 2154, 2155
Temporal lobe epilepsy, 245, 392, 1125, 1128, 1129, 1135, 1143–1154
Temporary radiation syndrome, 38
Tentorium cerebelli, 60, 129, 162, 180, 184, 185, 223, 252
Teratoma
    CT-contrast-enhanced, 1882
    CT-non contrast-enhanced, 1882
    general imaging findings, 1882
    immature teratoma, 1880–1882, 1885
    immunophenotype, 1888
    macroscopic features, 1884–1885
    mature teratoma, 1880, 1882, 1885
    microscopic features, 1885–1888
    MRI-flair, 1883
    MRI-T1, 1883
    MRI-T2, 1883
    MRI-T1 contrast-enhanced, 1884
    MR-spectroscopy, 1884
    proliferation markers, 1888
    teratoma with malignant transformation, 1880–1882, 1885
    ultrastructural features, 1888–1889
    WHO definition, 1880–1889
Terminal fields, 278, 290
Terminal vein, 150
Tesla (T), 10
Testicular tumor, 2094–2096, 2155
Tetranucleotide repeat disease, 851
Tetraspan, 99, 252
Thalamic aphasia, 417
Thalamic degeneration, 828, 857
Thalamic syndrome, 209
Thalamic system, 326, 352
Thalamocortical fascicle, 147
Thalamus
    anterior nuclear group, 305
    intralaminar nuclei, 305
    lateral geniculate body, 305
    medial geniculate body, 305
    medial nuclear group, 305
    reticular nucleus, 305
    ventrolateral nuclear group, 305
Thecoma, 2107, 2111
Therapy-induced leukoencephalopathies, 2119, 2128–2129
Therapy-induced secondary neoplasms, 2119, 2129
Therapy-induced vasculopathies, 2119
Thiamine deficiency, 1224, 1233, 1240
Thioflavin S, 85, 89, 839, 914, 916
Third visual complex, 333

Thorn-shaped astrocyte, 837, 976
Threads, 64, 65, 163, 228, 837, 844, 979, 983, 1042
Thrombin, 257, 441
Thrombolysis, 496, 614
Thrombosis, 542, 552, 569, 576, 585, 596, 609, 639, 778, 990, 997, 1368, 2126, 2128
Thymoma, 2155, 2157, 2158, 2170–2174
Thyroid transcription factor-1 (TTF1), 104, 108, 1767–1771, 1775–1777, 2060, 2062, 2067, 2069, 2070, 2084, 2095, 2099, 2102, 2113
Thyrotropin-releasing hormone, 370, 371
Tick-borne encephalitis (TBE), 693, 736–741
Tics, 416, 828, 858, 2158
Time-of-flight MR-angiography, 17
Tinnitus, 52, 208, 1663
Tissue destruction, 76, 83, 485, 493, 507, 583, 687, 757, 781, 1191, 1196, 1201, 1202, 1358, 1477, 1944
Tissue processing, 58, 78, 79
201TlCl, 54
T-lymphocyte, 105, 106, 527, 641, 647, 680, 685, 688, 714, 717–719, 740, 1082, 1088, 1092, 1101, 1113–1115, 1275, 1739, 1871, 1872, 1920, 1924, 1934, 1949, 2057, 2166, 2168
TNF, see Tumor necrosis factor
Togaviridae, 695, 696, 736
Toll-like receptor (TLR), 689, 690, 1090, 1168
    signaling pathway, 1913
Tonic-clonic seizures, 326, 367, 1122–1124, 1137, 1255, 2156
Tonic seizures, 1122, 2157
Topoisomerase IIα, 106–107, 1365
Torticollis, 416
Total anterior circulation syndrome, 474
Toti-or pluripotent stem cells, 1868
Touton giant cells, 1933, 1938, 1944, 1945
Touton-like multinucleated giant cells, 1933, 1944, 1947
Toxoplasma gondii, 107, 108, 700, 702, 714, 750–762
Toxoplasmosis, 451, 750, 751, 753, 755, 767, 1897
T-PA and vasodilation, 4
TR, see Repetition time
Tracer-kinetics, 31–32, 44, 1341, 1358, 1381, 1414, 1420
Tracts, 20, 125, 147, 148, 155, 156, 158, 159, 209, 306, 308, 310, 312, 313, 335, 350, 351, 357, 402, 420, 421, 708, 713, 856, 875, 977, 1207, 1213, 1217, 1218, 1235, 1269, 1316
Tractus corticospinalis, 156
Transactive response binding protein of 43 kDa (TDP43), 102, 108, 834, 844, 845, 849, 850, 852, 953–960, 966–968, 1042, 1046, 1049–1053, 1213, 1214
Transcortical motor aphasia (dominant hemisphere), 207, 405, 414, 420, 475
Transcortical sensory aphasia, 401, 407, 409, 414, 859
Transcranial direct current stimulation (tDCS), 402
Transcranial magnetic stimulation (TMS), 402
Transcription factors (TFs), 91, 92, 95, 248, 884, 1018, 1050, 1134, 1244, 1258, 1259, 1266, 1283, 1290, 1303, 1657, 1780, 1787, 1792, 1804, 1867, 1998

Transentorhinal, 859, 861, 918, 919, 941, 965
Transependymal edema, 444, 445, 447
Transferrin, 99, 1042
Transferrin (iron transport glycoprotein in the oligodendrocyte cell body), 252
Transforming growth factor (TGF) family, 370
Transient global ischemia, 456, 457
Transient ischemic attack (TIA), 473, 606, 626, 640, 988, 1912
Transition areas, 301
Transition zone (mesocortex), 269, 918
Translocase of outer mitochondrial membrane 40 homolog (TOMM40), 614, 895, 923
Transmantle sign, 1158, 1159
Transmissible mink encephalopathy (TME), 796, 797
Transmissible spongiform encephalopathies (TSE), 797, 845
Transmission electron microscopy, 108
Transsphenoidal approach, 1793
Transtentorial herniation, 430, 434, 436
Transversal magnetization, 10, 11
Transverse fissure, 129
Transverse myelitis, 1072, 1097, 1245, 1247
Trauma, 4, 30, 58, 59, 71, 74, 75, 188, 247, 436, 503, 514, 530, 533, 658, 736, 828, 846, 1125, 1129, 1131, 1132, 1153, 1158, 1168, 1185–1220, 1271, 1829, 1998
Traumatic axonal injury (TAI), 1187, 1188, 1207–1211
Traumatic brain injury (TBI), 245, 402, 428, 522, 1186–1192, 1214–1218
T1 relaxation time, 11, 13, 14
T2 relaxation time, 11, 13
Trematode, 750
Tremor, 49, 207, 209, 416, 417, 419, 420, 622, 658, 736, 819, 820, 828, 838, 843, 865, 932, 946, 947, 974, 984, 1001, 1002, 1054, 1060, 1073, 1093, 1212, 1800, 2174
Trichrome (Masson), 87
Trigonum of the hypoglossal nerve, 158
Trigonum of the vagal nerve, 158
Trinucleotide repeat disease, 826, 851
Trisomy 21, 856, 897
"Trojan Horse" hypothesis, 717
Trophoblast, 293, 1868, 1880
True ependymal rosette, 1274
Truncal imbalance, 419
Trypanosomiasis, 750
TSH, *see* Tumor-producing thyrotropin
TTP, 18, 477
Tuberal region, 306
Tuber cinereum, 153, 155
Tubercles, 162, 687
Tuberculoma, 666, 687
Tuberculosis, 656, 665, 666, 687–689, 715, 1131, 1871
Tuberous sclerosis, 1125, 1130, 1135, 1157, 1291
Tubular, 258, 775, 923, 979, 984, 1045, 1529, 1639, 1644, 1646–1648, 1685, 1873, 1875, 2005, 2063, 2070, 2088, 2094, 2107, 2113
Tubulin, 99, 228, 815, 837, 838, 840, 1007, 1012, 1179
Tubulin polymerization promoting protein (TPPP/p25), 99

Tufted astrocyte, 837, 976, 979
Tumor
 blush, 1716
 suppressor, 1267, 1282, 1290–1293, 1303, 1325, 1748, 1749, 1995
 suppressor gene, 1266, 1284, 1289–1291, 1319, 1321, 1349, 1364, 1399–1401, 1403, 1476, 1629, 1630, 1697, 1700–1703, 1747, 1748, 1787, 1788, 1792, 1974, 1994
Tumor necrosis factor (TNF), 248, 249, 648, 816, 1217, 1272, 1296, 1300, 1302, 1311–1313
Tumor necrosis factor-α (TNFα), 242, 247, 517, 567, 568, 690, 710, 846, 1092, 1168, 1306, 1315
Tumor-producing thyrotropin (TSH), 108, 1754, 1781, 1787, 1791, 1793, 1794, 1799, 1800, 1806, 1812
Tumor-progression, 1300, 1306, 1317, 1349, 1376, 1747–1749, 1997, 2084, 2131–2148, 2159
Tumor-promoting inflammation, 1280
Tunica adventitia, 255
Tunica media composed of, 255
"Two-hit hypothesis," 1266, 1290
"Two-hit" model, 1701
Type I oligodendrocytes, 245–246
Type II oligodendrocytes, 246
Type III oligodendrocytes, 246
Type IV oligodendrocytes, 246
Type I transmembrane glycoprotein, 100
Typical AD, 852, 896
Tyrosinase, 102, 2058, 2083, 2084
Tyrosine kinase with immunoglobulin like and EGF like domains 1 (TIE1), 259

U

Ubiquilin, 844, 968, 1050
Ubiquilin 2, 844, 968, 1049, 1050, 1052
Ubiquitin, 102, 108, 241, 830, 836, 838–840, 844, 856, 860, 863, 908, 911, 937, 956, 958–963, 966–968, 979, 983, 1007, 1015, 1028, 1033, 1042, 1046, 1050–1053
Ubiquitination, 1014–1016, 1310
Ubiquitin proteasome system (UPS), 102, 840, 842, 845, 941, 1051, 1052
Ulcerations, 538
Ulex europaeus I, 102, 103, 2058
Ulex europaeus agglutinin I, 100
Ultrasonography, 3, 4
UMN, *see* Upper motor neuron
Uncinate fascicle, 127, 147, 148
Unconditioned reflex, 122
Uncus, 137, 138, 142, 300, 434, 435, 918, 919
Undifferentiated high-grade pleomorphic sarcoma-malignant fibrous histiocytoma (MFH), 1979
Undifferentiated pleomorphic sarcoma/malignant fibrous histiocytoma, 1985
Unit membrane, 226, 227
Unlimited replicative potential, 1280
Unspecified nodular encephalitis, 700
Upper motor neuron (UMN), 334, 1037–1039

UPS, *see* Ubiquitin proteasome system
Upward transtentorial herniation, 436
Urinary incontinence, 207, 208, 404, 443, 449, 475, 879, 932, 1021
Urothelial carcinoma (transitional cell carcinoma), 2059, 2061, 2085, 2092
UV irradiation, 1266, 1285

V
Vacuolar leukoencephalopathy (VL), 702, 708
Vacuolar myelopathy (VM), 702, 708, 713, 1089
Valosin-containing protein (VCP), 850, 953, 956–959, 968, 1049, 1050, 1052
Vanishing white matter syndrome (VWM), 243
Variable proteinase-sensitive prionopathy (VPSPr), 797, 812
Varicella-zoster virus (VZV), 107, 641, 695, 697, 698, 702, 715
Varicosity formation, 1214
Varix of the vein of Galen, 577
Vascular cells, 568, 1969, 1979
Vascular channels, 13, 474, 578, 582, 583, 594, 1274, 1597, 1601, 1731, 1982
Vascular cognitive impairment (VCI), 614, 988, 989, 997–999
Vascular dementia (VaD), 640, 852–854, 901, 987–999
Vascular endothelial growth factor (VEGFs), 370, 519, 568, 1056, 1091, 1306, 1309, 1331, 1492, 1749, 1979, 1996, 1998, 2056, 2139, 2148
Vascular endothelial growth factor A (VEGF-A), 441, 1311–1313, 1657
Vascular endothelial growth factor B (VEGF-B), 441
Vascular hyalinization with luminal stenosis, 2126, 2128
Vascular occlusion, 641, 865, 987
Vasculitis
    Aspergillus arteritis, 635, 636
    infectious vasculitis, 635
    large vessel vasculitis, 635–638, 640, 644
    medium vessel vasculitis, 635–638
    non-infectious vasculitis, 635–637
    Rickettsial vasculitis, 635
    small vessel vasculitis, 635–639
    syphilitic aortitis, 635
Vasculogenesis, 1266, 1310
Vaso-active agents, 21, 441
Vasoactive intestinal peptide (VIP), 232, 233, 291, 292, 349, 370, 371, 836
Vasodilatory challenge, 52
Vasopressin, 230, 350, 370, 371, 384
Vasospasm, 9, 517, 1215, 1216, 1218
VCP, *see* Valosin-containing protein
VEGFs, *see* Vascular endothelial growth factor
Veins
    anterior pontomesencephalic veins, 215
    basal vein of Rosenthal, 212–214
    brachicephalic vein, 212
    brainstem/posterior fossa veins (infratentorial veins), 214
    central supratentorial veins, 213, 214
    cerebral veins, 211–214
    cervical veins, 213, 215
    cranial veins, 212, 213
    deep cerebral veins, 211, 212, 214
    deep (subependymal) cerebral veins, 212
    deep cervical veins, 213, 215
    deep middle cerebral vein, 212, 214
    deep paramedian veins, 214
    diploic veins, 212, 213, 215, 224
    dural sinuses, 17, 179, 182–186, 211, 212, 215, 1716
    emissary veins
        condylar emissary veins, 212
        internal carotid venous plexus, 213
        mastoid emissary veins, 212
        occipital emissary veins, 213
        parietal emissary veins, 212
        portal veins of pituitary gland, 213
        venous plexus of formane ovale, 213
        venous plexus of hypophyseal canal, 213
    extracerebral veins, 213, 215
    facial vein, 213, 215
    great cerebral vein of Galen, 213, 214
    inferior anastomotic vein of Labbé, 214
    inferior cortical veins, 214
    inferior vermian veins, 215
    internal cerebral veins, 212–214
    internal jugular vein, 185, 212, 213, 218, 223, 224
    medullary veins, 212, 214
    middle cortical veins, 214
    petrosal vein, 215
    posterior anastomotic vein of Labbé, 214
    precentral cerebellar vein, 215
    pterygoid vein, 213, 215
    retromandibular vein, 213, 215
    right cardiac atrium, 212
    septal veins, 212, 214
    subependymal veins, 212, 214
    superficial (cortical) cerebral veins, 211, 213
    superficial middle cerebral vein, 185, 212–214, 223, 224
    superior anastomotic vein of Trolard, 211, 213
    superior cortical veins, 213
    superior vena cava, 212
    superior vermian veins, 215
    thalamostriate veins, 212, 214
    vein of Galen, 184, 212, 223, 577, 1132
    vein of Labbé, 211, 214
    vertebral veins, 213, 215
Venous angioma, 577, 596
Venous drainage, 179, 211–224
Venous sinuses, 14, 179, 182, 212, 213, 222, 530, 533, 997, 1708, 1720
Ventral, occipito-temporal network, 291
Ventral stream, 332, 333, 357–361, 409
Ventral trigemino-thalamic tract, 342
Ventricle
    fourth ventricle, 72, 74, 169, 171, 174–176, 186, 250, 321, 677, 1022, 1077, 1224, 1229, 1276, 1492–1494, 1501, 1507, 1511, 1522, 1525, 1550, 1583–1585, 1613–1616, 1618

lateral ventricles
  anterior horn, 169, 171, 174, 175, 230, 320, 334, 958, 982, 1039, 1042, 1044, 1066, 1213
  central part, 169, 171, 174, 175, 177
  inferior horn, 138, 142, 144, 169, 171, 174–176, 303
  posterior horn, 150, 167, 169, 171, 174–177, 1100, 1524
  third ventricle, 14, 150, 151, 153, 155, 156, 167, 169, 171, 174–176, 204, 250, 444, 449, 450, 476, 616, 677, 838, 974, 1214, 1229, 1231, 1276, 1323, 1492, 1501, 1511, 1522, 1576, 1824, 1843–1852, 1866
Ventricular drainage, 441, 451, 1218
Ventricular obstruction, 1490
Ventricular system, 13, 74, 169–177, 249, 321, 322, 387, 443, 444, 449, 450, 466, 715, 828, 829, 861, 873, 901, 958, 1077, 1213, 1490, 1492, 1501, 1513, 1575, 1652
Ventriculomegaly, 444
Ventriculo-peritoneal shunt, 4, 451
Ventriculostomy, 451
Ventro-dorsal (v-d) stream, 333
Ventrolateral sulcus, 160, 162, 164
Venule, 254, 258, 259, 607, 613, 638, 1106, 1272
Verbal dyslexia, 209
Vermis, 72, 74, 76, 162–164, 204, 419, 1233, 1620, 1632
Verocay bodies, 1274, 1669, 1672, 1689
Vertebral body, 65, 2026
Vertebral spines, 65, 66
Vertebroplasty, 4
Vertigo, 52, 207, 208, 419, 475, 476, 622, 1073
Vesicles, 321, 372, 440, 848, 959, 1067, 1880
Vesicular transporters, 372, 1014, 1015
Vessel type, 636, 639, 844
Vestibular area, 158
Vestibulocerebellar tracts, 350
VGKC, see Voltage-gated potassium channel complex
Vif, 701
Vimentin, 96, 97, 102, 108, 241, 253, 815, 1158, 1162, 1164, 1166, 1168, 1341, 1364, 1394, 1396, 1418, 1420, 1476, 1480, 1496, 1501, 1510, 1529–1531, 1557, 1569, 1645, 1647, 1648, 1654, 1686, 1742, 1746, 1769, 1770, 1776, 1792, 1908, 1940, 1966, 1977, 1979, 1997, 2016, 2021, 2025, 2058, 2060–2062, 2075, 2088, 2099, 2104, 2107, 2113–2115
Vincristine, 1329, 1330, 1431, 1466, 1913
VIP, see Vasoactive intestinal peptide
Viral receptors, 698–699
Virchow-Robin spaces, 675, 853, 1269, 1935, 2050
Virus, 542, 693–741, 1071, 1089
Visceromotor, 122, 123
Viscerosensory, 122, 123
Visual agnosia, 407, 409, 413
Visual allesthesia, 408
Visual anosognosia, 407
Visual examination, 74
Visual field defects, 209, 417, 418, 421, 500, 658

Visual hallucinations, 209, 407, 410, 843, 932, 1002, 2155
Visual interpretation, 32, 45, 51, 2125
Visual loss, 421, 640, 818, 1267, 1779, 1793, 1817
Visual obscurations, 1267
Visual-spatial-perceptual dysfunction, 207
Visual system, 327, 328, 332, 359
Visual system-two stream hypothesis, 356–360
Visuospatial neglect, 207, 475
Vitamin B1 deficiency, 1233, 1240
Voltage-gated calcium channel (VGCC), 1092, 1134, 1135
  P/Q type, N-type, 1092, 2153, 2170, 2171, 2174
Voltage-gated Na+ channels, 1134
Voltage-gated potassium antibody syndromes, 2156–2158
Voltage-gated potassium channel complex (VGKC), 2157–2158, 2170, 2171, 2174
Voltammetry, 402
Vomiting, 38, 207, 208, 419, 476, 500, 520, 654, 658, 694, 736, 749, 751, 763, 773, 774, 862, 1098, 1106, 1186, 1267, 1490, 1813, 2155, 2173
von Hippel–Lindau (VHL) disease, 1291, 1956, 1967, 1974, 2102
Von Kossa, 89
Von Willebrand factor, 717, 1979
Voxel, 5, 6, 13, 19–21
Voxel-based morphometry, 402

W

Walker Warburg, 1132
Wallenberg syndrome, 208, 505
Warthin Starry, 89
Water, 5, 11, 13, 15–16, 19, 67, 78–80, 176, 241, 243, 244, 249, 259, 355, 356, 418, 427, 441, 471, 756, 768, 771, 802, 878, 1101
Watershed zone infarcts, 457
Weakness, 207, 208, 456, 474–476, 496, 558, 722, 826, 846, 847, 850, 862, 864, 988, 1038, 1039, 1055, 1073, 1106, 1212, 2152, 2176
Weber's syndrome, 209
Well-being, 869–875
Wernicke encephalopathy, 857, 1229–1231
Wernicke-Korsakoff encephalopathy, 244, 1228–1233
Wernicke-Korsakoff syndrome (WKS), 1223–1224, 1227, 1228
Wernicke's area, 410, 413
Wernicke speech center, 134
Western blot, 111–113, 797, 812, 816
Western equine encephalitis, 696, 737
White matter
  fiber systems, 19, 1178
  heterotopias, 1157, 1175–1176
White matter tauopathy with globular glial inclusions (WMT-GGI), 953, 956, 957, 964
WHO grading system, 1277
Wilson disease, 50, 244, 827, 865, 1130
Wnt signaling, 925, 1266, 1306, 1320, 1321, 1324, 1582, 1614, 1629
Wölke iron hematoxylin, 85
Word selection anomia, 409

X

Xanthomatous changes, 1386, 1529
Xantogranuloma of the sellar region, 1765
X-linked adrenoleukodystrophy, 864, 1035
X-ray(s)
    fan, 5
    tube, 5, 7
XTC, 1244, 1259

Y

Yeast, 774–776, 784, 790, 888
Yolk sac tumor
    immunophenotype, 1874, 1875
    macroscopic features, 1873
    microscopic features, 1874, 1875
    proliferation markers, 1875
    ultrastructural features, 1875
    WHO definition, 1873, 1875
Yttrium-90, 31, 1716

Z

Ziehl-Neelsen, 89, 688
Zonulae adherentes, 1343, 1496, 1501, 1510, 1604, 1648